GLOBAL PERSPECTIVES ON CHILDHOOD OBESITY
CURRENT STATUS, CONSEQUENCES AND PREVENTION

GLOBAL PERSPECTIVES ON CHILDHOOD OBESITY

CURRENT STATUS, CONSEQUENCES AND PREVENTION

Edited by

DEBASIS BAGCHI
University of Houston, College of Pharmacy, Houston, TX, USA

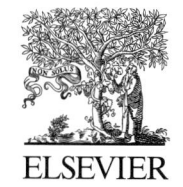

ELSEVIER

AMSTERDAM • BOSTON • HEIDELBERG • LONDON • NEW YORK • OXFORD • PARIS • SAN DIEGO
SAN FRANCISCO • SINGAPORE • SYDNEY • TOKYO

Academic Press is an imprint of Elsevier

Academic Press is an imprint of Elsevier
32 Jamestown Road, London NW1 7BY, UK
30 Corporate Drive, Suite 400, Burlington, MA 01803, USA
525 B Street, Suite 1800, San Diego, CA 92101-4495, USA

First edition 2011

Copyright © 2011 Elsevier Inc. All rights reserved with the exception of Chapter 7

Chapter 7 is in the Public Domain

No part of this publication may be reproduced, stored in a retrieval system or transmitted in any form or by any means electronic, mechanical, photocopying, recording or otherwise without the prior written permission of the publisher

Permissions may be sought directly from Elsevier's Science & Technology Rights Department in Oxford, UK: phone (+ 44) (0) 1865 843830; fax (+44) (0) 1865 853333; email: permissions@elsevier.com. Alternatively, visit the Science and Technology Books website at www.elsevierdirect.com/rights for further information

Notice
No responsibility is assumed by the publisher for any injury and/or damage to persons or property as a matter of products liability, negligence or otherwise, or from any use or operation of any methods, products, instructions or ideas contained in the material herein. Because of rapid advances in the medical sciences, in particular, independent verification of diagnoses and drug dosages should be made

British Library Cataloguing-in-Publication Data
A catalogue record for this book is available from the British Library

Library of Congress Cataloging-in-Publication Data
A catalog record for this book is available from the Library of Congress

ISBN: 978-0-12-374995-6

For information on all Academic Press publications
visit our website at elsevierdirect.com

Typeset by TNQ Books and Journals Pvt Ltd.
www.tnq.co.in

Printed and bound in United States of America

10 11 12 13 14 15   10 9 8 7 6 5 4 3 2 1

Working together to grow
libraries in developing countries

www.elsevier.com | www.bookaid.org | www.sabre.org

ELSEVIER   BOOK AID International   Sabre Foundation

Table of Contents

Contributors vii
Preface xi

I
EPIDEMIOLOGY AND PREVALENCE

1. Pediatric Obesity: A Pediatrician's Viewpoint 3
   Allison Collins and Rebecka Peebles
2. Salient Features on Child Obesity from the Viewpoint of a Nutritionist 13
   Bernard Waysfeld and Dominique Adele Cassuto
3. Developmental Trajectories of Weight Status in Childhood and Adolescence 21
   Samar Hejazi, V. Susan Dahinten, Pamela A. Ratner, and Sheila K. Marshall
4. The Measurement and Epidemiology of Child Obesity 31
   David S. Freedman, Cynthia L. Ogden, and Sarah E. Cusick
5. Good-Enough Parenting, Self-Regulation and the Management of Weight-Related Problems 43
   Moria Golan
6. Nursing Perspective on Childhood Obesity 57
   Cynthia Yensel and Carrie Tolman
7. Contemporary Racial/Ethnic and Socioeconomic Patterns in U.S. Childhood Obesity 71
   Gopal K. Singh and Michael D. Kogan
8. Prediabetes among Obese Youth 87
   Orit Pinhas-Hamiel and Phil Zeitler
9. Prediabetes and Type 2 Diabetes: An Emerging Epidemic among Obese Youth 95
   Kathryn Love-Osborne
10. Prevalence of the Metabolic Syndrome in U.S. Youth 107
    Sarah E. Messiah, Kristopher L. Arheart, Steven E. Lipshultz, and Tracie L. Miller

II
PATHOPHYSIOLOGY

11. Emerging Pathways to Child Obesity Starts from the Mother's Womb: A Prospective View 119
    Ashik Mosaddik
12. The Social, Cultural and Familial Contexts Contributing to Childhood Obesity 127
    Cathy Banwell, Helen Kinmonth, and Jane Dixon
13. Cardiovascular Risk Clustering in Obese Children 139
    Ram Weiss

14. A Link between Maternal and Childhood Obesity 147
    Siân Robinson
15. Is Prenatal Exposure to Maternal Obesity Linked to Child Mental Health? 157
    Alina Rodriguez
16. Sleep and Obesity in Children and Adolescents 167
    Amy Darukhanavala and Silvana Pannain
17. Cellular Remodeling during the Growth of the Adipose Tissue 183
    Coralie Sengenès, Virginie Bourlier, Jean Galitzky, Alexia Zakaroff-Girard, Max Lafontan, and Anne Bouloumié
18. Children Obesity, Glucose Tolerance, Ghrelin and Prader-Willi Syndrome 191
    Simonetta Bellone, Arianna Busti, Sara Belcastro, Gianluca Aimaretti, Gianni Bona, and Flavia Prodam
19. Insulin Resistance and Glucose Metabolism in Childhood Obesity 201
    Subhashini Yaturu and Sushil K. Jain
20. Insulin Resistance in Pediatric Obesity: Physiological Effects and Possible Diet Treatment 209
    Ulf Holmbäck
21. Role of Fatty Liver Disease in Childhood Obesity 221
    Valerio Nobili, Anna Alisi, and Melania Manco

III
PSYCHOLOGICAL AND BEHAVIORAL FACTORS

22. An Overview of Psychological Symptoms in Obese Children 233
    Lisa Y. Gibson
23. Childhood Obesity: Depression, Anxiety and Recommended Therapeutic Strategies 245
    Dana L. Rofey, Jessica J. Black, Jennifer E. Phillips, Ronette Blake, and KayLoni Olson
24. The Emotional Impact of Obesity on Children 257
    Robert E. Cornette
25. Psychiatric Illness, Psychotropic Medication and Childhood Obesity 265
    Lawrence Maayan and Leslie Citrome

IV
CONSEQUENCES

26. Childhood Obesity: Public Health Impact and Policy Responses 281
    Rogan Kersh and Brian Elbel

27. Childhood Obesity and Juvenile Diabetes 289
    Mikael Knip
28. Bone Health in Obesity and the Cross Talk between Fat and Bone 297
    Sowmya Krishnan and Venkataraman Kalyanaraman

V

PREVENTION AND TREATMENT

29. A Community-Level Perspective for Childhood Obesity Prevention 305
    Christina Economos and Erin Hennessy
30. School-Based Obesity-Prevention Programs 319
    Genevieve Fridlund Dunton, Casey P. Durand, Nathaniel R. Riggs, and Mary Ann Pentz
31. School-Based Obesity Prevention Interventions Show Promising Improvements in the Health and Academic Achievements among Ethnically Diverse Young Children 333
    Danielle Hollar, Sarah E. Messiah, Gabriela Lopez-Mitnik, T. Lucas Hollar, and Michelle Lombardo
32. School and Community-Based Physical Education and Healthy Active Living Programs: Holistic Practices in Hong Kong, Singapore, and the United States 345
    Ming-Kai Chin, Christopher R. Edginton, Mei-Sin Tang, Kia-Wang Phua, and Jing-Zhen Yang
33. Schools as "Laboratories" for Obesity Prevention: Proven Effective Models 359
    Michelle Lombardo, Danielle Hollar, T. Lucas Hollar, and Karen McNamara
34. Fitness and Fatness in Childhood Obesity: Implications of Physical Activity 371
    Sarah P. Shultz, Benedicte Deforche, Nuala M. Byrne, and Andrew P. Hills
35. Pharmacotherapy in Childhood Obesity 383
    Amélio F. Godoy-Matos, Erika Paniago Guedes, Luciana Lopes de Souza, and Mariana Farage
36. Beverage Interventions to Prevent Child Obesity 389
    Rebeccá Muckelbauer, Mathilde Kersting, and Jacqueline Müller-Nordhorn
37. Psychotherapy as an Intervention for Child Obesity 401
    Carl-Erik Flodmark
38. Childhood Obesity: Psychological Correlates and Recommended Therapeutic Strategies 411
    Jennifer E. Phillips, Ethan E. Hull, and Dana L. Rofey
39. Dietary Supplements in the Prevention and Treatment of Childhood Obesity 419
    Robert I-San Lin
40. The Role of Arginine for Treating Obese Youth 433
    Catherine J. McNeal, Guoyao Wu, Susie Vasquez, Don P. Wilson, M. Carey Satterfield, Jason R. McKnight, Hussain S. Malbari, and Mujtaba Rahman
41. Prevention of Childhood Obesity with Use of Natural Products 443
    Jin-Taek Hwang, Dae Young Kwon, and Joohun Ha

VI

COMMENTARY AND RECOMMENDATIONS

42. The Role of United States Law to Prevent and Control Childhood Obesity 455
    Jennifer L. Pomeranz
43. Childhood Obesity as an Amplifier of Societal Inequality in the United States 463
    Stanley J. Ulijaszek
44. Childhood Obesity, Food Choice and Market Influence 475
    Jane Kolodinsky, Amanda Goldstein, and Erin Roche
45. The Role of Media in Childhood Obesity 487
    Amy B. Jordan and Ariel Chernin
46. Evaluation and Management of Childhood Obesity in Primary Care Settings 495
    Goutham Rao
47. The Future Directions and Clinical Management of Childhood Obesity 501
    Clodagh S. O'Gorman, Jonathan Cauchi, Jill K. Hamilton, and Denis Daneman

Index 515

Contributors

Gianluca Aimaretti Endocrinology, Department of Clinical and Experimental Medicine, University of Piemonte Orientale, Novara, Italy

Kristopher L. Arheart Division of Pediatric Clinical Research, Department of Pediatrics, Department of Epidemiology and Public Health and University of Miami Leonard M. Miller School of Medicine, Miami, FL, USA

Cathy Banwell National Centre for Epidemiology and Population Health (NCEPH), College of Medicine, Biology and Environment, Australian National University Canberra, Australia

Sara Belcastro Division of Paediatrics, Department of Medical Science, University of Piemonte Orientale, Novara, Italy and Endocrinology, Department of Clinical and Experimental Medicine, University of Piemonte Orientale, Novara, Italy

Simonetta Bellone Division of Paediatrics, Department of Medical Science, University of Piemonte Orientale, Novara, Italy

Jessica J. Black University of Cincinnati, OH, USA

Ronette Blake Children's Hospital of Pittsburgh, PA, USA

Gianni Bona Division of Paediatrics, Department of Medical Science, University of Piemonte Orientale, Novara, Italy

Anne Bouloumié Institut National de la Santé et de la Recherche Médicale (INSERM), U858, Toulouse, France and Université Toulouse III Paul Sabatier, Institut de Médecine Moléculaire de Rangueil, Equipe n°1 AVENIR, France

Virginie Bourlier Institut National de la Santé et de la Recherche Médicale (INSERM), U858, Toulouse, France and Université Toulouse III Paul Sabatier, Institut de Médecine Moléculaire de Rangueil, Equipe n°1 AVENIR, France

Arianna Busti Division of Paediatrics, Department of Medical Science, University of Piemonte Orientale, Novara, Italy and Endocrinology, Department of Clinical and Experimental Medicine, University of Piemonte Orientale, Novara, Italy

Nuala M. Byrne Institute of Health and Biomedical Innovation, Queensland University of Technology, Australia

Dominique Adele Cassuto Hopital Pitié-Salpêtrière, Paris France

Jonathan Cauchi Division of Endocrinology, Department of Pediatrics, The Hospital for Sick Children and University of Toronto, Toronto, Ontario, Canada

Ariel Chernin University of Pennsylvania, PA, USA

Ming-Kai Chin School of Health, Physical Education and Leisure Services, University of Northern Iowa, Cedar Falls, Iowa, IA, USA

Leslie Citrome New York University School of Medicine, New York and Nathan S. Kline Institute for Psychiatric Research, New York, NY, USA

Allison Collins Department of Pediatrics, Stanford University School of Medicine, CA, USA

Robert E. Cornette Department of Nursing, Berea College, Berea, KY, USA

Sarah E. Cusick Division of Epidemiology and Community Health, School of Public Health, University of Minnesota, Minneapolis, MN, USA

V. Susan Dahinten School of Nursing, University of British Columbia, Vancouver, British Columbia, Canada

Denis Daneman Division of Endocrinology, Department of Pediatrics, The Hospital for Sick Children and University of Toronto, Toronto, Ontario, Canada

Amy Darukhanavala Department of Medicine, Section of Adult and Pediatrics, Endocrinology, Diabetes, and Metabolism, The University of Chicago, IL, USA

Benedicte Deforche Department of Human Biometry and Biomechanics, Faculty of Physical Education and Physiotherapy, Vrije Universiteit Brussel, Belgium

Jane Dixon National Centre for Epidemiology and Population Health (NCEPH), College of Medicine, Biology and Environment, Australian National University Canberra, Australia

Genevieve Fridlund Dunton Department of Preventive Medicine, University of Southern California, Alhambra, CA, USA

Casey P. Durand Department of Preventive Medicine, University of Southern California, Alhambra, CA, USA

Christina Economos John Hancock Research Center for Physical Activity, Nutrition, and Obesity Prevention, Gerald J. and Dorothy R. Friedman School of Nutrition Science and Policy, Tufts University, Medford, MA, USA

Christopher R. Edginton School of Health, Physical Education and Leisure Services, University of Northern Iowa, Cedar Falls, IA, USA

Brian Elbel NYU Wagner School, NY, USA and NYU Medical School, NY, USA

Mariana Farage Serviço de Metabologia do Instituto Estadual de Diabetes e Endocrinologia (IEDE/RJ), Rio de Janeiro, RJ, Brazil

Carl-Erik Flodmark Department of Pediatrics, Childhood Obesity Unit, University Hospital in Malmö, Malmö, Sweden

David S. Freedman Division of Nutrition, Physical Activity and Obesity, Centers for Disease Control and Prevention K-26, Atlanta, GA, USA

Jean Galitzky Institut National de la Santé et de la Recherche Médicale (INSERM), U858, Toulouse, France and Université Toulouse III Paul Sabatier, Institut de Médecine Moléculaire de Rangueil, Equipe n°1 AVENIR, France

Lisa Y. Gibson Telethon Institute for Child Health Research, Centre for Child Health Research, The University of Western Australia, Perth, Western Australia

Amélio F. Godoy-Matos Serviço de Metabologia do Instituto Estadual de Diabetes e Endocrinologia (IEDE/RJ), Rio de Janeiro, RJ, Brazil

Moria Golan Shahaf, Community Services for the Management of Weight-Related Problems, Tel Hai Academic College, Upper Galilee and School of Nutritional Sciences, the Hebrew University of Jerusalem, Israel

Amanda Goldstein University of Vermont, Department of Community Development and Applied Economics and the Food Systems Research Collaborative at the Center for Rural Studies, Burlington, VT, USA

Erika Paniago Guedes Serviço de Metabologia do Instituto Estadual de Diabetes e Endocrinologia (IEDE/RJ), Rio de Janeiro, RJ, Brazil

Joohun Ha Department of Biochemistry and Molecular Biology, Medical Research Center for Bioreaction to Reactive Oxygen Species and Biomedical Science Institute, School of Medicine, Seoul, Republic of Korea

Jill K. Hamilton Division of Endocrinology, Department of Pediatrics, The Hospital for Sick Children and University of Toronto, Toronto, Ontario, Canada

Samar Hejazi School of Nursing, University of British Columbia, Vancouver, British Columbia, Canada

Erin Hennessy John Hancock Research Center for Physical Activity, Nutrition, and Obesity Prevention, Gerald J. and Dorothy R. Friedman School of Nutrition Science and Policy, Tufts University, Medford, MA, USA

Andrew P. Hills Institute of Health and Biomedical Innovation, Queensland University of Technology, Australia

Danielle Hollar Department of Pediatrics, University of Miami Miller School of Medicine, Miami, FL, USA

T. Lucas Hollar Department of Government, Stephen F. Austin State University, Nacogdoches, TX, USA

Ulf Holmbäck Clinical Nutrition and Metabolism, Department of Public Health and Caring Sciences, Uppsala University, Uppsala, Sweden

Ethan E. Hull Children's Hospital of Pittsburgh, Pittsburgh, PA, USA

Jin-Taek Hwang Department of Biogeron Food Technology, Korea Food Research Institute, Kyongki-do, Republic of Korea

Sushil K. Jain Department of Pediatrics, Louisiana State University Health Sciences Center, Shreveport, LA, USA

Amy B. Jordan The Annenberg Public Policy Center, University of Pennsylvania, Philadelphia, PA, USA

Venkataraman Kalyanaraman Department of Medicine, University of Oklahoma Health Sciences Center, Harold Hamm Oklahoma Diabetes Center, Oklahoma City, Oklahoma and VA Medical Center, Oklahoma City, OK, USA

Rogan Kersh NYU Wagner School, New York City, NY, USA

Mathilde Kersting Research Institute of Child Nutrition, Dortmund, Germany

Helen Kinmonth National Centre for Epidemiology and Population Health (NCEPH), College of Medicine, Biology and Environment, Australian National University Canberra, Australia

Mikael Knip Hospital for Children and Adolescents and Folkhälsan Research Center, University of Helsinki, Helsinki, and Department of Pediatrics, Tampere University Hospital, Tampere, Finland

Michael D. Kogan U.S. Department of Health and Human Services, Health Resources and Services Administration, Maternal, and Child Health Bureau, Rockville, MD, USA

Jane Kolodinsky University of Vermont, Department of Community Development and Applied Economics and the Food Systems Research Collaborative at the Center for Rural Studies, Burlington, VT, USA

Sowmya Krishnan Department of Pediatrics, University of Oklahoma Health Sciences Center, Children's Medical Research Institute Diabetes and Metabolic Research Program, Harold Hamm Oklahoma Diabetes Center, Oklahoma City, OK, USA

Dae Young Kwon Department of Biogeron Food Technology, Korea Food Research Institute, Kyongki-do, Republic of Korea

Max Lafontan Institut National de la Santé et de la Recherche Médicale (INSERM), U858, Toulouse, France and Université Toulouse III Paul Sabatier, Institut de Médecine Moléculaire de Rangueil, Equipe n°1 AVENIR

Robert I-San Lin Chairman, the Certification Board for Nutrition Specialists, Irvine, CA, USA

Steven E. Lipshultz Division of Pediatric Clinical Research, Department of Pediatrics and University of Miami Leonard M. Miller School of Medicine, Miami, FL, USA

Anna Lisi Scientific Directorate, "Bambino Gesù" Children's Hospital and Research Institute, Rome, Italy

Michelle Lombardo The OrganWise Guys, Inc., Duluth, GA, USA

Luciana Lopes de Souza Serviço de Metabologia do Instituto Estadual de Diabetes e Endocrinologia (IEDE/RJ), Rio de Janeiro, RJ, Brazil

Gabriela Lopez-Mitnik University of Miami, Miller School of Medicine, Batchelor Children's Research Institute, Miami, FL, USA

Kathryn Love-Osborne Division of Pediatrics, Section of Adolescent Medicine, Denver Health and Hospitals and University of Colorado at Denver Health Sciences Center, Denver, CO, USA

Lawrence Maayan New York University School of Medicine, New York City, New York and Nathan S. Kline Institute for Psychiatric Research, Orangeburg, NY, USA

Hussain S. Malbari Department of Pediatrics, Scott & White Healthcare, Temple, TX, USA

Melania Manco Scientific Directorate, "Bambino Gesù" Children's Hospital and Research Institute, Rome, Italy

Sheila K. Marshall School of Social Work, University of British Columbia, Vancouver, British Columbia, Canada

Jason R. McKnight Faculty of Nutrition, Texas A&M University, College Station, TX, USA

Karen McNamara The OrganWise Guys, Inc., Duluth, GA, USA

Catherine J. McNeal Department of Pediatrics, Scott & White Healthcare, Temple, TX, USA

Sarah E. Messiah Division of Pediatric Clinical Research, Department of Pediatrics and University of Miami Leonard M. Miller School of Medicine, Miami, FL, USA

Tracie L. Miller Division of Pediatric Clinical Research, Department of Pediatrics and University of Miami Leonard M. Miller School of Medicine, Miami, FL, USA

Ashik Mosaddik Department of Pharmacy, Rajshahi University, Bangladesh, and Subtropical Horticulture Research Institute, Faculty of Biotechnology, Jeju National University, Jeju, Republic of Korea

Rebecca Muckelbauer Berlin School of Public Health, Charité University Medical Center, Berlin, Germany

Jacqueline Müller-Nordhorn Berlin School of Public Health, Charité University Medical Center, Berlin, Germany

Valerio Nobili Scientific Directorate, "Bambino Gesù" Children's Hospital and Research Institute, Rome, Italy

Clodagh S. O'Gorman Division of Endocrinology, Department of Pediatrics, The Hospital for Sick Children and University of Toronto, Toronto, Ontario, Canada

Cynthia L. Ogden National Center for Health Statistics, Centers for Disease Control and Prevention, Hyattsville, MD, USA

KayLoni Olson Children's Hospital of Pittsburgh, PA, USA

Silvana Pannain Department of Medicine, Section of Adult and Pediatrics, Endocrinology, Diabetes, and Metabolism, The University of Chicago, IL, USA

Rebecka Peebles Department of Pediatrics, Stanford University School of Medicine, Stanford, CA, USA

Mary Ann Pentz Department of Preventive Medicine, University of Southern California, Alhambra, CA, USA

Jennifer E. Phillips University of Pittsburgh, PA, USA

Kia-Wang Phua North Vista Primary School, Singapore

Orit Pinhas-Hamiel Pediatric Endocrinology and Diabetes, Sheba Medical Center, Tel-Hashomer, Ramat-Gan, 52621, Tel-Aviv University, Israel and Juvenile Diabetes Center, Maccabi Health Care Services, Israel

Jennifer L. Pomeranz Rudd Center for Food Policy and Obesity, Yale University, New Haven, CT, USA

Flavia Prodam Division of Paediatrics, Department of Medical Science, University of Piemonte Orientale, Novara, Italy and Endocrinology, Department of Clinical and Experimental Medicine, University of Piemonte Orientale, Novara, Italy

Mujtaba Rahman Department of Pediatrics, Scott & White Healthcare, Temple, TX, USA

Goutham Rao Weight Management and Wellness Center, Children's Hospital of Pittsburgh (of UPMC), University of Pittsburgh School of Medicine, Pittsburgh, PA, USA

Pamela A. Ratner School of Nursing, University of British Columbia, Vancouver, British Columbia, Canada

Nathaniel R. Riggs Department of Preventive Medicine, University of Southern California, Alhambra, CA, USA

Siân Robinson MRC Epidemiology Resource Centre, University of Southampton, United Kingdom

Erin Roche University of Vermont, Department of Community Development and Applied Economics and the Food Systems Research Collaborative at the Center for Rural Studies, Burlington, VT, USA

Alina Rodriguez Department of Psychology, Uppsala University, Sweden, Department of Epidemiology and Biostatistics, School of Public Health, Imperial College London, United Kingdom and MRC Social Genetic Developmental Psychiatry (SGDP), Institute of Psychiatry, King's College London, United Kingdom

Dana L. Rofey Children's Hospital of Pittsburgh, PA, USA

M. Carey Satterfield Faculty of Nutrition, Texas A&M University, College Station, TX, USA

Coralie Sengenès Institut National de la Santé et de la Recherche Médicale (INSERM), U858, Toulouse, France and Université Toulouse III Paul Sabatier, Institut de Médecine Moléculaire de Rangueil, Equipe n°1 AVENIR

Sarah P. Shultz Institute of Health and Biomedical Innovation, Queensland University of Technology, Australia

Gopal K. Singh U.S. Department of Health and Human Services, Health Resources and Services Administration, Maternal and Child Health Bureau, Rockville, MD, USA

Mei-Sin Tang Baptist (Sha Tin Wai) Lui Ming Choi Primary School, Hong Kong, China

Carrie Tolman Center for Healthy Weight and Nutrition, Nationwide Children's Hospital, Columbus, OH, USA

Stanley J. Ulijaszek Institute of Social and Cultural Anthropology, University of Oxford, United Kingdom

Susie Vasquez Department of Pharmacology, Scott & White Healthcare, Temple, TX, USA

Bernard Waysfeld Hopital Saint Michel, Paris, France

Ram Weiss Hadassah – Hebrew University School of Medicine, Braun School of Public Health and Community Medicine, Jerusalem, Israel

Don P. Wilson Division of Pediatric Endocrinology and Diabetes, Phoenix Children's Hospital, Phoenix, AZ, USA

Guoyao Wu Faculty of Nutrition, Texas A&M University, College Station, TX, USA

Jing-Zhen Yang Department of Community and Behavioral Health, College of Public Health, University of Iowa, Iowa City, IA, USA

Subhashini Yaturu Department of Endocrinology, Stratton VA Medical Center, Albany, New York; Albany Medical College, Albany, NY, USA

Cynthia Yensel Center for Healthy Weight and Nutrition, Nationwide Children's Hospital, Columbus, OH, USA

Alexia Zakaroff-Girard Institut National de la Santé et de la Recherche Médicale (INSERM), U858, Toulouse, France and Université Toulouse III Paul Sabatier, Institut de Médecine Moléculaire de Rangueil, Equipe n°1 AVENIR, France

Phil Zeitler Division of Endocrinology, Department of Pediatrics, The University of Colorado Denver, The Children's Hospital, Aurora, CO, USA

Preface

The major goal of *Global Perspectives on Childhood Obesity: Current Status, Consequences and Prevention* is to present the intricate aspects of the obesity paradigm, especially insights about the alarming upsurge of obesity in children, and its consequences on future generations and society. The book is designed to expand the reader's scope and opportunity to gain important information about childhood obesity in a way that is valuable to scientists, the public, and those in general health positions.

I believe in advocating an array of solutions for the worldwide epidemic of childhood obesity and want to make people more aware of the seriousness of our children's decline in health. The impact of childhood obesity reaches beyond the individual family and into the public arenas of social systems and government policy and programs. This book is a collection of insights, commentaries, and studies written by prestigious global representatives of the clinical, government, university, and industrial fields, and it addresses the current state of childhood obesity, strategies for its prevention and treatment, and its effects on the future for children and society.

The book starts with a section titled "Epidemiology and Prevalence," which consists of 10 chapters that provide insights, viewpoints, and perspectives from pediatricians, nurses, epidemiologists, and nutritionists, and it discusses the prevalence of obesity, metabolic syndrome, and diabetes, especially type 2 diabetes, in obese youth. The influence of contemporary racial, ethnic, and socioeconomic patterns on childhood obesity is demonstrated. Furthermore, the impact of good parenting and self-regulation in helping the management of weight-related problems is also extensively discussed.

The second section, "Pathophysiology," focuses on a broad spectrum of emerging areas, including the social, cultural, and familial contexts contributing to childhood obesity, and a link between maternal and childhood obesity. The other chapters highlight the association of childhood obesity with cardiovascular risk factors, the child's mental health, sleep, and cellular remodeling during the growth of the adipose tissues. Renowned experts from the field explore the association and link between pediatric obesity and insulin resistance, glucose metabolism, the hunger hormone "ghrelin," fatty liver disease, and Prader-Willi syndrome.

In the third section, "Psychological and Behavioral Factors," the diverse elements associated with childhood obesity, including depression, anxiety, and other emotional aspects, are extensively discussed by four eminent groups of researchers in these areas.

The fourth section, "Consequences," discusses the impacts of childhood obesity on juvenile diabetes, bone health, and public health and policy.

In the fifth section, "Prevention and Treatment," 12 worldwide groups of experts cover diverse strategies for averting or managing childhood obesity, including community efforts, school-based physical activity and nutrition curriculum, pharmacotherapy, psychotherapy, bariatric surgery, and the potential use of novel dietary supplements.

The sixth section, "Commentary and Recommendations," offers various approaches for preventing and controlling childhood obesity. The section explores healthy food choices for children, guidelines for primary care settings, the influence of the market, the role of media, and future strategies of clinical management.

Overall, these 47 chapters provide directional impact and strategies to the clinicians, scientists, and general public, especially parents. I believe this book can demonstrate our encompassed philosophies in the global perspectives on childhood obesity and its intervention.

The material in this book complements the information in my first obesity book, *Obesity: Epidemiology, Pathophysiology, and Prevention*, from CRC Press/Taylor & Francis. The first book did very well in the academic field, receiving high appreciation from the *Journal of the American Medical Association (JAMA)* and the *New England Journal of Medicine (NEJM)*, and I hope this second book will have the same recognition and success.

I offer my sincere regards and gratitude to all the eminent scientists, researchers, doctors, and authors who contributed to this book. Also, my special thanks go to Ms. Carrie Bolger and Ms. Nancy Maragioglio for their continued support, help, and cooperation.

Debasis Bagchi Ph.D., FACN, CNS, MAIChE
University of Houston, College of Pharmacy,
Houston, Texas

Dedication

To My Only Beloved Daughter Dipanjali

SECTION I

EPIDEMIOLOGY AND PREVALENCE

CHAPTER 1

Pediatric Obesity
A Pediatrician's Viewpoint

Allison Collins, Rebecka Peebles

Department of Pediatrics, Stanford University School of Medicine, Stanford, CA, USA

Pediatric obesity has rapidly become one of the leading international public health challenges. Since the 1980s, rates have more than doubled for preschool-aged children (2 to 5 years) and adolescents (12 to 19 years) and have more than tripled for school-aged children (aged 6-11 years) in the United States [1]. In Australia, a recent study showed a prevalence of overweight and obesity of 25% in children aged 2 to 18 years [2]. A study of Indonesian adolescents showed obesity rates of 10% [3]. In Spain, researchers have found rates of overweight and obesity in 4-year-olds of up to 32% in certain regions [4]. Worldwide, there are estimates that more than 22 million children under the age of 5 are obese, and one in ten children are overweight [5]. This demonstrates the tremendous scope of the pediatric obesity problem, which appears to affect almost all nations worldwide.

Childhood obesity involves both immediate and long-term risks to physical health, including diabetes, hypertension, liver disease, heart disease, and osteoarthritis, as well as significant psychosocial burdens among numerous other concerns [6]. Obese children have also been shown to have significantly lower health-related quality of life than children and adolescents who are normal weight, with ratings similar to children diagnosed with cancer [7].

Pediatricians play a particularly important role in pediatric obesity. As primary care providers, pediatricians are involved in a child's health from birth through adolescence, which gives them a unique role and involvement in the life of a child and family. Children generally see their pediatrician anywhere from one to ten-plus times a year, especially in the younger age groups. Pediatricians are already involved in regularly scheduled well-child visits dedicated to discussions of health, growth, development, nutrition, safety, and overall well-being. These visits also provide opportunities to form rapport with families and children. The pediatrician can become a key player in the field of pediatric overweight and obesity by becoming involved in prevention, screening and identification, treatment or referral, and community involvement to affect pediatric obesity at a higher level. This chapter focuses on these areas in detail.

PREVENTION

It has been shown that treating obesity is not only difficult and costly, but it is often ineffective [6]. Prevention in childhood is particularly important, as obesity in childhood often persists into adulthood [8]. Working with families to establish healthy eating and activity behaviors early in life is especially important in the prevention model. Starting at birth and continuing through adolescence, pediatricians should be teaching prevention strategies in their well-child visit exams. Although there are many possible prevention strategies, evidence-based target behaviors have been identified that are particularly relevant for the prevention of obesity (Table 1.1). Although it is often impossible to discuss all target behaviors at every visit because of time constraints, practitioners should choose a few felt to be most salient to their patients and incorporate these over multiple visits. Previsit screening questionnaires are often efficient ways of obtaining this information. Over time, it is important to discuss establishing these healthy nutrition and activity habits at a young age in order to prevent unhealthy habits from developing.

Prevention can begin as early as the prenatal period. Research has shown that maternal nutrition during pregnancy may establish future obesity patterns. Both overweight and obesity in the first trimester and excess

TABLE 1.1 Evidence-Based Target Behaviors to Prevent Obesity [14]

NUTRITION

Limiting sugar-sweetened beverages—including sodas, fruit drinks, energy drinks

Adequate fruits and vegetables (U.S. Department of Agriculture [USDA] currently recommends nine servings/day; serving size varies by age)

Decreased eating out, including fast food

Eating breakfast every morning

Encouraging family meals—parents and children sit down and eat together

Appropriate portion sizes for age (having models of food/cups to teach)

Adequate fiber in diet (age appropriate)

Breastfeeding at least 6 months

Reduce dieting behaviors (particularly in teens)

ACTIVITY

Limit screen time (TV, video games) to less than 2 hours/day (none for children under 2 years of age)

No TV in child's room

>1 hour of physical activity/day

---

pregnancy-related weight gain is associated with increased risk of child overweight at age 3 years [9]. Although the impact was greater for women that were overweight or obese to start with, the effect was also seen in normal weight women who gained an excessive amount of weight in pregnancy [9]. In addition, poor maternal weight gain and very low birth weight have also been associated with future childhood obesity, highlighting the impact of extremes in prenatal nutrition at both ends of the pregnancy spectrum [10]. This underscores the importance of working together with family medicine and obstetric practitioners on counseling mothers during pregnancy about establishing healthy lifestyles for themselves in order to prevent excess or poor weight gain during pregnancy. Early weight gain in infants can be another important warning sign. Rapid weight gain in infancy may substantially increase the risk of obesity later in life [11]. Pediatricians should monitor patients' growth patterns as a part of infant well-child checks and discuss any unusual trends with parents in a thoughtful manner.

SCREENING

Because of high rates of overweight and obesity and the seriousness of the disease, many organizations, such as the American Academy of Pediatrics, the Center for Disease Control (CDC), and the World Health Organization, recommend that pediatricians universally assess all children for obesity risk to improve early identification and management and highlight prevention [12, 13]. The screening should entail weight and height measurements of all patients. For patients 2 years and up, a body mass index (BMI) should be calculated using the following formula: body weight in kilograms/(height in meters) [2]. BMI should then be plotted on charts with percentiles specific for age and gender, as available by the CDC. A percentile BMI should be obtained from the chart, allowing the clinician to categorize the child into a BMI category: underweight is considered below the 5th percentile, normal weight, the 5th to 84th percentiles; overweight, the 85th to 94th percentiles; obese, the 95th to 99th percentiles; and morbidly obese is defined as greater than the 99th percentile or a BMI greater than 40 [14].

For patients younger than 2 years, the weight and length should still be plotted on a weight for length growth curve, specific for gender and age, and a percentile should be evaluated. For these young children, the rate of change of weight for length is particularly important. For example, if an infant is rapidly increasing in weight for length percentiles (i.e., crossing percentile lines), this could be a high-risk situation that would require further counseling, as discussed later.

In addition to determining BMI and appropriate weight categories, pediatricians should assess medical and behavioral risk factors for obesity in their patients (Table 1.2). This helps the clinician further differentiate the overall risks and assessments that will help in the identification stage, as discussed next.

IDENTIFICATION

The next step is identifying patients from the screening process at increased risk for future adverse health consequences, either because of their category

TABLE 1.2 Risk Evaluation [25]

MEDICAL RISKS

Family history: obesity, diabetes, heart disease, hypertension, hyperlipidemia [15]

Race (African American, American Indian, Hispanic at higher risk)

Current obesity-related medical conditions (Table 1.5)

BEHAVIORAL RISKS

Eating habits

Activity habits

Sedentary behavior habits

Dieting behaviors

of overweight or obesity or because they have concerning medical or behavioral risk factors. If a patient is underweight, further follow-up with investigation of potential malnutrition or underlying disease is likely warranted and is beyond the scope of this text. If a patient is normal weight, medical and behavioral risks together with a BMI growth trend should still be reviewed. If several medical or behavioral risk factors are present or if the patient's BMI has been continually trending upward, particularly if it has crossed more than two percentile lines, close observation (i.e., before the next year or 2-year scheduled exam) or a discussion of any problematic weight and health habits identified in screening should be considered. If a patient falls into the overweight category, the medical and behavioral risk and BMI curve trends need to be assessed.

Although the BMI is an efficient screening tool, it can improperly categorize people into the overweight or even obese category, particularly extreme athletes or muscular people [15]. In addition, there are also individuals who are overweight or obese by BMI screen but do not incur increased metabolic, cardiovascular, or mortality risk and thus might not be "overfat" [14] just as there are some patients in a normal weight range who are not physiologically or metabolically fit. Some pediatric patients may be above the 85th percentile for BMI their entire life but growing and thriving at a stable rate, and these individuals may therefore be at an appropriate weight for their age, height, and body composition. Thus, the clinician needs to remember that BMI is only a screening tool, and clinical judgment is still critical to the proper assessment of overall health and the creation of an appropriate treatment plan. Many overweight and most obese or morbidly obese children will merit further medical assessment. Both child and parental perspectives of weight category and their level of concern should be deduced, as this will help in formulating a treatment plan that the family will readily accept.

ASSESSMENT

A thorough medical assessment and exam is essential to a complete evaluation of current or future health risks potentially incurred from weight dysregulation. The history should review the onset of weight gain and any stressors or events surrounding them, eating behaviors and dietary habits, exercise and sedentary activities, followed by a review of symptoms, past medical history, family history, social history, physical exam, and any tests or labs that need to be done. These are discussed later in more detail, with the obesity-related aspects highlighted.

History of Weight Gain

The timing of when the patient or parent first noticed weight to be an issue is an important place to start. It is generally helpful to discuss infant and early childhood growth patterns. Any available past growth curves should be reviewed. If these are not available, asking the family to recall several prior weights in the past is useful in assessing whether the child's weight is stable over time or if it has been rapidly escalating. Learning about any prior feeding difficulties, especially in infancy, and whether the child was breast-fed is also helpful as breast-feeding can be protective [16], and early childhood feeding patterns and weight gain can sometimes set a trend for future difficulties. It is also important to ask what the patient and family perceive as the cause of the overweight/obesity (diet, activity, genes, etc.) as well how concerned they are about the problem. Determining the extent that weight impacts the child's life (social, school, daily living, etc.) and if any attempt has been made in the past, successful or not, for weight loss is helpful to the history [12].

Diet and physical activity should be assessed next. This can be accomplished in several ways, ranging from a survey the family fills out before the visit to a direct interview and assessment with a practitioner. Food and activity recall over a recent 24-hour period can be helpful in determining general trends in eating behaviors. A few key components should be included in a comprehensive food and activity assessment: hours of physical activity per day (including walking/biking to work, outside playtime, physical education at school); screen time per day (i.e., TV, computer, play station); availability of a TV, videogames, or computer in the child's bedroom; sugary beverage frequency (including soft drinks, juice drinks, juice, energy drinks, etc.); typical locations and frequency of dining out; fruit and vegetable servings per day; location of meals (e.g., in front of the TV, in bedroom, at table) and how often meals are eaten with the family; and a general idea of typical portion sizes [12]. As many young people show disordered or dysregulated eating at an early age, and these can predict future weight gain and comorbidity [17], all patients at risk for obesity and their parents should be asked if they skip meals in an average week or engage in binge-eating or purging behaviors, fasting, dieting, food hoarding or secretive eating in their room, diet pill or laxative use, and any night eating habits (waking up in the middle of the night to eat). If any of these behaviors are present, they may be the first and most critical targets to garner attention, often in conjunction with qualified mental health practitioners, as addressing other health behaviors without correcting underlying disordered eating patterns effectively may yield suboptimal results [18, 19].

Review of Systems

A thorough review of systems that are particularly geared at obesity-related complications is important for the evaluation. Table 1.3 outlines symptoms to review in addition to any other issues raised by the patient or family [14].

Past Medical History

Getting a detailed past medical history is important to a full assessment. Surgical history (possible tonsil and adenoidectomy, cholecystectomy, etc.), any behavioral issues or developmental problems that could indicate Prader-Willi or another genetic syndrome, and medication history (steroids, some anticonvulsants, some psychiatric drugs, or hormonal contraceptives can cause issues with weight control) should be included.

Family History

A detailed family history should be obtained. Race and ethnicity should be noted, as African American, American Indian, and Hispanic patients are at higher risk of obesity [20]. Direct and first extended family history should be taken, with special notes asking about obesity, diabetes mellitus type 2, premature cardiovascular disease (i.e., angina, atherosclerosis, or myocardial infarction <55 years for men, <65 years for women), hypertension, stroke, gallbladder disease, sleep apnea, hyperlipidemia, hypothyroidism, fertility and or menstrual issues (elucidating possible familial risk of polycystic ovarian syndrome), and bariatric surgery (all of these geared toward the patient's siblings, parents, grandparents, aunts, and uncles) [12].

Social History

Understanding the patient's social environment is often critical to developing appropriate treatment plans. For young children, this history is often obtained from parents, but in adolescents it is important to discuss a confidential social history. A basic history includes understanding the home environment. The marital and custodial status of parents, involvement of other caregivers, neighborhood safety, and meal planning and preparation are all important in understanding how behavior change may be implemented. In addition, taking the time to assess psychosocial risk factors such as symptoms of depression, anxiety, history of abuse, bullying, and drug and alcohol use are also critical to developing the most appropriate treatment plan for each child or adolescent [21].

Readiness for Change

Another important aspect of the assessment is the patient and parent's readiness for change, which can be assessed based on the Stages of Change model (Table 1.4). This model states that "for most persons, a change in behavior occurs gradually, with the patient moving from being uninterested, unaware or unwilling to make a change (precontemplation), to considering a change (contemplation), to deciding and preparing to make a change. Genuine, determined action is then taken and, over time, attempts to maintain the new behavior occur. Relapses are almost inevitable and become part of the process of working toward life-long change" [14, 22]. Gauging this can be done by asking the patient and family what they think or by using an

TABLE 1.3 Review of Systems of Obesity Assessment

RESPIRATORY
Shortness of breath
Snoring, apnea episodes while sleeping
Endocrine
Darkening of skin on neck/axillae/abdomen
Polyuria or nocturia
Polydipsia
GASTROINTESTINAL
Abdominal pain
Constipation
GYNECOLOGICAL
Irregular menses
Amenorrhea
NEUROLOGICAL
Headaches
DERMATOLOGICAL
Acne
ORTHOPEDIC
Back pain
Hip or knee pain
PSYCHIATRIC
Depression
Anxiety
Substance use
Binge eating
Purging
Bullying or being bullied

TABLE 1.4 Stages of Change [14, 22]

PRECONTEMPLATION STAGE

Patients do not even consider changing

Denial: does not believe it applies to self

Believes consequences are not serious

CONTEMPLATION STAGE

Patients are ambivalent about changing

Weighing benefits and costs of behavior

PREPARATION STAGE

Patients prepare to make a specific change

May experiment with small changes

Determination to change increases

ACTION STAGE

Patient ready to take definitive action

Desire for lifestyle change

MAINTENANCE

Patient maintains new behavior over time

RELAPSE

Patient experiences relapse to old behaviors

Normal part of process of change

"importance" or "confidence" ruler, where the patient rates both the importance of changing this behavior and the patient's confidence in his or her ability to change on a scale of one to ten. This information can be very helpful as you plan for the treatment stage and is particularly useful in a method called motivational interviewing that will be discussed later [14].

Physical Exam

A thorough physical exam should be performed, much as would be done for a yearly well-child exam. A height and weight should be obtained, as well as vital signs, including a blood pressure taken with appropriate cuff size, which typically necessitates having some larger adult cuffs available to ensure proper fitting. After plotting the percentile BMI, height, and weight, the systolic and diastolic blood pressure should also be compared to normative percentiles according to age, gender, and height percentile by using appropriate tables published by the National Heart, Lung, and Blood Institute (www.nhlbi.nih.gov/health/prof/heart/hbp/hbp_ped.htm). If the blood pressure is abnormal, it should be repeated, including a manual reading if not done the first time. Table 1.5 outlines other key physical exam findings to look for and what they might indicate.

Laboratory Assessment

There are some screening labs that are recommended to better assess patient's risks for comorbidities that are highly associated with overweight and obesity. If a patient falls into the overweight category (BMI 85% to 94%), a fasting lipid panel is recommended for children over 10 years of age [14]. If any risk factors are present, a fasting glucose, as partate aminotransferase (AST) and alanine aminotransferase (ALT) should also be measured. If a patient falls into the obesity category (BMI >95%), fasting lipids, fasting glucose, AST, and ALT should be done for all patients over the age of 10 years regardless of risk factors [14]. If any of these labs are abnormal, they should be discussed and followed at least every year with possible referral to a specialist. For example, if the AST or ALT levels are above 60 units/L on two occasions, referral to a pediatric gastroenterologist should be considered [14]. If labs are within normal limits, they should be repeated every 2 years. Other labs that also should be considered, although evidence and recommendations for these are mixed, include a fasting insulin level and hemoglobin A1C to screen for insulin resistance, a high-sensitivity C-reactive protein (CRP) to screen for inflammatory and cardiovascular risk, and a 25-OH vitamin D level, as the risk of deficiency is correlated with increasing BMI and can be associated with increased cardiovascular risk [23]. If the vitamin D level is <20 ng/mL, consider giving supplemental ergocalciferol either 5000 units daily for 2 to 3 months or 50,000 units every week for 8 weeks [24]. Other labs that may be done depending on the patient's symptoms and exam include complete blood count (CBC), blood urea nitrogen (BUN), and creatinine, free thyroxine (T4) and thyroid stimulating harmone (TSH), and Prader-Willi fluorescent in situ hybridization (FISH) probe (especially with concerns of developmental delay). Strong consideration should be given to screening for polycystic ovarian syndrome (PCOS) in postmenarchal females with obesity and menstrual irregularity or dysfunction, especially if they exhibit other signs or symptoms of either hyperandrogenism (i.e., acne, hirsutism) or hyperinsulinism; these labs would ideally include luteinizing hormone, follicle stimulating hormone, prolactin, free and total testosterone, DHEA-S, and sex hormone binding globulin. Although rare, late-onset congenital adrenal hyperplasia (CAH) and androgen-secreting tumors can sometimes present in this population and appear similar to PCOS clinically; as a result, if adrenal androgens are elevated screening for CAH with a 17-OH-progesterone level is warranted, and ultrasounds or magnetic resonance imaging (MRI) may be indicated if either ovarian or adrenal androgens are markedly elevated [19].

TABLE 1.5 Physical Examination Findings in Obesity Assessment and Possible Causes [14]

Growth	
Short stature (<25% for age)	Underlying endocrine or genetic condition
VITALS	
Elevated blood pressure	Hypertension if SBP or DBP >95% for sex, age, and height on three or more occasions [25]
SKIN	
Acanthosis nigricans	Increased risk of insulin resistance
Excessive acne	Polycystic ovarian syndrome
Hirsutism	Polycystic ovarian syndrome
Irritation or inflammation under pannus	Folliculitis; intertriginous infection
Violaceous striae	Cushing syndrome
Atrophic striae	Weight gain/loss
EYES	
Papilledema	Pseudotumor cerebri; cerebral tumor (less likely)
THROAT	
Tonsillar hypertrophy	Obstructive sleep apnea
NECK	
Goiter	Hypothyroidism
ABDOMEN	
Tenderness on palpation	GERD, gall bladder disease
Hepatomegaly	NAFLD
GENITOURINARY	
Delayed pubertal or Tanner stage	Genetic syndrome; can be due only to obesity
Undescended testicles	Prader-Willi syndrome
Clitoromegaly	Polycystic ovarian syndrome; congenital adrenal hyperplasia
EXTREMITIES	
Abnormal gait, hip, or knee pain	Slipped capital femoral epiphysis
Bowing of tibia	Blount disease
Small hands and feet	Genetic syndromes
Polydactyly	Genetic syndromes
Joint or back pain	Can be due solely to obesity
BACK	
Buffalo hump	Cushing's syndrome

Comorbidity Assessment

After a full history, physical exam, and initial laboratory assessment is complete, patients should be assessed for any comorbidities they might have associated with their overweight or obesity. Table 1.6 outlines common comorbidities. Depending on the severity of the comorbidity and the experience of the provider, further testing or referral to a pediatric specialist may be indicated. For example, if obstructive sleep apnea is suspected, a polysomnogram should be ordered. The more weight-related comorbidities the patient has, the more concerning the health risks, and the more aggressive the family/patient may need to be with interventions, as discussed in the treatment section that follows. In general, it is helpful to recall that these complications of obesity often cluster together, with insulin resistance being a central factor in many common comorbidities, such as obstructive sleep apnea, elevated inflammatory markers, diabetes, PCOS, hypertension, hyperlipidemia, and nonalcoholic fatty liver disease.

TREATMENT

Once patients have been identified and a full assessment has been done, a treatment plan should be made, based on each individual's risks, level of motivation, and resources. It should be recognized that obesity treatment is best conceptualized within a chronic care model,

TABLE 1.6 Comorbidities of Obesity

RESPIRATORY

Asthma

Obstructive sleep apnea

ENDOCRINE

Insulin resistance

Diabetes mellitus type 2

Dyslipidemia

Gynecomastia

CARDIOVASCULAR

Hypertension

Left ventricular hypertrophy

GASTROINTESTINAL

Nonalcoholic fatty liver disease (NAFLD)

Gallstones

Gastroesophageal reflux

Constipation

GYNECOLOGICAL

Irregular menses

Polycystic ovary syndrome

NEUROLOGICAL

Pseudotumor cerebri

DERMATOLOGICAL

Acne

Acanthosis nigricans

ORTHOPEDIC

Back pain

Blount's disease

Slipped capital femoral epiphysis

NUTRITION

Vitamin D deficiency

Iron-deficiency anemia

Hypercholesterolemia

Hypertriglyceridemia

PSYCHIATRIC

Depression

Anxiety

Disordered eating

as effective behavior and weight change can take time to implement. The primary goal of treatment is to create a healthier lifestyle in order to minimize risks of current or future morbidity and mortality. This means that the primary goal may not necessarily be weight loss, but weight stabilization or simply healthier habits. A staged approach has been recommended by the American Academy of Pediatrics in order to take into account that different patients will require different levels of intervention and support depending on responses to treatment, age, degree of obesity, health risks, and motivation, as outlined in Table 1.7 [14]. Weight goals have been suggested, depending on the patient's age and level of overweight or obesity, which is a general guideline to ensure healthy weight management, as outlined in Table 1.8. As previously outlined, for children under 2 years of age, weight for length and height should be plotted and the corresponding percentiles noted. If a child falls above the 85% for age/gender or if there is rapidly increasing growth in the weight for length curve (crossing more than two percentile lines in the past year), the parents should be given prevention counseling, but no weight loss or weight goals should be suggested [14].

For adolescents, an approach called motivational interviewing has also shown promise. This approach relies on the gradual creation of a treatment contract with the teen patient as an active participant in creating the plan. This approach relies on first assessing how important change is to the patient or family and then how confident they are that they can make these changes. The responses given are incorporated in a graduated, collaborative approach that creates a partnership between the patient and physician and allows for more effective implementation of behavior change over time. This approach requires minimal training and can allow impressive gains in treatment, although it does demand increased flexibility on the part of the practitioner in developing target treatment goals, which can be a challenge for pediatricians more comfortable with didactic or authoritative approaches to patient care [14, 22].

ADVOCACY

The pediatrician can play a key role in many critical obesity prevention and treatment efforts, not only with patients and families but also at a community and federal level. Barriers to addressing obesity are numerous in our culture, ranging from reduced physical education curricula, changes in the built environment that block healthy and safe behavior change within communities, and federal legislation that promote advertising and marketing choices that may worsen weight-related problems in children. Effective advocacy is imperative in working to change children's access to safe play spaces, healthy food options, physical activity in schools, and healthier communities. Pediatricians need to continue to make their voices heard in these public health forums.

TABLE 1.7 Stages of Obesity Treatment

STAGE 1: PREVENTION PLUS

Goal: Weight maintenance to improve BMI through basic healthy lifestyle eating and activity habits

Plan: Encourage the following habits:

Consume at least five servings of fruits and vegetables/day (serving size varies by age)

Eliminate or minimize sugar-sweetened beverages

Decrease television viewing to no more than 2 hours/day if >2 years, none if <2 years

Physical activity at least 1 hour/day (unstructured play for young children, unstructured or structured activities for older children such as sports, dance, walking, riding bike)

Less eating out and fast food, more meals at home

Eat at the table as a family at least five times/week

Consume a healthy breakfast every day

Involve the entire family in lifestyle changes

Allow child to self-regulate meals and avoid overly restrictive feeding behaviors

Help families tailor recommendations to their own cultural values

Tips on implementation

Families and providers work together to identify target behaviors that will work for the patient and family's circumstance

Use motivational interviewing techniques to elicit target behavior changes

Stepwise target behaviors (choose three at a time, modify depending on patient's level)

Follow-up visits should be scheduled based on individual case

If no improvement in BMI in 3 to 6 months, move onto stage 2

Location: Primary care office

STAGE 2: STRUCTURED WEIGHT MANAGEMENT

Goal: Weight maintenance or loss based on more targeted healthy lifestyle changes

Plan: Same as prevention plus, but with more support and structure

Planned diet or eating outline, emphasizing low-energy density foods, balanced diet—by dietitian or skilled clinician

Structured daily meals and snacks (three meals/day and one to two snacks/day)

Reduction in screen time to <1 hour/day

Planned, supervised physical activity for at least 1 hour/day

Monitoring behavior through logbooks

Planned reinforcement for achieving target behaviors

Tips on Implementation

Monthly office visits generally required

Group sessions can be effective and efficient way to implement

Some families need referral to counselor for parenting skills, motivation, or family conflict resolution

If no improvement in BMI in 3 to 6 months, move onto stage 3

Location: Primary care office with referrals as needed

STAGE 3: COMPREHENSIVE MULTIDISCIPLINARY INTERVENTION

Goal: Weight maintenance or loss based on more structured behavioral modification techniques

(*Continued*)

TABLE 1.7 Stages of Obesity Treatment—cont'd

Plan:

Structured program in behavioral modification with food monitoring, short-term diet and physical activity goal setting

Parental participation, especially with children <12 years

Evaluation of body measurements, diet, physical activity at regular intervals

Multidisciplinary team with experience in childhood obesity: behavioral counselor (social worker, psychologist, etc.), registered dietitian, exercise specialist, primary care provider

Frequent office visits: weekly visit for 2 to 3 months, then monthly

Tips on Implementation

Group visits can make the frequent visits more cost effective and beneficial

Commercial weight management program can be considered with the primary care doctor involved to screen the program to ensure healthy approach for age

If no improvement, consider stage 4

Location: Established pediatric weight management program

STAGE 4: TERTIARY CARE INTERVENTIONS

Goal: Weight loss based on intensive interventions beyond nutrition and activity changes in other stages

Plan: Options include the following:

Medications: potential use in teenagers; however, minimal effect; need medical supervision

    Sibutramine for patients 16 years and older—serotonin reuptake inhibitor

    Orlistat for patients 12 years and older—fat malabsorption

Very low-calorie diets: Restrictive diets generally not recommended for pediatric population but in certain extreme cases can be used under very close medical watch.

Bariatric surgery: gastric bypass and gastric banding

    Generally leads to substantial weight loss and improvement in medical conditions but also has significant risks and lifelong lifestyle change

    Requires careful evaluation presurgery and longtime psychological and nutrition support postsurgery

    Criteria [26]:

        BMI >35 kg/m^2 with comorbidities with significant short-term morbidity (DM2, moderate to severe OSA, severe NASH, pseudotumor cerebri)

        BMI >40 kg/m^2 with a medical condition (HTN, insulin resistance, glucose intolerance, dyslipidemia, mild to moderate OSA, significant impairment of quality of life or activities of daily living)

        BMI >50 kg/m^2

        Physical maturity (generally 13 years for girls, 15 years for boys)

        Emotional and cognitive maturity

        Weight loss efforts more than 6 months in behavior-based program

Location: Tertiary care pediatric weight management program

TABLE 1.8 Weight Goals [14]

BMI	2–5 years old	6–11 years old	12–18 years old
85th–94th percentile	Weight maintenance or slowed weight gain	Weight maintenance	Weight maintenance or gradual weight loss
95th–98th percentile	Weight maintenance	Gradual weight loss (no more than 1 pound/month)	Weight loss (no more than 2 pounds/week)
>99th percentile	Weight maintenance or weight loss of no more than 1 pound/month	Weight loss (no more than 2 pounds/week)	Weight loss (no more than 2 pounds/week)

CONCLUSION

Obesity is a serious condition, increasing in frequency and severity in children and adolescents. Pediatricians play an important role in initial prevention, treatment, and advocacy efforts. Comprehensive medical assessment of the obese child is important in directing the best overall treatment plan and assessing the urgency of intervention. Current national recommendations highlight a tiered approach to the treatment of overweight and obesity in this vulnerable population, with weight goals or maintenance highlighted when appropriate. Although typically this treatment is best conceptualized as a chronic care model, effective behavior change is possible and can improve overall and future health while reducing the risk of comorbidities.

References

1. Koplan JP, Liverman CT, Kraak VI. Preventing childhood obesity: health in the balance: executive summary. *J Am Diet Assoc* 2005;**105**:131–8.
2. Olds TS, Tomkinson GR, Ferrar KE, Maher CA. Trends in the prevalence of childhood overweight and obesity in Australia between 1985 and 2008. *Int J Obes (Lond)* 2009;**34**(1):57–66.
3. Collins AE, Pakiz B, Rock CL. Factors associated with obesity in Indonesian adolescents. *Int J Pediatr Obes* 2007:1–7.
4. Cattaneo A, Monasta L, Stamatakis E, et al. Overweight and obesity in infants and pre-school children in the European Union: a review of existing data. *Obes Rev* 2009.
5. Kosti RI, Panagiotakos DB. The epidemic of obesity in children and adolescents in the world. *Cent Eur J Public Health* 2006;**14**:151–9.
6. Lobstein T, Baur L, Uauy R. Obesity in children and young people: a crisis in public health. *Obes Rev* 2004;**5**(Suppl. 1):4–104.
7. Schwimmer JB, Burwinkle TM, Varni JW. Health-related quality of life of severely obese children and adolescents. *JAMA* 2003;**289**:1813–19.
8. Dietz WH. Health consequences of obesity in youth: childhood predictors of adult disease. *Pediatrics* 1998;**101**:518–25.
9. Olson CM, Strawderman MS, Dennison BA. Maternal weight gain during pregnancy and child weight at age 3 years. *Matern Child Health J* 2009;**13**:839–46.
10. Huang JS, Lee TA, Lu MC. Prenatal programming of childhood overweight and obesity. *Matern Child Health J* 2007;**11**(5):461–73.
11. Taveras EM, et al. Weight status in the first 6 months of life and obesity at 3 years of age. *Pediatrics* 2009;**123**(4):1177–83.
12. Krebs NF, et al. Assessment of child and adolescent overweight and obesity. *Pediatrics* 2007;**120**(Suppl. 4):S193–228.
13. *World Health Organization Global Strategy on Diet, Physical Activity, and Health* 2010; Available from: http://www.who.int/dietphysicalactivity/goals/en/
14. Barlow SE. Expert committee recommendations regarding the prevention, assessment, and treatment of child and adolescent overweight and obesity: summary report. *Pediatrics* 2007;**120**(Suppl. 4):S164–92.
15. Prentice AM, Jebb SA. Beyond body mass index. *Obes Rev* 2001;**2**(3):141–7.
16. Armstrong J, Reilly JJ. Breastfeeding and lowering the risk of childhood obesity. *Lancet* 2002;**359**(9322):2003–4.
17. Neumark-Sztainer DR, et al. Shared risk and protective factors for overweight and disordered eating in adolescents. *Am J Prev Med* 2007;**33**(5):359–69.
18. Neumark-Sztainer D. Preventing obesity and eating disorders in adolescents: what can health care providers do? *J Adolesc Health* 2009;**44**(3):206–13.
19. Peebles R. Adolescent obesity: etiology, office evaluation, and treatment. *Adolesc Med State Art Rev* 2008;**19**(3):380–405.
20. Taveras EM, et al. Racial/ethnic differences in early-life risk factors for childhood obesity. *Pediatrics* 2010;**125**(4):686–95.
21. Goldenring JM, Rosen DS. Getting into adolescent heads: an essential update Contemporary. *Pediatrics* 2004;**21**(1):64–90.
22. Zimmerman GL, Olsen CG, Bosworth MF. A 'stages of change' approach to helping patients change behavior. *Am Fam Physician* 2000;**61**(5):1409–16.
23. Reis JP, et al. Vitamin D Status and Cardiometabolic Risk Factors in the United States Adolescent Population. *Pediatrics* 2009.
24. Bordelon P, Ghetu MV, Langan RC. Recognition and management of vitamin D deficiency. *Am Fam Physician* 2009;**80**(8):841–6.
25. The fourth report on the diagnosis, evaluation, and treatment of high blood pressure in children and adolescent. *Pediatrics* 2004;**114**(2 Suppl, 4th Report):555–76.
26. Pratt JS, et al. Best practice updates for pediatric/adolescent weight loss surgery. *Obesity (Silver Spring)* 2009;**17**(5):901–10.

CHAPTER 2

Salient Features on Child Obesity from the Viewpoint of a Nutritionist

Bernard Waysfeld*, Dominique Adele Cassuto[†]

*Hopital Saint Michel, Paris, France and [†]Hopital Pitié-Salpétrière, Paris, France

The prevalence of child obesity has significantly increased in recent years [1, 2]. If the dietician or the nutritionist is challenged to explain this evolution, one could expect a dietary explication for this epidemic aspect. However, there is no international consensus or intervention study based on diet alone, or studies are not conclusive on the long-term effects on the body weight of children [3, 4]. Furthermore, the effects of different diets on weight reduction—such as low-fat, low-carbohydrate, high-protein, and low-glycemic index diets—have not been shown to have any superiority over other diets [4]. From the viewpoint of a nutritionist interested in the eating habits and eating disorders of children, the question is "What are the determinants and how can one intervene?" To answer this question, one needs to keep in mind the conundrum of preventing eating disorders without worsening obesity. According to the etiological nature of obesity, its importance, age, time of onset, personal and family psychological backgrounds, and different strategies can be proposed.

GENETIC AND FAMILY ASPECTS

Nutritionists are convinced that the family influences are not limited to genetic aspects [5, 6]. However, professionals are aware of their importance in child obesity (we shall not take into account genetic obesity). As Davidson has suggested, the child lives in an ecological nest box [5]. In the case of a child at risk of becoming overweight (including dietary, physical aspects, and sedentary behavior), the main characteristics can be explained by the influence of familial and school environment as well as a larger social environment (Figure 2.1).

There are consistent data to support that in noncontrolling conditions, children have the ability to self-regulate the amount of food or energy consumed. The energy needs of children differ from those of adults as a function of their rate of growth, particularly during adolescence, and gender.

Birch and her colleagues have performed studies revealing that children can adjust energy intake, both in short-term, single meal protocols and over 24-hour periods [7–9]. Children younger than 2 years may have some innate ability to self-regulate their intake by responding to internal cues for hunger and satiety. As children get older, these internal cues appear to be overridden by external factors, leading them to overeat in an environment that offers numerous opportunities to garner large portions of palatable food.

Influence of Family Life

Let us consider an example:

Mehdi, 12, has been referred by his school doctor as obese (187 pounds for 5.4 ft). He is the second in a family of four children. The eldest is very athletic and very thin, and the youngest are rather plump. Parents own a grocery store and come home late at night. The children are alone at dinnertime. The home is full of food, and children often come to look for dishes ready to be consumed in the store.

Everyone eats when and what he or she wants, often in his or her room watching television at the same time. This family is in danger. It does not seem possible to give Mehdi a diet. On the contrary, one can try to restore the ritual of meals, menus, and the like.

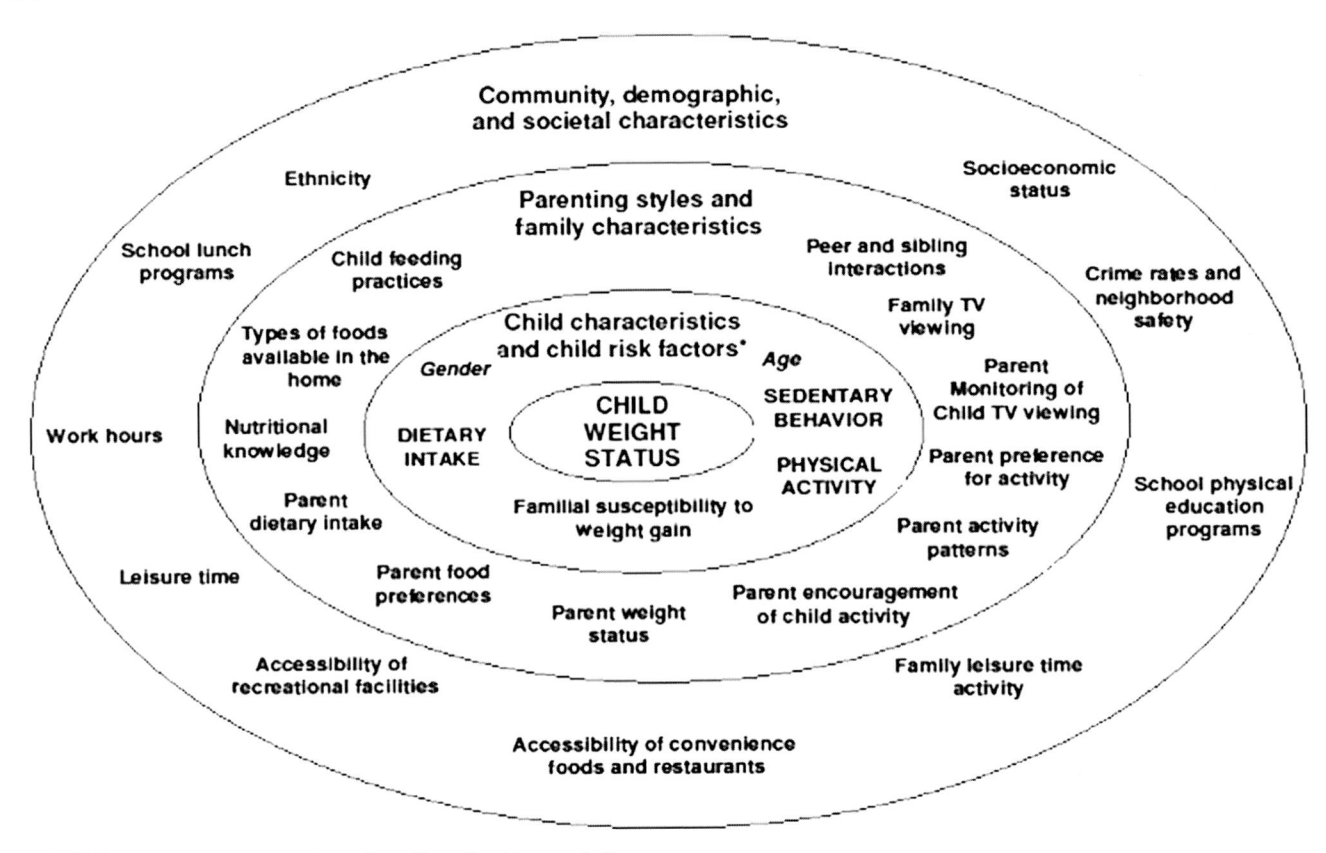

FIGURE 2.1 Child ecological nest box (from Davidson, ref. 5).

Children's dietary patterns are central in the development of overweight. Excess caloric intake will result in the storage of energy as fat [3, 4]. A preference for energy-dense foods may serve as a risk factor in becoming overweight if consumption of these foods leads to excessive fat and energy intake. Conversely, a preference for fruits and vegetables may serve as a protective factor. But the relationship between a preference for fruits and vegetables and a child's weight status has not yet been demonstrated [3].

The actual environment has been conceptualized as "obesogenic," promoting excessive food intake and sedentary behavior in many individuals. Research in adults has shown that there is a wide degree of interindividual variability in tolerance of overfeeding. Some research implicates poor self-regulation training when a child is overweight. Children who are predisposed to obesity may be more susceptible to the effects of excessive energy intake than children with no familial history of obesity [10–12].

Moreover, there is evidence of an association between larger portions and greater energy intake. Some authors found a link between meal portion size and increased body weight in children. The degree to which children are usually exposed to large portions may be the key for understanding the implication of portion size in overweight children [13]. Parents tend to judge the portion size on their belief about a child's appetite and are further influenced by the nutritional status of the given food [14]. Parents play a central role in determining how much food can be given, especially because they eat at the table the same meals with the whole family. All of these considerations can help clinicians to understand the child obesity epidemic.

IMPORTANCE OF COGNITIVE RESTRAINT IN CHILDREN

Sonia, 13, 143 pounds, 5.3 ft, almost obese for her age, was always at the top of the curve, but weight gain has increased recently. She is a very happy, edacious child who eats all types of food, including vegetables; she likes cooking too. On the other hand, she is not active and does not practice sports. She eats quickly, consumes large quantities of food, and nibbles when she can because she knows it is forbidden. Her mother is overweight. Her father, who gained weight when he stopped smoking, is concerned and irritated by his daughter's voracious appetite. Sonia is indeed hungry for a child of her age. Her mother forbids her to nibble, so she nibbles secretly after dinner and declares she needs to do this in order to be able to sleep. Her sister, 15, makes fun of her weight and complains when Sonia eats secretly.

Parents are often frustrated by children's reluctance to consume healthy foods and appear to be concerned by the quantities of food their children should be eating. In attempts to improve children's eating patterns, parents often use strong-arm child-feeding strategies: restricted access to palatable foods can particularly draw the child's attention and may cause overconsumption. Monitoring child feeding can be associated with a decrease in the child's ability to self-regulate [15, 16]. These strategies are counterproductive because they do not contribute to building longterm eating habits, even if they appear to be effective in the short term. The more the parents are invested in their own weight status, the more they will focus on their children's eating and weight [16].

Parents' concerns may become a self-fulfilling prophecy as excessive parental control is theorized to limit children's opportunities for learning self-control [16]. Deficits in children's self-regulation of energy intake as well as childhood overweight have been linked to self-reports of parents' disinhibition of feeding restraints [17].

Mothers showing self-reports with higher levels of dieting and impulsive eating have children who experienced greater difficulty in self-regulating energy intake. Thus, mothers can be considered as role model for inappropriate eating strategy behaviors [18, 19]. Cutting et al. reported a relationship in weight status between mothers and daughters that was mediated by maternal self-reports of disinhibition [19].

We know that among adults, cognitive restraint prevents food intake from being comforting, as adults cannot think positively about food items that are regarded as detrimental to weight control. In this case, the food item cannot create positive emotions but will be freighted with negative emotional associations such as anxiety, guilt, sadness, and anger. The restrained eater is thus led to go on consuming, vainly seeking a comfort he or she imagines without ever being able to experience it. The individual can never stop eating and will fail to regulate excess eating. This can be described as the cycle of cognitive restraint [20].

Factors Interfering with Cognitive Restraint

Stress

Psychosomatic theory proposes that eating in response to emotional distress rather than hunger is a cause of excessive weight gain. Dietary restraint occurs in children and may influence the effect of stress on eating.

Interpersonal stress increases snacking in high-dietary-restraint children, perhaps because of stress-induced disinhibition, although it decreases snacking in low-dietary-restrained children [21].

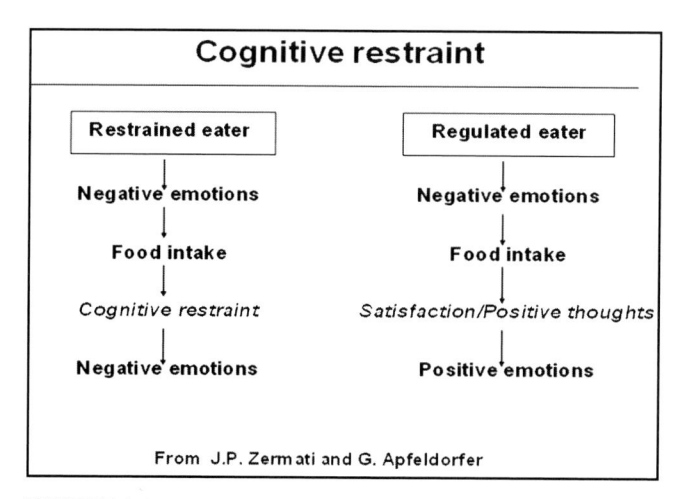

FIGURE 2.2 Cognitive restraint consequences.

Mother-Child Relationship

Mother-child relationship appears to be dramatically important, especially during the first year of life. Hilde Bruch was the first to describe the deleterious consequences of an inadequate attitude of some mothers [22]. If the mother, moved by the desire of doing her best, gave a systematic alimentary answer to all of her children's demands (love, sleep, anger, hunger, etc.), it may result in an alteration of the sensation of hunger for that child. In other words, the child and later the adult may feel hungry each time he or she is looking for love, sleep, or feels angry and not necessarily hungry. This motherly attitude occurs frequently, as food is the first item that can be given to the child and symbolizes the paradigm of exchange and relationship. Furthermore, it may be difficult for some mothers to say no overall when they are convinced they have to do something for their children [22, 23]. However, giving food in all circumstances will deeply disturb the natural signals of hunger and specific satiety, and it will not allow "an emotional tuning" between mother and child [24].

This may have long-term consequences. First, affective confusion will lead to excessive energy intake, food being considered at the same time as sweetness, love, anger, and so on. Second, this motherly behavior does not permit a good development of the child's own identity: the child will remain a continuation of the mother, lacking of insight. Third, the characteristic of the maternal answer does not permit a "right timing" of the alimentary sequence.

The normal sequence can be illustrated as follows:

Hunger → desire for food → food → pleasure (reward) (need) → lack (or craving) → (item) → pleasure (reward)

The force-feeding mother interferes in short-circuiting the time of "longing for" or desire and will thus compromise the affective future of the child [25, 26]. This may be the same with the *too-good mother* that Winnicott has described [27].

The process is not fundamentally different: driven by the intention of being a good mother, the too-good mother will anticipate the desires or demands of the child, and therefore the child will have no time left for craving foods that lead to a poor diet. In such conditions, the child (who is also the future adult) will have a tendency to show rebellion because he or she is longing for immediate satisfaction. Often these children, as well as many adults, react in a typical behavior, which can be expressed by the phrase "all or nothing." In other words, they do not bear any frustrations, and this intolerance may lead to constant disappointments. These inappropriate responses lead to abnormal weight gain if alimentary behavior is affected by this attitude.

The absent mother, though less described, appears to be the worst, when considering the future of children and the importance of eating disorders. One can easily understand that a baby or a young child facing an ailing feeding behavior will show a tendency to rush on food as much as possible, not knowing what the next day will provide. Food can also be considered as an equivalent of love, and facing the doubt of not being loved, these children may develop disruptive disorders; these eating disorders are the least serious among these psychopathic personalities. This could explain why eating disorders are predominant among girls, who target more in the interior of their body, than among boys, who show a greater investment in the exterior world.

Parental Styles

Birch et al. [18] proposed that the implications of inhibitory control for weight outcomes could interact with parenting, because optimal parenting strategies in many contexts depend on the child's behavioral style. In the developmental literature, this is referred to as *goodness of fit* [18, 19]. For example, intrusive parenting does not seem to be a good fit for children with a low level of self-regulation [28].

Anzman and Birch have shown that girls with lower inhibitory control at age 7 had higher body mass index (BMI), greater weight gain, and higher BMI at age 15 [29]. In this study, girls who perceived higher parental restriction exhibited the strongest inverse relationship between inhibitory control and weight status. Variability in inhibitory control could help identify individuals who are predisposed to obesity risk [29].

Studies suggest that parents who impose control on their children's eating may interfere with the child's ability to regulate food intake. This may potentially increase the risk for later eating disorders and obesity. On the contrary, parenting strategies that facilitate appropriate child autonomy enable the children to regulate their own eating behaviors. Strategies that decide how much the child wishes to eat have been found to be more effective in selecting adequate changes in the child's eating patterns [30–32, 34, 35]. Parental style and skills have been shown to predict children's BMI, fruit and vegetable intake, healthy eating, physical activity, and sedentary behavior [30]. This situation is frequently found in everyday clinical practice on overweight or obese children and children with a family history of obesity.

The family meals remain important; eating meals together allows the family to connect and communicate, even without words. The dining room is the scene of symbolic exchanges. The family meals, taken together, play a role in exchange, integration, and regulation.

OBESITY AND EATING DISORDERS

Aurélie, 20, wants to lose weight. She is overweight (187 pounds, 5.4 ft). Since puberty, she gained weight and underwent her first diet at the age of 13. She lost 10 kg in 2 months with a strict diet. She quickly regained her initial weight and did not stop putting on weight since that time. She tried many diets but remained in a yoyo ascending curve. She has cravings for sweet foods and occasionally gorges when she does not feel good. She has poor self-esteem, although she is a good student. These compulsions are clearly the consequences of the cognitive restraint secondary to numerous previous diets.

Dietary restraint is often implicated in the development and persistence of binge eating. Teenage girls who diet are more likely to gain weight and become obese than their nondieting peers [31].

Childhood or parental obesity has been shown to be a specific risk for the development of a binge eating disorder such as bulimia. A family context of weight concern and weight control sensitizes a child to its appearance and promotes dissatisfaction. Furthermore, the normalization of weight control may encourage overweight children and teenagers to attempt dietary restriction. We know that this behavior strongly reinforces weight and shape concerns.

Previous studies suggested an inverse association between body weight and self-esteem. We now know that body weight, when excessive, has a negative effect on self-esteem and the person will favor severe diets with cognitive restraint and, consequently, eating disorders [32].

PHYSICAL ACTIVITY

The nutritionist should encourage patients with a sedentary lifestyle and lack of activity to expend energy as well as to promote self-esteem and better eating behavior. Some authors have confirmed the negative effect of sedentary activities on self-esteem. They have emphasized healthy eating and active living in childhood to improve physical and mental health. Less activity, a more sedentary lifestyle, poor diets, and excess body weight are all risk factors for low self-esteem. Furthermore, signals of hunger and satiety are better recognized in an active lifestyle [32].

STRATEGIES

A recent article [36] proposed to answer the following question: What can healthcare providers do to prevent obesity and eating disorders in adolescents? The answers appear to be as follows:

1. Discourage unhealthy dieting.
2. Promote a positive body image.
3. Encourage more frequent and more enjoyable family meals.
4. Encourage the family to talk less about weight and do more at home to facilitate healthy eating and physical activity.
5. Assume that overweight teens have experienced weight mistreatments and address this issue with teens and their families [37–39].

Whereas most studies use dieting as a core part of lifestyle modification in the management of pediatric overweight, some researchers not only question the effectiveness of food restriction but also warn against the risks associated with dieting in this population. Thus, it can be difficult for children to comply with dieting behavior for a prolonged period, leading to negative self-perception and reduced self-esteem. Using a restricted meal plan may in some cases lead to an increase in weight gain in children who are already treated causing the suppression of hunger cues. Moreover, dieting may result in developing binge eating once food is available and increased preoccupation with food is no longer prohibited [34, 37].

These reservations have led in recent years to the development of a nondieting approach. Helping children attend to internal cues of hunger and satiety should be promoted as a productive child-feeding strategy and as an alternative to coercive or restrictive practices [12]. This approach has the additional advantage of removing the stigma of "being on a diet" and increasing the opportunity of the children to feel empowered and be able to have a choice, in contrast to feelings of incompetence that may arise if the youngsters fail to stick to their diet.

The Place of Parents

Current family-based behavioral pediatric weight-loss programs require parental involvement and necessary changes with the overweight child considered to be the main agent of change [30–35]. Golan et al. [33, 34] have suggested that parents, rather than their children, should be the main agent of change. Targeting parents only with a family health-centered approach has been associated with greater weight loss and higher consumption of healthy foods in overweight children. According to Satter's model, it is the parent's job to provide a healthy array of food at regularly scheduled opportunities; it is the child's choice to decide how much and whether he or she will consume the food that is offered [40]. One common strategy for controlling portions has been to serve smaller amounts and then allow second helpings if the child is still hungry.

It is possible to communicate to parents that they should help regulate what their children eat but that this restriction should be discreet instead of overt. For example, parents can control which foods are available in the home, thereby allowing children to choose within constraints and helping them to cultivate healthy habits.

Parents should care about what, how, and how much their children consume. For preadolescents, the role of parents is to provide foods low in energy density and to reduce the child's accessibility to foods that are high in energy density. One must therefore cook just enough to avoid too many temptations and adapt the portions to each child. The role of parents is to explain to children, disturbed by a strong sense of injustice, that the portions are based on one's age and level of physical activity.

Giving advice to parents based on studies by Golan showed a marked superiority to dealing only with parents and the absence of eating disorders 7 years later [33]. These results were largely superior to the ones where children were the therapeutic target themselves.

Thus, healthier eating strategies can be maintained throughout childhood and into adulthood. There is evidence that exposure to procedure familiarization leads to food preferences and acceptance, but in cases where discreet restriction may not be adequate, an additional approach that may be effective is to include setting limits, being sure to follow them with explanation and expressions of warmth.

Parents may be seen as role models for their children, and they may also provide an environment designed to reduce maladjusted eating-related attitudes and improve self-regulation and healthy behaviors.

CONCLUSION

The future of the obese children, even if they have obese parents, is not only determined by the genetic lottery. The roles of environment and behavior are crucial and prevention is essential. A healthy atmosphere contributes to helping the child learn to eat when he or she is hungry and provides adapted responses when the child is bored or just attracted by food lying on the table. Parents must specify the times reserved for meals or snacks; these moments authorize eating as much as the child wants with no food prohibited or limited. The child must also be taught not to eat between meals out of boredom. Boredom appears to be the first stage of nibbling, and this behavior is often associated with loneliness. Therefore, the child should not be left alone for a long time, especially during late afternoon, and parents must try to organize activities (inviting a friend, organizing studies). As a preventive measure, we should keep the following considerations in mind:

- We should not pursue impossible goals.
- To be slim is often to grow up without becoming fat with a decrease in BMI.
- A child may remain obese, but eating disorders must be avoided as much as possible.

Medical action should target the three goals of nutrition: respond to biological needs, allow pleasure, and be integrated in a social environment. If a child is at risk of becoming obese, the usual tendency is to advocate restriction. This strategy may have serious consequences. The enjoyment of food and eating in a convivial atmosphere is what matters first. Education is much more important than information. Information refers to tables, quantities, and concentrations, and parents and children cannot integrate it. Education refers to models, examples of which are more powerful than precepts built on rationale conceptions with no link to inner instincts and natural patterns. One must avoid bringing the child into the vicious circle of cognitive restraint leading to disinhibition. The child must be helped to eventually accept being plump; often at puberty. The management of the family is mandatory. It is counterproductive to prescribe to a child or to anyone a rule that will always be broken. Furthermore, it discredits the adult adviser and the rule itself.

It is possible to talk about nutrition with a child if the adult message is adapted to the age of the child and focuses on promoting health and fitness and not just being overweight. A child's self-esteem is fragile, and one should not overemphasize food choices and weight. The child needs help to grow and to love his or her body, even if the child is not the continuation of the parents' slimmer image. The child must experience good foods. These positive food contacts will be the first step toward improving the child's eating behavior. The final goal is to give the child consistent messages that can be seen as good benchmarks to those who apply them to themselves.

References

1. Lobstein T, Jackson-Leach R. Child overweight and obesity in the USA: prevalence rates according to IOTF definitions. *Int J Pediatr Obes* 2007;**2**(1):62–4.
2. Lobstein T, Frelut ML. Prevalence of overweight among children in Europe. *Obes Rev* 2003;**4**(4):195–200. Nov.
3. Latzer Y, Edmunds L, Fenig S, Golan M, Gur E, Hochberg Z, Levin-Zamir D, Zubery E, Speiser P.W, Stein D. Managing childhood overweight: behaviour, family, pharmacology, and bariatric surgery interventions. Obesity (Silver Spring) 2009;**17**(3):411–23. Mar.
4. Sacks FM, Bray GA, Carey VJ, Smith SR, Ryan DH, Anton SD, McManus K, Champagne CM, Bishop LM, Laranjo N, Leboff MS, Rood JC, de Jonge L, Greenway FL, Loria CM, Obarzanek E, Williamson DA. Comparison of weight-loss diets with different compositions of fat, protein, and carbohydrates. *N Engl J Med* 2009;**360**(9):859–73. Feb 26.
5. Davidson KK, Birch LL. Childhood overweight: a contextual model and recommendations for future research. *Obesity Rev* 2001;**2**:159–71.
6. Vauthier JM, Lluch A, Lecomte E, Artur Y, Herberth B. Family resemblance In energy and macronutrient Intakes: The Stanislas Family study. *Int J of Epidemiol* 1996;**25**(5):1030–7.
7. Birch LL, Deysher M. Caloric compensation and sensory specific satiety: evidence for self regulation of food intake by young children. *Appetite* 1986;**7**(4):323–31. Dec.
8. Johnson SL, McPhee L, Birch LL. Conditioned preferences: young children prefer flavors associated with high dietary fat. *Physiol Behav* 1991;**50**(6):1245–51. Dec.
9. Birch LL, Fischer JO. Development of eating behaviours among children and adolescents. *Pediatrics* 1998;**101**:539–49.
10. Hill C, Llewellyn CH, Saxton J, Webber L, Semmler C, Carnell S, van Jaarsveld CH, Boniface D, Wardle J. Adiposity and eating in the absence of hunger in children. *Int J Obes (Lond)* 2008;**32**(10):1499–505. Oct Epub Jul 22.
11. Birch LL, Fisher JO, Davison KK. Girls' learning to overeat: maternal use of restrictive feeding practices promotes eating in the absence of hunger. *Am J Clin Nutr* 2003;**78**(2):215–20. Aug.
12. Johnson SL, Birch LL. Parents' and children's adiposity and eating style. *Pediatrics* 1994;**94**(5):653–61. Nov.
13. Lioret S, Volatier JL, Lafay L, Touvier M, Maire B. Is food portion size a risk factor of childhood overweight? *Eur J Clin Nutr* 2009;**63**(3):382–91. Mar.
14. Croker H, Sweetman C, Cooke L. Mothers' views on portion sizes for children. *J Hum Nutr Diet* 2009;**22**(5):437–43. Oct.
15. Birch LL, Mc Phe, Shoba BC, Steiberg L, Krehbiel R. Clean up your plate: effects of child feeding practices on the conditioning of meal size. *Learning motivation* 1987;**18**:301–17.
16. Constanzo PE, Woody EZ. Domain specific parenting styles and their impact on the child's development of particular deviance: the example of obesity proneness. *J Soc Clin Psychol* 1985;**4**:425–45.

17. Hood MY, Moore LL, Sundarajan-Ramamurti A, Cupples LA, Elison RC. Parental eating attitudes and the development of obesity in children; The Framigham Children's Study. *Int J of Obesity* 2000;**24**:1319–25.
18. Birch LL, Fisher JO, Davison KK. Learning to overeat: maternal use of restrictive feeding practices promotes girls' eating in the absence of hunger. *Am J Clin Nutr* 2003;**78**(2): 215–20. Aug.
19. Cutting TM, Fisher JO, Grimm-Thomas K, Birch LL. Like mother, like daughter: familial patterns of overweight are mediated by mothers' dietary disinhibition. *Am J Clin Nutr* 1999;**69**(4):608–13. Apr.
20. Zermati JP, Apfeldorfer G. "Practical Consequences". In: R Ling Peter, editor. *Trends in Obesity Research*. New York: Nova Biomedical Books; 2004.
21. Roemmich JN, Smith JR, Epstein LH, Lambiase M. Stress reactivity and adiposity of youth. *Obesity Sep* 2007;**15** (9):2303–10.
22. Bruch H. Psychological aspects of overeating and obesity. *Psychosomatics* 1964;**5**:269–74. Sep-Oct.
23. Bruch H. Transformation of oral impulses in eating disorders: a conceptual approach. *Psychiatr Q* 1961;**35**:458–81. Jul.
24. Stern D. « *Le monde interpersonnel du nourrisson* », Paris, puf 1; 1989.
25. Waysfeld B. Psychological approaches to the obese. Mar 18. *Presse Med* 2000;**29**(10):556–63. Review. French.
26. Waysfeld B. « *Le poids et le moi* ». Paris: Armand Colin; 2003.
27. Winnicot, Donald W. Primary maternal preoccupation. In: *Collected papers, through paediatrics to psychoanalysis*. London: Tavistock Publications; 1956.
28. Johnson SL. Improving Preschoolers' self-regulation of energy intake. *Pediatrics* 2000;**106**(6):1429–35. Dec.
29. Anzman SL, Birch LL. Low inhibitory control and restrictive feeding practices predict weight outcomes. Nov. *J Pediatr* 2009; **155**(5):608-9.
30. Kremers SP, Brug J, de Vries H, Engels RC. Parenting style and adolescent fruit consumption. *Appetite* 2003;**41**(1):43–50. Aug.
31. Stein RI, Epstein LH, Raynor HA, Kilanowski CK, Paluch RA. The influence of parenting change on pediatric weight control. *Obes Res* 2005;**13**(10):1749–55. Oct.
32. Wang F, Veugelers PJ. Self-esteem and cognitive development in the era of the childhood obesity epidemic. *Obes Rev* 2008;**9** (6):615–23. Nov.
33. Golan M. Parents as agents of change in childhood obesity—from research to practice. *Int J Pediatr Obes* 2006;**1**(2):66–76. Review.
34. Enten RS, Golan M. Parenting styles and eating disorder pathology. *Appetite* 2009;**52**(3):784–7. Jun.
35. Robertson W, Friede T, Blissett J, Rudolf MC, Wallis M, Stewart-Brown S. Pilot of "Families for Health": community-based family intervention for obesity. *Arch Dis Child* 2008;**93**(11):921–6. Nov.
36. Neumark-Sztainer D. Preventing obesity and eating disorders in adolescents: what can health care providers do? *Adolesc Health* 2009;**44**(3):206–13. Mar.
37. Webber L, Hill C, Cooke L, Cornell S, Wordle J. Associations between child weight and maternal feeding styles are mediated by maternal perceptions concerns. *Eur J Clin Nutr* 2010 Mar;**64** (3):259–65. Epub 2010.
38. Hill AJ. Obesity and eating disorders. *Obes Rev* 2007;**8**(Suppl. 1): 151–5. Mar.
39. Hill AJ. Does dieting make you fat? *Br J Nutr* 2004;**92**(Suppl. 1): S15–18. Aug.
40. Satter E. The feeding relationship: problems and interventions. *J Pediatr* 1990;**117**(2 Pt 2):S181–9. Aug.

CHAPTER 3

Developmental Trajectories of Weight Status in Childhood and Adolescence

Samar Hejazi*, V. Susan Dahinten*, Pamela A. Ratner*, Sheila K. Marshall[†]

*School of Nursing, University of British Columbia, Vancouver, British Columbia, Canada and
[†]School of Social Work, University of British Columbia, Vancouver, British Columbia, Canada

DEVELOPMENTAL TRAJECTORIES OF WEIGHT STATUS IN CHILDHOOD AND ADOLESCENCE

The majority of children establish a consistent weight status early in their lives. Others change trajectories or grow into a particular pattern only at a certain age or stage in their development. Both normal weight and overweight status tend to persist, with fewer children changing weight status. For example, longitudinal studies have revealed that some children move from a normal weight category into overweight status or obesity and other children, albeit far fewer in number, move from an overweight status to a healthier weight. Additionally, the weight status of some children has been shown to fluctuate over time.

Various statistical approaches are available for conceptualizing, modeling, and studying the developmental trajectories of weight status in childhood and adolescence, particularly when the data provide repeated observations for individuals within the sample. Researchers have commonly relied on two measurements over time (i.e., time point to time point comparisons) to describe individual stability and change in weight status through the estimation of correlation or regression coefficients, or the computation of odds ratios. More advanced statistical methods such as growth curve modeling draw on multiple assessments of weight status and have allowed researchers to assess intraindividual growth over time and to identify aggregated patterns of development. Some growth curve modeling methods (e.g., multilevel models and latent growth analysis) have been used to describe the normative or average trajectory of children's weight status and to explore individual variation around the trajectory [1, 2]. Important developments in applied statistics also have enabled researchers to explore heterogeneity in developmental trajectories and to identify meaningful subgroups of people who follow distinct trajectories of development. These non-normative models, which do not assume homogeneity in the distribution of individual trajectories, rely on techniques such as growth mixture modeling [3], latent transition analysis [4], and group-based modeling of development [5].

In the following sections, we present the findings from a selection of research studies that applied longitudinal data analyses to understanding the developmental trajectories of weight status within childhood and adolescence, with a focus on studies that have measured weight status in terms of body mass index (BMI). Our review is organized with respect to three different approaches used in the field of obesity research to investigate developmental patterns or trajectories of weight status: tracking methods, normative growth curve methods, and non-normative growth curve methods. Each of these approaches provides researchers and healthcare professionals with valuable information for prevention and intervention purposes.

TRACKING OF WEIGHT STATUS IN CHILDHOOD AND ADOLESCENCE

In the field of obesity research, epidemiological studies have used repeated measures to assess the stability of weight status throughout childhood and adolescence and to identify children who are more likely to be overweight or obese at a later age. In addition to reporting the percentage of children who have maintained or changed their weight status over time, researchers using tracking methods generally report relationships between baseline weight status and follow-up weight status as correlation coefficients or odds ratios. Research evidence shows that most children maintain a stable weight status (normal weight or overweight[1]) over time with far fewer children changing weight status [6]. For example, stability has been shown to be as high as 85% with 72% of children maintaining normal weight within a 3-year follow-up period [7], with similar results reported by other studies [8–10].

Research findings suggest that overweight status, obesity, and high BMI, if present in early childhood, typically persist into adolescence [6, 11]. Our review of other recent literature identified findings similar to the systematic reviews of Singh et al. (2008) and Reilly et al. (2003) [6, 11]. We found that the percentage of children who were overweight or obese and maintained their weight status over time ranged from 54% [12] to 73% [7] when any two time points were compared. However, when tracking over several time points, the study by Nader et al. (2006) reported that 80% of children who had been overweight at any time during their elementary school years were overweight at age 12 years [13]. Lower percentages have been found when tracking stability at younger ages. For example, only 24% of overweight infants continued to be overweight at 4 years of age [14]. One of the factors that may influence persistence is the severity of overweight status, as some studies have shown greater stability of weight status at higher BMI levels [7, 15, 16]. However, it is not clear whether these observed differences in persistence were statistically significant.

Odds ratios are frequently reported in tracking studies to indicate the magnitude of risk of being overweight at a second time point, given the initial weight status. For example, a child who was classified as overweight between 5 and 10 years of age had 25 times greater odds of being classified as either overweight or obese 3 years later compared with a child who was of normal weight at baseline [7]. As with percentages indicating stability, reported odds ratios have varied widely across studies, with some evidence suggesting that relationships are stronger at older ages and, unsurprisingly, across shorter age intervals [11–13, 17, 18]. Children who were overweight (rather than normal weight) at 2.5 years were more likely to be classified as overweight when they were 6 or 9 years old (OR = 12.2 and OR = 4.9, respectively), but not when they were 12 or 15 years of age [12]. However, overweight status at 12 or 15 years was predicted by weight status at age 6 or 9 years. Another study found greater odds ratios for shorter age intervals [14].

There is evidence that some children change their weight status between measurements. Although not reported by all tracking studies, in general, a smaller percentage of children move from a higher to lower weight status, compared with those who move from a lower to higher weight status, whether measured by relative BMI standings [9] or normal/overweight status [7, 15]. Twice as many children moved from normal weight to overweight status between 6 and 15 years, compared with children who moved from overweight to normal weight status [12]. Only 4% of the total sample in Hesketh et al.'s (2004) study resolved to a normal weight from an unhealthy weight category within a 3-year interval [7].

Sex differences in the stability of weight status have been investigated in many tracking studies, but the results have been mixed and inconclusive [11]. Girls were less likely to stay in the same weight category compared with boys when followed from childhood through to adolescence (38% and 42%, with a weighted kappa (κ) = .29 and .33, respectively[2]) [16]. On the contrary, Hesketh et al. (2004) followed a similar age sample, but only to early adolescence, and failed to find a significant sex difference [7]. Imed et al. (2009) also failed to find sex differences in their 4-year follow-ups of 13- to 15-year-olds [9].

Findings from tracking studies of weight status have been shown to be influenced by the reference criteria used to categorize weight status. For example, Willows et al. (2007) found that, compared with the Centers for Disease Control and Prevention (CDC) cut-off criteria, the International Obesity Task Force (IOTF) underestimated weight stability in 2-year-old Canadian Cree children tracked over 3 years [10]. Using IOTF standards, 5% of the children who were normal weight at age 2 years were found to be obese at age 5 years, whereas 15% of children who were normal weight at 2 years of age were identified as obese at age 5 years under the CDC criteria.

In summary, evidence from tracking studies suggests a persistence of overweight status across childhood and adolescence but with considerable variation in the magnitude of the relationships observed, not unexpected given the variation in the methods applied. Studies have varied

---

[1]When referring to the tracking of normal weight versus overweight or obesity, we generally use the term overweight to represent both overweight status and obesity, unless indicated otherwise. Some (e.g., ref. 7) but not all studies (e.g., ref. 12) have distinguished between the two.

[2]The weighted kappa (κ) measures degree of agreement and can be interpreted as an intraclass correlation coefficient [19].

in the age and age span of the sample at baseline and in the intervals between measurements. However, more important, methodologists have shown that when two assessments of weight status are positively correlated, the probability of a study participant maintaining his or her position in an extreme ranking (e.g., the upper quartile of BMI or the obesity grouping) is greater than that of individuals in other positions; thus, findings should be interpreted cautiously, particularly when claims are made about the stability of obesity [20]. Finally, tracking studies provide limited information about the developmental trajectories of weight status in childhood and adolescence. Even when data are available from multiple time points, analytic procedures such as correlation analysis and the computation of odds ratios focus on a comparison of time point to time point data, in contrast to the simultaneous analysis of multiple time point data, as is done in growth curve modeling.

NORMATIVE GROWTH CURVE METHODS

Normative growth curve modeling has been used extensively in the study of childhood weight status to describe the average trends or trajectories of children's weight status and to explore individual variation around the normative or average trajectory. Statistical methods such as latent growth analysis, random regression models, multilevel models, and mixed linear models are used to identify individual trajectories and patterns of development at aggregated levels, based on an assumption of homogeneity in individual trajectories within the population or subpopulations. More specifically, such analyses provide estimates of both the mean level of the outcome of interest at a particular time point (the intercept) and mean rate of change over age or time (the slope). Growth curve modeling approaches may describe developmental change in terms of a continuous outcome measure such as BMI, or the probability of being in a particular condition (e.g., overweight versus normal weight) at a particular age, with change being modeled as a linear or nonlinear curve. The amount of unexplained variance in each parameter is also estimated and may be reduced or explained by the inclusion of time variant or time invariant predictors that are expected to yield individual or subgroup differences. Individual variation in the level or rate of change that is unexplained by predictors in the model is considered random error. Normative growth curve approaches require longitudinal outcome data with a minimum of three data collection points and can handle missing data and data collected at different intervals.

There has been extensive use of normative growth curve methods to investigate the developmental trajectories of weight status, with a focus on describing individual variation about the population mean trajectory and identifying predictors of that variation. Earlier work in this area typically modeled BMI, or weight category based on BMI, as the outcome measure. More recently, researchers have begun to model and compare trajectories for other measures of weight status, such as skin-fold thickness and fat mass index.

A common finding is that BMI increases steadily with age for both boys and girls, and among various ethnic/racial groups, including whites, blacks, Hispanics, and Asians [21–24]. However, there may be some sex differences in level of BMI at certain stages of development. For example, a longitudinal study of children from 5 to 17 years showed little sex difference in the level of BMI or rate of change, although the girls' BMI trajectory was significantly higher than that of the boys between the ages of 12 and 14 years [22]. Similar results were found in Wardle et al.'s (2006) study that followed children from early to middle adolescence (11 to 16 years). The girls' BMI level was found to be significantly higher, but with no difference in the rate of change [24].

Whereas BMI trajectories appear to be fairly linear in shape with little sex difference, developmental trajectories based on other measures of weight status are suggestive of nonlinear change and sex differences in both the level and rate of change. Trajectories based on peripheral skin fold measures showed a higher level for girls than boys from 5 to 17 years [22]. Additionally, the rate of increase was similar for boys and girls until age 11 years, but thereafter, peripheral skinfold thickness in boys decreased steadily. Other studies reported similar findings of sex differences in level of skinfold thickness [21, 25, 26]. Following the same sample of youth from 8 to 17 years, studies showed that the girls had higher levels of skinfold thickness and fat mass (respectively), with black girls showing the highest levels [21, 25]. In contrast, mean skinfold thickness was higher for non-black males compared with black males, suggesting an interaction between sex and ethnicity/race. The trajectories for skinfold thickness were clearly nonlinear [21], whereas the shape of the trajectories for fat mass index varied by sex [25]. In summary, the developmental trajectories of weight status obtained through normative growth curve modeling vary according to the measure of weight status used, with models based on BMI showing smaller sex differences and the most linear trajectories over time.

In addition to sex and ethnicity/race, family socioeconomic characteristics have been commonly included in the analysis of normative growth curve models [26–29], with similar results among studies. The rate of increase in weight status has been shown to be associated with lower family socioeconomic status. Low family income was associated with an accelerated weight gain in children followed from age 3 months to 6 years, and low parental education was linked with a faster rate of increase in waist circumference within a sample of children followed into adulthood [26, 28]. Also, in a sample of children followed from kindergarten through fifth grade, parental education was negatively associated with the level of BMI at kindergarten and with the rate of increase in BMI over time [27]. However, the relationships were weaker for Hispanic children compared with non-Hispanic children. Socioeconomic characteristics of the child's more distal environment also have been implicated in more rapid weight gain. For example, an investigation of the effects of neighborhood income levels in Canadian children followed from ages 2 to 3 years through to 10 to 11 years of age found that children living in the "most poor" neighborhoods showed a faster increase in BMI percentile relative to children living in a "middle" income neighborhood [29].

Earlier children's weight and parental weight also have been explored as predictors of children's weight and rate of change in weight status. For example, Silverwood et al. (2009) showed a relationship between the timing and extent of the BMI peak during infancy and later BMI z-scores for children between the ages of 5 and 13 years [23]. Infants with higher BMI at peak and later BMI peak were more likely to have higher BMI z-scores later in childhood. Parental weight has been shown to be linked to level and rate of change in children's BMI. Another study demonstrated that maternal prepregnancy weight was associated with children's weight status at age 4 years, although the relationship had not been significant at age 2 years [28]. Similarly, but using a female only sample, Francis, Ventura, Marini, and Birch (2007) showed that the rate of increase in BMI between the ages of 5 and 13 years was positively associated with parents' overweight or healthy weight status [30]. Several predictors that are commonly associated with level of weight, including sedentary behavior [31, 32] and activity levels [33], also have been investigated through growth curve modeling in relation to the rate of increase in weight status, with findings in the expected direction.

Normative growth curve modeling provides a powerful means of describing the average trajectories of weight status for known population subgroups, such as in identifying trajectories by sex and ethnicity/race. One clear finding in this subset of the literature is that, whereas BMI trajectories appear to be fairly linear in shape, rising over time with little sex difference, developmental trajectories based on other measures of weight status are suggestive of nonlinear change with sex differences in both the level and rate of change. Moreover, in contrast to BMI trajectories, some measures of weight status show a decline over time for certain sex-ethnicity/race groups of children. Normative growth curve methods also have been useful in showing the negative effects of low socioeconomic status on the rate of increase in weight status.

Although there are likely further important relationships to be revealed through normative growth curve methods, particularly through the modeling of time varying predictors, there are limitations to the use of traditional growth curve methods in informing our understanding of the developmental trajectories of weight status in childhood and adolescence. Normative growth curve methods are not equipped to model complex developmental trajectories in which individuals do not follow a common developmental process of growth [34]. Neither can these methods be used to reveal heterogeneity in the developmental trajectories of weight status that is not explained by predictor variables theorized to be influential and included within the model. Identifying different trajectories that may exist within "unknown" population subgroups requires other statistical approaches to growth curve modeling.

NON-NORMATIVE GROWTH CURVE METHODS

Non-normative growth curve methods are an advanced application of growth curve modeling used with longitudinal data to identify distinctive subgroups of individuals who follow distinctive trajectories [5, 35–37]. Group-based modeling, growth mixture modeling (GMM), and latent transitions analysis (LTA) are three approaches that consider the effects of unobserved or latent heterogeneity in populations and provide a robust method of estimating developmental trajectories. Although these procedures differ in important ways, they all estimate trajectory parameters for each individual and specify how these parameters vary throughout the sample [38–39]. Through these methods, researchers are able to identify groups of individuals that follow distinctive weight status trajectories, estimate the proportion of the population with a particular weight status trajectory, use the different trajectory groups to produce profiles of group members, and explore predictors of membership in specific trajectories.

Similar to traditional latent growth modeling, growth parameters (intercepts and slopes) are estimated as latent variables through repeated measures of a developmental process. However, non-normative modeling strategies assume that the population consists of distinct groups identified by their developmental trajectories rather than by known subgroup characteristics (e.g., sex or ethnicity/race). Accordingly, these methods draw on a multinomial modeling strategy rather than relying on a multivariate normal and continuous distribution function [40]. The estimation of these trajectories can be conducted through such software applications as Proc Traj (a SAS-based procedure) for group-based modeling (Jones, Nagin, & Roeder, 2001; Nagin, 2005), M-Plus, developed by Muthén and Muthén (1998–2007) and PROC LTA for latent trajectory analysis developed by Lanza, Lemmon, Schafer, and Collins (2008) and Lanza and Collins (2008) (SAS® 9.2/version 1.2.3 beta). In these modeling applications, cases are classified in a probabilistic manner and individuals are assigned to the group for which they have the highest probability of membership. Group-based methods, GMM, and LTA, offer significant advantages over traditional or normative growth curve modeling for studying overweight status because researchers can identify different trajectories of weight status that exist within the data and explore potential risk factors that may predict membership within the various trajectories.

We were able to identify six studies that applied non-normative growth curve methods to provide evidence of heterogeneity in the development of overweight status or obesity in childhood and adolescence (Table 3.1). Researchers have identified the occurrence of several distinctive patterns of weight status change across childhood and adolescence through group-based modeling [41, 42], GMM [43–45], and LTA [46]. In the following sections, we summarize key findings obtained through these methods. We first describe the distinct trajectories of weight status that have emerged from the data, beginning with trajectories that have shown a persistence of weight status over time—that is, those who have maintained either a normal weight or overweight status. This is followed by a description of trajectory groups showing variation in weight status over time (i.e., declining, rising, or fluctuating trajectories). We conclude this section with a presentation of predictors associated with trajectory group membership.

Distinct Trajectories of Weight Status

Six research studies have explored variations in the development of BMI in clustered and distinct groups through non-normative growth curve modeling; however, even with this small number of studies, contrasting and comparing the results is challenging because of differences in the ages and age intervals at which anthropometric assessments were reported or measured and in the reference cutoffs used to categorize the children's weight status. Further, the various studies handled potential sex differences in a variety of ways. One study's sample consisted solely of girls [45], four studies combined boys and girls in the trajectory analysis [42–44, 46], and one conducted sex-specific analyses [41]. Nonetheless, we observed the occurrence of four general types of weight status trajectory groups: (1) never overweight trajectories, (2) chronically overweight trajectories, (3) rising trajectories, and (4) declining trajectories.

Trajectories of stable weight status include groups of children who have maintained a normal weight trajectory (i.e., never overweight or obese) and those who have persisted in being overweight throughout a study period. Researchers have clearly identified that the most common trajectory subgroup is the never overweight group. This subgroup was observed in all six studies, irrespective of the ages sampled. However, with variation in the definition of overweight status and obesity, the age of the children studied, and the statistical method applied, estimates of the proportion of children and adolescents in the never overweight trajectory ranged from 60% to 84% [43, 45–46]. The second most common trajectory subgroup, chronic overweight, was observed in four studies only [42–45]. For example, 11% of children 2 to 12 years of age and 15% of children 9 to 16 years of age were estimated to belong to chronic overweight trajectories by Li et al. and Mustillo et al., respectively [42, 43].

Trajectories of weight status that have varied over time encompass groups of children whose BMI trajectories have risen, declined, or fluctuated across the study period. Four studies reported the presence of subgroups of children who moved into an overweight status from a normal, healthy weight at baseline, but the ages at which the children entered overweight status varied across the studies [41–43, 46]. The reverse pattern of declining from an overweight to normal weight status was also observed [41–42, 46]. Two studies, with similar ages at baseline and follow-up, reported that the decline in weight status occurred between the ages of 11 and 12 years [42, 45]. Within the rising and declining trajectories there also has been evidence of some fluctuation. For example, two of the three boys' trajectories fluctuated over time; one, "transient high BMI," went from normal to overweight and back to normal weight status; the other, "j-curve rise to obesity," fluctuated from an overweight to normal weight and back to overweight status [41]. Another study also found fluctuation, with one of the girls' subgroup trajectories ("delayed downward percentile crossing") showing a steep increase in BMI, followed by stabilization, and then a decline [45].

The trajectories that emerged through non-normative growth curve modeling have the potential to reveal critical ages at which change in weight status is likely to occur. However, with the exception of the two declining groups from Mustillo et al. (2003) and Ventura et al. (2009) studies, it is difficult to detect any consistency in the patterns of change within the six studies, possibly because of the variation in study design [42, 45]. For example, using same age samples (followed from 2 to 12 years), O'Brien et al. (2007) found that within the rising trajectory, children entered and maintained overweight status from 54 months on. Within the rising trajectory identified by Li et al. (2007), the increased

TABLE 3.1 Summary of Findings from Non-normative Growth Curve Methods

Study	Age (years)	Outcome variable	Trajectory groups	Percentage
Hejazi et al. [41]	2 to 8	BMI-Continuous	**Girls**	
			1. Stable-normal BMI	64%
			2. Accelerating rise to obesity	14%
			3. Early-declining BMI	8%
			4. Late-declining BMI	14%
			Boys	
			1. Stable-normal BMI	70%
			2. J-curve rise to obesity	11%
			3. Transient high BMI	19%
Li et al. [43]	2 to 12	BMI-Dichotomized	**Girls and Boys**	
			1. Never overweight	84%
			2. Early-onset overweight	11%
			3. Late-onset overweight	5%
Mustillo et al. (2003) [42]	9 to 16	BMI-Dichotomized	**Girls and Boys**	
			1. Never obese	73%
			2. Chronic obesity	15%
			3. Adolescent obesity	8%
			4. Childhood obesity	5%
Nonnemaker et al. [44]	12 to 17	BMI-Continuous	**Girls and Boys**	
			1. Low risk	44%
			2. Low-to-moderate risk	36%
			3. Moderate-to-high risk	16%
			4. High risk	4%
O'Brien et al. [46]	2 to 12	BMI-Continuous	**Girls and Boys**	
			1. Never overweight	60%
			2. Preschool overweight	19%
			3. Elementary overweight	10%
			4. Return to normal weight	7%
			5. Variable	4%
Ventura et al. [45]	5 to 15	BMI-Continuous	**Girls Only**	
			1. The 50th percentile tracking	37%
			2. The 60th percentile tracking	29%
			3. Upward percentile crossing	14%
			4. Delayed downward percentile	20%

probability of overweight status occurred after the children were 8 years old [43]. A methodological difference between the two studies is that a continuous measure of weight status was used in one study, and a dichotomized measure was used in the other.

In summary, the application of non-normative growth curve modeling has yielded evidence of heterogeneity in the developmental trajectories of weight status in childhood and adolescence. The studies suggest the occurrence of four general types of weight status trajectory groups, with the majority of children sustaining a normal weight trajectory. In studies that identified a trajectory of chronic overweight status, the trajectory accounted for a much smaller percentage of children. In addition, some studies identified groups of children who developed a pattern of overweight status only later in childhood. This raises the question of how such children (at risk for later overweight status) might be identified early so that preventive measures can be undertaken before overweight status presents. On the other hand, a small percentage of children were able to transition from an overweight to a healthful weight status, and understanding factors that precipitate such a decline is equally important for the development of interventions designed to facilitate the attainment and maintenance of a healthy weight status.

Predictors of Trajectory Membership

In the studies reviewed, predictors of membership in the various trajectories were most commonly identified through multivariate analysis (e.g., multinomial regression; multivariate analysis of variance; discriminant function analysis), with children belonging to the never obese trajectories typically used as the referent group. The predictors investigated in the studies were wide ranging, encompassing variables such as family socioeconomic factors (income, parental education, and single-parent status), child demographic characteristics (sex, race, and birth order), early life factors (birth weight and duration of breastfeeding), parental factors (maternal age, maternal weight status, and maternal gestational weight gain), child and parent behavior (fussy temperament, adolescent psychiatric disorders, child's sedentary behavior, parental smoking, and parental parenting practices), and others (metabolic health risks and early puberty). Most commonly, the predictors were measured only at the beginning of the trajectory period. Findings related to these factors are described later in the chapter; we present these findings as they relate to the types of weight status trajectory groups reported in the studies, the never obese, the chronically obese, the rising, and the declining trajectory groups.

The majority of studies have reported significant associations between family socioeconomic status and membership in the chronically overweight or rising trajectory groups, relative to other trajectory groups in the study [42–45, 47]. For example, the Hejazi (2007) study showed parental educational attainment was lower for girls in the "accelerating rise to obesity" group than for girls in the "stable-normal BMI" group and the "early and late declining BMI" groups [47]. Among the boys, those in the rising trajectories group ("j-curve obesity") were more likely to reside in homes with low family income and to have parents with lower educational attainment than those in the other two groups. Furthermore, compared with the never obese group, children belonging to the chronically obese group were significantly more likely to come from lower and middle income backgrounds (RR = 2.16) and to have parents with lower educational levels (RR = 2.34) [42]. Children's demographic characteristics [43, 44] and early life context [43, 45] also have been found to be associated with trajectories of chronic and rising to overweight status. In general, these results replicate findings from studies using other research designs and analytic methods.

Some studies included variables that have not been well established as predictors of overweight status. Unexpected associations between the rising trajectories group and parenting practices in the "j-curve obesity" boys group were more likely to have parents who self-reported lower levels of harmful and hostile parenting practices [47]. Further associations have been found between oppositional disorders, adolescent depressive disorders, and chronic overweight [42] and between fussy temperament and "accelerating rise to obesity" among girls [47].

Non-normative growth curve methods have the potential to advance our understanding of factors that influence weight status in that predictors are linked with specific trajectories of weight status over time. However, within the studies reviewed, only two variables were found to be predictive of declining trajectory groups, parental education and early puberty. Parental education was predictive of declining trajectories within two different studies, but in an unexpected direction. Children in the "childhood obesity" group (i.e., declining) were more likely to have parents with low levels of education than those in the "never obese" group [42]. Moreover, girls belonging to the "delayed downward percentile" had parents with lower educational attainment compared with girls in the two 'never obese' groups; they also showed earlier pubertal development than the "never obese" girls [45].

A possible explanation for the limited findings regarding predictors of declining trajectories (and possibly for the nonsignificant relationships shown for predictors of the other trajectories) might be that predictors have typically been measured only at the beginning of the trajectory period. This is important for two reasons. First, there may be a long lag period between assessment of the predictor and the onset of change in weight status. Second, measuring the predictor only once suggests that the predictor is time invariant (i.e., does not change over time). Although this is a logical assumption for some potentially influential characteristics (e.g., maternal gestational weight gain and child's birth weight), other characteristics such as family income and maternal depression may vary over time.

CONCLUSION

The objective of this chapter was to present findings from a selection of research studies that used longitudinal data analyses to understand the developmental trajectories of weight status within childhood and adolescence. Our review focused on three different approaches used to investigate developmental patterns or trajectories of weight status: tracking methods, normative growth curve methods, and non-normative growth curve methods. Studies using tracking methods involve time point to time point analysis, often through correlational methods or the expression of odds ratios. The more advanced statistical methods (i.e., normative and non-normative growth curve modeling) simultaneously use multiple or repeated assessments of weight status to describe the normative or average trajectory of children's weight status (in the case of normative modeling) or to explore heterogeneity in developmental trajectories (i.e., identify distinct subgroups), in the case of non-normative modeling.

The results that have been obtained from both tracking and non-normative methods suggest that children's weight status is best described through four general weight status patterns, the never overweight, the chronically overweight, and the rising and declining weight status patterns. Children with normal weight or overweight status tend to maintain their weight status over time, with relatively fewer children changing weight status. A child with healthful weight will most likely continue in the same weight status but is at risk for developing overweight. A child who is overweight will most likely continue to be overweight but may decline to a normal weight status. Tracking studies have generally focused on the persistence of overweight status, with fewer studies exploring variation in weight status over time. In contrast, studies using non-normative growth curve methods have focused on the identification of distinctive patterns of weight change over time and have been able to reveal, more explicitly, BMI trajectories that have risen, declined, or fluctuated across a study period. Although the results of both methodological approaches have indicated that, over time, the majority of children maintain a normal, healthful weight status, non-normative methods provide a more comprehensive evaluation of patterns of change and thus are considered stronger than tracking approaches. The statistical estimation of stability and change through the former approach is based on the simultaneous analysis of multiple assessments, whereas tracking methods, which by design focus on time point to time point comparisons, fragment the trajectories. For example, with tracking methods, children who are found to maintain an overweight status between time 2 and time 3 assessments will include those who were overweight at time 1, as well as those who were normal weight at time 1 but had become overweight by time 2; however, this variability will not be apparent in the time 2 to time 3 "overweight to overweight" trajectory.

In contrast to exploring distinctive patterns of weight status, studies using normative growth curve methods focus on describing average trajectories of weight status within a known population. Normative methods can only reveal subgroup differences in developmental trajectories when predictor variables are included in the model (and thus they must be known or hypothesized, a priori). As has been shown in tracking and non-normative growth curve studies, the majority of children follow a fairly stable trajectory of weight status, with most persisting in being of normal weight. Thus, it is not surprising that results from normative growth curve modeling of BMI data suggest that, on average, children's weight status increases only moderately with age within the overall population and within known subgroups (e.g., identified by ethnicity/race). In the application of normative methods, variation around the average or normative trajectory is generally considered to represent unexplained individual variation rather than the possibility of distinctive, alternative patterns of change in weight status. Accordingly, application of normative methods in the field of obesity research has tended to be for the purpose of describing the normative development of weight status in children and adolescents and exploring factors that may explain variation around the average trajectory. The results from normative methods are particularly informative when comparing trajectories of different measures of weight status. Whereas BMI trajectories appear to be fairly linear in shape with little sex difference, developmental trajectories based on other measures of weight status have been suggestive of nonlinear change with sex and ethnic differences in both the level and rate of change. Further, a more rapid increase in weight status has been shown to be associated with lower family socioeconomic status, parental overweight, and several additional predictors that are commonly associated with weight gain or weight status.

Researchers using non-normative methods have identified distinctive profiles of change in weight status that vary from the dominant normative growth profile. They also have identified predictors of chronic overweight status; for example, lower family socioeconomic status has been associated with the chronic overweight trajectory. However, what has been most informative in the use of these methods is the very finding that distinctive trajectories exist and that there are distinct subgroups in the population that vary from the normative growth profile even though the predictors or risk factors associated with these trajectories remain fully or partially unknown. That is, distinctive trajectories can be identified in the absence of known or hypothesized risk factors, which may motivate the quest for explanatory factors. Still, our understanding of the heterogeneity in the developmental trajectories of childhood weight status remains incomplete because researchers tend to follow samples over different age spans, making it difficult to draw conclusions about the ages at which a child or an adolescent is at greater risk for becoming overweight and to identify factors that influence such changes in weight status, particularly the time variant factors.

There are other perspectives that can be brought to the search for predictors of weight status trajectory membership. For example, rather than focusing on predictors of the chronic obesity trajectory, researchers could shift their attention to understanding factors that contribute to membership in the normal weight status trajectory or declining weight status, as well as factors that vary across trajectories. Researchers could also give increased attention to the effect of factors that may vary over time and ask whether exposure to certain conditions is more detrimental at particular ages.

The non-normative statistical techniques are a recent development and researchers should take advantage of the opportunity to build on what has been learned from the six studies reviewed here. Ideally, future studies should follow children from birth through adulthood to provide a more comprehensive understanding of the different ways some children develop obesity or reach obesity and then decline to normal weight status. Further research is needed to identify predictors of trajectory group membership; the research that has been completed has not been successful in providing a comprehensive explanation of the profiles of change in weight status that have been observed. The scope of study should be expanded to include unexplored factors, and to combine biological and social/behavioral risk factors to better understand the interactions. Researchers ought to consider the heterogeneity in the trajectories with an eye to enumerating the distinct profiles that occur in childhood and adolescence, their characteristics, their risk or protective factors, and their health and social outcomes to better understand both the normative and non-normative growth trajectories that exist in the population. Ultimately, different interventions and prevention strategies could be developed for individuals in different subgroups of growth or change in weight status.

References

1. Goldstein H. *Multilevel statistical models*. 3rd. ed. London: Arnold; 2003.
2. Raudenbush SW, Bryk AS. *Hierarchical linear models: Applications and data analysis methods*. 2nd ed. Newbury Park, CA: Sage; 2002.
3. Muthén B, Muthén LK. Integrating person-centered and variable-centered analyses: Growth mixture modeling with latent trajectory classes. *Alcoholism: Clinical and Experimental Research* 2000;**24**:882–91.
4. Collins LM, Lanza ST. *Latent class and latent transition analysis: with applications in the social, behavioral, and health sciences*. New York: Wiley; 2009.
5. Nagin DS. *Group-based modeling of development*. Cambridge, MA: Harvard University Press; 2005.
6. Reilly JJ, Methven E, McDowell ZC, Hacking B, Alexander D, Stewart L, et al. Health consequences of obesity. *Archives of Disease in Childhood* 2003;**88**:748–52.
7. Hesketh K, Wake M, Waters E, Carlin J, Crawford D. Stability of body mass index in Australian children: A prospective cohort study across the middle childhood years. *Public Health Nutrition* 2004;**7**:303–9.
8. Deshmukh-Taskar P, Nicklas TA, Morales M, Yang SJ, Zakeri I, Berenson GS. Tracking of overweight status from childhood to young adulthood: The Bogalusa Heart Study. *European Journal of Clinical Nutrition* 2006;**60**:48–57.
9. Imed H, Jihene MM, Hamida BH, Rafika G, Fatma L, Amel B, et al. Tracking of overweight among urban school children: A 4 years cohort study in Sousse Tunisia. *Journal of Public Health and Epidemiology* 2009;**1**:31–6.
10. Willows ND, Johnson MS, Ball GD. Prevalence estimates of overweight and obesity in Cree preschool children in northern Quebec according to international and US reference criteria. *American Journal of Public Health* 2007;**97**:311–16.
11. Singh AS, Mulder C, Twisk JWR, van Mechelen W, Chinapaw MJ. Tracking of childhood overweight into adulthood: A systematic review of the literature. *Obesity Reviews* 2008;**9**:474–88.
12. Johannsson E, Arngrimsson SA, Thorsdottir I, Sveinsson T. Tracking of overweight from early childhood to adolescence in cohorts born 1988 and 1994: Overweight in a high birth weight population. *International Journal of Obesity* 2006;**30**:1265–71.
13. Nader PR, O'Brien M, Houts R, Bradley R, Belsky J, Crosnoe R, et al. Identifying risk for obesity in early childhood. *Pediatrics* 2006;**118**:e594–601.
14. Mei Z, Grummer-Strawn LM, Scanlon KS. Does overweight in infancy persist through the preschool years? An analysis of CDC Pediatric Nutrition Surveillance System data. *Sozial- und Praventivmedizin* 2003;**48**:161–7.
15. Hesketh K, Carlin J, Wake M, Crawford D. Predictors of body mass index change in Australian primary school children. *International Journal of Paediatric Obesity* 2009;**4**:45–53.
16. Wang Y, Ge K, Popkin BM. Tracking of body mass index from childhood to adolescence: A 6-y follow-up study in China. *American Journal of Clinical Nutrition* 2000;**72**:1018–24.
17. Fuentes RM, Notkola IL, Shemeikka S, Tuomilehto J, Nissinen A. Tracking of body mass index during childhood: A 15-year prospective population-based family study in eastern Finland. *International Journal of Obesity and Related Metabolic Disorders* 2003;**27**:716–21.
18. Irigoyen M, Glassman ME, Chen S, Findley SE. Early onset of overweight and obesity among low-income 1- to 5-year olds in New York City. *Journal of Urban Health* 2008;**85**:545–54.
19. Fleiss JL. *Statistical methods for rates and proportions*. 2nd ed. New York: Wiley; 1981.
20. Wang Y, Wang X. How do statistical properties influence findings of tracking (maintenance) in epidemiologic studies? An example

21. Dai S, Labarthe DR, Grunbaum JA, Harrist RB, Mueller WH. Longitudinal analysis of changes in indices of obesity from age 8 years to age 18 years. Project HeartBeat!. *American Journal of Epidemiology* 2002;**156**:720−9.
22. Heude B, Kettaneh A, de Lauzon Guillain B, Lommez A, Borys JM, Ducimetière P, et al. Growth curves of anthropometric indices in a general population of French children and comparison with reference data. *European Journal of Clinical Nutrition* 2006;**60**:1430−6.
23. Silverwood RJ, De Stavola BL, Cole TJ, Leon DA. BMI peak in infancy as a predictor for later BMI in the Uppsala Family Study. *International Journal of Obesity* 2009;**33**:929−37.
24. Wardle J, Brodersen NH, Cole TJ, Jarvis MJ, Boniface DR. Development of adiposity in adolescence: Five year longitudinal study of an ethnically and socioeconomically diverse sample of young people in Britain. *BMJ* 2006;**332**:1130−5.
25. Eissa MA, Dai S, Mihalopoulos NL, Day RS, Harrist RB, Labarthe DR. Trajectories of fat mass index, fat free-mass index, and waist circumference in children: Project HeartBeat!. *American Journal of Preventive Medicine* 2009;**37**:S34−9.
26. Dekkers JC, Podolsky RH, Treiber FA, Barbeau P, Gutin B, Snieder H. Development of general and central obesity from childhood into early adulthood in African American and European American males and females with a family history of cardiovascular disease. *American Journal of Clinical Nutrition* 2004;**79**:661−8.
27. Balistreri K, Van Hook J. Socioeconomic status and body mass index among Hispanic children of immigrants and children of Natives. *American Journal of Public Health* 2009;**99**:2238−46.
28. Berkowitz RI, Stallings VA, Maislin G, Stunkard AJ. Growth of children at high risk of obesity during first 6 years of life: Implications for prevention. *American Journal of Clinical Nutrition* 2005;**81**:140−6.
29. Oliver L, Hayes M. Effects of neighbourhood income on reported body mass index: An eight year longitudinal study of Canadian children. *BMC Public Health* 2008;**8**:16.
30. Francis LA, Ventura AK, Marini M, Birch LL. Parent overweight predicts daughters' increase in BMI and disinhibited overeating from 5 to 13 Years. *Obesity* 2007;**15**:1544−53.
31. Danner F. A national longitudinal study of the association between hours of TV viewing and the trajectory of BMI growth among US children. *Journal of Pediatric Psychology* 2008;**33**:1100−7.
32. Henderson VR. Longitudinal associations between television viewing and body mass index among white and black girls. *Journal of Adolescent Health* 2007;**41**:544−50.
33. Pabayo R, Gauvin L, Barnett TA, Nikiéma B, Séguin L. Sustained active transportation is associated with a favorable body mass index trajectory across the early school years: Findings from the Quebec Longitudinal Study of Child Development birth cohort. *Preventive Medicine* 2009;**50**:S59−64.
34. Raudenbush SW. Comparing personal trajectories and drawing causal inferences from longitudinal data. *Annual Review of Psychology* 2001;**52**:501−25.
35. Muthén B. Latent variable analysis: Growth mixture modeling and related techniques for longitudinal data. In: Kaplan D, editor. *Handbook of quantitative methodology for the social sciences.* Thousand Oaks, CA: Sage; 2004. pp. 345−68.
36. Muthén B. Latent variable hybrids: Overview of old and new models. In: Hancock GR, Samuelsen KM, editors. *Advances in latent variable mixture models*. Charlotte, NC: Information Age Publishing; 2008.
37. Nagin DS. Analyzing developmental trajectories: A semi-parametric, group-based approach. *Psychological Methods* 1999;**4**:139−57.
38. Muthén B. The potential of growth mixture modelling. *Infant and Child Development* 2006;**15**:623−5.
39. Nagin DS, Tremblay RE. What has been learned from group-based trajectory modeling? Examples from physical aggression and other problem behaviors. *Annals of the American Academy of Political and Social Science* 2005;**602**:82−117.
40. Lacourse E, Nagin D, Tremblay RE, Vitaro F, Claes M. Developmental trajectories of boys' delinquent membership and facilitation of violent behaviors during adolescence. *Development & Psychopathology* 2003;**15**:183−97.
41. Hejazi S, Dahinten VS, Marshall SK, Ratner PA. Developmental pathways leading to obesity in childhood. *Health Reports* 2009;**20**:63−9.
42. Mustillo S, Worthman C, Erkanli A, Keeler G, Angold A, Costello EJ. Obesity and psychiatric disorder: Developmental trajectories. *Pediatrics* 2003;**111**:851−9.
43. Li C, Goran MI, Kaur H, Nollen N, Ahluwalia JS. Developmental trajectories of overweight during childhood: Role of early life factors. *Obesity* 2007;**15**:760−71.
44. Nonnemaker JM, Morgan-Lopez AA, Pais JM, Finkelstein EA. Youth BMI trajectories: Evidence from the NLSY97. *Obesity* 2009;**17**:1274−80.
45. Ventura AK, Loken E, Birch LL. Developmental trajectories of girls' BMI across childhood and adolescence. *Obesity* 2009;**17**:2067−74.
46. O'Brien M, Nader PR, Houts RM, Bradley R, Friedman SL, Belsky J, et al. The ecology of childhood overweight: A 12-year longitudinal analysis. *International Journal of Obesity* 2007;**17**:1469−78.
47. Hejazi S. *Temperament, parenting and the development of childhood obesity*. Unpublished doctoral dissertation. Vancouver, BC: University of British Columbia; 2007.

Suggested Readings

Jones BL, Nagin DS, Roeder K. A SAS procedure based on mixture models for estimating developmental trajectories. *Sociological Research and Methods* 2001;**29**:374−93.

Lanza ST, Collins LM. A new SAS procedure for latent transition analysis: Transitions in dating and sexual risk behavior. *Developmental Psychology* 2008;**44**:446−56.

Lanza ST, Lemmon DR, Schafer JL, Collins LM. *PROC LCA & PROC LTA user's guide*. University Park, PA: The Methodology Center, Pennsylvania State University; 2008.

Muthén LK, Muthén B. Mplus user's guide. Los Angeles: Muthén & Muthén; 2006.

Muthén LK, Muthén B. Mplus user's guide. Los Angeles: Muthén & Muthén; 1998−2007.

CHAPTER 4

The Measurement and Epidemiology of Child Obesity

David S. Freedman*, Cynthia L. Ogden†, Sarah E. Cusick‡

*Division of Nutrition, Physical Activity and Obesity, Centers for Disease Control and Prevention K-26, Atlanta, GA, USA, †National Center for Health Statistics, Centers for Disease Control and Prevention, Hyattsville, MD, USA and ‡School of Public Health, University of Minnesota, Minneapolis, MN, USA

INTRODUCTION

The prevalences of overweight (body mass index [BMI] of between 25 kg/m² and 29.9 kg/m²) and obesity (BMI ≥ 30 kg/m²) among adults have greatly increased throughout the world since the 1960s. In the United States, for example, the mean weights of adults increased by about 10 kg from 1960–1962 through 1999–2002, and over one third of U.S. adults are now considered to be obese [1, 2]. Although there are fewer countries with weight and height data for children, secular increases in overweight and obesity among children and adolescents appear to have accelerated between the 1980s and late 1990s [3], with the prevalences having substantially increased in many countries [4]. Based on data from various surveys [3] and from self-reports among adolescents in 34 countries [5], the prevalence of child obesity is particularly high in countries in North America, southwestern Europe, the eastern Mediterranean, and Great Britain.

The secular trends among children (ages, 2 to 19 years) in the United States (Figure 4.1) have been well documented, with the combined prevalence of overweight and obesity (BMI ≥ 85th percentile of the 2000 CDC growth charts or BMI ≥ 25 kg/m², left panel) having increased about three-fold (13% to 33%) between examinations conducted in 1963–1965 and 2003–2006. This increase was largely due to the almost four-fold increase in the prevalence of child obesity (BMI ≥ CDC 95th percentile or BMI ≥ 30 kg/m², middle panel). In contrast, the prevalence of overweight (BMI between the CDC 85th and 94th percentiles or a BMI between 25 and 29.9 kg/m²) increased about two-fold (9% to 16%, right panel). These trends in the United States have varied substantially by age and race-ethnicity, with the largest increases in obesity occurring among older children and among black and Mexican-American children [6], and about 28% of 12- to 19-year-old black girls were obese in 2003–2006 [7]. Furthermore, the prevalences of obesity and overweight among children in the United States are now similar, with about 16% of children in each of the two categories.

Comparing the prevalences of child overweight and obesity across countries and time periods, however, remains difficult. Most countries lack recent, representative data based on measured weights and heights, and comparisons are further complicated by the use of different classification criteria for overweight and obesity. Different cut-points and reference populations have been recommended by the International Obesity Task Force (IOTF) [8], the Centers for Disease Control (CDC) [9], and the World Health Organization (WHO) [10, 11]. The use of different classification systems can result in substantial, unanticipated differences in the prevalences of overweight and obesity [12]. For example, the estimated prevalence of obesity among 2- to 5-year-olds in the United States in 2003–2006 was 12% based on the CDC 95th percentile, but it was only 6% based on the IOTF cut-points.

Furthermore, almost all estimates of the prevalence of child obesity are based on BMI. Several investigators, however, have concluded that many children with excess body fatness do not have a high BMI (low sensitivity) [13–19], and this could result in underestimating

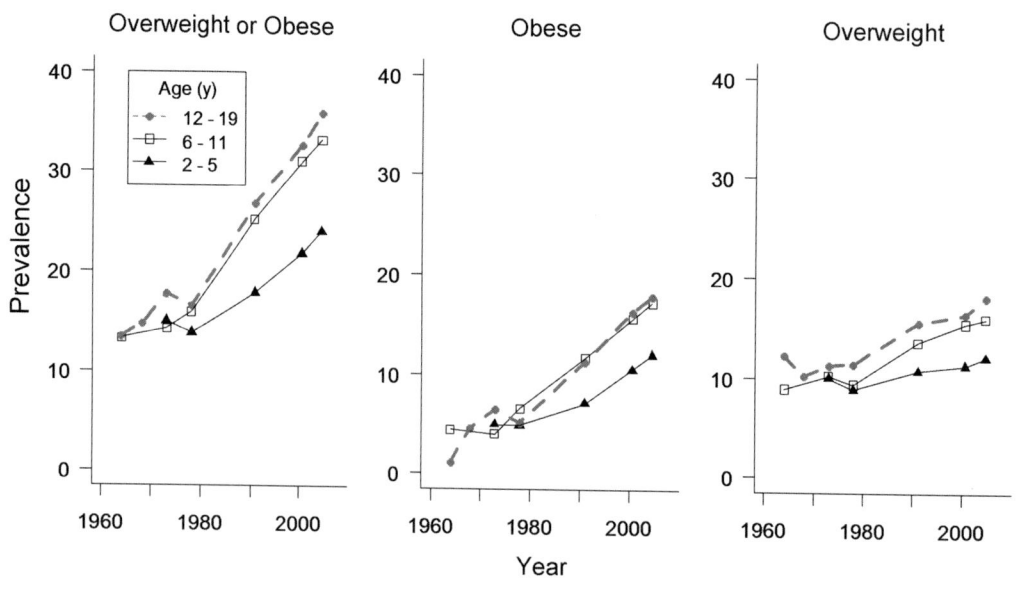

FIGURE 4.1 Prevalence of overweight and obesity (BMI-for-age ≥ CDC 85th percentile or BMI ≥ 25 kg/m^2, *left panel*), obesity (BMI-for-age ≥ CDC 95th percentile or BMI ≥ 30 kg/m^2, *middle panel*), and overweight (BMI-for-age between the 85th and 95th percentiles of the CDC reference population or BMI between 25 and 29.9 kg/m^2) among 2- to 19-year-olds in the United States. Data are from nine national studies conducted from 1963 through 2006. Two-year estimates for some studies have been combined into 4-year periods (1999–2002 and 2003–2006) to improve precision.

the actual prevalence of excess body fatness. Although there is some evidence that BMI-based comparisons may have underestimated the secular trends in excess body fatness among children [20], other results [21] indicate that BMI may be a more sensitive indicator of excess body fatness than is frequently asserted.

This review focuses on the classification of high levels of BMI and body fatness, the relation of BMI to body fatness among children, and the ability of a high BMI to identify children with excess body fatness. Many of the results are based on published data from the Pediatric Rosetta Study [21–23], but several are from unpublished analyses of this large data set.

BMI AND BODY FATNESS

The limitations of BMI, which does not distinguish between fat, skeletal, and muscle mass, are widely known [24]. Among children, the use of BMI is further complicated by the large changes in weight and height that occur during growth and development, resulting in the median BMI increasing by almost 50% between the ages of 5 and 19 years. Although the moderate, positive correlation between BMI and height among children has also led to concerns about the use of this index [25], the body fatness of children is positively correlated with height [26].

It is possible to account for the differences in BMI by sex and age by expressing a child's BMI relative to other children of the same sex and age [27]. The use of standard deviation (z) scores and percentiles for these relative BMI levels allows comparisons to be made between boys and girls as well as across age groups, but differences in z-scores and percentiles are not always easy to interpret. It should also be realized that even among children who have the same sex, age and BMI, there can be a wide range of levels of body fatness [28, 29].

BMI levels have also been calculated from self-reported or parent reported (for younger children) as simple, inexpensive, and rapid alternatives to weight and height measurements. However, several investigators have found that self-reported [30] and parent-reported [31] data for weight and height can lead to biased and imprecise estimates of BMI. Although various correction factors have been suggested to improve the accuracy of these reported data, the validity of these corrections is uncertain. BMI levels based on reported data will not be further discussed in this chapter.

Relation of BMI to Body Fatness

An ideal measure of body fatness would be accurate, precise, and accessible, and reference data would be widely available, but no existing measure satisfies all these criteria [32]. The four-compartment model, in which independent estimates of body density, body water, and bone are obtained, may be the most accurate [33, 34], but it is expensive, time consuming, and available at very few locations. In contrast, the speed and low operating costs of dual-energy x-ray absorptiometry (DXA) has led to its widespread use as a reference method.

Several large studies of children have incorporated DXA measurements, including ~7500 8- to 19-year-olds examined in the National Health and Nutrition Examination Survey (NHANES) between 1999 and 2004 [35], ~6900 children in the Avon Longitudinal Study of Parents and Children (ALSPAC) [36], and ~1200 children in the Pediatric Rosetta Study [21]. Whereas the NHANES sample is representative of the U.S. population, children in the Pediatric Rosetta Study were recruited through newspaper notices, announcements at schools and activity centers, and word of mouth [21]. Pregnant women residing in three health districts in Bristol, England, with an expected date of delivery between April 1991 and December 1992 were eligible to participate in ALSPAC, and more than 14,000 women were enrolled.

DXA estimates of body fatness are highly correlated with those from the four-compartment model, but DXA-estimated body fatness can be influenced by various characteristics, such as the level of body fatness as well as the equipment manufacturer and software [33, 37–41]. A systematic error in the estimation of body fatness by DXA could influence the observed screening performance of BMI in identifying children who have excess body fatness.

The relation of BMI to levels of percentage body fat, measured by DXA, among children has varied substantially across studies, with some investigators [42, 43] reporting only modest ($r < 0.50$) associations in some subgroups. These findings, however, may largely be due to the relative thinness of the examined children; BMI has been characterized as "almost useless" in assessing the body fatness of normal-weight children [37]. In contrast, among children who have BMI levels that are similar to those of the current U.S. population, regression models including BMI, age, and race-ethnicity as predictor variables have been found to be good predictors of body fatness [22], accounting for about 79% (boys) to 81% (girls) of the variability in percentage body fat. Of these characteristics, BMI was, by far, the most important predictor of body fatness (discussed later). The residual standard errors of the fitted regression models were 5% (boys) and 4% (girls), and the median, absolute difference between the observed (DXA) and predicted level of percentage body fat was 3%.

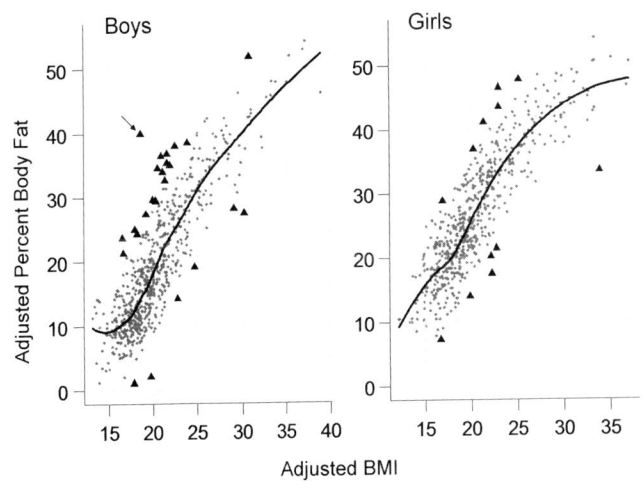

Figure 4.2 shows age-adjusted levels of percentage body fat versus BMI among boys (left panel) and girls (right panel). To account for race and age differences in percentage body fat and BMI, levels of these two characteristics were first regressed on age (using splines to allow for nonlinearity) and race (black versus other) within each sex. Residuals from these regression models were then added to the mean levels of BMI and percentage body fat; these adjusted levels of percentage body fat and BMI are shown for each of the 626 boys and 570 girls in the two panels. The solid lines are based on lowess (locally weighted scatterplot smoother) and show the relation of the (adjusted) level of BMI to the (adjusted) level of percentage body fat among boys and girls. Regression analyses incorporating cubic splines indicated that based on these adjusted levels, differences in BMI could account for 77% (boys) and 79% (girls) of the variability in levels of percentage body fat.

As seen by the small scatter around the fitted curves relative to the range of levels of percentage body fat, BMI was a good predictor of body fatness among most boys and girls. Most children who had a relatively high BMI (for their sex and age) also had a relatively high percentage body fat. However, there were children for whom the BMI-predicted level of body fatness was poor. The solid triangles in Figure 4.2 represent children with predicted levels of percentage body fat that differed by 10% or more from the DXA-calculated level

FIGURE 4.2 Adjusted levels of percentage body fat versus BMI among boys (left panel) and girls (right panel) among children in the Pediatric Rosetta Study. Levels of BMI and percentage body fat were first regressed on age and race (black versus other) within each sex, and residuals from these models were added to the sex-specific means to derive age-adjusted levels. Each point represents the adjusted level of percentage body fat and BMI of an individual child (n = 1196). The solid lines are based are based on lowess (locally weighted scatterplot smoother). The gray points represent children who have a prediction error of <10%, whereas the black triangles represent prediction errors of ≥10%. A boy with a prediction error of 25% is indicated by an arrow.

of percentage body fat. The largest difference was seen for a 9-year-old boy (indicated by a diagonal arrow in the left panel). This boy had a BMI of 17.4 kg/m² (about the 70th percentile of BMI-for-age in the CDC reference population), but his DXA-calculated percentage body fat was 43%; this was the 16th highest value of body fatness among the 626 examined boys.

Alternatives to BMI

Skinfold thickness measurements and bioelectrical impedance analysis (BIA) have been considered to be attractive alternatives to BMI in the estimation of body fatness, but both methods have limitations. As compared with BMI, skinfold thicknesses have been found to be more strongly associated with the body fatness of children in most [22, 37, 44–46] but not all [47] studies. However, the large measurement errors [48, 49] associated with skinfold thicknesses are problematic, there is little agreement on the optimal sites for these measurements, and these measurements are more intrusive than are those for weight and height.

BIA is another inexpensive and noninvasive method for assessing body composition, but its accuracy remains uncertain, and these measurements can be influenced by sex, age, and race-ethnicity [34]. Furthermore, comparisons with estimates of body fatness from reference methods have indicated that there can be substantial errors in BIA [37, 50, 51], and some investigators [37] have concluded that BIA estimates are less accurate than are skinfold thicknesses. Some studies have also indicated that the accuracy of BIA may be particularly low among overweight and obese adults [50, 51].

Despite the desire for more accurate estimates of body fatness, it is possible that BMI conveys most of the relevant information on metabolic risk. BMI has been found to be as strongly related to levels of various risk factors as are estimates of body fatness obtained from BIA or skinfold thicknesses in several cross-sectional studies of children [46, 52] and adults [53–55]. For example, an analysis of about 10,000 adults [54] indicated that body fatness estimates obtained from various BIA equations did not show stronger associations with levels of blood pressures, fasting glucose, lipids, or lipoproteins than did BMI. Furthermore, the BIA estimates that were most predictive of risk factor levels were the ones that were most strongly correlated ($r > 0.9$) with BMI. Levels of various metabolic risk factors have also been found to be related similarly to BMI and to DXA-estimated levels of body fatness among children [46, 56].

Somewhat similar results have been observed among 6866 children who were examined in the Bogalusa Heart Study [57]. Adjusted (for sex, age, and study period) levels of lipids, fasting insulin, and blood pressures were found to show similar associations with levels of BMI and skinfold (subscapular and triceps) thicknesses (Table 4.1). For example, among children under 12 years of age, correlations with levels of triglycerides were

TABLE 4.1 Adjusted[a] Correlations between the Adiposity Measures and Risk Factor Levels, Stratified by Age

Age (years)	N		BMI	Triceps	Skinfold thickness Subscapular	Skinfold sum[b]
≤12	3228	Triglycerides	0.35	0.32[c]*	0.34	0.35
		LDL cholesterol	0.17	0.15	0.15	0.16
		HDL cholesterol	−0.23	−0.19**	−0.21	−0.21
		Fasting insulin	0.48	0.41**	0.45**	0.45**
		SBP	0.42	0.37**	0.35**	0.37**
		DBP	0.34	0.31*	0.28**	0.31**
>12	3638	Triglycerides	0.31	0.28*	0.33	0.32
		LDL cholesterol	0.20	0.19	0.22	0.21
		HDL cholesterol	−0.20	−0.18	−0.19	−0.19
		Fasting insulin	0.44	0.38**	0.41**	0.42**
		SBP	0.18	0.11**	0.14**	0.13**
		DBP	0.09	0.06*	0.09	0.08

[a]Levels of the BMI, skinfold thicknesses and risk factors have been adjusted for sex, age, race, and study period.
[b]Sum of the triceps and subscapular skinfold thicknesses.
[c]P-values indicate whether the correlation between the risk factor and skinfold thickness is significantly different from the correlation between the risk factor and BMI; *$p < 0.01$, **$p < 0.001$.

r = 0.35 (for both BMI and the skinfold sum), whereas correlations with fasting insulin were r = 0.48 (BMI) and r = 0.45 (skinfold sum). Although the differences in the magnitudes of the observed correlations were relatively small, almost all comparisons indicated that BMI was at least as strongly associated with levels of the various risk factors as was the skinfold sum. Furthermore, in many cases, correlations with BMI were significantly (p < 0.01) stronger than the corresponding correlation with the skinfold sum. Neither skinfold thickness showed a significantly stronger association with levels of any risk factor than did BMI.

Relatively few longitudinal studies have compared the predictive abilities of BMI and more accurate estimates of body fatness for various health outcomes, but several investigators [58–61] have found that skinfold thickness measurements among adults provide little additional information for type 2 diabetes and cardiovascular disease. Although the limitations of BMI as an index of body fatness among children should be appreciated, it is possible that this simple index conveys most of the relevant information on obesity-related metabolic risk.

CLASSIFICATION SYSTEMS FOR HIGH LEVELS OF BMI AND BODY FATNESS

Classification of BMI

Although BMIs of 25 kg/m^2 (overweight) and 30 kg/m^2 (obesity) are used as cut-points among adults, the marked changes that occur in BMI levels with age make it necessary to specify a high BMI relative to children of the same sex and age. Furthermore, if BMI levels are expressed relative to levels from a reference population, one could then compare prevalences of overweight and obesity across populations and time periods. Unfortunately, several reference populations and cut-points have been proposed, complicating comparisons across studies.

The two most widely used classification systems for BMI levels among school-aged children are the 2000 CDC growth charts [9, 62] and the IOTF cut-points [8]. Both classifications are based on the cross-sectional distributions of BMI levels by sex and age in nationally representative samples, but the choices for the specific BMI cut-points (and the adult ages) for overweight and obesity, although reasonable, were somewhat arbitrary. The 85th and 95th percentiles (rather than other distributional cut-points) of BMI-for-age (and sex) were used as cut-points in the CDC growth charts [63, 64], whereas the IOTF linked BMIs of 25 and 30 kg/m^2 at age 18 years (rather than at some other adult age) to BMI levels at younger ages.

The CDC growth charts (for persons aged 2 to 19 years) were based on data from national (U.S.) surveys conducted from 1963–1965 to 1988–1994 [9, 62]. (Only data from 2- to 5-year-olds in the 1988–1994 survey were included in the construction of the BMI growth charts.) Although there is not complete agreement on the labels for the BMI categories, many investigators now classify children who have a BMI-for-age ≥ 95th P of this reference population as obese and children with a BMI-for-age between the 85th and 94th percentiles as overweight [65]. These two categories were originally termed "overweight" and "at-risk for overweight" [64].

An additional complication is that among older adolescents, the 85th percentile of BMI-for-age may be greater than 25 kg/m^2 (the adult cut-point for overweight), and the 95th percentile of BMI-for-age may be greater than 30 kg/m^2 (the adult cut-point for obesity). Therefore, it may be preferable to classify adolescents who have a BMI of 30 kg/m^2 or greater as obese even if their BMI-for-age is below the 95th percentile. Similarly, adolescents who have a BMI between 25 and 29.9 kg/m^2 should likely be considered overweight even if their BMI-for-age is below the 85th percentile. The use of both BMI values and BMI-for-age percentiles in the classification of overweight and obesity among older adolescents was recommended by a 2007 expert committee [66].

The IOTF cut-points were calculated using nationally representative data from six countries (Brazil, Great Britain, Hong Kong, the Netherlands, Singapore, and the United States) [8], and within each sample, BMIs of 25 kg/m^2 and 30 kg/m^2 at age 18 years were linked to levels at younger ages. (The U.S. data were identical to the data used to construct the CDC growth charts, except that the 1988–1994 data were excluded.) For example, because 30 kg/m^2 was the 96.7th percentile among boys in the United States at age 18 years, younger boys (2 to 17 years of age) in the United States who had a BMI at or above the 96.7th percentile for their age were considered to be obese. The resulting sex- and age-specific BMI cut-points for overweight and obesity were then averaged over the six countries.

Although the IOTF classification links the child cut-points to adult levels of overweight and obesity, the use of age 18 for the adult cut-points has important implications. Because BMI levels tend to increase with age among adults, if the cut-points had been based on the distribution of BMI levels at age 30 years (rather than age 18), the prevalences of adult overweight and obesity would have been greater, and the derived BMI cut-points among children would have been substantially lower. In addition, age-related changes in the BMI cut-points among children in Singapore appeared to differ substantially from the age differences in other countries.

Despite differences between these two classification systems [12], the IOTF-25 (overweight) and the CDC 85th percentile cut-points are very similar (particularly for girls) between the ages of 6 and 18 years (Figure 4.3). Therefore, the use of either of these classification systems would result in fairly similar prevalences of overweight among school-aged children. However, the IOTF-30 cut-points (upper gray lines) are substantially higher than the CDC 95th percentile, resulting in large differences in the prevalence of obesity. For example, the estimated prevalence of obesity among 6- to 11-year-olds in NHANES 2003−2006 is about 50% higher using the CDC 95th percentile (17%) than the IOTF-30 cut-points (12%). As Figure 4.3 shows, the IOTF-30 cut-points are fairly similar to the CDC 97th percentile among school-aged children.

A third classification system, the WHO childhood growth standards [67], was released in 2006 for children up to age 5 years. The goal was to describe how "children should grow," and these data represent a prescriptive growth reference for healthy infants and young children who grew up in relatively high-income environments and who were fed according to international recommendations. Infants and children in communities from six countries were included based on various selection criteria such as high socioeconomic status and an indication that at least 20% of mothers in the community would be willing to follow the study's feeding criteria. Individual exclusion criteria included maternal smoking during pregnancy and lactation, prematurity (<37 weeks), high gestational age (>42 weeks), multiple births, or an unwillingness to follow feeding criteria [68]. Subsequent to data collection, all measurements of weight-for-length more than three standard deviations (SDs) away from the overall study median (< 2 years of age) and more than 2 SDs (for > 2 years of age) were considered to be outliers and were excluded from the final sample [67].

For children 5 years of age and older, the WHO growth references are a reconstruction of the 1977 National Center for Health Statistics (NCHS)/WHO reference [11]. The reference population is based on thee U.S. surveys conducted from the mid-1960s to the mid-1970s, along with supplemental data from the WHO child growth standards for children younger than 5 years of age. The statistical methodology was similar to that used in the construction of the WHO standards for infants and young children [67].

A comparison of the sex- and age-specific cut-points for high BMI levels in the CDC, IOTF, and WHO data for children between 2 and 5 years of age is shown in Table 4.2. The WHO sample was thinner than either the IOTF or CDC samples, and the 1 SD (above the median) cut-points were lower than either the CDC 85th percentile or the IOTF-25 cut-points. (In a normal distribution, 1 SD is close to the 84th percentile.) The WHO 2 SD cut-points are slightly below the CDC 95th percentile at 24 months of age, but they approach the CDC 97th percentiles at older ages. A recent analysis [69] of children from NHANES 2003−2006 found that the use of the CDC 95th percentile or WHO 2 SD cut-points yielded fairly similar (overall) prevalences of obesity (9.6% and 8.5%, respectively) among 24- to 59-month-old children. The IOTF-30 cut-points are consistently higher than the other cut-points in this age range, and among 36- to 60-month-old boys, the IOTF cut-points are about 1 kg/m² higher than either the CDC 97th percentile or WHO 2 SD cut-points.

Although none of these BMI classifications systems was based on associations with disease outcomes, several analyses have shown that a high BMI relative to the CDC reference population is associated with increased body fatness, adverse levels of metabolic risk factors, and adult obesity [21, 70, 71]. Because the underlying associations are continuous, it is likely that similar associations would be observed with the IOTF or WHO classifications.

Classification of Excess Body Fatness

There is no agreement on the definition of excess body fatness among children. This classification would ideally be based on the risk of future disease, but it would be difficult to examine these longitudinal associations over periods of 50 or more years. In addition to

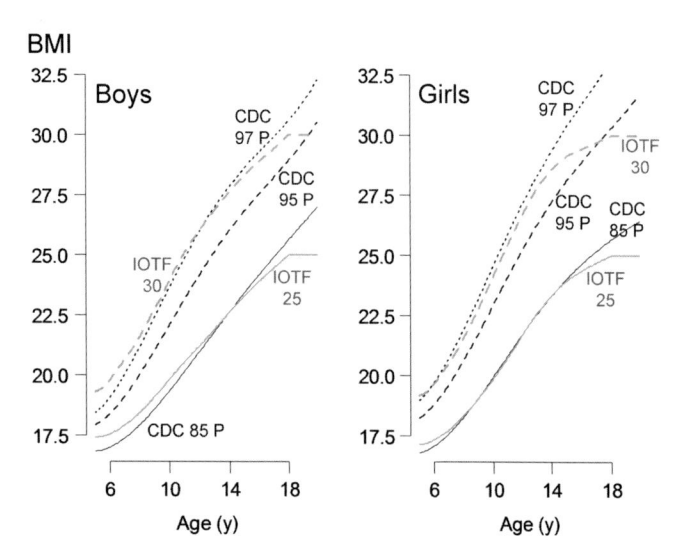

FIGURE 4.3 Comparison of the CDC and IOTF BMI cut-points for overweight (CDC 85th percentile and IOTF-25) and obesity (CDC 95th percentile and IOTF-30) among 5- to 19-year-olds. The CDC 97th percentile is also shown for comparison. The black lines represent the CDC cut-points; gray lines represent the IOTF cut-points. The IOTF cut-points end at age 18 years, and horizontal lines have been extended at BMIs of 25 (adult overweight) and 30 kg/m² (adult obesity). Among older adolescents, the CDC 85th percentile is greater than 25 kg/m² and the CDC 95th percentile is greater than 30 kg/m².

TABLE 4.2 Comparison of CDC, WHO, and IOTF BMI Cut-Points[a] among 2- to 5-Year-Olds

	Age (months)[c]	Overweight[b]			Obesity[b]			
		WHO 1 SD	CDC 85th P	IOTF 25	CDC 95th P	WHO 2 SD	CDC 97th P	IOTF 30
Boys	24	17.3	18.1	18.4	19.3	18.9	19.8	20.1
	30	17.1	17.7	18.1	18.7	18.6	19.1	19.8
	36	16.9	17.3	17.9	18.2	18.4	18.6	19.6
	42	16.8	17.1	17.7	18.0	18.2	18.3	19.4
	48	16.7	16.9	17.6	17.8	18.2	18.2	19.3
	54	16.6	16.8	17.5	17.8	18.2	18.3	19.3
	60	16.6	16.8	17.4	17.9	18.3	18.4	19.3
Girls	24	17.1	18.0	18.0	19.1	18.7	19.6	19.8
	30	16.9	17.5	17.8	18.6	18.5	19.0	19.6
	36	16.8	17.2	17.6	18.3	18.4	18.8	19.4
	42	16.8	16.9	17.4	18.1	18.4	18.6	19.2
	48	16.8	16.8	17.3	18.0	18.5	18.6	19.2
	54	16.8	16.8	17.2	18.1	18.7	18.8	19.1
	60	16.9	16.8	17.2	18.3	18.8	19.0	19.2

[a]*WHO cut-points are from the z-score tables at www.who.int/childgrowth/standards/bmi_for_age/en/index.html. CDC cut-points are from the BMI-for-age charts at www.cdc.gov/nchs/about/major/nhanes/growthcharts/datafiles.htm. IOTF cut-points are from Cole et al. [8].*
[b]*Within the 2 BMI categories (overweight and obesity), columns are generally arranged in ascending order of the suggested cut-points. For example, at most ages the CDC 85th percentile (2nd column) cut-points are higher than the WHO 1 SD cut-points, but lower than the IOTF 25 cut-points.*
[c]*The IOTF and WHO cut-points are given for exact ages, whereas the CDC cut-points are given for children whose age is the last completed month. For example, age 24 months corresponds to 730 (24 × 365.24) days in the WHO and IOTF cut-points, but it represents children who were between 24 months (730 days) and 24.9 months (760 days) of age in the CDC cut-points.*

the length of follow-up, these associations would be expected to be influenced by adult levels of body fatness, requiring multiple periodic examinations to be able to disentangle the effects of body fatness in childhood and adulthood. It should also be realized that even among adults, there is little agreement on the specific cut-points for excess body fatness [72].

Because of the lack of longitudinal data, some investigators have based cut-points for excess body fatness among children on cross-sectional associations with metabolic risk factors such as lipids, insulin, and blood pressure [73–75]. Of these classifications, the most widely used is based on the relation of percentage body fat estimated from skinfold thicknesses to adverse (upper quintile for a child's race, sex, and age) risk factor levels in the Bogalusa Heart Study [73, 76]. These investigators proposed cut-points for excess body fatness among 5- to 18-year-old children of 25% (boys) and 30% (girls); these cut-points did not vary by age.

Although it is appealing to use a single cut-point for classifying excess body fatness across all ages, this approach is unlikely to be optimal. A cut-point that does not vary by age cannot account for the normal changes in body fatness that occur during growth and

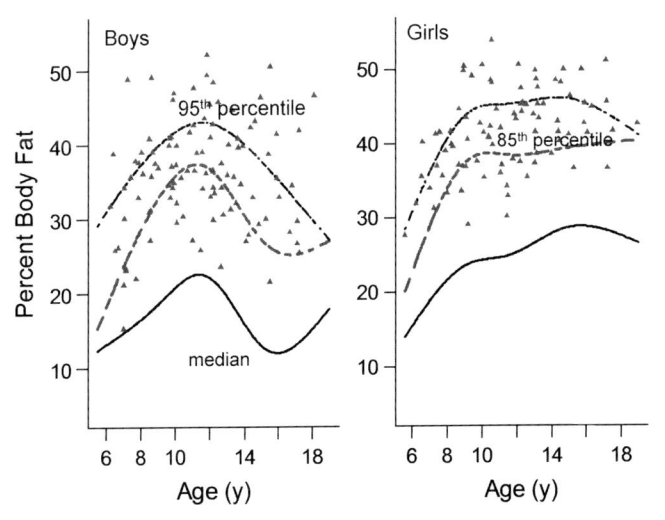

FIGURE 4.4 The 50th, 85th, and 95th percentiles of body fatness by age among boys *(left panel)* and girls *(right panel)* among children in the Pediatric Rosetta Study. Percentiles were estimated using quantile regression [86], and the gray triangles represent levels of percentage body fat among children who have a BMI at or above the 95th percentile of the CDC reference population. About 16% of the children had a BMI above the CDC 95th percentile, and another 17% had a BMI between the 85th and 94th percentiles.

development (Figure 4.4). For example, among girls in the Pediatric Rosetta Study, 30% body fat is about the 95th percentile among 7-year-olds, but is close to the 50th percentile among 14- to 18-year-olds (right panel). It seems unlikely that the health effects of 30% body fat would be similar in these two age groups. Furthermore, the underlying associations between body fatness and risk factor levels are continuous, making the selection of any cut-point somewhat arbitrary. Additional errors can arise when attempting to predict percentage body fat from published equations that incorporate skinfold thicknesses and estimates of body density. (These published equations, which were derived to provide the best fit in the original data, are likely to result in larger errors when applied to a different sample, particularly one that is studied decades later.) It has been suggested that it is preferable to leave skinfold thicknesses in raw form or to convert them to sex- and age-specific z-scores rather than using published equations to convert them to percentage body fat [77].

Despite the added complexity, it is probable that excess body fatness should be defined relative to a child's sex and age peers, in much the same way that BMI cut-points among children have been constructed. Various techniques have been used to derive sex- and age-specific percentiles (e.g., 85th and 95th) of body fatness [16, 78–80], as well as age-specific levels of percentage body fat that correspond to the body fatness of an 18-year-old with a BMI of 30 kg/m^2 [79, 81]. It is also possible to select cut-points for percentage body fat so that the prevalence (within sex and age categories) of children with excess body fatness is approximately equal to the prevalence of high levels of BMI [21].

ABILITY OF A HIGH BMI TO IDENTIFY CHILDREN WHO HAVE EXCESS BODY FATNESS

Several investigators have assessed the ability of a high BMI to identify children who have excess body fatness [16, 18, 19, 82], but the results are difficult to compare. There are differences in the methods (skinfolds, DXA, etc.) used to estimate body fatness, in the cut-points used to classify high levels of BMI and percentage body fat, and in the statistics used to summarize the screening performance of BMI. The accuracy of BMI as a screening tool has frequently been summarized by the (1) sensitivity (proportion of children with excess body fatness who have a high BMI), (2) positive predictive value (proportion with a high BMI who have excess body fatness), and (3) specificity (proportion without excess body fatness who do not have a high BMI). These measures, however, can be greatly influenced by the cut-points used for both BMI and body fatness.

Identification of Excess Body Fatness by BMI

It is frequently asserted that a high BMI is a specific, but not a sensitive, indicator of excess body fatness [13, 14, 16–19, 47, 83]. A low sensitivity, however, may simply indicate that the proportion of children who have a high BMI is lower than is the proportion of children considered to have excess body fatness; this can largely be due to the cut-points chosen for BMI and percentage body fat. For example, even if levels of BMI-for-age and percentage body fat were perfectly correlated when treated as continuous variables, if the prevalence of excess body fatness was two times higher than the prevalence of a high BMI, the sensitivity could never exceed 50%. Similarly, if the prevalence of a high BMI was three times that of excess body fatness, the maximum positive predictive value would be 33%. These differences in prevalences (high BMI versus excess body fatness) may account for many of the reports that have concluded that a high BMI is not a sensitive indicator of excess body fatness. Rather than indicating that many children with excess body fatness have normal levels of BMI, the observed low sensitivity may simply reflect the use of cut-points that result in a greater proportion of children having excess body fatness. Recent analyses of the NHANES 1999–2004 DXA data for 8- to 19-year-olds (n = 8821, including 1352 subjects who had imputed data) [84] emphasize that markedly different estimates of positive predictive value can be obtained using different cut-points for excess body fatness.

Analyses from the Pediatric Rosetta Project have indicated that a high BMI-for-age is a good indicator of excess body fatness [21, 23, 80], and the ability of BMI categories (based on the 85th and 95th CDC percentiles) to correctly identify children with excess body fatness is shown in Table 4.3. Of the 187 children that had a BMI ≥ CDC 95th percentile, 143 (76%, positive

TABLE 4.3 Classification of Children by Categories of both BMI-for-Age and Body Fatness

CDC BMI-for-age	Body Fatness Category[a]			
	Normal	Moderate	Elevated	Total
<85th percentile	740 (91)[b]	63 (8)	6 (1)	809
85th to 94th percentiles	65 (33)	97 (49)	38 (19)	200
≥ 95th percentile	3 (2)	41 (22)	143 (76)	187
Total	808	201	187	1196

[a]Body fatness categories were defined so that the number of children in each of the three categories would be equal to the number of children in the corresponding BMI-for-age category.
[b]Values in parentheses represent the percentage of children in the specified BMI category who were also in the specified category of body fatness.
Based on data from Freedman et al. [21].

predictive value) had excess body fatness. (Cut-points for percentage body fatness were selected so that the number of children in each of the three body fatness categories—within sex and age groups—would equal the number in each BMI category; these cut-points were based on levels of body fatness among children and adolescents who participated in the Pediatric Rosetta Study.) The estimated sensitivity was 76% (of the 187 children with elevated body fatness, 143 had a BMI $\geq$ 95th percentile), and the specificity was 96% (965 of the 1009 children without excess body fatness had a BMI below the 95th percentile). The kappa statistic (with disagreements weighted according to their squared distance from the diagonal) for the cross-classification of BMI and body fatness categories was 0.82, indicating good agreement between the two measures.

Although the Pediatric Rosetta Study was based on a convenience sample, these results are in agreement with those from 8- to 19-year-olds who had whole-body DXA scans in NHANES 1999−2004 [84]. In these analyses, it was found that about 79% of obese (BMI $\geq$ CDC 95th percentile) boys and 82% of obese girls had a percentage body fat that was equal to or greater than the 80th percentile. Furthermore, the estimates of the proportions of overweight (85th to 94th percentiles of BMI-for-age) children who had excess body fatness were also fairly similar: 19% in the Pediatric Rosetta Study [21] versus 26% to 29% in NHANES (based on the smoothed 80th percentile of percentage body fat) [84].

Because there are no widely agreed-upon cut-points for high levels of either BMI or percentage body fat, the screening accuracy of BMI can be better summarized by receiver operator characteristic (ROC) curves [85]. These curves are constructed by calculating the sensitivity and specificity at each possible cut-point of BMI-for-age among children in the Pediatric Rosetta Study, and they emphasize the inherent tradeoffs between sensitivity and specificity (Figure 4.5). (ROC analysis requires the percentage body fat be classified into two categories.) The area under the curve (AUC) can be interpreted as the probability that the BMI-for-age of a randomly selected child with excess body fatness is higher than the BMI-for-age of a child without excess body fatness; the maximum AUC is 1.0. Based on this statistic, BMI-for-age was a good indicator (AUC ~ 0.95) of excess body fatness in the Pediatric Rosetta Study.

As shown by the middle horizontal line in the two panels, the CDC 95th percentile of BMI-for-age had moderate sensitivity (75% to 79%) and very high specificity (95% to 96%) in detecting excess body fatness. The use of a higher BMI-for-age cut-point, such as the 97th percentile, results in a lower sensitivity, identifying only about 60% of the children who had had excess body

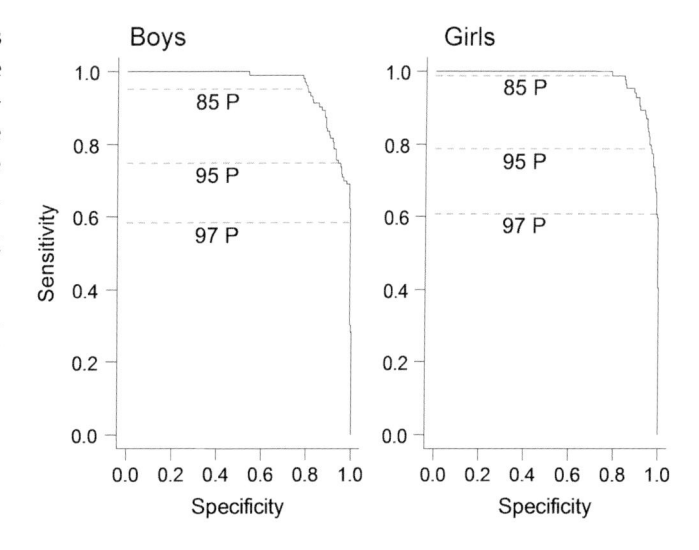

FIGURE 4.5 Estimated sensitivity and specificity of BMI-for-age in the prediction of excess body fatness among boys and girls in the Pediatric Rosetta Study. Each point along the curves represents the screening performance of a different BMI-for-age cut-point in the prediction of excess body fatness. The gray dashed lines give the sensitivity of three different BMI-for-age cut-points: the CDC 85th, 95th, and 97th percentiles. Note that specificity is plotted on the x-axis of the figure, whereas ROC curves typically have 1 minus specificity on this axis.

fatness. This reduction in sensitivity, based on the use of the CDC 97th percentile, did not result from the limitations of BMI but from using cut-points that result in a larger proportion of children having excess body fatness (15% to 16%) than having a high BMI (10%). An even higher BMI cut-point would further lower the sensitivity because even fewer children would be considered to have a high BMI. In contrast, lowering the BMI-for-age cut-point to the CDC 85th percentile (top gray line) increased the sensitivity to about 97%. Of the 187 children with excess body fatness, 181 had a BMI-for-age at or above the CDC 85th percentile; there were five misclassified boys and only one misclassified girl.

CONCLUSION

Based on levels of BMI, there have been marked increases in child obesity over the past few decades in most countries that have recent, representative data. BMI, however, is a measure of weight relative to height, and several investigators have concluded that a large proportion of children with excess body fatness do not have a high BMI (low sensitivity). However, after accounting for race and age differences, BMI levels among children are a fairly good predictor of body fatness in linear regression models, with BMI accounting for about 77% (boys) to 79% (girls) of the variability in percentage body fat.

The lack of agreement on the definition of excess body fatness complicates the assessment of BMI categories in correctly identifying children with excess body fatness. However, if body fatness cut-points are selected so that the prevalences of children with a high BMI and excess body fatness are approximately equal, a high BMI-for-age has moderately high (75% to 80%) sensitivity and high specificity (95%) in identifying children with excess body fatness. It should be realized, however, that the use of other cut-points for either body fatness or BMI can result in markedly different estimates of positive predictive value, sensitivity, and specificity.

Although BMI (even after adjustment for sex and age) can give an inaccurate indication of the body fatness of an individual child, it performs well as a screening tool for excess body fatness. It is therefore unlikely that the secular trends that have been reported in child obesity, along with prevalence differences across countries, would be substantially altered if more accurate estimates of body fatness were used. However, these trends and comparisons are hindered by the use of various classification systems and cut-points for overweight and obesity among children. It would be helpful if, in addition to the BMI cut-points that are used in the analyses, authors could report the prevalences of overweight and obesity based on one common set of cut-points.

References

1. Ogden CL, Fryar CD, Carroll MD, Flegal KM. Mean body weight, height, and body mass index, United States 1960–2002. *Adv Data*; 2004:1–17.
2. Ogden CL, Carroll MD, Curtin LR, McDowell MA, Tabak CJ, Flegal KM. Prevalence of overweight and obesity in the United States, 1999–2004. *JAMA* 2006;**295**:1549–55.
3. Jackson-Leach R, Lobstein T. Estimated burden of paediatric obesity and co-morbidities in Europe. Part 1. The increase in the prevalence of child obesity in Europe is itself increasing. *Int J Pediatr Obes* 2006;**1**:26–32.
4. Wang Y, Lobstein T. Worldwide trends in childhood overweight and obesity. *International Journal of Pediatric Obesity* 2006;**1**:11–25.
5. Janssen I, Katzmarzyk PT, Boyce WF, Vereecken C, Mulvihill C, Roberts C, Currie C, Pickett W. Comparison of overweight and obesity prevalence in school-aged youth from 34 countries and their relationships with physical activity and dietary patterns. *Obes Rev.* 2005;**6**:123–32.
6. Freedman DS, Khan LK, Serdula MK, Ogden CL, Dietz WH. Racial and ethnic differences in secular trends for childhood BMI, weight, and height. *Obesity (Silver Spring)* 2006;**14**:301–8.
7. Ogden CL, Carroll MD, Flegal KM. High body mass index for age among US children and adolescents, 2003–2006. *JAMA* 2008;**299**:2401–5.
8. Cole TJ, Bellizzi MC, Flegal KM, Dietz WH. Establishing a standard definition for child overweight and obesity worldwide: international survey. *BMJ* 2000;**320**:1240–3.
9. Kuczmarski RJ, Ogden CL, Grummer-Strawn LM, Flegal KM, Guo SS, Wei R, Mei Z, Curtin LR, Roche AF, Johnson CL. CDC growth charts: United States. *Adv Data*; 2000:1–27.
10. WHO Multicentre Growth Reference Study Group. *WHO Child Growth Standards: Length/height-for-age, weight-for-age, weight-for-length, weight-for-height and body mass index-for-age: Methods and development*. Geneva: World Health Organization. Available at, www.who.int/childgrowth/standards/technical_report/en/index.html; 2006.
11. de Onis M, Onyango AW, Borghi E, Siyam A, Nishida C, Siekmann J. Development of a WHO growth reference for school-aged children and adolescents. *Bull World Health Organ* 2007;**85**:660–7.
12. Flegal KM, Ogden CL, Wei R, Kuczmarski RL, Johnson CL. Prevalence of overweight in US children: comparison of US growth charts from the Centers for Disease Control and Prevention with other reference values for body mass index. *Am. J. Clin. Nutr.* 2001;**73**:1086–93.
13. Wellens RI, Roche AF, Khamis HJ, Jackson AS, Pollock ML, Siervogel RM. Relationships between the Body Mass Index and body composition. *Obes Res.* 1996;**4**:35–44.
14. Reilly JJ, Dorosty AR, Emmett PM. Identification of the obese child: adequacy of the body mass index for clinical practice and epidemiology. *Int J Obes Relat Metab Disord* 2000;**24**:1623–7.
15. Fu WP, Lee HC, Ng CJ, Tay YK, Kau CY, Seow CJ, Siak JK, Hong CY. Screening for childhood obesity: international vs population-specific definitions. Which is more appropriate? *Int J Obes Relat Metab Disord* 2003;**27**:1121–6.
16. Zimmermann MB, Gubeli C, Puntener C, Molinari L. Detection of overweight and obesity in a national sample of 6–12-y-old Swiss children: accuracy and validity of reference values for body mass index from the US Centers for Disease Control and Prevention and the International Obesity Task Force. *Am. J. Clin. Nutr.* 2004;**79**:838–43.
17. Neovius MG, Linne YM, Barkeling BS, Rossner SO. Sensitivity and specificity of classification systems for fatness in adolescents. *Am. J. Clin. Nutr.* 2004;**80**:597–603.
18. Wickramasinghe VP, Cleghorn GJ, Edmiston KA, Murphy AJ, Abbott RA, Davies PS. Validity of BMI as a measure of obesity in Australian white Caucasian and Australian Sri Lankan children. *Ann Hum Biol.* 2005;**32**:60–71.
19. Neovius M, Rasmussen F. Evaluation of BMI-based classification of adolescent overweight and obesity: choice of percentage body fat cutoffs exerts a large influence. The COMPASS study. *Eur J Clin Nutr* 2008;**62**:1201–7.
20. Wells JC, Coward WA, Cole TJ, Davies PS. The contribution of fat and fat-free tissue to body mass index in contemporary children and the reference child. *Int J Obes Relat Metab Disord* 2002;**26**:1323–8.
21. Freedman DS, Wang J, Thornton JC, Mei Z, Sopher AB, Pierson Jr RN, Dietz WH, Horlick M. Classification of body fatness by body mass index-for-age categories among children. *Arch Pediatr Adolesc Med* 2009;**163**:805–11.
22. Freedman DS, Wang J, Ogden CL, Thornton JC, Mei Z, Pierson RN, Dietz WH, Horlick M. The prediction of body fatness by BMI and skinfold thicknesses among children and adolescents. *Ann Hum Biol.* 2007;**34**:183–94.
23. Freedman DS, Ogden CL, Berenson GS, Horlick M. Body mass index and body fatness in childhood. *Curr Opin Clin Nutr Metab Care* 2005;**8**:618–23.
24. Prentice AM, Jebb SA. Beyond body mass index. *Obes Rev.* 2001;**2**:141–7.
25. Franklin MF. Comparison of weight and height relations in boys from 4 countries. *Am. J. Clin. Nutr.* 1999;**70**:157S–62S.

26. Freedman DS, Thornton JC, Mei Z, Wang J, Dietz WH, Pierson Jr RN, Horlick M. Height and adiposity among children. *Obes Res.* 2004;**12**:846–53.
27. Cole TJ. The LMS method for constructing normalized growth standards. *Eur J Clin Nutr* 1990;**44**:45–60.
28. Wells JC. A Hattori chart analysis of body mass index in infants and children. *Int J Obes Relat Metab Disord* 2000;**24**:325–9.
29. Freedman DS, Wang J, Maynard LM, Thornton JC, Mei Z, Pierson RN, Dietz WH, Horlick M. Relation of BMI to fat and fat-free mass among children and adolescents. *Int J Obes (Lond)* 2005;**29**:1–8.
30. Sherry B, Jefferds ME, Grummer-Strawn LM. Accuracy of adolescent self-report of height and weight in assessing overweight status: a literature review. *Arch Pediatr Adolesc Med* 2007;**161**:1154–61.
31. Akinbami LJ, Ogden CL. Childhood overweight prevalence in the United States: The impact of parent-reported height and weight. *Obesity* 2009;**17**:1574–80.
32. Cole TJ, Rolland-Cachera MF. Measurement and definition. In: Burniat W, Cole T, Lissau I, Poskitt EME, editors. *Child and adolescent obesity: causes, consequences, prevention and management.* Cambridge UK: Cambridge University Press; 2002. pp. 1–27.
33. Fields DA, Goran MI. Body composition techniques and the four-compartment model in children. *J. Appl. Physiol.* 2000;**89**:613–20.
34. Lee SY, Gallagher D. Assessment methods in human body composition. *Curr Opin Clin Nutr Metab Care* 2008;**11**:566–72.
35. National Center for Health Statistics. (2008) National Health and Nutrition Examination Survey: Technical Documentation for the 1999–2004 Dual Energy X-Ray Absorptiometry (DXA) Multiple Imputation Data files. Available at www.cdc.gov/nchs/data/nhanes/dxa/dxa_techdoc.pdf
36. Brion MA, Ness AR, Davey Smith G, Leary SD. Association between body composition and blood pressure in a contemporary cohort of 9-year-old children. *J Hum Hypertens* 2007;**21**:283–90.
37. Bray GA, DeLany JP, Volaufova J, Harsha DW, Champagne C. Prediction of body fat in 12-y-old African American and white children: evaluation of methods. *Am. J. Clin. Nutr.* 2002;**76**:980–90.
38. Wong WW, Hergenroeder AC, Stuff JE, Butte NF, Smith EO, Ellis KJ. Evaluating body fat in girls and female adolescents: advantages and disadvantages of dual-energy X-ray absorptiometry. *Am. J. Clin. Nutr.* 2002;**76**:384–9.
39. Sopher AB, Thornton JC, Wang J, Pierson Jr RN, Heymsfield SB, Horlick M. Measurement of percentage of body fat in 411 children and adolescents: a comparison of dual-energy X-ray absorptiometry with a four-compartment model. *Pediatrics* 2004;**113**:1285–90.
40. Williams JE, Wells JC, Wilson CM, Haroun D, Lucas A, Fewtrell MS. Evaluation of Lunar Prodigy dual-energy X-ray absorptiometry for assessing body composition in healthy persons and patients by comparison with the criterion 4-component model. *Am. J. Clin. Nutr.* 2006;**83**:1047–54.
41. Plank LD. Dual-energy X-ray absorptiometry and body composition. *Curr Opin Clin Nutr Metab Care* 2005;**8**:305–9.
42. Daniels SR, Khoury PR, Morrison JA. The utility of body mass index as a measure of body fatness in children and adolescents: differences by race and gender. *Pediatrics* 1997;**99**:804–7.
43. Bray GA, DeLany JP, Harsha DW, Volaufova J, Champagne CC. Evaluation of body fat in fatter and leaner 10-y-old African American and white children: the Baton Rouge Children's Study. *Am. J. Clin. Nutr.* 2001;**73**:687–702.
44. Sarria A, Garcia-Llop LA, Moreno LA, Fleta J, Morellon MP, Bueno M. Skinfold thickness measurements are better predictors of body fat percentage than body mass index in male Spanish children and adolescents. *Eur J Clin Nutr* 1998;**52**:573–6.
45. Sardinha LB, Going SB, Teixeira PJ, Lohman TG. Receiver operating characteristic analysis of body mass index, triceps skinfold thickness, and arm girth for obesity screening in children and adolescents. *Am. J. Clin. Nutr.* 1999;**70**:1090–5.
46. Steinberger J, Jacobs DR, Raatz S, Moran A, Hong CP, Sinaiko AR. Comparison of body fatness measurements by BMI and skinfolds vs dual energy X-ray absorptiometry and their relation to cardiovascular risk factors in adolescents. *Int J Obes (Lond)* 2005;**29**:1346–52.
47. Gaskin PS, Walker SP. Obesity in a cohort of black Jamaican children as estimated by BMI and other indices of adiposity. *Eur J Clin Nutr* 2003;**57**:420–6.
48. Ulijaszek SJ, Kerr DA. Anthropometric measurement error and the assessment of nutritional status. *Br. J. Nutr.* 1999;**82**:165–77.
49. WHO Multicentre Growth Reference Study Group. Reliability of anthropometric measurements in the WHO Multicentre Growth Reference Study. *Acta Paediatr Suppl.* 2006;**450**:38–46.
50. Pateyjohns IR, Brinkworth GD, Buckley JD, Noakes M, Clifton PM. Comparison of three bioelectrical impedance methods with DXA in overweight and obese men. *Obesity (Silver Spring)* 2006;**14**:2064–70.
51. Shafer KJ, Siders WA, Johnson LK, Lukaski HC. Validity of segmental multiple-frequency bioelectrical impedance analysis to estimate body composition of adults across a range of body mass indexes. *Nutrition* 2009;**25**:25–32.
52. Geiss HC, Parhofer KG, Schwandt P. Parameters of childhood obesity and their relationship to cardiovascular risk factors in healthy prepubescent children. *Int J Obes Relat Metab Disord* 2001;**25**:830–7.
53. Wannamethee SG, Shaper AG, Morris RW, Whincup PH. Measures of adiposity in the identification of metabolic abnormalities in elderly men. *Am. J. Clin. Nutr.* 2005;**81**:1313–21.
54. Willett K, Jiang R, Lenart E, Spiegelman D, Willett W. Comparison of bioelectrical impedance and BMI in predicting obesity-related medical conditions. *Obesity (Silver Spring)* 2006;**14**:480–90.
55. Hemmingsson E, Udden J, Neovius M. No apparent progress in bioelectrical impedance accuracy: Validation against metabolic risk and DXA. *Obesity (Silver Spring)* 2009;**17**:183–87.
56. Lindsay RS, Hanson RL, Roumain J, Ravussin E, Knowler WC, Tataranni PA. Body mass index as a measure of adiposity in children and adolescents: relationship to adiposity by dual energy x-ray absorptiometry and to cardiovascular risk factors. *J. Clin. Endocrinol. Metab.* 2001;**86**:4061–7.
57. Freedman DS, Katzmarzyk PT, Dietz WH, Srinivasan SR, Berenson GS. Relation of body mass index and skinfold thicknesses to cardiovascular disease risk factors in children: the Bogalusa Heart Study. *Am. J. Clin. Nutr.* 2009;**90**:210–16.
58. Warne DK, Charles MA, Hanson RL, Jacobsson LT, McCance DR, Knowler WC, Pettitt DJ. Comparison of body size measurements as predictors of NIDDM in Pima Indians. *Diabetes Care* 1995;**18**:435–9.
59. Spataro JA, Dyer AR, Stamler J, Shekelle RB, Greenlund K, Garside D. Measures of adiposity and coronary heart disease mortality in the Chicago Western Electric Company Study. *J Clin Epidemiol* 1996;**49**:849–57.
60. Yarnell JW, Patterson CC, Thomas HF, Sweetnam PM. Central obesity: predictive value of skinfold measurements for subsequent ischaemic heart disease at 14 years follow-up in the Caerphilly Study. *Int J Obes Relat Metab Disord* 2001;**25**:1546–9.
61. Kim J, Meade T, Haines A. Skinfold thickness, body mass index, and fatal coronary heart disease: 30 year follow up of the

Northwick Park heart study. *J Epidemiol Community Health* 2006;**60**:275–9.

62. Ogden CL, Kuczmarski RJ, Flegal KM, Mei Z, Guo S, Wei R, Grummer-Strawn LM, Curtin LR, Roche AF, Johnson CL. Centers for Disease Control and Prevention 2000 growth charts for the United States: improvements to the 1977 National Center for Health Statistics version. *Pediatrics* 2002;**109**:45–60.
63. Himes JH, Dietz WH. Guidelines for overweight in adolescent preventive services: recommendations from an expert committee. The Expert Committee on Clinical Guidelines for Overweight in Adolescent Preventive Services. *Am. J. Clin. Nutr.* 1994;**59**: 307–16.
64. Kuczmarski RJ, Flegal KM. Criteria for definition of overweight in transition: background and recommendations for the United States. *Am. J. Clin. Nutr.* 2000;**72**:1074–81.
65. Krebs NF, Himes JH, Jacobson D, Nicklas TA, Guilday P, Styne D. Assessment of child and adolescent overweight and obesity. *Pediatrics* 2007;**120**(Suppl. 4):S193–228.
66. Barlow SE. Expert committee recommendations regarding the prevention, assessment, and treatment of child and adolescent overweight and obesity: summary report. *Pediatrics* 2007;**120** (Suppl. 4):S164–92.
67. World Health Organization. (2006) WHO child growth standards: length/height-for-age, weight-for-age, weight-for-length, weight-for-height and body mass index-for-age. Methods and development. World Health Organization, Department of Nutrition for Health and Development. Available at www. who.int/childgrowth/standards/technical_report/en/index.html, Geneva
68. de Onis M, Garza C, Victora CG, Onyango AW, Frongillo EA, Martines J. The WHO Multicentre Growth Reference Study: planning, study design, and methodology. *Food Nutr Bull.* 2004;**25**:S15–26.
69. Mei Z, Ogden CL, Flegal KM, Grummer-Strawn LM. Comparison of the prevalence of shortness, underweight, and overweight among US children aged 0 to 59 months by using the CDC 2000 and the WHO 2006 growth charts. *J Pediatr* 2008;**153**:622–8.
70. Freedman DS, Mei Z, Srinivasan SR, Berenson GS, Dietz WH. Cardiovascular risk factors and excess adiposity among overweight children and adolescents: the Bogalusa Heart Study. *J Pediatr* 2007;**150**:12–7. e12.
71. Lambert M, Delvin EE, Levy E, O'Loughlin J, Paradis G, Barnett T, McGrath JJ. Prevalence of cardiometabolic risk factors by weight status in a population-based sample of Quebec children and adolescents. *Can J Cardiol* 2008;**24**:575–83.
72. WHO Expert Committee. (1995) Physical status: the use and interpretation of anthropometry. WHO technical report series (#854), Geneva, Switzerland, page 420
73. Williams DP, Going SB, Lohman TG, Harsha DW, Srinivasan SR, Webber LS, Berenson GS. Body fatness and risk for elevated blood pressure, total cholesterol, and serum lipoprotein ratios in children and adolescents. *Am J Public Health* 1992;**82**:358–63.
74. Dwyer T, Blizzard CL. Defining obesity in children by biological endpoint rather than population distribution. *Int J Obes Relat Metab Disord* 1996;**20**:472–80.
75. Higgins PB, Gower BA, Hunter GR, Goran MI. Defining health-related obesity in prepubertal children. *Obes Res.* 2001;**9**:233–40.
76. Lohman TG, Going SB. Assessment of body composition and energy balance. In: Lamb D, Murray R, editors. *Exercise, nutrition, and the control of body weight*. Carmel, Indiana: Cooper Publishing Group; 1998. pp. 61–99.
77. Wells JC, Fewtrell MS. Measuring body composition. *Arch Dis Child* 2006;**91**:612–17.
78. Lazarus R, Baur L, Webb K, Blyth F. Body mass index in screening for adiposity in children and adolescents: systematic evaluation using receiver operating characteristic curves. *Am. J. Clin. Nutr.* 1996;**63**:500–6.
79. McCarthy HD, Cole TJ, Fry T, Jebb SA, Prentice AM. Body fat reference curves for children. *Int J Obes (Lond)* 2006;**30**:598–602.
80. Mei Z, Grummer-Strawn LM, Wang J, Thornton JC, Freedman DS, Pierson Jr RN, Dietz WH, Horlick M. Do skinfold measurements provide additional information to body mass index in the assessment of body fatness among children and adolescents? *Pediatrics* 2007;**119**:e1306–13.
81. Taylor RW, Jones IE, Williams SM, Goulding A. Body fat percentages measured by dual-energy X-ray absorptiometry corresponding to recently recommended body mass index cutoffs for overweight and obesity in children and adolescents aged 3–18 y. *Am. J. Clin. Nutr.* 2002;**76**:1416–21.
82. Mei Z, Grummer-Strawn LM, Pietrobelli A, Goulding A, Goran MI, Dietz WH. Validity of body mass index compared with other body-composition screening indexes for the assessment of body fatness in children and adolescents. *Am. J. Clin. Nutr.* 2002;**75**:978–85.
83. Baumgartner RN, Heymsfield SB, Roche AF. Human body composition and the epidemiology of chronic disease. *Obes Res.* 1995;**3**:73–95.
84. Flegal, K.M., Ogden, C.L., Yanovski, J.A., Freedman, D.S., Shepherd, J.A., Graubard, B.I. and Borrud, L.G. High adiposity and high BMI-for-age in US children and adolescents by race-ethnic group. *Am. J. Clin. Nutr.* 2010;**91**:1020–26.
85. Fletcher RW, Fletcher SW. *Clinical Epidemiology: The Essentials*. Baltimore, Maryland: Lippincott Williams & Williams; 2005.
86. Koenker, R. (2009) Quantreg: Quantile Regression. R package version 4.38. Available at http://cran.r-project.org/web/packages/quantreg/index.html

CHAPTER 5

Good-Enough Parenting, Self-Regulation, and the Management of Weight-Related Problems

Moria Golan

Shahaf, Community Services for the Management of Weight-Related Problems, Tel Hai Academic College, Upper Galilee and School of Nutritional Sciences, the Hebrew University of Jerusalem, ISRAEL

INTRODUCTION

The world faces a substantial physical and emotional health burden caused by weight-related problems [1, 2]. Weight-related problems including obesity, disordered eating, and the broad spectrum of eating disorders increase the risk of poor health, low body image, low self-esteem, and low quality of life. All have extensive implications on family distress, individual well-being, and society economy.

With substantial international burdens of disease attributable to the obesogenic environment and the increase in childhood obesity, disordered eating behaviors, and eating disorders, the role of parents has perhaps never been more important [3]. Parents and healthcare providers' practices are challenged by the need to find a way to provide offspring and clients with *"good enough" parenting* so they will internalize self-regulation, prosocial coping skills, and the ability to take care of their well-being. Often parents find that in spite of their best intentions, the result is worsening the problem. This might be due to confusing messages and conflicting values that guide us all.

The evolution in society values and norms is a result of the socioeconomic and cultural changes following the Second World War. The postmodern society leans toward pluralism, democracy, religious freedom, consumerism, mobility, and increasing access to news and entertainment. It is also characterized by uncertainty, insecurity, and doubt, resulting in a society that has lost its faith in absolute truth and individuals have to choose what to believe. This is the context in which we all raise our children and advise our clients.

There is also a clear evolution in the organization of the family. There is a transformation from a typology of the merely patriarchal family to the nuclear family and a change from an adult-centered to a child-centered view, which is typical of our society [4].

Philosophers and psychologists supported this shifting toward a child-centered approach to have a better understanding of the child; improve the adult's educational and emotional behavior toward the child; and support child autonomy, curiosity, capabilities, achievements, fulfillment, and mainly well-being. However, good intentions are not enough.

In the past, parenthood was a result of following the familial pathway and functioning as a parent, according to what was seen in the close environment (parent's house, neighbors). Today, the phenomenon of educated parenthood is common in Western societies. In the modern era, parenting was intuitive and child health professionals guided parents by teaching them the general norms of development. In contrast, parenting in the postmodern world is perceived as a learned technique with specific strategies for dealing with particular issues. Nardone [5] suggested that the current increase in pathological behaviors among children and adolescents is a result of overapplied or oversimplified applications of all the new values, theories, and instructions. For many postmodern children, there is dual socialization by family and daycare providers and the child is required to make continuous adjustments between these spheres. Responsibilities may not be divided clearly between the home and daycare center. As a result, neither may provide some crucial aspects of child rearing such as helping the child develop the capacity to exercise self-control or social comportments such as table manners.

There is a consensus that a nurturing parenting style builds strong character and a sense of self-worth. Nevertheless, the type of parenting style and practices are controversial, mainly its application within different ethnic groups, different personal characteristics, and different social-demographic circumstances.

This chapter discusses the association between weight-related problems, self-regulation, and parenting. It first discusses the association between weight-related problems and self-regulation. Then it briefly reviews some of the self-regulation theories, the development of self-regulation skills, coping, and competence. Lastly, it reviews current knowledge about the components of parenting and their impact on coping, self-regulation, and weight-related problems.

WEIGHT-RELATED PROBLEMS AND SELF-REGULATION

Numerous theorists have posited that difficulties in self-regulation contribute to the development and maintenance of preoccupation with eating and food as well as other pathological behaviors including binge eating, starving, and substance use [6].

Weight-related problems are often the result of difficulties overcoming the temptations in our "obesogenic" environment (large amounts of palatable, high-caloric foods that are available at any place and at any time) [7]. Schachter [8] posited that obese individuals are hypersensitive to external cues, particularly cues that incite hunger and eating, and have a compromised capacity to self-regulate. Results from several studies implicate self-regulation failure in the development of overweight and obesity in youth and adults, primarily through its effects on dysregulated eating behavior [9, 10]. Francis and Susman [11] found that children who exhibited low self-regulation and a significantly higher body mass index (BMI) also had the most rapid gains in BMI from age 3 to 12 years. Their findings suggest that early childhood self-regulatory problems are important longitudinal predictors of weight problems in early adolescence, and self-regulation failure in behaviors appears to generalize to regulatory problems in the energy balance domain of development, as evidenced by higher weight status and more rapid weight gain. Impulsive behaviors such as overeating, excessive alcohol consumption, or drug abuse are thought to be performed without conscious judgment, characterized by acting on the spur of the moment, by an inability to focus on a specific task, and by a lack of adequate planning [12]. Additionally, personality factors, such as temperament, sensation seeking, or risk taking have been associated with impulsive behaviors [13].

Close examination of this literature reveals that promotion of self-regulation and decision-making skills is a major objective to foster child's well-being. There are also some indications that promoting self-regulation *and* decision-making skills via a school-based program demonstrated positive changes in attitudes toward self-regulation of appetitive behavior, actual food choices, and television viewing patterns [14].

Since the late 1990s, the cultural norms about appearance have also changed. The media is often blamed for the increasing incidence of eating disorders (EDs) on the grounds that media images of idealized (slim) physiques motivate people to attempt to achieve slimness themselves [15]. Many young women want to be socially accepted and, consequently, strive for a certain physical appearance [16]. Young girls often begin the treacherous cycle of diet and exercise by trying to win the affection and respect of their fathers. As with the culture of abundance, idealized media images are at best an underlying cause of EDs. Polivy and Herman [17] noted that while it is difficult to imagine an eating disorder developing without body dissatisfaction, the majority of individuals who are dissatisfied with their bodies never go on to develop an eating disorder. Accordingly, sociocultural models have been refined and developed to suggest specific vulnerability factors and psychological processes that may influence the extent to which these pressures affect women [18]. Overidentification with Western norms and values has been hypothesized as a reason for increased eating pathology [19]. Social comparison has also been shown to be related to uncertainty about the self as well as a desire for self-reassurance [20].

Increased anxiety is one of the consumptory society characteristics. Hypervigilance and attention bias were mentioned as key features of anxiety [21, 22]. As such, anxiety leads individuals to scan the environment excessively for any threatening stimuli, preferentially attending to threat when it is present. Individuals who are highly anxious about relationships may thus be considered to show increased hypervigilance (or social comparison) to others in their environment who they perceive as threatening. In addition, it is possible that these individuals will show an attention bias to idealized others who they are likely to view as more threatening (i.e., they are likely to show increased social comparison in an upward direction), which is likely, in turn, to increase body dissatisfaction and disordered eating. This finding is important as it suggests that if appearance based social comparison can be reduced in individuals who are highly anxious about relationships, their harmful behaviors may also be reduced.

Preoccupation with both food and thinness may provide an outlet for individual pathology. It may distract from emotional distress, as well as provide a space to practice self-control, which is often overly challenged in our society.

Maturity fears emerged as a significant predictor of both the incidence and number of impulsive behaviors [23]. Polivy and Herman [17] hypothesized that an individual need for control is an essential feature in the development of an eating disorder. Others suggested that control issues such as lack of control over the individual's life and emotions, lack of control in respect to growth and maturation, and an extreme need for self-control or control within the family setting are also common features in eating disorders [24]. Fairburn et al. [25] have suggested that the eating disorder patient need for general self-control becomes dominated by the need to have control over eating and weight and the preoccupation with controlling eating provides direct, tangible evidence for self-control.

These modern views were previously elaborated in the early psychoanalytic theory. Winnicott [26] mentioned the term "greed" as joining together the psychical and the physical, love and hate, what is acceptable and what is not acceptable to the ego. He suggested that greed is never met within the human being, even in an infant, in undisguised form, and that greediness, when it appears as a symptom, is always a secondary phenomenon, implying anxiety. Greed means to Winnicott something so primitive that it could not appear in human behavior except disguised and as part of a symptom complex. Careful history taking has had a profound effect on Winnicott's outlook, enlightening the clinical continuity of appetite disorders as they present themselves in earliest infancy, in childhood, in adolescence, and in adult life. Through analysis of older children and adults, he saw that there is no sharp dividing line between anorexia nervosa of adolescence, the inhibitions of feeding of childhood, the appetite disorders in childhood that are related to certain critical times, and the feeding inhibitions of infancy, even of earliest infancy.

Winnicott views appetite as an expression to different needs. First in the appreciation of oral function there comes the recognition of *oral instinct*. "I want to suck, eat, bite. I enjoy sucking, eating, biting. I feel satisfied after sucking, eating, biting."

Next comes *oral fantasy*. "When hungry I think of food, when I eat I think of taking food in. I think of what I like to keep inside, and I think of what I want to be rid of and I think of getting rid of it." Third comes a more sophisticated linking up of this theme of oral fantasy with the "inner world." The word "inner" in this term applies primarily to the belly and secondarily to the head and the limbs and any part of the body. The individual tends to place the happenings of fantasy inside and to identify them with the things going on inside the body. Winnicott wrote: "It is not much of a guess to say that in unconscious fantasy she had eaten good and bad people, and bits of people, and that according to the love and hate involved she has been enriched and burdened respectively with intensely sweet or terrifyingly grotesque objects in her inner world." Winnicott wrote about the internalization of good and bad objects, the "good internalized breast," the inhibition of greed, the continuum of feeding conditions in his experience and the "inner world." From Winnicott's point of view, *appetite becomes involved in defense against anxiety and depression*. Examples of crises in which appetite is affected are the birth of a new baby, loss of first nurse, removal from first home, first feeding with the two parents, attempts to induce self-feeding, introduction of solids or even simply of thickened feeds, and anxious reaction to breast biting. Thus, effective emotional skills, self-regulation, and self-control are major objectives in parenting.

SELF-REGULATION

The term "self-regulation" relates to the many cognitive processes that manage drives and emotions [27]. Self-control may be viewed as part of self-regulation.

Self-regulation from the social learning theory perspective looks at the triadic interaction among the person (e.g., beliefs about success), his or her behavior (e.g., engaging in a task), and the environment (e.g., feedback or impact on others) [28]. Self-regulation is the process by which an individual attempts to control these three (triadic) factors to reach a goal. Bandura's triadic model [27] assumes that people self-regulate their health through the use of self-care strategies, setting reasonable health goals, and monitoring feedback concerning the effectiveness of strategies in meeting their goals. People's perceptions of self-efficacy are also assumed to play a major role in motivating them to self-regulate their health functioning. Self-regulation involves self-observation, judgmental processes, and self-reaction. There are two main functions within the individual for self-regulation: monitoring (test) and controlling (operate). These two processes enable an individual to evaluate his or her current behavior in relation to a goal in order to decide whether to pursue further regulation or disengage from a goal (exit). Successful monitoring includes accurately assessing the discrepancy between current progress and a goal (which requires self-awareness), whereas successful behavioral control includes resisting temptation, altering behavior, or even maintaining behavior in light of environmental disturbances [29]. Studies had shown that exposure to temptations can undermine people's subsequent and self-regulatory functioning [30].

Self-control relates to emotions and affects as well as to urges and desires regulation [31]. Moreover, one should distinguish spontaneous, uncontrollable, and unintentional reactions, that follow exposure to unnoticed motivational stimuli versus reactions that follow a redefining or drawbacks of an existing goal, such as lowering one's standards for health [32]. Muraven and Baumeister [33] have suggested that if people are to be momentarily drawn toward temptations, then the temptation must be both immediately available and motivationally self-relevant. Thus, a restrained eater might find it harder to resist a temptation when it is available (a situation often occurred in healthy hungry subject when going shopping) and when he or she is hungry (as often happens in an anorexia binging type).

Frequent, extensive exposure to tempters may have lasting consequences for social self-regulation. For instance, meeting new people who simply resemble known tempters might trigger patterns of responding that are reminiscent of the way one typically behaves around the tempters. Such transference processes may create a cyclical problem in that those who were once tempted by others might eventually behave as tempters themselves. Chronic indulgers may also come to implicitly evaluate the quality of their relationships based on their relevance to the temptations [34], or they might unwittingly immerse themselves in social environments that only increase their exposure to tempters [35].

The ability to regulate and control our behaviors is a key accomplishment of the human species, yet the psychological mechanisms involved in self-regulation remain incompletely understood. Absence of self-regulation is often related to problems in interpersonal interaction, addiction, and mental diseases. Recent studies on the quality of self-regulation indicate that it is both a trait and an ability [6]. People with high self-regulation ability can control their impulses much easier than can people with low self-regulation ability, and the presence of temptation-related social cues increases the susceptibility to indulging in the temptation.

However, it is also the case that self-regulation can be trained: repeated acts of self-regulation enlarge the total pool of energy we have [33]. Current scientific knowledge proclaims that all the energy of a person is drawn from a single source [6]. One single act of self-regulation can have an effect on our behavior on a very different task, because we lack the energy that is necessary to control our impulses; this state is called ego depletion. It can be restored by rest and by positive affect. Thus, actions that give us self-satisfaction and a sense of self-worth are more likely to be pursued than actions that lead to self-censure.

Leander et al. [35] demonstrated that *contextual factors* can suppress a temptation's appeal. Relational distance and chronic self-regulatory tendencies can increase resistance to temptation. These findings are interesting because people may not always have a more important goal to pursue in temptation-laden social contexts, yet they may nonetheless benefit from the natural shielding provided by their chronic self-regulatory tendencies.

According to social cognitive theory, processes entailed in regulating one's health can be taught through social modeling, support, and feedback; gradually these external supports are withdrawn as one is able to self-regulate.

There is evidence that positive emotionality and negative emotionality induce different patterns of activation of the prefrontal cortex [36] and that this can affect levels of attention as well as self-regulation and self-control [37]. The fact that the same area of the brain is responsible for emotional control and for the metacognitive functions further supports the idea of the interconnection between social-emotional self-regulation and cognitive self-regulation [38].

Research suggests that if a neural system is repeatedly exercised, it, like a muscle, will blossom [39]. Consequently, current brain research supports the importance of the environment in the development of self-regulation.

For Vygotsky, self-regulation is a critical development signaling the emergence of a uniquely human set of competencies that lead to "higher mental functions" [40]. Vygotsky described self-regulated behaviors as deliberate, intentional, or volitional behaviors, as something that humans have control of acquiring higher mental functions allowing children to make a critical transition from being "slaves to the environment" to becoming "masters of their own behavior."

This process requires children to master specific cultural tools including language and other symbolic systems that they can use to gain control over their physical, emotional, and cognitive functioning. As it is true for all higher mental functions, children's self-regulatory abilities originate in social interactions and only later become internalized and independently used by children [41]. This means that self-regulation is not something that emerges spontaneously as the child matures but is instead taught formally or informally within the social context. In the case when none of the social contexts support the development of self-regulatory behaviors, children continue to operate as "slaves to the environment" being guided by ever-changing external stimulation and incapable of intentional actions.

For Vygotsky, three critical conditions are necessary for the development of self-regulatory behaviors in children. First, to develop any higher mental function children have to experience it on the shared (intersubjective) plane—it means that children need to have an opportunity to engage in other-regulation. Other-regulation implies that children act both as subjects of another person's regulatory behaviors (as is the case of many of their interactions with adults) and as actors regulating other person's behaviors (as might happen in the interaction with peers or younger children). A second necessary condition for the emergence of self-regulation is children's learning of specific cultural tools that would allow them to eventually use self-regulatory behaviors independently. Among the first of such tools that children develop is *self-talk* or *private speech*. When children engage in private speech to themselves, the same words that adults once used to regulate children's behaviors are now used by children themselves for the purposes of self-regulation. Studies of private speech have found a direct link between children's use of private speech and their self-regulatory abilities [42]. The last condition is young children's engagement in well-developed make-believe play. Play provides opportunities for children to practice self-regulatory components of multiple mental functions—from fulfilling their desires in a symbolic form while at the same time delaying gratification and beginning to develop reflective competencies while taking multiple perspectives [43].

Although the capacity to self-regulate may vary across domains within a person, there is evidence to suggest that the capacity to self-regulate is more trait than state [44]. In studies of young children, self-regulation measured in early childhood was linked to parent and teacher ratings of self-regulation or impulsivity later in life [45].

Self-control is fostered by being in a long-term positive relationship with an accountable person who communicates the value of this goal; working at self-control challenges carefully chosen to be at the correct level of difficulty for present skill; getting many positive models of the successful exercise of self-control; logging in many hours of practice where valued rewards are contingent upon greater and greater exercise of effort; learning that valued rewards can be obtained by effort, and thereby learning to enjoy effort; using fantasy rehearsal; learning compliance skills; learning verbal concepts (including a term for self-control itself) that affect the worldview in ways conducive to this skill; learning the art of self-instruction; learning to remove oneself from tempting stimuli, physically and mentally; and learning self-monitoring [46]. Self-regulatory competence is to some extent influenced by individual temperament, but, by definition, it includes skills that are developed during childhood and adolescence and may be promoted by intervention programs [47].

Emotional distress may therefore work against the usual pattern of *impulse control* because distress promotes a short-term focus, whereas impulse control requires a long-term one. A present-oriented desire to escape from emotional distress probably enhances the search for immediate sources of good feelings. Many of the common foci of self-regulatory restraints are activities that hold some promise of immediate pleasure: alcohol, drugs, high-calorie foods, illicit sex, extra sleep, expensive purchases, time-wasting games, and other entertainments.

Thus, there is a special connection between affect regulation and other spheres of self-control. Impulse control may fail because emotionally distraught people give primacy to affect regulation, which often is the case in weight-related problems [48].

COPING AND COMPETENCE

Like adults, children cope with challenges in prosocial, antisocial, or asocial ways [49]. When coping prosocially, they respond by resolving, or attempting to resolve, the challenge in a constructive manner, not only focusing on their own feelings and preferences but taking the constraints of the situation into account.

When coping antisocially, they attempt to resolve the challenge in an aggressive, destructive, or deceitful manner, or they deny any responsibility in seeking a solution to the challenge, often hurting others and themselves in the process.

When coping asocially, they respond by withdrawing from the situation and from others or by hurting themselves in an attempt to minimize or dismiss the stressful impact of the challenge [50].

The coping-competence model [49] assumes that all young children exhibit ways of coping that are precursors of antisocial and asocial conduct but serve an important role in survival and development. For example, crying signals the infant's need for affection, food, and protection. Avoidance of unfamiliar persons prevents one from getting into danger. In most cases, with repeated exposure to countless challenges coupled with consistent social support and guidance, as well as clear limits, older children and adults acquire predominantly prosocial ways of coping, even though they rely occasionally on antisocial and asocial strategies. All three ways of coping depend to a considerable extent on verbal and nonverbal communication. This communication can be with others or with oneself. More specifically, the coping-competence model assumes that the development of prosocial coping is linked closely to the mastery of effective communication skills [51].

PARENTING, COPING, AND SELF-REGULATION

Good parenting, as measured by different research-based scales, has been shown to build good self-control, which is important for the development of self-regulation [46]. A healthy environment, good-enough parenting, secured attachment, meta-emotion coaching, effective communication, appropriate parenting style, and practices that promote self-regulation and decision-making skills as well as self-confidence and the ability to filter negative messages are some of the protective factors associated with normal physical and emotional development as well as prevent psychopathology.

Healthy Environment

Caregivers generally have good knowledge of what foods children need for health, but for various reasons the application does not always reflect such knowledge usually because of barriers in parental implementation of their own responsibilities during mealtime [52]. Parents' main responsibilities during mealtimes are summarized in Satter's trust paradigm [53]: Parents provide structure (e.g., establishing regular mealtime and table rules), support, and opportunities (repeatedly offering new foods and physical activities initiatives). Children choose if and how much to eat from what parents provide.

In response to environmental temptations, Leander et al. [35] had shown that although the influence of temptations may be automatic, this influence is not invariant. Instead, their momentary appeal relies on several personal, interpersonal, and motivational factors. The authors demonstrated increased motivation toward temptations not just when situational cues suggested social support, but also when the temptation was appealing to the individual, when the source of the temptation was relationally close and thus readily relied on, among individuals who chronically failed to detect temptation-related social cues, and among individuals who were chronically motivated to disengage from their focal goals. Parents should provide an environment that not only minimizes one's exposure to temptations but also provides social contexts that promote alertness (rather than vigilance) against them.

Thus, parents should talk less about food and dieting and at the same time introduce a healthy environment with a moderate level of opportunities for unhealthy food temptation as well as a moderate level of exposure to dieting and the value of thinness [36].

Good-Enough Parenting

Emotion regulation starts while interacting with the primary caregivers. During the 1950s and 1960s, Winnicott viewed individual emotional development as a journey from "absolute dependence" to a "relative dependence" and "towards independence." Winnicott [37] symbolized the holding environment as the mother who acts as a holder for those feelings that threaten to overwhelm the immature baby—later on it will be developed into the self-regulation system. Moreover, the mother's capacity, or willingness, to create the setting in which the baby can experience his or her absolute helplessness by providing looking, reflecting, and recognizing (being seen, visible and invisible) is the origins of human mind and selfhood. The mother's face may well be an original source of reflection and recognition, helping to secure the distinctions between stillness and movement, animate and nonanimate, life and death. In losing sight of the mother's face the infant can lose her or himself; an ordinary anxiety of infantile life: no face, no reflection.

After the early stage of connection with the mother and illusions of omnipotence comes the stage of relative dependence (objective reality) where children realize their dependence and learn about loss. As the infant develops, the *good-enough mother* tries to provide what the infant needs, but she instinctively leaves a time lag between the demands and their satisfaction and progressively increases the time lags. Her failure to satisfy the infant's needs immediately induces the child to compensate for the temporary deprivation by mental activity and by understanding. The good-enough mother's "graduated failure of adaptation" teaches the infant to tolerate for increasingly longer periods both his or her ego needs and instinctual tensions [55].

The mother's gradual failure of adaptation is the sprout of the child's ego strength, the ability to contain frustration and develop self-regulation. The trick of the good-enough mother is to give the child a sense of loosening rather than the shock of being "dropped." This teaches children to predict and hence allows them to retain a sense of control as well as develop a healthy sense of independence. The feeling of safety that is endorsed first via the mother's warmth and reflections and later on through the validation and mentalization process held by the caretakers is the basis for the gradual process in which the child is able to take back and master his or her difficult feelings.

The good-enough mother stands in contrast with the "perfect" mother who satisfies all the needs of the infant on the spot, thus preventing him or her from developing a healthy self-regulation and self-control [56].

In the past few years, researchers have increasingly examined the relations of parental socialization style to children's dispositional control-related characteristics (e.g., self-regulation, impulsivity) and children's maladjustment [57, 58], as will soon be explored.

Secured Attachment

The balance between independence and relatedness to others is the foundations of child's growth [59]. Adequate protection during childhood as well as higher degree of freedom of communication between caregiver and infant supports the development of secured attachment. Bowlby [60, 61] accentuated the concept of attachment as central to understanding the origins of a child's tie to the mother. Most early observers focused on the anxiety displayed by infants and toddlers when threatened with separation from a familiar caregiver. *Attachment theory* suggests that only when one has established a secure base can one freely move away from one's parents [60, 61].

Secure attachment, a healthy form of attachment, is characterized by comfort with independence and closeness in relationships this is in contrast to the insecure attachments: avoidant and resistant. Avoidant attachment is characterized by preferring extreme distance from others in relationships, whereas resistant attachment is characterized by having an intense need to keep others in close proximity in relationships [62]. *Insecure attachment* has been associated with a number of negative outcomes, such as low self-esteem, lower academic achievement, and psychopathology, including eating disorders [63].

Eating problems may be viewed as an unconscious way to address the need for eliciting parental attention and delay the separation process through the risks involved in the behaviors inherent to the disorders as well as the occupation with food. Indeed, more individuals with eating disorders worried that they may see their mothers less when their symptoms subsided, as compared to their clinical counterparts [64].

The developing child must balance its need for autonomy with its need for security and belonging. Too much autonomy can leave the individual isolated and vulnerable, yet excessive closeness to the caregiver can interfere with learning to function independently.

Bowlby [62] identified five instinctual responses that protect the infant and young child from physical and psychological danger by summoning the primary object. These responses mature at various rates and serve the dual function of binding the child and the parent to each other. The specific behavioral responses include sucking, crying, smiling, clinging, and following. These reactions satisfy physical security and as the child matures, psychological security increasingly becomes the new goal. Several recent studies have examined eating disorders in terms of attachment phenomena. Kenny and Hart [65] found that the presence of an affectively positive and emotionally supportive parental relationship, in cooperation with parental fostering of autonomy, is inversely associated with weight preoccupation, bulimic behavior, and feelings of ineffectiveness.

It is also likely that patient may attempt to summon parental attention through Bowlby's concept of following. Through dangerous behaviors such as extreme binging, self-starvation, purging, and others, physically close encounters are frequently created between mother and daughter, thus potentially increasing both physical and psychological proximity. Generally, there is protest from the child concerning this degree of parental closeness; however, the child rarely accepts the solution of relinquishing symptoms in the service of greater autonomy. Instead, the symptoms generally persist or are exacerbated, until some type of clinical intervention is imposed. It is as if these eating disorder symptoms are a manifestation, representation, or reenactment of early infantile and childhood attempts to seek or maintain parental proximity.

Attachment theory has been widely used also to explain how individuals relate to themselves and to others. Bamford and Halliwell [66] suggested that individuals with high attachment anxiety tend to devaluate themselves and use others for reassurance or validation. This tendency may heighten their vulnerability to using others as a source of comparison in order to evaluate themselves. Such people tend to overly internalize social values such as thinness and following comparison. They are likely to show increased social comparison in an upward direction, which is likely, in turn, to increase body dissatisfaction and disordered eating.

Parents have a major role in being tuned in and addressing their child's apprehensions and anxieties as well as filtering out negative societal messages that can lead to extreme and harmful behaviors [67].

EFFECTIVE COMMUNICATION AND PROSOCIAL COPING

Effective communication—at home and, later, at school and in other social settings—consists of three interrelated processes in which language skills are paramount: information exchange, behavior influence, and problem solving [50]. As language becomes internalized, competent children and adolescents make increasing use of self-talk to describe and evaluate their own thoughts, feelings, and actions, as well as those of others, relying on all three processes of effective communication to plan and monitor their own behavior [68]. Through such communication, the developing child acquires the foundations of self-regulation on which affective, social, and achievement competence depend. As children learn to understand and use language, they are able to modify their behavior, first in response to immediate adult instructions and later through self-verbalizations and internalization of these instructions. With maturation, repeated practice, and authoritative guidance from trusted adults, children become increasingly capable of self-initiated planning and monitoring and show greater flexibility in their control strategies of self and others as a function of changing situational demands. Thus, with growing competence, self-regulation encompasses complex abilities much beyond compliance with immediate instructions, including "delay of gratification, control of impulses and affect, modulation of motor and linguistic activities, and the ability to act in accordance with social norms in the absence of external monitors" [69].

PARENTING STYLE

Parents try to foster a healthy lifestyle and good habits using different strategies for controlling their child's behaviors. Parenting style, according to Baumrind [70, 71], captures two important elements of parenting and revolves around issues of control: *parental responsiveness* (the extent to which parents address a child's needs, intentionally fostering individuality, self-regulation, and self-assertion) and *parental demandingness* (the claims parents make on children). According to Baumrind, authoritative parents provide balanced responsiveness, and demandingness—they are assertive but not intrusive and restrictive [72, 73].

Authoritarian parents tend to be highly directive with their children and value unquestioning obedience in their exercise of authority over their children. Authoritarian parenting style had been shown to have a negative relationship with children's psychosocial well-being [74], obesity [75], and eating disorders [76].

Permissive parents are more responsive than they are demanding. They essentially allow children to make their own decisions and regulate their own activities. Such parents may avoid setting boundaries and strict sedentary activity as is recommended by the American Academy of Pediatrics Committee [77]. Chen and Kennedy [23] suggested that a permissive parenting style is associated with greater food intake in Chinese American children. Because such a democratic parenting style may reflect unstructured parenting in the Chinese culture, children in a less structured family environment may not be able to self-regulate their food intake.

The impact of parental control on children's eating habits is an important area for investigation because children's fruit and vegetable consumption intake is consistently low and parents need to be informed about which feeding strategies are effective and which are counterproductive. Moreover, in response to the obesogenic environment, parents may attempt to limit children's consumption of "junk" or "unhealthy" foods by keeping these foods out of reach or by placing constraints on when and how much food may be consumed. Experimental studies have shown, however, that restrictive feeding practices increase children's preferences for restricted foods [78, 79], heighten responsiveness to the presence of palatable foods, and promote overeating when restricted foods are freely available [80, 81]. Moreover, mothers who reported exerting a greater degree of control over their child's food intake had children who demonstrated less ability to internally regulate energy intake. Furthermore, children who demonstrated less ability to self-regulate energy intake had higher body fat stores.

Thus, external parental control of the child's dietary intake and the imposition of stringent parental controls can potentiate preferences for high-fat, energy-dense foods limit children's acceptance of a variety of foods and disrupt children's regulation of energy intake by altering children's responsiveness to internal cues of hunger and satiety, thus indirectly fostering the development of excess adiposity in the child [10, 81]. This can occur when well-intentioned but concerned parents assume that children need help in determining what, when, and how much to eat and when parents impose child-feeding practices that provide children with few opportunities for self-control. Thus, parental insensitivity or unresponsiveness to feeding cues from the child might be counterproductive to the development of the child's ability to self-regulate and may have adverse consequences for the development of the child's food preferences and intake [82].

The child's social environment also might interfere with this self-regulation by instructing a child to finish the food on his or her plate, a practice that discourages one's response to bodily cues [80]. Johnson [83] reported that preschool children who were enrolled in a 6-week role-play exercise to make them aware of internal cues of hunger and satiety improved their self-regulation and ate less lunch after a high-calorie drink. Thus, social learning should be manifested to improve children's self-regulation.

Satter [53] suggested that healthcare providers and parents should rely on what she has referred to as a "trust" paradigm instead of the current "control" paradigm for understanding childhood obesity. She suggested a division of responsibility between parent and child in which it is the parent's responsibility to supply the child with a healthful array of foods and a supportive eating context, and it is the child's responsibility to decide when and how much to eat. In this model, it is assumed that children will eat the amount they need and that it is normal for some children to be overweight. Such feeding style—an authoritative feeding style—is one in which adults determine which foods are offered, and children determine the amount eaten. Kirschenbaum and Kelly [84] asserted that the trust model would most likely cause obese children additional failure. Enten and Golan asserted [85] that the effective way is neither extensive trusting nor extensive restricting around food, but rather the induction of self-regulation and self-control. This can be achieved in most cultures by applying an authoritarian parenting style engaging in an effective communication style.

Family Functioning

There are data indicating that poor family functioning, including difficulties with communication, parenting skills, parental distress, and psychopathology, is associated with pediatric obesity [86, 87]. Complex links have been described between family factors and interactions and children's eating patterns [3, 81]. Various theoretical perspectives have suggested that lack of control over the environment is associated with psychopathology [89]. The belief in a *powerful benevolent other*, who can prevent a negative outcome (e.g., a parent, an authority figure, or God) can act as a protective factor in the face of a perceived lack of one's own control over the environment [89] and thus decreases the risk of psychopathology. To help a child form an organized, clear, and stable internal world, parents should provide age-appropriate external boundaries. A well-structured environment promotes child trust, confidence, and strength of ego and exercises a child's self-control capacities. Later on the child will achieve interior boundaries on his or her own.

Overprotection is one of the pathological features of many families with weight-related problems. Overprotection often delays or even blocks the natural evolution of the young child who needs to become autonomous and independent in order to become an adult and take personal and social responsibilities. The increased prevalence of overprotection might be due to the shift from an adult-centered view to a child-centered view, which is typical of Western society [4].

Some cultures and individual houses still support this schema, being intolerant and using harsh punishment when children exhibit nonconformist behavior. Some of the children who are educated within an adult-centered approach might feel confused when they are exposed to the "outer world" or even dare to challenge this approach. Bryant-Waugh and Lask [90] reported on cases of anorexia nervosa in Asian children in the United Kingdom. They argued that the more traditional the family, the more the possibility of sociocultural conflict about such issues as arranged marriage, dress norms, contact with the opposite sex, and the role of females in cooking and at mealtimes. They believe that young people growing up in juxtaposition between two different cultures may experience confusion. DiNicola [91] has proposed a transcultural hypothesis that anorexia nervosa can be viewed as a "cultural change syndrome" whose onset may be triggered by conditions of sociocultural flux. Bulik [92] argued that stresses relating to immigration and acculturation may lead to the emergence of eating disorders in populations not previously considered at risk.

Overpermissiveness, in contrast to overprotection, is a pattern often driven by parental anxiety about being blamed for not providing their children with the perfect environment for individuality and creativity; hence, these parents endorse few rules and promote the child's self-esteem with an overdose of reinforcement. Such parents often relate to the child as if he or she were a consumer or a client with the main objective of making the child happier rather than helping the child to become a well-adjusted grownup: the child should not be annoyed.

This is in similarity to the overprotective parents who are driven by anxiety to be blamed for their lack of affection or for causing their child to have psychological problems. Thus, in order to avoid risk, parents fall into an opposite trap: they overprotect the child or lose their authority. The result is a happy child but a confused adolescent who finds the grownup lives too fast and challenging, who mistrusts himself and the adults' words, who is less self-regulated and less self-controlled, and who has more weight-related problems.

Structure is an important component in learning self-regulation. Lack of structure stresses children, and there is considerable evidence that structure around feeding is eroding. In the modern society, working mothers tend to cook less and children tend to eat by themselves and have their own money to buy food—a more democratic atmosphere with the tendency to promote the child's independence; the optimal ratio of control relative to freedom within the family increases [93].

There are indications that a structured mealtime is a valuable component in adopting regular eating habits and preventing eating disorders. When the family environment lacks control, adolescent girls tend to develop bulimia, hypothesized to be related to the lack of adequate control and self-regulation learned from the family [94].

Family meals appear to play an important role in promoting positive dietary intake among children. Whereas in the past, eating for children has generally been within a social context, such as the family meal, in the modern lifestyle, eating alone has become a common event. Unfortunately, the result of this independence is often that unhealthy nutritional patterns abound, including skipping meals and increased consumption of junk food [95]. Research suggests that when parents provide companionship at mealtime, establish a positive atmosphere, and model appropriate food-related behaviors, their children tend to have improved dietary quality [96, 97].

Modeling

Because most children do not normally think about health issues, adults have to communicate health-related values, either directly or indirectly through the behaviors they enact, if children are to develop healthy lifestyles as adults. For example, greater success can be achieved in getting children to eat well if adults engage children in discussions about healthy food, including information about food content, available choices among different foods with similar nutritional content, and the importance of eating well [98]. Through communication, adults can share their knowledge about health with children, correct children's misconceptions about health issues, encourage children to become critical consumers of health information, provide verbal assurances about children's abilities to enact healthy behaviors, and motivate children through proper incentives [98].

CONCLUSION AND FUTURE DIRECTIONS FOR PARENT PRACTICES

The ability to regulate and control our behaviors is a key accomplishment of the human species. It is both a trait and ability. Children's self-regulatory abilities originate in social interactions, and only later do the children internalize these abilities and use them independently.

Because self-regulation involves self-observation, judgmental processes, and self-reaction, parents and healthcare educators should strive to challenge children with these practices, implementing a "good enough" (not perfect) and regulated manner.

Contextual factors can suppress a temptation's appeal. Relational distance and chronic self-regulatory tendencies can increase resistance to temptation. The presence of temptation-related social cues increases the susceptibility to indulge in the temptation. Anxiety affects levels of attention as well as self-regulation and self-control and thus should be addressed rather than avoided.

The home environment is undoubtedly the most important setting in relation to shaping children's behaviors, as well as perceptions, self-esteem and self-efficacy, body image, and future weight-related problems. The development of prosocial coping is linked closely to the mastery of effective communication skills. Through communication, adults can share their knowledge about health with children, correct children's misconceptions about health issues, encourage children to become critical consumers of health information, provide verbal assurances about children's abilities to enact healthy behaviors, and motivate children through proper incentives. Parents with a tuned presence log in practices where valued rewards are contingent on greater and greater exercises of effort: learning that valued rewards can be obtained by effort, and thereby learning to enjoy effort; using fantasy rehearsal; learning compliance skills; learning verbal concepts (including a term for self-control itself) that affect the worldview in ways conducive to this skill; learning the art of self-instruction; learning to remove oneself from tempting stimuli, physically and mentally; and learning self-monitoring.

Absence of self-regulation is often related to problems in interpersonal interaction, addiction, and mental diseases, whereas people with high self-regulation ability can control their impulses much easier than people with low self-regulation ability.

To manage the broad spectrum of weight-related problems and to support self-regulation, decision-making skills, and self-control, the following guidelines are suggested:

1. Perfect parenting is the hindrance for a good-enough parenting.
2. Too much is often less. Excellent is the enemy of the very good.
3. A well-behaved child is not necessarily a self-regulated child.
4. Effective communication always works.

Parents are advised to do the following:

1. Foster self-regulation through modeling, educating, and logging into family games. Foster a positive and moderated reaction to internal needs. Parents have a major role in being tuned in and addressing their child's apprehensions and anxieties, validating the child's feelings while in emotional distress, providing empathy and verbalization, and encouraging self-talk to support decision-making skills and effective coping styles.
2. Avoid preoccupation with both food and thinness, which may provide an outlet for individual emotional distress, and nurture an exaggerated space to practice self-control. Prevent appetite from becoming involved in the child's defense against anxiety and

depression. Avoid social comparisons, mainly those based of appearance, and foster appropriate filtering out of negative external/social messages that can lead to extreme and harmful behaviors.

3. Foster healthy lifestyle habits by modeling healthy behaviors, providing a healthy environment with a positive atmosphere, establishing regular mealtimes and sleeping hours, and educating children about health practices while respecting their psychological space.

Environment can foster self-esteem by helping children recognize their own worth, cultural food practices, and family tradition; by teaching body satisfaction and a positive body image; and by modeling qualities that facilitate health-promoting behaviors. The best thing that parents can do when acting as role models is to demonstrate that healthy weight management is a reflection of self-care that includes positive food and activity behaviors that come from, and reinforce, a positive self-image.

References

1. Ferraro KF, Su YP, Gretebeck RJ, Black DR, Badylak SF. Body mass index and disability in adulthood: a 20-year panel study. *Am J Public Health* 2002;**92**:834—40.
2. Global Burden of Disease: Mental Disorders and Illicit Drug Use Expert Group, www.med.unsw.edu.au/gbdweb.nsf/page/home Accessed 28 July, 2009.
3. Golan M, Crow S. Parents are key players in the prevention and treatment of weight-related problems. *Nutr Rev* 2004;**62**:39—50.
4. Damon W. *Greater expectations: overcoming the culture of indulgence in our homes and schools*. New York: The Free Press; 1995.
5. Nardone G, Giannotti E, Rocchi R. *The evolution of family patterns and indirect therapy with adolescents*. London: Karnac Books; 2007.
6. Baumeister RF, Heatherton TF. Self-Regulation Failure: An Overview. *Psychol Inq* 1996;**7**:1—15.
7. Swinburn B, Egger G, Raza F. Dissecting obesogenic environments: the development and application of a framework for identifying and prioritizing environmental interventions for obesity. *Prev Med* 1999;**29**:563—70.
8. Schachter S. Obesity and eating: internal and external cues differentially affect the eating behavior of obese and normal subjects. *Science* 1986;**161**(843):751—6.
9. Fisher JO, Birch LL. Eating in the absence of hunger and overweight in girls from 5 to 7 y of age. *Am J Clin Nutr* 2002;**76**(1):226—31.
10. Johnson SL, Birch LL. Parents' and children's adiposity and eating style. *Pediatrics* 1994;**94**:653—61.
11. Francis LA, Susman EJ. Self-regulation and rapid weight gain in children from age 3 to 12 Years. *Arch Pediatr Adolesc Med* 2009;**163**(4):297—302.
12. Fishbach A, Shah JY. Self Control in Action: Implicit Dispositions toward Goals and Away from Temptations. *J Personal Soc Psychol* 2006;**90**:820—32.
13. Favaro A, Zanetti T, Tenconi E, Degortes D, Ronzan A, Veronese A, Santonastato. The relationship between temperament and impulsive behaviors in eating disordered subjects. *Eat Disord* 2005;**13**:61—70.
14. Riggs NR, Sakuma KK, Pent MA. Preventing risk for obesity by promoting self-regulation and decision-making skills. *Eval Rev* 2007;**31**(3):287—310.
15. Derenne JL, Beresin EV. Body image, media and eating disorders. *Acad Psychiatry* 2006;**30**:257—61.
16. Striegel-Moore RH. A feminist perspective on the etiology of eating disorders. In: Brownell KD, Fairburn CG, editors. *Eating disorders and obesity: A comprehensive handbook*. New York: Guilford Press; 1995. pp. 224—9.
17. Polivy J, Herman CP. Causes of eating disorders. *Ann Rev Psychol* 2002;**53**:187—213.
18. Dittmar H. Vulnerability factors and processes linking sociocultural pressure and body dissatisfaction. *J Soc Clin Psychol* 2005;**24**:1081—7.
19. Rathner G, Túry F, Szabo P, Geyer M, Rumfold G, Forgács A, Sollner W, Plottner G. Prevalence of eating disorders and minor psychiatric morbidity in Central Europe before the political changes in 1989: a cross-cultural study. *Psychol Med* 1995;**25**:1027—35.
20. Eurich TL & Byrne ZS. (2004). A closer look at social comparison orientation. Presented as a poster session for the 19th annual conference of the society for industrial and organizational psychology in Illinois, April 2nd—4th.
21. Mogg K, Bradley BP. A cognitive motivational analysis of anxiety. *Behav Res Ther* 1998;**36**:809—48.
22. Harvey AH, Watkins E, Mansell W, Shafran R. *Cognitive behavioural processes across psychological disorders: A transdiagnostic perspective to research and treatment*. Oxford: OUP; 2004.
23. Chen JL, Kennedy C. Family functioning, parenting style, and Chinese children's weight status. *J Family Nurs* 2004;**10**(2):262—79.
24. Surgenor J, HornPlumridge EW, Hudson SM. Anorexia nervosa and psychological control: A reexamination of selected theoretical accounts. *Eur Eat Disord Rev* 2002;**10**:85—101.
25. Fairburn CG, Doll HA, Welch SL, Hay PJ, Davies BA, O'Connor ME. Risk factors for binge eating disorder: A community-based, case-control study. *Arch Gen Psychiatry* 1998;**55**:425—32.
26. Winnicott DW. *Collected Papers. Through Paediatrics to Psycho-Analysis*. London: Tavistock Publications; 1958.
27. Bandura A. *Social foundations of thought and action: A social cognitive*. Englewood Cliffs, NJ: Prentice Hall; 1986.
28. Dweck CS, Leggett EL. A social-cognitive approach to motivation and personality. *Psychol Rev* 1988;**95**:256—73.
29. Barber LK, Munz DC, Bagsby PG, Grawitch M. When does time perspective matter? Self-control as a moderator between time perspective and academic achievement. *Pers Indiv Differ* 2009;**46**:250—3.
30. Baumeister RF, Bratslavsky E, Muraven M, Tice DM. Ego depletion: Is the active self a limited resource? *J Pers Soc Psychol* 1998;**74**:1252—65.
31. Linehan M, Lindenboim N. Skills Practice in Dialectical Behavior Therapy for Suicidal Women Meeting Criteria for Borderline Personality Disorder. *Cogn Behav Pract* 2007;**14**:147—56.
32. Fishbach A, Zhang Y. The Dynamics of Self-Regulation: When Goals Commit Versus Liberate. In: Wvnke M, editor. *"The Social Psychology of Consumer Behavior" (in the series Frontiers of Social Psychology)*. New York: Psychology Press; 2009. pp. 365—86.
33. Muraven M, Baumeister RF. Self-regulation and depletion of limited resources: does self-control resemble a muscle? *Psychol Bull* 2000;**126**:247—59.
34. Fitzsimons GM, Shah JY. How goal instrumentality shapes relationship evaluations. *J Pers Soc Psychol* 2008;**95**:319—37.
35. Leander NP, Shah JY, Chartrand TL. Moments of Weakness: The Implicit Context Dependencies of Temptations. *Pers Soc Psychol Bull* 2009;**35**:853.

36. Davidson RJ, Jackson DC, Kalin NH. Emotion, plasticity, context, and regulation: Perspectives from affective neuroscience. *Psychol Bull* 2000;**126**:890–909.
37. Davidson RJ. Perspectives on affective styles and their cognitive consequences. In: Dalgleish T, Power M, editors. *Handbook of Cognition and Emotion*. Chichester, England: Wiley; 1999. pp. 103–23.
38. Blair C. School readiness: Integrating cognition and emotion in a neurobiological conceptualization of children's functioning at school entry. *Am Psychol* 2002;**57**(2):111–27.
39. Bialystok E, Craik FIM, Grady C, Chau W, Ishii R, Gunji A, Pantev C. Effect of bilingualism on cognitive control in the Simon task: Evidence from MEG. *Neuroimage* 2005;**24**:40–9.
40. Zimmerman BJ, Schunk DH. Vygotskian view. In: Zimmerman BJ, Schunk DH, editors. *"Self-regulated learning and academic achievement"*. 2nd ed. Hillsdale, NJ: Lawrence Erlbaum; 1996. pp. 227–52.
41. Vygotsky L. Mind in society: The development of higher psychological processes. In: Cole M, John-Steiner V, Scribner S, Souberman E, editors. Cambridge, MA: Harvard University Press; 1978.
42. Winsler A, Diaz RM, Atencio DJ. Verbal Self-regulation over time in preschool children at risk for attention and behavior problems. *J Chil Psychol Psychiatry* 2000;**41**(7):875–86.
43. Vygotsky LS, Luria AR. Studies on the history of behavior: Age, primitive, and child. In: Golod VI, Knox JE, editors. Hillsdale, NJ: Lawrence Erlbaum; 1993.
44. Mischel W, Shoda Y, Rodriguez ML. Delay of gratification in children. *Science* 1989;**244**(4907):933–8.
45. Tremblay RE, Masse B, Perron D, Leblanc M, Schwartzman AE, Ledingham JE. Early disruptive behavior, poor school achievement, delinquent behavior, and delinquent personality: longitudinal analyses. *J Consult Clin Psychol* 1992;**60**(1):64–72.
46. Strayhorn Jr JM. Self-control: theory and research. *J Am Acad Child Adol Psychiatry* 2002;**41**(1):7–16.
47. Schunk DM, Zimmerman BJ. Social origins of self-regulatory competence. *Educ Psychol* 1997;**32**:195–208.
48. Stice DM, Bratslavsky E, Baumeister RF. Emotional distress regulation takes precedence over impulse control. *J Pers Soc Psychol* 2001;**80**(1):53–67.
49. Blechman EA, Prinz RJ, Dumas JE. Coping, competence, and aggression prevention. *Appl Prev Psychol* 1995;**4**:211–32.
50. Dumas JE, Prinz RJ, Smith EP, Laughlin J. The Early Alliance Prevention Trial: An integrated set of interventions to promote competence and reduce risk for conduct disorder, substance abuse, and school failure. *Clin Child Fam Psychol Rev* 1999;**2**(1):37–54.
51. Dumas JE. Home and school correlates of early at-risk status: A transactional perspective. In: Kronick RF, editor. *"At-risk youth: Theory, practice, reform"*. New York: Garland; 1997. pp. 97–117.
52. Hoerr S, Utech AE, Ruth E. Child control of food choices in Head Start families. *J Nutr Educ Behav* 2005;**37**(4):185–90.
53. Satter E. *Your child's weight, helping without harming*. Madison, WI: Kelcy Press; 2005. p. 16.
54. Neumark-Sztainer D. Eating in a weight-obsessed world: parenting teens with a healthy body and a healthy body image. *Int J Child Adol Health* 2008;**1**(4):313–32.
55. Winnicott DW. *The Piggle. An account of the psychoanalytic treatment of a little girl*. London: Hogarth Press; 1977.
56. Winnicott DW. *Playing and Reality*. London: Routledge; 1999.
57. Eisenberg N, Zhou Q, Losoya S, Fabes RA, Shepard SA, Murphy BC, et al. The relations of parenting, effortful control, and ego control to children's unregulated expression of emotion. *J Child Develop* **74**:875–95.
58. Kochanska G, Knaack A. Effortful control as a personality characteristic of young children: Antecedents, correlates, and consequences. *J Personal* 2003;**71**:1087–112.
59. Guisinger S, Blatt SJ. Individuality and relatedness. *Am Psychol* 1994;**49**:104–11.
60. Bowlby J. *Attachment and loss: Vol. 1. Attachment*. New York: Basic Books; 1969.
61. Bowlby J. *Attachment and loss: Vol. 2. Separation*. New York: Basic Books; 1973.
62. Bowlby J. *Attachment and loss: Vol. 3. Loss, sadness, and depression*. New York: Basic Books; 1980.
63. Sroufe L, Carlson E, Levy A, Egeland B. Implications of attachment theory for developmental psychopathology. *Develop Psycho* 1999;**11**:1–13.
64. Orzolek-Kronner C. The effect of attachment theory in the development of eating disorders: Can symptoms be proximity-seeking? *J Child Adol Soc Work* 2002;**19**(6):421–34
65. Kenny M, Hart K. The extent and function between parental attachment in eating disorders in an inpatient and a college sample. *J Counsl Psychol* 1992;**39**:521–6.
66. Bamford B, Halliwell E. Investigating the role of attachment in social comparison theories of eating disorders within a non-clinical female population. *Eur Eat Disord Rev* 2009;**17**(5):371–9.
67. Golan M. *The PATCH program – parental agency towards child's health, leaders guide*. Israel: Maxanna Press; 2008.
68. Greenberg MT, Kusche CA, Speltz ML. In: Cicchetti D, Toth SL, editors. *"Rochester Symposium on Developmental Psychopathology". Emotional regulation, self-control, and psychopathology: The role of relationships in early childhood*, Vol. 2. New York: Cambridge University Press; 1991. pp. 21–66.
69. Kopp CB. Young children's progression to self-regulation. In: Bullock M, editor. *"The development of intentional action: Cognitive, motivational, and interactive processes"*. Basel, Switzerland: Krager; 1991. pp. 38–54.
70. Baumrind D. The influence of parenting style on adolescent competence and substance use. *J Early Adoles* 1991;**11**:56–95.
71. Baumrind D. Effects of authoritative parental control on child behavior. *J Child Develop* 1966;**37**(4):887–907.
72. Baumrind D. Current patterns of parental authority. *Development Psychology Monograph* 1971;**4**:101–3.
73. Baumrind D. Patterns of parental authority and adolescent autonomy. *N ew Dir Child Adoles Dev* 2005;**108**:61–9.
74. Olvera-Ezzell N, Power TG, Cousins JH. Maternal socialization of children's eating habits: Strategies used by obese Mexican-American mothers. *Child Dev* 1990;**61**:395–400.
75. Wardle J, Sanderson S, Guthrie CA, Rapoport L, Plomin R. Parental Feeding Style and the inter-generational transmission of obesity risk. *Obes Res* 2002;**10**(6):453–62.
76. Enten SR, Golan M. Parenting styles and the eating disorder pathology. *Appetite* 2009;**52**(3):784–7.
77. American Academy of Pediatrics. Committee on Communications. Children, adolescents and television. *Pediatrics* 1995;**96**:786–7.
78. Birch LL. Effect of peer models' food model choices and eating behaviors on preschooler' food preferences. *J Child Dev* 1980;**51**:489–96.
79. Birch LL. Children's preferences for high-fat foods. *Nutr Rev* 1992;**50**:249–55.
80. Birch LL, Davison KK. Family environmental factors influencing the developing behavioral controls of food intake and childhood overweight. *Pediatric Clin North Am* 2001;**48**:893–907.
81. Birch LL, Fisher JO. Development of eating behaviors among children and adolescents. *Pediatrics* 1998;**101**:539S–49S.

REFERENCES

82. Birch LL, Marlin DW, Rotter J. Eating as the "means" activity in a contingency: effects on young children's food preferences. *J Child Dev* 1984;**55**:432–9.
83. Johnson SL. Improving preschoolers' self-regulation of energy intake. *Pediatrics* 2000;**106**:653–61.
84. Kirschenbaum DS, Kelly KP. Five reasons to distrust the trust model. *Obesity* 2009;**17**(6):1107–11.
85. Enten R, Golan M. Parenting Style and Weight Related Problems. *Nutr Rev* 2008;**66**(2):65–75.
86. Stunkard AJ, Wadden TA. Psychological aspects of severe obesity. *Am J Clin Nutr* 1992;**55**:524–32.
87. Tinsley BJ. *How children learn to be healthy.* New York: Cambridge University Press; 2003.
88. Wilkins SC, Kendrick OW, Stitt KR, Stinett N, Hammarkund VA. Family functioning is related to overweight in children. *J Am Diet Assoc* 1998;**98**:572–4.
89. Shapiro DH, Astin JA. *Control therapy: An integrated approach to psychotherapy, health, and healing.* New York: Wiley; 1998.
90. Bryant-Waugh R, Lask B. Anorexia nervosa in a group of Asian children living in Britain. *Br J Psychitry* 1991;**158**: 229–33.
91. DiNicola V. Anorexia multiform: self starvation in historical and cultural context. anorexia nervosa as a cultural reactive syndrome. *Transcultl Psychiatr Res Rev* 1990;**27**:4.
92. Bulik CM. Eating disorders in immigrants: two case reports. *Int J Eat Disord* 1987;**6**:133–41.
93. Benton D. Role of parents in the determination of the food preferences of children and the development of obesity. *Int J Obes* 2004;**28**:858–69.
94. Agras S, Hammer L, McNicholas F. A prospective study of the influence of eating-disordered mothers on their children. *Int J Eat Disord* 1997;**25**:253–62.
95. Graber JA, Brooks-Gunn J. Prevention of eating problems and disorders: including parents. *Eat Disord* 1996;**4**:348–63.
96. Stanek K, Abbott D, Cramer S. Diet quality and the eating environment. *J Am Diet Assoc* 1990;**90**:1582–4.
97. Gillman MW, Rifas-Shiman SI, Frazier AL, Rockett HR, Camargo CA, Field AE, et al. Family dinner and diet quality among older children and adolescents. *Arch Fam Med* 2000;**9**:235–40.
98. Rimal RN. Intergenerational transmission of health: the role of intrapersonal, interpersonal, and communicative factors. *Health Educ Behav* 2003;**30**(1):10–28.

CHAPTER 6

Nursing Perspective on Childhood Obesity

Cynthia Yensel, Carrie Tolman

Center for Healthy Weight and Nutrition, Nationwide Children's Hospital, Columbus, OH, USA

INTRODUCTION

Childhood obesity has become a global concern, no longer confined to westernized countries. Since the late 1970s, it is estimated that the threat of obesity has increased from 12% to more than 30% in developed countries, and from 2% to 12% in developing countries [1]. Of concern is the dramatic progression of obesity rates over the years. In 2003—2004, the National Health and Nutrition Examination Survey (NHANES) estimated that 17% of children and adolescents 2 to 19 years of age are overweight. It also found that obese adolescents had an 80% chance of being obese as adults, stressing the need for prevention and early treatment to prevent persistent obesity [2].

Nurses have historically been involved in health-promoting activities and preventive care. Current trends in healthcare have pushed for more preventive care, and the role of the nurse has been driven in this direction [3]. Nurses have a unique opportunity to positively affect the outcomes related to obesity in children, as they come into contact with children and families in a variety of settings, including outpatient clinics, primary care offices, home healthcare, hospitals, schools and other community settings [2]. Nurses must recognize the global scope of the obesity epidemic and how it has trickled down to the children of the world. Because they serve in a variety of settings and roles, nurses can use their expertise to identify children who are at risk for becoming obese, as well as those who are already overweight and obese. This can include screenings, not only for overweight status and obesity, but for obesity-related comorbidities as well. This requires knowledge of the health consequences related to obesity and their long-term effects. Nurses need to be aware of the factors directly influencing the risks for obesity, including environment and family issues. They need to have the tools to educate children and families and implement a treatment plan. This involves the identification of barriers for the children, their families, and the nurses themselves. All of this must incorporate cultural and ethnic awareness of the populations with which they work. Nurses also play an integral role in cultivating public policy around the topic of childhood obesity.

Factors Influencing Obesity

The complex interaction between family, genetics, environment, characteristics of the community and region, culture, and social behaviors has resulted in an energy imbalance. This has led to an increase in obesity rates, especially among children, resulting in an overall negative health impact. To positively impact the rising global obesity problem, these contributing factors need to be identified not only at the local level but also at the international level and addressed by the nursing community.

Genetics and Family

Numerous studies have demonstrated a familial tendency for obesity. The presence of parental overweight in one or both parents has been seen as a positive indicator for a child's risk for overweight [4]. When both parents are obese, the child has a 70% chance of becoming obese. If one parent is obese, the chance for the child to be obese is 50%. If neither parent is obese, the child has only a 10% chance of becoming obese [5]. It has been shown that 80% of obese adolescents aged 10 to 14 with at least one obese parent will become obese as adults [6]. Single overweight mothers have an increased risk of having a child who is overweight or obese [7]. McDonald, Baylin, Arsenault, Mora-Plazas, and Villamor (2009) found the number of overweight

Columbian children with an obese mother to be more than three and a half times greater than those children with a mother who was not obese [8]. Informing the parents that the father's weight can also be a predictor of the child's weight as they grow would be beneficial, as this has not been considered in the past.

Lifestyle and Environment

The built environment, with its endless availability of energy-dense nutrient-poor foods (EDNP), along with a sedentary lifestyle promoting decreased activity, has had a huge impact on children's health and well-being worldwide. Known factors that positively affect obesity include sedentary behaviors, skipping meals, and consuming high-fat meals, all of which have been seen frequently in teenage girls in Taiwan [3]. Kids are not eating many fruits and vegetables daily, having instead developed a preference for foods that are high in fat and sugar. Foods customary in the diets of many cultures, such as fruits, vegetables, and whole grains, are being replaced by EDNP foods, as seen, for example, in Latin American populations [8]. The high intake of juices, soda, sports drinks, and other high-calorie beverages are another factor contributing to weight gain in children and adolescents. These toxic food environments surround the child in all areas of life, including almost all high schools, three fourths of junior high schools, and fewer than half of elementary schools, with access to vending machines and snack shops that distribute nutrient-poor food choices [9]. Larger portion sizes, such as supersizing in the fast-food industry, have decreased the awareness of proper portion sizes and are contributing to weight gain [10]. Taiwan's eating patterns have changed because of the invasion of these westernized food preferences, in addition to the advertising of all types of fast foods and EDNP foods on television [11]. McDonald, Baylin, Arsenault, Mora-Plazas, Villamor (2009) found that frequency of food consumption in the form of snacking was identified as a positive influence on weight gain in Columbian children [8].

Society today is rich in conveniences that promote inactivity and decreased physical effort. Walking and riding a bike have been replaced with driving a car, riding buses, or using subway and train systems. Elevators and escalators have replaced the use of stairs. The amount of time spent watching TV, playing video games, and using the computer is another form of inactivity identified in the Taiwanese population [11]. In the United Kingdom, watching TV for more than 3 hours daily was a positive risk factor for overweight in 3-year-old children. Adolescents, and even younger children, frequently spend many hours per day listening to music and talking and texting on a cell phone, resulting in decreased energy expenditure.

Safety is a newly identified barrier to physical activity that parents have cited. There are fewer safe areas for play and travel through neighborhoods due to gang activity, drug dealers, drug dealings, crime, and violence. Racism was also identified as a factor keeping children and families from feeling safe to be physically active. This is seen increasingly in immigrant parents and children, who experience racism as they begin to develop relationships with peers and begin to assimilate into the community [12].

Cultural Beliefs

Cultural and ethnic differences in perception of weight are driving factors in the obesity epidemic. Some countries and cultures consider a person's larger size and sedentary lifestyle a sign of health and status [13]. For instance, in Latino culture, an overweight child is considered to be a sign of health and of the parents' wealth, thus weight gain is viewed positively [14]. A study in 2003 found more obese boys than girls between the ages of 7 to 9 in the Northeast region of Thailand, which may reflect the cultural acceptance for boys to have excess weight, but not girls. Weight is also affected by the change in diet and activity as families move from one country to another. The prevalence of obesity increases the longer immigrants live in the United States. This has been observed in both Hispanic and Asian Americans born in the United States, as they were twice as likely to be obese as compared to their counterparts born elsewhere or newly immigrated. This is evidence that ethnic differences are strongly influenced by environmental factors [15]. In the United States, Davidson and Kanfl (2006) found that African Americans did not view obesity as a health concern but found it to be socially acceptable, adding to attractiveness and improving self-assurance [16]. White Americans, on the other hand, viewed obesity as a negative attribute, being seen as unattractive and socially unacceptable, leading to poor body image and negative health consequences.

With all of this in mind, the nurse will need to be familiar with the cultural perspectives related to obesity, nutrition, and activity when counseling the family and child in order to have a positive impact on health promotion. It is crucial to explain how these factors negatively impact their health and the potential for developing comorbid conditions. Families that work with nurses who understand their culture and are like them will be more helpful in making changes because the nurses will understand the families' foods, families, cultures, and lifestyles [17]. These culturally sensitive nurses can be instrumental in helping families becoming more healthy by promoting trust and communication.

IMPACT OF CHILDHOOD OBESITY

A direct correlation between increasing body mass index (BMI) and health risk has been identified. Therefore, early identification and intervention of obesity and related comorbidities is essential. Obesity is a chronic condition that, if left untreated, increases the risk for comorbid conditions in most obese individuals. If these conditions are acquired during childhood and no intervention for the obesity is provided, there is greater likelihood that these negative health effects will persist into adulthood, significantly impacting morbidity and mortality [18].

The rise in childhood obesity and obesity-related comorbidities is significantly impacting healthcare spending. The cost of treating obesity and its related comorbidities has neared $150 billion [2]. This will only increase as children are diagnosed at younger ages and require long-term treatment of comorbidities previously seen only in adults. Families may experience this cost in direct and indirect ways, as they must find ways to pay for medical care. It is crucial that nurses assist in the identification and treatment of obesity and related comorbidities at a much younger age.

As healthcare professionals, nurses are seeing adult health consequences in the pediatric population. It is critical, then, that nurses and nurse practitioners educate themselves on the potential serious health consequences of obesity in children and find ways to prevent these conditions from persisting into adulthood. Basic nursing training may have included pediatric nursing skills, but it does not adequately prepare the nurse to address issues unique to the overweight and obese child. Developmentally appropriate care is critical when caring for children, despite the fact that they are faced with adult health issues [2].

Nearly every system within the body has the potential to be negatively impacted by overweight and obesity, especially if left unidentified and untreated. This brings to light the role of the nurse in identifying children at risk for such comorbidities and intervening at all levels, depending on practice setting. Many serious health conditions once thought to be found only in adults are being diagnosed in children at increasingly earlier ages and at alarming rates. The long-term effects of this have yet to be uncovered.

Screening for Obesity-Related Comorbid Conditions

Children identified as overweight (BMI 84th to 94th percentile) or obese (BMI equal to or greater than the 95th percentile) are at an increased risk for developing comorbidities [19]. Once a child is found to be overweight or obese, the nurse should begin the process of screening for comorbidities associated with the child's unhealthy weight. Nurses in a variety of settings can participate in gathering the necessary history and physical findings and may even be able to order diagnostic laboratory studies as further evaluation for comorbidities. A thorough family history that includes first- and second-degree relatives can identify children at increased risk due to familial health conditions such as dyslipidemia, diabetes, and cardiovascular disease, driving the need for additional evaluation. Review of systems in the obese child may also prompt the need for further investigation into comorbidities. Regular screening of vital signs, including height, weight, and blood pressure, can be accomplished by nurses in many settings, including schools, health departments, and medical offices. Advanced practice nurses then play a significant role in performing physical assessments that can identify physical signs indicative of comorbid conditions related to obesity [20].

Cardiovascular disease, a leading cause of death in adults, is already being observed in children at very young ages. Dyslipidemia is currently the most prevalent obesity-related comorbidity seen in children. Therefore, regular screening by a nurse or healthcare provider should be standard in this population of children. For dyslipidemia that does not respond to lifestyle changes, the nurse should facilitate a referral to a pediatric cardiologist for additional evaluation [2, 18, 20].

Overweight and obese children are already experiencing systolic and diastolic hypertension and should be screened at every clinic visit. To ensure accurate blood pressure readings, it is important for offices to be equipped with blood pressure cuffs of an appropriate size, including extra long adult cuffs and thigh cuffs [20].

Also disturbing is the presence of insulin resistance, impaired glucose tolerance, and type 2 diabetes in childhood [7]. Acanthosis nigricans (AN), a sign of insulin resistance, is being observed more frequently in obese children and adolescents of all races and ethnicities. AN is a thickening or a darkening of the skin found along the neckline and in the axillae, as well as in flexor aspects of the body, abdominal creases, under the breast line, and on the elbows, knees, knuckles and other skin surfaces related to increased serum insulin levels, and it can be a precursor to type 2 diabetes [21]. Nurses in many settings can be trained to screen for this sign of insulin resistance and facilitate additional screening for these at-risk children. This provides an opportunity for nurses to educate families about insulin resistance and the increased risk of developing type 2 diabetes in overweight and obese children at a young age. Insulin resistance may be present despite the absence of AN; therefore, a nurse should consider screening laboratory studies that include a serum insulin level, as well as a fasting blood glucose level and lipid profile.

Another health concern on the rise in children is nonalcoholic steatohepatitis, or fatty liver disease. Previously, cirrhosis was correlated most significantly with alcohol consumption [21]. However, because of the increase in obesity, alcohol has been surpassed by fatty liver infiltrates as the leading cause of cirrhosis [7]. A large, school-based study of obese high school seniors nationwide found nonalcoholic fatty liver disease to be most common in the Latino population [14]. Screening for fatty liver disease should include serum Alanine transaminase (ALT) and Aspartate transaminase (AST), which are likely to be elevated. Children with an ALT or AST twice the normal level should be referred to a pediatric gastroenterologist or hepatologist for further evaluation [20]. Ideally, weight loss is the best treatment for fatty liver infiltrates and may require a very low calorie diet.

Exacerbation of other gastrointestinal problems, including gallstones and gastroesophageal reflux, is seen in obese children. There is greater prevalence of gallstones in overweight and obese children, as well as in children experiencing rapid weight loss. Treatment for gallstones and reflux in obese children is no different from that in children of normal weight. It is important, however, for nurses to be aware of the increased presence of these conditions in this population of children [20].

Respiratory issues are common in overweight and obese children. Children with asthma may find it more difficult to be physically active if the asthma is not well controlled. This can exacerbate weight gain and further decrease their level of activity. School nurses especially can work with the child's family and healthcare provider to ensure proper asthma management to encourage regular participation in physical activity. The occurrence of obstructive sleep apnea is much higher in children who are severely obese and impacts health negatively in a number of ways, including hypertension and ventricular hypertrophy [20]. Nurses should screen for symptoms of snoring with or without apneic periods, fractured sleep patterns, and frequent fatigue, and they should assess for enlarged tonsils on physical exam. If present, a referral for a sleep study is recommended. If sleep apnea is identified on polysomnography in an obese child, weight loss is recommended. Other treatment options may include removal of tonsils and adenoids or implementation of continuous positive airway pressure (CPAP) therapy [20]. Both of these treatments may facilitate the needed weight loss.

One frequently overlooked area in obese children is the skin. Nurses, especially from the inpatient setting, play an important role in identifying children at risk of developing skin breakdown as a result of their weight [2, 20]. Obese children and their families need to understand the importance of thorough skin assessments and good hygiene to prevent skin complications. Nurses in the hospital setting can encourage regular movement or repositioning to avoid skin breakdown at pressure points [2]. Preventing tubes and catheters from finding their way under pressure points also aids in prevention of skin breakdown. In the outpatient setting, nurses should educate children and their families about proper skin care at home. The skin folds should be kept dry, especially after bathing, by patting, not rubbing, the area, as friction causes irritation and breakdown. Topical antifungal creams and antibiotic ointments may be needed if infection is suspected. Use of bactericidal soaps may be helpful. For severe infections, systemic antibiotic treatment may be warranted [20].

Other obesity-related health conditions include pseudotumor cerebri, orthopedic problems, precocious puberty, and polycystic ovarian syndrome [2, 20]. Nurses can be instrumental in evaluating and referring children to specialists capable of treating these conditions.

Overweight and obese children are at risk not only for medical consequences related to their unhealthy weight. Being overweight or obese has psychosocial implications, especially in children. Quality of life is often impaired as a result of being obese. Overweight and obese children frequently suffer from depression, anxiety, and low self-esteem [2]. These can lead to lifelong mental health issues if not identified and treated early. These mental health problems often present because children in this population are often teased or bullied. They also may perpetrate the bullying, resulting in negative consequences such as punishment at school. To avoid these situations, obese children often isolate themselves socially.

Sometimes the negative feelings come as a result of discrimination experienced because of the child's size. Inadequate seating to accommodate an obese child may lead to that child seeking home schooling to avoid the embarrassment of not being able to sit in the regular school desks. Driving can be a struggle for some children who do not fit safely in a car. Children of this weight find it difficult to find clothing that is in fashion in their size. These all lead to low self-esteem and poor self-image, which may lead children to indulge in risky behaviors to gain acceptance from their peers.

NURSE'S IDENTIFICATION OF AT-RISK CHILDREN

Nurses are an invaluable resource when it comes to screening children for overweight or obesity. They provide care in a number of settings where they come into contact with children, giving them unique opportunities to conduct important weight screenings. Nurses, however, must be well educated in the tools currently available for taking this measurement so they may accurately identify children who are overweight or obese.

Tools for Measurement

Body fatness can be measured by a number of different tools such as bioelectrical impedance analysis (BIA), dual-energy X-ray absorptiometry (DEXA), hydrodensitometry, and skinfold thickness. Although these tools are excellent for assessing excess body fat, they have limitations, including ease of availability, expense, and lack of expertise in their use. In some countries, the percentage-weight-for-height (PWH) is used to screen children for obesity. This tool is based on a population-specific reference value, using the individual's weight to desirable height [22, 23].

The most widely accepted measure to identify those who are overweight and obese is the BMI. It is easy to use and correlates fairly well with the percentage of body fatness; however, it does not take into consideration lean muscle mass or the pregnant female. The BMI may not be a reliable tool to accurately assess all children of different ethnic groups due to their body composition [4]. A lower BMI may be associated with chronic disease in some groups, as seen in the Asian population [22]. Because a global measure for the identification of children who are overweight and obese has been difficult to establish and has not been standardized worldwide, the actual number of children at risk may be underreported [22, 24]. Until a universal, standardized measure is established, the BMI is the accepted tool for the assessment of children for overweight and obesity.

Categorization of weight based on BMI is different for children than for adults. For adults, a BMI greater than or equal to 25 kg/m2 is defined as overweight. A BMI greater than or equal to 30 kg/m2 is defined as obese [25]. For children, the BMI category is based on age and gender. Children with a BMI greater than or equal to the 85th percentile for age and gender are considered overweight. Those with a BMI greater than or equal to the 95th percentile are considered obese [20]. For children aged 2 to 18, the age and gender-appropriate growth charts should be used for plotting these growth points. The BMI is not used for children under 2 years of age, instead, the gender-appropriate, weight-for-length growth chart is used to follow their growth more accurately.

The child's weight and height should be plotted and evaluated at each visit regardless of age. Careful inspection for the rate at which the child's weight begins to advance should occur. A weight crossing more than 2 percentiles on the weight curve should prompt the nurse to screen for behaviors that are impacting weight, particularly with physical activity and nutrition, and to intervene early on to slow continued weight gain. The BMI should also be calculated and evaluated at each visit, not only at yearly well-child visits, to identify any upward trend in weight as early as possible, as prevention is key.

Nurses can use the BMI in most settings, as they will most likely have access to a scale and a way to measure the child's height. Nurses may, however, lack the knowledge and experience for identification of obesity. Moyers, Bugle, and Jackson (2005) found that only a third of school nurses used the BMI to assess for obesity, with half of the nurses using "eye-ball analysis" and four nurses not screening for obesity at all [9]. When the BMI is not used as part of the child's evaluation, at-risk children may be overlooked and not identified for intervention. Discussing the BMI chart with families can be a useful way for the nurse to help the family understand the seriousness of the child's weight and how it relates to potential comorbid conditions. The nurse can then discuss making healthy lifestyle changes to improve the child's health and decrease the risk for comorbidities. Regardless of the measure used to identify overweight and obese children, the nurse needs to be familiar with the tool being used, understand how to use it accurately and effectively, and include it as part of the child's evaluation in any setting [9].

Because children spend the major part of their day in school, this is a primary setting where nurses can positively impact health outcomes [1]. School nurses already share other important health information with families, which makes them a primary source to share obesity information with families. These nurses would also be able to help families find access to healthcare. School nurses support incorporating school health services and using schools as primary sites for obesity prevention and intervention [26]. This may be problematic, however, as fewer than 40% of nurses obtain weight, height and BMI screenings, with only a third of them agreeing that schools would be responsible for reporting these findings to families [26]. The ratio of students and schools to nurses available may also present a difficulty in obtaining the required information on all students, as well as follow through with families of at-risk children.

Nurses in the pediatric primary care setting play a role in identifying children at risk for being overweight and obese. Nurses in the pediatric office should obtain weight and height, calculate BMI, and plot all measures accurately on the gender-specific growth chart as part of the well-child visit, as well as most visits in between, to evaluate for normal growth and development. Frequent assessment of these measures allows for early identification of rapid increases in weight, which can be addressed before the weight gain becomes significant. Educating parents using BMI at each well-child visit regarding healthy lifestyles, including age-appropriate portion sizes and physical activity, is an important task for nurses in this particular setting.

The nurse has overlooked hospitals as a resource for identification of obesity. Many children are hospitalized each year, either in a children's hospital, on a pediatric unit in an adult hospital, or on a general hospital floor. Regardless of the reason for the admission, there should be an evaluation for childhood overweight or obesity risk. In the hospital setting, it is important to identify overweight and obese children to ensure that they are provided with the best care. They may need special equipment, such as a bariatric bed, wheelchair, bedside commode, or linens and gowns to make their hospital stay more comfortable. Nurses are in an excellent position to facilitate obtaining the necessary supplies. It is also important to make sure the blood pressure cuff is of adequate size to provide accurate blood pressure readings during the stay. This may prevent the need for additional, even unnecessary medical treatment.

Nurses working in the community are a valuable resource when it comes to screening for overweight and obese children. Churches and community centers are often venues where children participate in activities and could benefit from having a nurse available to do occasional health screenings and provide recommendations for referral for further evaluation of children who fall into at-risk categories.

NURSE'S ROLE IN PREVENTION AND TREATMENT IMPLEMENTATION

With the escalating trend of childhood obesity worldwide, the nurse's role must not only include identification of at-risk children but the prevention and treatment of obesity as well. Nurses must intervene on the patient level, as well as through community and legislative routes. However, as with many other healthcare providers, nurses often feel ill prepared for this task. A survey of nurse practitioners (NPs) through the National Association of Pediatric Nurse Practitioners (NAPNAP) found that many felt unprepared to effectively prevent and treat overweight and obesity [27]. Larsen et al. (2006) found that, although many NPs are aware of the prevention guidelines for pediatric overweight and obesity, few used BMI for age to target children at risk for obesity [28]. For this reason, it is imperative that nurses in all settings become proficient in providing care for children during this pandemic of childhood obesity.

The education of nurses regarding the worldwide problem of childhood obesity must start as early as nursing school. Curriculum within the pediatric nursing rotation should incorporate evidence-based guidelines for identification and treatment of childhood obesity, in addition to overall health and wellness [29]. Beyond early nursing training, it is important for nurses to pursue other educational opportunities on current health topics such as childhood obesity. Brief training, for example on the Healthy Eating and Activity Together clinical practice guidelines, offered through NAPNAP, increased practitioner knowledge and confidence in using weight management topics [27]. Education must include strategies for prevention, with nutrition education as early as the prenatal period; treatment through nutrition, physical activity, and behavior modification; and, finally, community intervention and political activism to combat childhood obesity.

Prevention

Prevention is key in combating childhood obesity, because the likelihood of untreated obesity as a child increases the risk of carrying the excess weight into adulthood. It is easier to prevent children from becoming overweight than it is to correct the problem [30]. Promotion of early healthy lifestyles can prevent or reduce negative health outcomes and establish long-term healthy behaviors [31]. Education on the prevention of overweight and obesity needs to be ongoing, from the prenatal period into late adolescence, and can be facilitated by the nurse in a variety of settings. Three critical periods exist during which factors can influence the development of obesity in children [32]. The first is during the prenatal period and early infancy. The second occurs from 5 to 7 years of age, when a rebound of adiposity may exist. Adolescence is the last critical period when obesity may develop. Involving communities, parents, and children for input and feedback on strategies to address health concerns such as obesity is important for success [33].

Weight and obesity are significantly influenced by early availability of nutrients during pregnancy [32]. Nurses caring for pregnant mothers should begin to educate the mother on proper nutrition for herself and the baby. Education should focus on healthy eating and physical activity to ensure adequate, not excessive, weight gain during the pregnancy, and the importance of carrying the pregnancy to term. A study of Colombian schoolchildren by McDonald et al. (2009) found a positive association between maternal BMI and child weight. Children of obese mothers were more than 3.5 times likely to be overweight than children whose mothers were of a healthy weight [8]. When parents are educated early on regarding healthy nutrition and activity, children are less likely to be overweight or obese at age 3 years [32]. Women who are overweight or obese during pregnancy are at increased risk of gestational diabetes, which can, in turn, lead to infants with excessive birth weight. Excessive birth weight has been identified as a risk factor for overweight status or obesity during adulthood [33]. Prematurity or low birth weight may lead to childhood weight gain, particularly during the period of adiposity rebound, from ages 5 to 7 years [32]. Nurses should also provide education on the risk of smoking during pregnancy. Smoking during pregnancy can lead to small for gestational age infants, which then also predisposes them to being overweight or obese as they get older [4].

It is a well-documented fact that breast milk is the ideal food for infants. It provides the precise nutrients the infant needs to grow and develop during the first 6 months of life [34]. Children who are breast-fed are at much lower risk of becoming obese than children who are formula-fed. Breast-feeding has been shown to have a protective benefit for obesity and overweight, as seen in a cross-sectional study by von Kries et al. (1999) in southern Germany [35]. Infants who breast-feed over a longer period have a much lower risk of becoming overweight or obese [32]. The high protein and nitrogen makeup of formula may have an effect on metabolism, causing an increase in insulin and insulin-like growth factor -1 (IGF-1), which may result in increased weight gain. Breast-fed babies may also be more proficient in self-regulating their intake as compared to formula-fed babies, who may be more likely to overeat [36]. Nurses in prenatal, perinatal, and pediatric settings can influence the likelihood of breast-feeding through proper maternal education. It is important for nurses to promote breast-feeding at all stages and provide the necessary support to mothers. Referring mothers to lactation consultants for additional support can be beneficial for the nurse who is unfamiliar with breast-feeding technique and troubleshooting.

As the infant grows, nurses can teach parents about feeding strategies that will help the baby grow at a normal rate. Timing for the introduction of solid foods in the first year of life can impact an infant's risk of overweight and obesity as he or she gets older. For each month that solid food introduction is delayed, there may be a 0.1% reduction in the risk of overweight at 3 to 5 years of age [36]. The American Academy of Pediatrics (AAP) recommends exclusive breast or formula feeding until 6 months of age. Nurses can play a role in educating parents on when to start solid food and the portion sizes appropriate for a child of that age.

Because children are often overweight by the time they reach school, parents have identified the need for interventions for healthy lifestyles to occur before the school-age years. Early education regarding healthy lifestyles needs to be directed at the parents, as they are the parties responsible for providing healthy nutrition and encouraging physical activity. This can lead to more positive outcomes regarding weight [31]. Nurses can be effective in repeatedly addressing these issues with parents at well-child checkups. As the child grows, feeding behaviors should continue to be monitored, and the child should have adequate physical activity in many forms including age-appropriate play, sports, and other physical activities.

Adolescents are a group at high risk for overweight and obesity, which can then lead to negative health consequences. During the adolescent years, children are exploring self-identity and struggle with body image. Risk-taking behaviors such as unhealthy eating habits and a sedentary lifestyle contribute to this risk. These lifestyle choices can also lead to psychosocial issues within this population [3]. As they get older, adolescents often move from their pediatric office to a family practice for their primary care. Nurses in either setting need to be aware of the risks of overweight and obesity and should provide preventive education to the adolescent and parents, if they accompany them to appointments. School nurses are also instrumental with this age group in promoting healthy lifestyles [3].

TREATMENT OPTIONS

Moving beyond prevention, nurses need to be prepared to provide education regarding treatment options available for children identified as overweight and obese. Treatment, however, will vary depending on the degree of overweight and obesity and the presence and extent of comorbidities [16]. The goal for overweight and obese children who have not yet developed comorbid conditions is to maintain or slow their weight gain as they grow taller, allowing the BMI to normalize. For those children already exhibiting comorbidities related to weight, a more aggressive weight loss of 1 to 2 pounds per month is recommended [18, 20].

Before addressing weight loss with a family, the nurse must first assess the family's and child's readiness to make change. If they are not motivated to make the changes needed for weight loss, then everyone will be frustrated and no forward progress will be made. Assessment of motivation can be accomplished through motivational interviewing (MI), the principles of which rely on the notion that changes in behavior are affected more by the level of motivation to make change than by the mere provision of information regarding the change [37]. MI involves the child or parent, depending on the age of the child, and can be used to find out the family's priorities for weight loss, what goals they would like to set, and how to achieve them [20]. The nurse must recognize that motivation fluctuates over time and can reassess accordingly. MI requires instruction on how to use it successfully, and practice to become proficient, which may be barriers to using MI.

Lifestyle Changes

The goal in lifestyle changes to encourage weight loss must focus on energy balance, which takes into account how much energy through calories goes into the body and the amount of energy expended through physical activity [34]. Overweight and obesity interventions need to address not only the energy imbalance that exists in the overweight state through education regarding nutrition and physical activity, but also other behaviors that lead to a healthier weight [10, 18]. In general, children must consume fewer calories and increase physical activity to lose or maintain weight. It is helpful for the nurse to remind families that even small changes in nutrition and physical activity can have significant impact on weight [2]. The nurse should stress that parental role modeling with food selection and activity can positively or negatively affect the weight of a child; therefore, parental involvement is key in treating obese children [38]. Young children will often mimic the actions taken by their parents regarding food and activity [2]. Weight-loss interventions are more positively reinforced when parents model healthy lifestyle behaviors than when they just talk about these behaviors with their children [31]. Many times parents and children have a good understanding of what constitutes healthy nutrition and physical activity, but this knowledge is not always put into practice [31].

Nutrition

The first component in the weight-loss intervention is finding ways to reduce calories in the child's diet without compromising normal growth and development. Nurses are able to provide basic recommendations regarding nutrition, but they should be able to refer families to dietitians for more detailed nutrition guidelines as appropriate. Especially in younger children, the parents heavily influence nutrition, as they are responsible for the food that is brought into the home and how it is prepared [2]. Parents need to be educated on simple ways to reduce caloric intake, such as limiting high-calorie beverages like soda and juice. Offering age-appropriate portion sizes is a topic that nurses can quickly review with families at well-child visits. As time allows, nurses can teach parents about reading labels so they can be making healthier food choices for their children [18]. Nurses can encourage children to eat three structured meals a day and recommend an increase in consumption of fruits and vegetables daily. Having regular family meals is a factor in weight management. Using a food journal helps families and children to become more aware of the type and quantity of food being consumed daily. Parents should be discouraged from using food as a reward for good behavior, as this effects the perception of that food as more desirable [32]. Nurses can provide information regarding the nutrient value of foods and encourage parents to look for high-nutrient, low-energy dense foods. Food models are useful in helping children practice making healthy food choices [32].

Certain behaviors surrounding food can lead to overweight and obesity. Where food is consumed is an important factor in weight. Watching television while having a meal or snack can lead to overeating. The television acts as a distraction, overriding the body's natural sensation of satiety, which causes an overconsumption of calories and, therefore, weight gain. The nurse should encourage families to eat all meals and snacks in the kitchen without the distraction of the television to promote weight loss.

Food is often seen as a comfort measure or coping mechanism. Children sometimes eat out of emotion, such as happiness, boredom, depression, and stress. This eating as a result of nonphysical hunger cues also leads to overeating and weight gain. The nurse can help the child explore why this type of eating is occurring and, if necessary, make a referral to a behavioral health professional to address any underlying psychosocial issues contributing to the weight gain.

Physical Activity

Physical activity is a critical piece in the weight management strategy. In addition to expending calories, physical activity has many overall health benefits [2]. Exercise has been shown to improve insulin resistance and hypertension in children with those conditions [39]. It can also improve self-esteem and decrease psychological issues such as depression and anxiety [39]. Children who are physically active tend to be more physically active as adults.

Defining physical activity for parents can be a challenge that the nurse can address. There is often a lack of understanding of how much energy is required to burn off excess calories eaten, such that some children think that any activity, included playing the piano, for example, is sufficient to counteract calorie intake [31]. Parents need to understand that physical activity is not busyness, but activity that causes an increase in heart rate, more so than with merely playing. Physical activity should be planned so that it takes place daily and should include parents, depending on the child's age. A study in 2003 found that children's sedentary activities were closely related to their parents, reinforcing the need for parental modeling in lifestyle changes [12].

One of the greatest concerns for children today is the amount of screen time they encounter on a daily basis. This includes time spent watching television, playing videos games, computer use, and cell phone texting. The AAP recommends limiting screen time to no more than 2 hours per day, except for children under the age of 2 years, who should not watch any television [39]. Lanningham-Foster et al. (2006) found that replacing sedentary screen time with more active screen time increased energy expenditure more than two-fold [40].

Nurses are beneficial in assessing the amount of physical activity and screen time that children are experiencing regularly and make recommendations based on the findings. Currently, 30 to 60 minutes of moderate physical activity is recommended for most days of the week beyond gym class. The nurse should encourage participation from the entire family in the activities. Nurses should remind parents that activities should be fun and age appropriate, and they can include organized sports, outdoor free play, and personal fitness.

Pharmacological Treatment Options

Beyond lifestyle changes and behavioral modification, there are limited resources available for the treatment of overweight and obesity in children and adolescents. At this time, the Federal Drug Administration (FDA) has approved two weight-loss medications for use in adolescents. Both the AAP and the Endocrine Society have established recommendations regarding the use of medications for weight loss, including a level of maturity in the child, which would allow the child to understand the risks and benefits of the use of pharmacological agents for weight loss. These should only be considered if the child and family have undergone intensive weight management through lifestyle modification without success. This would include adolescents with a BMI at or above the 95th percentile or those with a BMI between the 85th and 94th percentile with significant comorbidities. It is recommended that only tertiary care providers prescribe these medications. Nurse practitioners in the primary care setting should refer these adolescents to an appropriate center for initiation of these medications. They should also reinforce the need to maintain lifestyle changes along with the medication to improve the likelihood of successful weight loss [41]. Weight loss in adolescents using medications was approximately 3 kg more than those with diet alone [20]. It is important to remember, though, that weight-loss medications should not be used alone. Successful weight loss requires combination therapy with medication as well as lifestyle changes with nutrition and physical activity [2].

Sibutramine, or Meridia, has been approved by the FDA for patients 16 years of age and older. Its mechanism of action is to inhibit the reuptake of serotonin and norepinephrine in the brain, which leads to more rapid satiety [2, 41]. Sibutramine plus behavioral therapy has shown a greater mean weight loss than with placebo. Significant improvements in BMI, triglyceride levels, High-density lipoprotein (HDL) cholesterol levels, insulin levels, and sensitivity have also been seen. Side effects include tachycardia, hypertension, insomnia, palpitations, anxiety, and depression. In the adolescent population, there is also an increased risk of suicidal ideation, as with other antidepressant medications [41]. It is crucial for nurses to assess patients using this medication for all of the conditions previously discussed.

Orlistat, which is FDA approved for use in children 12 years of age and older, acts to inhibit pancreatic and gastric lipases, enzymes responsible for fat absorption. It prevents the absorption of fats by as much as 30%. This, however, is responsible for the most common adverse effects, including oily stools, abdominal discomfort, and flatulence. The oily stool is most often the reason patients discontinue orlistat. There may also be malabsorption of fat-soluble vitamins. Nurses following patients using orlistat should make sure the patient is taking a daily multivitamin to prevent this. A randomized control trial in adolescents found a significant decrease in BMI, waist circumference, and body with orlistat than with placebo. It is available over the counter as Alli and in prescription dose as Xenical. Because orlistat should be taken with meals, it may be a difficult treatment for an adolescent as this would necessitate taking medication at school [41].

Surgical Weight-Loss Options

For adolescents who have not had successful weight loss with lifestyle changes or weight-loss medication, bariatric surgery may be an option. Bariatric surgery leads to significant weight loss and often improvement in obesity-related comorbidities [20]. This is still a relatively new procedure in this age group, therefore long-term effects are yet unknown [2]. There are currently two procedures commonly used in adolescents: gastric bypass and adjustable gastric banding. Both procedures provide a restrictive component by creating a small stomach pouch, which leads to early satiety and, as a result, decreased caloric intake. Gastric bypass provides the additional component of malabsorption of nutrients in the small intestine. The sleeve gastrectomy, a restrictive procedure, is currently being considered as another option. None of these procedures, however, is a cure for chronic obesity. Bariatric surgery is a tool that must be utilized along with changes in nutrition, physical activity, and eating behavior.

The International Pediatric Endosurgery Group has established bariatric surgery candidate selection guidelines [41]. Criteria for the ideal bariatric candidate, however, vary by institution. It is generally accepted that adolescents be considered for bariatric surgery if they have a BMI of 40 kg/m^2 with the presence of comorbidities, or a BMI of 50 kg/m^2 [20, 41]. The adolescent should have reached physical maturity, which is generally thought to be age 13 years for females and

15 years for males. There also needs to be a significant degree of cognitive and emotional maturity. For this reason, psychological evaluation is very important in the candidate selection process.

In the primary care setting, the nurse practitioner can refer patients who may be good surgical candidates to centers performing bariatric surgery. Knowing this resource is available more widely adds to the NP's arsenal of weight-loss treatment options for the obese adolescent. Nurse practitioners may also play an active role in the 6-month preoperative medically managed weight-loss attempts required by most insurance companies and surgical programs. It is important to remember that successful bariatric surgery requires management by a multidisciplinary team, which should include the primary NP, both preoperatively and postoperatively. NPs in the primary care setting should maintain regular follow-up with these patients to continue managing comorbidities and monitoring vitamin levels, especially in the post-bypass patient. The NP should be aware of potential postoperative complications such as pulmonary embolus, wound infection or dehiscence, incisional hernia, anastomotic leaks, and vitamin deficiency and should help the patient seek immediate treatment from the surgical team. Another concern is the psychological impact of bariatric surgery, particularly in this already emotionally vulnerable population. Social eating situations can become a challenge in the adolescent; therefore, helping the adolescent adjust to a new way of eating requires ongoing care. The NP should also continue to monitor the adolescent for adherence to lifestyle changes for weight-loss success. Ensuring that the patient takes a daily multivitamin and calcium is crucial to stave off potential vitamin deficiency. The NP can also assess for adequate daily protein intake. It would be helpful for the NP to consult with the bariatric team to determine long-term management needs [41].

Nurses as Advocates for Childhood Obesity Policy

Beyond being aware of the increasing trend of childhood obesity globally, nurses need to take an active role in advocating for public policy that addresses this important issue. Nurses serve as advocates for our youngest patients, who rely on adults to provide an environment that promotes healthy living. Nurses, overall, are a trusted group within the community. Using this connection with families and the communities in which they work, nurses can have a significant impact on obesity prevention and treatment [42]. With nursing presence in settings such as schools, community health centers, pediatric offices, and hospitals, nurses bring a unique point of view and are in an excellent position to influence public policy for the prevention and treatment of childhood obesity [42, 43]. It is important to be aware of current public policy and any pending legislation regarding the childhood obesity. Nurses should contact local legislators involved with healthcare policy and work with professional nursing organizations to push for more awareness of the obesity epidemic and the need for action [44]. With the increasing cost of healthcare related to obesity and its comorbidities, nurses must advocate for public policy that addresses the prevention of obesity in settings such as schools, where children spend the majority of their day. School nurses are well positioned to fight for funding for increased obesity screening in schools. They can also advocate to keep physical education in school curricula and to work with communities to encourage physical activity in children. In collaboration with nutrition services and policy makers, nurses can work to ensure healthy food for school breakfast and lunch programs, which often provide most of a child's daily nutrition intake. Legislation regarding children's media exposure is also an arena for nurses to tackle. Children are bombarded daily with unhealthy food choices, which can easily influence what they are eating. Limiting a child's exposure to such potent messages is a critical piece in fighting obesity in this population. Sweden, for instance, prohibits the food industry from using cartoon characters to market food to children [7]. The nurse's role in the political arena is endless and can be powerful in influencing policy and legislation.

BARRIERS TO SUCCESSFUL TREATMENT

Many barriers have been identified when addressing obesity issues. Story et al. (2002) identified the most common barriers as lack of support services, parent involvement, and patient motivation [45]. Barriers to obesity management exist not only with children and their families, but with healthcare providers as well. Strategies for overcoming these barriers need to be defined in order to move forward with the prevention and treatment of obesity in children.

Provider Barriers and Healthcare Bias

Nurse practitioners themselves have identified the lack of time allowed for a visit as a barrier, with the visit time spent with patients decreasing by half in the past 13 years [46]. Half of the NPs identified lack of reimbursement as a major barrier to addressing obesity. Without sufficient reimbursement for obesity management, NPs are less likely to incorporate this into their care for patients. Practitioners also did not feel proficient when addressing behavioral techniques, family conflicts, or parenting strategies related to childhood obesity.

Providing education on these strategies, as well as obesity assessment and training in undergraduate and graduate nursing programs, would be beneficial. Continuing educational training for providers would be a useful tool in obesity management. Not being proficient in using techniques such as motivational interviewing to assess readiness for change is another barrier when addressing obesity. Workshops, seminars, and online training would be beneficial for obesity training for all healthcare providers [45].

Some of the barriers include biases held by healthcare providers about obese patients. Just under 37% of overweight children were informed that they were overweight by their clinician. Parents of children 2 to 11 years of age were less frequently informed that their child was overweight, where adolescents between 16 to 19 years of age were more frequently informed that they were overweight [38]. This is troubling because early intervention is instrumental in addressing and managing overweight children. Nurses have been found to have negative attitudes toward obese patients. They often feel obese individuals are lazy, lacking self-control and motivation for lifestyle changes. Almost 69% of British nurses related the obesity to being noncompliant with dietary and activity interventions. Nurses were frustrated with patients' noncompliance with weight-loss interventions, leading the nurses to feel that obesity management is futile [45, 47]. In one study, fewer than 22% of nurses felt they were effective in helping an individual to achieve weight loss. Obese individuals reported feelings of obesity bias by almost half of the nurses they encountered in one study [47]. Even bariatric surgery individuals reported bias from medical professionals. Nurses need to overcome their biases in order to help these children and families seeking medical care. Some medical providers have used scare tactics to motivate children and families to make lifestyle changes, going so far as to tell families not to get routine immunizations because it won't be effective due to the child's excessive weight. It is critical for nurses to face their bias toward obese individuals and implement behavioral changes in themselves so they can care for these patients more effectively and compassionately.

Unfortunately, as a result of healthcare bias and previous negative experiences with healthcare, obese patients frequently avoid medical care. This is detrimental to this population considering the considerable risk of comorbidity they are faced with. These patients fail to seek medical care because they are embarrassed to undress for physical exams because of their size. The medical office may not be accommodating to obese patients in the equipment available. It is important to assess the office environment for obese-friendly equipment, such as adequate seating, appropriate sized gowns, scales that are capable of obtaining an accurate weight, and blood pressure cuffs large enough to obtain an accurate blood pressure. Staff should be trained to be sensitive to obese patients and understand if the patient chooses not to be weighed at each visit. Again, motivational interviewing can be effective in assessing the child's or family's readiness to even discuss weight issues.

Parent Perception of Child's Weight

Parental identification of child's weight as a health risk and the parents' readiness for change is essential for successful weight loss [37]. If the parents do not understand their child's weight status and the significance of associated health risks, it will be more difficult for the nurse to address and implement a plan for healthy lifestyle interventions. Parents often underestimate the weight of their child, with girls being more frequently identified as overweight than boys. Many times, mothers identified their child's weight status in reference to physical limitations and social factors, not by the growth chart [38]. Mothers who are overweight are more likely not to see their child as obese, as seen by Women, Infants, and Children (WIC) providers who found that most of the mothers with overweight preschoolers in their program did not see their children as being overweight in any way [48].

The nurse who is aware of these factors will be better prepared to work with these families. Many families and children are not concerned with their weight because they look like everyone else in the family or feel that large size is an important feature. Clinicians must address the child's weight status with families at each visit, being sensitive to the family's perceptions of the weight. The parents may not have been educated on their child's weight and the potential for negative health consequences. The BMI growth chart is an ideal tool for educating the family regarding weight concerns. The nurse should be aware, however, that parents may not want to admit that their child is overweight. When implementing healthy intervention recommendations, the nurse must take these considerations into account in order to improve the rate of success.

Language and Cultural Barriers

As cultures immigrate and immerse in new societies, a basic understanding of these cultures will be critical in caring for these individuals. It is important to understand that culture's perception of weight in order to address the health risks associated with being overweight or obese. If the family members do not believe that their child is overweight, they are less likely to understand the need for lifestyle changes. This may have a negative impact on the child's overall health.

There is a strong need to have nurses that are culturally and linguistically competent, even being of the same culture or community, to facilitate the communication of healthy lifestyle choices. Being aware that a community is not composed exclusively of one culture also will be helpful to the nurse when addressing health issues. Nurses who are familiar with the culture of the community will be better suited to help families apply lifestyle changes that will promote weight loss; these nurses will also be able to present information on nutrition and physical activity in a culturally sensitive manner [17]. Nurses within these communities can lead by example, such as by preparing ethnic foods in healthier ways or by promoting physical activity by being active themselves. Culturally sensitive nurses will be instrumental in communicating with and developing tools and strategies to help families of diverse cultures to understand health-related consequences and to implement healthier lifestyle changes.

CONCLUSION

With the growing epidemic of childhood obesity, nurses are uniquely positioned to positively impact obesity prevention and treatment. Nurses come into contact with children in many settings, including schools, primary care offices, and hospitals. They have a responsibility in all settings to identify children who are at risk for becoming overweight or obese and ensuring that families are well educated regarding health promotion strategies to prevent further progression of obesity into the adult years. The challenge is to make sure nurses are, themselves, educated on the current obesity trends in children and recommendations available so they are as effective as possible in addressing this issue with families. Understanding the screening tools used to identify overweight and obese children is critical to early intervention, in hopes of reducing the likelihood of developing comorbidities related to the obesity. Nurses need to be aware of barriers to treatment, and they need a method of overcoming these obstacles in order to have a positive impact on health outcomes. Finally, nurses should take an active role in public health policy to focus more attention on the need for obesity prevention and treatment in children.

References

1. Flynn MAT, McNeil DA, Maloff B, Mutasingwa D, Wu M, Ford C, Tough SC. Reducing obesity and related chronic disease risk in children and youth: A synthesis of evidence with "best practice" recommendations. The International Association for the Study of Obesity, *obesity reviews* 2006;**7**(suppl. 1):7–66.
2. Gallagher Camden G. A captive condition: Childhood obesity. *Nursing Management* 2009;**40**(2):25–31.
3. Chen MY, Huang LH, Wang EK, Cheng NJ, Hsu CY, Hung LL, Shiao YJ. The effectiveness of health promotion counseling for overweight adolescent nursing students in Taiwan. *Public Health Nursing* 2001;**18**:350–6.
4. Hawkins SS, Cole TJ, Law C, the Millennium Cohort Study Child Health Group. An ecological systems approach to examining risk factors from early childhood overweight: Findings from the UK Millennium Cohort Study. *J Epidemiol Community Health* 2009;**63**:147–55.
5. Yensel CS, Preud'Homme D, Curry DM. Childhood obesity and insulin resistant-syndrome. *Journal of Pediatric Nursing* 2004;**19**:238–46.
6. Zametkin AJ, Zoon CK, Klein HW, Munson S. Psychiatric aspects of child and adolescent obesity: A review of the past 10 years. *FOCUS: The Journal of Lifelong Learning in Psychiatry* 2004;**2**(4):625–41.
7. Ben-Sefer E, Ben-Natan M, Ehrenfeld M. Childhood obesity: Current literature, policy and implications for practice. *International Nursing Review* 2009;**56**:166–73.
8. McDonald CM, Baylin A, Arsenault JE, Mora-Plazas M, Villamor E. Overweight is more prevalent than stunting and is associated with socioeconomic status, maternal obesity, and a snacking dietary pattern in school children from Bogota, Colombia. *The Journal of Nutrition* 2009;**139**:370–6.
9. Moyers P, Bugle L, Jackson E. Perceptions of school nurses regarding obesity in school-age children. *The Journal of School Nursing* 2005;**21**:86–93.
10. Paoletti J. Tipping the scales what nurses need to know about the childhood obesity epidemic. *RN* 2007;**11**:35–41.
11. Hsieh P, FitzGerald M. Childhood obesity in Taiwan: Review of the Taiwanese literature. *Nursing and Health Sciences* 2005;**7**:134–42.
12. Snethen JA, Beauchamp Hewitt J, Petering DH. Addressing childhood overweight: Strategies learned from one Latino community. *Journal of Transcultural Nursing* 2007;**18**:366–72.
13. Milligan F. Child obesity 1: Exploring its prevalence and causes. *Nursing Times* 2008;**104**:26–7.
14. Harrington S. Overweight in Latino/Hispanic adolescents: Scope of the problem and nursing implications. *Pediatric Nursing* 2008;**34**:389–94.
15. Kumanyika SK. Environmental influences on childhood obesity: Ethnic and cultural influences in context. *Physiology & Behavior* 2008;**94**:61–70.
16. Davidson M, Knafl KA. Dimensional analysis of the concept of obesity. *Journal of Advanced Nursing* 2006;**54**:342–50.
17. Parker S. *Fighting childhood obesity in minority communities*. Retrieved March 7, 2009, from, www.minoritynurse.com/obesity/fighting-childhood-obesity-minority-communities; 2005.
18. Harbaugh BL, Jordan-Welch M, Bounds W, Blom L, Fisher W. Nurses and families rising to the challenge of overweight children. *The Nurse Practitioner* 2007;**32**:31–4.
19. Nsiah-Kumi PA, Ariza AJ, Mikhail LM, Feinglass J, Binns HJ. Family history and parents' beliefs about consequences of childhood overweight and their influence on children's health behaviors. *Academic Pediatrics* 2009;**9**:53–9.
20. Barlow SE, the Expert Committee. Expert committee recommendations on the prevention, assessment, and treatment of child and adolescent overweight and obesity. *Pediatrics* 2007;**120**:S164–92.
21. Burke JP, Hale DE, Hazuda HP, Stern MP. *Diabetes Care* 1999;**22**:1655–9.

22. Yoo S, Lee S-Y, Kim K-N, Sung E. Obesity in Korean pre-adolescent school children: Comparison of various anthropometric measurements based on bioelectrical impedance analysis. *International Journal of Obesity* 2006;**30**:1086−90.
23. Fu WPC, Lee HC, Ng CJ, Tay YK, Kau CY, Seow CJ, Siak JK, Hong CY. Screening for childhood obesity: International vs. population-specific definitions. Which is more appropriate? *International Journal of Obesity* 2003;**27**:1121−6.
24. Wang Y, Lobstein T. Worldwide trends in childhood overweight and obesity. *International Journal of Pediatric Obesity* 2006;**1**:11−25.
25. World Health Organization. *Obesity and overweight fact sheet.* Retrieved June 19, 2009, from, www.who.int/mediacentre/factsheets/fs311/en/print.html; 2006.
26. Kubik MY, Story M, Davey C. Obesity prevention in schools: Current role and future practice of school nurses. *Preventative Medicine* 2007;**44**:504−7.
27. Gance-Cleveland B, Sidora-Arcolea K, Keesing H, Gottesman MM, Brady M. Changes in nurse practitioners' knowledge and behaviors following brief training on the Healthy Eating and Activity Together (HEAT) guidelines. *Journal of Pediatric Health Care* 2009;**23**(4):222−30.
28. Larsen L, Mandleco B, Williams M, Tiedeman M. Childhood obesity: Prevention practices of nurse practitioners. *Journal of the American Academy of Nurse Practitioners* 2006;**18**:70−9.
29. Ben-Sefer E. The childhood obesity pandemic: Promoting knowledge for undergraduate nursing students. *Nurse Education in Practice* 2009;**9**:159−65.
30. Wofford LG. Systematic Review of childhood obesity prevention. *Journal of Pediatric Nursing* 2008;**23**(1):5−19.
31. Hesketh K, Waters E, Green J, Salmon L, Williams J. Healthy eating, activity and obesity prevention: A qualitative study of parent and child perceptions in Australia. *Health Promotion International* 2005;**20**:19−26.
32. Sothern MS, Gordon ST. Prevention of obesity in young children: A critical challenge for medical professionals. *Clinical Pediatrics* 2003;**42**:101−11.
33. Williams C.L. Childhood obesity: New epidemic of an old disease. Retrieved June 20, 2009, from www.nestle-infantnutrition.com/clinicaltopics/artilces.aspx?articleId=B30E3026-B382-49D7-95D0-E1
34. Heinzer MM. Obesity in infancy: Questions, more questions, and few answers. *Newborn and Infant Nursing Reviews* 2005;**5**:194−202.
35. von Kries R, Koletzko B, Sauerwald T, von Mutius E, Barnert D, Grunert V, von Voss H. Breast feeding and obesity: Cross sectional study. *BMJ* 1999;**319**:147−50.
36. Hediger ML, Overpeck MD, Kuczmarski RJ, Ruan WJ. Association between infant breastfeeding and overweight in young children. *Journal of the American Medical Association* 2001;**285**:2453−60.
37. Söderlund LL, Nordqvist C, Angbratt M, Nilsen P. Applying motivational interviewing to counseling overweight and obese children. *Health Education Research* 2009;**24**:442−9.
38. De La O A, Jordan KC, Ortiz K, Moyer-Mileur LJ, Stoddard G, Friedrichs M, Cox R, Carlson EC, Heap E, Mihalopoulos NL. Do parents accurately perceive their child's weight status? *Journal of Pediatric Health Care* 2009;**23**:216−21.
39. American Academy of Pediatrics Council on Sports Medicine and Fitness & Council on School Health. Policy statement: Active healthy living: Prevention of childhood obesity through increased physical activity. *Pediatrics* 2006;**117**:1834−42.
40. Lanningham-Foster L, Jensen TB, Foster R, Redmond AB, Walker BA, Heinz D, Levine JA. Energy expenditure of sedentary screen time compared with active screen time for children. *Pediatrics* 2006;**118**:e1831−5.
41. Woo T. Pharmacotherapy and surgery treatment for the severely obese adolescent. *Journal of Pediatric Health Care* 2009;**23**(4):206−12.
42. Tao H, Glazer G. Legislative: Obesity from a health issue to a political and policy issue. *Online Journal of Issues in Nursing;*. Available, www.nursingworld.org/mainmenucategories/ANAmarketplace/ANAperiodicals/OJIN/Columns/Legislative/Obesity; 2005. Accessed September 9, 2009.
43. Sheehan NC, Yin L. Childhood obesity: Nursing policy implications. *Journal of Pediatric Nursing* 2006;**4**:308−10.
44. Henry LL, Royer L. Community-based strategies for pediatric nurses to combat the escalating childhood obesity epidemic. *Pediatric Nursing* 2004;**30**:162−4.
45. Story MT, Neumark-Stzainer DR, Sherwood NE, Holt K, Sofka D, Trowbridge FL, Barlow SE. Management of child and adolescent obesity: Attitudes, barriers, skills and training needs among health care professionals. *Pediatrics* 2002;**110**:210−14.
46. Briscoe JS, Berry JA. Barriers to weight loss counseling. *The Journal for Nurse Practitioners* 2009;**5**:161−7.
47. Puhl RM, Heure CA. The stigma of obesity: A review and update. *Obesity* 2009;**17**:941−64.
48. Chamberlin LA, Sherman SN, Jain A, Powers SW, Whitaker RC. The challenge of preventing and treating obesity in low-income, preschool children. *Archives of Pediatric Adolescent Medicine* 2002;**156**:662−8.

CHAPTER 7

Contemporary Racial/Ethnic and Socioeconomic Patterns in U.S. Childhood Obesity

Gopal K. Singh, Michael D. Kogan

U.S. Department of Health and Human Services, Health Resources and Services Administration, Maternal and Child Health Bureau, Rockville, MD, USA

INTRODUCTION

The prevalence of childhood obesity has increased dramatically in the United States, with the rate having risen more than three-fold since the mid 1970s [1–6]. Increases in obesity prevalence have been marked across all gender, race, and socioeconomic groups [1]. Because of a relatively high prevalence, a rapidly increasing trend, and the existence of large social-group disparities, childhood obesity is not only recognized as a major public health problem in the United States, but it has emerged at the forefront of the national health policy and research agenda [2–4, 6]. Monitoring obesity levels among different population subgroups and examining the role of socioeconomic and behavioral influences in obesity disparities represent an important research and policy focus [2–4, 6].

National prevalence estimates of childhood obesity are routinely available by age, gender, and race/ethnicity in the United States [1, 5]. Whereas childhood obesity estimates for non-Hispanic whites, blacks, and Hispanics are well documented, prevalence for other major ethnic groups in the United States, such as American Indians/Alaska Natives, Asians, Hawaiians, and Pacific Islanders, is less well known [1, 3–5]. Differences in childhood obesity rates by socioeconomic status (SES) have also been analyzed, albeit to a lesser extent [1, 3, 4, 6–8]; however, most studies have focused on the difference in obesity risks between poor and nonpoor children [1, 7, 8]. Analysis of inequalities in obesity prevalence according to a wider range of socioeconomic variables such as household income, education, and employment status is much less common [3, 4].

The analysis of racial/ethnic and SES disparities in childhood obesity is important for several reasons. First, obesity has been identified as one of the 10 leading health indicators for the nation, and reducing or eliminating racial and socioeconomic inequalities in health is one of the major goals of the national health initiative, *Healthy People 2010* [9]. However, social inequalities in health, disease, and mortality have not only remained substantial in the United States but have also increased over the past several decades [1, 4, 10–12]. Inequalities in chronic disease risk factors such as smoking, obesity, physical inactivity, and poor diet have contributed greatly to the persistence or widening of the social gradient in health [4, 10, 11]. Second, a contemporary analysis of ethnic and SES disparities is important in that it could help identify key population subgroups who are or remain at high risk of childhood obesity and who, therefore, can be targeted for obesity prevention programs [3, 6]. Third, documenting disparities between the least and most advantaged ethnic and socioeconomic groups can tell us the extent to which reductions in obesity prevalence can be achieved.

Note: The views expressed are the authors' and not necessarily those of the Health Resources and Services Administration or the U.S. Department of Health and Human Services.

The main objectives of this study are (1) to provide the latest estimates of obesity and overweight prevalence among U.S. children and adolescents aged 6 to 17 years from detailed racial/ethnic and socioeconomic groups using two large, nationally representative health surveys and data systems, (2) to examine racial/ethnic and socioeconomic gradients in childhood obesity and overweight risks after controlling for behavioral and neighborhood characteristics, and (3) to examine whether socioeconomic influences on childhood obesity vary across major racial and ethnic groups in the United States.

DATA AND METHODS

We used two different national health surveys to examine racial/ethnic and SES patterns in childhood obesity. These data systems and the measurement of dependent and independent variables are described next.

The 2007 National Survey of Children's Health (NSCH)

The data for in-depth analyses of racial/ethnic and SES disparities in childhood obesity came from the 2007 NSCH [13, 14]. This survey was conducted by the U.S. Centers for Disease Control and Prevention's (CDC) National Center for Health Statistics (NCHS), with funding and direction from the Health Resources and Services Administration's Maternal and Child Health Bureau [14]. The purpose of the NSCH is to provide national and state-specific prevalence estimates for a variety of children's health and well-being indicators [14]. It also includes an extensive array of questions about the family, including parental health, stress and coping behaviors, family activities, and parental concerns about their children [13, 14].

The 2007 NSCH was a telephone survey conducted between April 2007 and July 2008 [14]. It has a sample size of 91,642 children from birth through 17 years of age, including a sample of about 1800 children per state [14]. In the NSCH, a random-digit-dial sample of households with children <18 years of age was selected from each of the 50 states and the District of Columbia. One child was selected from all children in each identified household to be the subject of the survey. Interviews were conducted in English, Spanish, and four Asian languages. The respondent was the parent or guardian who knew the most about the child's health status and healthcare. The interview completion rate, measuring the percentage of completed interviews among known households with children, was 66% [14]. Substantive and methodological details of the 2007 NSCH are described elsewhere [14].

For the NSCH analysis, the dependent variables were the binary outcomes of overweight and obesity defined as body mass index (BMI) at or above the gender- and age-specific 85th and 95th percentile BMI cutoff points from the 2000 CDC growth charts, respectively [1–6, 15]. BMI in the NSCH was calculated from parent-reported children's height and weight data. Note that the overweight category (BMI ≥85th percentile) includes obese children (BMI ≥95th percentile). Analysis of obesity and overweight differentials was carried out for 44,101 children aged 10 to 17 years in 2007. Information on BMI was not available for children under age 10 in the 2007 public-use NSCH dataset [14].

Based on previous research, we considered the following sociodemographic and behavioral covariates of childhood obesity: age (10 to 11, 12 to 14, 15 to 17 years), gender, race/ethnicity (non-Hispanic white, non-Hispanic black, Hispanic, mixed race, American Indian/Alaska Native, Asian, Hawaiian/Pacific Islander, and other), household composition (two-parent biological or stepfamilies, single-mother, and other), metropolitan/nonmetropolitan residence, household poverty status measured as a ratio of family income to poverty threshold (<100%, 100% to 199%, 200% to 399%, ≥400%), parental education (<12, 12, 13 to 15, ≥16 years), household employment (employed or unemployed), social capital, perceived neighborhood safety (safe or unsafe), the amount of television viewing (<1, 1, 2, ≥3 hours/day), recreational computer use (<1, 1 to 2, ≥3 hours/day), and physical activity (0, 1 to 2, 3 to 4, ≥5 days/week) [2–4, 6, 7, 16, 17]. The measurement of social capital, a composite index, is described next. All other covariates were measured as shown in Table 7.1.

Social capital was defined by an index that measured parents' perceived level of neighborhood social support and combined four variables capturing social cohesion, trust, and reciprocity [3, 6, 18]. The four variables related to the following items: (1) people in this neighborhood help each other out; (2) we watch out for each other's children in this neighborhood; (3) there are people I can count on in this neighborhood; and (4) if my child was playing outside and got hurt or scared, there are adults nearby who I trust to help my child. The response codes for each of the four items ranged from 1 (*definitely agree*) to 4 (*definitely disagree*) and were summed to create a simple index that ranged in its value from 4 to 16, denoting highest to lowest levels of social capital. These variables were also factor analyzed, and the high factor loadings ranging from 0.81 to 0.86 confirmed the existence of a single scale [3, 6]. The reliability coefficient, Chronbach's alpha, for the index was 0.86. The social capital index scores were grouped into the following four categories: 4, 5 to 7, 8 to 10, and ≥11.

TABLE 7.1 Obesity (BMI ≥ 95th Percentile) Prevalence (Weighted %) and Odds among U.S. Children Ages 10–17 Years by Racial/Ethnic, Socioeconomic, Demographic, and Behavioral Characteristics: The 2007 National Survey of Children's Health (N = 44,101)

Characteristic	Prevalence %	SE	Age-gender adjusted OR	95% CI		Fully adjusted OR	95% CI	
Total population	16.37	0.49						
RACE/ETHNICITY								
Non-Hispanic White	12.86	0.49	1.70	0.86	3.36	1.55	0.72	3.35
Non-Hispanic Black	23.86	1.22	3.77	1.90	7.47	2.49	1.14	5.47
Hispanic	23.42	1.86	3.66	1.81	7.41	2.65	1.23	5.70
Non-Hispanic mixed race	14.16	1.86	1.90	0.91	3.96	1.57	0.68	3.65
Other	13.37	1.93						
American Indian	22.99	3.29	3.44	1.60	7.41	2.84	1.18	6.84
Asian	8.66	2.68	1.00	reference		1.00	reference	
Hawaiian/Pacific Islander	20.88	9.68	2.94	0.68	12.79	3.08	0.63	15.18
HIGHEST HOUSEHOLD OR PARENTAL EDUCATION LEVEL, YEARS								
<12	30.43	2.57	4.25	3.24	5.58	2.52	1.89	3.36
12	20.92	1.10	2.54	2.13	3.03	1.91	1.57	2.33
13–15	17.93	0.99	2.05	1.72	2.45	1.69	1.41	2.01
16+	9.74	0.52	1.00	reference		1.00	reference	
HOUSEHOLD POVERTY STATUS (RATIO OF FAMILY INCOME TO POVERTY THRESHOLD)								
Below 100%	27.37	1.56	3.43	2.73	4.30	2.23	1.67	2.98
100–199%	21.15	1.31	2.48	1.99	3.09	1.87	1.48	2.38
200–399%	14.51	0.78	1.52	1.23	1.87	1.34	1.09	1.66
At or above 400%	9.96	0.73	1.00	reference		1.00	reference	
HOUSEHOLD EMPLOYMENT STATUS[a]								
Employed	15.11	0.49	1.00	reference		1.00	reference	
Unemployed	26.05	1.92	2.00	1.61	2.49	1.56	1.22	2.00
CHILD'S AGE, YEARS								
10–11	22.75	1.15	1.95	1.63	2.32	2.23	1.84	2.69
12–14	15.64	0.77	1.22	1.03	1.44	1.22	1.03	1.45
15–17	13.30	0.71	1.00	reference		1.00	reference	
GENDER								
Male	19.19	0.69	1.54	1.34	1.78	1.70	1.46	1.98
Female	13.50	0.68	1.00	reference		1.00	reference	
HOUSEHOLD COMPOSITION								
Two-parent biological	13.60	0.55	1.00	reference		1.00	reference	
Two-parent stepfamily	19.11	1.81	1.56	1.21	2.00	1.29	0.98	1.68
Single mother	21.89	1.24	1.87	1.58	2.22	1.18	0.95	1.46
Other family type	19.11	1.37	1.54	1.26	1.88	1.15	0.92	1.45

(Continued)

TABLE 7.1 Obesity (BMI ≥ 95th Percentile) Prevalence (Weighted %) and Odds among U.S. Children Ages 10–17 Years by Racial/Ethnic, Socioeconomic, Demographic, and Behavioral Characteristics: The 2007 National Survey of Children's Health (N = 44,101)—cont'd

Characteristic	Prevalence %	SE	Age-gender adjusted OR	95% CI		Fully adjusted OR	95% CI	
PLACE OF RESIDENCE								
Metropolitan	16.19	0.56	1.00	reference		1.00	reference	
Nonmetropolitan	17.27	0.77	1.08	0.94	1.03	1.16	1.01	1.34
PRIMARY LANGUAGE SPOKEN AT HOME								
English	15.55	0.47	1.00	reference		1.00	reference	
Any other language	24.68	2.49	1.79	1.35	2.37	1.13	0.75	1.71
SOCIAL CAPITAL INDEX								
4 (highest)	14.13	0.74	1.00	reference		1.00	reference	
5–7	15.02	0.68	1.10	0.94	1.29	0.93	0.79	1.11
8–10	18.68	1.36	1.41	1.14	1.75	1.06	0.85	1.32
11+ (lowest)	26.48	2.58	2.29	1.71	3.07	1.24	0.89	1.73
PERCEIVED NEIGHBORHOOD SAFETY[b]								
Safe	15.53	0.51	1.00	reference		1.00	reference	
Unsafe	22.27	1.61	1.61	1.32	1.97	1.04	0.84	1.29
TELEVISION WATCHING (NO. OF HOURS PER DAY)[c]								
<1	11.03	0.89	1.00	reference		1.00	reference	
1	13.69	0.87	1.28	1.02	1.61	1.13	0.89	1.43
2	17.68	0.97	1.70	1.36	2.12	1.37	1.10	1.72
3 or more	22.57	1.11	2.31	1.85	2.88	1.52	1.19	1.93
COMPUTER USE FOR PURPOSES OTHER THAN SCHOOL WORK (NO. OF HOURS PER DAY)[d]								
<1	15.34	0.42	1.00	reference		1.00	reference	
1–2	15.43	0.45	1.12	0.95	1.30	1.08	0.92	1.26
3 or more	19.07	1.65	1.53	1.23	1.92	1.24	0.96	1.58
PHYSICAL ACTIVITY (NO. OF DAYS PER WEEK)[e]								
0	19.73	1.38	1.84	1.50	2.26	1.37	1.10	1.72
1–2	19.25	1.48	1.67	1.35	2.07	1.36	1.10	1.68
3–4	17.28	1.09	1.36	1.14	1.63	1.32	1.09	1.59
5 or more	14.24	0.61	1.00	reference		1.00	reference	

[a] A dichotomous variable denoting whether or not someone in the household was employed at least 50 weeks out of the past 52 weeks.
[b] Based on the question, "How often do you feel the child is safe in your community or neighborhood: never, sometimes, usually, or always?"
[c] Based on the question, "On an average school day, how much time (hours) does the child usually watch TV, watch videos, or play video games?"
[d] Based on the question, "On an average school day, how much time (hours) does the child use a computer for purposes other than schoolwork?"
[e] Based on the question, "During the past week, on how many days did the child exercise or participate for at least 20 minutes that made him/her sweat and breathe hard, such as basketball, soccer, running, or similar aerobic activities?"
SE = standard error; OR = odds ratio; CI = confidence interval. The chi-square test for independence between each covariate (except metro/nonmetro residence) and obesity prevalence statistically significant at $p<.05$.

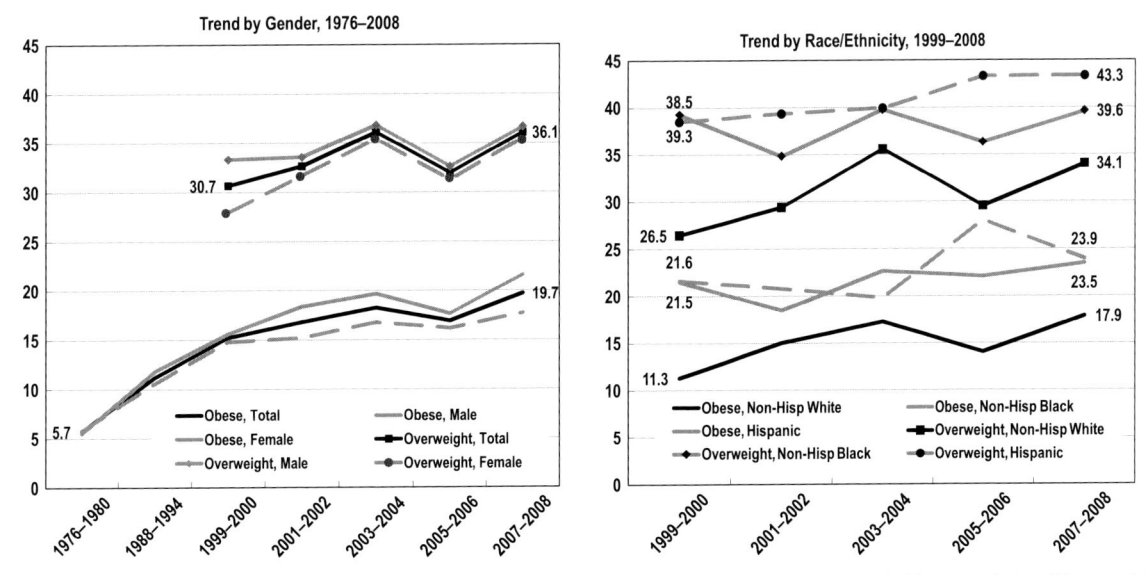

FIGURE 7.1 Race- and gender-specific trends in obesity and overweight prevalence (%) among U.S. children aged 6 to 17 years, 1976–2008.

The National Health and Nutrition Examination Survey (NHANES)

We also used the measured height and weight data for children aged 6 to 17 years from the NHANES to calculate BMI and to define binary outcomes of obesity and overweight using the BMI cutoff points described earlier [1, 19]. Since the mid 1970s, the NHANES surveys have been conducted periodically by the NCHS to obtain data on chronic disease prevalence and risk factors such as obesity, smoking, hypertension, cholesterol levels, diet, and nutritional factors [1, 19]. Beginning in 1999, the NHANES became a continuous annual survey using a complex, stratified, multistage probability clustered sample design, collecting data for a representative sample of the U.S. civilian population. The NHANES data are based on clinical examinations, selected medical and laboratory tests, and in-home person interviews [1, 19].

For the analysis presented in Table 7.4 (presented later in the chapter), we pooled 6 years of the NHANES data from 2003 through 2008, although we also analyzed 1999–2000 and 2001–2002 data for race and gender-specific trends shown in Figure 7.1. The overall response rate in the NHANES for both interview and examination components was at least 76% in each of the five waves, 1999–2000, 2001–2002, 20003–2004, 2005–2006, and 2007–2008 [1, 19]. Substantive and methodological details of the NHANES are described elsewhere [1, 19].

We conducted multivariate analyses of the 2003–2008 NHANES data for 7510 children aged 6 to 17 years for whom BMI information was available. The covariate analysis of the NHANES data is somewhat limited because of a lack of data on detailed demographic and behavioral covariates of childhood obesity. We considered four covariates for the NHANES analysis: child's age (6 to 9, 10 to 11, 12 to 14, 15 to 17), gender, race/ethnicity (non-Hispanic white, non-Hispanic black, Hispanic, and all other ethnic groups), and household poverty status (<100%, 100% to 199%, 200% to 399%, and ≥400% of poverty level). Unlike the NSCH, American Indians/Alaska Natives, Asians, Hawaiians/Pacific Islanders, and mixed-race children were not identified as separate groups in the NHANES.

Statistical Analysis

Prevalence (%) of childhood obesity and overweight were computed for all racial/ethnic and socioeconomic groups. The χ^2 statistic was used to test the overall association between each covariate and obesity or overweight prevalence. To estimate obesity and overweight differentials by race/ethnicity and socioeconomic factors, we fitted two sets of logistic regression models keeping in mind the causal sequencing of the covariates with obesity [3, 4, 6]. The first set of models presents age- and gender-adjusted odds of obesity and overweight associated with each sociodemographic or behavioral factor. The second set of models in the NSCH analysis consists of full models showing the net effects of race/ethnicity, SES, and demographic factors after adjusting for differences in physical activity and sedentary behaviors. To account for the complex sample designs of the NSCH and NHANES, SUDAAN software was used to conduct all statistical analyses [20].

RESULTS

Trends in Obesity and Overweight Prevalence

In addition to the analysis of the 1999–2008 NHANES data, we used published statistics from the 1976–1980 and 1988–1994 NHANES to describe long-term trends in childhood obesity [1]. The prevalence of obesity among children aged 6 to 17 increased sharply between 1976 and 2008 for the total child population as well as for male and female children (Fig. 7.1). The obesity prevalence for male children quadrupled from 5.5% in 1976–1980 to 21.6% in 2007–2008; for female children, the obesity prevalence tripled during the same period. The average annual rate of increase in obesity prevalence was 4.5% for male children and 3.8% for female children. Between 1999 and 2008, the obesity prevalence increased by 58% for non-Hispanic white children aged 6 to 17, 9% for black children, and 11% for Hispanic children. The overweight prevalence for non-Hispanic white children rose by 29% from 26.5% in 1999–2000 to 34.1% in 2007–2008.

Disparities in Socioeconomic Conditions and Obesity-Related Behaviors

In this section, we describe sociodemographic characteristics and obesity-related health behaviors of U.S. children according to their race/ethnicity and household socioeconomic status by using data from the 2007 NSCH. Socioeconomic conditions vary greatly across children in various racial/ethnic groups (Fig. 7.2). In 2007, approximately 19% of U.S. children under 18 years of age lived below the poverty line. At least one-third of Hispanic, black, and American Indian/Alaska Native children lived below the poverty line compared with 9% of non-Hispanic white children and 10% of Asian children. Children in ethnic-minority and socially disadvantaged groups were generally more likely to live in neighborhoods with unfavorable physical or built environmental characteristics. In 2007, 26% of black children and 23% of Hispanic children lived in unsafe neighborhoods as compared with 8% of non-Hispanic white children. About 20% to 30% of black and Hispanic children

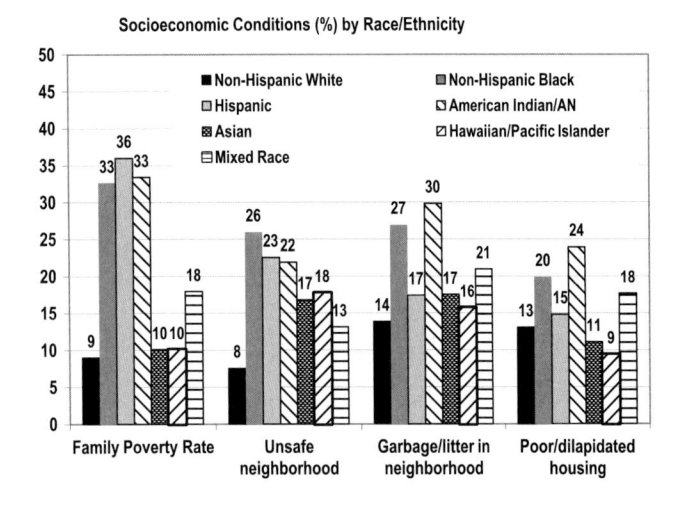

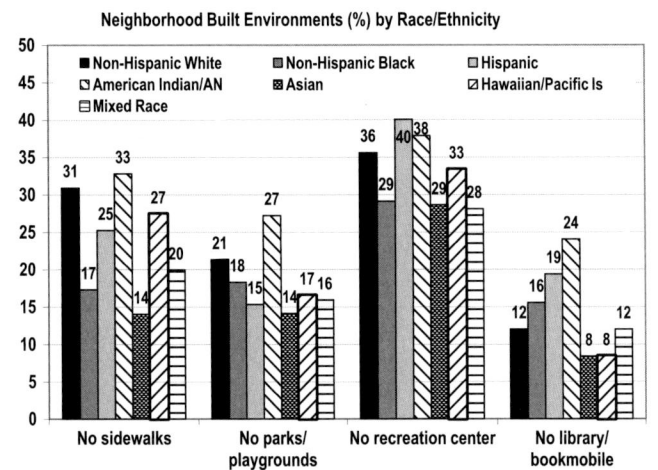

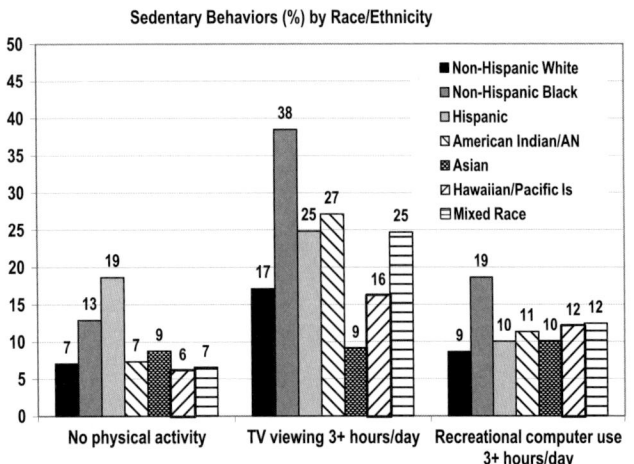

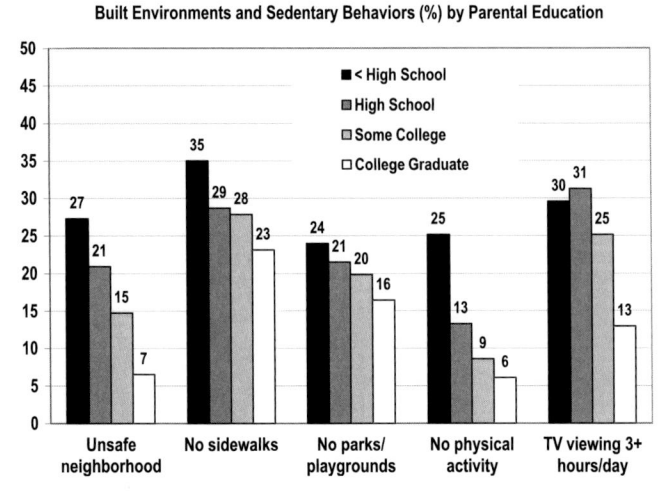

FIGURE 7.2 Socioeconomic conditions and obesity-related behaviors of U.S. children according to race/ethnicity and parental education: The 2007 National Survey of Children's Health (N = 91,532).

lived in neighborhoods with litter/garbage on streets or sidewalks or in neighborhoods with poor/dilapidated housing compared with 14% of non-Hispanic white children. About 27% of children of parents without a high school diploma lived in unsafe neighborhoods as compared with 7% of children whose parents had a college degree. About 35% of children from low-education households did not have neighborhood access to sidewalks or walking paths and 24% had no access to parks/playgrounds, compared with 23% and 16% of children from high-education households, respectively (Fig. 7.2).

Ethnic-minority children were generally more likely to engage in sedentary behaviors than non-Hispanic white children. Nineteen percent of Hispanic children and 13% of black children were physically inactive compared with 7% of non-Hispanic white children. Thirty-eight percent of black children, 27% of American Indian/Alaska Native children, and 25% of Hispanic children watched television ≥3 hours/day compared with only 9% of Asian children. Furthermore, children from lower SES households were considerably more likely to be physically inactive, watch higher amounts of daily television, and engage in higher levels of recreational computer use than children from higher SES groups. Household income gradients in the built environmental characteristics and obesity-related behaviors were similar to those for parental education (data not shown).

Racial/Ethnic and Socioeconomic Disparities in Obesity and Overweight Risks

Table 7.1, based on the analysis of the 2007 NSCH, shows substantial racial/ethnic and socioeconomic inequalities in obesity and overweight prevalence for children aged 10 to 17 years. In 2007, 16.4% of U.S. children were obese and 31.6% were overweight. The obesity prevalence was highest among non-Hispanic black children (23.9%), followed by Hispanic children (23.4%), American Indian/Alaska Native children (23.0%), Hawaiian/Pacific Islander children (20.9%), mixed-race children (14.2%), and Asian children (8.7%). The overweight prevalence ranged from a low of 18.4% for Asian children to a high of 44.3% for Hawaiian/Pacific Islander children; 41% of black and Hispanic children were overweight (Table 7.2).

The obesity and overweight prevalence increased significantly in relation to decreased levels of household income and education, neighborhood social capital, perceived neighborhood safety, physical activity, and increased levels of television viewing and recreational computer use. The prevalence was also significantly higher among children from single-parent and non-English-speaking households and from higher unemployment households (Tables 7.1 and 7.2). Specifically, the obesity prevalence for children with parents <12 years of education was 30.4% in 2007, 3.1 times higher than the prevalence (9.7%) for children whose parents had a college degree. The obesity prevalence for children living below the poverty line was 27.4%, 2.7 times higher than the prevalence (10.0%) for children with family income exceeding 400% of the poverty threshold (Table 7.1). Nearly half of all children in low-education and low-income stratum were overweight, compared with less than 23% of children in high-education or high-income stratum (Table 7.2).

Tables 7.1 and 7.2 also show age-gender-adjusted and fully adjusted odds of obesity and overweight, respectively. In 2007, black and Hispanic children had about two-fold higher odds of obesity and overweight than non-Hispanic white children. After adjusting for age and gender, Hispanic, non-Hispanic black, and American Indian/Alaska Native children had 3.4 to 3.8 times higher odds of obesity and 3.0 to 3.5 times higher odds of overweight than Asian children. Children of mixed ethnicity and Hawaiian/Pacific Islander children had 2.6 and 3.9 times higher odds of being overweight than Asian children, respectively.

Age- and gender-adjusted socioeconomic gradients in obesity and overweight were quite pronounced in 2007 (Tables 7.1 and 7.2). Children whose parents had <12 and 12 years of education had, respectively, 325% and 154% higher odds of obesity than children whose parents had a college degree. Income gradients were quite steep as well. Children living below the poverty line had 243% higher odds of obesity and 187% higher odds of being overweight than children with family income exceeding 400% of the poverty threshold. Children from higher-unemployment households had 100% and 54% higher odds of obesity and overweight, respectively.

Racial/ethnic and socioeconomic gradients in obesity and overweight risks persisted and remained substantial even after taking into account behavioral factors (fully adjusted models of Tables 7.1 and 7.2). Black, Hispanic, and American Indian/Alaska Native children had 2.5 to 2.8 times higher adjusted odds of obesity and overweight than their Asian counterparts. Children in the lowest income and education households had at least 123% higher adjusted odds of being obese and at least 71% higher adjusted odds of being overweight than children in the highest income and education households. Children from unemployed households had 56% higher adjusted odds of obesity than children from employed households.

Behavioral factors contributed significantly to disparities in childhood obesity and overweight even after controlling for ethnic and socioeconomic characteristics. Children who watched television ≥3 hours/day had 52% higher odds of obesity and 54% higher odds of

TABLE 7.2 Overweight (BMI ≥85th Percentile) Prevalence (Weighted %) and Odds among U.S. Children Ages 10–17 Years by Racial/Ethnic, Socioeconomic, Demographic, and Behavioral Characteristics: The 2007 National Survey of Children's Health (N = 44,101)

Characteristic	Prevalence %	SE	Age-gender adjusted OR	95% CI		Fully adjusted OR	95% CI	
Total population	31.64	0.59						
RACE/ETHNICITY								
Non-Hispanic White	26.84	0.60	1.76	1.11	2.79	1.60	0.95	2.68
Non-Hispanic Black	41.12	1.46	3.46	2.16	5.55	2.46	1.44	4.20
Hispanic	40.96	2.13	3.41	2.09	5.57	2.77	1.64	4.70
Non-Hispanic mixed race	34.80	2.67	2.57	1.54	4.28	2.11	1.19	3.73
Other	26.72	2.47						
American Indian	38.22	3.83	2.96	1.69	5.18	2.46	1.32	4.59
Asian	18.45	3.54	1.00	reference		1.00	reference	
Hawaiian/Pacific Islander	44.32	11.11	3.85	1.50	9.88	4.07	1.66	9.97
HIGHEST HOUSEHOLD OR PARENTAL EDUCATION LEVEL, YEARS								
<12	47.39	2.67	3.17	2.52	4.00	2.11	1.64	2.71
12	38.25	1.34	2.17	1.88	2.50	1.75	1.49	2.06
13–15	34.17	1.11	1.78	1.56	2.03	1.52	1.33	1.74
16+	22.78	0.77	1.00	reference		1.00	reference	
HOUSEHOLD POVERTY STATUS (RATIO OF FAMILY INCOME TO POVERTY THRESHOLD)								
Below 100%	45.07	1.68	2.87	2.43	3.39	2.11	1.69	2.62
100–199%	37.98	1.46	2.17	1.85	2.54	1.73	1.45	2.06
200–399%	30.44	1.05	1.51	1.31	1.75	1.36	1.18	1.58
At or above 400%	22.33	0.86	1.00	reference		1.00	reference	
HOUSEHOLD EMPLOYMENT STATUS								
Employed	30.51	0.61	1.00	reference		1.00	reference	
Unemployed	40.08	2.02	1.54	1.28	1.84	1.20	0.97	1.48
CHILD'S AGE, YEARS								
10–11	39.92	1.28	1.85	1.61	2.13	2.13	1.84	2.47
12–14	31.73	0.96	1.29	1.14	1.46	1.32	1.16	1.5
15–17	26.60	0.90	1.00	reference		1.00	reference	
GENDER								
Male	34.49	0.80	1.32	1.19	1.47	1.40	1.25	1.58
Female	28.73	0.86	1.00	reference		1.00	reference	
HOUSEHOLD COMPOSITION								
Two-parent biological	28.66	0.74	1.00	reference		1.00	reference	
Two-parent stepfamily	31.91	1.84	1.21	1.00	1.45	0.97	0.8	1.17
Single mother	39.20	1.35	1.67	1.46	1.91	1.11	0.94	1.31
Other family type	34.33	1.76	1.34	1.12	1.59	0.99	0.82	1.2

(Continued)

TABLE 7.2 Overweight (BMI ≥85th Percentile) Prevalence (Weighted %) and Odds among U.S. Children Ages 10–17 Years by Racial/Ethnic, Socioeconomic, Demographic, and Behavioral Characteristics: The 2007 National Survey of Children's Health (N = 44,101)—cont'd

Characteristic	Prevalence %	SE	Age-gender adjusted OR	95% CI		Fully adjusted OR	95% CI	
PLACE OF RESIDENCE								
Metropolitan	31.12	0.68	1.00	reference		1.00	reference	
Nonmetropolitan	34.28	0.94	1.16	1.04	1.28	1.21	1.08	1.35
PRIMARY LANGUAGE SPOKEN AT HOME								
English	30.77	0.58	1.00	reference		1.00	reference	
Any other language	40.45	2.77	1.53	1.20	1.95	0.98	0.69	1.38
SOCIAL CAPITAL INDEX								
4 (highest)	28.48	0.95	1.11	0.98	1.25	0.98	0.86	1.11
5–7	30.17	0.88	1.31	1.11	1.55	1.03	0.87	1.23
8–10	34.07	1.55	2.20	1.75	2.76	1.34	1.02	1.76
11+ (lowest)	45.70	2.61	1.00	reference		1.00	reference	
PERCEIVED NEIGHBORHOOD SAFETY								
Safe	30.64	0.62	1.00	reference		1.00	reference	
Unsafe	38.24	1.82	1.43	1.22	1.69	0.96	0.8	1.15
TELEVISION WATCHING (NO. OF HOURS PER DAY)								
<1	23.27	1.21	1.00	reference		1.00	reference	
1	28.68	1.11	1.33	1.12	1.58	1.23	1.03	1.46
2	33.98	1.10	1.67	1.42	1.97	1.45	1.22	1.72
3 or more	39.18	1.26	2.11	1.78	2.50	1.54	1.28	1.86
COMPUTER USE FOR PURPOSES OTHER THAN SCHOOL WORK (NO. OF HOURS PER DAY)								
<1	30.34	0.87	1.00	reference		1.00	reference	
1–2	30.60	0.88	1.11	0.99	1.25	1.07	0.95	1.21
3 or more	35.55	1.78	1.49	1.25	1.78	1.20	0.99	1.46
PHYSICAL ACTIVITY (NO. OF DAYS PER WEEK)								
0	35.95	1.85	1.71	1.43	2.05	1.37	1.14	1.65
1–2	36.18	1.77	1.62	1.37	1.93	1.43	1.20	1.70
3–4	33.51	1.22	1.36	1.20	1.55	1.33	1.15	1.52
5 or more	28.30	0.75	1.00	reference		1.00	reference	

SE = standard error; OR = odds ratio; CI = confidence interval. The chi-square test for independence between each covariate and overweight prevalence statistically significant at $p < .05$.

being overweight than those who watched television <1 hour/day. Children who did not engage in any vigorous physical activity had 37% higher odds of obesity or overweight than those who exercised ≥5 days/week.

Household income, education, and employment were all significantly related to obesity and overweight risks among children in each of the major racial/ethnic groups (Table 7.3). Income and education gradients in obesity and overweight risks were larger for Hispanic and non-Hispanic white children than for black children. The SES gradients were steepest for children in the residual ethnic category "all other races"; children in this ethnically heterogeneous group had more than six-fold higher odds of obesity in the low-education category than their counterparts in the high-education category. Moreover, within each SES stratum, important ethnic disparities exist. Note, for example,

TABLE 7.3 Joint Effects of Race/Ethnicity and Household Socioeconomic Status on Obesity and Overweight Prevalence and Odds among U.S. Children Ages 10–17 Years: The 2007 National Survey of Children's Health

	Obesity (BMI ≥ 95th percentile)					Overweight (BMI ≥ 85th percentile)				
	Prevalence		Age-sex adjusted			Prevalence		Age-sex adjusted		
	%	SE	OR	95% CI		%	SE	OR	95% CI	
RACE/ETHNICITY* HOUSEHOLD POVERTY STATUS										
Non-Hispanic White										
<100% of poverty level	20.82	1.68	2.72	2.08	3.54	39.75	2.26	2.48	2.00	3.07
100–199% of poverty level	20.17	1.72	2.63	2.03	3.41	35.77	1.77	2.10	1.76	2.50
200–399% of poverty level	12.38	0.73	1.45	1.17	1.80	26.54	1.00	1.35	1.16	1.56
At or above 400% of poverty level	8.77	0.69	1.00	reference		20.93	0.84	1.00	reference	
Non-Hispanic Black										
<100% of poverty level	28.89	2.56	2.20	1.39	3.49	44.96	2.72	1.90	1.31	2.77
100–199% of poverty level	22.79	2.33	1.66	1.04	2.65	42.88	3.15	1.81	1.22	2.69
200–399% of poverty level	23.83	2.22	1.68	1.08	2.63	40.46	2.62	1.57	1.08	2.30
At or above 400% of poverty level	16.33	2.42	1.00	reference		31.76	3.64	1.00	reference	
Hispanic										
<100% of poverty level	32.86	3.71	2.60	1.11	6.07	51.06	3.87	2.61	1.43	4.77
100–199% of poverty level	24.38	3.76	1.73	0.73	4.12	39.20	4.07	1.61	0.87	2.97
200–399% of poverty level	16.97	3.38	1.05	0.42	2.66	39.54	4.39	1.60	0.85	3.03
At or above 400% of poverty level	16.67	5.34	1.00	reference		28.97	5.41	1.00	reference	
All other										
<100% of poverty level	25.50	5.55	3.74	2.01	6.96	42.82	5.26	3.02	1.84	4.95
100–199% of poverty level	14.63	2.80	1.87	1.08	3.25	34.99	4.33	2.18	1.38	3.44
200–399% of poverty level	13.48	2.64	1.68	0.95	2.97	30.88	3.72	1.74	1.11	2.71
At or above 400% of poverty level	8.22	1.19	1.00	reference		19.90	2.15	1.00	reference	
RACE/ETHNICITY* PARENTAL EDUCATION										
Non-Hispanic White										
Less than high school	24.01	2.66	3.73	2.74	5.06	41.24	3.15	3.03	2.32	3.95
High school	19.59	1.36	2.71	2.18	3.36	36.79	1.58	2.39	2.04	2.8
Some college	14.22	1.04	1.84	1.48	2.28	29.47	1.19	1.71	1.48	1.97
College graduate	8.48	0.54	1.00	reference		20.07	0.70	1.00	reference	
Non-Hispanic Black										
Less than high school	31.77	4.29	2.06	1.3	3.27	48.63	4.38	1.78	1.18	2.68
High school	22.09	1.99	1.27	0.89	1.83	37.95	2.46	1.16	0.84	1.59
Some college	27.26	2.26	1.59	1.11	2.29	45.96	2.55	1.53	1.11	2.1
College graduate	19.12	2.27	1.00	reference		36.55	3.08	1.00	reference	
Hispanic										
Less than high school	33.32	4.72	3.43	1.77	6.65	50.18	4.86	2.19	1.27	3.78
High school	24.48	3.45	2.28	1.23	4.23	42.75	4.24	1.68	1.00	2.83
Some college	22.66	3.67	2.01	1.05	3.87	39.80	3.92	1.47	0.88	2.44
College graduate	12.89	2.92	1.00	reference		31.51	4.52	1.00	reference	

(Continued)

TABLE 7.3 Joint Effects of Race/Ethnicity and Household Socioeconomic Status on Obesity and Overweight Prevalence and Odds among U.S. Children Ages 10–17 Years: The 2007 National Survey of Children's Health—cont'd

	Obesity (BMI ≥ 95th percentile)					Overweight (BMI ≥ 85th percentile)				
	Prevalence		Age-sex adjusted			Prevalence		Age-sex adjusted		
	%	SE	OR	95% CI		%	SE	OR	95% CI	
All other										
Less than high school	28.89	6.09	6.08	3.24	11.42	45.72	6.63	3.50	2.00	6.14
High school	16.73	3.58	2.99	1.67	5.36	36.82	4.76	2.46	1.52	3.99
Some college	17.36	3.31	2.91	1.67	5.07	34.20	4.06	1.90	1.17	3.08
College graduate	6.64	0.90	1.00	reference		20.82	2.51	1.00	reference	
RACE/ETHNICITY* HOUSEHOLD EMPLOYMENT STATUS										
Non-Hispanic White										
Employed	20.93	2.31	1.00	reference		34.26	2.51	1.00	reference	
Unemployed	12.17	0.50	1.96	1.46	2.62	26.21	0.61	1.49	1.19	1.87
Non-Hispanic Black										
Employed	28.31	3.06	1.00	reference		43.28	3.42	1.00	reference	
Unemployed	22.87	1.32	1.35	0.98	1.86	40.59	1.62	1.15	0.86	1.53
Hispanic										
Employed	32.49	5.06	1.00	reference		46.87	5.20	1.00	reference	
Unemployed	21.38	1.96	1.80	1.06	3.05	39.64	2.34	1.35	0.85	2.16
All other										
Employed	24.43	6.89	1.00	reference		38.20	6.45	1.00	reference	
Unemployed	11.89	1.30	2.46	1.14	5.32	28.11	2.07	1.58	0.86	2.89

approximately two-fold higher obesity prevalence among Hispanic children (16.7%) and black children (16.3%) than among non-Hispanic white children (8.8%) in the highest income category, or a two-fold black/white difference in obesity prevalence among children of college graduates (Table 7.3).

The NHANES analysis shows significantly higher obesity and overweight prevalence in 2007–2008 among Hispanic and black children aged 6 to 17 years than among non-Hispanic white children (Table 7.4). As mentioned earlier, detailed racial/ethnic disparities could not be shown for the NHANES because of lack of detailed ethnic information. Similar to the NSCH analysis, the income gradients in the NHANES-based obesity prevalence were quite pronounced. Even after adjusting for age, gender, and race/ethnicity, children aged 6 to 17 years living below the poverty line had 100% higher odds of obesity and 62% higher odds of being overweight than children with family incomes exceeding 400% of the poverty threshold. Even after adjusting for income differences, Hispanic children aged 6 to 17 years had 36% to 40% higher odds of obesity and overweight and black children had 32% higher odds of obesity than their non-Hispanic white counterparts.

CONCLUSION

Using two large, nationally representative health surveys, we have documented considerable racial/ethnic and socioeconomic disparities in U.S. childhood obesity. The NSCH data show that 16.4% of U.S. children aged 10 to 17 years (i.e., 5.2 million children) were obese in 2007, which suggests an increase of 10% in prevalence or 570,000 additional obese children aged 10 to 17 since the 2003 NSCH [3, 4, 6]. An overweight prevalence of 31.6% in 2007 meant that more than 10 million children aged 10 to 17 years were obese or overweight—an additional 512,000 overweight children since the 2003 NSCH [4]. The 2007–2008 NHANES data show a current obesity prevalence of 19.7% and an overweight prevalence of 36.1% for children aged 6 to 17. The number of obese

TABLE 7.4 Obesity and Overweight Prevalence (Weighted %) and Odds among U.S. Children Ages 6–17 Years by Race/Ethnicity and Sociodemographic Characteristics: The 2003–2008 National Health and Nutrition Examination Survey (N = 7,510)

Characteristic	Prevalence %	SE	Age-gender adjusted OR	95% CI		Fully adjusted model OR	95% CI	
OBESITY (BMI ≥ 95TH PERCENTILE)–BASED ON MEASURED HEIGHT AND WEIGHT DATA								
Total population	18.28	0.89						
RACE/ETHNICITY								
Non-Hispanic White	16.36	1.34	1.00	reference		1.00	reference	
Non-Hispanic Black	22.73	0.89	1.51	1.22	1.87	1.32	1.06	1.64
Hispanic	23.90	1.05	1.61	1.27	2.05	1.40	1.12	1.77
Other	11.12	1.52	0.64	0.48	0.87	0.63	0.47	0.83
HOUSEHOLD POVERTY STATUS (RATIO OF FAMILY INCOME TO POVERTY THRESHOLD)								
Below 100%	22.48	1.23	2.30	1.81	2.92	2.00	1.57	2.54
100–199%	20.75	1.56	2.08	1.58	2.73	1.89	1.43	2.50
200–399%	18.95	1.29	1.84	1.44	2.36	1.79	1.40	2.28
At or above 400%	11.38	1.12	1.00	reference		1.00	reference	
CHILD'S AGE, YEARS								
6–9	17.29	1.25	0.91	0.72	1.14	0.85	0.67	1.07
10–11	19.45	1.43	1.04	0.81	1.35	1.01	0.77	1.33
12–14	18.29	1.58	0.97	0.75	1.25	0.94	0.73	1.21
15–17	18.74	1.27	1.00	reference		1.00	reference	
GENDER								
Male	19.62	1.08	1.20	1.03	1.40	1.21	1.03	1.42
Female	16.89	1.03	1.00	reference		1.00	reference	
OVERWEIGHT (BMI ≥ 85TH PERCENTILE)–BASED ON MEASURED HEIGHT AND WEIGHT DATA								
Total population	34.69	1.07						
RACE/ETHNICITY								
Non-Hispanic White	33.03	1.63	1.00	reference		1.00	reference	
Non-Hispanic Black	38.60	1.14	1.28	1.08	1.51	1.17	0.99	1.37
Hispanic	42.23	1.40	1.49	1.24	1.81	1.36	1.14	1.62
Other	21.52	1.96	0.56	0.43	0.73	0.54	0.42	0.70
HOUSEHOLD POVERTY STATUS (RATIO OF FAMILY INCOME TO POVERTY THRESHOLD)								
Below 100%	39.00	1.31	1.81	1.52	2.15	1.62	1.36	1.93
100–199%	37.44	1.90	1.70	1.37	2.10	1.57	1.26	1.96
200–399%	36.39	2.01	1.62	1.29	2.02	1.58	1.26	1.99
At or above 400%	26.33	1.52	1.00	reference		1.00	reference	
CHILD'S AGE, YEARS								
6–9	32.40	1.58	0.90	0.76	1.06	0.86	0.73	1.01
10–11	40.10	1.59	1.25	1.03	1.52	1.23	1.01	1.50
12–14	33.88	1.84	0.96	0.80	1.14	0.94	0.79	1.11
15–17	34.86	1.51	1.00	reference		1.00	reference	

(Continued)

TABLE 7.4 Obesity and Overweight Prevalence (Weighted %) and Odds among U.S. Children Ages 6–17 Years by Race/Ethnicity and Sociodemographic Characteristics: The 2003–2008 National Health and Nutrition Examination Survey (N = 7,510)—cont'd

Characteristic	Prevalence %	SE	Age-gender adjusted OR	95% CI		Fully adjusted model OR	95% CI	
GENDER								
Male	35.34	1.29	1.06	0.93	1.20	1.06	0.93	1.21
Female	34.02	1.27	1.00	reference		1.00	reference	

SE = standard error; OR = odds ratio; CI = confidence interval. The chi-square test for independence between each covariate and obesity or overweight prevalence (except for age-obesity and gender-overweight) was statistically significant at p < .05.

children aged 6 to 17 years increased from 6.9 million in 1999–2000 to 9.3 million in 2007–2008, whereas the number of obese or overweight children aged 6 to 17 grew from 14.1 million in 1999–2000 to 17.1 million in 2007–2008.

Large racial/ethnic disparities exist in obesity and overweight prevalence among U.S. children. Although black and Hispanic children have higher obesity rates than non-Hispanic white children, analysis of detailed ethnic disparities indicates that black, Hispanic, Hawaiian/Pacific Islander, and American Indian/Alaska Native children have three to four times higher odds of obesity and overweight than Asian children. Almost one in four black, Hispanic, or American Indian/Alaska Native children is obese, compared with fewer than one in ten of Asian American children. The overweight prevalence for black, Hispanic, and Hawaiian/Pacific Islander children currently exceeds 40%.

Substantial disparities in U.S. childhood obesity also exist according to household income, education, and employment status. Children from low-income and low-education households have 3 times higher prevalence and 3.4 to 4.3 times higher odds of obesity than children from high SES groups. Nearly half of all children in the lowest SES group are overweight, compared with one in four children in the highest SES group.

The socioeconomic gradients in obesity and overweight prevalence are not just limited to differences between the highest and lowest SES groups. Instead, the gradient in obesity and overweight risks extends progressively downward from the poor through the lower middle class, upper middle class, and to the most affluent group. The excess obesity burden is therefore shared greatly by children and families in the middle SES groups who make up more than half of the child population or households.

Race/ethnicity and SES are not only powerful and independent determinants of childhood obesity, but they also jointly influence the obesity risk in children in a significant manner. Stratified analyses show substantial SES gradients (main effects) in obesity and obesity risks among children in all major racial/ethnic groups. The joint or interaction effect of race/ethnicity and SES is quite striking and indicates a much wider social disparity than when either race or SES is considered as an individual covariate. For example, a four-fold higher prevalence in obesity can be noted for Hispanic and black children from low-income and low-education households compared with affluent non-Hispanic white children.

The marked racial/ethnic and socioeconomic disparities in childhood obesity shown in our study are consistent with those observed previously [1, 3–8]. Increased obesity prevalence has been noted for black and Hispanic children, and substantial inverse socioeconomic gradients in childhood obesity have been observed not only for the United States but also for the United Kingdom, Canada, Australia, and other industrialized countries [1, 3–8, 16–17, 21–26]. Indeed, recent analyses of the NSCH and NHANES data have shown rising socioeconomic inequalities in obesity among U.S. children (4, 8). Although the magnitude of SES gradients in the United Kingdom is not as pronounced as those for the United States, socioeconomic inequalities in childhood obesity have also increased over time for the United Kingdom [4, 21].

The recent increase in the overall obesity and overweight prevalence among U.S. children has been partly attributed to increases in the proportion of the socially disadvantaged groups as the percentage of households with Hispanic children and low-income, high-unemployment, and non-English speaking households grew between 2003 and 2007 [4]. Additionally, a more rapid increase in the obesity prevalence among Hispanic children and among children from lower SES backgrounds has been cited as a major factor in the rise of social inequalities in U.S. childhood obesity [4].

Although sociodemographic and behavioral factors considered here accounted for some of the racial/ethnic and SES disparities in childhood obesity and overweight prevalence, substantial ethnic and SES differentials remain even after the multivariate adjustment. What might account for the residual differences? Regular physical activity and healthy diet are considered two important proximate factors in obesity prevention

[2, 16]. Although we did consider physical activity as a covariate, certain dietary factors, which we were unable to consider because of lack of data, might partly account for the racial/ethnic and socioeconomic differentials. Contrary to expectation, our analysis of the NHANES data showed lower total calorie (kcal) and fat intake among both youth and adults in lower SES groups and in such ethnic-minority groups as blacks and Hispanics [19]. However, some studies have found higher consumption of lower-quality diets and energy-dense foods and lower intakes of fruits and vegetables among blacks and lower SES groups [27−29]. The apparent inconsistency in ethnic and socioeconomic disparities in total energy intake and fat intake and in the corresponding obesity risks may be due to methodological problems that characterize cross-sectional studies of diet and obesity [16]. Most dietary information based on self-reports tends to underestimate energy intake and other nutrients, and such underreporting is greater among obese or overweight people [16]. Longitudinal studies are needed to accurately assess the significance of dietary influences on obesity risks among various ethnic and SES groups.

A few limitations of our study should be noted. First, the childhood obesity and overweight measure in the NSCH was based on parental reports of children's height and weight, which may not accurately reflect the true prevalence. However, previous research has indicated parental or self-reported height and weight data as a valid and reliable indicator of childhood and adolescent obesity [30, 31]. Furthermore, recent comparisons of the NSCH and NHANES data as well as the estimates from the two surveys presented here show a fairly close correspondence between parent-reported and measured obesity and overweight estimates for children aged 10 to 17 [3, 4, 6]. Second, because of lack of data in the NSCH or NHANES, we were unable to consider additional individual- and community-level covariates, such as children's dietary patterns and parental obesity status, and direct or area-based measures of the neighborhood social environment, including access to recreation facilities, outdoor parks, playgrounds and other amenities for physical activity, modes of transportation and vehicular traffic congestion, and availability of fast-food outlets and restaurants [2−4, 6, 32]. Differences in these factors may partially explain the substantial ethnic and SES inequalities in childhood obesity reported here. Third, because of small sample sizes and confidentiality protection of individual records, both the NSCH and NHANES do not identify specific Hispanic subgroups (e.g., Mexicans [NSCH], Cubans, Puerto Ricans, and Central/South Americans) and major Asian subgroups (such as Chinese, Asian Indians, Filipinos, Japanese, Koreans, Vietnamese, and Cambodians) who are extremely heterogeneous in their socioeconomic, behavioral, and health characteristics and who are, therefore, expected to also differ in their childhood obesity patterns.

The United States has one of the highest rates of childhood obesity in the industrialized world [17]. Existence of large racial/ethnic and socioeconomic inequalities in obesity, as shown here, has been mentioned as one of the major reasons for its unfavorable international standing [3]. Monitoring disparities in U.S. childhood obesity across major racial/ethnic and socioeconomic groups is therefore vital in tracking progress toward achieving the broad *Healthy People 2010* objectives of reducing and ultimately eliminating health inequalities and in evaluating the impact of specific policy interventions in reducing childhood obesity [3, 4, 9]. Marked racial/ethnic and socioeconomic inequalities shown here indicate the potential for a considerable reduction in U.S. childhood obesity. However, the continued existence of, or increase in, the obesity disparities is likely to exacerbate health inequalities among both children and adults. Prevention programs for reducing disparities in childhood obesity should not only include behavioral interventions aimed at reducing children's physical inactivity levels and limiting their television viewing and recreational screen time but should also include social policy measures aimed at improving the broader social and physical environments that create obesogenic conditions that put children at risk for poor diet, physical inactivity, and other sedentary activities [2, 3, 6].

References

1. National Center for Health Statistics. *Health, United States, 2008 with Special Feature on the Health of Young Adults*. Hyattsville, MD: US Department of Health and Human Services; 2009.
2. Koplan JP, Liverman CT, Kraak VA, editors. *Preventing Childhood Obesity: Health in the Balance. Institute of Medicine*. Washington, DC: The National Academies Press; 2005.
3. Singh GK, Kogan MD, van Dyck PC, Siahpush M. Racial/ethnic, socioeconomic, and behavioral determinants of childhood and adolescent obesity in the United States: analyzing independent and joint associations. *Ann Epidemiol* 2008;**18**(9):682−95.
4. Singh GK, Siahpush M, Kogan MD. Rising social inequalities in US childhood obesity, 2003−2007. *Ann Epidemiol* 2010;**20**(1):40−52.
5. Ogden CL, Carroll MD, Curtin LR, McDowell MA, Tabak CJ, Flegal KM. Prevalence of overweight and obesity in the United States, 1999−2004. *JAMA* 2006;**295**(13):1549−2850.
6. Singh GK, Kogan MD, van Dyck PC. A multilevel analysis of state and regional disparities in childhood and adolescent obesity in the United States. *J Community Health* 2008;**33**(2):90−102.
7. Wang Y, Beydoun MA. The obesity epidemic in the United States − gender, age, socioeconomic, racial/ethnic, and geographic characteristics: a systematic review and meta-regression analysis. *Epidemiol Rev* 2007;**29**:6−28.
8. Miech RA, Kumanyika SK, Setler N, Link BG, Phelan JC, Chang VW. Trends in the association of poverty with overweight among US adolescents, 1971−2004. *JAMA* 2006;**295**(20):2385−93.

REFERENCES

9. US Department of Health and Human Services. *Healthy People 2010: Understanding and Improving Health*. 2nd ed. Washington, DC: US Government Printing Office; 2000.
10. Singh GK, Siahpush M. Widening socioeconomic inequalities in US life expectancy, 1980–2000. *Int J Epidemiol* 2006;**35**(4):969–79.
11. Singh GK. Area deprivation and widening inequalities in US mortality, 1969–1998. *Am J Public Health* 2003;**93**(7):1137–43.
12. Braveman P, Egerter S. *Overcoming Obstacles to Health*. Princeton, NJ: Robert Wood Johnson Foundation; 2008.
13. National Center for Health Statistics. *The National Survey of Children's Health (NSCH), 2007: the public use data file*. Hyattsville, MD: US Department of Health and Human Services 2009. Available at: www.cdc.gov/nchs/about/major/slaits/nsch07.htm (Accessed June 1, 2009).
14. Blumberg SJ, Foster EB, Frasier AM, Satorius J, Skalland BJ, Nysse-Carris KL, et al. Design and operation of the National Survey of Children's Health, 2007. *Vital Health Stat* 2009;1. Forthcoming. Available at: ftp://ftp.cdc.gov/pub/Health_Statistics/NCHS/slaits/nsch07/2_Methodology_Report/NSCH_Design_and_Operations_052109.pdf (Accessed October 9, 2009).
15. Kuczmarski RJ, Ogden CL, Guo SS, Grummer-Strawn LM, Flegal KM, Mei Z, et al. 2000 CDC growth charts for the United States: methods and development. *Vital Health Stat* 2002;**11**(246):1–190.
16. Branca F, Nikogosian H, Lobstein T, editors. *The Challenge of Obesity in the WHO European Region and the Strategies for Response*. Copenhagen: Denmark:WHO Regional Office for Europe; 2007.
17. Janssen I, Katzmarzyk PT, Boyce WF, Vereecken C, Mulvihill C, Roberts C, et al. Comparison of overweight and obesity prevalence in school-aged youth from 34 countries and their relationships with physical activity and dietary patterns. *Obes Rev* 2005;**6**(2):123–32.
18. Kawachi I, Kim D, Coutts A, Subramanian SV. Commentary: reconciling the three accounts of social capital. *Int J Epidemiol* 2004;**33**(4):682–90.
19. National Center for Health Statistics. *The National Health and Nutrition Examination Survey (NHANES), 1999–2008 Public Use Data Files*. Hyattsville, MD: US Department of Health and Human Services 2009. Available at: www.cdc.gov/nchs/nhanes/nhanes_questionnaires.htm (Accessed October 9, 2009).
20. SUDAAN. *Software for the Statistical Analysis of Correlated Data, Release 9.0.1*. Research Triangle Park, NC: Research Triangle Institute; 2005.
21. Jotangia D, Moody A, Stamatakis E, Wardle H. *Obesity Among Children Under 11*. London, UK: National Centre for Social Research; 2005.
22. Stamatakis E, Primatesta P, Chinn S, Rona R, Falascheti E. Overweight and obesity trends from 1974 to 2003 in English children: what is the role of socioeconomic factors. *Arch Dis Child* 2005;**90**(10):999–1004.
23. Willms JD, Tremblay MS, Katzmarzyk PT. Geographic and demographic variation in the prevalence of overweight Canadian children. *Obesity Research* 2003;**11**(5):668–73.
24. Oliver LN, Hayes MV. Neighborhood socio-economic status and the prevalence of overweight Canadian children and youth. *Can J Public Health* 2005;**96**(6):415–20.
25. Booth ML, Wake M, Armstrong T, Chey T, Hesketh K, Mathur S. The epidemiology of overweight and obesity among Australian children and adolescents 1995–97. *Aus NZ J Pub Health* 2001;**25**(2):162–9.
26. Langnase K, Mast M, Muller MJ. Social class differences in overweight of prepubertal children in northwest Germany. *Intl J Obes Relat Metab Disord* 2002;**26**(4):566–72.
27. Darmon N, Drewnowski A. Does social class predict diet quality? *Am J Clin Nutr* 2008;**87**(5):1107–17.
28. Kant AK, Graubard BI, Kumanyika SK. Trends in black-white differentials in dietary intakes of U.S. adults, 1971–2002. *Am J Prev Med* 2007;**32**(4):264–72.
29. Kant AK, Graubard BI. Secular trends in the association of socio-economic position with self-reported dietary attributes and biomarkers in the US population: National Health and Nutrition Examination Survey (NHANES) 1971–1975 to NHANES 1999–2002. *Public Health Nutrition* 2005;**10**(2):158–67.
30. Goodman E, Hinden BR, Khandelwal S. Accuracy of teen and parental reports of obesity and body mass index. *Pediatrics* 2000;**106**(1):52–8.
31. Brener ND, McManus T, Galuska DA, Lowry R, Wechsler H. Reliability and validity of self-reported height and weight among high school students. *J Adolesc Health* 2003;**32**(4):281–7.
32. Booth KM, Pinkston MM, Poston WSC. Obesit and the built environment. *J Am Diet Assoc* 2005;**105**(5 Suppl. 1):S110–17.

CHAPTER 8

Prediabetes among Obese Youth

Orit Pinhas-Hamiel*, Phil Zeitler[†]

*Pediatric Endocrinology and Diabetes, Sheba Medical Center, Tel-Hashomer, Ramat-Gan, 52621, Tel-Aviv University, Israel and Juvenile Diabetes Center, Maccabi Health Care Services and [†]Division of Endocrinology, Department of Pediatrics, The University of Colorado Denver, The Children's Hospital, Aurora, CO, USA

INTRODUCTION

Prediabetes is an intermediate state reflecting early abnormalities of glucose metabolism when the criteria do not fit the diagnosis of diabetes. The term is used both for children with clear type 1 diabetes who were identified very early in the disease course, have hyperglycemia and positive antibodies, but do not fulfill the criteria for diabetes, and for children with a suggestive clinical picture of pending type 2 diabetes mellitus (T2DM). The focus of this chapter is only on pre-T2DM.

DEFINITIONS

Diabetes is diagnosed either through random serum glucose > 200 mg/dL in the presence of symptoms of diabetes (polyuria, polydipsia, weight loss) or on the basis of an oral glucose tolerance test (OGTT) in asymptomatic patients. In the absence of symptoms, the diagnosis of diabetes by OGTT must be confirmed on a separate day. Criteria for the diagnosis of diabetes based on OGTT established by the American Diabetes Association (ADA) include the following:

1. A fasting plasma glucose (FPG) concentration of ≥126 mg/dL (7 mmol/L) after an overnight fast of at least 8 hours
2. A plasma glucose concentration of ≥200 mg/dL (11.1 mmol/L) 2 hours after a 1.75 g/kg (maximum dose 75 grams) oral glucose load given in the morning after an overnight fast.

The progression from normal glucose metabolism to type 2 diabetes mellitus (T2DM) involves intermediate states that reflect early abnormalities of glucose metabolism but do not meet the ADA established criteria for diabetes. These states have been given the name "prediabetes" because of the presumption that they represent a high-risk for progression to overt diabetes.

Prediabetes includes subjects who have the following conditions:

1. *Impaired fasting glucose (IFG)*. Plasma glucose concentration of 100 to 125 mg/dL (5.6 to 6.9 mmol/L) after an overnight fast of at least 8 hours.
2. *Impaired glucose tolerance (IGT)*. Plasma glucose concentration of 140 to 199 mg/dL (7.8 to 11 mmol/L) 2 hours after a 1.75 g/kg (maximum dose 75 grams) oral glucose load given in the morning after an overnight fast.
3. *Both*. IFG/IGT

Pathophysiology

The Zucker fatty rat (fa/fa; ZR) is considered a model for prediabetes. These animals have a genetic defect in the leptin receptor, which results in obesity and insulin resistance. In response, the endocrine pancreas of ZR undergoes adaptive and compensatory changes. Measurement of the time course of the pathological changes by histological analysis of the pancreatic islet in combination with changes in metabolic parameters is an effective way to reveal disease progression [1]. In this model, a loss in glucose tolerance occurs first and is accompanied by impaired islet histology, changes in beta-cell mass, and impaired islet function. Thus, early expression of insulin resistance and glucose intolerance in ZR results in morphological and functional changes of pancreatic islets, despite their ability to maintain normoglycemia.

Studies of the early metabolic defects leading to the development of T2DM in youth have been limited. In a recent study, the appearance of an early defect in β-cell function was suggested as the underlying cause for the development of IGT and T2DM in obese youth [2]. Genetic predisposition, compounded by environmental factors such as increased caloric intake, is suggested as mechanism underlying this progressive decline in β-cell function. In a longitudinal cohort study in overweight and obese Hispanic adolescents with a family history of T2DM, persistent prediabetes was associated with compromised beta cell function and with a lower than expected and decreasing acute insulin response to glucose, indicating decreased β-cell function, along with greater accumulation of visceral fat over time [3].

Screening Tests for the Diagnosis of Prediabetes and Their Value

A fasting plasma glucose is recommended by the American and Canadian Diabetes Associations for screening obese young people for prediabetes. The International Society for Pediatric and Adolescent Diabetes (ISPAD) recommends testing for IFG, IGT, and diabetes in children with body mass index (BMI) between the 85 and 95th percentiles who have a family history of cardiovascular disease and/or signs of insulin resistance and in all children with a BMI greater than the 95th percentile [4].

The usefulness of these screening approaches in youth is not clear. First, it appears that testing by fasting plasma glucose alone is less effective than fasting plasma glucose combined with an OGTT. Indeed in a 2-year prospective longitudinal study among 172 obese children aged 5 to 18, 8.7% of participants screened positive for prediabetes with the fasting plasma glucose test alone, whereas 24.3% screened positive for prediabetes when the screening procedure included a 2-hour OGTT combined with the fasting plasma glucose compared ($P < 0.01$) [5].

Second, there are substantial questions regarding the reliability of the tests. Libman and colleagues reported that the OGTT in at-risk obese adolescents is poorly reproducible, with the agreement between a first and second OGTT performed within 1 month of each other being only 22% for IFG and 27% for IGT [6]. Of interest, though, those adolescents with discordant OGTT results were more likely to have evidence for subtle abnormalities in glucose metabolism, suggesting that, even if they do not reproducibly meet specific criteria, adolescents who have at least one abnormal OGTT likely have early dysfunction of glucose metabolism.

Further evaluation of this group of adolescents may provide greater insight into the evolution of frank diabetes in adolescents.

Until more information is available, the evidence reviewed here suggests that the value of an OGTT for the diagnosis of glucose dysregulation in an asymptomatic adolescent is too limited to support recommendations for using OGTT as a screening tool for T2DM and for prediabetes. Given the low prevalence of frank undiagnosed T2DM (discussed later), even among high-risk individuals, a large number of OGTTs would have to be performed to identify a single case that was not clinically apparent. Finally, the poor reproducibility of the OGTT implies that the identification of abnormal glucose regulation on a single test is unreliable and, therefore, repeated testing would be required. A much deeper appreciation of the likely outcome of extensive screening for diabetes and a clearer understanding of risk among adolescents is necessary before truly useful guidelines can be developed.

EPIDEMIOLOGY OF DIABETES AND PREDIABETES

In the General Population of Children and Adolescents

The prevalence and incidence of T2DM in youth has been established in numerous reports from around the world and has been reviewed elsewhere [7], and the remaining reeports were population studies. In population studies, silent cases of T2DM among children and adolescents appear to be rare. In a nationally representative sample of 915 U.S. adolescents aged 12 to 19 years examined in the 1999–2000 National Health and Nutrition Examination Survey (NHANES), no cases of T2DM were identified. The prevalence of IFG was 7.0% and was higher in boys than in girls [8]. Similarly, in a study at 12 middle schools around the United States, 1740 eighth graders, of whom 49% had BMI greater than the 85th percentile, underwent fasting and 2-hour postload glucose determinations. Diabetes by fasting criteria was identified in only 0.4%, and following a glucose load, only 0.1% had diabetes [9]. IFG was present in 40.5%, and following a glucose load, only 2% had IGT [9]. Of note, the presence of impaired fasting glucose was not a strong predictor of diabetes by OGTT in this sample. Furthermore, the findings vary greatly among age groups, degree of obesity, and ethnic origin. Therefore, the prevalence of IFG and IGT has been studied mainly in at-risk groups, based on obesity or family of T2DM or birth following a pregnancy complicated by diabetes.

Among Obese Children (Table 8.1)

In a multiethnic cohort of 167 obese children and adolescents in the United States, IGT was detected in 25% of obese children aged 4 to 10 years and 21% of 112 obese adolescents (11 to 18 years of age) [10]. In Germany, among 520 obese subjects (237 boys and 283 girls; mean age of 14 ± 2 years [range 8.9 to 20.4 years]), IFG was detected in 3.7% and IGT in 2.1% of the patients [11]. In Greece, among 117 obese children and adolescents 12.1 ± 2.7 years old the overall prevalence of IGT was 14.5% (prepubertal subjects 9% and pubertal subjects 18%), none had T2DM [12]. In Italy, among 100 obese children and adolescents (mean age of 10.1 ± 2.7 years), none of the subjects had IFG or diabetes, whereas 4% of obese patients had IGT [13]. In Turkey, from a total of 196 obese children, 6.6% had an abnormal fasting glucose concentration and 18% had IGT [14]. In Spain, among 95 obese children and adolescents aged 4 to 16 years, the prevalence of IGT was 7.4% [15]. Among 427 asymptomatic obese children from Argentina with a mean age of 10.7 ± 3.5, IGT was present in 7% [16]. In central Mexico, among 1238 children 6 to 13 years of age the prevalence of prediabetes was 5.7% [17]. In Israel, among 234 obese patients ranging from 5 to 22 years of age, IGT was present in 13.5%. Taken together, these data show a wide variation in the prevalence of prediabetes in obese children, likely secondary to variations in age, ethnicity, and severity of obesity.

Prevalence in Those with Family History of T2DM

The influence of family history and obesity on glucose intolerance was studied among 105 children and adolescents aged 10 to 18 years (mean age of 13.3 ± 2.5 years). Children and adolescents were divided into three groups according to positive family history of T2DM and obesity. The prevalence of prediabetes (either IGT of IFG) was 15.2% in the whole group, whereas it was 25.5% in obese children who also had a positive family history of T2DM [18]. Recent data from the SEARCH study have now extended these findings by exploring diabetes diagnosis among African American, Hispanic, and non-Hispanic white youth from the SEARCH cohort who had a parent with diabetes [19]. Adolescents with T2DM were almost nine times more likely to have a parent with either T1DM or T2DM than youth with T1DM.

Prevalence in Those with Gestational Diabetes Mellitus (GDM)

Studies have tried to analyze the effect of gestational diabetes, separately from family history of T2DM, obesity, and increased gestational weight gain on offspring. Recent data from the SEARCH Case-Control Study [20] show that youth with T2DM were almost six times more likely than nondiabetic control youth to have been exposed to maternal diabetes *in utero* (odds ratio [OR] 5.7 [95% confidence interval (CI) 2.4–13.4]) and 2.8 times more likely (95% CI 1.5–5.2) to be exposed to obesity *in utero*. Interestingly, correction for the BMI of the youth substantially attenuated this association, suggesting that at least part of the effect of the *in utero* environment is mediated by changes in body composition of the youth. Furthermore, T2DM was diagnosed nearly 2 years earlier among those exposed to diabetes *in utero* than among those whose mothers' diabetes was diagnosed later, whereas there was no such effect on the

TABLE 8.1 Prevalence of Prediabetes and Silent T2DM in Obese Subjects

Place	No of obese subjects	Age	IGT (%)	IFG (%)	Silent T2DM%
United States	55	4–10	25		
	112	11–18	21		4
Argentina	427		7		1.6
Mexico	1238	6–13		5.7	0
Israel	234	5–22	13.5		0.4
Greece	117	5–19 (12.1 ± 2.7) Prepubertal pubertal	9% 18%		0
Turkey	196	7–18	18	6.6	3
Germany	520	8.9–20.4	2.1	3.7	1.5
Italy	100	3–16 (10.1 ± 2.7)	4	0	0
Spain	95	4–16	7.4		0

age at diagnosis of T1DM. As in the Pima studies, the presence of diabetes in the father before the child's birth was not associated with age at diagnosis.

In a study of the prevalence of IGT in offspring of mothers whose pregnancies were complicated by gestational diabetes mellitus (GDM) at a mean age of 9.1 years, 6.9% (5/72) had abnormal glucose metabolism (four children had IGT and one had T2DM) [21]. In another study of women with pregestational diabetes (either type 1 and T2DM) and gestational diabetes, IGT was reported in 36% of offspring of those with gestational diabetes and was associated with elevated amniotic fluid insulin *in utero* [22].

Finally, the influence of both family history of T2DM and GDM was studied among 150 overweight Latino children [23]. IGT was present in 28% of children with a family history of T2DM and was similar across obesity groups, but it was higher in children exposed to GDM (41%).

WHOM TO SCREEN?

Which children have an increased risk and should be screened for prediabetes? Guidance from the literature in identifying those individuals for whom further testing is most likely to yield clinically relevant results is limited. Reinehr et al. studied potential predictors, such as history of T2DM in parents and grandparents, degree of overweight, age, pubertal stage, birth weight, hypertension, dyslipidemia, acanthosis nigricans, and abdominal obesity. The only risk factors for prediabetes were parental diabetes, pubertal stage, and extreme obesity [24]. Another particularly high-risk population to target for screening described recently is overweight siblings of children previously diagnosed with T2DM; siblings had four times greater odds of having abnormal glucose tolerance compared with unrelated overweight children [9].

In a study of 84 obese, insulin-resistant, predominantly Hispanic adolescents undergoing OGTT [25], all 10 (100%) subjects with IGT had fasting triglycerides $\geq$ 150 mg/dl. The likelihood ratio for IGT with fasting triglycerides $\geq$ 150 was 3.1. More important, the negative predictive value for a normal fasting triglyceride was 100% in this cohort. If confirmed in a larger cohort with more diverse ethnicity, measurement of serum triglycerides may be useful in identifying patients who need no further testing.

Additional at-risk groups have been described. In a study of adolescents prescribed a combination antipsychotic therapy, antidepressants, and mood stabilizers, the odds of developing T2DM were higher for girls, adolescents aged 13 years or older, those exposed to multiple antipsychotics (OR 2.36; 95% CI, 1.13–4.92), and those on long-term treatment with antipsychotic [26]. Finally, girls diagnosed with polycystic ovary syndrome (PCOS) have more insulin resistance, IGT and T2DM than their non-PCOS counterparts [27].

Considering both previous consensus recommendations and the preceding studies in adolescents, populations at high risk for the development of diabetes who may be appropriate for targeted screening may include those with the following conditions:

- Marked obesity
- Family history of diabetes in parents and siblings
- History of gestational diabetes
- Puberty
- Increased serum triglycerides
- Polycystic ovary syndrome
- Treatment with antipsychotics

Although hypertension and low concentrations of high-density lipoprotein cholesterol are part of the metabolic syndrome, their role as markers for screening for prediabetes has not been well studied.

PROGRESSION OF PREDIABETES

Among adults, prediabetes raises short-term absolute risk of T2DM; the cumulative incidence of diabetes for subjects with both IFG and IGT was 64.5% compared with 4.5% for those with normal glucose levels at baseline [28]. The odds ratios for diabetes, adjusted for age, sex, and follow-up duration, were 10.0 (95% CI, 6.1–16.5), 10.9 (95% CI, 6.0–19.9), and 39.5 (95% CI, 17.0–92.1), respectively, for those having isolated IFG, isolated IGT, and both IFG and IGT.

There are no population studies regarding the rate of progression to diabetes in children and adolescents. However, there are several clinical studies among obese subjects. Weiss et al. have demonstrated that glucose tolerance status in obese children is highly dynamic and can deteriorate rapidly. Over about 2 years of follow-up, about 10% of subjects initially classified as normal glucose tolerance developed IGT and 24% of subjects initially classified as IGT developed overt T2DM. Severely obese children, particularly of African American descent, had a higher risk of developing T2DM [29]. The evolution of β-cell function, insulin sensitivity, and glucose tolerance was studied in a multiethnic group of 60 obese adolescents over the course of approximately 30 months. At baseline, all 60 subjects had normal glucose tolerance (NGT). IGT developed in 23% and those who progressed to IGT had relatively poorer β-cell function at baseline [2].

Changes in glycemic status were examined in 128 overweight and obese Hispanic adolescents at high risk of developing T2DM with a family history of

T2DM. Participants were evaluated annually for 4 years with an OGTT. During this period, no participants developed T2DM, 40% never had prediabetes, 47% had intermittent prediabetes with no clear pattern over time, and 13% had persistent prediabetes. At baseline, those with persistent prediabetes had lower β-cell function and higher intraabdominal adipose tissue. Thus, in children at high risk of type 2 diabetes, the presence of prediabetes is highly variable from year to year, with a small fraction of at-risk adolescents having persistent prediabetes [3].

TREATMENT OF PREDIABETES

Interestingly, adolescents diagnosed with overt T2DM often present with microvascular complications. This may suggest either a long-standing period of undiagnosed T2DM or that in the progression from normal glucose tolerance to frank diabetes these subjects were already subjected to the toxicity of elevated glucose concentrations. Despite the possible contribution of the prediabetic state to existence of diabetes-related complications, few studies have examined the management of children and adolescents with prediabetes, and no evidence-based recommendations are available. However, it seems reasonable that the preferred treatment approach in children and adolescents would be intensive lifestyle management, given its safety.

LIFESTYLE

Currently there are several studies designed and implemented to explore prevention of the growing numbers of children and adolescents being diagnosed with T2DM. For example, the HEALTHY primary prevention was planned to moderate risk factors for T2DM with an intervention consisting of four integrated components: (1) changes in the quantity and nutritional quality of food and beverage offerings throughout the total school food environment; (2) physical education class lesson plans and accompanying equipment to increase both participation and number of minutes spent in moderate-to-vigorous physical activity; (3) brief classroom activities and family outreach vehicles to increase knowledge, enhance decision-making skills, and support and reinforce youth in accomplishing goals; and (4) communications and social marketing strategies to enhance and promote changes through messages, images, events, and activities [30].

Although there are numerous prevention projects for obesity, only limited studies have examined the prevention of transition to IGT and T2DM. One of these is a 7-month community-based nonpharmacological lifestyle intervention to prevent/reduce the risk of developing diabetes and its complications in a resource-poor village in Tamil Nadu, India. The prevalence of prediabetes in youth aged 10 to 17 years was 5.1%. Intervention successfully reduced FBG levels by 17% in youth with IFG ($P = 0.014$). Intervention also lowered waist circumference, hip circumference, thigh circumference, and waist hip ratio ($P = 0.001$) although BMI increased. Educational intervention was successful in reducing some of the obesity parameters and improving dietary patterns of individuals with prediabetes and diabetes [31].

PHARMACOTHERAPY IN PREDIABETES

Currently, there are no pharmacological therapies that have been approved by the U.S. Food and Drug Administration for the prevention of diabetes in adults, nor are there any approved pharmacological options for use in children or adolescents. Thus, any decision to implement pharmacological therapy for prediabetes, and specifically in children/adolescents, is off-label and requires careful judgment regarding the risks and benefits of each specific agent in each individual patient.

Although a number of controlled randomized clinical trials have demonstrated that pharmacological agents, such as metformin, can lead to substantial delay or reduction in progression to T2DM in high-risk adults, reviewed in [32], there have been no studies to date specifically examining pharmacological approaches to reducing the progression of high-risk adolescents to overt diabetes. The numbers of children with IGT remains limited, and available data suggest that the progression to diabetes in these children over the short periods of time characteristic of clinical trials is relatively low, making the design and execution of such studies challenging. In a small study of 29 obese adolescents aged 12 to 19 years, metformin caused a decline of 0.12 standard deviation in BMI in study participants (-1.3% from baseline) and a 5.5% reduction in serum leptin in girls. In contrast, BMI and serum leptin rose 2.3% and 16.2%, respectively, in the placebo group during the 6-month treatment period. Metformin caused a progressive decline in fasting blood glucose (from a mean of 84.9 to 75.1 mg%) and a reduction in fasting insulin levels (from 31.3 to 19.3 microU/mL). In contrast, fasting glucose levels in the placebo group rose slightly from 77.2 to 82.3 mg%, and fasting insulin levels did not change [33]. In a more recent, larger randomized, placebo-controlled 6-month trial in 85 high-risk adolescents, metformin was associated with modest improvements in BMI, fasting glucose and glucose tolerance, particularly in females. However, the study was not designed nor powered to demonstrate prevention of progression to diabetes [34].

In a recent meta-analysis of randomized controlled trials, the efficacy of metformin in reducing BMI and cardiometabolic risk in obese children and adolescents without diabetes was summarized. Metformin appears to be moderately efficacious in reducing BMI and insulin resistance in hyperinsulinemic obese children and adolescents in the short term. Larger, longer-term studies in different populations are needed to establish its role in the treatment of overweight children [35].

CONCLUSION

Prediabetes in children and adolescents is relatively newly identified entity that needs to be further studied in terms of efficient screening approaches, populations at risk, progression rates to frank T2DM, and treatment. However, despite the challenges in the reliability of screening tests among youth and despite the fact that clear screening and treatment guidelines are still lacking, the relatively high progression rates to diabetes and, more important, the evidence that prediabetes itself is a high-risk state for cardiovascular disease means that it will be critical to define and develop intensive evaluation and intervention strategies for these high-risk youth.

References

1. Augstein P, Salzsieder E. Morphology of Pancreatic Islets: A Time Course of Pre-diabetes in Zucker Fatty Rats. Methods Mol.Biol 2009;**560**:159—89.
2. Cali' AM, Man CD, Cobelli C, Dziura J, Seyal A, Shaw M, Allen K, Chen S, Caprio S. Primary Defects in Beta-Cell Function Further Exacerbated by Worsening of Insulin Resistance Mark the Development of Impaired Glucose Tolerance in Obese Adolescents. Diabetes Care 2008;**32**:456—61.
3. Goran MI, Lane C, Toledo-Corral C, Weigensberg MJ. Persistence of pre-diabetes in overweight and obese Hispanic children: association with progressive insulin resistance, poor beta-cell function, and increasing visceral fat. Diabetes 2008;**57**:3007—12.
4. Rosenbloom AL, Silverstein JH, Amemiya S, Zeitler P, Klingensmith GJ. ISPAD Clinical Practice Consensus Guideline 2006—2007. Type 2 diabetes mellitus in the child and adolescent. Pediatr Diabetes 2008;**9**:512—26.
5. Kermode-Scott B. Fasting plasma glucose is inadequate screening test for prediabetes in obese youth. BMJ 2008;**337**:a488.
6. Libman IM, Barinas-Mitchell E, Bartucci A, Robertson R, Arslanian S. Reproducibility of the oral glucose tolerance test in overweight children. J Clin.Endocrinol.Metab 2008;**93**:4231—7.
7. Pinhas-Hamiel O, Zeitler P. The global spread of type 2 diabetes mellitus in children and adolescents. J Pediatr 2005;**146**:693—700.
8. Williams DE, Cadwell BL, Cheng YJ, Cowie CC, Gregg EW, Geiss LS, Engelgau MM, Narayan KM, Imperatore G. Prevalence of impaired fasting glucose and its relationship with cardiovascular disease risk factors in US adolescents, 1999—2000. Pediatrics 2005;**116**:1122—6.
9. Baranowski T, Cooper DM, Harrell J, Hirst K, Kaufman FR, Goran M, Resnicow K, The Stopp-T2D Prevention Study Group. Presence of diabetes risk factors in a large U.S. eighth-grade cohort. Diabetes Care 2006;**29**:212—17.
10. Sinha R, Fisch G, Teague B, Tamborlane WV, Banyas B, Allen K, Savoye M, Rieger V, Taksali S, Barbetta G, Sherwin RS, Caprio S. Prevalence of impaired glucose tolerance among children and adolescents with marked obesity 1. N Engl J Med 2002;**346**:802—10.
11. Wabitsch M, Hauner H, Hertrampf M, Muche R, Hay B, Mayer H, Kratzer W, Debatin KM, Heinze E. Type II diabetes mellitus and impaired glucose regulation in Caucasian children and adolescents with obesity living in Germany. Int.J Obes. Relat Metab Disord 2004;**28**:307—13.
12. Xekouki P, Nikolakopoulou NM, Papageorgiou A, Livadas S, Voutetakis A, Magiakou MA, Chrousos GP, Spiliotis BE, Dacou-Voutetakis C. Glucose dysregulation in obese children: predictive, risk, and potential protective factors. Obesity. (Silver.Spring) 2007;**15**:860—9.
13. Valerio G, Licenziati MR, Iannuzzi A, Franzese A, Siani P, Riccardi G, Rubba P. Insulin resistance and impaired glucose tolerance in obese children and adolescents from Southern Italy. Nutr. Metab Cardiovasc.Dis 2006;**16**:279—84.
14. Atabek ME, Pirgon O, Kurtoglu S. Assessment of abnormal glucose homeostasis and insulin resistance in Turkish obese children and adolescents. Diabetes Obes.Metab 2007;**9**:304—10.
15. Tresaco B, Bueno G, Moreno LA, Garagorri JM, Bueno M. Insulin resistance and impaired glucose tolerance in obese children and adolescents. J Physiol Biochem 2003;**59**:217—23.
16. Mazza CS, Ozuna B, Krochik AG, Araujo MB. Prevalence of type 2 diabetes mellitus and impaired glucose tolerance in obese Argentinean children and adolescents. J Pediatr Endocrinol.Metab 2005;**18**:491—8.
17. Aradillas-Garcia C, Malacara JM, Garay-Sevilla ME, Guizar JM, Camacho N, Cruz-Mendoza E, Quemada L, Sierra JF. Prediabetes in rural and urban children in 3 states in Mexico. J Cardiometab. Syndr 2007;**2**:35—9.
18. Babaoglu K, Hatun S, Arslanoglu I, Isguven P, Bas F, Ercan O, Darendeliler F, Bundak R, Saka N, Gunoz H, Bereket A, Memioglu N, Neyzi O. Evaluation of glucose intolerance in adolescents relative to adults with type 2 diabetes mellitus. J Pediatr Endocrinol.Metab 2006;**19**:1319—26.
19. Pettitt DJ, Lawrence JM, Beyer J, Hillier TA, Liese AD, Mayer-Davis B, Loots B, Imperatore G, Liu L, Dolan LM, Linder B, Dabelea D. Association between maternal diabetes in utero and age at offspring's diagnosis of type 2 diabetes. Diabetes Care 2008;**31**:2126—30.
20. Dabelea D, Mayer-Davis EJ, Lamichhane AP, D'Agostino Jr R, Liese AD, Vehik KS, Narayan KM, Zeitler P, Hamman RF. Association of intrauterine exposure to maternal diabetes and obesity with type 2 diabetes in youth: the SEARCH Case-Control Study. Diabetes Care 2008;**31**:1422—6.
21. Malcolm JC, Lawson ML, Gaboury I, Lough G, Keely E. Glucose tolerance of offspring of mother with gestational diabetes mellitus in a low-risk population. Diabet.Med 2006;**23**:565—70.
22. Silverman BL, Rizzo TA, Cho NH, Metzger BE. Long-term effects of the intrauterine environment. The Northwestern University Diabetes in Pregnancy Center. Diabetes Care 1998;**21**(Suppl. 2):B142—9.
23. Goran MI, Bergman RN, Avila Q, Watkins M, Ball GD, Shaibi GQ, Weigensberg MJ, Cruz ML. Impaired glucose tolerance and reduced beta-cell function in overweight Latino children with a positive family history for type 2 diabetes. J Clin.Endocrinol. Metab 2004;**89**:207—12.
24. Reinehr T, Wabitsch M, Kleber M, de Sousa G, Denzer C, Toschke AM. Parental diabetes, pubertal stage, and extreme obesity are the main risk factors for prediabetes in children and

25. Love-Osborn K, Butler N, Gao D, Zeitler P. Elevated fasting triglycerides predict impaired glucose tolerance in adolescents at risk for type 2 diabetes. *Pediatr Diabetes* 2006;**7**:205—10.
26. McIntyre RS, Jerrell JM. Metabolic and cardiovascular adverse events associated with antipsychotic treatment in children and adolescents. *Arch Pediatr Adolesc Med* 2008;**162**:929—35.
27. Nur MM, Newman IM, Siqueira LM. Glucose Metabolism in Overweight Hispanic Adolescents With and Without Polycystic Ovary Syndrome. *Pediatrics* 2009 [ePub ahead of print].
28. de Vegt F, Dekker JM, Jager A, Hienkens E, Kostense PJ, Stehouwer CD, Nijpels G, Bouter LM, Heine RJ. Relation of impaired fasting and postload glucose with incident type 2 diabetes in a Dutch population: The Hoorn Study. *JAMA* 2001;**285**: 2109—13.
29. Weiss R, Taksali SE, Tamborlane WV, Burgert TS, Savoye M, Caprio S. Predictors of changes in glucose tolerance status in obese youth. *Diabetes Care* 2005;**28**:902—9.
30. Hirst K, Baranowski T, DeBar L, Foster GD, Kaufman F, Kennel P, Linder B, Schneider M, Venditti EM, Yin Z. HEALTHY study rationale, design and methods: moderating risk of type 2 diabetes in multi-ethnic middle school students. *Int.J Obes. (Lond)* 2009;**33**(Suppl. 4):S4—20.
31. Balagopal P, Kamalamma N, Patel TG, Misra R. A community-based diabetes prevention and management education program in a rural village in India. *Diabetes Care* 2008;**31**: 1097—104.
32. Zeitler P, Pinhas-Hamiel O. Prevention and screening for type 2 diabetes in youth. In: Dabelea D, Klingensmith GJ, editors. *Epidemiology of pediatric and Adolescent Diabetes*. New York: Informa Healthcare; 2008. pp. 201—16.
33. Freemark M, Bursey D. The effects of metformin on body mass index and glucose tolerance in obese adolescents with fasting hyperinsulinemia and a family history of type 2 diabetes. *Pediatrics* 2001;**107**:E55.
34. Love-Osborn K, Sheeder J, Zeitler P. The addition of metformin to a lifestyle intervention in obese insulin-resistant adolescents. *J Pediatr* 2008;**152**:817—22.
35. Park MH, Kinra S, Ward KJ, White B, Viner RM. Metformin for obesity in children and adolescents: a systematic review. *Diabetes Care* 2009;**32**:1743—45.

CHAPTER 9

Prediabetes and Type 2 Diabetes
An Emerging Epidemic among Obese Youth

Kathryn Love-Osborne

Division of Pediatrics, Section of Adolescent Medicine, Denver Health and Hospitals and University of Colorado at Denver Health Sciences Center, Denver, CO, USA

INTRODUCTION

An increase in pediatric overweight and obesity has been observed worldwide. A large, school-based survey of 13 European countries, Israel, and the United States of almost 30,000 13- and 15-year-old adolescents showed the highest prevalence of obesity in youth from the United States. Almost 30% of American youth were overweight or obese, followed by youth from Ireland, Greece, and Portugal. The lowest prevalence of overweight was found in Lithuania at approximately 20% [1].

The global increase in pediatric obesity has contributed to an increase in the diagnosis of type 2 diabetes mellitus (T2DM), which has now been reported worldwide. Diabetes is defined as fasting plasma glucose (FPG) ≥ 7.0 mmol/l (126 mg/dl) or 2-hour post glucose challenge plasma glucose ≥ 11.1 mmol/l (200 mg/dl). Recently, glycosylated hemoglobin (HbA1c) $\geq 6.5\%$ has been recommended to diagnose diabetes in adults. Estimating prevalence of diabetes in youth is difficult because many studies report center-based results and may not report comparable information. Many large population-based studies included both type 1 (T1DM) and type 2 (T2DM).

GLOBAL T2DM PREVALENCE REPORTS

Japan has been conducting urine glucose screening in school children since 1975. Almost 10 million children have been screened. Glycosuria on first screening is reported in 0.05% to 0.1% of primary school children and 0.12% to 0.2% of junior high school children. Through this program, 236 children, of which 189 were junior high school students, have been diagnosed with T2DM. The overall incidence of T2DM is estimated to be 2.55/100,000/year during 1975–2000. In junior high students the rate increases to 6.27/100,000/year [2]. Interestingly, the frequency of T2DM diagnosed by this screening program has not changed significantly since 1974 and was actually lowest in the most recent screening period of 2001–2004.

The SEARCH for Diabetes in Youth study involved six centers in the United States of youth with physician-diagnosed diabetes. More than 6000 youth < 20 years of age with diabetes, and 769 cases of T2DM were identified. Based on this study, the overall prevalence of T2DM in youth aged 10 to 19 was estimated at 0.42 cases per 1000 [3]. Total diabetes prevalence was estimated at 0.79 cases per 1000 in children under 10 years of age and 2.8 per 1000 in 10- to 19-year-old youth. In the younger age group, >80% of diabetic children and adolescents were classified as T1DM regardless of ethnicity.

In the 10 to 19 year age group, the proportion of diabetics with T2DM varied by ethnicity. In non-Hispanic whites, 6% of diabetics had T2DM for a prevalence of 0.18 cases per 1000 [4]. In Hispanic American diabetic youth, 22% had T2DM with a prevalence of 0.48/1000. T2DM exceeded T1DM in Hispanic female adolescents aged 15 to 19 years [5]. In Asian and Pacific Islander diabetic youth, 40% had T2DM with a prevalence of T2DM of 0.52/1000 [6]. In African American diabetic youth, 33% had T2DM with a prevalence of T2DM of 1.06/1000 [7]. The highest prevalence of T2DM was in American Indian youth, with 76% of diabetics classified as T2DM, a prevalence of 1.74 cases per 1000 youth. Among the subgroup of Navajo adolescents aged 15 to 19, 1 in 359 had diabetes, with a prevalence of 2.78 per 1000, and 1 in 2542 developed diabetes annually [8].

ADDITIONAL T2DM REPORTS FROM CENTERS AND UNIQUE POPULATIONS

An increase in T2DM incidence has been reported in children globally. In a pediatric center in Thailand, the percentage of new diabetic cases in children that were diagnosed as T2DM rose from 5% from 1987 to 1996, to 18% from 1997 to 1999, to 28% from 2003 to 2004 [9].

India has also reported an increase in T2DM, with 26.7% of 434 children with diabetes diagnosed as T2DM in one center and another center reporting 8% of diabetic children < 18 years with T2DM [10].

The increase in T2DM diagnosis was reported in the early 1990s at many centers in the United States [11, 12]. One group reported an increase in percentage of youth under age 19 with T2DM from 4% before 1992 to 16% in 1994. Among older youth 10 to 19 years of age, T2DM accounted for 33% of new diabetes diagnosed in 1994 [13]. A review of T2DM among North American children and adolescents showed a prevalence per 1000 ranging from 7.2 in an Ohio population of white and African American 10- to 19-year-olds to 8 in a California population of whites, Hispanics, African Americans, and Asian Americans aged 0 to 16 years to as high as 50.9 in Pima Indians aged 15 to 19 years. Although the majority of patients in clinic-based studies were African American or Hispanic, 17% to 31% of pediatric patients diagnosed with T2DM were white. The majority of these patients had a family history of T2DM [14].

A cross-sectional survey of children aged 4 to 19 years in an aboriginal community in Canada evaluated 719 children (82% of the school) [15]; 64% of girls and 60% of boys had a body mass index (BMI) > 85%, with 40% of girls and 34% of boys > 95%. Diabetes was identified in eight children. All were female, and only one was normal weight. The prevalence of diabetes in females with BMI > 95% was 4.3%.

The United Kingdom reports a prevalence of T2DM under age 16 as 0.21/100,000 overall, with a higher prevalence of 1.42/100,000 in South Asian children [16].

PREDIABETES PREVALENCE IN YOUTH

Prediabetes is defined as either impaired fasting glucose (IFG) or impaired glucose tolerance (IGT) or both. The definition of IFG is currently plasma glucose $\geq$ 5.6 mmol/l (100 mg/dl) and $\leq$ 7.0 mmol/l (126 mg/dl) [17]. Before 2003, IFG was defined as glucose $\geq$ 6.1 mmol/l (110 mg/dl) and $\leq$ 7.0 mmol/l (126 mg/dl). Unless specified as "pre-2003 criteria," the current definition of IFG will be used. IGT is defined as serum glucose 2 hours after a glucose load of $\geq$ 7.8 mmol/l (140 mg/dl) and $\leq$ 11.1 mmol/l (200 mg/dl). The new adult guidelines define prediabetes as HbA1c 5.7–6.4%.

A large, school-based study in Iran of 4811 students aged 6 to 18 years showed fasting glucose > 100 mg/dl in 4.1% of subjects. The prevalence was only 1% in students < 10 years of age but increased in older subjects. In this population, the prevalence of BMI > 85% was 17% [18].

A study of 1083 Polish children aged 8 to 19 reported 4.6% to be obese and 17.8% overweight; 229 overweight or obese and 83 normal-weight children had fasting glucose values checked. IFG was present in 16.7% of obese children. Subjects with IFG underwent an oral glucose tolerance test (OGTT); 7% of obese children were found to have IGT. The authors estimated prevalence of IFG of 6.7/1000 and IGT 3/1000 for the entire population [19].

A study of 1238 Mexican children aged 6 to 13 identified no cases of T2DM, but 5.7% of children had IFG [20].

2501 U.S. students, aged 9 to 20 years, mean age 14.3 years, were evaluated for glucose intolerance [21]; 35% were overweight or obese. IFG was found on initial screening in 175 subjects (11%). 890 students (36%) underwent an oral glucose tolerance test (OGTT) due to initial IFG or additional risk factors for T2DM. Of interest, only 29 subjects had IFG on the second test. This finding underscores the difficulty of using a single fasting specimen to accurately categorize abnormal glucose metabolism. IGT only was present in 0.3% of subjects, and both IFG and IGT were present in 0.2%. "Near diabetes" (defined as either fasting glucose > 7.0 mmol/L/126 mg/dl or 2-hour glucose > 11.1 mmol/L/200 mg/dl, but not confirmed as diabetes) was present in 0.3%. One student was diagnosed with T2DM.

A study of 1496 U.S. adolescents aged 12 to 19 years from the 1999–2002 National Health and Nutrition Examination Survey (NHANES) showed 12% to have IFG > 100 mg/dl [22]; 15% of obese adolescents, 14% of overweight adolescents, and 9% of normal-weight adolescents had IFG. IFG was twice as common in boys as in girls. The 2005–2006 NHANES survey interviewed 2288 adolescents [23]; 7 adolescents reported having diabetes, 2 using insulin, 2 using oral medications, and 3 not using any medications. A total of 871 adolescents had fasting glucose testing, 90% of whom underwent an OGTT; 29% of the adolescents studied were overweight or obese. Previously undiagnosed diabetes was identified in 2 subjects. IFG was present in 13.1% and IGT in 3.4% of all subjects. Among overweight teens, 14.9% had IFG and 3.6% had IGT. Among obese teens, 22.7% had IFG and 9.5% had IGT. Obese adolescents with hyperinsulinemia (defined as fasting insulin > 13.8 uU/ml) had a significantly higher prevalence of both IFG and IGT. Among obese youth without hyperinsulinemia, only 1.2% had IGT versus 9.9% in youth with hyperinsulinemia. Youth with two or more out of four (not including glucose criteria) metabolic syndrome (MetS) criteria (Table 9.1) also had a higher prevalence of prediabetes, a 2.7-fold higher rate than those with no criteria. Prediabetes was more common in boys than girls. Non-Hispanic blacks had the lowest incidence of prediabetes, with Mexican American having the highest incidence.

A large U.S. study conducted in 12 middle schools of 1740 students (mean age 13.6 years, 53% Hispanic, 23% African American, 15% Caucasian, 2% Native American, and 7% other) collected data on BMI and performed laboratory testing for diabetes [24]. Results showed that 49% of students had a BMI > 85% (20% 85—95% and 29% > 95%); 40% of students had IFG, and 36% had fasting insulin levels > 30 uU/ml. Of students with BMI > 95%, 47% had IFG and 72% had elevated fasting insulin levels; 2.3% of students had IGT; 0.9% of normal-weight students, 3.4% of overweight students, and 4.1% of obese students; 3% of students had a hemoglobin A1c > 6%.

A retrospective chart review study done in a primary care U.S. setting of 7710 patients revealed a prevalence of T2DM (0.2%), IFG (0.2%) and IGT (3.1%) in a population of youth aged 10 to 19 years with 45% of patients that met the American Diabetes Association (ADA) criteria for diabetes screening being tested [25].

CENTER-BASED STUDIES AND UNIQUE POPULATIONS

A study on glucose intolerance examined 710 obese Italian children (aged 6 to 18 years) of European origin, mean BMI 35 kg/m2. Of these, 54% had a family history of diabetes, one child was identified with diabetes, and 4.2% were identified with IGT [26].

A German study of 520 obese Caucasian children and adolescents aged 9 3—20 years, mean 14 years were studied for glucose intolerance [27]. T2DM (defined in this study as fasting glucose > 110 mg/dl and/or 2-hour glucose > 200 mg/dl) was present in 1.5%; three fourths of these patients were not previously diagnosed. IFG was present in 3.7% and IGT in 2.1%. Family history of a parent with diabetes and BMI z-score > 2.5 were associated with increased risk for glucose dysregulation.

A European study of 491 obese children and adolescents aged 7 to 18 years had fasting glucose and insulin levels checked. Only 12 subjects (2½%) had IFG (pre-2003 definition). An oral glucose tolerance test was also performed on 102 subjects with either abnormal fasting glucose or additional risk factors

TABLE 9.1 Metabolic Syndrome Criteria

	WHO criteria, insulin resistance or altered glucose metabolism plus two or more additional criteria	Modified NCEP criteria, three or more of the following	IDF criteria, elevated waist circumference plus two or more additional criteria	Modified Cook criteria for adolescents, three or more of the following
Obesity or Abdominal Obesity	BMI > 30 kg/m^2 and/or waist/hip ratio > 0.9 male/0.85 female	Waist circumference > 102 cm male > 88 cm female	Waist circumference > 94 cm male > 80 cm female	BMI or waist circumference > 95% for age and sex
Blood Pressure	> 140/90 mg Hg	> 130/85	> 130/85	> 90% for age, sex, and height
Triglycerides	> 150 mg/dl (> 1.7 mmol/l)	> 150 mg/dl (> 1.7 mmol/l)	> 150 mg/dl (> 1.7 mmol/l)	> 110 mg/dl (> 1.2 mmol/l)
HDL	< 35 mg/dl male (< 0.90 mmol/l) < 39 mg/dl female (< 1.0 mmol/l)	< 40 mg/dl male (< 1.03 mmol/l) < 50 mg/dl female (< 1.29 mmol/l)	< 40 mg/dl male (< 1.03 mmol/l) < 50 mg/dl female (< 1.29 mmol/l)	< 40 mg/dl (< 1.03 mmol/l)
Glucose, Other	Microalbuminuria > 20 mg/min	Fasting glucose > 100 mg/dl (> 5.6 mmol/l)	Fasting glucose > 100 mg/dl (> 5.6 mmol/l) 2-hour glucose > 140 mg/dl (> 7.8 mmol/l) or diagnosed diabetes	Fasting glucose > 100 mg/dl (> 5.6 mmol/l) 2-hour glucose > 140 mg/dl (> 7.8 mmol/l) or diagnosed diabetes

such as family history of T2DM, hyperlipidemia, or acanthosis nigricans. Mean BMI of this group was 33.3 kg/m^2 for males and 34.2 for females. Of these 102, 36% had IGT and 6% had T2DM; 88% of subjects with abnormal glucose tolerance and 66% of subjects with T2DM were Caucasian [28].

A study of 22 overweight and 234 obese Israeli children and adolescents aged 5 to 22 showed IGT in 13.5% and previously undiagnosed diabetes in one subject. Subjects with IGT had higher (but still normal) fasting glucose levels and significantly higher fasting triglyceride levels (157 mg/dl versus 117 mg/dl) than subjects with normal glucose tolerance (NGT) [29].

A U.S. center administered oral glucose tolerance tests to 439 obese, 31 overweight, and 20 normal-weight youth (aged 4 to 20 years) [30]. The group was ethnically diverse with 41% white, 31% black, and 27% Hispanic youth. IGT was found in 3% of overweight, 14.4% of moderately obese, and 19.9% of severely obese (BMI z-score > 2.5) youth. This trend in increasing prevalence IGT with worsening obesity was observed in all ethnic groups.

Canadian Aboriginal youth aged 6 to 18 years (N = 192, 19% BMI 85% to 95%, 26% > 95%) were studied for glucose intolerance. Of these, 60% had a positive family history of diabetes. IFG was present in 19% and IGT in 5%. IFG was twice as common in boys as in girls. Of the 10 subjects with IGT, only 50% had IFG [31]. Another Canadian study of 719 children aged 4 to 19 found 19 to have IFG. The prevalence of IFG was highest in overweight children, 6.3% in boys and 3.5% in girls [15].

LONGITUDINAL STUDIES IN ADULTS

The San Antonio Heart Study was a population-based study of T2DM and cardiovascular disease. The study enrolled 2941 nondiabetic Mexican American and non-Hispanic white adults. 59% completed 7 to 8 years of follow-up. Diabetes was diagnosed in 11%; 13.7% in Mexican Americans and 6.4% in whites. Incident diabetes was associated with Mexican ethnicity, BMI, and fasting insulin. IGT and MetS (National Cholesterol Education Program definition) were more sensitive at predicting diabetes incidence. Lowering the fasting glucose cutoff to > 5.4 mmol/l improved the predictive discrimination of MetS so that it was similar to IGT in predicting diabetes. Subjects meeting MetS criteria had a six-fold higher risk of developing diabetes [32].

In a group of 319 adult Pima Indians, 48 subjects (15%) progressed to T2DM during 6 years of follow-up. Subjects that progressed to diabetes had higher fasting and 2-hour insulin levels than subjects that maintained NGT [33]. Of another group of 254 Pima Indian adults with NGT, 31% developed IGT at 4½-year follow-up [34]. Of 145 adults with IGT at baseline, 44% developed diabetes at 5½-year follow-up. Both insulin resistance and insulin secretory dysfunction were independent predictors of worsening glucose tolerance.

A large study in western Finland followed more than 2000 non-diabetic adults for 6 years [35]; 6% of subjects developed T2DM. Predictors of diabetes included family history of diabetes, BMI, elevated waist-to-height ratio, and beta cell function. The combination of IFG, BMI > 30 kg/m2, and family history of diabetes had a hazard ratio of 3.7 for predicting diabetes.

A study followed 13,000 young men aged 26 to 45 years (mean age 32 years) in the Israel Defense Forces for a mean of almost 6 years. All subjects had normal fasting glucose (NFG) at baseline. Diabetes developed in 1.5%. Elevated triglycerides over 150 mg/dl, family history of diabetes, increasing fasting glucose (within the normal range), and BMI were independently associated with development of diabetes. In obese subjects (BMI > 30 kg/m2) with baseline fasting glucose > 90 mg/dl (5.0 mmol/l), the incidence of diabetes was 5.7% [36].

In one study, 872 American adults, 580 with NGT and 292 with IGT at baseline, were followed for 5 years [37]; 16% developed diabetes at follow-up; 8% of NGT and 33% of IGT subjects developed T2DM. Five risk factors were identified, including high triglycerides > 150 mg/dl, low HDL < 40 mg/dl, hypertension > 140/90, IGT, and high plasminogen activator inhibitor > 28 ng/ml. The incidence of diabetes increased linearly with the number of risk factors, ranging from 5% in subjects with no risk factors to 50% in those with all five risk factors.

LONGITUDINAL STUDIES IN YOUTH

Pacific Island communities such as Nauru and Tuvalu have reported high rates of T2DM in youth. Prevalence of T2DM in youth is reported at 0.6 to 1%, with IGT prevalence of 3.5% to 5.1%. 8- to 29-year-old subjects first seen in 1976 were followed for 11 years for development of IGT or T2DM. The cumulative incidence of abnormal glucose tolerance (IGT or T2DM) consistently increased with each quartile of fasting insulin, reaching 23% in those subjects in the fourth quartile of fasting insulin at baseline [38].

A cohort of 1491 black and white 9- to 10-year-old U.S. adolescent girls was followed for 10 years. Study retention was excellent at 85%. BMI data were available on 955 girls at both baseline and 10-year follow-up, and fasting glucose data were available at year 10. IFG (pre-2003 criteria) was present at year 10 in 3% of black adolescents and 1.3% of white adolescents. Seven black girls developed diabetes, for a 1.4% incidence rate;

only one of these girls was not overweight or obese. Baseline BMI predicted development of IFG in black girls, but the rate of BMI increase predicted development of IFT in white girls [39].

A study of 117 ethnically diverse obese U.S. children and adolescents (4 to 18 years) evaluated progression to diabetes over a mean of 20 months. Of these, 33 subjects had IGT at baseline. Eight subjects, all with IGT and meeting criteria for metabolic syndrome at baseline, developed T2DM during the study period (24% of those with IGT at baseline). Those that developed diabetes had a higher baseline BMI but similar measures of insulin resistance at baseline. They also gained more weight, whereas the 15 subjects with IGT that reverted to NGT maintained BMI during the follow-up period. During the follow-up period, 8 subjects (10%) with baseline NGT developed IGT [40].

The Bogalusa Heart Study is a longitudinal study of black and white U.S. children [41]. It consists of cross-sectional surveys of coronary artery disease risk factors among biracial children and young adults in Louisiana. Almost 2000 subjects were followed during childhood (4 to 11 years), adolescence (12 to 18 years), and adulthood (19 to 44 years). The average age at baseline was 10.9 years and the average age at last follow-up was 32 years. Subjects with diabetes at baseline were excluded. At follow-up, 60 subjects (3%) developed T2DM and 4.5% developed IFG. Subjects that developed T2DM had higher BMI, triglycerides, glucose, and insulin and lower HDL cholesterol from childhood through adulthood than those that maintained normoglycemia.

AMERICAN DIABETES ASSOCIATION (ADA) GUIDELINES FOR SCREENING

The ADA recommends screening youth for T2DM if they have a body mass index (BMI) > 85% for age and gender and at least two additional risk factors for the development of T2DM: ethnic minority (American Indian, African American, Hispanic, Asian/Pacific Islander), family history (first or second degree) of diabetes, or other evidence of insulin resistance (hypertension, polycystic ovarian syndrome, acanthosis nigricans, dyslipidemia). The recommended test is a fasting plasma glucose level or a 2-hour plasma glucose level [42]. As previously noted, adult recommendations have changed to use HbA1c for screening purposes.

A study in Texas of 1076 ethnically diverse 10- to 12-year-old students found that 23% met ADA criteria for screening. The percentage of students at risk for T2DM based on these criteria was 27% of Mexican American youth, 28% of African American youth, 8% of Asian youth, and 5% of white youth [43].

RISK FACTORS IDENTIFIED FOR PEDIATRIC T2DM

Family History

As in adult T2DM, family history plays an important role in risk of developing diabetes. The Bogalusa Heart Study evaluated 1338 black and white U.S. young adults; 23% of the subjects reported having a parent with diabetes. In all, 1.6% of those studied were diagnosed with IFG (pre-2003 criteria, N = 7) or diabetes (N = 15, 9 of which were previously undiagnosed). Offspring of diabetic parents had higher triglycerides and glucose after adjusting for BMI and waist circumference than young adults without a family history of diabetes. These differences were greater among blacks than whites in the study [44].

A study of 317 Mexican children aged 10 to 14 years identified family history of diabetes by direct measurement of parental laboratory values [45]; 18% of children were overweight and 23% obese. IGT was identified in 15% of subjects, 23% in those with a family history of diabetes, hypertension, or obesity and 11% in those with no family history. In addition, 41% of subjects with IGT had a normal weight but a positive family history. Children with a family history were more likely to exhibit hyperinsulinemia, defined as fasting insulin > 16 uIU/ml. All of the normal-weight or overweight children with hyperinsulinemia had a family history of T2DM, hypertension, or obesity, and 63% of the obese children with hyperinsulinemia had a positive family history.

One concern about the reliability of family history is that family members, especially fathers, may not have been screened for diabetes and thus may be undiagnosed. A small study of family members of 11 adolescents diagnosed with T2DM confirmed this finding. A known history of T2DM was present in 45% of mothers and 36% of fathers. During the study, an additional 27% of fathers were diagnosed with diabetes [46].

Insulin Resistance

A study of 207 overweight Latino U.S. children aged 8 to 13 with a family history of T2DM showed 12% to have IFG and 25% to have IGT [47]. Males were more likely than females to have IFG. There were no differences in BMI between children in the NFG and IFG groups. IFG children had 15% lower disposition index, an index of beta cell function, and higher fasting insulin levels.

Race/Ethnicity

Although the increase in T2DM has been observed in all ethnic groups, T2DM risk is higher in ethnic minorities. Early U.S. studies reported T2DM rates in African

American youth to be out of proportion to the general population [12, 13]. Other minority groups were reported to have increased prevalence of T2DM than in the surrounding population [48]. Although T2DM is prevalent in African American youth, the prevalence of IFG has been reported to be lower in African American youth than in Hispanic youth [22].

Pima Indian youth have a high incidence of diabetes. A longitudinal study followed 529 children, 936 adolescents aged 10 to 14, and 653 adolescents aged 15 to 19 for 5 years. Twenty-two children were diagnosed with T2DM (7.5/1000 person-years), 45 young adolescents (9.2/1000 person-years), and 53 older adolescents (16.4/1000 person-years); 33% of subjects had at least one parent with onset of diabetes prior to 30 years of age. The incidence of diabetes for youth with a diabetic parent was 24.1/1000 person-years [49].

Gender

Many studies of youth have shown boys to have higher rates of IFG, typically twice as common as in girls [22]. However, in the SEARCH population of youth with T2DM, prevalence was higher among females in black, Asian Pacific Islander, and American Indian adolescents [3].

Obesity

Early studies identified obesity as a risk factor for T2DM in youth. Most but not all youth with T2DM are obese, emphasizing the importance of considering other risk factors in addition to obesity. A longitudinal study of 181 obese youth demonstrated that increasing beta cell demand and the degree of obesity at baseline were independently related to elevated glucose levels over time [50]. The change in degree of obesity over time was not related to hyperglycemia.

In other studies, the combination of obesity and family history of diabetes has been shown to impact diabetes risk. For example, 155 adults in one study that had both parents with T2DM and a control group of 186 adults without a family history of parental diabetes were followed for an average of 13 years [51]. At baseline, offspring of diabetic parents after controlling for obesity had higher fasting and stimulated insulin levels and slower glucose removal rates than control subjects. Also, 16% of offspring of diabetic parents developed diabetes during the follow-up period, eight times the rate expected for the age of the population studied. For normal-weight subjects, the fasting insulin level did not vary by family history. In obese subjects, fasting insulin levels were dramatically higher (approximately double) in offspring of diabetic parents compared with obese controls.

Maternal Diabetes

Maternal diabetes has been shown to increase the risk for abnormal glucose metabolism in youth [52, 53]. In a study of 88 offspring of women with diabetes (including T1DM, T2DM, and gestational diabetes or GDM), the prevalence of IGT during adolescence was associated with amniotic fluid insulin (AFI) at 32 to 38 weeks gestation. The prevalence of IGT at 10 to 16 years was 19.5% and was not associated with the etiology of the mother's diabetes. Seventeen subjects > 10 years of age had IGT with one having T2DM. Of adolescents that had normal AFI during gestation, only 3.7% had IGT, whereas 33.3% of adolescents with elevated AFI had IGT. This study suggests that not only the history of maternal diabetes but the adequacy of glucose control during the pregnancy can be deemed important in determining risk. A study of 150 overweight or obese Hispanic youth aged 8 to 13 years with a family history (first- or second-degree relative) of diabetes showed 28% to have IGT [52]. None of the subjects had IFG. Of subjects whose mother had gestational diabetes (GDM), 41% had IGT.

Acanthosis Nigricans (AN)

A study of Mexican American children aged 10 to 12 years identified by ADA criteria to be at risk for T2DM (N = 61) and their siblings (N = 78) were evaluated. Children with acanthosis nigricans were shown to be heavier, with significantly higher fasting insulin levels and fasting triglyceride levels. Insulin levels were > 15 uU/ml in 84% of subjects with AN, with a mean of 30 uU/ml. However, even in the children without AN, 38% had elevated insulin levels [43].

Elevated Waist Circumference (WC)

The Bogalusa Heart Study demonstrated that within given BMI categories, subjects with elevated waist circumferences were observed to have twice the incidence of high triglyceride levels, high insulin levels, and the metabolic syndrome as in the low WC group. Fasting glucose levels were significantly higher in high WC compared with low WC subjects in the normal-weight and overweight categories, but not in the obese category [54]. Normal values have been suggested for waist circumference in samples of American youth [55].

Weight Gain

A longitudinal study of 17 adult Pima Indians who deteriorated from NGT to IGT to diabetes showed the time interval from NGT to diabetes to be a mean of

5 years. Compared with subjects that maintained NGT, subjects that developed diabetes gained more weight (14% versus 7%) during the follow-up period and had higher baseline fasting insulin levels [56].

PRESENTATION

As in adults, youth with T2DM are more likely to be diagnosed by routine screening than youth with T1DM. For example, 35% to 40% of youth with T2DM in the SEARCH study were identified through routine screening. When symptoms of diabetes do occur, symptoms are present in similar percentages of patients as those reported with T1DM (abdominal pain, dizziness, headache, nocturia, polydipsia, polyphagia, polyuria, vaginal yeast infection, and visual disturbance) with the exception of weight loss, which is less often present in patients with T2DM than T1DM [11].

Youth with T2DM may present with diabetic ketoacidosis (DKA); in one series of 9- to 18-year-old patients with DKA, 9 (13%) were diagnosed with T2DM. Of these, 7 of 9 did not require insulin at 1-year follow-up [57]. A study of 50 youth with T2DM in Arkansas showed DKA to be present at diagnosis in 25% [58].

SCREENING FOR T2DM IN PRIMARY CARE

Although current guidelines in the United States advocate for using fasting plasma glucose as a screen for T2DM in youth, practitioners do not often follow these guidelines. A retrospective chart review of 7710 youth aged 10 to 19 years evaluated whether patients meeting ADA criteria for screening had been screened [25]. Findings showed that 18% of patients were overweight and 24% obese. Of the 672 subjects who met the criteria for screening, 45% were screened. The most common screening test was a random plasma glucose level (87%). In an office-based setting, most patients are not fasting and may not be willing or able to return fasting. In addition, as previously discussed, fasting glucose values are not well reproducible [21].

In 2009, new recommendations were made by an expert committee to consider using glycosylated hemoglobin (HgbA1c) as diagnostic criteria for diabetes in adults [59]. This recommendation was supported in 2010 by the ADA. Data are presented that indicate that complications from retinopathy begin to increase with HgbA1c values > 6% (42 mmol/mol) and increase more sharply at values > 6.5% (48 mmol/mol). The reliability and reproducibility of HgbA1c has improved over the past decade, making this test more useful as a screening test. Because the HgbA1c is a measure of glucose values over the past 3 to 4 months, this test may more accurately reflect patients at increased risk for long-term comorbidities and may lead to less repeat testing. HgbA1c has been shown to reliably predict T2DM in obese children as well [60]. In the entire cohort of 468 obese youth (mean age 12.8, BMI 34.4 kg/m2), HgbA1c of 5.7% or greater was 86% sensitive and 85% specific for detecting T2DM. In a subgroup of 193 insulin resistant obese youth, HgbA1c of 6% had a sensitivity of 99% and a specificity of 96% for detecting T2DM.

COMPLICATIONS OF T2DM

As in adults, youth with T2DM are at increased risk for hypertension, nephropathy, retinopathy, dyslipidemia, nonalcoholic fatty liver disease (NAFLD), cardiovascular disease, psychiatric disorders, polycystic ovarian syndrome, and orthopedic problems [61].

Because of the younger age at onset of T2DM, youth are more likely to suffer from complications at some point during their lifetime. Japanese studies have found that the incidence of nephropathy for patients diagnosed with diabetes under 30 years of age was higher in T2DM than T1DM patients (44% versus 20%), despite patients with T2DM having lower A1c levels [62]. The study included 278 patients with T2DM diagnosed at 10 to 19 years. Of these patients, the mean age at follow-up was 27.6 years.

FOLLOW-UP FOR YOUTH WITH T2DM

A study of 129 German and Austrian children with T2DM showed significant (60%) rates of subjects that were lost to follow-up from specialized diabetes centers [63]. Lifestyle intervention alone was not often useful for long-term metabolic control of diabetes.

PREVENTION

Adult studies have shown lifestyle modification to be beneficial in preventing T2DM [64, 65]. The Finnish Diabetes Prevention Study showed a 58% reduction in the incidence of diabetes in the intervention group which consisted of individualized counseling aimed at weight reduction, lowered fat intake, increased fiber intake, and increased physical activity [66]. Specifically evaluating physical activity, those subjects who increased moderate to vigorous or strenuous leisure-time physical activity were 65% less likely to develop diabetes. The Diabetes Prevention Program found an intensive lifestyle modification program to be superior to metformin in preventing T2DM in adults with IGT. The benefits of lifestyle over metformin were less pronounced in younger patients. These types of studies have not been conducted in at-risk youth.

CONCLUSIONS AND SUGGESTED APPROACHES TO SCREENING

As the number of overweight and obese youth increases, primary care providers are faced with making the decision of whom to test, what tests to order, and how often they should screen their patients. The ADA suggests screening overweight or obese children with two additional risk factors for T2DM every 2 years with a fasting glucose. However, based on the literature, it is clear that not all risk factors are equal in predicting risk for development of T2DM. For example, although family history of diabetes is generally considered to be either first- or second-degree relative, a child with a first-degree relative with T2DM is at higher risk for developing diabetes than a child with a second-degree relative with T2DM [45]. Thus, a child that is not overweight but has multiple other risk factors may deserve screening.

IDENTIFIED RISK FACTORS FOR T2DM

- Obese > overweight > normal weight
- Family history of T2DM: GDM > first-degree relative > second-degree relative > negative FH
- Race/ethnicity: American Indian > African American > Pacific Islander > Hispanic > White
- Signs of insulin resistance (acanthosis nigricans, hypertension, dyslipidemia, polycystic ovarian syndrome)

Screening Strategy for T2DM in Youth

	Screen	Consider screening
BMI	>95%	>85% + one risk factor Normal + two risk factors
Family History	GDM or first-degree relative + one risk factor	Second degree + one risk factor
Race/Ethnicity	Ethnic minority + one risk factor	White + two risk factors
Signs of Insulin Resistance	All	

WHICH TESTS TO USE?

In addition to T2DM screening, youth identified to be at risk for T2DM should also be screened for dyslipidemia and for nonalcoholic fatty liver disease (NAFLD) [67].

Considerations in deciding which tests to use include cost, convenience, and reproducibility. Some tests may be inexpensive but if many patients require follow-up testing, this may not be the most cost-effective screening approach.

Diabetes

Concerns with using a fasting glucose to screen for T2DM have been discussed. IFG is not highly reproducible and patients may not be willing or able to return for fasting tests. Random glucose values are difficult to interpret unless they are in the diabetic range. Recent recommendations to use HgbA1c for T2DM screening may prove to be a useful tool for pediatric providers, although the long-term predictive value of this test has not been studied in youth at risk for T2DM [17]. Although the cost of the HgbA1c is typically higher than that of a serum or fingerstick glucose, the use of HgbA1c may significantly decrease the need for repeat testing including oral glucose tolerance testing. A HgbA1c value > 6.5% is considered diagnostic for diabetes in adults.

Hyperlipidemia

The optimal screening test for dyslipidemia is a fasting lipid panel [68]. If lipid panels are ordered non-fasting, triglyceride values in particular may be falsely elevated. On the other hand, it may be reasonable to screen with a random cholesterol level in patients at risk for T2DM in order to increase the number of patients who are screened. Borderline values for total cholesterol 170 to 200 mg/dl or elevated values 200 to 240 mg/dl can be followed with a fasting lipid panel done 2 to 3 months after initiation of lifestyle change. More significant elevations of total cholesterol > 240 mg/dl may require confirmation with a fasting lipid panel.

Nonalcoholic Fatty Liver Disease (NAFLD)

Although both aspartate aminotransferase (AST) and alanine aminotranferase (ALT) are recommended as screening for NAFLD, ALT is more commonly elevated in the 1½ to 3 times the upper limit of normal in NAFLD [69]. Thus, it is reasonable for initial screening of at-risk youth to start with ALT alone in the interest of cost containment. Elevated ALT levels < 3 times the upper limit of normal can be followed in 2 to 3 months with a full liver panel. Higher elevation of ALT may require additional evaluation.

	Fasting (ideal)	Random
Diabetes	HgbA1c	HgbA1c
Dyslipidemia	Lipid panel	Cholesterol
NAFLD	Liver panel	ALT

HOW OFTEN TO TEST?

Although the ADA recommends testing at-risk youth every 2 years, the addition of the HgbA1c may help providers prioritize which patients may need more frequent screening. Patients with a HgbA1c value in the 5.7% to 6.4% should be re-tested in 3–6 months. An additional consideration may be changes in BMI over time; patients with significant increases in BMI may require more frequent screening. Patients with completely normal laboratory tests who maintain or lose weight could potentially be screened less frequently.

CONCLUSION

With T2DM clearly now a pediatric disease, providers of children are charged with screening at-risk youth for not only T2DM but dyslipidemias and NAFLD in addition to multiple other comorbidities of obesity. With a clearer understanding of risk factors for T2DM in youth, pediatric providers have in important role in identifying these young people in an attempt to modulate the long-term complications of this chronic disease.

References

1. Lissau I, Overpeck MD, Ruan WJ, Due P, Holstein BE, Hediger ML. Body mass index and overweight in adolescents in 13 European countries, Israel, and the United States. Arch Pediatr Adolesc Med 2004;158(1):27–33.
2. American Diabetes Association. Diagnosis and Classification of Diabetes Mellitos. Diabetes Care 2010;33(Suppl. 1):S62–9.
3. Liese AD, D'Agostino Jr RB, Hamman RF, et al. The burden of diabetes mellitus among US youth: prevalence estimates from the SEARCH for Diabetes in Youth Study. Pediatrics 2006;118(4):1510–18.
4. Bell RA, Mayer-Davis EJ, Beyer JW, et al. Diabetes in non-Hispanic white youth: prevalence, incidence, and clinical characteristics: the SEARCH for Diabetes in Youth Study. Diabetes Care 2009;32(Suppl. 2):S102–11.
5. Lawrence JM, Mayer-Davis EJ, Reynolds K, et al. Diabetes in Hispanic American youth: prevalence, incidence, demographics, and clinical characteristics: the SEARCH for Diabetes in Youth Study. Diabetes Care 2009;32(Suppl. 2):S123–32.
6. Liu LL, Yi JP, Beyer J, et al. Type 1 and type 2 diabetes in Asian and Pacific Islander U.S. youth: the SEARCH for Diabetes in Youth Study. Diabetes Care 2009;32(Suppl. 2):S133–40.
7. Mayer-Davis EJ, Beyer J, Bell RA, et al. Diabetes in African American youth: prevalence, incidence, and clinical characteristics: the SEARCH for Diabetes in Youth Study. Diabetes Care 2009;32(Suppl. 2):S112–22.
8. Dabelea D, DeGroat J, Sorrelman C, et al. Diabetes in Navajo youth: prevalence, incidence, and clinical characteristics: the SEARCH for Diabetes in Youth Study. Diabetes Care 2009;32(Suppl. 2):S141–7.
9. Santiprabhob J, Weerakulwattana P, Nunloi S, et al. Etiology and glycemic control among Thai children and adolescents with diabetes mellitus. J Med Assoc Thai 2007;90(8):1608–15.
10. Mohan V, Jaydip R, Deepa R. Type 2 diabetes in Asian Indian youth. Pediatr Diabetes 2007;8(Suppl. 9):28–34.
11. Carrel AL, Clark RR, Peterson SE, Nemeth BA, Sullivan J, Allen DB. Improvement of fitness, body composition, and insulin sensitivity in overweight children in a school-based exercise program: a randomized, controlled study. Arch Pediatr Adolesc Med 2005;159(10):963–8.
12. Pihoker C, Scott CR, Lensing SY, Cradock MM, Smith J. Non-insulin dependent diabetes mellitus in African-American youths of Arkansas. Clin Pediatr (Phila) 1998;37(2):97–102.
13. Pinhas-Hamiel O, Dolan LM, Daniels SR, Standiford D, Khoury PR, Zeitler P. Increased incidence of non-insulin-dependent diabetes mellitus among adolescents. J Pediatr 1996;128(5 Pt 1):608–15.
14. Fagot-Campagna A, Pettitt DJ, Engelgau MM, Burrows NR, Geiss LS, Valdez R. Type 2 diabetes among North American children and adolescents: an epidemiologic review and a public health perspective. J Pediatr 2000;136:664–72.
15. Young TK, Dean HJ, Flett B, Wood-Steiman P. Childhood obesity in a population at high risk for type 2 diabetes. J Pediatr 2000;136(3):365–9.
16. Ehtisham S, Hattersley AT, Dunger DB, Barrett TG. First UK survey of paediatric type 2 diabetes and MODY. Arch Dis Child 2004;89(6):526–9.
17. Genuth S, Alberti KG, Bennett P, et al. Follow-up report on the diagnosis of diabetes mellitus. Diabetes Care 2003;26(11):3160–7.
18. Kelishadi R, Gheiratmand R, Ardalan G, et al. Association of anthropometric indices with cardiovascular disease risk factors among children and adolescents: CASPIAN Study. Int J Cardiol 2007;117(3):340–8.
19. Mazur A, Grzywa M, Malecka-Tendera E, Telega G. Prevalence of glucose intolerance in school age children. Population based cross-sectional study. Acta Paediatr 2007;96(12):1799–802.
20. Aradillas-Garcia C, Malacara JM, Garay-Sevilla ME, et al. Prediabetes in rural and urban children in 3 states in Mexico. J Cardiometab Syndr 2007;2(1):35–9.
21. Dolan LM, Bean J, D'Alessio D, et al. Frequency of abnormal carbohydrate metabolism and diabetes in a population-based screening of adolescents. J Pediatr 2005;146(6):751–8.
22. Duncan GE. Prevalence of diabetes and impaired fasting glucose levels among US adolescents: National Health and Nutrition Examination Survey, 1999–2002. Arch Pediatr Adolesc Med 2006;160(5):523–8.
23. Li C, Ford ES, Zhao G, Mokdad AH. Prevalence of pre-diabetes and its association with clustering of cardiometabolic risk factors and hyperinsulinemia among U.S. adolescents: National Health and Nutrition Examination Survey 2005-2006. Diabetes Care 2009;32(2):342–7.
24. Baranowski T, Cooper DM, Harrell J, et al. Presence of diabetes risk factors in a large U.S. eighth-grade cohort. Diabetes Care 2006;29(2):212–17.
25. Anand SG, Mehta SD, Adams WG. Diabetes mellitus screening in pediatric primary care. Pediatrics 2006;118(5):1888–95.

26. Invitti C, Guzzaloni G, Gilardini L, Morabito F, Viberti G. Prevalence and concomitants of glucose intolerance in European obese children and adolescents. *Diabetes Care* 2003;**26**(1):118−24.
27. Wabitsch M, Hauner H, Hertrampf M, et al. Type II diabetes mellitus and impaired glucose regulation in Caucasian children and adolescents with obesity living in Germany. *Int J Obes Relat Metab Disord* 2004;**28**(2):307−13.
28. Wiegand S, Maikowski U, Blankenstein O, Biebermann H, Tarnow P, Gruters A. Type 2 diabetes and impaired glucose tolerance in European children and adolescents with obesity−a problem that is no longer restricted to minority groups. *Eur J Endocrinol* 2004;**151**(2):199−206.
29. Shalitin S, Abrahami M, Lilos P, Phillip M. Insulin resistance and impaired glucose tolerance in obese children and adolescents referred to a tertiary-care center in Israel. *Int J Obes (Lond)* 2005;**29**(6):571−8.
30. Weiss R, Dziura J, Burgert TS, et al. Obesity and the metabolic syndrome in children and adolescents. *N Engl J Med* 2004;**350**(23):2362−74.
31. Zorzi A, Wahi G, Macnab AJ, Panagiotopoulos C. Prevalence of impaired glucose tolerance and the components of metabolic syndrome in Canadian Tsimshian Nation youth. *Can J Rural Med* 2009;**14**(2):61−7.
32. Lorenzo C, Okoloise M, Williams K, Stern MP, Haffner SM. The metabolic syndrome as predictor of type 2 diabetes: the San Antonio heart study. *Diabetes Care* 2003;**26**(11):3153−9.
33. Weyer C, Hanson RL, Tataranni PA, Bogardus C, Pratley RE. A high fasting plasma insulin concentration predicts type 2 diabetes independent of insulin resistance: evidence for a pathogenic role of relative hyperinsulinemia. *Diabetes* 2000;**49**(12):2094−101.
34. Weyer C, Tataranni PA, Bogardus C, Pratley RE. Insulin resistance and insulin secretory dysfunction are independent predictors of worsening of glucose tolerance during each stage of type 2 diabetes development. *Diabetes Care* 2001;**24**(1):89−94.
35. Lyssenko V, Almgren P, Anevski D, et al. Predictors of and longitudinal changes in insulin sensitivity and secretion preceding onset of type 2 diabetes. *Diabetes* 2005;**54**(1):166−74.
36. Tirosh A, Shai I, Tekes-Manova D, et al. Normal fasting plasma glucose levels and type 2 diabetes in young men. *N Engl J Med* 2005;**353**(14):1454−62.
37. D'Agostino Jr RB, Hamman RF, Karter AJ, Mykkanen L, Wagenknecht LE, Haffner SM. Cardiovascular disease risk factors predict the development of type 2 diabetes: the insulin resistance atherosclerosis study. *Diabetes Care* 2004;**27**(9):2234−40.
38. Zimmet PZ, Collins VR, Dowse GK, Knight LT. Hyperinsulinaemia in youth is a predictor of type 2 (non-insulin-dependent) diabetes mellitus. *Diabetologia* 1992;**35**(6):534−41.
39. Klein DJ, Aronson FL, Harlan WR, et al. Obesity and the development of insulin resistance and impaired fasting glucose in black and white adolescent girls: a longitudinal study. *Diabetes Care* 2004;**27**(2):378−83.
40. Weiss R, Taksali SE, Tamborlane WV, Burgert TS, Savoye M, Caprio S. Predictors of changes in glucose tolerance status in obese youth. *Diabetes Care* 2005;**28**(4):902−9.
41. Nguyen QM, Srinivasan SR, Xu JH, Chen W, Berenson GS. Changes in risk variables of metabolic syndrome since childhood in pre-diabetic and type 2 diabetic subjects: the Bogalusa Heart Study. *Diabetes Care* 2008;**31**(10):2044−9.
42. American Diabetes Association. Type 2 diabetes in children and adolescents. *Diabetes Care* 2000;**23**(3):381−9.
43. Urrutia-Rojas X, Menchaca J, Wadley W, et al. Cardiovascular risk factors in Mexican-American children at risk for type 2 diabetes mellitus (T2DM). *J Adolesc Health* 2004;**34**(4):290−9.
44. McClain MR, Srinivasan SR, Chen W, Steinmann WC, Berenson GS. Risk of type 2 diabetes mellitus in young adults from a biracial community: the Bogalusa Heart Study. *Prev Med* 2000;**31**(1):1−7.
45. Rodriguez-Moran M, Guerrero-Romero F. Hyperinsulinemia in healthy children and adolescents with a positive family history for type 2 diabetes. *Pediatrics* 2006;**118**(5):e1516−22.
46. Pinhas-Hamiel O, Standiford D, Hamiel D, Dolan LM, Cohen R, Zeitler PS. The type 2 family: a setting for development and treatment of adolescent type 2 diabetes mellitus. *Arch Pediatr Adolesc Med* 1999;**153**(10):1063−7.
47. Weigensberg MJ, Ball GD, Shaibi GQ, Cruz ML, Goran MI. Decreased beta-cell function in overweight Latino children with impaired fasting glucose. *Diabetes Care* 2005;**28**(10):2519−24.
48. Jones KL. Non-insulin dependent diabetes in children and adolescents: the therapeutic challenge. *Clin Pediatr (Phila)* 1998;**37**(2):103−10.
49. Franks PW, Hanson RL, Knowler WC, et al. Childhood predictors of young-onset type 2 diabetes. *Diabetes* 2007;**56**(12):2964−72.
50. Weiss R, Cali AM, Dziura J, Burgert TS, Tamborlane WV, Caprio S. Degree of obesity and glucose allostasis are major effectors of glucose tolerance dynamics in obese youth. *Diabetes Care* 2007;**30**(7):1845−50.
51. Warram JH, Martin BC, Krolewski AS, Soeldner JS, Kahn CR. Slow glucose removal rate and hyperinsulinemia precede the development of type II diabetes in the offspring of diabetic parents. *Ann Intern Med* 1990;**113**(12):909−15.
52. Goran MI, Bergman RN, Avila Q, et al. Impaired glucose tolerance and reduced beta-cell function in overweight Latino children with a positive family history for type 2 diabetes. *J Clin Endocrinol Metab* 2004;**89**(1):207−12.
53. Silverman BL, Metzger BE, Cho NH, Loeb CA. Impaired glucose tolerance in adolescent offspring of diabetic mothers. Relationship to fetal hyperinsulinism. *Diabetes Care* 1995;**18**(5):611−17.
54. Janssen I, Katzmarzyk PT, Srinivasan SR, et al. Combined influence of body mass index and waist circumference on coronary artery disease risk factors among children and adolescents. *Pediatrics* 2005;**115**(6):1623−30.
55. Fernandez JR, Redden DT, Pietrobelli A, Allison DB. Waist circumference percentiles in nationally representative samples of African-American, European-American, and Mexican-American children and adolescents. *J Pediatr* 2004;**145**(4):439−44.
56. Weyer C, Bogardus C, Mott DM, Pratley RE. The natural history of insulin secretory dysfunction and insulin resistance in the pathogenesis of type 2 diabetes mellitus. *J Clin Invest* 1999;**104**(6):787−94.
57. Sapru A, Gitelman SE, Bhatia S, Dubin RF, Newman TB, Flori H. Prevalence and characteristics of type 2 diabetes mellitus in 9−18 year-old children with diabetic ketoacidosis. *J Pediatr Endocrinol Metab* 2005;**18**(9):865−72.
58. Scott CR, Smith JM, Cradock MM, Pihoker C. Characteristics of youth-onset noninsulin-dependent diabetes mellitus and insulin-dependent diabetes mellitus at diagnosis. *Pediatrics* 1997;**100**(1):84−91.
59. International Expert Committee report on the role of the A1C assay in the diagnosis of diabetes. *Diabetes Care* 2009;**32**(7):1327−34.
60. Shah S, Kublaoui BM, Oden JD, White PC. Screening for type 2 diabetes in obese youth. *Pediatrics* 2009;**124**(2):573−9.
61. Pinhas-Hamiel O, Zeitler P. Acute and chronic complications of type 2 diabetes mellitus in children and adolescents. *Lancet* 2007;**369**:1823−31.
62. Yokoyama H, Okudaira M, Otani T, et al. Higher incidence of diabetic nephropathy in type 2 than in type 1 diabetes in early-onset diabetes in Japan. *Kidney Int* 2000;**58**(1):302−11.

REFERENCES

63. Reinehr T, Schober E, Roth CL, Wiegand S, Holl R. Type 2 diabetes in children and adolescents in a 2-year follow-up: insufficient adherence to diabetes centers. *Horm Res* 2008;**69**(2):107–13.
64. Laaksonen DE, Lindstrom J, Lakka TA, et al. Physical activity in the prevention of type 2 diabetes: the Finnish diabetes prevention study. *Diabetes* 2005;**54**(1):158–65.
65. Diabetes Prevention Program Research Group. Reduction in the incidence of type 2 diabetes with lifestyle intervention or metformin. *JAMA* 2002;**346**(6):393.
66. Lindstrom Ericksson JG, Valle TT, Aunola S, Cepaitis Z, Hakumaki M. Prevention of diabetes mellitus in subjects with impaired glucose tolerance in the Finnish diabetes prevention study: results from a randomized clinical trial. *J Am Soc Nephrol* 2003;**14**(S):108.
67. Barlow SE. Expert committee recommendations regarding the prevention, assessment, and treatment of child and adolescent overweight and obesity: summary report. *Pediatrics* 2007;**120**(Suppl. 4):S164–92.
68. Daniels SR, Greer FR. Lipid screening and cardiovascular health in childhood. *Pediatrics* 2008;**122**(1):198–208.
69. Marchesini G, Brizi M, Morselli-Labate AM, et al. Association of nonalcoholic fatty liver disease with insulin resistance. *Am J Med* 1999;**107**(5):450–5.

CHAPTER 10

Prevalence of the Metabolic Syndrome in U.S. Youth

Sarah E. Messiah [*,‡], Kristopher L. Arheart [*,†,‡], Steven E. Lipshultz [*,‡], Tracie L. Miller [*,‡]

[*] Division of Pediatric Clinical Research, Department of Pediatrics, [†] Department of Epidemiology and Public Health and [‡] University of Miami Leonard M. Miller School of Medicine, Miami, FL, USA

INTRODUCTION

Not long ago, the terms "metabolic syndrome" and "child" would not have been mentioned in the same sentence. However, an entirely different scenario is rapidly unfolding before our society and our healthcare system. Deeply rooted in the current childhood obesity epidemic are both the components of metabolic syndrome (elevated blood pressure and glucose levels, hypertriglyceridemia, low High-density lipoprotein (HDL) cholesterol levels, and central adiposity) and the syndrome itself (three or more of these components in the same individual). Children are being diagnosed with metabolic syndrome at increasingly younger ages, including some as young as 8 years old [1]. The longer-term consequences of childhood obesity and its metabolic changes are now just starting to emerge [2–4].

Childhood overweight is a major public health problem, not only in the United States but worldwide. Virtually no age group is left unscathed; currently, one in four U.S. children *under the age of 5* is overweight [5]. Even more alarming is the fact that the latest U.S. pediatric obesity prevalence estimates for all children aged 2 to 18 for the first time now included levels of *morbid obesity* (a body mass index percentile for age and sex at or above the 97th percentile), whereas previous reports only included up to the 95th percentile (cut off for obese) [5]. However, the latest news is that morbidity associated with childhood obesity is occurring at younger ages and is associated with adult diseases, including adult-onset obesity [3], atherosclerotic cardiovascular disease, and diabetes [6–9].

Specifically, autopsy results from the Pathobiological Determinants of Atherosclerosis in Youth (PDAY) study and the Bogalusa Heart Study have revealed that the atherosclerotic process begins in childhood [7, 10–13].

Identifying children who are at risk for metabolic syndrome has remained elusive and controversial. Much of the controversy surrounding the syndrome in children is its definition. Definitions of pathological processes are typically based on end points. The difficulty in defining these cardiovascular risk factors in childhood is that most children have not reached the end point (atherosclerotic cardiovascular disease) [14–16]. Thus, there is technically no single, widely accepted operational definition of metabolic syndrome in children. This confusion has led to more than 50 different definitions being proposed in the pediatric literature. Most of these definitions are based on a modified adult definition [17] proposed by Cook et al. [16] and include the following components in variation: (1) waist circumference greater than the 90th percentile for age, sex, and ethnicity; (2) a fasting glucose level greater than 100 mg/dL; (3) a blood pressure (systolic or diastolic) greater than the 90th percentile for age and height; (4) fasting triglyceride levels greater than 110 mg/dL; and (5) HDL cholesterol less than 40 mg/dL.

The challenge in pediatrics lies in the difficulty of arriving at an appropriate threshold for each risk factor that takes into account age and sex as well as continuous growth, the onset of puberty, and perhaps ethnic background. This challenge has led several groups, including ours, to employ percentiles adjusted for age and sex. This approach then raises the issue of what percentile maximizes both sensitivity and specificity and what historical cohort is used to derive these thresholds: one before the current obesity epidemic, perhaps as far back as NHANES I or II, or one that is current and potentially skewed toward higher values?

In this chapter, we summarize the national prevalence estimates of metabolic syndrome in U.S. youth based on various definitions that employ either a clinical threshold value for each component or a percentile threshold based on some combination of age, sex, and ethnicity. The national estimates are followed by a summary of large, key regional studies. We present this information because the authors are aware that literally hundreds of small clinical studies have estimated the prevalence of metabolic syndrome in youth, and summarizing them all is beyond the scope of this chapter.

ESTIMATING THE POPULATION-BASED PREVALENCE OF METABOLIC SYNDROME IN CHILDREN AND ADOLESCENTS

The National Health and Nutrition Examination Survey (NHANES) is the primary data source for monitoring the prevalence of overweight and obesity in the United States, as well as all components of metabolic syndrome in those aged 12 and older. Also, since 1960, NHANES anthropometry data has been used to determine obesity levels in the United States [18]. NHANES surveys used a stratified, multistage probability design to capture a representative sample of the civilian noninstitutionalized U.S. population. The major objectives of NHANES are (1) to estimate the number and percent of persons in the U.S. population and designated subgroups with selected diseases and risk factors; (2) to monitor trends in the prevalence, awareness, treatment, and control of selected diseases; (3) to monitor trends in risk behaviors and environmental exposures; (4) to analyze risk factors for selected diseases; (5) to study the relationship between diet, nutrition, and health; (6) to explore emerging public health issues and new technologies; (7) to establish a national probability sample of genetic material for future genetic research; and (8) to establish and maintain a national probability sample of baseline information on health and nutritional status.

Although the NHANES III (1988–1994) survey was designed to be nationally representative for either 3 or 6 years of data collection, since 1999 the survey has been conducted biannually and since 2007 annually, and it is designed to identify annually a nationally representative sample. The NHANES data include demographic, survey, and laboratory information. Demographic and survey information are collected in a home interview, and all laboratory and physical examination data are collected at a medical visit scheduled at a separate time.

One of the unique advantages to using the NHANES data to generate prevalence estimates is the sampling weights created by the National Center for Health Statistics. The purpose of weighting the NHANES sample data is to permit the analysis of estimates that would have been obtained if the entire sampling frame had been surveyed—in this case, every child in the United States. Weighting takes into account several features of the surveys: the specific probabilities of selection for the individual domains that were oversampled (in both the 1999–2000 and 2001–2002 surveys, Mexican Americans and blacks were oversampled), as well as nonresponse and differences between the sample and the total population.

NHANES III PREVALENCE ESTIMATES

The first attempts to estimate the prevalence of metabolic syndrome at a population-based level used the NHANES III data [16]. One group of authors defined metabolic syndrome threshold criteria based on the National Cholesterol Education Program's (NCEP) Adult Treatment Panel III adult definition because these criteria had never before been formally defined or applied in children or adolescents [16]. The authors stated that in developing a definition for metabolic syndrome in adolescents [19], they considered reference values from the NCEP Pediatric Panel report [20], the American Diabetes Association's statement on type 2 diabetes in children and adolescents [21], and the updated Task Force report on the diagnosis and management of hypertension in childhood [19], as well as on Adult Treatment Panel III [22].

Youth with a waist circumference at or above the 90th percentile value for age and sex were defined as having abdominal obesity. Elevated systolic or diastolic blood pressures were defined as a value at or above the 90th percentile for age, sex, and height, as defined by the National High Blood Pressure Education Program [19]. The NCEP *Report of the Expert Panel on Blood Cholesterol Levels in Children and Adolescents* [20] was used to establish the criteria for cholesterol level abnormalities. The range of 35 to 45 mg/dL (0.91 to 1.16 mmol/L) was given for borderline-low HDL cholesterol levels for all sexes and ages. In children aged 10 to 19 years, a borderline high range for triglyceride levels was given as 90 to 129 mg/dL (1.02 to 1.46 mmol/L). Therefore, the midpoint value for HDL cholesterol [≤40 mg/dL (≤1.03 mmol/L)] was used as a 10th percentile value, and the midpoint value for triglycerides [≥110 mg/dL

(≥1.24 mmol/L)] was taken as the 90th percentile value for age. The reference value for elevated fasting glucose was taken from the American Diabetes Association guideline of 110 mg/dL or higher (≥6.1 mmol/L) [21].

On the basis of these threshold criteria, these authors estimated that nearly 1 million adolescents aged 12 to 19 in the United States during the late 1980s and the first half of the 1990s, or about 4% of the population of that age, have signs and symptoms of metabolic syndrome [16]. They also found three or more components of the syndrome in 29% of children classified as overweight by the Centers for Disease Control percentile definition (>95th percentile), in 7% of at-risk adolescents (between the 85th and 95th percentile of body mass index), and in 0.1% of children with a body mass index (BMI) below the 85th percentile. The prevalence of one and two components of the syndrome was 41% and 14%, respectively. The most common abnormalities were high triglycerides and low high-density lipoprotein (HDL) cholesterol levels. In contrast, the prevalence of high fasting glucose was relatively low at 1.5%.

A second analysis of the same data set (NHANES III) among the same age group also extrapolated the threshold definition from adult criteria, but it differed slightly. Triglyceride and HDL thresholds were taken from equivalent pediatric percentiles [23]. This analysis also defined hyperglycemia using the Adult Treatment Panel III threshold but used a different criterion for waist circumference based on the adult threshold of the 70th percentile [24]. As in the previous analysis, the National Heart, Lung, and Blood Institute's National High Blood Pressure Education Program recommended threshold of the 90th percentile for age, sex, and height was used to define elevated systolic or diastolic blood pressure.

This second analysis showed that low HDL, hypertriglyceridemia, and central obesity were common but that elevated blood pressure and glucose were not. The authors reported that 10% of all U.S. children aged 12 to 19 years and almost one third of overweight and obese children had metabolic syndrome. Moreover, two thirds of all adolescents had at least 1 metabolic component.

The metabolic syndrome definition implemented by the first group used more restrictive lipid and abdominal waist circumference thresholds, which ultimately led to the lower prevalence estimates in adolescents (4%). Translating their definition into pediatric percentiles, an HDL level of 40 mg/dL represents the 10th to the 25th percentile in boys and the 10th to the 15th percentile in girls, lower than the adult 40th percentile. The higher triglyceride threshold of 110 mg/dL represents the 85th to the 95th pediatric percentile, also higher than the adult 75th to 85th percentile used by the second group. Additionally, the first group used an abdominal circumference threshold of the 90th percentile whereas the second group used the 75th percentile.

Regardless of their discrepancies in defining metabolic syndrome, these two analyses were the first population-based attempts to identify metabolic syndrome risk in youth. Each analysis indicated that a substantial percentage of U.S. adolescents may be at substantially heightened risk for metabolic syndrome in adulthood and the subsequent risks for type 2 diabetes and premature coronary artery disease, and they ultimately laid the foundation for future NHANES analyses, particularly in light of the obesity epidemic of the past 20 to 30 years.

LATER NHANES PREVALENCE ESTIMATES

In the time between the publication of the first NHANES III national prevalence estimates and later NHANES samples, namely 1999 and beyond, several smaller clinical studies estimated the prevalence of metabolic syndrome among specific groups of children, such as children in ethnic groups or those who were obese. For example, Cruz et al. [25] showed that 30% of overweight Hispanic youth had metabolic syndrome, Weiss et al. [26] reported that 39% of moderately obese and 50% of severely obese youth had metabolic syndrome, and Goodman et al. [27], using the adult NCEP criteria, found that 4.2% of adolescents met these criteria.

Analysis of the NHANES 1999–2002 combined data showed that the prevalence of metabolic syndrome among all U.S. 12- to 19-year-olds ranged from 2% to 9.4%, depending on the definition used. Among obese adolescents, the prevalence varied from 12.4% to 44.2%. In the group of obese teens, applying the definition by Cruz [25] produced a prevalence of 12.4%, whereas applying a different definition by Caprio et al. [27] produced a rate of 14.1%. None of the normal weight or overweight teens met either definition. Applying the definition by Cook [16] produced a prevalence rate of 7.8% in overweight teens and 44% in obese teens. The adult definition of metabolic syndrome produced a prevalence rate of 16% in overweight teens and 26% in obese teens.

More recently, an analysis of the NHANES 1999–2006 combined data estimating the prevalence of metabolic syndrome among 12- to 19-year-olds [28] used a definition by Ford et al. [29] that included having three or more of the following five characteristics: a waist circumference above the 90th percentile for age and sex according to the 1988–1994 NHANES III data [30]; either a systolic or a diastolic blood pressure in the 90th percentile for height, age, and sex [31]; a triglyceride concentration of 110 mg/dL or greater (to convert to millimoles per liter, multiply by 0.0113); an HDL-cholesterol concentration of 40 mg/dL or less; and a glucose concentration of 100 mg/dL or greater (to convert to millimoles per liter, multiply by 0.0555). The authors reported that 8.6% of the sample had metabolic syndrome, and approximately half of the participants had at least one component. Prevalence was higher in boys (10.8%) than in girls (6.1%), and in Hispanic (11.2%) and non-Hispanic white (8.9%) adolescents than in non-Hispanic black adolescents (4.0%). In non-Hispanic black girls, the prevalence of a large waist circumference was high (23.3%), but no one individual component dominated its diagnosis in non-Hispanic blacks of either sex. Elevated waist circumference, abnormal (high) fasting triglyceride levels, and low HDL serum cholesterol concentrations were the most prevalent components in Hispanic and white adolescents of both sexes, whereas elevated glucose concentrations were prominent among Hispanic and non-Hispanic white boys.

Given the ensuing obesity epidemic among increasingly younger children, we analyzed the 1999–2004 NHANES dataset for 8- to 14-year-olds [1]. We had two objectives. The first was to determine the prevalence of metabolic syndrome components (using one crude and one ethnicity- and sex-adjusted profile) among two specific age groups, 8- to 11-year-olds and 12- to 14-year-olds. The second objective was to examine the relationship between body mass index (BMI) and the prevalence and distribution of the presence of three or more metabolic syndrome components among adolescents in the same age groups. We created two profiles to compare in our analysis: (1) a crude profile similar to that used in the NHANES III analysis [16] that included single, nonadjusted threshold points to define elevated blood lipids, waist circumference, and blood glucose, and (2) an age-, sex-, and ethnicity-adjusted profile. All individual component threshold values were based on national standardized norms and were similar to those reported by others [32, 33].

Fasting Glucose. On the basis of the American Diabetes Association criteria, a fasting glucose level of 100 mg/dL or higher was considered to be abnormal for both the crude and adjusted profiles [34]. Fasting (>8 hours but < 24 hours) glucose data were available for 12- to 14-year-olds only, and the appropriate fasting glucose-specific, 4-year weights were applied. When analyzing the combined 4-year data set, the correct sampling weights must be used to produce unbiased estimates. In terms of fasting glucose specifically, appropriate sample weights have been calculated to reflect both the additional stage of sampling and the additional nonresponse (if any) for the subsample. These weights differ from the full examination weight, and the revised weights were used for statistical estimation.

Systolic and diastolic blood pressure. To define crude and adjusted threshold values of normal systolic and diastolic blood pressure adjusted for sex and age, we used the 90th percentile values. These values are proposed by the Update on the Task Force for High Blood Pressure in Children and Adolescents (a working group on hypertension control in children and adolescents from the National High Blood Pressure Education Program [31]). Blood pressure was considered to be abnormal if either systolic or diastolic values were abnormal.

Triglyceride. The 90th percentile values adjusted for sex and ethnicity (non-Hispanic black, non-Hispanic white, and Mexican American) from the NHANES III (1988–1994) findings in 12- to 14-year-olds were used for the adjusted profile [35]. As in previous studies, one normal-abnormal triglyceride threshold value of 110 mg/dL was used as the threshold for the crude profile [16]. Triglyceride values are not available for children younger than 12 in the NHANES data and were therefore not included in the analysis in this age group.

High-density lipoprotein cholesterol. The adjusted profile HDL cholesterol threshold value was the 10th percentile adjusted for age and ethnicity (non-Hispanic black, non-Hispanic white, and Mexican American) from NHANES III (1988–1994) data [35]. For the crude profile, an HDL cholesterol value of 40 mg/dL or greater was considered abnormal [16].

Waist circumference. The adjusted profile used the 75th percentile threshold value for waist circumference based on data from NHANES III, adjusted for age, sex, and ethnicity [30]. We used this threshold percentile to be consistent with the well-accepted adult criteria of metabolic syndrome risk factors [36] and another pediatric study of NHANES [37] and to provide some contrast to the crude profile. Additionally, because this analysis included young adolescents, we chose a conservative percentile for this profile to be as sensitive as possible and therefore, to identify all children who may be in the earliest stages of chronic disease. As in the NHANES III analysis [16], the crude profile used the 90th percentile of this sample as the abnormal threshold value.

Body mass index. We used the Centers for Disease Control weight classifications for youth using BMI [defined as weight (kg)/height (m)^2] [36] percentiles ranges: underweight (< 5th percentile), normal weight (> 5th to < 85th percentiles), overweight (> 85th to < 95th percentiles), and overweight/obese (> 95th percentile). As in adults, BMI is an imperfect indicator of adiposity in children. However, because BMI is nonlinear in children, BMI percentiles and not absolute BMI thresholds must be used to evaluate weight [38, 39].

We found that the prevalence of metabolic syndrome among children as young as 8 years old ranged from 2% to 9%, using two age-, sex-, and ethnicity-adjusted definitions [1]. Using a similar (crude) profile for comparison purposes, we found at least three metabolic syndrome components in 9% of 12- to 14-year-olds (about twice the 4% reported by Cook et al. [16]) and in 44% of those who are overweight (again, about twice the 29% reported by Cook). This relative doubling of the prevalence of obesity and overweight in the early 2000s has been reported elsewhere [40–42], yet few have reported associated cardiovascular disease risk factors, particularly in large numbers of 8- to 11-year-olds. Regrettably, our data showed that the prevalence of overweight in the younger children was similar to that of the older children.

Our higher prevalence rates may be the result of classification differences; namely, our use of the 75th percentile as a threshold for waist circumference for the adjusted profile rather than the 90th percentile as used in other studies [16]. Interestingly, the authors [30] who generated the standardized waist circumference threshold values for the U.S. pediatric population that we used stated:

> Based on these values, the careful attention to children and adolescents with waist circumference values that fall on the 75th and 90th percentile, according to their ethnic classification and sex, becomes important in the identification—and prevention—of children at risk for various comorbidities, including cardiovascular disease, hyperinsulinemia, and type II diabetes. (p 443.)

On the basis of their recommendations, on previous authors' [37] use of the 75th percentile as a threshold for waist circumference, and on the probability that these 75th percentile values are similar to those of the 90th percentile only 20 years earlier as a result of the current obesity epidemic, our goal with this work was to help move the field forward by presenting an analysis that differed from previous studies yet still addressed the lack of a consensus for a definition of metabolic syndrome in children.

One of the unique features of this study is that it took advantage of the previous NHANES III to generate appropriately adjusted threshold values based on age, sex, and race-ethnicity to define metabolic syndrome in children and applied this information to the 1999–2002 NHANES data. The definition, validity, and long-term importance of metabolic syndrome, particularly among children, are controversial [43–45]. As our and other analyses show, the threshold values used to define metabolic syndrome among children greatly influence estimates of its prevalence. Similarly, our study shows that crude and adjusted threshold values often provided different estimates of risk for these children, even among 8- to 11-year-olds; an age group that has received little attention. The extent to which these threshold values will truly predict adverse outcomes in these children can only be determined with longitudinal follow-up studies. Furthermore, longitudinal studies would be able to determine whether or not the most common metabolic syndrome components identified in this paper do in fact result on adult-onset disease.

The primary limitation of this analysis was not having fasting glucose values and appropriate weights available to analyze triglycerides for the 8- to 11-year-old children. Creating the appropriate weights for the triglyceride subsample in children younger than 12 years old would allow for comparisons across age groups. Thus, our data likely underestimate the true prevalence of metabolic syndrome in this age group because we were not able to analyze this important component. Finally, we did not have Tanner values that would have allowed us to analyze how the onset of puberty affects the presence or onset of metabolic syndrome. This subject warrants further investigation.

OTHER REGIONAL-BASED SAMPLE ESTIMATES

As stated previously, describing the smaller clinic-based prevalence estimates of metabolic syndrome in children and adolescents is beyond the scope of this chapter. This issue becomes more complicated given the large number of definitions of the syndrome. One exhaustive literature review on the pediatric definitions of the syndrome found at least 27 articles with 46 definitions of the syndrome, most of them unique [46]. The following section summarizes a few of the better-known and larger cohort studies in the United States.

The Bogalusa Heart Study [47], a regional, longitudinal study of cardiovascular disease risk factors in black and white children aged 5 to 17 years old, defined metabolic syndrome as having four components greater than the 75th percentile for age and sex derived from their own population data. Based on this definition, the prevalence of metabolic syndrome was 4% among white children and 3% among black children [48].

Similarly, the Cardiovascular Risk in Young Finns Study [49], another large multicenter study of risk factors for heart disease in children and young adults, found the prevalence to be 4% among children aged 6 to 18 years old.

Goodman et al. [50] determined the prevalence of metabolic syndrome among adolescents by using definitions from the NCEP's Adult Treatment Panel III and World Health Organization (WHO) guidelines. The WHO definition requires either insulin resistance, hyperglycemia, or known diabetes. In addition to this requirement for WHO-defined metabolic syndrome, two of three other risk factors had to be present: hypertension, dyslipidemia (hypertriglyceridemia or low HDL cholesterol), and central obesity (a high waist circumference, or a BMI ≥ 30). In contrast, to have NCEP-defined metabolic syndrome, three of five possible risk factors had to be present, including hypertension, low HDL cholesterol, hypertriglyceridemia, hyperglycemia, or high waist circumference. Risk-factor thresholds were those used for adults, except in relation to obesity, which was defined by the established and widely used epidemiological definition in adolescence of a BMI at or above the 95th percentile. The study analyzed a school-based, cross-sectional sample of 1513 black, white, and Hispanic teenagers who had a fasting morning blood sample drawn and a physical examination. The prevalence of metabolic syndrome was 4.2% by the NCEP definition and 8.4% by the WHO definition. The syndrome was found almost exclusively among obese teens, for whom the prevalence was 20% by the NCEP definition and 39% by the WHO definition.

ETHNICITY AND THE PREVALENCE OF METABOLIC SYNDROME

An analysis of NHANES III found that the prevalence of metabolic syndrome was highest among Hispanic (6% to 13%) and lowest among black adolescents (2% to 3%), with white adolescents in between (5% to 11%) [16, 37]. Smaller clinical studies have estimated the prevalence to be between 4% and 9% in preadolescents and adolescents and also reported higher prevalence rates in minorities than in whites [51–53]. Collectively, the authors of these studies concluded that the higher prevalence among Hispanic youth can most likely be attributed to their overall higher rates of overweight and obesity. Similarly, studies among U.S. adults have reported that the prevalence of metabolic syndrome is higher among Hispanics (31.9%) and lower among black adults (21.6%) than among white adults (23.8%) [54].

Paradoxically, although the prevalence of obesity among black and non-Hispanic black adolescents in the United States is also high (21%), they tend to have a lower prevalence of the syndrome [16, 47, 48] when a definition similar to that used by the NCEP Adult Treatment Panel III is applied. Some have hypothesized that this paradox may result from the fact that black youth (like adults) have lower triglycerides and higher HDL cholesterol levels than do their white counterparts, even though they have higher blood pressure [47]. These findings suggest that the impact of obesity on the components of metabolic syndrome may vary by ethnic group.

A recent American Heart Association scientific statement calls for research to determine whether there are racial and ethnic differences in the overall prevalence, mechanisms, and pathways to metabolic syndrome in children and adolescents [55]. This research should eventually help guide pediatric clinical practice by clarifying the predictive value of using an ethnic-specific definition or a one-definition-fits-all approach to metabolic syndrome.

PATHOPHYSIOLOGY AND SECULAR TRENDS

The concept of metabolic syndrome in childhood can easily diverge into two different and, at times, opposing views. Epidemiologically, the literature indicates quite clearly that this cluster of abnormal risk factors exists in both clinic and population-based samples and is highly prevalent in the obese. However, the pathophysiological view suggests that this association is not so clear. For example, some have questioned the advantage of naming a syndrome that includes several different components. Instead, should each individual risk factor be treated independently? On the other hand, should a different set of criteria be based on racial-ethnic background? The literature consistently shows that certain ethnic groups display elevated risk factors at baseline.

Although a consensus has been reached in defining metabolic syndrome in adults [56], controversy nevertheless remains concerning the actual underlying causal factors. Currently, the most accepted hypothesis supported by prospective studies is that obesity and insulin resistance are the key underlying factors in the syndrome [57, 58], and both have been explored in children using both cross-sectional and prospective studies [52, 59]. In the Cardiovascular Risk in Young Finns Study, one the first studies to explore childhood predictors of metabolic syndrome, fasting insulin at baseline was related to the development of the syndrome after a 6-year follow-up of 1865 children and adolescents 6 to 18 years old. Baseline insulin concentration was higher in children who subsequently developed metabolic syndrome, lending support to the theory that insulin resistance precedes the development of the syndrome in childhood [49].

More recently, the Bogalusa Heart Study explored the relationship of childhood obesity (as measured by BMI) and insulin resistance (as measured by fasting insulin levels) on the risk of developing metabolic syndrome as an adult [60]. Researchers followed 718 children aged 8 to 17 at baseline for an average of 11.6 years. They defined metabolic syndrome as having four of the following: a BMI, fasting insulin, systolic or mean arterial blood pressure, and a triglycerides/HDL ratio in the highest quartile for age, sex, ethnicity, and study year. The highest childhood BMI and insulin quartiles were significantly related to the incidence of risk-factor clustering in adulthood. More specifically, children in the top quartile for BMI and insulin versus those in the bottom quartile were 11.7 and 3.6 times, respectively, more likely to develop the clustering of factors that defines metabolic syndrome as adults. A high childhood BMI was significantly associated with adult onset of the syndrome, even after adjusting for childhood insulin levels, suggesting that childhood-onset obesity can predict the development of metabolic syndrome in adulthood.

Despite differences in the definition of metabolic syndrome in the studies reviewed here, overall findings suggest that both obesity and insulin resistance contribute to the development of the syndrome during childhood. Among those children who are overweight or obese, insulin resistance is likely more important than overall adiposity in the development of the syndrome. Therefore, the accumulation of visceral fat, as opposed to subcutaneous abdominal fat or, alternatively, increased ectopic fat, may be important in the pathophysiology of the disorder. For example, Cruz and colleagues [52] reported that visceral fat, in addition to total fat, is an important contributor to differences in insulin sensitivity among overweight Hispanic youth with a family history of type 2 diabetes.

Indeed, identifying children at the earliest stages of chronic disease should be the goal of clinical practice, yet no guidelines have been established for defining metabolic syndrome risk or appropriate individual component threshold values among young adolescents. If children are identified early in the disease process, lifestyle or clinical interventions can be instituted when they are potentially more effective. Only continued longitudinal follow-up of well-characterized pediatric cohorts into adulthood will provide sufficient information to define appropriate age-, sex-, and race- or ethnicity-specific cardiovascular risks in childhood.

The current epidemic of obesity and increased prevalence of type 2 diabetes mellitus in adolescents with its attendant consequences is a clinical and public health priority because interventions that target cardiometabolic risk in youth are more easily instituted than are those to modify behaviors later, when deleterious health habits are established [20]. However, given the current prevalence of childhood and adolescent obesity, it is unlikely that this major public health problem can be managed solely in clinical settings. Rather, public health strategies must be integrated into home and family, school, and community-based settings. Currently, the United States allocates substantially more resources to the adult obesity epidemic than to preventive strategies among children and adolescents. Clearly, prevention strategies for both age groups must take into account the causal factors of obesity that begin in childhood.

FUTURE PROJECTIONS

For the first time in decades, the life expectancy of Americans is projected to *decrease* as a consequence of obesity alone [61]. Furthermore, given the current obesity epidemic among adolescents, it is most likely that in a decade the country will be dealing with a young adult population facing potential chronic disease. Yet, we do not know the potential life-long consequences of being obese and having metabolic syndrome as a child. Learning more about how eating and physical activity patterns develop through infancy, childhood, and adolescence and how they track into adulthood should improve the effectiveness of obesity prevention strategies and interventions.

Clearly, the current adolescent obesity epidemic, if left to continue on into adulthood, will indirectly affect all Americans because it undoubtedly will take a heavy toll on the healthcare system. For example, a December 2004 report from Feinberg School of Medicine at Northwestern University in Chicago found that for men, the total average annual Medicare charges for those not overweight were $7205, for the overweight they were $8390, for the obese they were $10,128, and for the severely obese they were $13,674. The total average annual charges for women in the same four categories were, respectively, $6224, $7653, $9612, and $12,342. The annual average Medicare charges for severely obese men were $6469 *more* than for nonoverweight men and for severely obese women; annual average charges were $5618 *more* than for women not overweight [62].

Secular trends and longitudinal studies have shown that cardiometabolic disease risk factors that are present in childhood predict adult disease. The Princeton Lipid Research Clinics follow-up study showed that over 30 years, the risk for cardiovascular disease was nine times as high, and that for type 2 diabetes mellitus was four times as high, in children with metabolic syndrome than in children without the syndrome, after adjusting for age, sex, ethnicity, and family history [63]. This same study reported that differences between adults with and without metabolic syndrome first occurred at ages 8 and 13 for BMI and at ages 6 and 13 for waist circumference in boys and girls, respectively [64]. The authors concluded that children with BMI and waist circumference values exceeding the established criterion values are at increased risk for the adult metabolic syndrome.

CONCLUSION

The possibility of becoming obese is greater than ever for U.S. children and adolescents. If current prevalence trends continue, our children will grow up to be the most obese generation of adults in U.S. history, faced at increasingly younger ages with the onset of chronic conditions, such as metabolic syndrome, which in turn will lead to chronic and costly outcomes, such as diabetes and cardiovascular disease. However, even more troubling is that before reaching adulthood, as we have clearly shown here, large proportions of overweight and obese children are already experiencing substantial medical effects related to their overweight in the form of metabolic syndrome.

References

1. Messiah SE, Arheart K, Luke B, Lipshultz SE, Miller TL. Relationship between body mass index and metabolic syndrome risk factors among US 8 to 14 year olds, 1999–2002. *J Pediatr* 2008;**153**(2):215–21.
2. Morrison JA, Friedman LA, Gray-McGuire C. Metabolic syndrome in childhood predicts adult cardiovascular disease 25 years later: the Princeton Lipid Research Clinics Follow-up Study. *Pediatrics* 2007;**120**(2):340–5.
3. Morrison J, Friedman L, Wang P, Glueck C. Metabolic syndrome in childhood predicts adult metabolic syndrome and type 2 diabetes mellitus 25 to 30 years later. *J Pediatr* 2007;**152**(2):201–6.
4. Sun SS, Liang R, Huang TT-K, et al. Childhood obesity predicts adult metabolic syndrome: the Fels Longitudinal Study. *J Pediatr* 2008;**152**(2):191–200. Epub 2007 Oct 3.
5. Ogden CL, Carroll MD, Flegal KM. High body mass index for age among US children and adolescents, 2003–2006. *JAMA* 2008;**299**(20):2401–5.
6. Whitaker R, Wright J, Pepe M, Seidel K, Dietz W. Predicting obesity in young adulthood from childhood and parental obesity. *N Engl J Med* 1997;**337**(13):869–73.
7. Newman III WP, Freedman DS, Voors AW, et al. Relation of serum lipoprotein levels and systolic blood pressure to early atherosclerosis: the Bogalusa Heart Study. *N Engl J Med* 1986;**314**(3):138–44.
8. Baker J, Olsen L, Sorenson T. Childhood body-mass index and the risk of coronary heart disease in adulthood. *N Engl J Med* 2007;**357**(23):2329–37.
9. Bibbins-Domingo K, Coxson P, Pletcher M, Lightwood J, Goldman L. Adolescent overweight and future coronary heart disease. *N Engl J Med* 2007;**357**(23):2371–9.
10. Duncan GE, Li SM, Zhou XH. Prevalence and trends of a metabolic syndrome phenotype among U.S. adolescents, 1999–2000. *Diabetes Care* 2004;**27**(10):2438–43.
11. Berenson GS, Srinivasan SR, Bao W, Newman III WP, Tracy RE, Wattigney WA. Association between multiple cardiovascular risk factors and the early development of atherosclerosis. Bogalusa Heart Study. *N Engl J Med* 1998;**338**(23):1650–6.
12. McGill Jr HC, McMahan CA, Zieske AW, Malcom GT, Tracy RE, Strong JP. Effect of nonlipid risk factors on atherosclerosis in youth with favorable lipoprotein profile. Pathobiological Determinants of Atherosclerosis in Youth (PDAY) Research Group. *Circulation* 2001;**103**(11):1546–50.
13. McGill Jr HC, McMahan CA, Malcolm GT, Oalmann MC, Strong JP. Effects of serum lipoproteins and smoking on atherosclerosis in young men and women. The PDAY Research Group. Pathobiological Determinants of Atherosclerosis in Youth. *Arterioscler Thromb Vasc Biol* 1997;**17**(1):95–106.
14. Gorter PM, Olijhoeck JK, Graf van der Y, Algra A, Rabelink TJ, Visseren FLJ, Study Group SMART. Prevalence of the metabolic syndrome in patients with coronary heart disease, cerebrovascular disease, peripheral arterial disease or abdominal aortic aneurysm. *Atherosclerosis* 2004;**173**:363–9.
15. Isomaa B, Almgren P, Tuomi T, et al. Cardiovascular morbidity and mortality associated with the metabolic syndrome. *Diabetes Care* 2001;**24**(4):683–9.
16. Cook S, Weitzman M, Auinger P, Nguyen M, Dietz WH. Prevalence of a metabolic syndrome phenotype in adolescents: findings from the third National Health and Nutrition Examination Survey, 1988–1994. *Arch Pediatr Adolesc Med* 2003;**157**:821–7.
17. National Institutes of Health. *The Third Report of the National Cholesterol Education Program Expert Panel on Detection, Evaluation, and Treatment of High Blood Cholesterol in Adults (Adult Treatment Panel III)*. Bethesda, MD: National Institutes of Health; NIH Publication 01-3670; 2001.
18. Flegal KM, Carroll MD, Ogden CL, Johnson CL. Prevalence and trends in obesity among US adults, 1999–2000. *JAMA* 2002;**288**(14):1723–7.
19. National High Blood Pressure Education Program Working Group on Hypertension Control in Children and Adolescents. Update on the 1987 Task Force Report on High Blood Pressure in Children and Adolescents: a working group report from the National High Blood Pressure Education Program. *Pediatrics* 1996;**98**(4 pt 1):649–58.
20. National Cholesterol Education Panel. *Report of the Expert Panel on Blood Cholesterol Levels in Children and Adolescents*. Bethesda, MD: National Institutes of Health. NIH Publication No. 91-2732; 1991.
21. Type 2 diabetes in children and adolescents. American Diabetes Association. *Diabetes Care* 2000;**23**:381–9. Doi: 10.2337.
22. National Cholesterol Education Program. *Detection, Evaluation, and Treatment of High Blood Cholesterol in Adults (Adult Treatment Panel III): Full Report*. Bethesda, Md: National Institutes of Health. NIH publication No. 01-3670; 2001.
23. The Lipid Research Clinics Program Epidemiology Committee. Plasma lipid distributions in selected North Am populations: the Lipid Research Clinics Program Prevalence Study. *Circulation* 1979;**60**:427–39.
24. Zhu S, Wang Z, Heshka S, et al. Waist circumference and obesity-associated risk factors among whites in the third National Health and Nutrition Examination Survey: clinical action thresholds. *Am J Clin Nutr* 2002;**76**:743–9.
25. Cruz ML, Weigensberg MJ, Huang TT, Ball G, Shaibi GQ, Goran MI. The metabolic syndrome in overweight Hispanic youth and the role of insulin sensitivity. *J Clin Endocrinol Metab* 2004;**89**:108–13.
26. Weiss R, Dziura J, Burgert T, et al. Obesity and the metabolic syndrome in children and adolescents. *N Engl J Med* 2004;**350**:2362–74.
27. Caprio S. Definitions and pathophysiology of the metabolic syndrome in obese children and adolescents. *Int J Obes (Lond)* 2005;**29**(Suppl. 2):S24–5.
28. Johnson WD, Kroon JJ, Greenway FL, Bouchard C, Ryan D, Katzmarzyk PT. Prevalence of risk factors for metabolic syndrome in adolescents: National Health and Nutrition Examination Survey (NHANES), 2001–2006. *Arch Pediatr Adolesc Med* 2009;**163**(4):371–7.
29. Ford ES, Li C, Cook S, Choi HK. Serum concentrations of uric acid and the metabolic syndrome among US children and adolescents. *Circulation* 2007;**115**(19):2526–32.
30. Fernandez JR, Redden DT, Pietrobelli A, Allison DB. Waist circumference percentiles in nationally representative samples of African-American, European-American, and Mexican-American Children and Adolescents. *J Pediatr* 2004;**145**:439–44.

31. National High Blood Pressure Education Program Working Group on High Blood Pressure in Children and Adolescents. The fourth report on the diagnosis, evaluation, and treatment of high blood pressure in children and adolescents. Pediatrics 2004;114: 555–76.
32. Chi CH, Wang Y, Wilson DM, Robinson TN. Definition of metabolic syndrome in preadolescent girls. J Pediatr 2006;148:788–92. e2.
33. Freedman DS, Mei Z, Srinivasan SR, Berenson GS, Dietz WH. Cardiovascular risk factors and excess adiposity among overweight children and adolescents: the Bogalusa Heart Study. J Pediatr 2007;150:12–17. e2.
34. American Diabetes Association. Clinical practice recommendations 2002. Diabetes Care 2002;25:S1–147.
35. Hickman TB, Briefel RR, Carroll MD, Rifkind BM, Cleeman JI, Maurer KR, et al. Distributions and trends of serum lipid levels among United States children and adolescents ages 4-19 years: data from the Third National Health and Nutrition Examination Survey. Prev Med 1998;27:879–90.
36. Morrison JA, Friedman LA, Gray-McGuire C. Metabolic syndrome in childhood predicts adult cardiovascular disease 25 years later: the Princeton Lipid Research Clinics Follow-up Study. Pediatrics 2007;120(2):340–5.
37. de Ferranti SD, Gauvreau K, Ludwig DS, Neufeld EJ, Newburger JW, Rifai N. Prevalence of the metabolic syndrome in American adolescents: findings from the Third National Health and Nutrition Examination Survey. Circulation 2004;110: 2494–7.
38. Centers for Disease Control and Prevention. BMI—Body Mass Index: BMI for Children and Teens. Available at, www.cdc.gov/nccdphp/dnpa/bmi/bmi-for-age.htm; 2006. Accessed 1/7/10.
39. The Centers for Disease Control and Prevention. National Health and Nutrition Examination Survey: Laboratory Procedures Manual; 2001. Available at, www.cdc.gov/nchs/data/nhanes/lab1-6.pdf; 2001. Accessed 1/7/10.
40. Institute of Medicine. Preventing Childhood Obesity. Health in the Balance. Washington, DC: National Academy Press; 2004.
41. Ogden CL, Carroll MD, Curtin LR, McDowell MA, Tabak CJ, Flegal KM. Prevalence of overweight and obesity in the United States, 1999–2004. JAMA 2006;295:1549–55.
42. The Surgeon General's Call to Action to Prevent and Decrease Overweight and Obesity. 2001. Rockville, MD: Public Health Service, Office of the Surgeon General. Available from: U.S. Government Printing Office, Washington, D.C.
43. Grundy SM, Cleeman JI, Daniels SR, et al. Diagnosis and management of the metabolic syndrome. An American Heart Association/National Heart, Lung, and Blood Institute Scientific Statement. Circulation 2005;112:2735–52.
44. Kahn R. The metabolic syndrome (emperor) wears no clothes. Diabetes Care 2006;29(7):1693–6.
45. Grundy SM. Does the metabolic syndrome exist? Diabetes Care 2006;29:1689–92.
46. Ford ES, Chaoyang L. Defining the MS in children and adolescents: will the real definition please stand up? J Pediatr 2008; 152(2):160–4.
47. Chen W, Bao W, Begum S, Elkasabany A, Srinivasan SR, Berenson GS. Age-related patterns of the clustering of cardiovascular risk variables of syndrome X from childhood to young adulthood in a population made up of black and white subjects: the Bogalusa Heart Study. Diabetes 2000;49(6):1042–8.
48. Chen W, Srinivasan SR, Elkasabany A, Berenson GS. Cardiovascular risk factors clustering features of insulin resistance syndrome (syndrome X) in a biracial (black-white) population of children, adolescents, and young adults: the Bogalusa Heart Study. Am J Epidemiol 1999;150:667–74.
49. Raitakari OT, Porkka KV, Ronnemaa T, et al. The role of insulin in clustering of serum lipids and blood pressure in children and adolescents. The Cardiovascular Risk in Young Finns Study. Diabetologia 1995;38:1042–50.
50. Goodman E, Daniels SR, Morrison J, Huang B, Dolan LM. Contrasting prevalence of and demographic disparities in the World Health Organization and National Cholesterol Education Program Adult Treatment Panel III definitions of metabolic syndrome among adolescents. J Pediatr 2004;145:445–51.
51. Rodriguez-Moran M, Salazar-Vazquez B, Violante R, Guerrero-Romero F. Metabolic syndrome among children and adolescents aged 10-18 years. Diabetes Care 2004;27:2516–17.
52. Cruz ML, Weigensberg MJ, Huang TT, Ball G, Shaibi GQ, Goran MI. The metabolic syndrome in overweight Hispanic youth and the role of insulin sensitivity. J Clin Endocrin Metab 2004;89:108–13.
53. Cossrow N, Falkner B. Race/ethnic issues in obesity and obesity-related comorbidities. J Clin Endocrinol Metab 2004;89(6):2590–4. Review.
54. Ford ES, Giles WH, Dietz WH. Prevalence of the metabolic syndrome among US adults: findings from the third National Health and Nutrition Examination Survey. JAMA 2002;287(3): 356–9.
55. Steinberger J, Daniels SR, Eckel RH, et al. Progress and challenges in metabolic syndrome in children and adolescents. A Scientific Statement from the American Heart Association Atherosclerosis, Hypertension, and Obesity in the Young Committee of the Council on Cardiovascular Disease in the Young; Council on Cardiovascular Nursing; and Council on Nutrition, Physical Activity, and Metabolism. Circulation 2009; 119(4):628–47. Epub 2009 Jan 12.
56. Lakka HM, Laaksonen DE, Lakka TA, et al. The metabolic syndrome and total and cardiovascular disease mortality in middle-aged men. JAMA 2002;288:2709–16.
57. Reaven GM. Relationship between insulin resistance and hypertension. Diabetes Care. 14 Suppl 1991;4:33–8.
58. Reaven GM. Dietary therapy for non-insulin-dependent diabetes mellitus. N Engl J Med 1988;319(13):862–4.
59. Sinaiko AR, Jacobs Jr DR, Steinberger J, et al. Insulin resistance syndrome in childhood: associations of the euglycemic insulin clamp and fasting insulin with fatness and other risk factors. J Pediatr 2001;139(5):700–7.
60. Srinivasan SR, Myers L, Berenson GS. Predictability of childhood adiposity and insulin for developing insulin resistance syndrome (syndrome X) in young adulthood: the Bogalusa Heart Study. Diabetes 2002;51(1):204–9.
61. Olshansky SJ, Passaro DJ, Hershow RC, et al. A potential decline in life expectancy in the United States in the 21st century. N Engl J Med 2005;352(11):1138–45.
62. Daviglus ML, Liu K, Yan LL, et al. Relation of body mass index in young adulthood and middle age to Medicare expenditures in older age. JAMA 2004;292(22):2743–9.
63. Huang TT, Nansel TR, Belsheim AR, Morrison JA. Sensitivity, specificity, and predictive values of pediatric metabolic syndrome components in relation to adult metabolic syndrome: the Princeton LRC follow-up study. J Pediatr 2008;152(2):185–90.
64. Morrison JA, Friedman LA, Gray-McGuire C. Metabolic syndrome in childhood predicts adult cardiovascular disease 25 years later: the Princeton Lipid Research Clinics Follow-up Study. Pediatrics 2007;120(2):340–5.

SECTION II

PATHOPHYSIOLOGY

CHAPTER

11

Emerging Pathways to Child Obesity Starts from the Mother's Womb
A Prospective View

Ashik Mosaddik

Department of Pharmacy, Rajshahi University, Bangladesh, and Subtropical Horticulture Research Institute, Faculty of Biotechnology, Jeju National University, Jeju, Republic of Korea, e-mail: mamosaddik@yahoo.com

INTRODUCTION

In the past, when someone thought of obesity, a child was rarely the first thing to come to mind. Children were highly active little creatures who never seemed to slow down. Sadly, times have changed. According to the National Center for Chronic Disease and Health Promotion [1], "The prevalence of overweight among children aged 6 to 11 more than doubled in the past 30 years, going from 7% in 1980 to 18.8% in 2004. The rate among adolescents aged 12 to 19 more than tripled, increasing from 5% to 17.1%" [1]. Those are some scary numbers! Obesity in itself is an awful thing to deal with as a child. By examining more than 120,000 children under age 6 in Massachusetts over 22 years, Gillman's research group [2] found that the prevalence of overweight children increased from 6.3% to 10%, a 59% jump (based on weight and height measures documented in medical records). The proportion of children at risk of becoming overweight grew from 11.1% to 14.4% overall, a 30% jump. Infants from birth to 6 months of age, an age group seldom studied before, had particularly surprising results. Of all the age groups studied, these infants had the greatest jump in risk of becoming overweight, at 59%, and the number of overweight infants increased by 74%. "This information is important to public health because previous studies show that accelerated weight gain in the first few months after birth is associated with obesity later in life," noted Gillman [2]. He added, "These results show that efforts to prevent obesity must start at the earliest stages of human development, even before birth."

Therefore, from as early on as the development of the fetus, the risk of obesity can be evaluated. At the beginning of life, nutritional intake in humans is controlled by innate biological systems and internal signals; later on, the learning processes determine cognitive structures about food and nutrition, strongly influencing eating habits. It is important to identify all the factors that have an influence on childhood obesity and intervene with prevention programs. For this chapter, the various web databases were consulted to provide a prospective view of recent literature concerning obesity before birth. Particular importance is given to the influence exerted by parents. This discussion explores child obesity from the beginning of pregnancy. The nutritional or non-nutritional nature of the factors involved is also considered. Thus, this chapter can be a useful guide for public health professionals to detect the most critical periods for the onset of childhood obesity and to identify the target to which the intervention of primary prevention should be addressed.

BACKGROUND ON FACTORS OF CHILD OBESITY

Obesity is a pathology that has a multifactor etiology. Genetics and environment interact and play various roles in different socioeconomic realities, establishing a disease with high prevalence [3] in industrialized countries and in developing countries where a process of westernization is occurring. To institute prevention programs and treatment interventions against obesity, a deep knowledge of the underlying factors is required. Many of these factors are preventable or modifiable, which represents the phase where it is still possible to intervene and avoid the onset of the pathology.

The study of the effect of the factors involved is complicated and difficult. Some of these factors have convincing evidence for a positive relationship with obesity, others are probable or possible factors, and confounders often influence their effect. It is clear, in fact, that the risk of developing obesity starts early in life, even as early as during fetal development. At the beginning of life, various biological processes lead to the acquisition of cognitive structures, attitudes, and beliefs about food and nutrition, which are influenced mostly by parents and have a particular importance in the control of nutritional intake in adulthood [4].

INVOLVEMENT OF GENETICS IN CHILD OBESITY

Genetics involves in interact and modulate fat tissue accumulation, leading to obesity at an early age. Many studies performed on couples with twins or on obese parents and their children have confirmed the extreme importance of genetics in conditioning the fatty tissue deposition in children [5, 6]. There are some monogenic forms of obesity, in which genes play a major role in their development, but these are rare. The most common form of obesity is polygenic and involves a combination of genetic individual variants that are exposed to the so-called obesogenic environment (where exercise and diet represent the main factors). Exercise and diet can increase the relative risk to develop the disease [7, 8] without showing a cause-effect relationship. A recent report by the Human Obesity Gene Map consortium counts more than 240 genes that are able to modulate body weight and adiposity [9] through the regulation of food intake, energy expenditure, lipid and glucose metabolism, adipose tissue development, and inflammation processes. The presence of one or both overweight parents represents a higher risk of obesity in their children [10]. A genetically related factor is sex, with a predisposition in females to be overweight in all the ages. The race as well seems to determine some differences in weight status: for example, black and Hispanic populations have a higher risk of obesity compared to white populations [11]. Other research has been performed on the resting metabolic rate to establish a possible difference between obese and nonobese children. Such studies did not show any significant differences, per unit of fat-free mass, between the obese and normal-weight pediatric population [12], even after weight reduction [13].

FACTORS INVOLVED DURING FETAL LIFE (NUTRITIONAL)

The Predictive Adaptive Response

The connection metabolically linking the child to the mother starts in fetal life and is influential in establishing obesity in childhood [14—17]. A model has been developed [18] to illustrate the way the fetus selects a range of homeostatic responses that are proper for afterbirth life, in relation to the information obtained *in utero*. The postnatal environment that is expected and the real one that is encountered determine the so-called predictive adaptive response. The fetus that expects a nutritionally poor postnatal environment will choose a model of development proper for that nutritionally poor postnatal range, whereas the fetus expecting a nutritionally rich postnatal environment adopts different models. The pattern underlines that it is the difference between the nutrition of prenatal and postnatal environments that determines the pathological risk, rather than the absolute level of nutrition.

Undernutrition of Pregnant Women

The hypothesis that intrauterine undernutrition, as well as undernutrition during early childhood, could lead to obesity (mainly visceral) in adulthood has to be considered valid [19]. Some Indian children, who are generally exposed to the nutritional restraints of the mother, have at birth a low height, relatively low skeletal muscle, and a high quantity of central fat mass [20]. For this reason, the nutritional transition described by the Popkin group [21] could place children from developing countries in the position of having a higher risk of becoming obese. The mother's nutrition and dimension at birth are inversely related to central obesity in adolescence [22]. It is possible to induce the typical symptoms of metabolic syndrome, to which obesity is an associated condition, by manipulating the mother's nutrition with her exposure to synthetic glucocorticoids [23, 24]. It can be observed in newborn babies who develop hyperleptinemia, hyperphagia, central obesity, and low muscular mass [14, 16]. Also in similar experiments, some changes in the hypothalamic peptides that regulate appetite and a preference for fatty foods consumption have been reported [17].

Hypercaloric Nutrition of Mothers in the Third Trimester of Pregnancy

The formation of hypothalamic centers that are responsible for appetite and satiety regulation starts in the fetus during the first to second trimester of pregnancy. In the third trimester, the number of fat cells starts to increase. This is a critical period, because excessive caloric intake can stimulate an overproduction of fat cells. Thus, overeating by the mother can lead to a higher transfer of nutrients to the fetus through the placenta and induce permanent changes in appetite, neuroendocrine function, and energy metabolism [25]. Moreover, a hyperglycemic diet of the fetus is a risk condition for adult obesity. Recently, *Science Daily* (April 15, 2009) reported that mothers who snack on high Glycaemic Index (GI) foods like chocolate and white bread during later pregnancy may give birth to heavier babies with a greater risk of childhood obesity [26].

High-Fat Diet in Pregnancy

In 2008, Chang and coworkers [27] suggest that mothers who were fed a high-fat diet during pregnancy had higher levels of appetite-stimulating proteins in their brains. This increase started when the offspring were in the womb (from day 6 of gestation) and lasted up to 15 days after birth. The high-fat diet seemed to stimulate the nerve cells in certain regions of the brain to divide more often and to develop into cells that produced appetite-stimulating proteins. In addition, recently it was reported that a high-fat diet led to cardiovascular problems by triggering the release of high levels of stress hormones in the developing fetus [28].

Excessive Protein Intake by Pregnant Women

The higher local availability of proteins for the fetus could negatively influence the future child's metabolism. In fact, to protect the brain tissue from visceral and somatic growth, some changes can occur and alter the metabolic pattern, which could lead to the development of obesity in the child [29]. In addition, epidemiological evidence suggests that *in utero* exposure as well as early postnatal life exposure to imbalanced nutrition are both related to a greater propensity to become obese in later life. Rodent and sheep models of metabolic programming of obesity by early life nutrition include maternal low and high dietary protein and energy or food intake as well as high-fat diets. Underlying mechanisms of altered energy balance in programmed offspring are associated with disturbances of ontogeny of hypothalamic feeding circuits, leptin and glucocorticoid action, which have long-lasting effects on food intake, energy expenditure, and fat tissue metabolism [30].

Leptin Level in Early Life

A new animal study [31] revealed that obesity might be hard-wired into the brain from birth, and this will make some people more prone to put on weight than others do. In the study, obese rats had faulty brain wiring that impaired their response to the hunger-suppressing hormone leptin that is produced by fat tissue and acts as a signal to the brain about the body's energy status. It is understood that the brain calibrates the need for food intake based in part on leptin levels, and obesity-prone brains are insensitive to these leptin signals, so there are defects in the brain circuits that relay leptin signals throughout the hypothalamus [32]. Thus, leptin plays roles in neuroendocrine, reproductive, hematopoietic, and metabolic regulation, but its role in the regulation of energy balance, in which it influences both food intake and energy expenditure, remains the subject of the most intensive research.

Junk Food Intake during Pregnancy

Healthy eating habits should start during the fetal life of an individual, so future mothers need to be aware that pregnancy is not the time to overindulge on sugary-fatty treats. Eating large quantities of junk food when pregnant and breast-feeding could be causing irreversible damage to unborn children and could send them on the road to obesity and early onset of diabetes [33]. This study also found that rats fed on a diet high in processed foods such as doughnuts and crisps during pregnancy and lactation gave birth to offspring that over ate and had a preference for foods rich in fat, sugar, and salt compared with rats on a regular diet.

Intake of Dietary Toxic Substances in Pregnant Women

There are only a few studies showing a correlation between toxic substances of food and the effects on the fetal endocrine system. It was hypothesized that the fetus could undergo negative effects from food toxins added to a lack of dietary micronutrients, and this could be a condition that would increase the risk of adiposity [34].

FACTORS INVOLVED DURING FETAL LIFE (NON-NUTRITIONAL)

Mother's Weight at the Beginning and at the End of Pregnancy

Many studies show that the mother's obesity at the beginning of pregnancy is a risk factor for the onset of childhood obesity [35]. This is not only due to genetic reasons but also because a mother's obesity increases the transfer of nutrients through the placenta, which can induce permanent changes in appetite and energy metabolism. On January 26, 2010, Wiley-Blackwell published that obesity during pregnancy more than doubles the risk of obesity in children at 22 to 4 years of age.

Also, the risk of obesity in children born to obese mothers may extend into their adolescence, with the risk of obesity during adulthood being greater among obese children [36].

Pregnant Women Who Smoke

The substances contained in tobacco and the accumulations of nicotine in the fecundated ovule disturb the normal implantation of the fecundated ovule in the uterus. Smoking delays the growth of the fetus because the blood reaching the growing fetus contains less oxygen and has instead carboxyhemoglobin and other toxic substances liberated from the combustion of tobacco. Moreover, nicotine increases the catecholamine level, which causes the constriction of veins taking blood to the child and alters the structure of the placenta. In this way, the risk of having a child with low birth weight or having a premature birth increases. Both conditions are tightly related to the increase of the risk of developing obesity [37]. One can speculate that smoke acts through a metabolic imprinting on the system controlling hunger and satiety [38]. A cohort study in six Bavarian communities, during the 1999–2000 suggested that maternal smoking during pregnancy might be a risk factor for childhood obesity. The prevalence of overweight and obesity, expressed as percentages, increased in the following order: never smoked (overweight: 8.1, 95% obesity: 2.2, 95%); less than 10 cigarettes daily (overweight: 14.1, 95% obesity: 5.7, 95%); and 10 or more cigarettes daily (overweight: 17.0, 95%, obesity: 8.5, 95%), respectively [39].

Pathologies in Pregnant Women

Some diseases in pregnant women can be significant factors of child obesity: diabetes type 2 and phlogistic chronic intestinal diseases (putrefactive processes, constipation, and food intolerances [34]. Overweight women with poor glucose control or diabetes tend to give birth to inappropriately large babies that have fetal macrosomia. An excess of adipose tissue can account for the greater weight of the baby, with a possible limitation in lean tissue growth [40, 41]. Mothers with gestational diabetes mellitus (GDM) may be more likely to have high birth weight babies because the maternal-fetal glucose metabolism and maternal hyperglycemia during pregnancy are altered [42]. These can lead to excess fetal insulin—a growth hormone for the fetus—which can lead to high birth weight (generally, infants weighing more than 4000 g are considered to have high birth weight). Research shows that the risk of childhood obesity rises in tandem with a pregnant woman's blood sugar level and that untreated gestational diabetes nearly doubles a child's risk of becoming obese by age 5 to 7. The study also shows for the first time that by treating women with gestational diabetes, the child's risk of becoming obese is significantly reduced [43].

HIDDEN CHEMICALS THAT TRIGGER OBESITY DURING PREGNANCY

Exposure in the womb to common chemicals used to make everything from plastic bottles to pizza box liners may program a person to become obese later in life. One of the chemicals is called bisphenol A (BPA), found in polycarbonate plastics. Research has suggested it leaches from plastic food and drink containers [44]. A team at Tufts University in Massachusetts found that when rats were exposed to bisphenol-a early in their pregnancy, female mice offspring were fatter even though they ate the same foods and amounts and were as active as the mice whose mothers weren't exposed to BPA. A similar effect occurred with perfluorooctanoic acid, a grease-proofing agent used in products such as microwave popcorn bags [45]. Tributylin—another chemical used in boat paint, plastic food wrap, and as a fungicide on crops—may trigger obesity as well as child obesity [46]. These chemicals appear to disrupt the endocrine system by altering gene and metabolic function involved in weight gain. Studies on mice showed that exposed to even tiny amounts of these chemicals during development were fatter when they grew older compared with mice not exposed to the compounds [45]. The findings suggest that some people may be programmed to obesity before birth and underscore the need to identify biomarkers scientists can use to identify people at risk, the researchers said. In addition, researchers had discovered that when phthalates are absorbed into the body and act as endocrine disruptors, obesity levels rise in mice. This study is the first one to link endocrine disruptors to human obesity. Such types of hidden chemicals also accumulate over many years in humans and are passed from mother to fetus during the most sensitive period of brain development [47].

PREVENTION OF CHILD OBESITY BEFORE BIRTH

Now obesity is an issue that is everyone's responsibility to try and combat. President Obama [36] has stated that childhood obesity is "one of the most urgent health issues that we face in this country." On February 9, 2010, ABC's *Good Morning America* featured First Lady Michelle Obama, who is launching an initiative titled "Let's Move!" to combat childhood obesity [36]. But where to start? Although currently there are lots of programs and social movements, such as food habit or physical exercise starting during preschool in many different countries, this movement should start in early life even before the birth, and some of the preventive measures can be summarized as follows:

1. It is important to maintain a healthy balanced diet both during pregnancy and after the baby is born. Pregnant women will have different dietary requirements than women who are not pregnant, and they may need to eat more or less of certain foods to support the healthy development of their baby.
2. Before and during pregnancy, women should avoid high-fat food and reduce excessive protein intake to create a suitable womb for a nonobese baby. Moreover, pregnant women should follow advice from their doctors and midwives about their diet.
3. During pregnancy and especially in the third trimester of pregnancy, women should avoid hypercaloric food or high GI food like chocolate, rice, or white bread that may contribute to adult obesity in later life.
4. At the beginning and end of pregnancy, the mother should try to maintain a normal body weight, because the mother's weight gain itself is a risk factor for the onset of child obesity. In addition, overweight is directly correlated to high blood glucose or GDM. To prevent maternal overweight and gestational diabetes, early diagnosis, treatment, and monitoring of GDM are important for a child's future weight. Weight management programs to assist women of childbearing age are needed too.
5. Pregnant women and all parents should avoid eating large quantities of junk food and processed food, which could cause irreversible damage to their unborn baby and lead to offspring obesity and related complications.
6. Everyone, including pregnant women, should not take in dietary toxic substances in order to reduce the risk of adiposity. By reducing our intake of animal fat, we can reduce toxic threats as well as risks for heart disease and child obesity (as "bio-accumulating" chemicals are found mainly in animal fat). Moreover, high-mercury-containing fish such as tuna should be limited during pregnancy and lactation.
7. During pregnancy, women should avoid plastic contaminated food and drinks including vegetables treated with pesticides that sometimes cause the onset of obesity for the unborn baby. It's always better to consume organic food and vegetables.
8. Pregnant women should stop or reduce smoking and alcohol consumption during pregnancy or before planning to become pregnant. These two harmful behaviors are closely correlated for developing obesity and other diseases.
9. To prevent child obesity, it's better for pregnant women, particularly obese pregnant women who want to lose weight, to practice healthy eating habits. It is well known that eating more fibrous food (e.g., oatmeal), vegetables (e.g., cucumber), spices (e.g., turmeric), and fruits such as citrus, pear, grapes; drinking lots of water daily; and participating in physical activity help to reduce weight gain and suppress the growth of fatty tissue.
10. An alternative approach to healthcare can be a good way to prevent child obesity, such as yoga and positive thinking. Yogic practices can be beneficial during pregnancy; some of these practices focus on preventive and building up immunity against obesity and diseases, the maintenance of good health, longevity, and, above all, mental sanity. Yoga says, "What a fetus learns in the womb cannot be learned on the earth"[48].

CHANGE THE ATTITUDE, CHANGE THE TREND

We can't change our genes, but we can change our lifestyle pattern and outlook on life. First, we must change our attitude so we can change the trend of child obesity. Today, advanced science and cutting-edge technology have proved that the unborn baby can not only listen and feel but can also respond by its own way. More than 60% of brain development occurs in the intra-uterine period. In addition, the eating habits of unborn babies and developing infants can be programmed by their mothers' food choices [33]. Therefore, pregnant women should think wisely about changing eating habits and lifestyle patterns so that the seed of obesity cannot be planted in the womb. Second, pregnancy should always be planned instead of occurring by accident. A woman may not realize that she is pregnant until after she has missed a period. By this time, the fetus could have been developing for 4 to 8 weeks. Therefore, a woman should eat the right things, stop smoking, and avoid alcohol some weeks before she becomes pregnant. As rapid weight-loss dieting is very harmful during pregnancy, excess weight should be lost before conception. Third, parents should change the traditional notion of a bubbly-doubly baby to that of a slim, healthy baby. Every pregnant woman should hope for a healthy baby and should reject the concept that "I am eating for two"; rather she should think, "I am eating for a healthy baby," because when the pregnant woman thinks in this way, her mind and body will be more prepared for the coming baby and her mind will automatically guide her to do what is best for the unborn child. Fourth, a special initiative must be taken so that the general physician and pediatrician can counsel women during the prepartum, pregnancy, and postpartum periods and inform women about their own risks of overweight as well as their child's risk to become obese. In addition, it is now essential to add an obese class to help students recognize obesity early in the usual practice of weight measurement and scale of child growth. Finally, parents should serve as models for the coming baby, as they provide their children with both genes and environments. Overweight parents may pass on genes that predispose their children to becoming overweight, as well as lifestyle patterns, attitudes, and habits that also contribute to child obesity. Therefore, parents must adopt a "do as I do" not "do as I say" motto with their children, even before they are blessed with a child. Otherwise it will be difficult to change the current trends leading to obesity.

CONCLUSION

In recent years, childhood obesity has become a worldwide issue. The list of negative outcomes associated with its occurrence is constantly increasing and, simultaneously, we are learning or experimenting with various methods, techniques, and steps for introducing a different program for prevention and intervention. At the same time, many antiobese campaigns have been launched at both government and nongovernment levels. Although there is still much to learn about the causes and outcomes associated with childhood obesity, current empirical information has proposed a provocative new phenomenon, which suggest that child obesity begins much earlier than previously believed. In these circumstances, awareness before birth is the best prevention. However, enormous efforts must to be applied to obesity research by academic and industrial scientists, and we have to change our attitude to combat this global epidemic.

References

1. Ogden CL, Carroll MD, Curtin LR, McDowell MA, Tabak CJ, Flegal KM. Prevalence of overweight and obesity in the United States. *Journal of American Medical Association* 2006;**295**: 1549–55.
2. Kim J, Peterson KE, Scanlon KS, Fitzmaurice GM, Must A, Oken E, Shiman SLR, Edwards JWR, Gillman MW. Trends in Overweight from 1980 through 2001 among preschool-aged children enrolled in a Health Maintenance Organization. *Obesity* 2006;**14**:1107–12.
3. World Health Organization. *Obesity, Preventing and managing the global epidemic*. Geneva: World Health Organization; 1998.
4. Tabacchi G, Giammanco S, Guardia ML, Giammanco M. A review of the literature and a new classification of the early determinants of childhood obesity: from pregnancy to the first years of life. *Nutrition Research* 2007;**27**:587–604.
5. Stunkard AJ, Sorensen TIA, Hanis C, Teasdale TW, Chakraborty R, Schull WJ, Schulsinger F. An adoption study of human obesity. *New England Journal of Medicine* 1986;**314**: 193–8.
6. Bouchard C, Tremblay A, Despres JP. The response to long-term overfeeding in identical twins. *New England Journal of Medicine* 1990;**322**:1477–82.
7. Bray GA, Bouchard C, James WPT. *Handbook of obesity*. New York: Marcel Dekker; 1998.
8. Hill JO, Peters JC. Environmental contributions to the obesity epidemic. *Science* 1998;**280**:1371–4.
9. Rankinen T, Zuberi A, Chagnon YC, Weisnagel SJ, Argyropoulos G, Walts B, Pérusse L, Bouchard C. The human obesity gene map: the 2005 update. *Obesity (Silver Spring)* 2006; **14**:529–644.
10. Reilly JJ, Armstrong J, Dorosty AR, Emmett PM, Ness A, Rogers I, Steer C, Sherriff A. Early life risk factors for obesity in childhood: cohort study. *British Medical Journal* 2005;**330**: 1357–63.
11. Strauss RS, Pollack HA. Epidemic increases in childhood overweight. *Journal of American Medical Association* 2001;**286**: 2845–8.
12. Bandini L, Schoeller DA, Dietz W. *Proceedings of the congress news in childhood nutrition*. Bethesda, MD, 1992. p. 123.
13. Zwiauer KFM, Mueller T, Widhalm. K. Resting metabolic rate in obese children before, during and after weight loss. *International Journal of Obesity* 1992;**16**:11–16.
14. Vickers MH, Breier BH, Cutfield WS, Hofman PL, Gluckman PD. Fetal origins of hyperphagia, obesity and hypertension and its postnatal amplification by hypercaloric nutrition. *American Journal of Physiology and Endocrinology Metabolism* 2000;**279**: E83–7.
15. Vickers MH, Breier BH, McCarthy D, Gluckman PD. Maternal under nutrition leads to lethargy and hyperphagia combined with increased hepatic lipid accumulation, reduced muscle mass and obesity in offspring. *Pedestrian Research* 2003;**53**:39A.
16. Vickers MH, Breier BH, McCarthy D, Gluckman PD. Sedentary behaviour during postnatal life is determined by the prenatal environment and exacerbated by postnatal hypercaloric nutrition. *American Journal of Physiology* 2003;**285**:R271–3.
17. Bellinger L, Lilley C, Langley-Evans SC. Prenatal exposure to a low protein diet programs a preference for high fat foods in the rat. *Pediatric Research* 2003;**53**:38A.
18. Gluckman PD, Hanson MA. The developmental origins of the metabolic syndrome. *Trends Endocrinology Metabolism* 2004;**15**: 183–7.
19. Godfrey KM, Barker DJ. Fetal nutrition and adult disease. *American Journal of Clinical Nutrition* 2000;**71**(Suppl. 5): 1344S–1352S.
20. Yajnik CS. The insulin resistance epidemic in India: foetal origins, later lifestyle, or both? *Nutrition Review* 2001;**59**:1–9.
21. Popkin BM, Richards MK, Montiero CA. Stunting is associated with overweight in children of four nations that are undergoing the nutrition transition. *Journal of Nutrition* 1996;**126**:3009–16.
22. Barker M, Robinson S, Osmond C, Barker DJP. Birth weight and body fat distribution in adolescent girls. *Archives of Disable Child* 1997;**77**:381–3.
23. Bertram CE, Hanson MA. Animal models and programming of the metabolic syndrome. *Brazilian Medical Bulletin* 2001;**60**: 103–21.
24. Brawley L, Poston L, Hanson MA. Mechanisms underlying the programming of small artery dysfunction: review of the model using low protein diet in pregnancy in the rat. *Archives of Physiological Biochemistry* 2003;**111**:23–35.

25. Whitaker RC, Dietz WH. Role of the prenatal environment in the development of obesity. *Journal of Pedestrian* 1998;**132**: 768–76.
26. Smith NA, Mc Auliffe FM, Quinn K, Longergan P, Evans ACO. Transient high glycaemic intake in the last trimester of pregnancy increases offspring birth weight and postnatal growth rate in sheep. *British Journal of Obstetrics and Gynecology* 2009;**116**: 975–83.
27. Chang GQ, Gaysinskaya V, Karatayev O, Leibowitz SF. Maternal High-Fat Diet and Fetal Programming: Increased Proliferation of Hypothalamic Peptide-Producing Neurons That Increase Risk for Overeating and Obesity. *The Journal of Neuroscience* 2008;**28**: 12107–19.
28. Kirk SL, Samuelsson AM, Argenton M, Dhonye H, Kalamatianos T, Poston L, Taylor PD, Coen CW. Maternal obesity induced by diet in rats permanently influences central processes regulating food intake in offspring. *PLoS ONE* 2009;**4**:5870.
29. Jackson AA, Langley-Evans SC, McCarthy HD. Nutritional influences in early life upon obesity and body proportions. In: James WPT, Shaper G, editors. *Origins and consequences of obesity. CIBA Foundation Symposium no. 201*. Chichester (West Sussex): John Wiley & Sons; 1996. pp. 407–35.
30. Metges CC. Early Nutrition and Later Obesity: Animal Models Provide Insights into Mechanisms. In: Koletzko B, et al., editors. *Early Nutrition Programming and Health Outcomes in Later Life*. Obesity and Beyond: Springer Science, The Netherlands; 2009. p. 105.
31. Bouret SG, Gorski JN, Patterson CM, Chen S, Levin BE, Simerly RB. Hypothalamic Neural Projections Are Permanently Disrupted in Diet-Induced Obese Rats. *Cell Metabolism* 2008;**7**: 179–85.
32. Dallongeville J, Fruchart JC, Auwerx J. Leptin, a pleiotropic hormone: physiology, pharmacology, and strategies for discovery of leptin modulators. *Journal of Medicinal Chemistry* 1998;**41**: 5337–52.
33. Bayol SA, Farrington SJ, Stickland NC. A maternal "junk food" diet in pregnancy and lactation promotes an exacerbated taste for "junk food" and a greater propensity for obesity in rat offspring. *British Journal of Nutrition* 2007;**98**:843–51.
34. Di Tullio G. Eating errors in the pathogenesis of childhood obesity. *La Medicina Biologica* 2003;**4**:33–40.
35. Rossner S, Ohlina A. Maternal body weight and relation to birth weight. *Acta Obstet Gynecol Scand* 1990;**69**:475–8.
36. Walters MR, Taylor JS. *The potential consequences of maternal obesity*. Wiley-Blackwell. available from *Science Daily* in, www. sciencedaily.com/releases/2010/01/100120121558.htm; (Jan 26, 2010).
37. Ong KK, Ahmed ML, Emmett PM, Preece MA, Dunger DB. Association between postnatal catch-up growth and obesity in childhood: prospective cohort study. *British Medical Journal* 2000;**320**:967–71.
38. Bergmann KE, Bergmann RL, von Kries R, Böhm O, Richter R, Dudenhausen JW, Wahn U. Early determinants of childhood overweight and adiposity in a birth cohort study: role of breast-feeding. *International Journal of Obesity* 2003;**27**:162–72.
39. Kries RV, Toschke AM, Koletzko B, Slikker Jr W. Maternal Smoking during Pregnancy and Childhood Obesity. *American Journal of Epidemiology* 2002;**156**:954–61.
40. Catalano PM, Thomas A, Huston-Presley L, Amini SB. Increased fetal adiposity: a very sensitive marker of abnormal *in utero* development. *American Journal of Obstetrics and Gynecology* 2003; **189**:1698–1704.
41. Durnwald C, Huston-Presley L, Amini S, Catalano P. Evaluation of body composition of large-for-gestational-age infants of women with gestational diabetes mellitus compared with women with normal glucose tolerance levels. *American Journal of Obstetrics and Gynecology* 2004;**191**:804–8.
42. Gillman MW, Rifas-Shiman S, Berkey CS, Field AE, Colditz GA. Maternal Gestational Diabetes, Birth Weight, and Adolescent Obesity. *Pediatrics* 2003;**111**:221–6.
43. Hillier TA, Pedula KL, Schmidt MM, Mullen JA, Charles MA, Pettitt DJ. *Childhood Obesity and Metabolic Imprinting: The ongoing effects of maternal hyperglycemia Diabetes Care* 2007;**30**: 2287–92.
44. U.S. National Institute of Environmental Health Sciences (2007) Available from www2.canada.com/edmontonjournal/health/story.html?id=2b026a0c–f6e2-4aa8-899c-ee3ed918121f. (March 28, 2010).
45. Chemicals and obesity- one culprit is Bisphenol-A (2007) available from www.ditch-diets-live-light.com/chemicals-and-obesity.html. (March 28, 2010).
46. Protecting your child from toxic threats to brain development (2007) available from www.brainy-child.com/article/toxic-threats-to-brain-development.htm (March 19, 2010).
47. Landrigan PL. Child obesity is linked to chemicals in plastics. Available from , http://cityroom.blogs.nytimes.com/2009/04/17/child-obesity-is-linked-to-chemicals-in-plastics/?emc=eta1. (March 19, 2010).
48. Yago-Garbh Sankan (Educating the fetus in the womb). Available from http://thebestarticles.com/modules/AMS/article.php?staryid=227. (March 28, 2010).

CHAPTER 12

The Social, Cultural and Familial Contexts Contributing to Childhood Obesity

Cathy Banwell, Helen Kinmonth, Jane Dixon

National Centre for Epidemiology and Population Health (NCEPH), College of Medicine, Biology and Environment, Australian National University Canberra, Australia

INTRODUCTION

"[T]here is credible evidence suggesting that cultural norms within Western societies contribute to lifestyles and behaviors associated with risk factors of chronic diseases" [1]. On the topic of obesity, Fernandez-Armesto [2] wrote that it is "a cultural revolution with obvious economic roots."

Rising levels of childhood obesity signal that massive cultural changes have occurred since the 1960s and 1970s. These in tandem with other worldwide transformations such as increased urbanization, economic growth, modernization, and globalization of food markets [3] have led to an almost universal acceleration in the prevalence of obesity including childhood obesity [4]. In developed countries, obesity is the most common child health problem with most developing countries now following a similar trajectory. Childhood obesity raises the risk of diseases, preconditions, and complications across cardiovascular, neurological, endocrine, musculoskeletal, psychosocial, pulmonary, renal, and gastrointestinal systems, along with a raised risk of adult morbidity and mortality [5].

The complexity of childhood obesity lies in the distal, social, and environmental determinants that influence what children eat and how much they move [6]. Candib [7 p. 552] suggested that childhood obesity is best thought of as "a syndemic, a complex and widespread phenomenon in population health produced by multiple reinforcing conditions." Accompanying environmental and biological determinants, sociocultural norms and practices have a role in influencing childhood obesity.

CULTURES AND CHILDHOOD

Among the multiple definitions of "culture" [8], the term can encompass all facets of society or can be quite narrowly associated with the ephemeral practices. The most inclusive definitions generally discuss the complex of behaviors, ideas, and values that constitute the conduct of the human condition. Keesing [9 p. 383] linked social structures with culture but differentiated them:

> A culture is an organized system of knowledge, more or less shared by individuals, that enables them to communicate, share meanings, and do things together towards common ends. Social structure is the network of social relations among the actors on the social stage, in contrast to the scripts they follow and understandings they share.

Here, we lean toward an encompassing view of culture, proposing that it infuses all aspects of childhood obesity, including social and familial components. Indeed, childhood obesity cannot be understood or successfully responded to without accounting for sociocultural and familial contexts because "strategies of action are cultural products" [10 p. 284]. Cultural factors operate across and within populations such as nations and societies, ethnic, linguistic, tribal or other social groups and within even smaller subgroups, such as those associated with status, religion, or a particular shared interest. Traditionally, through the discipline of anthropology, the exploration of sociocultural factors has occurred in non-Western, small, bounded, social groups, but increasingly these factors are considered relevant when grappling with the health problems of complex, modern societies.

Childhood usually refers to the age and stage between infancy and either puberty or adulthood. Under the United Nations Convention on the Rights of the Child, any human being under the age of 18 is a child. However, it is clear that how childhood is constituted and the age period it is associated with varies enormously in history and culture [11, 12]. The concept of childhood did not exist until the late Middle Ages in Europe according to some [13]. Sociological debates on the constitution of childhood pertain to obesity in several ways. First, they draw attention to how notions of childhood shape children's agency and autonomy in legal, social, and family life. In preindustrial societies, children were often treated as property and their energy could be harnessed. Over the 20th century in Western societies, infant mortality declined, families had fewer offspring, and children became precious, with the concept of a childhood seen as something to be protected and differentiated from adulthood. Recently, in modern Western societies, concern is again being expressed that the innocence and naivety of childhood is being eroded as children are being sexualized and converted to consumerism at earlier ages [14]. Second, notions of childhood, intersected with gender and ethnicity among other factors, have had profound influence on how active children are, their freedom to move, and what, when, and where they eat. Questions of children's vulnerability, autonomy, and adult responsibilities for their care play out in their body size. Implicit in much writing on childhood obesity is the primary role of parental (ir)responsibility. The baton of responsibility is passed from government and business, who insist that parents, usually mothers, say no to children's demands, and back again when parents demand that governments intervene to limit big businesses' ability to promote food, drink, toys, and other products to children [14]. At a more abstract level, sociologists point to the way in which Western societies understand that "childhood happiness secures adulthood happiness" [12 p. 415], and in this context adult aspirations for body size are projected upon children.

Figure 12.1 provides a template for the way culture is operationalized interactively cross-nationally, within societies, and within families to produce population-wide childhood obesity. The black headings form the basis of this chapter and the white headings are acknowledged as important but of less relevance.

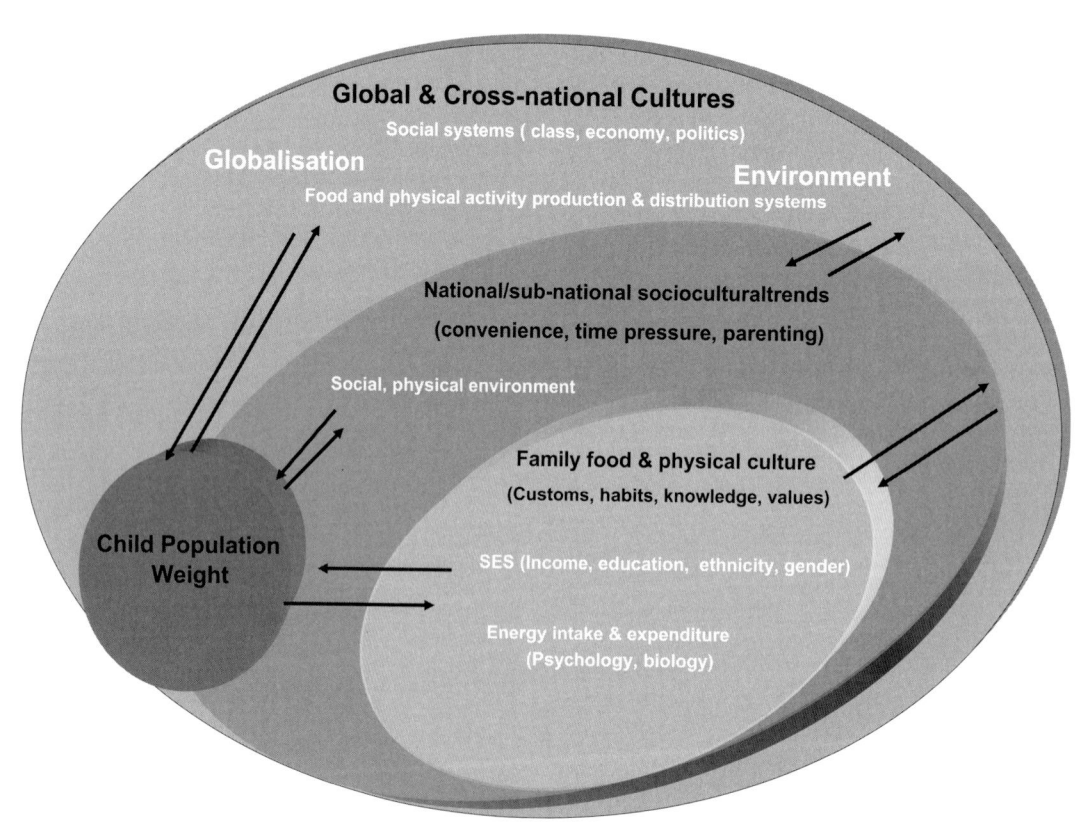

FIGURE 12.1 Sociocultural and familial contexts of childhood obesity.

This figure is an adaptation of a complex model of obesity [15].

CULTURED BODIES IN THE GLOBAL CONTEXT

Adopting a broad view of culture encourages an understanding of childhood obesity as culturally, socially, and biologically determined. In many premodern societies where food was scarce or required substantial effort to collect or produce, a well-covered body signified health, wealth, status, and (among women) fecundity. A comparison of ethnographies of non-Western societies shows that in most, plumpness (but not extreme heaviness) was considered beautiful among women, whereas in men size and muscle bulk were generally valued [16]. Even in recent times, many of the societies where weight was valued display levels of obesity that cannot be explained by economic or environmental factors alone. World Health Organization (WHO) cross-country comparisons show that Polynesian countries have the highest levels of obesity, followed by Middle Eastern countries (some less affluent such as Egypt and others like Saudi Arabia), and the United States of America. Japan and Korea rank quite low in terms of obesity. In Middle Eastern countries in particular, women far outstrip men in levels of obesity. For example, 18% of men and 39% of women are obese in Egypt [17].

Globalization has resulted in populations of developing countries being subjected to contradictory forces including images of Western, high-status, slim adults, particularly women, and the increasing availability of mass-produced, energy-dense foods and modern technologies. In wealthy Western countries, as more effort and capital [18] is required to resist obesogenic forces, increasing status is attached to slimness, particularly for women, and higher levels of obesity are associated with more disadvantaged groups [19]. As these Western trends gain traction in developing countries the cultural value attached to large bodies will probably decrease [20, 21].

International biomedical health disseminates modern Western ideals of body size for babies, children, and adults around the world via mass media, contributing to the normalization and standardization of body sizes. Although difficulties abound in scientifically assessing children's weight during their early years, the World Health Organization has developed standard growth charts for children less than 5 years of age to be used globally. Mothers and health officials are expected to produce babies and children that conform to them, and deviations from the expected pattern are identified and labeled. As a WHO background report states, "The new WHO Child Growth Standards show how every child in the world *should* grow" [22].

Little has been written about the cultural valuing of children's body size in non-Western societies. Generally, where food is scarce, thin babies and children signify a health risk, and their images are sometimes used to represent famines, war, and other major catastrophes, whereas well-covered babies are considered better able to withstand childhood diseases. Although much attention has been given to reducing childhood malnutrition and disease, there is now increasing concern about the prevalence of childhood overweight and obesity in most developed countries [23]. In developing countries, childhood undernourishment and overnourishment can coexist. There is likely to be a cultural lag in which adults continue to value heavy babies as healthier well after the threat of child mortality has diminished.

Perceptions of appropriate children's body size are somewhat influenced by adult weight. During the 20th century in the United States, plump children were considered attractive and most childrearing advice focused on encouraging children to eat more, whereas in France where the adult population is slimmer, less emphasis is placed on weight [24]. However, in the United States as girls get older, the messages were reversed and they were expected to restrict their diets and model their body size on slim women [24], whereas boys were not. In the United States, girls as young as 9 express a desire to lose weight [25]. A contributory factor is that the major sport in the United States is football, which requires a bulky, masculine body; by contrast, in France, popular sports such as cycling and soccer favor slight but muscular bodies [24].

However, in countries where plump women represent wealth and status, girls are encouraged to put on weight once they reach puberty [26]. Childhood obesity experts note that because parents often do not recognize that their children are overweight or obese, they do not attempt to modify their children's diet or weight status [27]. Perceptions of body size are influenced by ethnicity (or identification with a group on the basis of "biology, history, cultural orientation and practice, language, religion and lifestyle" [28 p. 1071]), which is regarded as one of the primary risk factors for obesity. Although research on weight differences between ethnic migrant populations and the population of the host country focuses on different food practices, some difference is due to a preference for a particular body size. African American girls and women continue to value a larger body size in defiance of white American women's aspirations to slimness [29]. Campos rather polemically argued that in the United States, "the disgust the thin upper classes feel for the fat lower classes has nothing to do with mortality statistics, and everything to do with feelings of moral superiority" [30 p. 68]. There is also increasing evidence that a gulf is growing between an acceptable body size defined by health experts on the basis of body mass index (BMI) and the BMI of most of the population supported by a countervailing trend to resist stigmatizing discourses around obesity, otherwise known in the United States as the "size acceptance movement" [31].

THE IMPORTANCE OF CHILDHOOD AND CLASS

Tastes in food and other primary pleasures are formulated during childhood [32] when individuals become enculturated and socialized. Children's tastes, preferences, and practices or the durable disposition to act in particular ways, labeled habitus [32], are developed during this time although they can be altered by later experiences over the life course [33]. Bourdieu suggested that it is taste and preference for food that is the strongest and most durable "mark of infant learning" [32 p. 79] and like other cultural preferences and practices become embedded through (family) upbringing and education [32]. Furthermore, much of what is learned unconsciously or semiconsciously in childhood endures into adulthood and is then passed to the future generations. Such tastes and preferences are associated with class-based cultures that dispose people to value particular styles of food and body forms. Thus, French working-class bodies are large and strong and need to consume plentiful and nutritious food. According to Bourdieu [32 p.190] "the body is the most indisputable materialization of class taste." But the importance of class in influencing dispositions varies across societies, with some arguing that in Australia, for example, class is not such a determining factor [34].

ENERGY IN AND ENERGY OUT: FOOD CONSUMPTION AND PHYSICAL ACTIVITY

The predominant ethnomedical model of the body in obesity research [35 p. 48] employs a "figurative language of combustion," in which energy absorbed must be balanced by energy expended and both are calculated. An ecological perspective, for example, the obesogenic environment [36] is much broader but ultimately reflects the understanding that children's body size derives from social and cultural practices influencing their energy flows. By practices we refer to embedded, embodied, relatively unconscious dispositions toward action that reflect individuals' social position and identity [32]. Our understanding is that practices, related to food consumption and physical activity, inform each other. For example, in hunter-gatherer societies, intense activity was required to obtain food, and a large meal was followed by a period of relative slothfulness. In modern times, the relationship between food consumption and activity is attenuated and will be discussed separately in this chapter, although they are interrelated both in practice and in body size. One of the recent strategies to combat obesity has been to encourage individuals to reflexively self-monitor their energy consumption and expenditure and for parents to do it for their children.

CULINARY CULTURES AND FOOD CONSUMPTION PRACTICES

A wide diversity of culinary cultures and food consumption practices exist across societies that have an impact on what children eat and their body size. They include types of foodstuffs and quantities, cooking and serving techniques, the elementary structure of meals and nonmeals [37], their timing and ordering throughout the day, commensality, seasonality, and the influence of festivals and special events on foods, all of which are subject to regional variations reflecting local habits. Furthermore, many have symbolic meanings sometimes reflecting relations of power, social distinction, and linkages [38, 39]. Food cultures often display underlying principles such as equilibrium of colors, flavors (spicy or bland), or understandings of medicinal elements such as the proper balance between heating and cooling foods in countries such as China [40] or the consideration of the regulation of other elements in Thailand [41] and India [42]. In Western countries such as Australia, health experts advise adherence to a food pyramid displaying the appropriate mix of proteins, carbohydrates, fiber, and nutrients. Religion plays a large part in some societies, proscribing some foods or food combinations, as in Judaism or Islam [43] or in Hinduism, which decrees, at least in theory, which caste members can eat with each other [42]. Catholics were expected to fast by eating fish rather than meat on Fridays. In many societies, religious festivals provide an opportunity to feast or consume special foods. However, although modernism and the secular trends described in the following discussion are weakening many of the traditions associated with culinary cultures the underlying structures of meals remain durable.

As long as there is enough food to fulfill nutritional requirements, premodern and non-Western diets are generally considered to be healthier than modern, Western ones, partially because irrespective of where they are sourced, they usually contain less meat, refined carbohydrates, and fats. Popkin's universal theory of the nutrition transition [44] proposes that as developing countries become wealthier and modernize, they embrace aspects of Western diets that include a greater consumption of meat, refined carbohydrates, and fats with a corresponding increase in diet-related conditions, such as obesity, diabetes, and cardiovascular disease. Others have shown how the role of global economic forces and the spread of foods like sugar [45], the growth of multinational corporations [46], and the impacts of technology (freezers, refrigerators, canneries) have played a role in changing global diets. However, global and local food systems intersect unevenly so that local and traditional foods often coexist with industrial food systems [47].

In middle-income countries such as Thailand [48], China [40], and Brazil [49], the nutrition transition is occurring rapidly. However, a few societies are attempting to protect their traditional food cultures. Japan, while exemplifying many of the characteristics of the global food system [50], introduced dietary guidelines in 2000 and in 2005 and followed them with the *Basic Act on Shokuiku,* which promotes education about eating by focusing on maintaining cultural food traditions [51]. South Korea has encouraged its citizens through a concerted campaign to maintain a traditional low-fat, high-vegetable diet. It has lower obesity levels and higher vegetable consumption than many Western and Asian countries [52]. France is notable both for its culinary culture and its comparatively low level of obesity in adults and children [38]. Grignon and Grignon [53] described the durability of the basic French meal structure (breakfast, lunch, dinner) despite major social changes such as industrialization, urbanization, and increasing wealth. The French eat smaller portions, eat more slowly, eat more often socially, and snack less than Americans. Furthermore, French environments encourage more physical activity than American ones. These sociocultural values that produce slimmer French bodies can be summarized as a cultural orientation toward moderation rather than excess, a focus on food quality rather than quantity, and a disposition toward taking pleasure in lived experiences rather than seeking comfort or convenience by making life less strenuous [38].

Our discussion about the influence of culinary culture on body size is predicated on the idea that generally, children participate in the same food culture as their families, as an inherent component of the enculturation and socialization process described by Bourdieu and others. However, in some cultures and among particular social groups this is not always the case. Children may be exempted from fasts such as Ramadan or other food restrictions. In British, upper-middle, social classes, children dined at a different time from adults, usually in the nursery, and ate bland food [54]. Children are also pivotal in both cultural continuity and change. They are often targeted by the advertising and education industries as a way of introducing new practices into family consumption patterns. In modern China the importance of the child is related to China's single-child policy and is signaled by preferential food treatment. Chinese children's power to shape family eating patterns is growing, and they have become expert food consumers, introducing new ideas about nutrition. Their weight has also increased [40]. However, a recent study in northeast Thailand found that about half the teenagers in the study valued their local (healthy) cuisine and felt that with some assistance it could be used to stem the increasing popularity of Western fast food among young people [55]. In Western countries where much research has been directed at food advertising to children, their role as implementers of change family food practices has been noted [56, 57]. In both France and the United States, generational differences were observed in attitudes to food [58].

THE CULTURE OF PHYSICAL ACTIVITIES

WHO has written that "successful implementation of physical activity promotion strategies will depend on whether cultural ties, groups and customs, as well as family ties, gender roles, social norms, languages and dialects have been taken into account" [59]. Again sociocultural factors are important in determining what activities are valued and considered appropriate in different societies. Generally, the freedom to move and use physical space reflects power hierarchies. Thus, it is that the activities of children, women, and poorer or marginalized members of society are controlled. In the past, the restrictions on upper-class women's physical activities in Western societies and elsewhere were supported by fashion (such as long dresses and tight corsets in European societies, and in China by bound feet) that effectively reinforced cultural expectations about women's activities. There has been a long history of the physical energy and activity levels of the lower or poorer classes being alienated (as slaves, serfs, child soldiers) and used for the benefit of the more powerful. Just how naturalized these hierarchies become is illustrated by an article written in the 1980s asking why U.S. girls do not throw like boys. The author and others [60, 61] argued that the reason lies in cultural expectations, training, and other practices rather than in biophysical form as is widely believed.

Currently, cultural and ethnic differences can be seen in the activities that women can freely undertake. For example, when commenting on the prevalence of overweight among Egyptian women it was noted that it is not acceptable for Egyptian women to "practice sports, exercise or even walk for a distance," and in undertaking household tasks many women now have access to modern labor-saving devices [19]. Pakistani and Indian women living in the United Kingdom, when encouraged to exercise to manage type 2 diabetes, state that the family obligations come first, that they do not felt comfortable going out on their own, or that they are ashamed to expose their bodies in public places such as gyms or swimming pools [62]. Restrictions are placed on women's activities in combination with high-calorie diets to fatten women in societies where large female body shapes are desirable [26].

In most societies there appears to be a period in children's lives when they do not have to conform to gender, class, or other expectations and are free to choose (within limits) their own activities, which are often described as play. Although multiple theories abound concerning the meaning and significance of play in children's development, of particular interest to childhood obesity is the early theory that play is a way for children to expend surplus energy not required for survival activities [63]. In this regard they are considered different from adults who are required to expend all their energy on productive activities. Usually once children reach a certain age, the schooling and other training processes absorb some of this surplus energy and time. In modern societies, concern is expressed over the shift in children's play from energy-expending activities to more sedentary ones involving the indoor use of screens (such as TV and the computer), partially in response to the trends described next. Thus, where once children were considered naturally active and adults often attempted to curb or direct their energies, efforts are now being made by adults worldwide, as evidenced by the WHO quotation presented earlier, to encourage children to be more active to prevent obesity.

NATIONAL SOCIOCULTURAL TRENDS INFLUENCING BODY WEIGHT

As in other Western countries, Australian children's weight remained relative stable for much of the 20th century but started trending sharply upward around the 1970s and 1980s. On the basis of these trends, it is estimated that within 30 years children will have a prevalence of overweight of 60%, similar to Australian adults [64]. This is likely because there is very little difference between the lifestyles of children and adults, in terms of both their dietary and physical activity patterns [64]. In a recent Delphi study on obesity in Australia, out of 50 experts in the field, 10 suggested increased time pressure as the social change that "contributed most to the rise in obesity over the last half century" with time ranking in the top seven factors, along with convenience around food and activity, and changing family dynamics [65—67]. These three factors—time pressure and busyness, convenience [68] and child-centered parenting as part of family dynamics [69]—have a particularly strong cultural component. They affect other modern and modernizing societies to a greater or lesser degree as they appear in global economies in which deregulated markets demand flexible labor forces and nonroutine work schedules, which have an impact on family life.

Busyness and time pressure are highly context specific but are experienced when individuals and families undertake too many activities to fit comfortably in a day. They are understood to arise from the expansion of working hours (for both men and women); the juggling of complex family schedules related to work, school, and leisure; and increasing travel time as Australian cities expand outward and traffic becomes heavier [70]. Technological innovations such as mobile phones can both alleviate and exacerbate busyness by demanding instant responses and permitting an intensification of scheduling while also being employed to fix scheduling problems. In the early part of the 20th century, convenience was about comfort; now it is about the reordering of time. Convenience "relaxes the constraints upon an individual's trajectory through time and space" [71]. The experience of time pressure leads families to choose conveniently accessible, pre-prepared foods, which are sometimes more energy dense than home-cooked meals made from raw ingredients. Many foods and other goods have been adapted to a child's eye view of convenience. Thus, the advertising and availability of energy-dense foods are often located close to schools or entertainment sites for children (sometimes in vending machines), making such food conveniently accessible to them. Time pressure leads people to become reliant on convenient forms of automobile travel, which is believed to be quicker and more flexible than the more energy-demanding forms of transport such as walking, cycling, or taking mass transport [72]. Children are chauffeured to school and other activities as part of women's cultural valuation of being a good mother [73], including keeping children safe from perceived dangers such as strangers and pedestrian accidents. Individuals feel that they do not have time to participate in social and healthy physical activities [67].

A somewhat different sociocultural trend is that of child-centered parenting, which has developed in the 1960s and 1970s in Western countries in tandem with a modern view of childhood as discussed earlier. In Australia as in many developed countries, the role of children has changed from "economic utility" to "economic liability" [76]. As each generation has fewer children, more is financially invested in those children and their development has become a growing concern of government, health authorities, the media, and industries specific to child development, food, and physical activity [82]. Children are understood to be vulnerable, requiring from good parents a high investment of time, energy, and knowledge to help them progress through a competitive and tough world. Value is placed on children's autonomy and the development of their abilities to discriminate and choose. As discussed later, this sometimes acts to produce children who are both open to market forces and are able to influence family dining patterns, food choices, and other social and physical activities. However, the perception of children as vulnerable has led to many of their physical activities such as free play outside the home being restricted and to the commercialization of alternative forms of children's play such as computer games, TV viewing, and scheduled sporting activities. When taken overall, these changes have resulted in many children leading less active lives and consuming more energy-dense foods.

FAMILIAL CONTEXTS OF CHILDHOOD OBESITY

Since the 1960s, families, especially in Australia and other developed countries, have changed in structure, function, and culture as populations moved through four major transitions: demographic, epidemiological, technological, and nutrition [44, 80]. All four, but mainly the latter two changes, fueled by economic growth, have especially contributed to a global growth in obesogenic environments [75, 81]. Aspects of these transitions have been major drivers of change in family food and physical activity, specifically, lower fertility; lower child mortality; longer life expectancy; labor-saving devices; the affordability, accessibility, and marketing of energy-dense foods; mothers entering the paid workforce; and the deregulation of labor markets. In Australia as in other developed countries, these changes have generated a cultural transition within families as they struggle to embody cultural expectations and to mediate some of the most severe aspects of the growing obesogenic environment.

Understanding the causes, prevention, and treatment of childhood obesity at a population level requires an understanding of familial contexts, as these are important influences on what children eat and how they move. Increasingly researchers are using systems approaches or cultural frameworks to understand the construction of meaning and dynamic interaction of all aspects of childhood obesity, often as these play out at the family level [99–101]. Family food and activity cultures are dynamic. They evolve as children are socialized into the (reflexive or not) practices and preferences of parents and as children act to influence (reflexively or not) those practices and preferences [56, 57]. They evolve as sociocultural aspects, such as the deregulation of job markets, influence the practices and preferences of both parents and children, for example, in valuing convenient food over healthy food. Finally, they evolve through feedback as family cultures influence sociocultural aspects and these changed aspects then influence family cultures. For example, the density of fast-food outlets within suburban areas differs according to the socioeconomic status (SES) of those areas [69, 77]. Family practices and preferences drive demand, markets respond by supply, and the supply then influences family practices and preferences.

Studies using a cultural framework, such as Kaufman and Karpati's 2007 [78] study of Latino families in New York, do not focus on one aspect of behavior but explore the complex web of social factors that underpin children's consumption and activity patterns. Such studies reveal the dynamic and systemic nature of family and show how everyday decisions on what children eat and what activity they undertake are generated both within families and by mediation of wider sociocultural influences, such as the national structuring of welfare payments [79]. Understanding the meaning, from a mother's perspective, as she adds sugary, chocolate flavoring to her overweight toddler's bottle of reduced-fat milk [78] cannot be underestimated in trying to effect change within that family culture, either through changes to distal, sociocultural aspects, such as TV advertising of junk food to children, or through more proximate aspects, such as parental feeding practices or health literacy.

Next we look briefly at the three sociocultural aspects explored previously at a national level—time pressure, convenience, and child-centered parenting—and set out some of the ways these aspects are mediated within family cultures around the food and physical activity of children.

RUNNING AND JUGGLING: TIME PRESSURE, CONVENIENCE, AND CHILD-CENTERED PARENTING

Strazdins [83] has suggested that time is often thought of as an individual resource, but for families time refers to household time. In Australia, fathers have held steady on their household time, over the past 40 years, but studies of the work/family balance show a severe drop in the time women in paid work (who remain the primary care givers of children) have to realize family food and activity practices that are of low obesity risk [76, 83, 84]. Working mothers have less time and energy to engage in behaviors such as monitoring children's food intake, preparing family meals, restricting children's screen viewing, and encouraging outdoor or active play [85].

In the movement of a mother into the paid workforce, a family, at least for some meals and activities, loses the knowledge and services of a domestic food and physical activity specialist who has a deep and abiding interest in the long-term health of family members. Since the late 1980s in Australia women have increased their workforce participation—55% in 2006 up from 48% in 1992—and increased the average time spent on paid work—up by an hour and 45 minutes per week over this time, but they have not compensated for this increase by reducing household time (including caring for children) but by reducing their own leisure time [84]. In 2006, the total average time spent by women in paid and household work differed according to employment level [84]. Women who work full-time (with children under 15 years of age and whose male partner works full-time) work the longest average household time (74 hours per week) compared to women who work part-time (70 hours) or were not in paid employment (66 hours). Taking paid employment hours out of these figures shows how much more time on average women who are not employed spend on households (between 1 and 32 hours) [84]. At a population level, families are losing their food and activity specialists to the paid labor market. The price for such positive effects as increased household income, financial independence for women, and increased national productivity is a decrease in healthy family practices and preferences such as home-prepared food and high-energy, unstructured play for children [86].

Often the market is used to fill the gap in family food and activity provision and does so without consideration for family members' long-term health. Moodie and colleagues [87 p. 133] have suggested that "contemporary market forces heavily favor behaviors for short-term preferences (i.e., overconsumption and underactivity) over long-term preferences (i.e., healthy weight) and this is especially true for children." This is described as a market failure as consumer's long-term health is suggested to be in the interest of the market [87]. Huang and Yaroch [88] have taken a different approach in suggesting that markets do not have a sufficient interest in the long-term health of customers unless this wins them profit. They suggest a practical response to this would be working with markets to regulate some obesogenic aspects of the marketplace while ensuring a level playing field of opportunity for all industry players. As the market remains relatively unregulated and time pressure on parents increases, engaging in behavior such as purchasing unhealthy food to save time, effort, and money is also increasing [85].

Despite this growing "convenience" trend of "eating out" and pre-prepared meals, O'Dea [89 p. 67] has suggested that children still consider parents to be "the gatekeepers of the family food supply and that parents act as important role models for children's eating behaviors." This suggests that what happens within the home, within the context of family food and activity culture, remains an essential influence on childhood obesity. In a recent UK study examining the relationship between mothers' full-time or part-time work hours and the behavior of their 5-year-old children, Sherburne Hawkins and colleagues [86] found these children were more likely to drink sweetened beverages between meals, have over 2 hours of screen-based activity, and be driven to school than children whose mothers had never been employed. These children were also less likely to primarily eat fruit/vegetables between meals or eat three or more portions of fruit daily. Yet not all 5-year-olds of full-time or part-time working mothers are obese. Cultural studies of families with full-time or part-time working mothers would be useful to understand the effect of different levels of time poverty, the meaning of time poverty constructed by families, and how such time constraints are mediated through different family practices and preferences around food and physical activity.

In Australia, since the late 1960s, a cultural norm of intensive mothering has evolved with mainly women, as the primary caregivers of children, expected to dedicate time and effort to children's needs and wishes, over the very time period that women have moved into the paid workforce [76]. Government and expert pressure in child development and broader cultural expectations have been of low control or permissive parenting to produce autonomous, resilient children [76]. However, exercising little control over what children eat along with unhealthy feeding practices such as the linking of food to reward is associated with overweight and obesity in children and can lead to a lower nutritional content of food consumed [90, 91]. When parents do not set or keep boundaries as part of their parenting practice around food, children may find it difficult to self-regulate or set their own boundaries [90]. A study by Hoerr and others [92] found permissive feeding styles such as these are associated with higher body mass index (BMI), and they were found to be more prevalent among Hispanic families and perhaps more influential among African American families of limited income with 3- to 5-year-old children. Rather than creating autonomous, independent children, the outcome of permissive feeding styles, encouraged by wider sociocultural pressure, is that sometimes the children are highly influenced by media with little ability to self-regulate around either food or physical activity.

In a cultural study by Maubach [93], parents in New Zealand report they want to provide good food for their families but juggling competing demands can mean nutritional information on food products is not considered in purchasing food and that parents have trouble articulating the reasons they assess food as healthy or unhealthy. The competing demands fall around time, accommodating the food preferences of their children, and conflict avoidance. Parents employed strategies such as "shopping without their children if possible, making sure children were not hungry if they were present, avoiding certain aisles in the store, and moving through the store swiftly" [93 p. 299]. This meant parents had less time to gather information on the food they purchased and had little opportunity to either socialize children to being aware of what they buy or to teach them how to read nutritional information. The pressure to use a child-centered approach to parenting, time pressure, and the valuing of convenience should be considered obesogenic, sociocultural factors that growing numbers of families find difficult to mediate in their quest to produce autonomous, resilient, healthy, and normal-weight children.

CONCLUSION: INTERVENING IN SOCIOCULTURAL AND FAMILIAL CONTEXTS OF CHILDHOOD OBESITY

Extensive research on the social and environmental factors influencing childhood obesity over the past few decades offers a rich, biomedical, and social etiology [6, 75] that has not translated into successful prevention or treatment at the population level. The isolated efforts of single academic disciplines researching obesity and the lack of a meta-model have hampered this process [20]. In recognition of the sociocultural complexity of this disorder, the Institute of Medicine [94 p. 15] concluded the report *Progress in Preventing Childhood Obesity* with the statement that "a succinct assessment of the nation's progress in preventing childhood obesity is not feasible given the diverse and varied nature of America's communities and population." In the United Kingdom, Butland [6] supported the concept of a "family of obesities" and recommended the use of systemic, multilevel, and tailored interventions for long-term, population-level success in prevention and treatment.

In developed countries, many interventions to prevent and treat childhood obesity are based around single behaviors, targeted at the individual level, use either the child or parent as the unit of measurement [74, 95], and seldom use the home or community as a setting [96]. Overall, interventions for children provide elements but no synthesis or "best practice model" for the prevention and treatment of childhood obesity [96]. Limited numbers of interventions for children as a population subgroup may contribute to outcomes such as low efficacy, unknown sustainability, sometimes poor evaluation, and on occasion an association with increased underweight [96–98].

To break the obesity/research nexus—the correlation of increasing research knowledge with increasing prevalence of obesity—researchers are moving toward the use of multidisciplinary models and theoretical paradigms such as systems theory, cultural studies, and cultural epidemiology to explore more complex, dynamic, cultural contexts, interrelationships, and networks [20, 99–101]. Studies and interventions based on in-depth understanding of the social and cultural context have the potential to harness cultural components, such as social support, that are important in eliciting long-term behavioral change [74]. Often associated with ethnic or other population-minority research, cultural frameworks are being extended for use on "own culture" or mainstream cultures, especially at the community and family level.

Other childhood health risks like injury evoke a societal response in the form of legislation (e.g., for car seats or swimming pool fences) with little complaint. Childhood obesity differs in that it is often treated as an individual problem for which parents are responsible. Instead it should be regarded in a similar manner to injury prevention, to require legal, economic, and environmental changes [102] as well as intervention in culture that pertains to the individual but in fact "refers to aggregates" [103]. Defining cultural factors is challenging, making the task more complex. When Western governments attempt cultural interventions they often attract pejorative descriptors such as nanny state or cultural imperialism [104], even as advertisers and other cultural intermediaries are becoming increasingly sophisticated in their efforts to encourage the valuing of overconsumption, or short-term pleasures over long-term health benefits.

As discussed, global cultural change has already occurred, and childhood obesity can be seen as an unintended consequence. The question then becomes how to respond. With regard to smoking, some argue that it was lay observations and local action that initiated interest by health specialists. This later led to the legal restrictions placed on the accessibility and availability of smoking that resulted in a cultural shift in Western countries whereby the practice was denormalized among the middle and upper classes [105]. As we have noted, Japan and Korea are implementing laws and educational strategies to support the valuing of their traditional food cultures, with the aim of preventing obesity and other diet-related health risks. It seems that cultural changes can be initiated and sustained at various levels of society, although they are often slow to embed and somewhat unpredictable. Rozin and others [38 p. S112] have observed that we may need to plan our environments so that we are more active and with regard to food "focus on quality and pleasure rather than quantity and convenience." We follow his lead in advocating such cultural changes through "government-inspired effort, in partnership with all sectors, [which] is required to encourage debate about the societal management of time pressure, the unintended consequences of holding convenience in such high regard, and the styles of parenting that might protect children against weight gain. In particular, we argue a case for a re-orientation of Australian society that takes time poverty as seriously as financial poverty, and re-values household food preparation and more active forms of transport" [106 p. 1].

References

1. Thomas SB, Fine MJ, Ibrahim SA. Health disparities: The importance of culture and health communication. *Am J Public Health* 2004;**94**:2050.
2. Fernandez-Armesto F. How gluttony went out of fashion. *New Statesman* 2002;**16**:75–7. December.
3. World Health Organization. *Fact Sheet: Overweight & Obesity*, www.who.int/dietphysicalactivity/media/en/gsfs_obesity.pdf; 2003. Accessed: 17 Dec 2009.
4. Wang Z, Hoy W, McDonald S. Body mass index in Aboriginal Australians in remote communities. *Aust N Z J Public Health* 2000;**24**:570–5.
5. Ebbeling CB, Pawlak DB, Ludwig DS. Childhood obesity: Public-health crisis, common sense cure. *Lancet* 2002;**360**:473–82.
6. Butland B, Jebb S, Kopelman P, McPherson K, Thomas S, Mardell J, Parry V. *"Tackling obesities: Future choices—Project report"*. London: Government Office for Science; 2007.
7. Candib LM. Obesity and diabetes in vulnerable populations: reflection on proximal and distal causes. *Ann Fam Med* 2007;**5**:547–56.
8. Lester R. Commentary: Eating disorders and the problem of "culture" in acculturation. *Cult Med Psychiatry* 2004;**28**:607–15.
9. Keesing R. *"Cultural Anthropology: A Contemporary Perspective"*. New York: Holt, Rinehart & Winston; 1981.
10. Swidler A. Culture in action: Symbols and strategies. *Am Sociol Rev* 1986;**51**:273–86.
11. Beck J, Jenks C, Keddie N, Young M. Childhood as a social construct. In: Beck J, Jenks C, Keddie N, Young M, editors. *"Toward a Sociology of Education"*. United Kingdom: Collier Macmillan; 1976. pp. 5–6.
12. Shanahan S. Lost and found: The sociological ambivalence toward childhood. *Ann Rev Sociol* 2007;**33**:407–28.
13. Aries P. Centuries of Childhood. In: Beck J, Jenks C, Keddie N, Young M, editors. *"Towards a Sociology of Education"*. United Kingdom: Collier Macmillan; 1976. pp. 37–47.
14. Linn S. *"Consuming kids: The hostile takeover of childhood"*. USA: The New Press; 2004.
15. Beaty M, Baker C, Banwell C, Barnett G, Berry H, Dixon J, Dyball R, Friel S, Griffin A, Proust K. (2007). "Complexity and the obesity epidemic," The 8th Asia-Pacific Complex Systems Conference, Surfers Paradise, Queensland, Australia.
16. Brown P. Culture and the evolution of obesity. *Hum Nat* 1991;**2**:31–57.
17. World Health Organization. *Global Database on Body Mass Index Graphs*, http://apps.who.int/bmi/index.jsp; 2010. Accessed: Jan 2010.
18. Offer A. Body weight and self-control in the United States and Britain since the 1950s. *Soc Hist Med* 2001;**14**:79–106.
19. Treloar C, Porteous HF, Kasniyah N, Lakshmanudu M, Sama M, Sja'bani M, Heller R. The cross cultural context of obesity: An INCLEN multicentre collaborative study. *Health Place* 1999;**5**:279–86.
20. Ulijaszek S. Seven models of population obesity. *Angiology* 2008;**59**:34S–8S.
21. Bordo S. *"Unbearable Weight: feminism, western culture and the body"*. Berkeley and Los Angeles: University of California Press; 2003.
22. World Health Organization. *WHO Child Growth Standards: Backgrounder 2*, www.who.int/childgrowth/2_why.pdf; 2006. Accessed: Jan 2010.
23. Wang Y, Lobstein T. Worldwide trends in childhood overweight and obesity. *Int J Pediatr Obes* 2006;**1**:11–25.
24. Stearns P. Children and weight control. In: Sobal J, Maurer D, editors. *"Weighty Issues. Fatness, thinness and social problems"*. New York: Aldine De Gruyter; 1999. pp. 11–30.
25. Thompson SH, Corwin SJ, Sargent RG. Ideal body size beliefs and weight concerns of fourth-grade children. *Int J Eat Disord* 1997;**21**:279–84.
26. Rguibi M, Belahsen R. Fattening practices among Moroccan Saharawi women. *East Mediterr Health J* 2006;**12**:619–24.
27. Jansen W, Brug J. Parents often do not recognize overweight in their child, regardless of their socio-demographic background. *Eur J Public Health* 2006;**16**:645–7.
28. Pearce N, Foliaki S, Sporle A, Cunningham C. Genetics, Race, Ethnicity and Health. *Br Med J* 2004;**328**:1070–2.
29. Molloy BL, Herzberger SD. Body image and self-esteem: A comparison of African-American and Caucasian women. *Sex Roles* 1998;**38**:631–43.
30. Campos P. *The Obesity Myth. "Why America's obsession with weight is hazardous to your health"*. New York: Gotham Books; 2004.
31. Sobal J, Maurer D. Body weight as a social problem. In: Sobal J, Maurer D, editors. *"Weight Issues"*. New York: Aldine De Gruyter; 1999. pp. 3–6.
32. Bourdieu P. *"Distinction: A social critique of the judgement of taste"*. London: Routledge & Kegan Paul; 1984.
33. Sobal J, Bisogni C, Devine C, Jastran M. In: Shepherd R, Raats M, editors. *"The psychology of food choice"*. A conceptual model of the food choice process over the life course, Vol III. Cambridge, MA: CABI; 2006. pp. 1–17.
34. Turner BS, Edmunds J. The Distaste of Taste: Bourdieu, cultural capital and the Australian postwar elite. *J Consum Cult* 2002;**2**:219–39.
35. Ferzacca S. Lived food and judgments of taste at a time of disease. *Med Anthropol* 2004;**23**:41–67.
36. Egger G, Swinburn B. An "ecological" approach to the obesity pandemic. *Br Med J* 1997;**315**:477–80.
37. Douglas M. *"In the active voice"*. London: Routledge & Kegan Paul; 1982.
38. Rozin P. The meaning of food in our lives: A cross-cultural perspective on eating and well-being. *J Nutr Educ Behav* 2005;**37**:S107–12.
39. Counihan C, Van Esterik P, editors. *"Food and Culture: A Reader"*. 2nd ed. New York: Routledge; 2008.
40. Klein J. Chinese Meals: diversity and change. In: Meiselman H, editor. *"Meals in Science and Practice"*. Oxford, Cambridge, New Delhi: Woodhead Publishing; 2009. pp. 452–82.

41. Seubsman S, Suttinan P, Dixon J, Banwell C. Thai meals. In: Meiselman H, editor. *"Meals in science and practice"*. Oxford, Cambridge, New Delhi: Woodhead Publishing; 2009. pp. 413–51.

42. Sen C. Indian Meals. In: Meiselman H, editor. *"Meals in Science and Practice"*. Oxford, Cambridge, New Delhi: Woodhead Publishing; 2009. pp. 394–412.

43. Douglas M. Deciphering a Meal. In: Counihan C, Van Esterik P, editors. *"Food and Culture: A Reader"*. 2nd ed. New York: Routledge; 2008. pp. 44–53.

44. Popkin BM, Du S. Dynamics of the nutrition transition toward the animal foods sector in China and its implications: A worried perspective. *J Nutri* 2003;**133**:3898S–906S.

45. Mintz S. Time, sugar and sweetness. In: Counihan C, Van Esterik P, editors. *"Food and Culture: A Reader"*. 2nd ed. New York: Routledge; 2008. pp. 91–103.

46. Hawkes C. Uneven dietary development: linking the policies and processes of globalization with the nutrition transition, obesity and diet-related chronic diseases. *Global Health* 2006;**2**:4.

47. Wilk R, editor. *"Fast Food/Slow Food: The cultural economy of the global food system"*. Lanham: Altamira Press; 2006.

48. Kosulwat V. The nutrition and health transition in Thailand. *Public Health Nutr* 2002;**5**:183–9.

49. Deliza R, Casotti L. Brazilian Meals. In: Meiselman H, editor. *"Meals in Science and Practice"*. Oxford, Cambridge, New Delhi: Woodhead Publishing; 2009. pp. 377–93.

50. Bestor T. Kaiten-zushi and Konbini. In: Wilk R, editor. *"Fast Food/Slow Food. The Cultural Economy of the Global Food System"*. Lanham: Altamira Press; 2006. pp. 115–30.

51. Melby MK, Utsugi M, Miyoshi M, Watanabe S. Overview of nutrition reference and dietary recommendations in Japan: Application to nutrition policy in Asian countries. *Asia Pac J Clin Nutr* 2008;**17**:394–8.

52. Lee M-J, Popkin B, Kim S. The unique aspects of the nutrition transition in South Korea: the retention of healthful elements in their traditional diet. *Public Health Nutr* 2002;**5**:197–203.

53. Grignon C, Grignon C. French Meals. In: Meiselman H, editor. *"Meals in Science and Practice"*. Cambridge, New Delhi: Woodhead Publishing Oxford; 2009. pp. 343–58.

54. Murcott A. Family Meals: A thing of the past?. In: Caplan P, editor. *"Food, Health and Identity"*. London and New York: Routledge; 1997. pp. 32–69.

55. Seubsman S-A, Kelly M, Yuthapornpinit P, Sleigh S. Cultural resistance to fast-food consumption? A study of youth in North Eastern Thailand. *Int J Consum Stud* 2009;**33**:669–75.

56. Coveney J. The government of the table: Nutrition expertise and the social organisation of family food habits. In: Germov. J, Williams L, editors. *"A sociology of food and nutrition: The social appetite"*. Melbourne: Oxford University Press; 1999. pp. 259–75.

57. Dixon J, Banwell C. Heading the table: Parenting and the junior consumer. *Br Food J* 2004;**106**:181–93.

58. Rozin P, Kurzer N, Cohen A. Free associations to "food": The effects of gender, generation, and culture. *J Res Pers* 2002;**36**:419–41.

59. World Health Organisation. *A guide for population-based approaches to increasing levels of physical activity: Implementation of the WHO global strategy on diet, physical activity and health*, www.who.int/dietphysicalactivity/physical-activity-promotion-2007.pdf; 2007. Accessed: Jan 2010.

60. Young I. Throwing like a girl: A phenomenology of feminine body comportment motility and spatiality. *Hum Stud* 1980;**3**:137–56.

61. Fallow J. Throwing Like a Girl. *Atlantic Monthly* 1996;**278**:84–7.

62. Lawton J, Ahmad N, Hanna L, Douglas M, Hallowell N. 'I can't do any serious exercise': barriers to physical activity amongst people of Pakistani and Indian origin with Type 2 diabetes. *Health Educ Res* 2006;**2**:43–54.

63. Verenikina I, Harris P, Lysaght P. Child's play: computer games, theories of play and children's development. In: *"ACM International Conference Proceedings Series"*, Vol. 98. Darlinghurst: Australian Computer Society, Inc; 2003. pp. 99–106.

64. Norton K, Dollman J, Martin M, Harten N. Descriptive epidemiology of childhood overweight and obesity in Australia: 1901-2003. *Int J Pediatr Obes* 2006;**1**:232–8.

65. Broom DH, Strazdins L. The Harried Environment: Is time pressure making us fat?. In: Dixon J, Broom DH, editors. *"The Seven Deadly Sins of Obesity: how the modern world is making us fat"*. Sydney: UNSW Press; 2007. pp. 35–45.

66. Broom DH, Dixon J. Introduction: Seven modern environmental sins of obesity. In: Dixon J, Broom DH, editors. *"The Seven Deadly Sins of Obesity: how the modern world is making us fat"*. Sydney: UNSW Press; 2007. pp. 1–19.

67. Banwell C, Hinde S, Dixon J, Sibthorpe B. Reflections on expert consensus: A case study of the social trends contributing to obesity. *Eur J Public Health* 2005;**15**:564–8.

68. Ulijaszek S. Obesity: a disorder of convenience. *Obes Rev* 2006;**8**:183–7.

69. Dixon J, Banwell C, Broom D, Davies A, Hattersley L, Hinde S, Strazdins L. *"Inquiry into Obesity in Australia: Submission from the National Centre for Epidemiology and Population Health"*. Canberra: Australian National University; 2008.

70. Strazdins L, Broom D, Banwell C, Griffin A, Korda R, Dixon J, Shipley M, Paoloucci F, Esler M, Glover J. (under revision) Time scarcity: Another health inequity? *Environ Plan A*.

71. Warde A, Shove E, Southerton D. *"Convenience, schedules and sustainability (draft paper for ESF workshop on sustainable consumption)"*. Lancaster: Department of Sociology, Lancaster University; 1998.

72. Hinde S. *Road rules: a Bourdieuian analysis of the social reproduction of health inequalities and transport practices in Melbourne. Unpublished PhD thesis*. Canberra: Australian National University; 2008.

73. Dowling R. Cultures of mothering and car use in suburban Sydney: a preliminary investigation. *Geoforum* 2000;**31**:345–53.

74. Gruber KJ, Haldeman LA. Using the family to combat childhood and adult obesity. *Prev Chronic Dis* 2009;**6**:1–10.

75. Popkin BM, Mendez M. The rapid shifts in stages of the nutrition transition: The global obesity epidemic. In: Kawachi I, Wamala S, editors. *"Globalization and Health"*. Oxford: Oxford University Press; 2007. pp. 68–80.

76. Banwell C, Shipley M, Strazdins L. The pressured parenting environment. In: Dixon J, Broom DH, editors. *"The Seven Deadly Sins of Obesity: How the modern world is making us fat"*. Sydney: UNSW Press; 2007. pp. 46–63.

77. Reidpath DD, Burns C, Garrard J, Mahoney M, Townsend M. An ecological study of the relationship between social and environmental determinants of obesity. *Health Place* 2002;**8**:141–5.

78. Kaufman L, Karpati A. Understanding the socio-cultural roots of childhood obesity: Food practices among Latino families of Bushwick, Brooklyn. *Soc Sci Med* 2007;**64**:2177–88.

79. Schubert L. Household food strategies and the reframing of ways of understanding dietary practices. *Ecol Food and Nutr* 2008;**47**:254–79.

80. Omran AR. Extract from The Epidemiologic Transition: A theory of the epidemiology of population change 1971. *Bull World Health Organ* 2001;**79**:161–70.

81. Swinburn B, Ley S, Carmichael H, Plank L. Body size and composition in Polynesians. *Int J Epidemiol* 1999;**23**:1178–83.

82. Conveney J. *"Food, morals and meaning: The pleasure and anxiety of eating"*. Londres: Routledge, Oxon; 2006.
83. Strazdins L, Loughrey B. Too busy: Why time is a health and environmental problem. *NSW Public Health Bull* 2007;**18**:219–21.
84. Australian Bureau of Statistics. *Australian Social Trends, March 2009*. Canberra: Australian Government; 2009.
85. Gable S, Lutz S. Household, parent, and child contributions to childhood obesity. *Fam Relat* 2000;**49**:293–300.
86. Sherburne Hawkins SS, Cole TJ, Law C. Examining the relationship between maternal employment and health behaviours in 5-year-old British children. *J Epidemio Community Health* 2009;**63**:999–1004.
87. Moodie R, Swinburn B, Richardson J, Somaini B. Childhood obesity—a sign of commercial success, but a market failure. *Int J Pediatr Obes* 2006;**1**:133–8.
88. Huang TT, Yaroch AL. A public-private partnership model for obesity prevention [letter to the editor]. *Prev Chronic Dis* 2009;**6**:1–2.
89. O Dea JA. Improving adolescent eating habits and prevention of child obesity: Are we neglecting the crucial role of parents? *Nutr Diet* 2005;**62**:66–8.
90. Blissett J, Haycraft E. Are parenting style and controlling feeding practices related? *Appetite* 2008;**50**:477–85.
91. Dalton S. *"Our overweight children: what parents, schools, and communities can do to control the fatness epidemic"*. Berkeley: University of California Press; 2005.
92. Hoerr SL, Hughes SO, Fisher JO, Nicklas TA, Liu Y, Shewchuk RM. Associations among parental feeding styles and children's food intake in families with limited incomes. *Int J Behav Nutr Phys Act* 2009;**6**:55–61.
93. Maubach N, Hoek J, McCreanor T. An exploration of parents' food purchasing behaviours. *Appetite* 2009;**53**:297–302.
94. Koplan JP, Liverman CT, Kraak VI, Wisham SL. *"Progress in preventing childhood obesity: how do we measure up?"*. Washington (DC): The National Academies Press; 2007.
95. Golan M, Weizman A, Apter A, Fainaru M. Parents as the exclusive agents of change in the treatment of childhood obesity. *Am J Clin Nutr* 1998;**67**:1130–5.
96. Flynn MAT, McNeil DA, Maloff B, Mutasingwa D, Wu M, Ford C, Tough SC. Reducing obesity and related chronic disease risk in children and youth: a synthesis of evidence with 'best practice' recommendations. *Obes Rev* 2006;**7**:7–66.
97. Doak CM, Visscher TL, Renders CM, Seidell JC. The prevention of overweight and obesity in children and adolescents: a review of interventions and programmes. *Obes Rev* 2006;**7**: 111–36.
98. Stice E, Shaw H, Marti CN. A meta-analytic review of obesity prevention programs for children and adolescents: the skinny on interventions that work. *Psychol Bull* 2006;**132**:667–91.
99. Dixon J, Banwell C. Theory driven research designs for explaining behavioural health risk transitions: The case of smoking. *Soc Sci Med* 2009;**68**:2206–14.
100. Galea S, Riddle M, Kaplan GA. Causal thinking and complex system approaches in epidemiology. *Int J Epidemiol*; 2009. Advance Access published October 9, 2009.
101. Leischow SJ, Milstein B. Systems thinking and modeling for public health practice. *Am J Public Health* 2006;**96**:403–5.
102. Schwartz M, Puhl R. Childhood obesity: a societal problem to solve. *Obes Rev* 2003;**4**:57–71.
103. Dressler W. Commentary: Taking culture seriously in health research. *Int J Epidemiol* 2006;**35**:258–9.
104. Førde O. Is imposing risk awareness cultural imperialism? *Soc Sci Med* 1998;**47**:1155–9.
105. Chapman S. *"Public health advocacy and tobacco control. Making smoking history"*. Oxford: Blackwell Publishing; 2007.
106. Dixon J, Banwell C, Broom DH, Davies A, Hattersley L, Hinde S, Strazdins L. *"Submission from the National Centre for Epidemiology and Population Health, Australian National University: Inquiry into obesity in Australia"*. Canberra: The Standing Committee on Health & Ageing, Australian Government; 2008.
107. Kjellstrom T, Hinde S. Car culture, transport policy, and public health. In: Kawachi I, Wamala SP, editors. *"Globalization and Health"*. New York: Oxford University Press; 2007. pp. 98–121.
108. Food and Agriculture Organization of the United Nations. The nutrition transition and obesity. www.fao.org/FOCUS/E/obesity/obes2.htm. Accessed: Jan 2010.

CHAPTER 13

Cardiovascular Risk Clustering in Obese Children

Ram Weiss

Hadassah — Hebrew University School of Medicine, Braun School of Public Health and Community Medicine, Jerusalem, Israel

The metabolic syndrome, also known as "the insulin resistance" syndrome and "syndrome X" describes a cluster of cardiovascular risk factors that have been shown to predict the development of cardiovascular disease (CVD) [1, 2] and type 2 diabetes (T2DM) [3]. As depicted by its name, this syndrome is characterized by the consequences of peripheral insulin resistance [4]. These metabolic characteristics represent a normal physiological adaptation induced by the resistance of specific insulin responsive tissues (mainly muscle) to the peripheral action of insulin. The clinical utility of defining this syndrome in adults and in children has been debated, as some propose that from a clinical standpoint, using each component of the syndrome individually has comparable clinical and predictive outcomes. This debate has important clinical implications, yet it is imperative to indicate that the underlying physiology that leads to the typical metabolic milieu characteristic of individuals with peripheral insulin resistance has common features in all ages and is postulated to be the driving force of the development of accelerated atherogenesis and altered glucose metabolism in susceptible individuals. Insulin resistance can be induced by different metabolic stimuli during the life course such as transient peripheral insulin resistance induced during pubertal development in adolescents [5], pregnancy in females of childbearing age [6], aging per se, and consumption of specific dietary components [7]. As part of a normal adaptive response to overcome peripheral insulin resistance, several mechanisms are activated to increase circulating insulin concentrations resulting in hyperinsulinemia. The tissue-specific metabolic response to this adaptation has common features regardless of age. The clinical manifestations of this adaptation (i.e., hyperinsulinemia) may rely on the length of exposure to it and on the susceptibility of the individual, yet the biomarkers of its presence exist at all ages.

PATHOPHYSIOLOGY OF THE INSULIN RESISTANCE SYNDROME IN CHILDHOOD

Several factor analyses of components of the insulin resistance syndrome have been performed in cohorts of adults [8—9] and of children [10—11] in order to shed light on the typical associations observed between its individual elements. These studies revealed that obesity and its related peripheral insulin resistance seem to cluster with the majority of the clinically used components of the syndrome yet also cluster with additional elements, such as increased fibrinolysis, endothelial dysfunction, and subclinical inflammation that seem to be part of the typical metabolic milieu of the insulin-resistant individual yet are not routinely assessed or clinically utilized for treatment decisions of for risk stratification. The conclusion of the majority of these analyses performed in children is that obesity, tightly associated with insulin resistance, is the common feature that is associated with the presence of the routinely measured cardiovascular risk factors (Figure 13.1). Importantly, insulin resistance per se probably does not provide a complete mechanistic explanation for the development of all the components of the syndrome. Indeed, the contribution of different fat depots, by way

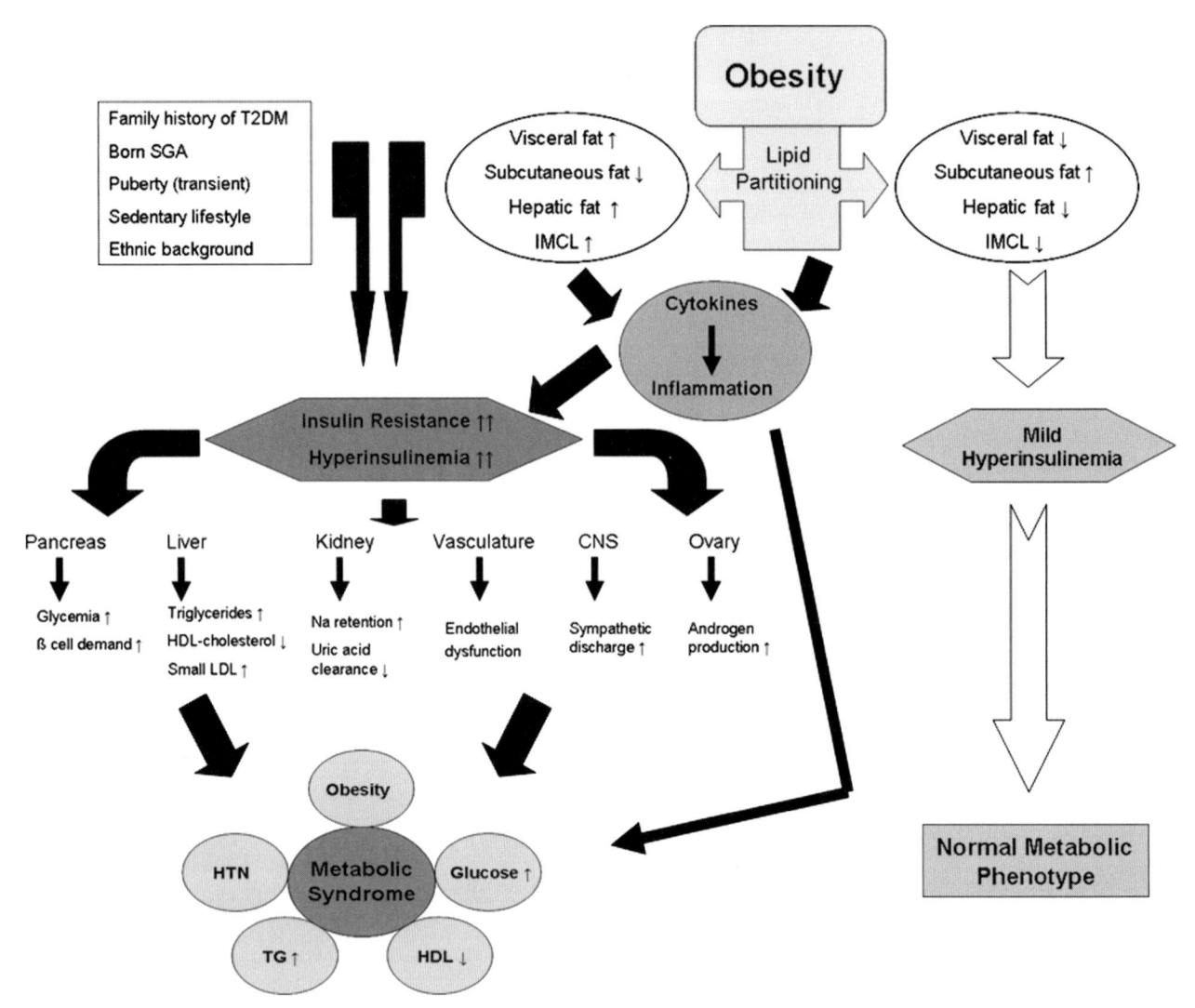

FIGURE 13.1 The metabolic impact of obesity in children is largely determined by the lipid partitioning pattern. A phenotype characterized by low visceral and ectopic lipid deposition in muscle (IMCL) and liver results in a low degree of insulin resistance. This is compensated by mild hyperinsulinemia, and the metabolic characteristics remain normal. On the other hand, increased visceral and ectopic fat along with its related subclinical inflammation and typical adipocytokine profile result in significant insulin resistance. Other contributing factors may further exacerbate this degree of insulin resistance (such as being born small for gestational age (SGA) or of specific ethnic backgrounds) or represent a priori reduced insulin sensitivity that is worsened by lipid deposition (offspring of patients with diabetes). Significant insulin resistance results in severe hyperinsulinemia, which activates several other insulin-responsive tissues and metabolic pathways to respond to the elevated insulin concentrations. The metabolic result of these responses is cardiovascular risk clustering, namely the metabolic syndrome.

of secretion of unique adipocytokines and of inflammatory cytokines, may have an additional role in the development of early atherogenesis. It has been shown in adults that adipose tissue is an important determinant of a low-level, chronic inflammatory state reflected by mildly elevated levels of interleukin-6 and C-reactive protein [12]. Such a low-level, chronic inflammatory state may induce insulin resistance and endothelial dysfunction and thus link the latter phenomena with obesity and cardiovascular disease. Moreover, fat surrounding blood vessels may accelerate atherogenesis by way of local secretion of the aforementioned inflammatory cytokines, thus inducing a paracrine, also suggested as the "vasocrine" effect [13].

It is important to indicate though that the presence of obesity or even severe obesity in a child does not necessarily indicate that significant insulin resistance is present and therefore does not imply that clustering of cardiovascular risk factors necessarily exists. Indeed, some severely obese children can be extremely insulin sensitive [14]. On the other hand, some may possess other cardiovascular risk factors that are not necessarily associated with obesity or insulin resistance such as certain heritable dyslipidemias [15]. The relation of obesity and peripheral insulin resistance is dependent more on the lipid distribution (or "lipid partitioning") in specific fat depots rather than on the absolute amount of fat per se. Different lipid depots have distinct metabolic characteristics that are reflected by their adipocytokine and cytokine secretion profile [16], sensitivity to hormones typically affecting adipose tissue (such as norepinephrine or insulin) as well as anatomical blood supply and drainage (portal versus systemic) [17]. Indeed, increased visceral fat accumulation in obese children has been associated with increased insulin resistance [18] and with the clustering of cardiovascular risk factors as well as with worsening of each one of them individually [19]. Some obese children tend to demonstrate a unique lipid-partitioning pattern characterized by a large visceral fat depot along with a relatively smaller subcutaneous fat depot. This lipid partitioning profile is associated with an adverse metabolic profile in comparison to those with larger subcutaneous fat depots, even when the latter have greater BMI and percentage body fat and may thus be seemingly "more obese" [20].

Lipid deposition in insulin responsive tissues, such as muscle and liver, represents another determinant of the sensitivity of these tissues to the metabolic effects of insulin. Intramyocellular lipid deposition is negatively correlated with peripheral insulin sensitivity and has been demonstrated to be increased in offspring of patients with T2DM and in obese children with impaired glucose tolerance [21]. The effect of lipid within the myocyte on insulin signal transduction is probably mediated by several fatty acid derivatives such as fatty acyl coA and ceramide that inhibit the insulin signaling cascade. Altered insulin signaling in muscle results in reduced glucose transporter 4 (GLUT-4) trafficking to the myocyte membrane and thus to lower glucose uptake by the cell. Similarly, hepatic fat accumulation is strongly associated with obesity and with hepatic resistance to the action of insulin in the context of metabolic pathways related to glucose metabolism. The liver governs glucose metabolism in the fasting state, and the muscle governs glucose metabolism in the post absorptive state, thus hepatic insulin resistance has a stronger impact on fasting glucose levels and on the early postabsorptive suppression of hepatic gluconeogenesis following a meal, whereas muscle lipid deposition may have a greater impact on postprandial glucose disposal. Although both tissues develop insulin resistance in association with increased lipid deposition, the pathophysiology of the effects of fat within the hepatocyte probably is not solely related to accumulation of fatty acid derivatives but also to inflammatory processes and increased oxidative stress, both induced by the influx of cytokines and other metabolites by the portal circulation.

The normal adaptive response to peripheral insulin resistance consists of increased insulin secretion by the beta cells along with reduced insulin clearance by the liver. The result of these two adaptive responses is increased circulating insulin levels (hyperinsulinemia). The ensuing hyperinsulinemia, at least at early stages of this metabolic adaptation, overcomes the tissue-specific insulin resistance within the pathways related to glucose metabolism and represents an adequate allostatic response, yet it carries a "metabolic price" of mildly increased circulating glucose levels along with a continuous burden on the beta cells to secrete adequate amounts of insulin [22, 23]. The mild increase in glucose levels serves as a major, yet probably not the only, signal to the beta cells to continuously up-regulate insulin secretion (the beta cell does not "sense" peripheral insulin sensitivity and needs a circulating signal to regulate its rate of insulin secretion).

Importantly, other metabolic pathways within the liver that are not involved in glucose metabolism or other insulin responsive tissues that do not share the pattern of increased lipid deposition within them, such as the kidney or the ovary, maintain their baseline insulin sensitivity levels yet are now exposed to hyperinsulinemia. This exposure results in a normal response of these tissues to elevated insulin levels and manifests as increased sodium retention [24] and reduced uric acid clearance by the kidney [25] and by increased androgen production by the ovary [26]. Insulin may also induce an activation of the sympathetic nervous system [27] and impact the metabolism and secretion of proinflammatory cytokines as well as coagulation mediators from adipose tissue [28]. Similarly, other metabolic pathways within the liver, specifically those related to lipoprotein metabolism, maintain their baseline insulin sensitivity (unlike those pathways related to glucose metabolism) and thus respond to the elevated insulin levels in a pattern that creates the typical dyslipidemia characteristic of insulin-resistant individuals. Some suggest that hepatic deposition of lipid does not necessarily result from an increased influx of free fatty acids induced by increased visceral fat and elevated concentration of circulating free fatty acids but is a "normal" response to elevated circulating insulin levels leading to increased local de novo lipogenesis and thus that hepatic steatosis is part of the result and not one of the culprits of the adverse metabolic phenotype characteristic of insulin-resistant individuals.

In summary, peripheral tissue resistance to the action of insulin, specifically in metabolic pathways related to glucose metabolism, results in a compensatory hyperinsulinemia. The exposure of metabolic pathways and tissues that were not affected by obesity or local lipid deposition and maintained their original sensitivity to insulin results in a metabolic profile characterized by the presence of dyslipidemia (specifically elevated triglycerides, low High Density Lipoprotein (HDL)-cholesterol, and the presence of small Low Density Lipoprotein (LDL) particles), elevated blood pressure, and altered glucose metabolism (that may manifest as impaired fasting glucose, impaired glucose tolerance, or overt diabetes). In addition, pro-inflammatory cytokines and factors related to hyper-coagulability may be present at increased levels. The clustering of some or all of these factors results in accelerated atherogenesis leading to later cardiovascular disease and in continuous beta cell stress that in some genetically prone individuals may result in beta cell failure and hyperglycemia (an individual contributor to accelerated atherogenesis). Thus, obesity and insulin resistance, each one independently and together synergistically, may contribute to the development of early atherogenesis and the appearance of cardiovascular risk factors early in the life course.

Cardiovascular Manifestations of Obesity and Insulin Resistance

The long-term effect of cardiovascular risk clustering is overt cardiovascular disease. Although some of the risk factors (such as dyslipidemia and dysglycemia) may contribute to accelerated atherogenesis, others (such as hypertension) may have significant adverse hemodynamic effects of the structure and functionality of the heart and blood vessels. Insulin resistance per se is linked mechanistically to several mechanisms that may result in blood pressure elevation, yet in large-scale studies, when insulin sensitivity is assessed using surrogate indices derived from fasting samples (such as Homeostatic Model Assessment-Insulin Resistance (HOMA-IR), which correlates marginally with clamp derived peripheral insulin sensitivity measures), it provides only a limited explanation for the increased prevalence of hypertension in people with the insulin resistance syndrome. The relationship between insulin resistance and hypertension is associated with several mechanisms, including effects on sodium reabsorption in the kidney as mentioned previously. This renal effect seems not to be consistent in all subjects and has been shown to be more substantial in Caucasians than in African Americans [29]. Insulin has an acute vasodilatory effect when infused intravenously [30], yet after several hours this effect is diminished and a compromised reactive dilatation is manifested in nonobese insulin-sensitive individuals. Thus, exposure to prolonged hyperinsulinemia, as commonly experienced by insulin-resistant individuals, can result in altered endothelial function presenting as a reduced posthyperemic dilatation [31]. In insulin-resistant individuals, the acute vasodilatory effect of insulin may be diminished [32] while the renal effect on sodium reabsorption seems to be preserved. Elevated circulating free fatty acids, characteristic of insulin-resistant individuals, probably have an independent vasoconstrictive effect as well in insulin-sensitive as well as in insulin-resistant individuals [33]. A central effect of elevated circulating insulin levels is the activation of the sympathetic nervous system that may result in blood pressure elevation.

Obesity has many independent adverse effects on the hemodynamic characteristics, structure, and function of the cardiovascular system [34]. In obese individuals, total blood volume and cardiac output are increased, resulting in a greater cardiac workload. Specifically, at any given level of activity, the cardiac workload is greater for obese subjects. Thus, obese individuals have a greater cardiac output along with a lower level of peripheral resistance per given degree of arterial pressure. To achieve greater cardiac output, obese individuals must mainly increase their stroke volume but also their heart rate via sympathetic activation. These compensatory responses lead to a shift to the left of the Frank-Starling curve, manifesting as an increased cardiac workload [35]. Thus, obese individuals are more likely to be hypertensive than their nonobese counterparts, and further weight gain is typically associated with slight yet significant increases in arterial pressure.

Activation of the rennin-angiotensin-aldosterone system (RAAS) has been suggested to play an active role in obesity-related hypertension. The RAAS regulates intravascular volume as well as vascular tone. Concentrations of angiotensin converting enzyme (ACE) and circulating angiotensinogen tend to be higher in obese individuals [36]. Studies in rodents have shown that angiotensinogen produced by adipocytes plays a role in local adipose tissue differentiation, yet it can be released into the bloodstream and create classical systemic endocrine effects. This suggests that elevated angiotensinogen levels may be associated with hypertension in obese patients as a result of increased release from fat depots [37]. Furthermore, local activation of renal RAAS can cause increased renal sodium reabsorption and a typical hypertensive shift of pressure-induced natriuresis [38]. Aldosterone levels are typically higher in obese subjects and are associated with abdominal obesity assessed by CT scanning and insulin resistance assessed by the euglycemic hyperinsulinemic clamp. Indeed, reduction of blood pressure induced by weight loss in obese adolescents is correlated with the reduction of plasma aldosterone levels [39].

The association of obesity with a subclinical inflammation may provide another mechanism that affects systemic blood pressure. A significant correlation exists between degree of obesity and concentration of interleukin − 6 (IL-6) and c reactive protien (CRP) levels [40]. A low-grade inflammatory state may play a role in increasing blood pressure [41]. Weight loss in obese adults is associated with a decrease in blood pressure. The average decrease in blood pressure is 1 to 4 mm Hg systolic and 1 to 2 mm Hg diastolic per kilogram of weight reduction as normalization of blood pressure [42]. In obese children, mixed results have been published regarding the effects of moderate weight loss on blood pressure levels [43, 44]. On the other hand, significant weight loss following bariatric surgery in obese adolescents has been shown to significantly reduce blood pressure [45]. Of note, after the weight loss has ceased, the persistent effect of weight loss on blood pressure may not always be encountered, specifically in adults in which hypertension was long standing [46].

DEFINING THE INSULIN RESISTANCE SYNDROME IN CHILDREN

The insulin resistance syndrome in children has several definitions used by various research groups [47, 48] and the use of different definitions in the same children may result in different outcomes [49]. The recently published consensus definition [50] utilizes waist circumference, a surrogate of abdominal obesity, as the body habitus component, thus reflecting the paramount importance of intraabdominal fat for the development of specific cardiovascular risk factors. Questions have been raised regarding the clinical utility of such definitions in adults [51] and in children [52], and some experts advocate addressing individual risk factors in their clinical context. Regardless of this controversy, it must be emphasized that cardiovascular risk factors such as elevated fasting glucose or elevated triglycerides represent continuous parameters that signify continuous risk, not necessarily in a linear fashion. For example, while increasing BMI during childhood, even within the normal BMI range, represents a continuous risk factor for the development of coronary heart disease in adulthood [53], severely obese children may have a significantly worse metabolic phenotype in comparison to moderately obese children [54]. A seemingly "upper normal" fasting glucose level in the context of obesity in young adulthood may signify future risk of developing type 2 diabetes [55]. Similarly, the triglyceride level in late adolescence and its change within a brief follow-up of ~5 years can predict the development of diabetes [56] and of coronary heart disease [57], even when both measurements are within the seemingly "normal" range. Thus, regardless of the definition used, one must remember that cardiovascular risk clustering in childhood and adolescence is not strictly a dichotomous diagnosis and that all these factors have a continuum that may have clinical implications even when it is below predetermined diagnostic thresholds.

CLINICAL RELEVANCE

Cardiovascular risk factors present in childhood have been shown to be associated with overt atherosclerosis in children as well as in young adults. Using the landmark Bogalusa cohort study, Berenson et al. [58] have shown by studying coronary arteries and aortas from autopsies that among the cardiovascular risk factors, body mass index, systolic and diastolic blood pressure, and serum concentrations of total cholesterol, triglycerides, low-density lipoprotein cholesterol, and high-density lipoprotein cholesterol, as a group, were strongly associated with the extent of lesions in the aorta and coronary arteries (r = 0.70; P < 0.001). Moreover, the additive effect of multiple risk factors on the extent of atherosclerosis was quite evident. Subjects with zero, one, two, three, or four risk factors had, respectively, 19.1%, 30.3%, 37.9%, and 35% of the intimal surface covered with fatty streaks in the aorta (P for trend = 0.01). The comparable figures for the coronary arteries were 1.3%, 2.5%, 7.9%, and 11.0%, respectively, for fatty streaks (P for trend = 0.01) and 0.6%, 0.7%, 2.4%, and 7.2% for collagenous fibrous plaques (P for trend = 0.003).

Most published studies regarding the clinical impact and correlates of cardiovascular risk factor clustering in childhood utilize surrogates of early atherogenesis, such as vascular functional characteristics. Children who meet criteria of the metabolic syndrome have been shown to have increased aortic stiffness [59], whereas associations with endothelial dysfunction (a surrogate of an early accelerated atherogenic process) show mixed results [60, 61]. Regardless of the definitions used and independent of specific threshold values, the presence of cardiovascular risk factors in childhood and adolescence tracks into adulthood and is associated with the presence of subclinical atherosclerosis in young adulthood [62, 63]. Although the stability of the diagnosis of the metabolic syndrome (i.e., of clustering of such markers beyond a specific threshold) in non-obese children is questionable [64], the stability of the syndrome in obese children (i.e., those at greatest risk to develop it) is tightly linked to dynamics in the degree of obesity (i.e., to weight changes) and insulin sensitivity [65]. Thus, in those at greatest risk, cardiovascular risk clustering seems to be stable and probably carries its adverse metabolic impact continuously.

CONCLUSION

These observations highlight the importance of primary and secondary prevention of the progression of early cardiovascular risk factors in children and adolescents. As the presence of some of these risk factors tends to track from childhood to adulthood, primary prevention of their development or early reversal of their presence in childhood are of paramount importance. Interventions ranging from diet-induced weight loss and increased physical activity to bariatric surgery have been attempted in obese children with the presence of cardiovascular risk factors or overt disease such as T2DM. Such interventions have shown that the absolute level of cardiovascular risk factors related to obesity and to insulin resistance can be reduced [66] and that presence of T2DM can be eliminated [67]. As such interventions are expensive and labor intensive, selection of those obese youth who may benefit most from them is crucial. Measures such as risk factor clustering (metabolic syndrome definitions) and its dynamics over time can serve as selection and follow-up tools for such patients.

References

1. Gami AS, Witt BJ, Howard DE, Erwin PJ, Gami LA, Somers VK, Montori VM. Metabolic syndrome and risk of incident cardiovascular events and death: a systematic review and meta-analysis of longitudinal studies. *J Am Coll Cardiol* 2007;**49**(4): 403—14.
2. Pyorala M, Miettinen H, Halonen P, Laakso M, Pyorala K. Insulin resistance syndrome predicts the risk of coronary heart disease and stroke in healthy middle-aged men: the 22-year follow-up results of the Helsinki Policemen Study. *Arterioscler Thromb Vasc Biol* 2000;**20**:538—44.
3. Cornier MA, Dabelea D, Hernandez TL, Lindstrom RC, Steig AJ, Stob NR, Van Pelt RE, Wang H, Eckel RH. The metabolic syndrome. *Endocr Rev* 2008;**29**(7):777—822.
4. Reaven GM. Role of insulin resistance in human disease. *Diabetes* 1988;**37**:1595—607.
5. Goran MI, Gower BA. Longitudinal study on pubertal insulin resistance. *Diabetes* 2001;**50**(11):2444—50.
6. Leturque A, Hauguel S, Ferré P, Girard J. Glucose metabolism in pregnancy. *Biol Neonate* 1987;**51**(2):64—9.
7. Lutsey PL, Steffen LM, Stevens J. Dietary intake and the development of the metabolic syndrome: the Atherosclerosis Risk in Communities study. *Circulation* 2008;**117**(6):754—61.
8. Sakkinen PA, Wahl P, Cushman M, Lewis MR, Tracy RP. Clustering of procoagulation, inflammation, and fibrinolysis variables with metabolic factors in insulin resistance syndrome. *Am J Epidemiol* 2000;**152**(10):897—907.
9. Hanley AJ, Festa A, D'Agostino Jr RB, Wagenknecht LE, Savage PJ, Tracy RP, Saad MF, Haffner SM. Metabolic and inflammation variable clusters and prediction of type 2 diabetes: factor analysis using directly measured insulin sensitivity. *Diabetes* 2004;**53**(7):1773—81.
10. Meigs JB, D'Agostino Sr RB, Wilson PW, Cupples LA, Nathan DM, Singer DE. Risk variable clustering in the insulin resistance syndrome: the Framingham Offspring Study. *Diabetes* 1997;**46**:1594—600.
11. Li C, Ford ES. Is there a single underlying factor for the metabolic syndrome in adolescents? A confirmatory factor analysis. *Diabetes Care* 2007;**30**(6):1556—61.
12. Goodman E, Dolan LM, Morrison JA, Daniels SR. Factor analysis of clustered cardiovascular risks in adolescence: obesity is the predominant correlate of risk among youth. *Circulation* 2005;**111**(15):1970—7.
13. Weiss R, Dziura J, Burgert TS, Tamborlane WV, Taksali SE, Yeckel CW, Allen K, Lopes M, Savoye M, Morrison J, Sherwin RS, Caprio S. Obesity and the metabolic syndrome in children and adolescents. *N Engl J Med* 2004;**350**(23):2362—74.
14. Yudkin JS, Stehouwer CD, Emeis JJ, Coppack SW. C-reactive protein in healthy subjects: associations with obesity, insulin resistance, and endothelial dysfunction: a potential role for cytokines originating from adipose tissue? *Arterioscler Thromb Vasc Biol* 1999;**19**(4):972—8.
15. Yudkin JS, Eringa E, Stehouwer CD. "Vasocrine" signalling from perivascular fat: a mechanism linking insulin resistance to vascular disease. *Lancet* 2005;**365**(9473):1817—20.
16. Weiss R, Taksali SE, Dufour S, Yeckel CW, Papademetris X, Cline G, Tamborlane WV, Dziura J, Shulman GI, Caprio S. The "obese insulin-sensitive" adolescent: importance of adiponectin and lipid partitioning. *J Clin Endocrinol Metab* 2005;**90**(6):3731—7.
17. Kwiterovich Jr PO. Recognition and management of dyslipidemia in children and adolescents. *J Clin Endocrinol Metab* 2008;**93**(11):4200—9.
18. Matsuzawa Y, Funahashi T, Nakamura T. Molecular mechanism of metabolic syndromeX: Contribution of adipocytokines adipocyte-derived bioactive substances. *Annals New Accademy of Sciences* 2000;(892):146—54.
19. Wajchenberg BL. Subcutaneous and visceral adipose tissue: their relation to the metabolic syndrome. *Endocr Rev* 2000;**21**(6):697—738.
20. Cruz ML, Bergman RN, Goran MI. Unique effect of visceral fat on insulin sensitivity in obese Hispanic children with a family history of type 2 diabetes. *Diabetes Care* 2002;**25**(9):1631—6.
21. Bacha F, Saad R, Gungor N, Janosky J, Arslanian SA. Obesity, regional fat distribution, and syndrome X in obese black versus white adolescents: race differential in diabetogenic and atherogenic risk factors. *J Clin Endocrinol Metab* 2003;**88**(6):2534—40.
22. Taksali SE, Caprio S, Dziura J, Dufour S, Calí AM, Goodman TR, Papademetris X, Burgert TS, Pierpont BM, Savoye M, Shaw M, Seyal AA, Weiss R. High visceral and low abdominal subcutaneous fat stores in the obese adolescent: a determinant of an adverse metabolic phenotype. *Diabetes* 2008;**57**(2):367—71.
23. Weiss R, Dufour S, Taksali SE, Tamborlane WV, Petersen KF, Bonadonna RC, Boselli L, Barbetta G, Allen K, Rife F, Savoye M, Dziura J, Sherwin R, Shulman GI, Caprio S. Prediabetes in obese youth: a syndrome of impaired glucose tolerance, severe insulin resistance, and altered myocellular and abdominal fat partitioning. *Lancet* 2003;**362**(9388):951—7.
24. Stumvoll M, Tataranni PA, Stefan N, Vozarova B, Bogardus C. Glucose allostasis. *Diabetes* 2003;**52**(4):903—9.
25. Weiss R, Cali AM, Dziura J, Burgert TS, Tamborlane WV, Caprio S. Degree of obesity and glucose allostasis are major effectors of glucose tolerance dynamics in obese youth. *Diabetes Care* 2007;**30**(7):1845—50.
26. Rocchini AP, Katch V, Kveselis D, Moorehead C, Martin M, Lampman R, Gregory M. Insulin and renal sodium retention in obese adolescents. *Hypertension* 1989;**14**(4):367—74.
27. Facchini F, Chen YD, Hollenbeck CB, Reaven GM. Relationship between resistance to insulin-mediated glucose uptake, urinary uric acid clearance, and plasma uric acid concentration. *JAMA* 1991;**266**(21):3008—11.
28. Dunaif A. Insulin resistance and the polycystic ovary syndrome: mechanism and implications for pathogenesis. *Endocr Rev* 1997c;**18**(6):774—800.
29. Anderson EA, Hoffman RP, Balon TW, Sinkey CA, Mark AL. Hyperinsulinemia produces both sympathetic neural activation and vasodilation in normal humans. *J Clin Invest* 1991;**87**(6): 2246—52.

30. Van Gaal LF, Mertens IL, De Block CE. Mechanisms linking obesity with cardiovascular disease. *Nature* 2006;**444**(7121):875−80.
31. Barbato A, Cappuccio FP, Folkerd EJ, Strazzullo P, Sampson B, Cook DG, Alberti KG. Metabolic syndrome and renal sodium handling in three ethnic groups living in England. *Diabetologia* 2004;**47**:40−6.
32. Steinberg HO, Brechtel G, Johnson A, Fineberg N, Baron AD. Insulin-mediated skeletal muscle vasodilation is nitric oxide dependent. A novel action of insulin to increase nitric oxide release. *J Clin Invest* 1994;**94**:1172−9.
33. Arcaro G, Cretti A, Balzano S, Lechi A, Muggeo M, Bonora E, Bonadonna RC. Insulin causes endothelial dysfunction in humans: sites and mechanisms. *Circulation* 2002;**105**(5):576−82.
34. Tooke JE, Hannemann MM. Adverse endothelial function and the insulin resistance syndrome. *J Intern Med* 2000;**247**:425−31.
35. Tripathy D, Mohanty P, Dhindsa S, Syed T, Ghanim H, Aljada A, Dandona P. Elevation of free fatty acids induces inflammation and impairs vascular reactivity in healthy subjects. *Diabetes* 2003;**52**:2882−7.
36. Alpert MA. Obesity cardiomyopathy: pathophysiology and evolution of the clinical syndrome. *Am J Med Sci* 2001;**321**:225−36.
37. Messerli FH, Nunez BD, Ventura HO, Snyder DW. Overweight and sudden death: increased ventricular ectopy in cardiomyopathy of obesity. *Arch Intern Med* 1987;**147**:1725−8.
38. Cooper R, McFarlane-Anderson N, Bennett FI, et al. ACE, angiotensinogen and obesity: a potential pathway leading to hypertension. *J Hum Hypertens* 1997;**11**(2):107−11.
39. Massiera F, Bloch-Faure M, Ceiler D, et al. Adipose angiotensinogen is involved in adipose tissue growth and blood pressure regulation. *FASEB J* 2001;**15**(14):2727−9.
40. Hall JE, Brands MW, Henegar JR. Mechanisms of hypertension and kidney disease in obesity. *Ann N Y Acad Sci* 1999;**892**:91−107.
41. Rocchini AP, Katch VL, Grekin R, Moorehead C, Anderson J. Role for aldosterone in blood pressure regulation of obese adolescents. *Am J Cardiol* 1986;**57**(8):613−18.
42. Weiss R, Dziura J, Burgert TS, Tamborlane WV, Taksali SE, Yeckel CW, Allen K, Lopes M, Savoye M, Morrison J, Sherwin RS, Caprio S. Obesity and the metabolic syndrome in children and adolescents. *N Engl J Med* 2004;**350**(23):2362−74.
43. Frohlich M, Imhof A, Berg G, Hutchinson WL, Pepys MB, Boeing H, Muche R, Brenner H, Koenig W. Association between C-reactive protein and features of the metabolic syndrome: a population-based study. *Diabetes Care* 2000;**23**:1835−9.
44. Schotte DE, Stunkard AJ. The effects of weight reduction on blood pressure in 301 obese patients. *Arch Intern Med* 1990;**150**:1701−4.
45. Reinehr T, de Sousa G, Toschke AM, Andler W. Long-term follow-up of cardiovascular disease risk factors in children after an obesity intervention. *Am J Clin Nutr* 2006;**84**(3):490−6.
46. Savoye M, Shaw M, Dziura J, Tamborlane WV, Rose P, Guandalini C, Goldberg-Gell R, Burgert TS, Cali AM, Weiss R, Caprio S. Effects of a weight management program on body composition and metabolic parameters in overweight children: a randomized controlled trial. *JAMA* 2007;**297**(24):2697−704.
47. Inge TH, Miyano G, Bean J, Helmrath M, Courcoulas A, Harmon CM, Chen MK, Wilson K, Daniels SR, Garcia VF, Brandt ML, Dolan LM. Reversal of type 2 diabetes mellitus and improvements in cardiovascular risk factors after surgical weight loss in adolescents. *Pediatrics* 2009;**123**(1):214−22.
48. Sjostrom CD, Peltonen M, Wedel H, Sjostrom L. Differentiated long-term effects of intentional weight loss on diabetes and hypertension. *Hypertension* 2000;**36**:20−5.
49. Druet C, Dabbas M, Baltakse V, Payen C, Jouret B, Baud C, Chevenne D, Ricour C, Tauber M, Polak M, Alberti C, Levy-Marchal C. Insulin resistance and the metabolic syndrome in obese French children. *Clin Endocrinol* 2006;**64**(6):672−8.
50. de Ferranti SD, Gauvreau K, Ludwig DS, Neufeld EJ, Newburger JW, Rifai N. Prevalence of the metabolic syndrome in American adolescents: findings from the Third National Health and Nutrition Examination Survey. *Circulation* 2004;**110**(16):2494−7.
51. Lee S, Bacha F, Gungor N, Arslanian S. Comparison of different definitions of pediatric metabolic syndrome: relation to abdominal adiposity, insulin resistance, adiponectin, and inflammatory biomarkers. *J Pediatr* 2008;**152**(2):177−84.
52. Zimmet P, Alberti G, Kaufman F, Tajima N, Silink M, Arslanian S, Wong G, Bennett P, Shaw J, Caprio S. The metabolic syndrome in children and adolescents. International Diabetes Federation Task Force on Epidemiology and Prevention of Diabetes. *Lancet* 2007;**369**(9579):2059−61.
53. Kahn R, Buse J, Ferrannini E, Stern M. American Diabetes Association; European Association for the Study of Diabetes. The metabolic syndrome: time for a critical appraisal: joint statement from the American Diabetes Association and the European Association for the Study of Diabetes. *Diabetes Care* 2005;**28**(9):2289−304.
54. Brambilla P, Lissau I, Flodmark CE, Moreno LA, Widhalm K, Wabitsch M, Pietrobelli A. Metabolic risk-factor clustering estimation in children: to draw a line across pediatric metabolic syndrome. *Int J Obes (Lond)* 2007;**31**(4):591−600.
55. Baker JL, Olsen LW, Sørensen TI. Childhood body-mass index and the risk of coronary heart disease in adulthood. *N Engl J Med* 2007;**357**(23):2329−37.
56. Freedman DS, Mei Z, Srinivasan SR, Berenson GS, Dietz WH. Cardiovascular risk factors and excess adiposity among overweight children and adolescents: the Bogalusa Heart Study. *J Pediatr* 2007;**150**(1):12−17.
57. Tirosh A, Shai I, Tekes-Manova D, Israeli E, Pereg D, Shochat T, Kochba I, Rudich A. Israeli Diabetes Research Group. Normal fasting plasma glucose levels and type 2 diabetes in young men. *N Engl J Med* 2005;**353**(14):1454−62.
58. Tirosh A, Shai I, Bitzur R, Kochba I, Tekes-Manova D, Israeli E, Shochat T, Rudich A. Changes in triglyceride levels over time and risk of type 2 diabetes in young men. *Diabetes Care* 2008;**31**(10):2032−7.
59. Tirosh A, Rudich A, Shochat T, Tekes-Manova D, Israeli E, Henkin Y, Kochba I, Shai I. Changes in triglyceride levels and risk for coronary heart disease in young men. *Ann Intern Med* 2007;**147**(6):377−85.
60. Berenson GS, Srinivasan SR, Bao W, Newman 3rd WP, Tracy RE, Wattigney WA. Association between multiple cardiovascular risk factors and atherosclerosis in children and young adults. The Bogalusa Heart Study. *N Engl J Med* 1998;**338**(23):1650−6.
61. Iannuzzi A, Licenziati MR, Acampora C, Renis M, Agrusta M, Romano L, Valerio G, Panico S, Trevisan M. Carotid artery stiffness in obese children with the metabolic syndrome. *Am J Cardiol* 2006;**97**:528−31.
62. Lee S, Gungor N, Bacha F. Arslanian S Insulin resistance: link to the components of the metabolic syndrome and biomarkers of endothelial dysfunction in youth. *Diabetes Care* 2007;**30**(8):2091−7.
63. Mimoun E, Aggoun Y, Pousset M, Dubern B, Bouglé D, Girardet JP, Basdevant A, Bonnet D, Tounian P. Association of arterial stiffness and endothelial dysfunction with metabolic syndrome in obese children. *J Pediatr* 2008;**153**(1):65−70.

64. Berenson GS, Srinivasan SR, Bao W, Newman III WP, Tracy RE, Wattigney WA. Association between multiple cardiovascular risk factors and atherosclerosis in children and young adults: the Bogalusa Heart Study. *N Engl J Med* 1998;**338**:1650−6.
65. Mahoney LT, Burns TL, Stanford W, Thompson BH, Witt JD, Rost CA, Lauer RM. Coronary risk factors measured in childhood and young adult life are associated with coronary artery calcification in young adults: the Muscatine Study. *J Am Coll Cardiol* 1996;**27**:277−84.
66. Goodman E, Daniels SR, Meigs JB, Dolan LM. Instability in the diagnosis of metabolic syndrome in adolescents. *Circulation* 2007;**115**(17):2316−22.
67. Weiss R, Savoye M, Shaw M, Caprio S. Obesity dynamics and cardio-vascular risk factor stability in obese adolescents. *Ped Diab* 2009;**10**(6):360−7.

CHAPTER

14

A Link between Maternal and Childhood Obesity

Siân Robinson
Medical Research Council Epidemiology Resource Centre, University of Southampton, United Kingdom

BACKGROUND

The number of overweight and obese children has risen dramatically during the past two decades. Although the prevalence is higher in economically developed countries, this is a worldwide trend, and an estimated 155 million school-aged children are currently either overweight or obese [1, 2]. A recent study shows that a third of school-aged children in the United States have a body mass index (BMI) at or above the 85th percentile [3], while projections in Europe indicate that 37% of schoolchildren are expected to be overweight by 2010 [4]. As body composition "tracks" from early life, many of today's overweight children are likely to remain overweight throughout their lives [5].

Childhood obesity is recognized as a major health problem. This has led to widespread research efforts to understand the factors involved in its etiology [6], including the role of the "obesogenic" environment and the importance of unhealthy dietary behaviors and patterns of physical activity. There have been dramatic environmental changes that have paralleled the rise in obesity in children, such as the greater availability of energy-dense foods, promotion of fast foods, and increases in the proportion of time spent in sedentary activities [2, 7]. Excess body weight is the result of a mismatch of energy intake to energy need over a long period, and it is likely that these changes in the environment are major contributors to the rising proportion of children who are in positive energy balance. However, despite the undoubted importance of these factors in contributing to gains in adiposity, it is important to recognize that not all children within a population become overweight. Understanding variations between individuals in the way that they interact with their environment, and the extent to which these interactions predispose some children to gain excess weight from early life will be key to developing future strategies to prevent obesity.

The child's immediate environment is its home and family—and this is also the context within which diet and health behaviors are learned. Because obesity tends to run in families [8], this has led to a focus on the family both in terms of understanding its etiology as well as the opportunities it provides for prevention and treatment [9, 10]. As family influences on obesity are evident even in young children [11], there is increasing interest in understanding the importance of the environment in very early life, as this may be a critical period when the risk of development and persistence of overweight and obesity is increased [12]. In children, intrauterine life, infancy, and the preschool period around the time of the adiposity rebound have all been considered as possible periods when the long-term regulation of energy balance is permanently "programmed" [12, 13]. This chapter considers some of the early life determinants of childhood obesity but focuses particularly on the link between obesity and overweight in mothers and their children, and the role of the prenatal environment.

OBESITY AND THE FAMILY

Body Mass Index

Many studies have documented familial concordance in overweight and obesity [5, 13–15], and cross-sectional data show that the BMI of parents and children are correlated. In 12,000 men and women in the 1958 British birth cohort study, the coefficients for BMI between parents and children ranged from 0.15 to 0.25 between the ages of 7 and 33 years [16]. Studies of younger children have yielded comparable findings; for example, the coefficient for parent-child BMI among 3306 children aged 5 to 7 years studied in the Kiel Obesity Prevention Study was 0.27 [17]. However, concordance in parent-child BMI may not be evident in very early childhood. In a comparison of children born to overweight or lean mothers, Berkowitz and colleagues found no difference in body size between the two groups of children studied when they were infants. The children born to overweight mothers gained weight more rapidly in early childhood, but differences between the groups were only evident from year 4 [18].

Overweight and Obesity

The parent-offspring BMI association translates into a marked increase in risk of obesity for children born to overweight parents. Recent findings from the UK Millennium Cohort Study of 13,188 children aged 3 years show that parental overweight is already evident as a risk factor for childhood overweight (father: adjusted odds ratio 1.45 [95% confidence interval 1.28, 1.63]; mother: adjusted odds ratio 1.37 [1.18, 1.58]) [15] and that this risk is further increased when both parents are overweight (adjusted odds ratio 1.89 [1.63, 2.19]). There are more striking effects of parental overweight and obesity on risk of childhood overweight at older ages. For example, in a study of children aged 4½ years, the risk of childhood overweight doubled (OR 2.1 [1.3, 3.6]) if one parent was overweight and tripled (OR 3.2 [1.7, 5.8]) when both were [11]. This compares with a study of children aged 7 years where the risk of being obese more than doubled if either parent had a BMI above 30 kg/m^2 (father: adjusted odds ratio 2.54 [1.72, 3.75]; mother: adjusted odds ratio 4.25 [2.86, 6.32]), but notably the risk was increased 10-fold for children in families where both parents were obese (adjusted odds ratio 10.44 [5.11, 21.32]) [13].

Parental overweight is therefore a key risk factor for childhood overweight. The concordance in body composition indicates that there are common influences that result in overweight and obesity in parents and their children. These shared determinants of obesity are likely to be both genetic and environmental.

THE GENETIC BASIS OF CHILDHOOD OBESITY

Our understanding of the genetic contribution to BMI and obesity in children is developing rapidly, and a number of candidate genes have been identified that are linked to variability in body composition across the population. However, the role of genotype is complex as less than 10% of childhood obesity has been attributed to single gene defects [19], and it is likely that genetic effects on body weight regulation result from a large number of genes each exerting small effects [20].

Evidence of Heritability of Body Composition

Clear evidence of the importance of genetic influences in the etiology of obesity has come from studies of twins. In 1986, Stunkard and colleagues showed in a comparison of adults who had been reared by biological or adoptive parents that their weight class was strongly related to BMI in their biological parents but that there was no association with BMI in their adoptive parents [21]. Since then a number of genetic studies of monozygotic and dizygotic twins have been carried out, yielding estimates of heritability of BMI ranging from 55% to 85% [20]. Interestingly, recent estimates have not changed substantially, even though the environment has become more obesogenic [20]. The genetic contribution to the regulation of BMI may differ across the life course, although there are few longitudinal twin studies that address this possibility. In a recent study of male twin pairs from birth to 18 years, there was little change in heritability estimates from the age of 1 year onward [22]. In contrast, UK studies of twins have shown relatively lower estimates of heritability of BMI at 4 years, when compared with older children [20, 23].

Genetic Makeup and Predisposition to Gain Weight

The mechanisms that underpin the genetic effects on body weight regulation are not known, although a number of recent papers have begun to address behavioral and dietary differences that are linked to genotype. In terms of the regulation of body weight, there may be genetic influences both on energy intake and on expenditure that affect sensitivity to changes in energy balance and susceptibility to weight gain [24]. A variety of aspects of dietary behavior have recently been shown to be heritable in children, including food neophobia [25], rate of eating [26], and satiety responsiveness [27].

To date, the gene that has received the most attention is the *FTO* gene that has been linked with obesity in genome-wide association studies, and common variants have been associated with higher body weight in both adults and children [28]. As *FTO* expression in the brain is greatest in areas of the hypothalamus that are associated with feeding, it may act through effects on appetite or satiety [29]. Consistent with this possibility, children carrying the higher risk allele have been shown to have reduced satiety [30] and greater energy intake when compared with other children [31, 32], but it is uncertain whether the *FTO* genotype influences individual preference for energy-dense foods [31, 33]. Although the *FTO* gene explains about 1% of variability in BMI [28], these studies provide new and important insights into the heritable influences that impact on body weight regulation in children.

As much as 90% of the tracking of BMI in children has been attributed to genetic factors, leading the conclusion that childhood BMI is under strong genetic control [22]. In comparison, the contributions of variations in early environment and the role of the family in influencing the development of childhood obesity and overweight appear relatively small [21]. At the same time, the rapid increases in prevalence of obesity seen in the past two decades point to the importance of changing environmental influences in the etiology of obesity. For example, clear evidence of the impact of the environment on the development of obesity comes from studies of second and third generation U.S. immigrants, where obesity rates among adolescents have been shown to be more than twice that of their first generation parents [34].

It is clearly difficult to disentangle the influences of shared genes and shared environment when considering parent-child concordance in obesity [2]. It is possible that the statistical models used to determine heritability rates underestimate the role of environmental factors in the regulation of body weight [35]. They may make untenable assumptions about the expected similarity in the environments of monozygotic and dizygotic twins, and importantly, they ignore the environmental influence of intrauterine experiences [36, 37]. Additionally, estimates of the effects of the shared environment are dependent on variability in the environments of the populations studied [38] and therefore may not be generalizable [2]. Although it may not be possible to determine the exact proportion of childhood obesity attributable to genes or to the environment, it is most likely that obesity in parents and children is linked through the effects of shared genes and shared environmental influences, with important effects on gene-environment interactions [39].

Early environmental influences are therefore very important in determining a child's risk of gaining excess weight. But to understand the link between maternal and child obesity, the early environment needs to be considered both in prenatal and in early postnatal life.

THE ROLE OF THE PRENATAL ENVIRONMENT

Prenatal life may be a critical period for the development of childhood obesity [40, 41]. Consistent with this proposition, there is now considerable evidence that maternal influences on the intrauterine environment play an important role in the "programming" of postnatal body composition [42].

Maternal Obesity

A number of longitudinal studies have looked at the influence of maternal weight around the time of pregnancy on the risk of overweight and obesity in the offspring. A consistent finding across these studies is that maternal overweight and obesity are strong predictors of obesity in the child. For example, in a large retrospective cohort study of 8494 children aged 2 to 4 years who were enrolled in the WIC program (Special Supplemental Nutrition Program for Women, Infants and Children), maternal obesity in early pregnancy (BMI $\geq$ 30 kg/m^2) more than doubled the risk of obesity in the children. By 4 years of age, 24.1% of the children born to mothers who had been obese in early pregnancy were also obese, compared with 9.0% of children born to mothers of normal body weight (BMI $\geq$ 18.5 and < 25 kg/m^2) [43].

These findings are comparable with data from the National Longitudinal Survey of Youth, in which 3022 children were followed up when they were 2 to 3 years, 4 to 5 years and 6 to 7 years of age [44]. The longitudinal design of this study enabled the authors to compare the effects of influences acting on childhood overweight at the different ages studied. At each age, maternal obesity (BMI $\geq$ 30 kg/m^2) was associated with an increased risk of overweight in the children. A key finding was that for the children studied at older ages, the greatest risk of being overweight was if the child had been overweight at the previous measurement. Thus, two thirds of the children who were overweight at 6 to 7 years had been overweight on at least one of the previous measurement occasions; likewise, three quarters of the children of normal weight at 6 to 7 years had been of normal weight throughout the study. A second key finding was that the influence of maternal obesity on childhood overweight increased substantially at older ages. However, conditioning on the previous weight in these analyses made small differences to the estimate of effects of maternal obesity on the risk of offspring overweight. The authors suggest that the effect of maternal obesity on childhood overweight not only is the result of an early persistent propensity to obesity, but it also affects the dynamics of the development of childhood overweight [44].

There are limitations in the use of BMI as an index of adiposity in children [41]. However, recent studies using direct measures of fat mass, determined by dual x-ray absorptiometry have shown associations that are consistent with the BMI data, as greater adiposity has been demonstrated among children whose mothers had a higher BMI before pregnancy [45]. Although each of these studies showed effects of maternal BMI on offspring adiposity that were independent of other factors, it is not possible to determine the extent to which there are direct effects of maternal overweight acting in prenatal life that influence the pattern of postnatal weight gain, or whether maternal overweight simply acts as an indicator of an obesogenic postnatal environment. In this respect, evidence of differences in body composition at birth may be important. For example, in a study of 448 neonates, adiposity, determined by dual x-ray absorptiometry, was greater in those born to mothers who had larger fat stores [46]—thus there are links between maternal and offspring body composition that are evident before shared environmental influences act in postnatal life.

An important consideration in understanding the influence of maternal obesity on the offspring comes from the comparison of effects with those of paternal obesity. Direct effects of maternal obesity acting in intrauterine life should result in a relatively greater correspondence in BMI between mother and child, when compared with that of father and child. There is some evidence that this is the case [13, 17], but few studies have made formal comparisons of the magnitude of effects, and the evidence is not conclusive [37, 47, 48]. Using data from the Avon Longitudinal Study of Parents and Children, Davey Smith and colleagues have shown that at 7 years maternal BMI appeared to have a greater influence on child BMI than paternal BMI, but that the size of the difference between mothers and fathers was small, and there was no evidence of any marked difference in the strength of association in terms of risk of obesity [37]. The authors concluded that in this population the influence of maternal BMI was not meaningfully greater than that of paternal BMI. In contrast, in a follow-up of an Australian cohort of 3340 parent-offspring trios at the age of 14 years, the maternal-offspring BMI association was stronger than the paternal-offspring association, suggesting a direct influence of maternal obesity acting in prenatal life [47].

Kral and colleagues published an important study that may provide insights into the direct effects of maternal obesity in 2006 [49]. In this study, the prevalence of obesity was compared in children aged 2 to 18 years who were born to 113 obese mothers before or after they had weight loss surgery. The prevalence of overweight and obesity among 45 children born before maternal surgery was 60%, compared with a prevalence of 35% among 172 children who were born after surgery. These data suggest that obesity surgery had prevented the transmission of obesity to the offspring, and they provide strong support for a direct influence of maternal obesity acting on the intrauterine environment that has long-term effects on the offspring and their regulation of body weight.

Gestational Weight Gain

The optimal pattern of gestational weight gain is not known. In 1990 the U.S. Institute of Medicine (IOM) report concluded that gestational weight gain was an important determinant of fetal growth and set guidelines for weight gain in women of different BMI [50]. However, gestational weight gain is often outside the recommended ranges, even in the United States where the IOM guidelines are promoted [51, 52]. Excessive gestational weight gain is common and there is evidence that prevalence is increasing [53]. This has raised concerns about its consequences, including long-term effects it may have on the offspring [53, 54].

A number of studies have described an effect of gestational weight gain on offspring body composition. For example, among 1044 mother-child pairs studied in Project Viva, child overweight at the age of 3 years was associated with greater gestational weight gain (OR 1.30, 95% CI: 1.04, 1.62 for each 5 kg weight gained) [52]. Adjustment for a range of confounding factors, including glucose tolerance and duration of breast-feeding, made little difference to this finding, but adjustment for parental BMI strengthened the association (OR 1.66, 95% CI: 1.31, 2.12). Using the 1990 IOM recommended ranges of weight gain, 51% of mothers in this cohort gained excess weight, 35% adequate weight, and 14% inadequate weight. When compared with children whose mothers had an inadequate weight gain in pregnancy, children whose mothers had adequate or excessive weight gains had a higher BMI at the age of 3 years, and their risk of being overweight at this age was increased four-fold.

Oken and colleagues have also shown effects of gestational weight gain on offspring overweight in older children, aged 9 to 14 years [55]. Before taking account of maternal BMI, a U-shaped relationship was described between gestational weight gain and adolescent adiposity, such that higher rates of obesity were observed in adolescents born to mothers in the lowest and highest categories of weight gain. This is consistent with findings from the Nurses Health Study II where low and high gestational weight gains were both associated with obesity in the daughters studied at the age of 18 years [56]. However, the role of maternal BMI differed between these studies. In the younger population, adjustment for maternal BMI changed the association, resulting in a positive linear relationship between gestational weight gain and child BMI. In contrast, the U-shaped relationship found in older adolescents was not changed by taking account of maternal BMI [56]. An important finding from the Nurses Health Study II was that there was an interactive effect of weight gain and maternal BMI, as the association between low and high gestational weight gain and obesity in the daughter was modest among women of normal weight but more marked among mothers who were overweight before pregnancy.

The optimal pattern of gestational weight gain has yet to be defined. Not all studies have shown an effect of weight gain on adiposity in the offspring [43, 45], and further studies are needed to determine how variations in the pattern and the amount of weight gained in pregnancy impact on childhood body composition.

Maternal and Fetal Overnutrition

The epidemiological evidence that points to direct effects of maternal obesity suggests that it causes permanent programmed changes in the fetus that result in a predisposition to gain weight in postnatal life. A proposed mechanism to explain the link between excess weight in the mother and offspring is that the fetus is overnourished (the "fetal overnutrition" hypothesis) because of exposure to high maternal plasma concentrations of glucose, free fatty acids, and amino acids [40, 47]. In postnatal life, there may be permanent consequences of prenatal overnutrition, which include effects on appetite control, neuroendocrine function, and energy metabolism—with lifelong consequences for the offspring's ability to regulate energy balance and body weight.

Support for the fetal overnutrition hypothesis and evidence of the influence of variations in substrate supply on risk of offspring obesity comes from studies of women who have poor glycemic control in pregnancy. In diabetic women, increased circulating concentrations of glucose and amino acids cause greater fetal secretion of insulin and insulin-like growth factors, leading to stimulated growth of fetal adipose tissue [57], and fasting glucose concentration has been shown to be a strong predictor of fat mass in the offspring [58]. Gestational diabetes is associated with greater adiposity in the offspring at birth [59] and in early childhood [60], and it may increase the risk of later obesity [42]. Clear evidence of the importance of the effects of diabetes on the intrauterine environment has come from a study of children born to Pima Indian women. Among Pima children who were born to women who developed diabetes, BMI was greater in those who were born after the diagnosis, when compared with their siblings who were born before [61]. Notably, there were no associations with a diagnosis of paternal diabetes, highlighting the importance of the effects of the intrauterine environment, rather than genetic effects, on the development of postnatal body composition.

An effect of maternal glycemia on offspring body composition may not be restricted to women who have gestational diabetes. For example, in a follow-up study of 7609 women with normal glucose tolerance at initial screening, Hillier and colleagues [62] showed that increasing maternal glycemia was associated with a greater risk of obesity in the children, even among children of normal birthweight. Importantly, in children born to women who fulfilled the criteria for gestational diabetes, the relationship between maternal glycemia and offspring obesity was lost if the mother received treatment.

Glycemic control is also affected by the mother's diet in pregnancy. A significant influence is the glycemic index (GI) of the diet, which has been shown to relate to maternal glycosylated hemoglobin and to plasma glucose levels following a glucose load [63]. Consistent with these findings, a low GI diet has been associated with a lower weight at birth [63], and dietary interventions to change GI in pregnancy have resulted in differences in fetal growth. In an intervention using dietary counseling, Moses and colleagues found that babies born to women who had a high GI diet were heavier than those born to women who had a low GI diet, and there was a 10-fold difference in the proportion of large-for-gestational-age (LGA) between the groups [64]. In a small follow-up of these infants, LGA was associated with greater weight at 22 months, but maternal diet group in pregnancy was not predictive of offspring size at this age [65]. Further data are needed to determine the long-term effects of the glycemic index of the maternal diet on body composition in the offspring.

The possibility that fetal overnutrition results in programmed changes in body composition in the offspring is supported by the findings of animal studies in which maternal diet has been manipulated in pregnancy [66]. Although it may not be clear how these experimental findings relate to human pregnancy, they provide proof that altering the intrauterine environment can permanently change offspring physiology—including body composition. For example, in a study of rats, offspring born to mothers fed a "junk" food diet during pregnancy and lactation, based on cakes, biscuits, potato crisps, marshmallows, cheese, and chocolate bars, had greater adiposity. They also had an exacerbated preference for fatty, sugary, and salty foods, suggesting that the junk food diet fed to mothers had caused permanent changes in appetite regulation in the offspring that resulted in hyperphagia and a propensity to gain weight [67]. Experimental studies show that a number of animal models that alter maternal nutrition result in obesity in the offspring [68]. Although the mechanisms are not known, there is some evidence that suggests there are common pathways that include programmed effects on the hypothalamus and appetite regulation, glucocorticoid signaling, and altered adipocyte development [68].

In some of the experimental studies that have demonstrated effects of manipulation of maternal diet on offspring body composition, these have been dependent on the offspring being challenged with high-energy diets in postnatal life [66]. Thus, the predisposition to gain excess weight is caused by prenatal experience, but this predisposition only becomes evident when the postnatal environment enables, or promotes, positive energy balance in the offspring.

MATERNAL OBESITY AND THE FAMILY ENVIRONMENT

The home environment is recognized to have an important role in the development of childhood obesity [69]. However, families vary in their patterns of diet and physical activity, and there are marked differences in its obesogenicity [70]. Maternal obesity may impact directly on the nature of children's diets and levels of physical activity, but it is also likely to have indirect effects, arising from the modeling of behavior. This is important as eating behaviors, including a tendency to overeat, show stability throughout childhood, suggesting that children have characteristic ways of interacting with their food environments that persist over time [71].

Shared Dietary Habits

A number of studies have examined familial similarities in eating patterns [72]. In most families, women still have the primary responsibility for feeding children [73] and there is strong evidence of links between maternal food choice and children's diets. The influence of maternal choice may be evident very early in life. For example, in a UK study of infants, the primary influence on their dietary patterns at 12 months of age was the quality of the mother's own diet [74]. Studies of older children suggest that the influence of maternal food choice on children's eating patterns persists [75, 76], and mothers' and children's dietary intakes are correlated. Maternal influence on the child's food environment is therefore of key importance in determining food preferences and dietary behavior [43, 77].

This influence may differ in women who are obese. One way to address this issue is to compare the dietary behaviors of children who were born to obese or lean mothers and who differ in their risk of becoming obese. For example, in a study of children aged 3 to 6 years, Kral and colleagues have shown that the high-risk children tended to overconsume food, when compared with the low-risk children [78]. Other studies have confirmed an "overeating-type" eating style in young children from obese families [79], but they have also shown that high-risk children may differ in their food preferences, showing a greater preference for fatty foods [79, 80] and a lower liking for vegetables [79].

Differences in dietary behavior among children who are born to obese mothers may be seen as evidence of gene-environment interactions. However, it is also possible that variation in prenatal experience may determine or condition a child's response to environmental influences acting in postnatal life. In terms of food choice, there are experimental data that provide clear evidence of programmed effects on appetite and food preferences [67, 68], although we currently know little about this in humans. Maternal undernutrition has been associated with changes in food choice in the offspring, as men and women who were exposed to the Dutch famine in early gestation have been shown to have a preference for fatty foods and to be more likely to consume a high-fat diet when compared with those exposed in later gestation [81]. However, it is not known whether there are comparable programmed effects on dietary behavior in the offspring that result from maternal overnutrition. Further data are needed to identify the effects of prenatal and early postnatal experience on food preference and food choice, and to determine their roles in the etiology of childhood obesity.

Shared Patterns of Physical Activity

Although a high-energy intake may be the main determinant of a high body weight in childhood [82], sedentary activity is also linked to the development of obesity [2]. In common with influences on diet, there are familial effects on patterns of physical activity, such that some "obesogenic" families have high levels of dietary intake and low levels of physical activity [70], and there is some evidence that children of obese parents are less active [83] and have a greater preference for sedentary activities [79]. A comparison of twins aged 4 to 10 years suggests that the familial resemblance in physical activity is explained principally by the effects of the shared environment and is unlikely to be strongly determined by genetic factors [84]. It is not known whether there are effects of prenatal experience on level of physical activity in postnatal life. However, experimental studies indicate that this could be possible, as rat offspring born to undernourished mothers have been shown to be more sedentary in postnatal life than offspring born to mothers that were fed ad libitum [85].

Maternal Obesity and Breast-feeding

In addition to influences of maternal obesity on dietary behavior and physical activity, there are many other differences in the characteristics of lean and obese women that could have implications for body weight regulation in their children. One factor is the duration of breast-feeding. There is some evidence that breast-feeding may be protective, as a number of studies have shown that breast-fed children are less likely to be obese, and there is a dose-response relationship with duration of feeding [86]. One possibility is that breast-feeding has an influence on appetite control, as infants learn to regulate their energy intake and to recognize satiety signals more effectively than infants who are fed formula milk. However, breast-feeding duration is often shorter in obese women [87, 88]—an effect that is attributed to difficulties in producing milk [87]. Early termination of breast-feeding among obese women has even been described in a sociocultural context in which breast-feeding is strongly supported [89]. The importance of the protective effects of breast-feeding has still to be defined, but it is of concern that children who are already at a higher risk of obesity are also less likely to be breast-fed [87] and to be breast-fed for a shorter period [88, 89].

THE LINK BETWEEN MATERNAL AND CHILD OBESITY: PUBLIC HEALTH IMPLICATIONS

The rapid increases occurring in childhood obesity threaten the long-term health of a generation. Obesity is therefore a major public health problem, and preventative strategies are urgently needed to halt the rise in prevalence.

Effects of Maternal Obesity on Future Generations

Studies of young children have identified factors that are associated with risk of becoming overweight. This chapter has outlined evidence showing that one of the key risk factors is being born to overweight parents. A number of epidemiological studies point to the particular importance of maternal obesity—that it affects the child's predisposition to gain weight as well as the dynamics of weight gain in childhood [44]. Although it is recognized that maternal obesity is linked to obesity in the child through shared genetic and environmental influences acting in early childhood, we also need to consider whether there are direct effects of maternal obesity acting in prenatal life that affect body composition in the offspring. Consistent with this suggestion, animal studies confirm that experimental manipulation of the intrauterine environment and fetal nutrition can result in permanent programmed changes in offspring body composition.

Ebbeling and colleagues have highlighted the importance of programmed effects of maternal obesity on children's body composition, as it raises the possibility that the current obesity epidemic could accelerate through successive generations [90]. Furthermore, this acceleration would occur independently of any other genetic or environmental changes taking place. If the higher levels of obesity seen in today's mothers cause programmed changes in body composition and increases in obesity in their daughters, this would increase the risk of obesity in the following generation in a "feed-forward" mechanism [37]. Such an effect would be expected to contribute to a widening of inequalities in obesity prevalence and obesity-related ill health [91] and has obvious implications for the developing world, where increases in obesity are occurring alongside the nutrition transition. Although it may not be straightforward to extrapolate from findings of studies carried out in the developed world, the possibility of a feed-forward mechanism that will accelerate obesity prevalence is alarming and could have dire consequences for future health in these populations [92].

Developmental Perspectives and Prevention of Childhood Obesity

Although our understanding of the role of early environment in the etiology of childhood obesity is just beginning, there is already enough evidence to show the need for a developmental perspective in considering strategies for its prevention. This approach recognizes the cumulative effects of early exposures on the development of overweight in children [93]—including the possibility of programmed effects arising from variations in fetal experience that predispose the offspring to gain weight in postnatal life. Standard approaches to obesity prevention have been disappointing, and targeted interventions toward key periods of development, particularly in early life, may be more effective in reducing subsequent risks of adult obesity [92]. For example, the greatest benefits may come from family interventions that target young children born to obese mothers [5]. Early life interventions may have the potential not only to change an individual's lifetime risk of obesity but also to impact on obesity risk in subsequent generations.

Implications for Advice to Young Women

Evidence of developmental influences on obesity is new, and it is not yet the basis for advice to young women. However, there are implications of the existing findings that could be disseminated. Health promotion efforts commonly link obesity to degenerative conditions and may therefore lack relevance for young adults. As a result, young women may be largely unaware that being overweight or obese has consequences for fetal development. Maternal obesity is a modifiable risk factor, and policies and interventions are needed that support young women and encourage them to have a healthy body weight before pregnancy. This may require a new approach to promoting health in young women, as recent UK data show little evidence of women changing health behaviors in order to prepare for pregnancy [94].

Future studies will define the public health impact of developmental influences on childhood obesity [95]. Although the mechanisms remain to be elucidated, it is already evident that obesity in today's mothers is clearly linked to obesity in their children. It should therefore be a public health priority to ensure that young women understand the importance of having a healthy body weight, both for their own health as well as for that of their children [43].

References

1. International Association for the Study of Obesity (2009). www.iotf.org/childhoodobesity.asp
2. Lobstein T, Baur L, Uauy R for IASO International Obesity TaskForce. Obesity in children and young people: a crisis in public health. Obes Rev 2004;5(Suppl. 1):4–85.
3. Ogden CL, Carroll MD, Flegal KM. High body mass index for age among US children and adolescents, 2003–2006. JAMA 2008;299:2401–5.
4. Jackson-Leach R, Lobstein T. Estimated burden of paediatric obesity and co-morbidities in Europe. Part 1. The increase in the prevalence of child obesity in Europe is itself increasing. Int J Pediatr Obes 2006;1:26–32.
5. Whitaker RC, Wright JA, Pepe MS, Seidel KD, Dietz WH. Predicting obesity in young adulthood from childhood and parental obesity. N Engl J Med 1997;337:869–73.
6. Goran MI. Metabolic precursors and effects of obesity in children: a decade of progress, 1990-1999. Am J Clin Nutr 2001;73:158–71.
7. Procter KL. The aetiology of childhood obesity: a review. Nutr Res Rev 2007;20:29–45.
8. Bouchard C. Obesity in adulthood: the importance of childhood and parental obesity. N Engl J Med 1997;337:926–7.
9. Agras WS, Hammer LD, McNicholas F, Kraemer HC. Risk factors for childhood overweight: a prospective study from birth to 9.5 years. J Pediatr 2004;145:20–5.
10. Gruber KJ, Haldeman LA. Using the family to combat childhood and adult obesity. Prev Chronic Dis 2009;6:A106.
11. Dubois L, Girard M. Early determinants of overweight at 4.5 years in a population-based longitudinal study. Int J Obes 2006;30:610–17.
12. Dietz WH. Overweight in childhood and adolescence. N Engl J Med 2004;350:855–7.
13. Reilly JJ, Armstrong J, Dorosty AR, Emmett PM, Ness A, Rogers I, Steer C, Sherriff A, ALSPAC Study Team. Early life risk factors for obesity in childhood: cohort study. BMJ 2005;330:1357–63.
14. Danielzik S, Czerwinski-Mast M, Langnase K, Dilba B, Muller MJ. Parental overweight, socio-economic status and high birth weight are the major determinants of overweight and obesity in 5-7 y-old children: baseline data of the Kiel Obesity Prevention Study (KOPS). Int J Obes 2004;28:1494–502.
15. Hawkins SS, Cole TJ, Law C, MCS Child Health Group. An ecological systems approach to examining risk factors for early childhood overweight: findings from the UK Millenium Cohort Study. J Epidemiol Community Health 2009;63:147–55.
16. Lake JK, Power C, Cole TJ. Child to adult body mass index in the 1958 British birth cohort: associations with parental obesity. Arch Dis Child 1997;77:376–81.
17. Danielzik S, Langnase K, Mast M, Spethmann C, Muller MJ. Impact of parental BMI on the manifestation of overweight 5–7 year old children. Eur J Nutr 2002;41:132–8.
18. Berkowitz RI, Stallings VA, Maislin G, Stunkard AJ. Growth of children at high risk of obesity during the first 6 y of life: implications for prevention. Am J Clin Nutr 2005;81:140–6.
19. Farooqi IS, O'Rahilly S. Genetics of obesity in humans. Endocr Rev 2006;27:710–18.
20. Wardle J, Carnell S, Haworth CM, Plomin R. Evidence for a strong genetic influence on childhood adiposity despite the force of the obesogenic environment. Am J Clin Nutr 2008;87:398–404.
21. Stunkard AJ, Sorensen TI, Hanis C, Teasdale TW, Chakraborty R, Schull WJ, Schulsinger F. An adoption study of human obesity. N Engl J Med 1986;314:193–8.
22. Silventoinen K, Pietilainen KH, Tynelius P, Sorensen TI, Kaprio J, Rasmussen F. Genetic and environmental factors in relative weight from birth to age 18: The Swedish Young Male Twins Study. Int J Obes 2007;31:615–21.
23. Koeppen-Schomerus G, Wardle J, Plomin R. A genetic analysis of weight and overweight in 4-year-old twin pairs. Int J Obes 2001;25:838–44.
24. Bouchard C, Tremblay A. Genetic influences on the response of body fat and fat distribution to positive and negative energy balances in human identical twins. J Nutr 1997;127:943S–7S.
25. Cooke LJ, Haworth CM, Wardle J. Genetic and environmental influences on children's food neophobia. Am J Clin Nutr 2007;86:428–33.
26. Llewellyn CH, van Jaarsveld CH, Boniface D, Carnell S, Wardle J. Eating rate is a heritable phenotype related to weight in children. Am J Clin Nutr 2008;88:1560–6.
27. Carnell S, Haworth CM, Plomin R, Wardle J. Genetic influence on appetite in children. Int J Obes 2008;32:1468–73.
28. Frayling TM, Timpson NJ, Weedon MN, Zeggini E, Freathy RM, Lindgren CM, Perry JR, Elliott KS, Lango H, Rayner NW, Shields B, Harries LW, Barrett JC, Ellard S, Groves CJ, Knight B, Patch AM, Ness AR, Ebrahim S, Lawlor DA, Ring SM, Ben-Shlomo Y, Jarvelin MR, Sovio U, Bennett AJ, Melzer D, Ferrucci L, Loos RJ, Barroso I, Wareham NJ, Karpe F, Owen KR, Cardon LR, Walker M, Hitman GA, Palmer CN, Doney AS, Morris AD, Smith GD, Hattersley AT, McCarthy MI. A common variant in the *FTO* gene is associated with body mass index and predisposes to childhood and adult obesity. Science 2007;316:889–94.
29. Wardle J, Llewellyn C, Sanderson S, Plomin R. The *FTO* gene and measured food intake in children. Int J Obes 2009;33:42–5.
30. Wardle J, Carnell S, Haworth CM, Farooqi S, O'Rahilly S, Plomin R. Obesity associated genetic variation in *FTO* is associated with diminished satiety. J Clin Endocrinol Metab 2008;93:3640–3.
31. Cecil JE, Tavendale R, Watt P, Hetherington MM, Palmer CN. An obesity-associated *FTO* gene variant and increased energy intake in children. N Engl J Med 2008;359:2558–66.
32. Timpson NJ, Emmett PM, Frayling TM, Rogers I, Hattersley AT, McCarthy MI, Davey Smith G. The fat mass- and obesity-associated locus and dietary intake in children. Am J Clin Nutr 2008;88:971–8.

33. Johnson L, van Jaarsveld CH, Emmett PM, Rogers IS, Ness AR, Hattersley AT, Timpson NJ, Davey Smith G, Jebb S. Dietary energy density affects fat mass in early adolescence and is not modified by *FTO* variants. *PloS One*; 2009. 4 e4594.
34. Popkin BM, Udry JR. Adolescent obesity increases significantly in second and third generation US immigrants: the National Longitudinal Study of Adolescent Health. *J Nutr* 1998;**128**: 701–6.
35. Segal NL, Feng R, McGuire SA, Allison DB, Miller S. Genetic and environmental contributions to body mass index: comparative analysis of monozygotic twins, dizygotic twins and same-age unrelated siblings. *Int J Obes* 2009;**33**:37–41.
36. Phillips DIW. Twin studies in medical research: can they tell us whether diseases are genetically determined? *Lancet* 1993;**341**: 1008–9.
37. Davey Smith G, Steer C, Leary S, Ness A. Is there an intrauterine influence on obesity? Evidence from parent-child associations in the Avon Longitudinal Study of Parents and Children (ALSPAC). *Arch Dis Child* 2007;**92**:876–80.
38. Musani SK, Erickson S, Allison DB. Obesity: still highly heritable after all these years. *Am J Clin Nutr* 2008;**87**:275–6.
39. Pomeroy J, Soderberg AM, Franks PW. Gene-lifestyle interactions and their consequences on human health. *Med Sport Sci* 2009;**54**: 110–35.
40. Whitaker RC, Dietz WH. Role of prenatal environment in the development of obesity. *J Pediatr* 1998;**132**:768–76.
41. Wells JC, Chomtho S, Fewtrell MS. Programming of body composition by early growth and nutrition. *Proc Nutr Soc* 2007;**66**: 423–34.
42. Huang JS, Lee TA, Lu MC. Prenatal programming of childhood overweight and obesity. *Matern Child Health J* 2007;**11**:461–73.
43. Whitaker RC. Predicting preschooler obesity at birth: the role of maternal obesity in early pregnancy. *Pediatrics* 2004;**114**:e29–36.
44. Salsberry PJ, Reagan PB. Dynamics of early childhood overweight. *Pediatrics* 2005;**116**:1329–38.
45. Gale CR, Javaid MK, Robinson SM, Law CM, Godfrey KM, Cooper C. Maternal size in pregnancy and body composition in children. *J Clin Endocrinol Metab* 2007;**92**:3904–11.
46. Harvey NC, Poole JR, Javaid MK, Dennison EM, Robinson S, Inskip HM, Godfrey KM, Cooper C, Aihie Sayer A, SWS Study Group. Parental determinants of neonatal body composition. *J Clin Endocrinol Metab* 2007;**92**:523–6.
47. Lawlor DA, Davey Smith G, O'Callaghan M, Alati R, Mamun AA, Williams GM, Najman JM. Epidemiologic evidence for the fetal overnutrition hypothesis: findings from the Mater-University Study of Pregnancy and its Outcomes. *Am J Epidemiol* 2007;**165**:418–24.
48. Kivimaki M, Lawlor DA, Davey Smith G, Elovainio M, Jokela M, Keltikangas-Jarvinen L, Viikari JS, Raitakari OT. Substantial intergenerational increases in body mass index are not explained by the fetal overnutrition hypothesis: the Cardiovascular Risk in Young Finns Study. *Am J Clin Nutr* 2007;**86**:1509–14.
49. Kral JG, Biron S, Simard S, Hould FS, Lebel S, Marceau S, Marceau P. Large maternal weight loss from obesity surgery prevents transmission of obesity to children who were followed for 2 to 18 years. *Pediatrics* 2006;**118**:e1644–9.
50. Institute of Medicine. *Nutrition during pregnancy*. Washington DC: National Academy Press; 1990.
51. Abrams B, Altman SL, Pickett KE. Pregnancy weight gain: still controversial. *Am J Clin Nutr* 2000;**71**:1233S–41S.
52. Oken E, Taveras EM, Kleinman KP, Rich-Edwards JW, Gillman MW. Gestational weight gain and child adiposity at age 3 years. *Am J Obstet Gynecol* 2007;**196**:322.e1–8.
53. Muktabhant B, Lumbiganon P, Ngamjarus C. Interventions for preventing excessive weight gain during pregnancy. *Cochrane Database of Systematic Reviews* 2008;(Issue 2). Art. No.: CD007145. DOI: 10.1002/14651858.CD007145.
54. Rasmussen KM, Yaktine AL, editors. *Weight gain during pregnancy: re-examining the guidelines*. Washington DC: National Academies Press; 2009.
55. Oken E, Rifas-Shiman SL, Field AE, Frazier AL, Gillman MW. Maternal gestational weight gain and offspring weight in adolescence. *Obstet Gynecol* 2008;**112**:999–1006.
56. Stuebe AM, Forman MR, Michels KB. Maternal-recalled gestational weight gain, pre-pregnancy body mass index and obesity in the daughter. *Int J Obesity* 2009;**33**:743–52.
57. Simmons R. Perinatal programming of obesity. *Semin Perinatol* 2008;**32**:371–4.
58. Catalano PM, Thomas A, Huston-Presley L, Amini SB. Increased fetal adiposity: a very sensitive marker of abnormal in utero development. *Am J Obstet Gynecol* 2003;**189**:1698–704.
59. Catalano PM, Thomas A, Huston-Presley L, Amini SB. Phenotype of infants of mothers with gestational diabetes. *Diabetes Care* 2007;**30**:S156–60.
60. Wright CS, Rifas-Shiman SL, Rich-Edwards JW, Taveras EM, Gillman MW, Oken E. Intrauterine exposure to gestational diabetes, child adiposity and blood pressure. *Am J Hypertens* 2009;**22**: 215–20.
61. Dabelea D, Hanson RL, Lindsay RS, Pettit DJ, Imperatore G, Gabir MM, Roumain J, Bennett PH, Knowler WC. Intrauterine exposure to diabetes conveys risk for type 2 diabetes and obesity. *Diabetes* 2000;**49**:2208–11.
62. Hillier TA, Pedula KL, Schmidt MM, Mullen JA, Charles MA, Pettitt DJ. Childhood obesity and metabolic imprinting. The ongoing effects of maternal hyperglycemia. *Diabetes Care* 2007;**30**: 2287–92.
63. Scholl TO, Chen X, Khoo CS, Lenders C. The dietary glycemic index during pregnancy: influence on infant birth weight, fetal growth, and biomarkers of carbohydrate metabolism. *Am J Epidemiol* 2004;**159**:467–74.
64. Moses RG, Luebcke M, Davis WS, Coleman KJ, Tapsell LC, Petocz P, Brand-Miller JC. Effect of a low-glycemic-index diet during pregnancy on obstetric outcomes. *Am J Clin Nutr* 2006;**84**: 807–12.
65. Moses RG, Luebcke M, Petocz P, Brand-Miller JC. Maternal diet and infant size 2y after the completion of a low-glycemic-index diet in pregnancy. *Am J Clin Nutr* 2007;**86**:1806.
66. Robinson SM, Godfrey KM. Feeding practices in pregnancy and infancy: relationship with the development of overweight and obesity in childhood. *Int J Obes* 2008;**32**(Suppl. 6):S4–10.
67. Bayol SA, Farrington SJ, Stickland NC. A maternal "junk food" diet in pregnancy and lactation promotes an exacerbated taste for "junk food" and a greater propensity for obesity in rat offspring. *Br J Nutr* 2007;**98**:843–51.
68. Taylor PD, Poston L. Developmental programming of obesity in mammals. *Exp Physiol* 2007;**92**:287–98.
69. Strauss RS, Knight J. Influence of the home environment on the development of obesity in children. *Pediatrics* 1999;**103**:e85–92.
70. Krahnstoever Davison K, Lipps Birch L. Obesigenic families: parents' physical activity and dietary intake patterns predict girls' risk of overweight. *Int J Obes* 2002;**26**:1186–93.
71. Ashcroft J, Semmler C, Carnell S, van Jaarsveld CHM, Wardle J. Continuity and stability of eating behaviour traits in children. *Eur J Clin Nutr* 2008;**62**:985–90.
72. van der Horst K, Oenema A, Ferreira I, Wendel-Vos W, Giskes K, van Lenthe F, Brug J. A systematic review of environmental correlates of obesity-related dietary behaviours in youth. *Health Educ Res* 2007;**22**:203–26.
73. Savage JS, Fisher JO, Birch LL. Parental influence on eating behavior. *J Law Med Ethics* 2007;**35**:22–34.

74. Robinson S, Marriott L, Poole J, Crozier S, Borland S, Lawrence W, Law C, Godfrey K, Cooper C, Inskip H, SWS Study Group. Dietary patterns in infancy: the importance of maternal and family influences on feeding practice. *Br J Nutr* 2007;**98**: 1029–37.
75. Oliveria SA, Ellison RC, Moore LL, Gillman MW, Garrahie EJ, Singer MR. Parent-child relationships in nutrient intake: the Framingham Children's Study. *Am J Clin Nutr* 1992;**56**:593–8.
76. Vereecken CA, Keukelier E, Maes L. Influence of mother's educational level on food parenting practices and food habits of young children. *Appetite* 2004;**43**:93–103.
77. Birch LL, Fisher JO. Development of eating behaviors among children and adolescents. *Pediatrics* 1998;**101**:539–49.
78. Kral TJ, Stunkard AJ, Berkowitz RI, Stallings VA, Brown DD, Faith MS. Daily food intake in relation to dietary energy density in the free-living environment: a prospective analysis of children born at different risk of obesity. *Am J Clin Nutr* 2007;**86**: 41–7.
79. Wardle J, Guthrie C, Sanderson S, Birch L, Plomin R. Food and activity preferences in children of lean and obese parents. *Int J Obes* 2001;**25**:971–7.
80. Fisher JO, Birch LL. Fat preferences and fat consumption of 3- to 5-year-old children are related to parental adiposity. *J Am Diet Assoc* 1995;**95**:759–64.
81. Lussana F, Painter RC, Ocke MC, Buller HR, Bossuyt PM, Roseboom TJ. Prenatal exposure to the Dutch famine is associated with a preference for fatty foods and a more atherogenic lipid profile. *Am J Clin Nutr* 2008;**88**:1648–52.
82. Swinburn BA, Jolley D, Kremer PJ, Salbe AD, Ravussin E. Estimating the effects of energy imbalance on changes in body weight in children. *Am J Clin Nutr* 2006;**83**:859–63.
83. Klesges RC, Eck LH, Hanson CL, Haddock CK, Klesges LM. Effects of obesity, social interactions and physical environment on physical activity in preschoolers. *Health Psychol* 1990;**9**: 435–49.
84. Franks PW, Ravussin E, Hanson RL, Harper IT, Allison DB, Knowler WC, Tataranni PA, Salbe AD. Habitual physical activity in children: the role of genes and environment. *Am J Clin Nutr* 2005;**82**:901–8.
85. Vickers MH, Breier BH, McCarthy D, Gluckman PD. Sedentary behaviour during postnatal life is determined by the prenatal environment and exacerbated by postnatal hypercaloric nutrition. *Am J Physiol* 2003;**285**:R271–3.
86. Arenz S, Ruckerl R, Koletzko B, von Kries R. Breast-feeding and childhood obesity: a systematic review. *Int J Obes* 2004;**28**: 1247–56.
87. Hilson JA, Rasmussen KM, Kjolhede CL. Maternal obesity and breast-feeding success in a rural population of white women. *Am J Clin Nutr* 1997;**66**:1371–8.
88. Oddy WH, Li J, Landsborough L, Kendall GE, Henderson S, Downie J. The association of maternal overweight and obesity with breastfeeding duration. *J Pediatr* 2006;**149**:185–91.
89. Baker JL, Michaelsen KF, Sorensen TI, Rasmussen KM. High prepregnant body mass index is associated with early termination of full and any breastfeeding in Danish women. *Am J Clin Nutr* 2007;**86**:404–11.
90. Ebbeling CB, Pawlak DB, Ludwig DS. Childhood obesity: public health crisis, common sense cure. *Lancet* 2002;**360**:473–82.
91. Law C, Power C, Graham H, Merrick D. Obesity and health inequalities. *Obes Rev* 2007;**8**(Suppl. 1):19–22.
92. Lawlor DA, Chaturvedi N. Treatment and prevention of obesity: are there critical periods for intervention? *Int J Epidemiol* 2006;**35**: 3–9.
93. Esposito L, Fisher JO, Mennella JA, Hoelscher DM, Huang TT. Developmental perspectives on nutrition and obesity from gestation to adolescence. *Prev Chronic Dis* 2009;**6**:A93.
94. Inskip HM, Crozier SR, Godfrey KM, Borland SE, Cooper C, Robinson SM, SWS Study Group. Women's compliance with nutrition and lifestyle recommendations before pregnancy: general population cohort study. *BMJ* 2009;**338**:b481.
95. Gillman MW, Rifas-Shiman SL, Kleinman K, Oken E, Rich-Edwards JW, Taveras EM. Developmental origins of childhood overweight: potential health impact. *Obesity (Silver Spring)* 2008;**16**:1651–6.

CHAPTER 15

Is Prenatal Exposure to Maternal Obesity Linked to Child Mental Health?

Alina Rodriguez

Department of Psychology, Uppsala University, Sweden; Department of Epidemiology and Biostatistics, School of Public Health, Imperial College London, United Kingdom; MRC Social Genetic Developmental Psychiatry (SGDP), Institute of Psychiatry, King's College London, United Kingdom

This chapter considers whether neurodevelopmental disturbances in children can be programmed *in utero* via exposure to maternal obesity. If the association is causal, the prenatal period represents a critical window of opportunity for prevention. Therefore, understanding possible mechanisms that may account for this association need to be evaluated and are the focus of this chapter.

Fetal brain development is dependent on maternal energy supply [1]. Until recently, researchers have concentrated exclusively on low maternal weight before or during pregnancy as a risk factor for child neurobehavioral disturbance, particularly as mediated via low birth weight. For example, several studies have found an association between schizophrenia in adult offspring of women who were exposed to famine during pregnancy. Significant associations have been found for women who had inadequate weight gain during pregnancy or for women who conceived during the peak of famine and thus had a greater likelihood of having lower prepregnancy body mass index (BMI) [2–4]. However, it is difficult to disentangle the effect of maternal weight from the potential effect of stress when using historical epidemiological methods.

Although low prepregnancy BMI is a strong predictor of adverse pregnancy outcomes, current attention has shifted to maternal overweight and obesity at the time of pregnancy because of the "obesity epidemic" in developed as well as in developing nations [5–6]. The prevalence of women entering pregnancy overweight or obese is high across Europe, the United States, and Asia [7]. A recent report from Sweden showed that approximately 35% of women in 1999–2000 entered pregnancy overweight or obese [8]. This trend in high maternal prepregnancy BMI is on the rise, as evidence from the United States shows at least a 43% increase in the prevalence of maternal obesity at the beginning of pregnancy in 2002–2003 as compared to 1993–1994 [9].

An early follow-up study by Neggers and coworkers (2003) examined neurodevelopment in 355 children at the age of 5 years [10]. The original study was on zinc supplementation during pregnancy. The sample consisted of low-income African American women and women with high BMI were overrepresented, making it possible for the authors to examine maternal obesity as a predictor of child neurodevelopment. After adjustment for a number of relevant environmental factors including daycare and home quality as well as an indicator of maternal IQ (mother's receptive language skills), the authors found a strong and statistically significant association between increasing maternal prepregnancy BMI and decreasing scores for general IQ and nonverbal scores in the 5-year-olds. The main caveat of this study is its limited generalizability owing to the small sample size and consisting of only families in poverty.

A more recent study examining predictors of intellectual disability comes from the Northern Finland Birth Cohorts (NFBC), which are prospective longitudinal studies of mental and physical health. These are two large-scale cohorts that include approximately 99% of pregnancies in the target region with expected dates of birth in 1966 (Rantakallio, 1969) and 1986 (Jarvelin et al., 1993), N = 12,058 and N = 9432 live births, respectively [11, 12]. The aim of the study was to explore the relative importance and impact of maternal sociodemographic characteristics during pregnancy in relation to risk for intellectual disability in children and to ascertain whether any changes occurred across the two time points [13]. The authors found that leanness in the NFBC 1966 and obesity in the NFBC 1986 cohorts were associated with elevated risk of intellectual disability and concluded that weight outside the optimal region, in either direction, posed heightened risk for children's cognitive development.

Two prospective, large-scale Nordic studies have specifically examined behavior problems in children as a function of maternal prepregnancy BMI. The first study combined data from three Nordic prospective pregnancy-offspring cohorts, NFBC 1986, Aarhus Birth Cohort from Denmark, and the First Child in the Family from Sweden with a total sample size of 12,556 [14]. Information on maternal BMI was collected from the prenatal medical charts, and teachers assessed the behavior of children aged 7 to 12 years. The findings showed that core symptoms of attention deficit hyperactivity disorder (ADHD) (i.e., inattention and hyperactivity) were associated with maternal overweight and obesity, which remained significant after adjustment for a variety of possibly confounding factors (gestational weight gain, smoking during pregnancy, gestational age, birth weight, infant sex, maternal age, maternal education, and family structure at follow-up). Although this study was well powered, the main drawback was inclusion of only a few core symptoms of ADHD that had been assessed in all three cohorts, as opposed to the full range of symptoms.

The second Nordic study examining child behavior was carried out in Sweden [8] and aimed to address questions that remained from the previous Nordic investigation [14]. A similar method was used here: prospective, longitudinal data, maternal prepregnancy BMI was abstracted from the prenatal medical chart, and mothers and daycare providers (mostly preschool teachers) reported on child behavior and emotion. This study set out to investigate the association between maternal prepregnancy BMI and child behavior in 5-year-olds in light of three possible alterative explanations, namely maternal distress, familial heritability (mothers' and fathers' ADHD symptoms), and child's current weight status. Maternal obesity was positively associated with self-reported depression symptoms, and lower education was more common among women who were overweight or obese. The results showed a robust association between maternal prepregnancy overweight/obesity and child ADHD symptoms, in particular inattention, as reported by teachers after control for these possible explanatory variables as well as other potential confounders. Moreover, this study reported a novel finding linking maternal prepregnancy weight to difficulties with emotion in children.

Children of mothers who had been obese before pregnancy were more likely to have difficulties with negative emotions. Here too some significant associations were found for maternal underweight (BMI <19.99) and child behavior difficulties.

Taken together, these studies offer a unified picture and point to the possibility that maternal nonoptimal weight and especially overweight/obesity are related to child neurodevelopmental disturbances. However, studies that have systematically addressed this link are few in number; therefore, more studies using varied approaches including direct assessment of behavior problems and a variety of confounders are necessary to better understand the nature of the association and will shed light on the mechanisms that underlie it. What are possible mechanisms that underlie the link between maternal overweight/obesity and child behavior problems? This chapter starts off first by providing a short overview of common behavioral disturbances in children. Second, the concept of fetal programming is introduced briefly. Third, several biologically plausible mechanisms are considered. These mechanisms by no means represent an exhaustive list of possibilities but rather represent only a selection. The chapter finishes with a short discussion of confounding factors.

BEHAVIOR PROBLEMS IN CHILDREN

Inattention, hyperactivity, and impulsivity are commonly seen in children. However, when these behaviors are developmentally inappropriate and pervasive, then they are characteristic of ADHD. ADHD is the most widespread problem in child and adolescent psychiatry with an estimated prevalence of 5% worldwide [15]. Difficulties associated with ADHD and its symptoms are numerous and include poor scholastic performance [16] as well as difficulties with peers and socioemotional relationships in general [17]. Children with ADHD often follow a sustained negative developmental trajectory. Besides the profound consequences of ADHD for the individual and family, society also pays a heavy price including increased risk of criminality among those with comorbid conduct disorder and high cost of healthcare [18]. Individuals with ADHD show deficits in executive functioning, such as poor memory, inhibition, difficulty planning, and problems with self-regulatory processes [19]. Thus, the scope of the problems associated with ADHD and its high prevalence makes it a public health concern. Although child behavior problems, including ADHD, have been the focus of intense research, so far no preventable actions are available, partly because the causes of ADHD are not well delineated.

CONCEPT OF PRENATAL PROGRAMMING

Neurodevelopmental disorders such as ADHD are complex with multiple pathways contributing to their etiology. It has been proposed that disturbances in fetal development can alter the individual's health and disease over the life course [20]. This concept in terms of potential perturbations to fetal brain development has also been applied to mental health [21]. Experimental data using animal models provide strong evidence in support for fetal programming [22]; however, its effects in humans are only beginning to be understood. Epidemiological studies of humans point to common maternal lifestyle factors during pregnancy such as stress and smoking as environmental exposures potentially linked with child behavioral symptoms, hence supporting prenatal programming theory [23, 24]. One study calculated that 15% of the attributable load of ADHD is due to prenatal stress exposure [25]. As described earlier, maternal obesity is an environmental exposure during prenatal development that has been associated with child behavior problems.

The picture is yet more complex, as genetic predisposition in mothers can increase the risk of pregnancy stress or obesity, thus, associations may be carried in part or entirely by genetic transmission [26–28]. The etiology of child behavior problems is complex and multifactorial with genes ascribed a major portion of the variance [29]. However, neither genes nor environment operate in isolation but rather in a complex interplay [30]. As illustrated in Figure 15.1, human mental health development is multifaceted allowing also for postnatal social environments to ameliorate or exacerbate prior vulnerabilities. Therefore, it is of particular strategic importance to identify modifiable environmental causal risk factors, especially during pregnancy when the critical periods of central nervous system development take place during a short time frame. The public health value in terms of prevention is enormous.

POTENTIAL MECHANISMS LINKING MATERNAL OBESITY AND CHILD BEHAVIOR PROBLEMS

A few biological plausible mechanisms are discussed next.

Leptin

The recognition that adipose tissue is not inert came with the discovery of leptin [31]. Leptin is a hormone synthesized in adipose tissue according to fat stores; it regulates food intake and energy balance by signaling metabolic status to the brain. Both in nonpregnant and pregnant states, increasing BMI is related to increasing levels of leptin [32, 33]. Leptin has a major role in the reproductive system, including implantation and fetal growth [34]. There is evidence pointing to diminished oocyte quality in relation to high leptin levels [35]. Leptin is also involved in pathology with increased levels seen in preeclamptic and diabetic women. Further, leptin is involved in numerous complex systems including the neuroendocrine and as such is regulated by glucocorticoids [36]. Data point to the involvement of leptin in mood disturbances including depression and stress [37, 38]. In sum, heightened leptin levels reflect

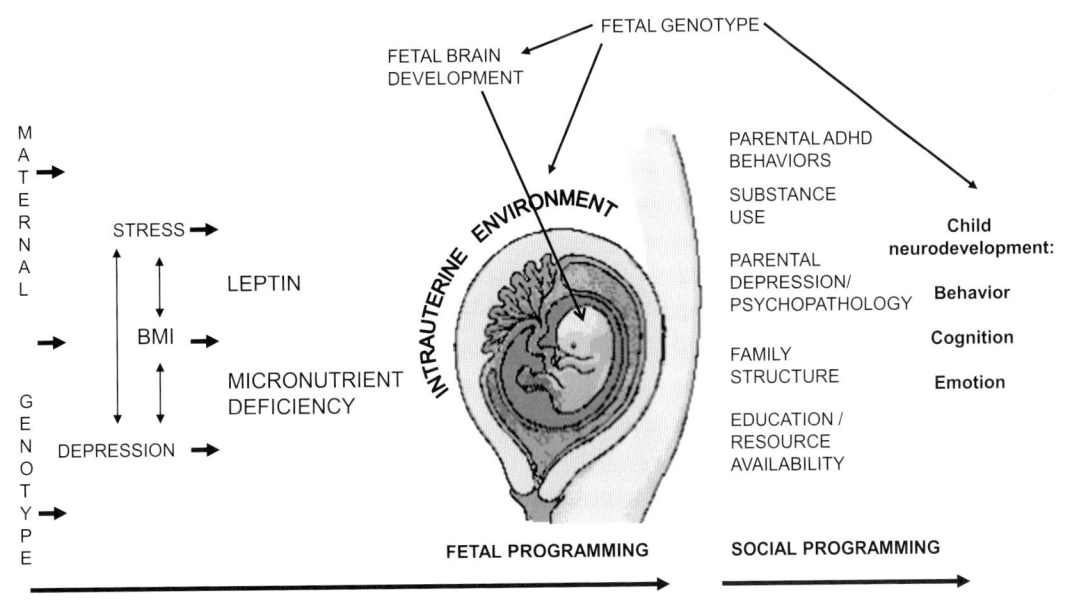

FIGURE 15.1 Potential pathways of child neurodevelopment.

adiposity, reproductive dysfunction, and mood disturbance, hence, pathways that could be potentially linked to fetal brain development.

The placenta also synthesizes leptin and is involved in fetal growth and brain development. High levels of leptin have been found to facilitate synaptic plasticity in the hippocampus, which is key for memory and learning and is rich in leptin receptors as reported by Walker et al. [39]. These researchers, however, did not study leptin administration during *in utero* development but rather injected leptin directly into the neonatal rats. Similarly, in vitro administration of leptin to hippocampal cells demonstrated that leptin induces long-term morphological changes in dendrites by increasing the number and motility of dendritic filopodia and ultimately increasing synaptic connections [40].

In this case it would be expected that increased levels of leptin would have a beneficial effect on fetal brain development. However, it is widely accepted that many obese people develop leptin resistance [41, 42]. Thus, it may be that leptin signaling in obese mothers to their fetuses is suboptimal. It has been suggested that leptin may be an environmental cue to the fetus signaling the nutritional status of the mother and consequently the rate of growth [43]. Obesity in mothers could perhaps disturb placental synthesis of leptin, but research is limited on placental changes in relation to maternal obesity. A recent study in the baboon, closely related to the human species, shows morphological changes in the placenta of obese animals [44].

Diet and Nutrition: Animal Models

The nutritional environment is pivotal for the developing fetal brain. Preimplantation embryos are sensitive to their nutritive environment as indicated by findings from experimental studies [45]. Because even the best cultures represent suboptimal environments for the embryo, Ecker and colleagues (2004) attributed cultures' inadequacy as instrumental in bringing about metabolic and gene expression changes in mice [46]. Furthermore, they found mice exposed to culture for an extended amount of time showed long-term effects on behavior, such as impaired spatial memory, locomotor activity, and anxiety. The authors speculated that these behavioral consequences were due to perturbations in the hippocampus, which is involved in these functions.

Deficient nutritive or caloric environments are well known to disturb brain development. At the other extreme, animal models are also being used to investigate the potential effect of excess availability of calories during prenatal development. In one study, adult offspring of dams fed a modestly high fat diet (similar to what would be found in humans) were found to have increased neurogenesis and synaptic plasticity in the hippocampus [47]. However, the opposite was true in two very recent investigations where mice were fed high-fat diets (up to 60% of calories from fat). Niculescu and Lupu (2009) demonstrated divergent development of hippocampal neurons during embryogenesis for offspring of dams who had been on a high-fat diet before and during pregnancy as compared to offspring of dams exposed to control diet [48]. Moreover, they reported reduction in cortical neurogenesis and neuronal differentiation in the fetal hippocampus. Further, another study found using a similar model, but in offspring nearing adulthood (postnatal day 70), that progenitor cells of the hippocampus were reduced [49]. Interestingly, they speculated that oxidative stress may reduce the viability of hippocampal neural progenitor cells. The results from these studies are very interesting and help to pinpoint the neural substrates of behavioral disturbances, although they did not measure behavior directly. Samuelson and colleagues (2008) designed an experiment focusing on metabolic outcomes in mice born to obese dams before and during pregnancy, but they also observed behavior. They reported that experimental animals showed significantly reduced activity in comparison to controls [50]. The hope is that the next studies will include both examinations of the brain as well as behavior in offspring exposed to maternal obesity *in utero*.

Results from these studies are fascinating and point to a proof of principle (i.e., exposure to maternal obesity *in utero* affects brain development in the offspring). However, the exact mechanisms are yet to be delineated as well as the link to behavioral measures. It is also important to consider the limitations associated with animal models, such as differential rate of prenatal brain development in comparison to humans, who have a long gestation and consequently much greater brain development before birth in comparison to rodents. Another limitation is that alterations in dietary composition to achieve higher fat content may induce an imbalance in the recommended proportions of other nutrients. Thus, this dietary quality difference makes it difficult to disentangle whether the association is due to exposure to high fat per se or whether it is due to micronutrient imbalance. This point, however, is relevant not only for animal models but also concerns studies of humans.

Micronutrients: Human Studies

Overweight and obesity, although closely related to overeating, paradoxically are not related to adequate nutrition in humans. Recent findings from the National Health and Nutrition Examination Survey III (N = 16,191), a large representative population-based cohort from the United States, show that overweight and obese people are more likely to be at higher risk of having low levels of micronutrients [51]. Further, they reported that the association was particularly pronounced in reproductive women who were more likely to have low levels of multiple micronutrients (including folate). Results converge from two recent reports specifically targeted at women's food quality during pregnancy. Pregnant women in North Carolina (Pregnancy, Infection, and Nutrition cohort, N = 2394) and in Massachusetts (Project Viva cohort, N = 1777) were found to have poorer diet quality as prepregnancy BMI increased [52, 53]. Recently, use of folate supplementation was found to be related to BMI among pregnant women in The Netherlands, such that higher BMI was associated with a lower likelihood of using supplementation [54].

Epigenetics and Dietary Methyl Donors

Epigenetics refers to the processes that regulate how and when certain genes are expressed or silenced. In contrast to the DNA sequence, which is stable, epigenetic processes are highly dynamic and react to environmental cues. Nonetheless, epigenetic changes can be conserved during cell replication and therefore may have a lifelong impact on the individual. This flexibility and ability to react to environmental influences is an adaptable yet vulnerable feature. Prenatal development, particularly during embryogenesis, is especially critical because DNA synthesis is high and epigenetic regulation of gene expression is needed for normal tissue differentiation and development. Epigenetic alterations have been proposed as one molecular mechanism mediating environmental risks during prenatal development to neurodevelopmental disturbances observable in childhood [55].

The DNA molecule is tightly packed to form chromosomes and DNA is wrapped tightly around proteins called histones. DNA expression is altered by either allowing or preventing accessibility to the DNA of the factors involved in transcription [56]. Methylation is an enzymatic process in the cell nucleus that can directly turn off gene expression, resulting in gene silencing in the short and long term [57].

Folate and choline are considered methyl donors because of their importance in the methylation process [58]. Metabolism of these two essential nutrients interact, making it difficult to differentiate the actions of one versus the other, particularly because disturbance in the metabolic pathway of one methyl donor elicits compensatory alterations in other methyl donors [59].

Both nutrients are required for neurogenesis in the brain and spinal cord. Lack of sufficient dietary intake of folate and choline can perturb development by allowing accumulation of toxic levels of homocysteine (because of a lack of clearing), altering DNA synthesis, and disturbing methylation reactions [58]. Choline is critical because it influences stem-cell and progenitor-cell proliferation and apoptosis (programmed cell death), thereby altering structure and function of the brain permanently [60]. Besides the well-known beneficial effects of folate for preventing neural tube defects, folate and choline have been implicated in the development of the hippocampus in rodents by increased progenitor-cell proliferation, dendritic spine density, and reduced apoptosis [61–63]. Further, offspring of dams fed high-choline diets during gestation show signs of reduced neurodegenerative processes in late life, suggesting that permanent changes resulted [62]. This may be due to the finding that the cells that proliferate and migrate seem to be particularly sensitive to choline deficiency [63]. Because the hippocampus is involved in learning and memory, these findings are significant in terms of the potential for programming behavioral and cognitive problems, including those related to ADHD. Indeed, using a learning paradigm Lamoureux and colleagues (2008) showed attention in rats was related to prenatal choline exposure [64]. Experiments conducted by Wong-Goodrich and coworkers (2008) demonstrated that the effect of prenatal choline on learning is complex [65]. These authors showed that to a certain extent learning was conditional on both prenatal and current choline supply. Rats exposed to prenatal choline supplementation as well as supplemented diets in adulthood outperformed all other groups, although under conditions of deficiency in adulthood the prenatally supplemented rats' performance deteriorated more than others.

Folate and Choline in Humans

Indeed maternal folate during pregnancy is related to methylation in children [66]; however, tissue-specific methylation (e.g., in the hippocampus) is impossible to test in humans. Results from a community-based prospective cohort from the Netherlands (N = 4214) showed a protective association between folate supplementation during early pregnancy and behavior problems in toddlers [54]. In contrast, an earlier study examining folate plasma levels, measured during several time points in pregnancy, was not linked to performance on neurodevelopmental tasks in 5-year-olds [67]. This study was conducted during the time that a mandate for fortification of common foods with folate was implemented. The authors believed that this limited variation in their sample and that none of the women were severely deficient. It may be the case that a threshold must be reached before the effects of folate on child neurodevelopment are measurable. Moreover, by studying only a socioeconomically deprived group of African American women (N = 589), the effect of folate, which may be small, may have been overshadowed by the expected large impact of poverty [67]. Wehby and Murray (2008) used data from the large United States based cohort (N = 6774) National Maternal and Infant Health Survey (NMIHS) that links vital records with data from maternal questionnaires [68]. Child development questions were designed as screeners and assessed by mothers. The authors found that folate supplementation during pregnancy was associated with better scores on their measure of overall child developmental risk and gross-motor development, although the former association was statistically significant only among African American children. This lack of consistency in findings raises questions concerning not only the sensitivity of instruments to detect effects but also whether genetic differences in folate synthesis and consequently the need for supplementation differs across the racial groups. Because folate and choline metabolism and function are intertwined, choline is expected to also be related to brain development. However, a study examining IQ in children as a function of maternal serum concentrations of free and total choline during pregnancy found no association with visuospatial processing and memory measures [69]. Further investigation is indeed necessary, particularly because the results of these studies taken together are mixed. A meta-analysis would be very informative, especially if an array of micronutrients were to be assessed.

Impact of Genes

The need for choline and folate increases dramatically during pregnancy. Even though premenopausal women are able to synthesize folate, dietary intake is necessary to ensure optimal development of the offspring [58]. The need for dietary methyl donors differs individually and stems from common variations in the DNA sequence in terms of a single-nucleotide polymorphism (SNP) in MTHFR gene (C677T), which influences folate metabolism and consequently methylation. The mutation (TT) is associated with reduced function and consequently greater need for dietary folate intake. This variation is common and afflicts about 13% of populations of European descent [70]. A meta-analysis of six studies examining the C677T polymorphism found that the TT mutation was associated with elevated risk of schizophrenia [71]. Until now, only one study has examined maternal folate intake during pregnancy and child neurobehavior [72]. These authors assessed child neurodevelopment (N = 253) with the Bayley Scales and found that deficient folate intake by the mother during the first trimester was associated with poorer development only among children whose mothers carried the TT mutation. These finding highlight the potential for a gene-environment interaction previously highlighted in the etiology of ADHD [28].

Besides examining the association with methyl donor deficiency, maternal obesity before pregnancy in general has only rarely been examined in relation to epigenetic alterations in children. Gemma and colleagues (2009) studied umbilical cord methylation in the human newborn and found that methylation of a key gene related to the metabolic syndrome (PPARGCIA) was related to maternal BMI before pregnancy [73]. Although this was a small study, the findings are interesting and provide preliminary evidence that the association between maternal BMI and offspring methylation status can be linked in humans. Nonetheless, the mechanism for this link remains to be established, as well as a link to behavioral end points.

The risks for both obesity and ADHD are known to run in families. There may be a common genetic pathway underlying both overweight/obesity and predisposition to poor mental health, which suggests certain genes may have pleiotropic effects. Frayling and colleagues (2007) offered the first clear-cut evidence that common variations in the FTO gene strongly contribute to obesity, a finding that has since been replicated [74]. If obesity and ADHD are linked, it may be via impulsive behavior and overeating. Indeed, the variants in the FTO have been linked to reported eating behaviors in youths [75, 76]. Further the FTO-risk genotype was associated with reactions to stress in adolescents [77].

The gene identification process involved in ADHD since the late 1990s has been relatively fruitful by screening genetic variants that lie within or close to genes that regulate neurotransmitter systems, mainly dopamine and serotonin pathways [78, 79]. However, according to a review, differences across the various published data sets were apparent [80], but the source of this variation is currently unknown. One possible source could be exposure to various environmental risks that either heighten or lessen the effect of genes, particularly those related to prenatal exposures.

Observations that obesity is more prevalent among persons with serious mental illness [81] and that psychopathology predicts overweight and obesity over the course of up to 20 years [82–84] lend support to the idea that genes related to mental health are also related to obesity. ADHD has been mainly linked to dysfunction in dopaminergic and serotonergic systems in genetic studies [85, 86]. In a study of overeating women with seasonal affective disorder, overweight and obesity were linked to both dopamine-4 receptor gene and retrospective reports of women's ADHD symptoms in childhood [87]. A small study found evidence for variations in the serotonin transporter gene (5-HTT) relating to both obesity and impulsivity, an important aspect of ADHD [88]. Taken together, genetic predisposition could account for both maternal weight and ADHD symptoms, which could be inherited by offspring. Genetic analysis or at least data on parental psychopathology is necessary to fully answer the question of whether exposure to maternal obesity is associated to child behavior problems via a common genetic link.

CONFOUNDING FACTORS

Is the association between exposure to maternal prepregnancy obesity and child neurodevelopmental problems causal or is the association simply spurious and caused by other factors?

Maternal Distress

Maternal distress is an obvious potential confounding factor because obesity has been previously related to mental health problems [89]. Besides the potential pleiotropic effects of genes increasing risk of both mental health disorders and obesity, it is possible that prenatal exposure to neuroendocrine changes related to maternal perceived stress or depression is the causal agent. One of the hypothesized mechanisms is through hypothalamic-pituitary-adrenal (HPA) axis dysfunction [90]. Both stress and depression during pregnancy have been linked to child behavior problems including ADHD symptoms in a growing body of research [91, 92]. Stress can precipitate depression, and both states are characterized by altered cortisol levels. Stressful events trigger the HPA-axis and results in cortisol secretion (a glucocorticoid). The postulated mode of action by which maternal distress negatively affects fetal brain development is through the HPA-axis and cortisol, although the mechanisms are still poorly understood.

Perceived stress is related to caloric intake and ingestion of "comfort food" [93], which is nutritionally poorer than the recommended diet. Moreover, a recent review suggests that depression symptoms during pregnancy are associated with deficiencies in various nutrients including folate, but this connection needs further assessment as there were a number of methodological limitations in the studies [94]. Nutritional deficiencies and depressed mood may very well be reciprocally related, but they may also be additive in their detrimental effect on fetal development as well as their tendency to interfere in postnatal development [95]. Nonetheless, the study by Rodriguez (2010) specifically testing this hypothesis showed that adjustment for maternal stress and depression symptoms (during pregnancy and concurrent) did not significantly attenuate the association between prenatal maternal obesity and ADHD symptoms and emotional problems in the child [8]. This suggests that maternal obesity and maternal distress may potentially be operating through separate mechanisms to influence fetal brain development.

Socioeconomic Status (SES)

Obesity, maternal distress, nutrient deficiencies, and so on often co-occur in the context of poverty. Low SES in turn has been associated with mental health in general [96] and child behavior problems [97, 98]. Poor diet during pregnancy related to poverty contributes to inequalities in pregnancy outcome, which in turn can be a risk factor for later behavior problems [99]. Albeit disparity in obesity by SES groups has diminished over time according to a report by the National Health and Nutrition Examination Surveys (NHANES) over a span of three decades in the United States and points to a high prevalence of obesity in the high SES groups as well [100]. Low SES is likely to contribute to poor fetal and postnatal development through numerous pathways; therefore, it may be difficult to disassociate this effect in human studies.

Gestational and Perinatal Complications

Prepregnancy obesity is not only a risk for the pregnant woman but also for her child. Rising prepregnancy BMI is associated with gestational diabetes, preeclampsia, labor complications, and adverse birth outcomes [7, 101]. In this case, it may not be maternal obesity per se that accounts for the association to neurodevelopmental difficulties in the child, but rather gestational or perinatal complications may be the causal factor. This hypothesis is relatively easy to test in a large pregnancy cohort where information on complications are available; however, such a study has not yet been reported.

CONCLUSION

Are we able to answer the question of causality in regard to whether neurodevelopmental disturbances in children can be programmed *in utero* via exposure to maternal obesity? This chapter outlined a few, albeit a nonexhaustive list, of plausible biological mechanisms that could underlie the association; however, the answer is clearly *no* at this time. For all pathways discussed here (i.e., leptin, nutrition, epigenetic, and genetic), much more research is needed before solid conclusions can be reached and used to guide public health policy. These mechanisms, along with others that were excluded from this chapter due to space constraints, are biologically plausible and not mutually exclusive, and thus multiple pathways may link exposure to maternal obesity *in utero* with later child neurodevelopmental disturbance. Determining the exact causal pathways remains a challenge and is important for prevention and treatment development of child mental health.

Acknowledgements

The author has no financial relationships to disclose. The author was in part funded by a grant from VINNMER (P32925−1). Please address correspondence to: Alina Rodriguez, Dept. of Psychology, Uppsala University, Box 1225, SE 751 42 Uppsala. Sweden; Email: Alina.Rodriguez@psyk.uu.se

References

1. Hay Jr WW, Sparks JW. Placental, fetal, and neonatal carbohydrate metabolism. *Clin Obstet Gynecol* 1985;**28**:473−85.
2. Susser ES, Lin SP. Schizophrenia after prenatal exposure to the Dutch Hunger Winter of 1944−1945. *Arch Gen Psychiatry* 1992;**49**:983−8.
3. Susser ES, Neugebauer R, Hoek HW, Brown AS, Lin S, Labovitz D, Gorman JM. Schizophrenia after prenatal famine. Further evidence. *Arch Gen Psychiatry* 1996;**53**:25−31.
4. St. Clair D, Xu M, Want P, Yu Y, Fang Y, Zhang F, Zheng X, Gu N, Feng G, Sham P, He L. Rates of adult schizophrenia following prenatal exposure to the Chinese famine of 1959−1961. *JAMA* 2005;**294**:557−62.
5. Hedley AA, Ogden CL, Johnson CL, Carroll MD, Curtin LR, Flegal KM. Prevalence of Overweight and Obesity Among US Children, Adolescents, and Adults, 1999−2002. *JAMA* 2004;**291**:2847−50.
6. Haslam DW, James WPT. Obesity. *Lancet* 2005;**366**:1197−209.
7. Cnattingius S, Lambe M. Trends in smoking and overweight during pregnancy: prevalence, risks of pregnancy complications, and adverse pregnancy outcomes. *Semin Perinatol* 2002;**26**:286−95.
8. Rodriguez A. Maternal pre-pregnancy obesity and risk for inattention and negative emotionality in children. *Journal of Child Psychology and Psychiatry* 2010;**51**:134−43.
9. Kim SY, Dietz PM, England L, Morrow B, Callaghan WM. Trends in pre-pregnancy obesity in nine states, 1993−2003. *Obesity (Silver Spring)* 2007;**15**:986−93.
10. Neggers YH, Goldenberg RL, Ramey SL, Cliver SP. Maternal prepregnancy body mass index and psychomotor development in children. *Acta Obstetricia et Gynecologica Scandinavica* 2003;**82**:235−40.
11. Rantakallio P. Groups at risk in low birth weight infants and perinatal mortality. *Acta Paediatr Scand* 1969;**193**(suppl):1−71.
12. Jarvelin MR, Hartikainen-Sorri AL, Rantakallio P. Labour induction policy in hospitals of different levels of specialisation. *Br J Obstet Gynaecol* 1993;**100**:310−15.
13. Heikura U, Taanila A, Hartikainen AL, Olsen P, Linna SL, von Wendt L, Jarvelin MR. Variations in prenatal sociodemographic factors associated with intellectual disability: a study of the 20-year interval between two birth cohorts in northern Finland. *Am J Epidemiol* 2008;**167**:169−77.
14. Rodriguez A, Miettunen J, Henriksen TB, Olsen J, Obel C, Taanila A, Ebeling H, Linnet KM, Moilanen I, Jarvelin MR. Maternal adiposity prior to pregnancy is associated with ADHD symptoms in offspring: evidence from three prospective pregnancy cohorts. *Int J Obes (Lond)* 2008;**32**:550−7.
15. Polanczyk G, de Lima MS, Horta BL, Biederman J, Rohde LA. The worldwide prevalence of ADHD: A systematic review and metaregression analysis. *Am J Psychiatry* 2007;**164**:942−8.
16. Rodriguez A, Jarvelin MR, Obel C, Taanila A, Miettunen J, Moilanen I, Henriksen TB, Pietilainen K, Ebeling H, Kotimaa AJ, Linnet KM, Olsen J. Do inattention and hyperactivity symptoms equal scholastic impairment? Evidence from three European cohorts. *BMC Public Health* 2007;**7**:327.
17. Klassen AF, Miller A, Fine S. Health-related quality of life in children and adolescents who have a diagnosis of attention-deficit/hyperactivity disorder. *Pediatrics* 2004;**114**:e541−7.
18. Matza LS, Paramore C, Prasad M. A review of the economic burden of ADHD. *Cost Eff Resour Alloc* 2005;**3**:5.
19. Nigg JT. Neuropsychologic theory and findings in attention-deficit/hyperactivity disorder: The state of the field and salient challenges for the coming decade. *Biological Psychiatry* 2005;**57**:1424−35.
20. Barker D. Fetal origins of coronary heart disease. *British Medical Journal* 1995;**311**:171−4.
21. Schlotz W, Phillips DIW. Fetal origins of mental health: Evidence and mechanisms. *Brain, Behavior, and Immunity* 2009;**23**:905−16.
22. Weinstock M. The potential influence of maternal stress hormones on development and mental health of the offspring. *Brain Behav Immun* 2005;**19**:296−308.
23. Linnet KM, Dalsgaard S, Obel C, Wisborg K, Henriksen TB, Rodriguez A, Kotimaa A, Moilanen I, Thomsen PH, Olsen J, Jarvelin MR. Maternal lifestyle factors in pregnancy risk of attention deficit hyperactivity disorder and associated behaviors: review of the current evidence. *Am J Psychiatry* 2003;**160**:1028−40.
24. Rodriguez A, Bohlin G. Are maternal smoking and stress during pregnancy related to ADHD symptoms in children? *Journal of Child Psychology and Psychiatry* 2005;**46**:246−54.
25. Talge NM, Neal C, Glover V. Antenatal maternal stress and long-term effects on child neurodevelopment: how and why? *Journal of Child Psychology and Psychiatry* 2007;**48**:245−61.
26. Thapar A, Langley K, Asherson P, Gill M. Gene-environment interplay in attention-deficit hyperactivity disorder and the importance of a developmental perspective. *British Journal of Psychiatry* 2007;**190**:1−3.
27. Rutter M, Moffitt TE, Caspi A. Gene-environment interplay and psychopathology: multiple varieties but real effects. *Journal of Child Psychology and Psychiatry* 2006;**47**:226−61.
28. Rodriguez A. The impact of prenatal risk factors in ADHD: A potential for Gene x Environment interactions. *Psychiatry* 2008;**7**:516−19.
29. Biederman J, Faraone SV. Attention-deficit hyperactivity disorder. *The Lancet* 2005;**366**:237.
30. Moffitt TE, Caspi A, Rutter M. Strategy for investigating interactions between measured genes and measured environments. *Arch Gen Psychiatry* 2005;**62**:473−81.
31. Zhang Q, Wang Y. Trends in the Association between Obesity and Socioeconomic Status in U.S. Adults: 1971 to 2000. *Obes Res* 2004;**12**:1622−32.
32. Chan JL, Mantzoros CS. Role of leptin in energy-deprivation states: normal human physiology and clinical implications for hypothalamic amenorrhoea and anorexia nervosa. *Lancet* 2005;**366**:74−85.
33. Hendler I, Blackwell SC, Mehta SH, Whitty JE, Russell E, Sorokin Y, Cotton DB. The levels of leptin, adiponectin, and resistin in normal weight, overweight, and obese pregnant women with and without preeclampsia. *American Journal of Obstetrics and Gynecology* 2005;**193**:979−83.
34. Domali E, Messinis IE. Leptin in pregnancy. *J Matern Fetal Neonatal Med* 2002;**12**:222−30.
35. Wattanakumtornkul S, Damario MA, Stevens Hall SA, Thornhill AR, Tummon IS. Body mass index and uterine receptivity in the oocyte donation model. *Fertil Steril* 2003;**80**:336−40.
36. Leal-Cerro A, Soto A, Martinez MA, Dieguez C, Casanueva FF. Influence of cortisol status on leptin secretion. *Pituitary* 2001;**4**:111−16.

37. Kishi T, Elmquist JK. Body weight is regulated by the brain: a link between feeding and emotion. *Molecular Psychiatry* 2005;**10**:132–46.
38. Lu XY, Kim CS, Frazer A, Zhang W. Leptin: a potential novel antidepressant. *Proc Natl Acad Sci U S A* 2006;**103**:1593–8.
39. Walker CD, Long H, Williams S, Richard D. Long-lasting effects of elevated neonatal leptin on rat hippocampal function, synaptic proteins and NMDA receptor subunits. *J Neurosci Res* 2007;**85**:816–28.
40. O'Malley D, MacDonald N, Mizielinska S, Connolly CN, Irving AJ, Harvey J. Leptin promotes rapid dynamic changes in hippocampal dendritic morphology. *Molecular and Cellular Neuroscience* 2007;**35**:559–72.
41. Banks WA. The blood-brain barrier as a cause of obesity. *Curr Pharm Des* 2008;**14**:1606–14.
42. Bence KK, Delibegovic M, Xue B, Gorgun CZ, Hotamisligil GS, Neel BG, Kahn BB. Neuronal PTP1B regulates body weight, adiposity and leptin action. *Nat Med* 2006;**12**:917–24.
43. Macajova M, Lamosova D, Zeman M. Role of Leptin in Farm Animals: a Review. *Journal of Veterinary Medicine Series A* 2004;**51**:157–66.
44. Farley D, Tejero ME, Comuzzie AG, Higgins PB, Cox L, Werner SL, Jenkins SL, Li C, Choi J, Dick Jr EJ, Hubbard GB, Frost P, Dudley DJ, Ballesteros B, Wu G, Nathanielsz PW, Schlabritz-Loutsevitch NE. Feto-placental Adaptations to Maternal Obesity in the Baboon. *Placenta* 2009;**30**:752–60.
45. Watkins AJ, Papenbrock T, Fleming TP. The preimplantation embryo: handle with care. *Semin Reprod Med* 2008;**26**:175–85.
46. Ecker DJ, Stein P, Xu Z, Williams CJ, Kopf GS, Bilker WB, Abel T, Schultz RM. Long-term effects of culture of preimplantation mouse embryos on behavior. *Proc Natl Acad Sci U S A* 2004;**101**:1595–600.
47. Walker CD, Naef L, d'Asti E, Long H, Xu Z, Moreau A, Azeddine B. Perinatal maternal fat intake affects metabolism and hippocampal function in the offspring: a potential role for leptin. *Ann N Y Acad Sci* 2008;**1144**:189–202.
48. Niculescu MD, Lupu DS. High fat diet-induced maternal obesity alters fetal hippocampal development. *International Journal of Developmental Neuroscience* 2009;**27**:627–33.
49. Tozuka Y, Wada E, Wada K. Diet-induced obesity in female mice leads to peroxidized lipid accumulations and impairment of hippocampal neurogenesis during the early life of their offspring. *Faseb J* 2009;**23**:1920–34.
50. Samuelsson AM, Matthews PA, Argenton M, Christie MR, McConnell JM, Jansen EH, Piersma AH, Ozanne SE, Twinn DF, Remacle C, Rowlerson A, Poston L, Taylor PD. Diet-induced obesity in female mice leads to offspring hyperphagia, adiposity, hypertension, and insulin resistance: a novel murine model of developmental programming. *Hypertension* 2008;**51**:383–92.
51. Kimmons JE, Blanck HM, Tohill BC, Zhang J, Khan LK. Associations between body mass index and the prevalence of low micronutrient levels among US adults. *MedGenMed* 2006;**8**:59.
52. Laraia BA, Bodnar LM, Siega-Riz AM. Pregravid body mass index is negatively associated with diet quality during pregnancy. *Public Health Nutrition* 2007;**10**:920–6.
53. Rifas-Shiman SL, Rich-Edwards JW, Kleinman KP, Oken E, Gillman MW. Dietary Quality during Pregnancy Varies by Maternal Characteristics in Project Viva: A US Cohort. *Journal of the American Dietetic Association* 2009;**109**:1004–11.
54. Roza SJ, van Batenburg-Eddes T, Steegers EA, Jaddoe VW, Mackenbach JP, Hofman A, Verhulst FC, Tiemeier H. Maternal folic acid supplement use in early pregnancy and child behavioural problems: The Generation R Study. *British Journal of Nutrition* 2010;**103**:445–52.
55. Mill J, Petronis A. Pre- and peri-natal environmental risks for attention-deficit hyperactivity disorder (ADHD): the potential role of epigenetic processes in mediating susceptibility. *J Child Psychol Psychiatry* 2008;**49**:1020–30.
56. Jacob S, Moley KH. Gametes and embryo epigenetic reprogramming affect developmental outcome: implication for assisted reproductive technologies. *Pediatr Res* 2005;**58**:437–46.
57. Mehler MF. Epigenetic principles and mechanisms underlying nervous system functions in health and disease. *Prog Neurobiol* Oct 18 2008;**86**(4):305–41.
58. Zeisel SH. Importance of methyl donors during reproduction. *Am J Clin Nutr* 2009;**89**:673S–677.
59. Zeisel SH. Epigenetic mechanisms for nutrition determinants of later health outcomes. *Am J Clin Nutr* 2009;**89**:1488S–93S.
60. Zeisel SH. Choline: critical role during fetal development and dietary requirements in adults. *Annu Rev Nutr* 2006;**26**:229–50.
61. Meck WH, Williams CL. Metabolic imprinting of choline by its availability during gestation: implications for memory and attentional processing across the lifespan. *Neurosci Biobehav Rev* 2003;**27**:385–99.
62. Meck WH, Williams CL, Cermak JM, Blusztajn JK. Developmental periods of choline sensitivity provide an ontogenetic mechanism for regulating memory capacity and age-related dementia. *Front Integr Neurosci* 2007;**1**:7.
63. Niculescu MD, Craciunescu CN, Zeisel SH. Dietary choline deficiency alters global and gene-specific DNA methylation in the developing hippocampus of mouse fetal brains. *FASEB J* 2006;**20**:43–9.
64. Lamoureux JA, Meck WH, Williams CL. Prenatal choline availability alters the context sensitivity of Pavlovian conditioning in adult rats. *Learn Mem* 2008;**15**:866–75.
65. Wong-Goodrich SJ, Glenn MJ, Mellott TJ, Blusztajn JK, Meck WH, Williams CL. Spatial memory and hippocampal plasticity are differentially sensitive to the availability of choline in adulthood as a function of choline supply in utero. *Brain Res* 2008;**1237**:153–66.
66. Steegers-Theunissen RgP, Obermann-Borst SA, Kremer D, Lindemans J, Siebel C, Steegers EA, Slagboom PE, Heijmans BT. Periconceptional Maternal Folic Acid Use of 400 µg per Day Is Related to Increased Methylation of the IGF2 Gene in the Very Young Child. *PLoS One* 2009;**4**:e7845.
67. Tamura T, Goldenberg RL, Chapman VR, Johnston KE, Ramey SL, Nelson KG. Folate Status of Mothers During Pregnancy and Mental and Psychomotor Development of Their Children at Five Years of Age. *Pediatrics* 2005;**116**:703–8.
68. Wehby G, Murray J. The effects of prenatal use of folic acid and other dietary supplements on early child development. *Maternal and Child Health Journal* 2008;**12**:180–7.
69. Signore C, Ueland PM, Troendle J, Mills JL. Choline concentrations in human maternal and cord blood and intelligence at 5 y of age. *Am J Clin Nutr* 2008;**87**:896–902.
70. Botto LD, Yang Q. 5, 10-Methylenetetrahydrofolate Reductase Gene Variants and Congenital Anomalies: A HuGE Review. *Am J Epidemiol* 2000;**151**:862–77.
71. Lewis SJ, Zammit S, Gunnell D, SmithGeorge D. A meta-analysis of the MTHFR C677T polymorphism and schizophrenia risk. *Am J Med Genet B Neuropsychiatr Genet* 2005;**135B**:2–4.
72. del Rio Garcia C, Torres-Sanchez L, Chen J, Schnaas L, Hernandez C, Osorio E, Portillo MG, Lopez-Carrillo L. Maternal MTHFR 677CT genotype and dietary intake of folate and vitamin B12: their impact on child neurodevelopment. *Nutritional Neuroscience* 2009;**12**:13–20.
73. Gemma C, Sookoian S, Alvarinas J, Garcia SI, Quintana L, Kanevsky D, Gonzalez CD, Pirola CJ. Maternal pregestational

BMI is associated with methylation of the PPARGC1A promoter in newborns. *Obesity* 2009;**17**:1032–9.
74. Frayling TM, Timpson NJ, Weedon MN, Zeggini E, Freathy RM, Lindgren CM, Perry JR, Elliott KS, Lango H, Rayner NW, Shields B, Harries LW, Barrett JC, Ellard S, Groves CJ, Knight B, Patch AM, Ness AR, Ebrahim S, Lawlor DA, Ring SM, Ben-Shlomo Y, Jarvelin MR, Sovio U, Bennett AJ, Melzer D, Ferrucci L, Loos RJ, Barroso I, Wareham NJ, Karpe F, Owen KR, Cardon LR, Walker M, Hitman GA, Palmer CN, Doney AS, Morris AD, Smith GD, Hattersley AT, McCarthy MI. A Common Variant in the FTO Gene Is Associated with Body Mass Index and Predisposes to Childhood and Adult Obesity. *Science* 2007;**316**:889–94.
75. Wardle J, Carnell S, Haworth CMA, Farooqi IS, O'Rahilly S, Plomin R. Obesity Associated Genetic Variation in FTO Is Associated with Diminished Satiety. *J Clin Endocrinol Metab* 2008;**93**:3640–3.
76. Stutzmann F, Cauchi S, Durand E, Calvacanti-Proenca C, Pigeyre M, Hartikainen AL, Sovio U, Tichet J, Marre M, Weill J, Balkau B, Potoczna N, Laitinen J, Elliott P, Jarvelin MR, Horber F, Meyre D, Froguel P. Common genetic variation near MC4R is associated with eating behaviour patterns in European populations. *Int J Obes* 2009;**33**:373–8.
77. Pausova Z, Syme C, Abrahamowicz M, Xiao Y, Leonard GT, Perron M, Richer L, Veillette S, Smith GD, Seda O, Tremblay J, Hamet P, Gaudet D, Paus T. A common variant of the FTO gene is associated with not only increased adiposity but also elevated blood pressure in French Canadians. *Circ Cardiovasc Genet* 2009;**2**:260–9.
78. Asherson P. Attention-Deficit Hyperactivity Disorder in the post-genomic era. *Eur Child Adolesc Psychiatry* 2004;**13**(Suppl. 1): I50–70.
79. Brookes K, Xu X, Chen W, Zhou K, Neale B, Lowe N, Anney R, Franke B, Gill M, Ebstein R, Buitelaar J, Sham P, Campbell D, Knight J, Andreou P, Altink M, Arnold R, Boer F, Buschgens C, Butler L, Christiansen H, Feldman L, Fleischman K, Fliers E, Howe-Forbes R, Goldfarb A, Heise A, Gabriels I, Korn-Lubetzki I, Johansson L, Marco R, Medad S, Minderaa R, Mulas F, Muller U, Mulligan A, Rabin K, Mommelse N, Sethna V, Sorohan J, Uebel H, Psychogiou L, Weeks A, Barrett R, Craig I, Banaschewski T, Sonuga-Barke E, Eisenberg J, Kuntsi J, Manor I, McGuffin P, Miranda A, Oades RD, Plomin R, Roeyers H, Rothenberger A, Sergeant J, Steinhausen HC, Taylor E, Thompson M, Faraone SV, Asherson P. The analysis of 51 genes in DSM-IV combined type attention deficit hyperactivity disorder: Association signals in DRD4, DAT1 and 16 other genes. *Molecular Psychiatry* 2006;**11**:934–53.
80. Curran S, Mill J, Sham P, Rijsdijk F, Marusic K, Taylor E, Asherson P. QTL association analysis of the DRD4 exon 3 VNTR polymorphism in a population sample of children screened with a parent rating scale for ADHD symptoms. *Am J Med Genet* 2001;**105**:387–93.
81. Dickerson FB, Brown CH, Kreyenbuhl JA, Fang L, Goldberg RW, Wohlheiter K, Dixon LB. Obesity among individuals with serious mental illness. *Acta Psychiatrica Scandinavica* 2006;**113**:306–13.
82. Hasler G, Pine DS, Gamma A, Milos G, Ajdacic V, Eich D, Rossler W, Angst J. The associations between psychopathology and being overweight: a 20-year prospective study. *Psychol Med* 2004;**34**:1047–57.
83. Hasler G, Pine DS, Kleinbaum DG, Gamma A, Luckenbaugh D, Ajdacic V, Eich D, Rossler W, Angst J. Depressive symptoms during childhood and adult obesity: the Zurich Cohort Study. *Molecular Psychiatry* 2005;**10**:842–50.

84. Mamun AA, O'Callaghan MJ, Cramb SM, Najman JM, Williams GM, Bor W. Childhood Behavioral Problems Predict Young Adults' BMI and Obesity: Evidence From a Birth Cohort Study. *Obesity* 2009;**17**:761–6.
85. Biederman J. Attention-deficit/hyperactivity disorder: a selective overview. *Biol Psychiatry* 2005;**57**:1215–20.
86. Quist JF, Barr CL, Schachar R, Roberts W, Malone M, Tannock R, Basile VS, Beitchman J, Kennedy JL. The serotonin 5-HT1B receptor gene and attention deficit hyperactivity disorder. *Mol Psychiatry* 2003;**8**:98–102.
87. Levitan RD, Masellis M, Lam RW, Muglia P, Basile VS, Jain U, Kaplan AS, Tharmalingam S, Kennedy SH, Kennedy JL. Childhood inattention and dysphoria and adult obesity associated with the dopamine D4 receptor gene in overeating women with seasonal affective disorder. *Neuropsychopharmacology* 2004;**29**:179–86.
88. Camarena B, Ruvinskis E, Santiago H, Montiel F, Cruz C, Gonzalez-Barranco J, Nicolini H. Serotonin transporter gene and obese females with impulsivity. *Mol Psychiatry* 2002;**7**:829–30.
89. Simon GE, Von Korff M, Saunders K, Miglioretti DL, Crane PK, van Belle G, Kessler RC. Association between obesity and psychiatric disorders in the US adult population. *Arch Gen Psychiatry* 2006;**63**:824–30.
90. Ellman LM, Schetter CD, Hobel CJ, Chicz-DeMet A, Glynn LM, Sandman CA. Timing of fetal exposure to stress hormones: Effects on newborn physical and neuromuscular maturation. *Developmental Psychobiology* 2008;**50**:232–41.
91. O'Connor TG, Heron J, Golding J, Glover V. Maternal antenatal anxiety and behavioural/emotional problems in children: a test of a programming hypothesis. *J Child Psychol Psychiatry* 2003;**44**:1025–36.
92. Rodriguez A, Waldenstrom U. Fetal origins of child non-right-handedness and mental health. *J Child Psychol Psychiatry* 2008;**49**:967–76.
93. Dallman MF, Pecoraro N, Akana SF, La Fleur SE, Gomez F, Houshyar H, Bell ME, Bhatnagar S, Laugero KD, Manalo S. Chronic stress and obesity: a new view of "comfort food". *Proc Natl Acad Sci U S A* 2003;**100**:11696–701.
94. Leung BMY, Kaplan BJ. Perinatal Depression: Prevalence, Risks, and the Nutrition Link—A Review of the Literature. *Journal of the American Dietetic Association* 2009;**109**(9):1566–75.
95. Wachs TD. Models linking nutritional deficiencies to maternal and child mental health. *Am J Clin Nutr* 2009;**89**:935S–9S.
96. WHO, The world health report 2001—mental health: new understanding, new hope. Geneva: World Health Organization; 2001.
97. Forssman L, Bohlin G, Lundervold AJ, Taanila A, Heiervang E, Loo S, Jarvelin MR, Smalley S, Moilanen I, Rodriguez A. Independent contributions of cognitive functioning and social risk factors to symptoms of ADHD in two Nordic populations-based cohorts. *Dev Neuropsychol* 2009;**34**:721–35.
98. Singh GK, Kogan MD, Van Dyck PC, Siahpush M. Racial/ethnic, socioeconomic, and behavioral determinants of childhood and adolescent obesity in the United States: analyzing independent and joint associations. *Ann Epidemiol* 2008;**18**:682–95.
99. Haggarty P, Campbell DM, Duthie S, Andrews K, Hoad G, Piyathilake C, McNeill G. Diet and deprivation in pregnancy. *Br J Nutr* 2009;**102**:1487–97.
100. Zhang Y, Proenca R, Maffei M, Barone M, Leopold L, Friedman JM. Positional cloning of the mouse obese gene and its human homologue. *Nature* 1994;**372**:425–32.
101. Catalano PM, Ehrenberg HM. The short- and long-term implications of maternal obesity on the mother and her offspring. *BJOG: An International Journal of Obstetrics and Gynaecology* 2006;**113**:1126–33.

CHAPTER 16

Sleep and Obesity in Children and Adolescents

Amy Darukhanavala, Silvana Pannain

Department of Medicine, Section of Adult and Pediatrics, Endocrinology, Diabetes, and Metabolism,
The University of Chicago, IL, USA

INTRODUCTION

Over the past few decades childhood and adolescent obesity have increased significantly worldwide. Genetic factors alone cannot explain the rapid and alarming increase of excess weight in children. Such phenomena since the late 1970s likely reflects behavioral, environmental, and social factors such as more time spent watching television or using the computer, decreased physical activity, and probably increased energy intake [1–3] and the interaction of the gene pool with these factors. Important changes in lifestyle have taken place during the past few decades, which have affected both adults and children. Particularly, a decline of habitual sleep duration among children and adolescents has been observed [4–6], which parallels the increase of overweight. The occurrence in parallel of these two phenomena has raised the question of a possible role of short sleep in the expanding epidemic of obesity [7], and since the late 1980s epidemiology and in laboratory studies have explored the link between short sleep and risk of obesity. Additionally, the increased prevalence and severity of obesity in children has led to an increase in sleep disorders related to excess weight, such as the obstructive sleep apnea syndrome (OSAS) and the hypoventilation syndrome. Although compelling literature both in the adult and pediatric population demonstrates a causative role of obesity on obstructive sleep apnea (OSA), more recent studies have began to suggest an inversed causative relationship between obesity and OSA such that OSA may play a potentiating role in weight gain.

In the following sections, we first review the epidemiological studies that have shown an association between short sleep and obesity in children and adolescents. We later examine the laboratory studies in adults that have analyzed the effect of sleep restriction on the neurohormonal control of appetite, and we formulate hypotheses on the possible mechanisms linking short sleep and the risk of obesity. Finally, we briefly review the pediatric sleep disorders that are related to obesity and propose that one of the common sleep disorders, OSA, may contribute to the epidemic of obesity.

PREVALENCE OF OBESITY AND SHORT SLEEP IN CHILDREN AND ADOLESCENTS

Prevalence of Obesity

Within the past few decades, the prevalence of obesity in children has increased so significantly that the World Health Organization has declared it a global epidemic. The National Health and Nutrition Examination Survey (NHANES), conducted in 2007–2008, found that 17% of children 2 to 19 years old were obese (defined as body mass index (BMI) ≥ 95th percentile for-age growth chart) [8]. This is triple the 5% to 6% estimation of the NHANES II (1976–1980). Twelve percent of children are considered more severely obese (≥97% BMI) [8], outnumbering those affected by childhood cystic fibrosis, HIV, juvenile diabetes, and cancer combined. Similar trends have been observed in many countries throughout the world [9–12]. Obese children and adolescents are likely to become obese adults [13–14] and to develop a variety of comorbidities such as diabetes, cardiovascular disease, OSAS, polycystic ovarian syndrome, nonalcoholic fatty liver disease, orthopedic disorders, pseudotumor cerebri, and psychological dysfunction [15–16]. As obesity rates in children reached record levels, an interest in the role of behavioral risk factors, including sleep curtailment, has been the topic of recent research studies.

Many factors play a role in the development of obesity. It is assumed that polygenic factors, combined with poor behavioral and environmental factors, contribute to the epidemic of childhood obesity [17–18]. Although twin and adoption studies have indicated that genetic factors have a significant role in obesity predisposition, the rapid increase in obesity over the past few decades cannot be explained by a change in the genetic pool alone but rather by the interaction of the preexisting genetic pool with environmental, socioeconomic, and demographic factors [19–20]. If genetic factors confer susceptibility to obesity, the environment may modulate the phenotypic expression [19]. The rapid behavioral and environmental changes that have occurred in modern society are likely to have contributed to the changes in the phenotypic expression of obesity [12, 21–22]. Excess prepackaged and processed food, an overabundance of fast food, ready availability of sweetened drinks, increased portion sizes, decreased family meals, and an increasingly sedentary lifestyle may all contribute to the problem [12, 22–23]. It is estimated that 25% of children between the ages of 8 and 16 spend about 4 hours a day watching television, whereas physical activity and sports are on the decline at school [24–26].

Prevalence of Short Sleep in Children and Adolescents

The hectic pace of the modern world has negatively affected the lives of children and adolescents not only through poor diet and exercise habits but also through poor sleep habits. There is increasing concern of decreased sleep times in children [4–6]. Different ages have different sleep requirements [27]. On average, as a child ages, sleep requirement declines, although substantial individual variability exists at all ages. In general, children younger than 5 years old require at least 11 hours of sleep a day and children 5 to 10 years of age need at least 10 hours [28]. Children and adolescents over 10 years of age need 9 or more hours of sleep a day [29].

Unfortunately, few studies exist with age-specific reference values from infancy through adolescence with large study populations. Most studies examined a small number of children, limited age groups, or did not analyze the interindividual variability. As a result, complete normative data on children's sleep duration as a function of chronological age is not well established. A longitudinal prospective study conducted by Iglowstein et al. followed 493 subjects using structured sleep-related questionnaires at 1, 3, 6, 9, 12, 18, and 24 months after birth and then at annual intervals until 16 years of age. Total sleep duration decreased from an average of 14.2 hours (STDEV: 1.9 hours) at 6 months of age to an average of 8.1 hours (STDEV: 0.8 hours) at 16 years of age (Fig. 16.1) [30]. Although normative sleep duration data are scarce, it is recognized that sleep duration has decreased significantly in the pediatric population and that generally accepted sleep requirements are not being met [31–32].

The study further compared three birth cohorts (in 1974, 1979, and 1986) and noted a decreasing trend of the mean total sleep duration across the cohorts in infants and young children and continuing up to adolescence. Although laboratory studies have assessed that sleep need does not change substantially across adolescence (9 hours in 10- to 17-year-olds), a 2006 survey conducted by the U.S. National Sleep Foundation's "Sleep in Adolescents Poll" showed that self-reported average sleep durations was under 9 hours in this age group and decreased from 8.4 hours at ages 11 to 12 years to only 6.9 hours by ages 17 and 18 years. More than half of the respondents reported feeling tired and sleepy during the day [33]. If sleep need in adolescents has been estimated at approximately 9 hours per night [29–30, 34], modern-day U.S. adolescents appears to run a significant sleep debt.

Another study by Snell et al. showed that although the majority of children achieved appropriate sleep over the weekend, on weekdays 13% of children aged 3 to 7 years slept less than 9 hours; 11% of children aged 8 to 12 years slept less than 8 hours, and 6% of children aged 13 to 18 years slept less than 7 hours [35]. Although young children went to sleep later, wake time remained unchanged. Sleep deprivation observed in preadolescents and adolescents is in part the result of environmental and social factors including excessive homework or after-school activities, active social lives, video or computer games, late-night television, or early start school times. Adolescents are more at risk of chronic sleep deprivation as the early school time conflicts with the natural delay of the circadian control of sleep propensity that is typical of this age [34, 36].

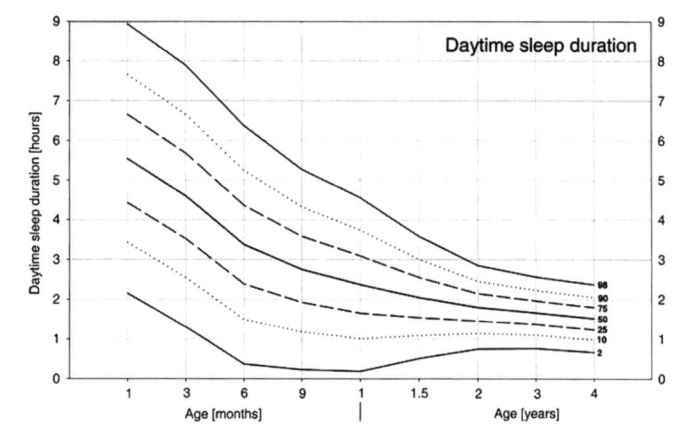

FIGURE 16.1 Percentiles for total sleep duration per 24 hours from infancy to adolescence (Adapted from Iglowstein, I., et al., Sleep duration from infancy to adolescence: reference values and generational trends. Pediatrics, 2003, 111(2): 302–307.)

Sleep, like physical activity and diet, plays an important role in the growth, maturation, and health of children and adolescents. It is well known that decreased sleep duration has immediate negative effects on the pediatric population, including behavioral problems, poor concentration [37–39], and an increased susceptibility to illness [40]. Given the nation's pediatric obesity epidemic and the concomitant shortened sleep duration, researchers have begun investigating the correlation between recent trends in increased obesity and sleep problems [4–5, 41–42]. In adults, multiple epidemiology association studies and laboratory intervention studies have suggested that sleep curtailment may contribute to obesity through a variety of mechanisms, which include changes in appetite-regulating hormones, eating patterns and caloric intake, and possibly physical activity and energy expenditure. Although a parallel epidemiological literature is available in children, similar laboratory studies do not currently exist because enforced sleep curtailment on the pediatric population would not be deemed appropriate. Conclusions of a possible impact of short sleep duration on the risk of obesity in children are derived either from epidemiological association studies in children or adolescents or by extrapolations from adult laboratory studies.

EPIDEMIOLOGICAL EVIDENCE OF A LINK BETWEEN SLEEP LOSS AND OBESITY

In adults sleep curtailment has been linked to the risk of weight gain in multiple epidemiological and a few laboratory studies. In children and adolescents similar and often large-scale epidemiological studies have been conducted and demonstrated an increased prevalence and incidence of obesity if sleep is restricted. Overall the findings of the pediatric studies are more robust than the adult studies, suggesting that the relationship between sleep duration and weight may weaken with age [43]. The studies in children and adolescents are summarized in Table 16.1 and Table 16.2 and described in detail here. The majority of these studies have been cross-sectional in design and sleep measures were obtained by self-report. Although the studies were conducted in different countries and cultures, they consistently demonstrate a significant association between short sleep and the risk of obesity.

Epidemiology Studies in Children

Up to the date of this publication, 16 studies have examined the relationship between sleep and obesity specifically in children. The studies are summarized in Table 16.1. A limitation shared by most of these studies is that they are cross-sectional in design and sleep duration is self-reported. The earliest of these studies published in 1992 by Locard et al. is a case-controlled study examining the relationship between sleep duration and risk of obesity in approximately a thousand French 5-year-old children (327 cases versus 704 controls) [44]. The authors looked at environmental factors related to lifestyle that could be associated with obesity at age 5. Obesity at this age predicts approximately 50% of cases of obesity by ages 10 and 12. The analysis found that short sleep duration had a dose effect relationship with obesity at age 5, even after adjusting for a highly predictive confounding factor such as parental overweight. In 2002, Von Kries et al. confirmed a dose-response effect in a larger German cohort of similar age in which the prevalence of overweight (BMI > 90th percentile) and obesity (BMI > 97th percentile) decreased with increased duration of sleep [45]. Specifically, after controlling for other lifestyle factors, the prevalence of obesity was 5.4% in the children who slept ≤10 hours versus 2.1% in children who slept ≥11.5 hours. Similarly, a Japanese study of more than 8000 children aged 6 to 7 years found an inverse dose-response relationship between hours of sleep and obesity, after adjusting for age, sex, parental obesity, physical activity, TV watching, and snacking [46]. One weakness of this study is that the analysis was not controlled for low socioeconomic status, often associated with obesity [47] and possibly with decreased sleep hours [48].

The "Quebec en Forme" project on 422 Canadian children aged 5 to 10 also confirmed the dose-response effects of sleep duration on the risk of childhood weight and obesity after adjusting for age, sex, parental obesity, and other risk factors [49]. A Portuguese study of 4390 school children aged 7 to 9 was the first to examine gender differences [48]. Although for the entire cohort, children who slept more had a decreased risk of overweight and obesity, when the data were analyzed by gender, a significant association with short sleep duration was only found for the obese boys and the overweight girls. Four additional cross-sectional studies conducted in four different countries further suggest that the association between short sleep and obesity spans different countries, cultures, and ethnicities [50–54]. One of these studies, conducted in Brazil on 6- to 10-year-old children, is unique because it measures obesity by percentage body fat rather than the BMI [52]. It is considered that percentage body fat may be a more specific measure of adiposity than BMI.

In one retrospective and cross-sectional study, Lumeng et al. assessed sleep hours and weight in 785 children in third and sixth grade. The study found that for every additional hour of sleep in sixth grade, the child was 20% less likely to be overweight. In addition,

TABLE 16.1 [a] Summary of the Findings from Studies Looking at the Association between Sleep and Obesity in Children

Author	Sample size	Study design	Country	Age (years)	Sleep assessment	Summary of findings
Locard et al. [44]	1031♂♀	Cross-sectional	France	5	Parents reported sleep duration	Risk of OB:<10 h OR = 4.9 10–11 h OR = 2.8 11–12 h OR = 2.0 >12 h Reference
Sekine et al. [46]	8941♂♀	Cross-sectional	Japan	6–7	Parents reported sleep duration	Risk of OB<8 h OR 2.9 8–9 h OR 1.9 9–10 h OR 1.49 >10 h Reference
Ben Slama et al. [50]	167♂	Cross-sectional	Tunisia	6–10	Parents reported sleep duration	Sleep duration of <8 h associated with increased obesity risk
Von Kries et al. [45]	6862♂♀	Cross-sectional	Germany	5–6	Parents reported sleep duration	Prevalence of OB:<10 h = 5.4% 10.5–11 h = 2.8% >11.5 h = 2.1%
Hui et al. [51]	343♂♀	Cross-sectional	Hong Kong	Mean 6.7	Parents reported sleep duration	Multivariate OR of overweight (BMI > 92nd percentile)< 9 h OR: 1.0) 9–11 h OR: 0.54 > 11 h OR: 0.31
Giugliano et al. [52]	97♂♀	Cross-sectional	Brazil	6–10	Self-reported sleep duration	Percentage of body fat inversely correlated to hours of sleep (r = −0.278, p < 0.02)
Agras et al. [56]	150♂♀	Prospective 9.5 y	United States	Birth	Parents reported sleep duration	Children OW at 9 y slept 30 min. less at 3–5 y
Padez et al. [48]	4411♂♀	Cross-sectional	Portugal	7–9.7	Parents reported sleep duration	OR of overweight 8 h Reference 9–10 h: 0.46 >11 h: 0.44 OR of Obesity 8 h Reference 9–10 h: 0.44 >11 h OR: 0.39
Reilly et al. [2]	6426♂♀	Prospective 7 y	United Kingdom	Birth	Parents reported sleep duration	Risk of obesity at age 7 with sleep duration at age 3:<10.5 h OR: 1.57 10.5–10.9 h OR: 1.31 11–11.9 h OR: 0.94 >12 h OR: Reference
Eisenmann et al. [53]	6324♂♀	Cross-sectional	Australia	7–15	Self-reported sleep duration	Risk of OW/OB *Boys*:<8h OR: 3.8–9 h OR: 1.8 3–9–10h OR: 1.6 10 h Reference *Girls*:No change
Chaput et al. [49]	422♂♀	Cross-sectional	Canada	5–10	Parents reported sleep duration	Risk of OW/OB 8–10 h OR = 3.4 10.5–11.5 h OR = 1.42 12–13 h = Reference c
Dieu et al. [54]	670♂♀	Cross-sectional	Vietnam	4–6	Parents reported sleep duration	Prevalence ratio OW/OB of 0.85 for longer sleep duration
Lumeng et al. [29]	785♂♀	Cross-sectional retrospective	United States	9–12	Parents reported sleep duration	1 h additional sleep at 12y = OR OW 0.81 h additional sleep at 9y = OR OW 0.60 at 12
Snell et al. [35]	1441♂♀	Longitudinal	United States	8–13.6	Parents reported sleep duration (sleep diaries)	1 h additional sleep at 8y = 5.3% decrease in likelihood of OW at 13.6y

[a]In each study the risk of obesity in relationship to sleep time is expressed as odds ratio or prevalence of obesity (%), unless those data were not available. Studies are listed by year of publication.
Abbreviations: odds ratio (OR); overweight (OW); obesity (OB); years (y); hours (h); ♂ male; ♀ female

TABLE 16.2 [a] Summary of the Findings from Studies Looking at the Association between Sleep and Obesity in Adolescents

Author	Sample size	Study design	Country	Age (years)	Sleep assessment	Summary of findings
Gupta et al. [58]	383♂♀	Cross-sectional	United States	11–16	Wrist Actigraphy	For every hour of increased sleep, OR of OB decreases by 80%
Benefice et al. [59]	40♀	Cross-sectional	Senegal	13	Accelerometer	1 kg/m2 increase in BMI associated with 6.85 min decrease in sleep duration
Knutson et al. [60]	4486♂♀	Cross-sectional	United States	13–18	Self-reported sleep duration	♂ Sleep duration predicted OW (OR 0.9, p = 0.04) ♀: no effect
Chen et al. [62]	656♂♀	Cross-sectional	Taiwan	13–18	Self-reported sleep duration	Higher frequency of adequate sleep (6–8 h on >4 weekdays) associated with 1.74 OR of non-OB
Seicean et al. [63]	509♂♀	Cross-sectional	United States	14–17		OR of OB <5 h OR: 7.65; 5–6 h OR: 2.8; 6–7 h OR: 2.55; 7–8 h OR: 1.38> 8 h: Reference
Yu et al. [61]	500 twins♂♀	Cross-sectional	China	10–20	Self-reported sleep duration	♂: no significant association sleep duration and measures of adiposity♀; U shaped relationship, most notable for ≥ 14 y

[a]In each study the risk of obesity in relationship to sleep time is expressed as odds ratio or prevalence of obesity (%), unless those data were not available. Studies are listed by year of publication.
Abbreviations: odds ratio (OR); overweight (OW); obesity (OB); years (y); hours (h); ♂ male; ♀ female

for every additional hour of sleep in third grade, the child was 40% less likely to be overweight in sixth grade, independent of the child's weight in third grade [29]. Three prospective studies have been conducted in children thus far. These studies examined the risk factors early in life that were associated with obesity later in childhood. The largest study conducted by Reilly et al. [2] analyzed a data set from the Avon Longitudinal Study of Parents and Children conducted in the United Kingdom [55]. More than 8000 children of both genders were followed prospectively from birth to age 7. The authors examined 25 putative early life risk factors for obesity and, using multivariate analysis, found that only birth weight, parental obesity, sleep duration, and television viewing were independently associated with the risk of obesity in the entire cohort. A smaller study by Agras et al. [56] on 150 U.S. children also found that short sleep duration as reported by parents at age 3 to 5 predicted the risk of being overweight at age 9.5. More recently, Snell et al. published data on a sample of approximately 1400 children from a larger American longitudinal database [35]. The authors showed that children who get less sleep tend to weigh more 5 years later. When the association between sleep duration and BMI was examined by age groups, an extra hour of sleep cut the likelihood of being overweight from 36% to 30% in children aged 3 to 8, and from 34% to 30% in those aged 8 to 13 [35].

Epidemiology Studies in Adolescents

Although adolescents are a population that may be at particular risk of chronic partial sleep loss [57], only six studies are available at this time that look at the relationship between sleep duration and the risk of overweight and obesity in this age group. The studies are summarized in Table 16.2. Unique in the methodology are the Heartfelt study [58] and a smaller subsequent study by Benefice et al. [59] as both adopted more objective measures of sleep other than self-reported sleep duration. The Heartfelt study [58] used 24-hour wrist actigraphy to estimate sleep duration and sleep disturbance in 383 11- to 16-year-old boys and girls. Findings demonstrated that in adolescents, sleep duration is negatively associated with obesity so that for each hour of sleep loss, the chance of obesity is increased by 80%. Sleep disturbance, but not sleep duration, appeared to be weakly associated with decreased physical activity, which suggests that sleep disturbance could indirectly affect the risk of obesity by a reduction in daytime physical activity. Benefice et al. [59] objectively measured sleep duration with an accelerometer worn for 3 days and 4 consecutive nights by 40 13- to 14-year-old Senegalese girls. The authors found that sleep duration was reduced by 6.85 minutes for every 1 kg/m2 increase in BMI. Because this study was run in rural Africa, they hypothesized that the increased sleep length in thinner girls would occur to spare energy.

Although cross-sectional studies cannot address the causal direction between sleep duration and weight, the dominant hypothesis is that short sleep duration leads to increased weight through mechanisms that are not yet fully understood. Benefice et al. suggested that the inverse relationship could be true at least in a developing country [59]. Knutson et al. examined a data set of 4486 American teenagers from the National Longitudinal Study of Adolescent Health, mean age 16.6 years [60]. When analyzed by gender, each hour increase in self-reported sleep duration was associated with a 10% reduction in risk of being overweight in boys, but the same effect was not found in girls. In contrast, Yu et al., in a study of 500 twins, showed that short sleep duration was associated with higher adiposity in females but not in males [61].

Both groups of researchers commented that these sex-differences may be explained by gender-specific physiology changes that accompany puberty. The novelty in the study by Yu et al. is that they introduced body composition by Duel Energy X-ray Absorptiometry scan and waist circumference as additional measures of adiposity and show that these measures have a stronger inverse relationship with short sleep than BMI [61]. Furthermore, this is the only study showing a U-shaped relationship between sleep duration and adiposity in adolescents so that both short (<8 hours) and long sleep duration (≥9 hours) in girls tended to have higher adiposity measures than 8 to 8.9 hours. Chen et al. found in a study of 656 Taiwanese school teenagers (mean age 15.0 years) that overall 54% reported getting less than adequate sleep on school days, defined in this study as 6 to 8 hours per night on more than 4 weekdays per week [62]. Middle school adolescents had a higher frequency of adequate sleep compared to high school. Furthermore, after controlling for gender and school grade, the frequency of obtaining adequate sleep was directly associated with normal-weight (P < 0.001), healthy behaviors, including a healthy diet, regular exercise, and a lower incidence of doctor and hospital visits [62].

Seican et al.'s cross-sectional study assessed lifestyle and sleep behaviors in 529 students from Ohio in the United States (mean age 15.6 ± 1.23) [63]. As much as 90% of students reported less than 8 hours average sleep time, and 19% reported less than 6 hours of sleep per night on school nights. Sleep duration appeared to have a dose effect on the likelihood of being overweight. Compared with students sleeping >8 hours, the age and gender-adjusted odds ratio of being overweight was 8.53 (95% Confidence Interval (CI): 2.26, 32.14) for those who slept <5 hours (P = 0.0036), 2.79 (95% CI :1.03, 7.55) for those who slept 5 to 6 hours, 2.81 (95% CI 1.14, 6.91) for those with 6 to 7 hours of sleep, and 1.29 (95% CI 0.52, 3.26) for those getting 7 to 8 hours of sleep.

In summary, multiple studies published in less than two decades support the hypothesis of an association between short sleep and increased BMI in children and adolescents. The consistent findings from studies spanning multiple countries and continents suggest that the association is independent of culture or ethnicity. A few studies in the pediatric population have attempted to identify the causal pathway linking sleep duration to obesity. Von Kries et al. found no relationship between habitual sleep duration and caloric intake [45]. Gupta et al. and Benefice et al. estimated activity levels and found no relationship between sleep duration and physical activity [58–59]. In general while cross-sectional studies strongly suggest an association, they do not inform on the direction of causality. More longitudinal and interventional studies are needed to uncover a causative role of short sleep duration on the risk of obesity.

The finding of a U-shaped relationship between sleep duration and obesity in the study by Yu et al. in the adolescents is concordant to a similar finding in four epidemiological studies in adults [64–67]. When trying to understand the significance of this U-shaped relationship, it must be taken in consideration that sleep duration is based on self-report. Are self-reported long sleepers truly getting that much sleep or are they just spending longer hours in bed trying to sleep? The latter would reflect poor sleep quality, which could be caused by sleep disordered breathing, insomnia or depression, conditions that are more frequent in adolescents and adults than in children. One alternative explanation is that long sleep leads to less time for physical activity and therefore the association between long sleep and obesity would not persist when adjusting for physical activity. At this time there is no known physiological mechanism to explain how too much sleep could lead to obesity. Without more objective measures of sleep duration and quality and without more mechanistic laboratory studies, it is premature to say that long sleep has unfavorable effects on weight.

LABORATORY EVIDENCE FOR A LINK BETWEEN SLEEP LOSS AND OBESITY

Although multiple epidemiological studies have pointed to an association between sleep loss and the increased risk of obesity in the pediatric population, the direction of causality and the underlying mechanisms are still unclear. The effect of sleep on metabolism and hormonal circadian rhythms in adults and children has been known for several years [68], whereas the discovery of the orexin system has provided the first clue of a molecular mechanism that links sleep to feeding [69–71]. To date there have been only few prospective intervention studies that attempt to explain the relationship between sleep loss and feeding, and these have been exclusively in adults in the laboratory setting. No laboratory studies exist at this time in children because of the ethical restrictions of imposing curtailed sleep on the pediatric population [72]. In this section we review the results of these studies. In the next section we attempt to formulate a hypothesis on molecular mechanisms linking sleep loss and the risk of weight gain, and we will assume that such mechanisms act both in the adult and in the pediatric populations.

The pioneer laboratory studies by Spiegel et al. looked at the impact of recurrent partial sleep deprivation in healthy young men [73, 74] and demonstrated a disruption of the neuroendocrine regulation of appetite as the levels of the anorexigenic hormone leptin were markedly decreased throughout the 24-hour cycle [73, 74], whereas the levels of the orexigenic factor ghrelin were found to be increased [74]. The changes in appetite regulation in the sleep debt condition were paralleled by an increase in the peripheral sympathetic nervous activity [74]. Scores of hunger, global appetite, and food preferences revealed increased hunger and appetite (particularly for calorie-dense foods with high carbohydrate content such as sweets, salty snacks, and starchy foods) when the subjects were sleep deprived [73]. These findings suggest that if exposed to *ad libitum* food the subjects, under sleep restriction, would have increased their food intake and possibly gained weight over time. A more recent study in healthy young adults estimated that after four nights of restricted sleep, participants ate in average 460 ± 196 more kcal from a *ad libitum* buffet as compared to the eating behavior that occurred after baseline sleep [75]. A sleep restriction study of 14 nights demonstrated an increased consumption of carbohydrates and calories mostly from snacks, particularly in the evening and overnight; however, it did not show changes in serum leptin and ghrelin levels [76].

In general, since the seminal publication by Spiegel et al. [74], a handful of laboratory studies of total or partial sleep restriction have been reproduced exclusively in adults and have reported variable results on hunger, food intake, and leptin and ghrelin levels [75–79]. The different results may be attributed to difference in the study design such as the duration of the sleep restriction protocol (few versus several days) and the calorie intake during the leptin and ghrelin measurements (controlled calorie restriction in the early studies [74] versus *at libitum* intake in more recent studies [76, 78]). One may postulate that the effect of sleep restriction on the neuroendocrine regulation of appetite mostly manifests in conditions of calorie restriction with a decrease in serum leptin, an increase in serum ghrelin, an increase in hunger, and possibly a decrease in energy expenditure. In this way sleep restriction could undermine the success to a low-calorie diet by decreasing the compliance to the dietary regimen and its efficacy.

In summary, data emerging from the laboratory studies in adults indicate that reduced sleep duration may increase the risk of weight gain and obesity via a decrease in leptin, an increase in ghrelin, and an overall increase in hunger. Limited evidence from population studies support a role of leptin in the link between short sleep and BMI [80–81]. Similar studies have not been reproduced in the pediatric population, but it is conceivable that the same mechanisms through which sleep loss affects metabolism and the increased risk of obesity in adults could operate in children and adolescents. A review of the regulation of body fat and the connection between sleeping, feeding, and metabolism is provided next as a background to formulate some hypotheses.

PUTATIVE MECHANISMS LINKING SLEEP LOSS AND THE RISK OF WEIGHT GAIN AND OBESITY

Neuroendocrine Regulation of Energy Balance and the Potential Impact of Sleep Loss

Body fat stores are regulated by a complex physiological process involving cross-talk between the periphery and the brain, a process that ultimately affects the balance between energy intake and expenditure. Figure 16.2 provides a schematic representation of the cross-talk between brain and periphery, which regulates energy homoeostasis. Figure 16.3 summarizes some of the main pathways connecting sleep-wake and energy homeostasis and identifies putative targets for the adverse impact of sleep restriction.

The orexin system likely plays a key role in the interaction between sleeping and feeding. It is now known that the orexin-producing neurons are the origin of an extensive and divergent projection system innervating numerous structures in the central nervous system (CNS) including all the components of the ascending arousal system and the entire cortex [82]. This system is involved in the regulation of many functions such as sleep-wakefulness, locomotor activity, feeding, thermoregulation, and neuroendocrine and cardiovascular control [83]. The orexins (or hypocretins) are two distinct neuropeptides (orexin A and B) synthesized mainly by neurons in the lateral hypothalamus area (LHA) and perifornical area (PFA) (Fig. 16.2), a region classically referred to as the "feeding center." This notion stimulated the in vivo studies in rodents that demonstrated the central role of the orexins in the link between sleep-wake cycle and feeding. Orexins induce and support arousal and promote feeding, particularly at a time when normal food intake is low [83] (Fig. 16.3). Proper maintenance of wakefulness is crucial for food search and intake, and the orexins represent the molecular basis of this vital interaction. Orexigenic neurons are firing during the wake period and are inactive during non-Rapid Eye Movement (non-REM) sleep also referred to as slow wave sleep because of the direct inhibition by GABA-ergic hypothalamic neurons [84].

As represented in Figures 16.2 and 16.3, the activity of the orexigenic neurons in the control of energy

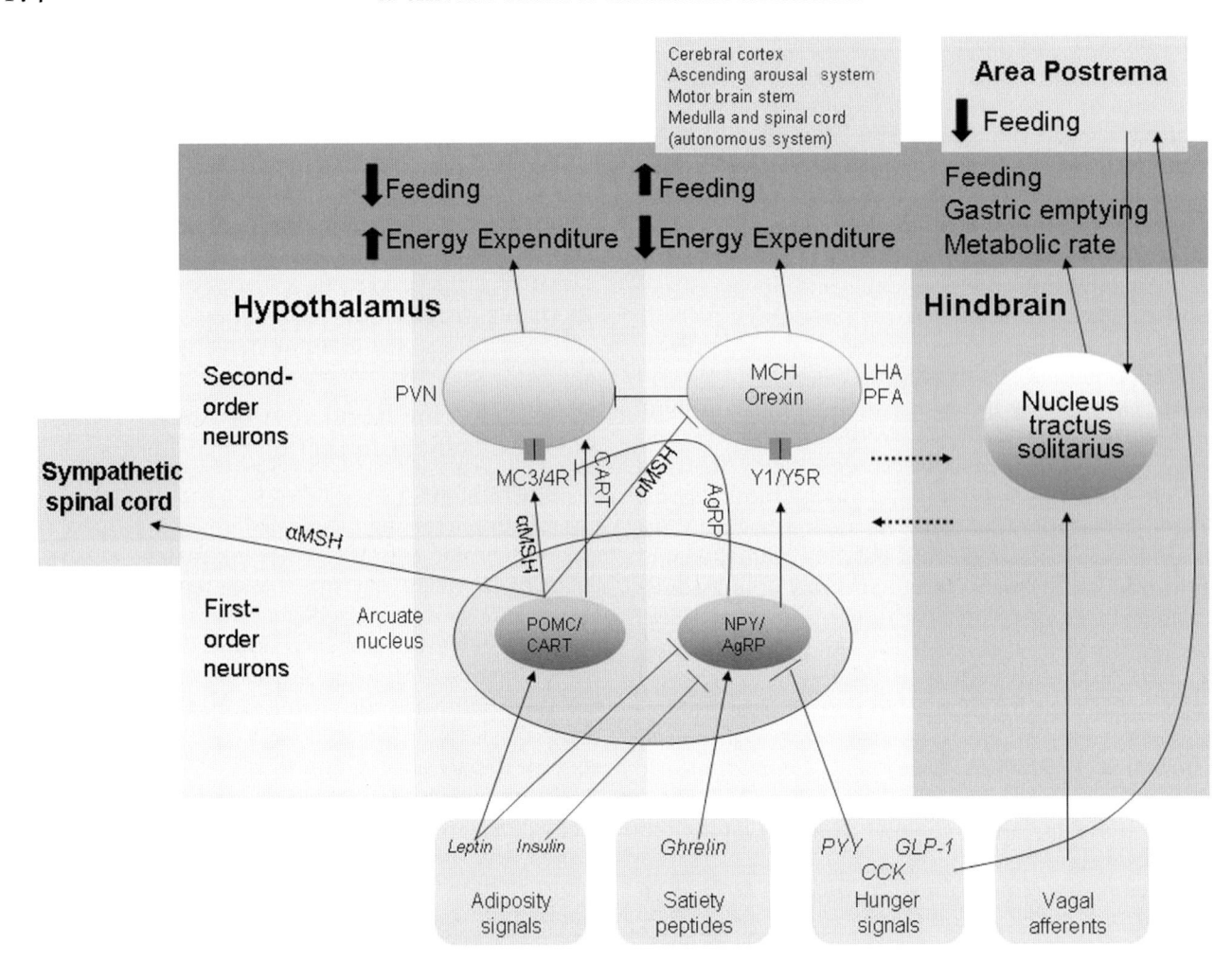

FIGURE 16.2 Schematic representation of the cross-talk between the periphery and the brain, which regulate energy homeostasis. The orexins synthesized by neurons in the lateral hypothalamus area (LHA) and perifornical area (PFA) have direct appetite-stimulating effects in part mediated by stimulation of NeuroPeptide Y (NPY) neurons in the arcuate nucleus (ARC). The ARC is a key region in the central homeostatic control of appetite and contains the "first-order" neurons where afferent signals from the periphery are integrated with central stimuli in a neuronal response. Among the afferent peripheral signals are leptin and ghrelin. Leptin acts in the ARC to stimulate anorexigenic and simultaneously inhibit orexigenic neurons. In contrast, ghrelin stimulates appetite, partly by activating NPY neurons in the ARC. The first-order neurons project then to "second-order" neurons, which are made up of neurons in the PVN and the orexin producing neurons in the lateral hypothalamus area (LHA) and perifornical area (PFA).

homeostasis is regulated by peripheral metabolic cues. During starvation, orexin neurons may be disinhibited by low levels of the anorexigenic hormone leptin and low glucose levels [84] and are excited by the orexigenic hormone ghrelin [85]. Peripheral metabolic cues, including glucose, leptin, cholecystokinin, and ghrelin, might also influence the activity of the orexin neurons via vagal afferents to the Nucleus Tractus Solitarius (NST) (Fig. 16.2). The orexins conversely have direct appetite-stimulating effects in part mediated by an increase in the activity of NeuroPeptide Y (NPY) neurons in the arcuate nucleus (ARC) in the hypothalamus. The ARC is a key region in the central homeostatic control of appetite and contains both appetite-promoting neurons (NPY and agouti-related peptide [AgRP] neurons) and appetite-inhibiting neurons (pro-opiomelanocortin [POMC] and cocaine- and amphetamine-related transcript [CART] neurons) (Fig. 16.2). These neurons in the ARC represent the "first-order" neurons in the hypothalamus where afferent signals from the periphery are integrated with central stimuli in a neuronal response. Among the afferent peripheral signals are again leptin, a 142-amino-acid peptide secreted by adipocytes, and ghrelin, released mainly by the stomach. Leptin acts in the ARC to stimulate anorexigenic and simultaneously inhibit orexigenic neuronal activity. In contrast, ghrelin stimulates appetite, partly by activating NPY neurons in the ARC [86]. The "first-order" neurons project then to "second-order" neurons, which are made up of neurons in the hypothalamic paraventricular nucleus (PVN) and the orexin producing neurons in the lateral

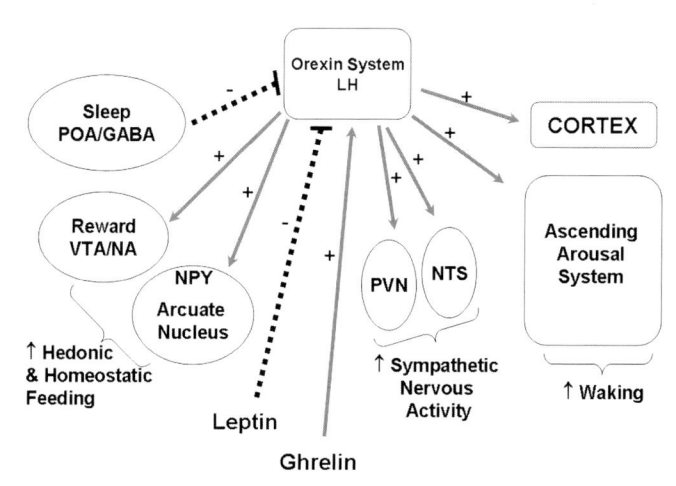

FIGURE 16.3 Schematic of the orexin system. The orexigenic neurons play a major role in the maintenance of arousal by activating the ascending arousal system and the entire cerebral cortex. Orexin activity is also involved in the regulation of feeding by acting on the arcuate nucleus, the nucleus tractus solitarius (NTS), the paraventricular nucleus (PVN), and on the ventro-tegmental area (VTA) and nucleus accumbens (NA) and by increasing sympathetic activity which will in turn inhibit leptin release and stimulate ghrelin release. Lower leptin and higher ghrelin levels will act in concert to further activate orexin neurons resulting in an increased drive for both homeostatic and nonhomeostatic food intake. (Adapted from S Pannain et al., Sleep loss, obesity and diabetes: prevalence, association and emerging evidence for causation. Obesity and Metabolism, 2008, 4(1): 28–41.)

The multiple roles of the orexin system in the control of sleep-wake regulation, homeostatic and hedonic feeding, and sympathetic nervous activity that are schematically illustrated in Figure 16.3 provide a framework to develop hypotheses on the mechanisms linking sleep loss and obesity. The maintenance of extended wakefulness against the homeostatic pressure for sleep requires an overactivation of the orexin neurons, which leads to cortical activation, maintenance of activity in the ascending arousal system, and inhibition of the sleep-active centers in the preoptic area. Such up-regulation of the orexin system could be mediated by the stimulation of the sympathetic nervous system. Indeed, protracted activity in the ascending arousal system will result in increased sympathetic nervous activity, which is consistent with the findings of the studies of sleep deprivation [73, 92]. Increased sympathetic nervous activity will in turn inhibit leptin release and stimulate ghrelin release, in concordance with the effects of short sleep on the peripheral levels of both hormones observed in human studies [65, 73–74, 81]. Lower leptin levels and higher ghrelin levels may act in concert to activate orexin neurons, resulting in an increased drive for both homeostatic and nonhomeostatic food intake. The direct impact of lower leptin and higher ghrelin levels on the orexin system could be heightened by their synergetic appetite-promoting effects on neuronal centers in the ARC.

hypothalamus area (LHA) and perifornical area (PFA). However, the system is redundant as there is also evidence that leptin and ghrelin directly affect the orexin system, with leptin-inhibiting and ghrelin-stimulating orexinergic activity, respectively [87–88] (Fig. 16.3).

Consistent with the fact that sympathetic nervous activity is higher during wake than during sleep, the orexin activity is associated with increased sympathetic tone, an effect mediated in part through the stimulation of neurons in the NTS and the PVN [87]. An orexin effect on sympathetic activity could explain the changes in sympathovagal balance reported in laboratory studies of sleep restriction in humans [73, 89]. The NTS integrates peripheral vagal afferent signals with satiety signals from the area postrema and directly modulates the activity of first-order neurons in the ARC and second-order neurons in the PVN, zona incerta, PFA, and the lateral hypothalamic area (LHA) [86] (Figs. 16.2 and 16.3).

Recently, a role for the orexin system in reward processing and addiction has been demonstrated as suggested by the finding that orexin producing neurons in the LHA send dense projections to the dopaminergic ventro-tegmental area (VTA) and nucleus accumbens (NA) [90–91], regions that are important in the hedonic control of food intake.

Peripheral Signals of Energy Balance and the Potential Impact of Sleep Loss

As described earlier, the state of wakefulness maintained by the orexin system is associated with increased sympathetic nervous activity. Increased peripheral sympathetic tone in sleep deprivation may in turn inhibit leptin release and stimulate ghrelin release, consistent with the effects of short sleep on the peripheral levels of both hormones observed in adults [65, 73, 74, 81]. Additionally, both acute total deprivation and partial sleep deprivation in healthy individuals are associated with an increase in serum C-reactive protein (CRP) concentrations [93]. It has been suggested that CRP is a leptin binding protein [94] and increased CRP levels as seen in obesity have been proposed as a possible mechanism of leptin resistance. In a similar fashion, CRP increase seen in sleep loss may reduce the amount of free leptin available to penetrate the blood-brain barrier and promote satiety. The combination in the sleep deprivation condition of the reduced leptin levels possibly secondary to increased sympathetic activity with the increased leptin-binding capacity secondary to higher CRP levels might lead to a larger negative impact on energy balance than that of the leptin reduction alone.

Energy Expenditure and the Potential Impact of Sleep Loss

It is also possible that sleep loss has an adverse effect on energy expenditure, which has an important role in the control of body weight and adiposity. The amount of total daily energy expenditure (TEE) is divided into three components: (1) *resting metabolic rate* (RMR, 60% of TEE) defined as the energy expenditure of an individual under basal conditions (at rest, fasting the morning after sleep); (2) *thermic effects of meal* (TEM 10% of TEE), which includes the energy expenditure involved in digestion, absorption metabolism, and storage of food; (3) *activity-related energy expenditure* (AEE, 30% of TEE), which involves all volitional and nonvolitional activities. For most individuals, AEE is not accounted by physical exercise but rather by low-moderate intensity activities of daily living such as sitting, standing, walking, and other occupational, volitional, and spontaneous activities together referred to as nonexercise activity thermogenesis (NEAT) [95]. AEE is the most variable component of TEE, has a major weight in the energy balance equation, and is critical for long-term weight maintenance Whether sleep loss has an impact on TEE possibly mediated by a decrease in reduced voluntary activity or other component of NEAT has not been directly studied.

Subjects with sleep problems or excessive daytime sleepiness have reported a significant reduction in their energy and the level of physical activity [96–97], which could decrease overall AEE. Subjective sleepiness and fatigue increase immediately and significantly with sleep deprivation [98]; however, it is not clear if these would affect volitional or nonvolitional daily activities or other components of TEE or if the effect would be different in children and adults.

There is an overall paucity of studies both in adults and children that have tried to answer these questions. Data from the Nurses' Health Study showed a different body weight but no difference in voluntary activity levels measured in the women sleeping ≤6 hours per day versus those sleeping 7 hours per day [99]. Both physical activity and BMI were not independently associated with sleep duration or sleep efficiency in approximately 700 early-middle aged adults participating in the Coronary Artery Risk Development in Young Adults (CARDIA) study [100]. In contrast, in participants to the Third National Health and Nutrition Examination Survey, self-reported fatigue was associated with a higher body mass index, higher waist circumference, and a reduced likelihood of getting recommended levels of physical activity [101]. In adolescents, two independent studies estimated sleep, BMI, and activity levels and found no relationship between sleep duration and physical activity [58–59]. A study in 6 to 19.9-year-old children reported a decrease in RMR with short sleep in boys but not in girls [102]. Thermoregulation may also be affected by short sleep. In our knowledge only one study has examined the effect of total sleep deprivation on core body temperature and reported a statistically significant drop in response to sleep loss [103].

At this time the few studies available in humans suggest that there may be an overall decrease in energy expenditure with short sleep. However, further studies are required to determine the exact relationship between sleep restriction and energy expenditure.

Behavior and Potential Impact of Sleep Loss

Although hormonal and neuroendocrine changes associated with sleep restriction in children may be responsible for increased food intake or decreased energy expenditure, it is possible that behavioral changes and poor parent-child dynamics may occur with sleep-deprived children, which may contribute to weight gain.

It is well known that children with sleep loss in early childhood show tiredness, hyperactivity, attention difficulties, cognitive disruptions, and poor impulse and emotional control [104–105]. Insufficient sleep may induce similar behavioral, cognitive, and mood impairments in children and adolescents [106] when sleep restriction is self-imposed because of excessive exposure to TV or video games, early school wake times, or an overinvolvement in social life or school-related activities or sports. From a behavioral standpoint, there are a few hypotheses as to why sleep-deprived children may overeat. It is possible that parents may use food to pacify sleep-deprived, irritable, and behaviorally unregulated children. These children may also request food more often and overeat to quell feelings of anxiety and depression, which can accompany sleep deprivation. These children may simply have more time available to eat and may ingest an additional meal or snack every day, which they ordinarily would not if they were sleeping an appropriate amount. The same parents who report less control over their child's intake may also be less strict about their child's bedtime. At this time, there are no studies available that have formally examined the eating behaviors or the parent-child dynamic in sleep-deprived children.

In summary, only few mechanistic studies in a small number of subjects are available at this time to explain the relationship between short sleep duration and the risk of obesity. Hence, research is warranted for further larger laboratory studies to better elucidate the central and peripheral mechanisms that react to chronic sleep loss and measure the effect of recurrent sleep curtailment on the components of human energy intake and expenditure. One has to recognize the limitations of the laboratory environment that does not reflect real free-living conditions, and one challenge may present when trying to translate the findings from short-term, well-controlled laboratory studies in a small number of subjects to the lifetime trajectory of weight gain observed in large populations. Laboratory studies should be complemented by studies in real-life conditions over longer period of follow-up with close monitoring of sleep duration and quality and objective measures of energy intake and expenditure.

SLEEP DISORDERS AND OBESITY IN CHILDREN

Obstructive Sleep Apnea Syndrome

The increase in both the prevalence of obesity in the pediatric population and its severity has translated into a corresponding increase in the prevalence of the obesity-associated morbidities, and among those, childhood obstructive sleep apnea syndrome (OSAS) has become widely recognized as a common disorder with potential serious clinical implications. Although compelling evidence points to obesity as a major risk factor for OSAS in children and adults, a possible reverse causation has begun to emerge from more recent studies suggesting that OSAS could contribute to obesity.

The prevalence of the obstructive sleep apnea (OSA) is estimated to be 3% in the overall 2- to 8-year-old pediatric population [107]. Obesity in children is an important predisposing factor to obstructive sleep apnea. A study conducted in China, which directly compared obese and lean children aged 7 to 11 years, showed that OSA was prevalent in 32.6% of children who were obese compared to 4.5% in normal-weight children [108]. Furthermore, the Cleveland Family study of 4- to 18-year-olds found that obese children are at 4.6-fold increased risk for sleep OSA than normal-weight children [109].

Whereas OSAS, the main component of obstructive types of sleep disordered breathing (SDB), is characterized by recurrent events of partial or complete upper airway obstruction resulting in a disruption of normal ventilation and sleep, obstructive SDB is considered an entire continuum that also encompasses upper airway resistance syndrome (sleep fragmentation in the absence of blunt apneas and abnormalities in gas exchange) and primary snoring, a relatively more benign expression of abnormal upper airway resistance [110]. True OSA manifests with noisy breathing, paradoxical chest and abdominal motion, retractions, witnessed apnea, or cyanosis. Daytime symptoms can include mouth breathing, difficulty in waking up, daytime sleepiness, moodiness, hyperactivity, and cognitive problems [111, 112]. Indeed reports that behavior problems, cognitive deficits, and poor academic performance in children improve after successful treatment of OSA suggest causation [113–115]. The most severe cases of OSA may lead to systemic hypertension, pulmonary hypertension and cor pulmonale, developmental delay, and even sudden death [116].

It is suggested that because of excess neck fat, obesity decreases the size and increases the collapsibility of the pharyngeal airway [117]. Also, increased adiposity in the abdominal wall and cavity reduces intrathoracic volume, which leads to poor oxygen reserves and increased work of breathing while asleep [118]. More recently studies have looked at the relationship among OSA, obesity, and the metabolic syndrome and have suggested a potentiating role of OSAS for obesity. If sleep deprivation (short sleep duration) appears to be a risk factor for obesity, OSAS—which is associated with sleep fragmentation, overall sleep loss, and daytime sleepiness—could also represent an independent risk factor for weight gain, which subsequently further worsens OSAS. Although the exact mechanism of how OSAS may contribute to obesity is not fully understood, emerging studies suggest that OSAS causes a complex interaction of behavioral changes, leptin resistance, and possibly increased ghrelin levels leading to increased appetite.

Many of the behaviors (low self-esteem, externalization disorders) and diseases (insulin resistance and systemic inflammation) associated with childhood OSAS have also been implicated in the risk of obesity. Children who manifest high levels of anger/frustration or clinically meaningful behavior problems are at increased risk of becoming overweight [56, 119]. Although no studies at this time have linked behavioral problems in a causal association between OSA and overweight, it is plausible that a vicious cycle exists where increased externalizing behavior and low self-esteem lead to overweight, which results in OSA, which may worsen behavioral problems and consequently cause weight gain.

OSA may promote further weight gain in overweight obese children by a decrease in physical activity or an increase in unhealthier eating habits. Reduced physical activity has been demonstrated in one study of adults with OSAS [120]. OSA could directly affect appetite regulation with the result of increased caloric intake. A prospective study by Phillips et al. in obese males newly diagnosed with SDB and similarly obese controls showed that subjects with SDB had gained weight in the year preceding the diagnosis and had higher leptin levels than expected by their percentage of body fat [121]. More recent studies confirmed similar higher leptin levels in OSA patients [122–124]. A study of humans at high altitude suggested that hypoxia may lead to increased leptin levels and could be a possible mechanism for the increased levels seen in SDB [125]. It is known that obesity leads to ineffective elevation of circulating leptin because of peripheral and central leptin resistance [126, 127]. Adults with OSAS have high levels of leptin and sympathetic activity [116, 128], which points to OSA as a condition of leptin resistance and a tendency for weight gain and cardiovascular dysfunction. Multiple intervention studies in adults demonstrated a decrease in leptin levels in patients treated with CPAP [129–134]. One study showed that 2 days of CPAP treatment were sufficient to significantly decrease ghrelin levels in patients with OSA [134]. To date, one study in children with metabolic syndrome demonstrated that SDB is associated with increased leptin levels, which significantly decrease after treatment with CPAP [135].

In summary, studies on adults and children suggest that OSA contributes to the leptin resistance observed in obesity. OSAS could therefore affect energy homeostasis by decreasing leptin signaling, which would result in increased food intake and decreased energy expenditure. In parallel, higher ghrelin levels would lead to increased hunger and caloric intake. The studies described did not measure rating of hunger, and food preferences or intake. One of the abnormalities of sleep architecture seen in OSAS is reduced non-REM, or "deep" sleep. Preliminary data showed that experimental suppression of non-REM sleep without affecting sleep duration in young healthy adults leads to increase hunger for calorie-dense foods with high carbohydrate content, particularly in the afternoon and evening hours [136]. In parallel to these early findings in the adults, a study in 5- to 9-year-old obese children with and without OSA demonstrated that children with OSA ate 2.2 times more fast food and less healthy food such as fruits and vegetables, and they were 4.2 times less likely to be involved in organized sports [137]. Furthermore, OSA severity positively correlated with plasma ghrelin levels.

In summary, it appears that in sleep deprivation, OSAS and obesity may interact in a complex relationship and ultimately exacerbate the severity and consequences of one another.

Obesity Hypoventilation Syndrome

The Pickwickian syndrome, also known as the obesity hypoventilation syndrome (OHS), is defined as obesity, sleep-disordered breathing and awake arterial hypercapnia (PaCO2 > 45 mmHg) in the absence of other causes of hypoventilation. The hypoventilation component of OHS should be considered a diagnosis of exclusion until other causes of hypoventilation are evaluated, such as pulmonary disease, chest wall deformities, severe hypothyroidism, or neuromuscular disease. Other central hypoventilation syndromes, such as congenital central hypoventilation syndrome or Arnold-Chiari type II malformations, should also be considered. Patients affected present with hypersomnolence, fatigue, and headaches and are at increased risk of cardiopulmonary failure and pulmonary hypertension [138, 139].

The pathogenesis of alveolar hypoventilation in morbidly obese patients is complex and likely multifactorial. There are several physiological mechanisms that can lead to hypercapnia: an increased load on the respiratory system because of obesity, an impaired central response to hypoxemia and hypercapnia, the presence of sleep-disordered breathing, and impaired neurohormonal responses (leptin resistance) [116, 140–142]. Sleep-disordered breathing is considered necessary for the diagnosis of OH, and can take two forms. The first and by far the most common type is OSA, and the second is central hypoventilation. OSA is well established as one of the causes of hypercapnia because in most patients with OHS the treatment of sleep-disordered breathing leads to the resolution of daytime hypercapnia.

Treatment of Obstructive Sleep Apnea and the Obesity-Hypoventilation Syndromes

Management of OSA and hypoventilation syndrome in children includes positive airway pressure (PAP) for short-term management and weight loss for long-term management. PAP can be used as continuous PAP (CPAP) and bilevel PAP. CPAP is often sufficient to treat OHS by relieving OSA. If hypoxemia persists despite adequate resolution of the obstructive respiratory events with CPAP, noninvasive ventilation in the form of bi-level PAP with or without supplemental oxygen is necessary [138–139]. Tracheostomy with or without nocturnal ventilation may be necessary in cases of PAP failure or poor adherence to PAP therapy [138].

Weight loss, although a difficult process, may be ultimately the most effective management for OSA and OHS. Recent studies showed that weight loss, both spontaneous [143] as well as from bariatric surgery [144], has a high success rate in relieving OSA in the pediatric population, but at this time there are no large studies in adults and in children that examine the role of weight loss and weight reduction surgery in the treatment of OHS.

CONCLUSION

Although it is ironic that a reduction in the most sedentary activity of all—sleep—should be associated with weight gain, strong evidence exists of an association between short sleep and obesity in children and adolescents. At this time no direct causal evidence has been established. Further prospective studies are needed to confirm an effect of sleep loss on the risk of obesity. More interventional laboratory studies should be performed to analyze the hormonal changes that occur in sleep deprivation. Field intervention studies would then be needed to prove that the laboratory findings are indeed reproducible in free-living conditions. Studies should also aim to investigate the role of age, gender, and genetic differences in the interaction between sleep loss and obesity risk. The association between increased BMI and short sleep has important implications for those concerned with the current pediatric obesity epidemic. Overweight children suffer from a poor quality of life and are more likely to become overweight adults with a wide range of physical and social health problems [145]. Additionally there is compelling literature that excessive weight is associated with an increased risk of sleep problems and some early evidence that sleep disorders, specifically OSA, may worsen weight problems.

Despite these associations and the increasing prevalence of long-term sleep deprivation in children, the 2004 Sleep in America Poll [146] found that only 38% of parents with school-aged children reported that their child's doctor asked about sleep habits. Although there is a need for further research in these areas, the evidence to date warrants that clinicians who work with overweight children evaluate their sleep habits and initiate discussions about appropriate bed and wake times and sleep hygiene. Additionally, public health officials and members of the medical community should institute policies that promote healthier lifestyles, including urging school districts to avoid very early school start times and urging parents to put their children to bed at an earlier hour. The effects of additional sleep may prove to be a relatively low-cost strategy to reduce childhood obesity and the related cardiometabolic risk.

References

1. Crespo CJ, et al. Television watching, energy intake, and obesity in US children: results from the third National Health and Nutrition Examination Survey, 1988–1994. *Arch Pediatr Adolesc Med* 2001;**155**(3):360–5.
2. Reilly JJ, et al. Early life risk factors for obesity in childhood: cohort study. *BMJ* 2005;**330**(7504):1357.
3. Berkey CS, et al. Activity, dietary intake, and weight changes in a longitudinal study of preadolescent and adolescent boys and girls. *Pediatrics* 2000;**105**(4):E56.
4. McLaughlin Crabtree V, et al. Cultural influences on the bedtime behaviors of young children. *Sleep Med* 2005;**6**(4):319–24.
5. Beebe DW, et al. Sleep in overweight adolescents: shorter sleep, poorer sleep quality, sleepiness, and sleep-disordered breathing. *J Pediatr Psychol* 2007;**32**(1):69–79.
6. Spilsbury JC, et al. Sleep behavior in an urban US sample of school-aged children. *Arch Pediatr Adolesc Med* 2004;**158**(10):988–94.
7. Keith SW, et al. Putative contributors to the secular increase in obesity: exploring the roads less traveled. *Int J Obes (Lond)* 2006;**30**(11):1585–94.
8. Ogden CL, et al. Prevalence of high body mass index in US children and adolescents, 2007–2008. *JAMA* 2010;**303**(3):242–9.
9. Silventoinen K, et al. Trends in obesity and energy supply in the WHO MONICA Project. *Int J Obes Relat Metab Disord* 2004;**28**(5):710–18.
10. Wang Y, Monteiro C, Popkin BM. Trends of obesity and underweight in older children and adolescents in the United States, Brazil, China, and Russia. *Am J Clin Nutr* 2002;**75**(6):971–7.
11. Luo J, Hu FB. Time trends of obesity in pre-school children in China from 1989 to 1997. *Int J Obes Relat Metab Disord* 2002;**26**(4):553–8.
12. Ebbeling CB, Pawlak DB, Ludwig DS. Childhood obesity: public-health crisis, common sense cure. *Lancet* 2002;**360**(9331):473–82.
13. Serdula MK, et al. Do obese children become obese adults? A review of the literature. *Prev Med* 1993;**22**(2):167–77.
14. Whitaker RC, et al. Predicting obesity in young adulthood from childhood and parental obesity. *N Engl J Med* 1997;**337**(13):869–73.
15. Daniels SR, et al. Overweight in children and adolescents: pathophysiology, consequences, prevention, and treatment. *Circulation* 2005;**111**(15):1999–2012.
16. Smith JC, et al. Coexisting health problems in obese children and adolescents that might require special treatment considerations. *Clin Pediatr (Phila)* 1999;**38**(5):305–7.
17. Must A, et al. Long-term morbidity and mortality of overweight adolescents. A follow-up of the Harvard Growth Study of 1922 to 1935. *New England Journal of Medicine* 1992;**327**(19):1350–5.
18. Abraham S, Collins G, Nordsieck M. Relationship of childhood weight status to morbidity in adults. *HSMHA Health Rep* 1971;**86**(3):273–84.
19. Barsh GS, Farooqi IS, O'Rahilly S. Genetics of body-weight regulation. *Nature* 2000;**404**(6778):644–51.
20. Friedman JM. Modern science versus the stigma of obesity. *Nature Medicine* 2004;**10**(6):563–9.
21. Hill JO, et al. Obesity and the environment: where do we go from here? *Science* 2003;**299**(5608):853–5.
22. de Onis M, Blossner M. Prevalence and trends of overweight among preschool children in developing countries. *Am J Clin Nutr* 2000;**72**(4):1032–9.
23. Andersen RE, et al. Relationship of physical activity and television watching with body weight and level of fatness among children: results from the Third National Health and Nutrition Examination Survey. *JAMA* 1998;**279**(12):938–42.
24. Gordon-Larsen P, McMurray RG, Popkin BM. Determinants of adolescent physical activity and inactivity patterns. *Pediatrics* 2000;**105**(6):E83.
25. Flegal K, Troiano R. Changes in the distribution of body mass index of adults and children in the US population. *International Journal of Obesity and Related Metabolic Disorders* 2000;**24**(7):807–18.
26. Kaufman FR, Lustig RH, Vigersky R. Patient guide to the prevention and management of pediatric obesity. *J Clin Endocrinol Metab* 2008;**93**(12):2. p following 4989.
27. Szymczak JT, et al. Annual and weekly changes in the sleep-wake rhythm of school children. *Sleep* 1993;**16**(5):433–5.
28. Gulliford MC, et al. Sleep habits and height at ages 5 to 11. *Arch Dis Child* 1990;**65**(1):119–22.

29. Lumeng JC, et al. Shorter sleep duration is associated with increased risk for being overweight at ages 9 to 12 years. Pediatrics 2007;**120**(5):1020−9.
30. Iglowstein I, et al. Sleep duration from infancy to adolescence: reference values and generational trends. Pediatrics 2003;**111**(2):302−7.
31. Kahn A, et al. Sleep problems in healthy preadolescents. Pediatrics 1989;**84**(3):542−6.
32. Sadeh A, Gruber R, Raviv A. The effects of sleep restriction and extension on school-age children: what a difference an hour makes. Child Dev 2003;**74**(2):444−55.
33. Foundation NS. *2006 Sleep in America Poll: Highlights and Key Findings*, www.sleepfoundation.org; 2006.
34. Carskadon MA, Acebo C. Regulation of sleepiness in adolescents: update, insights, and speculation. Sleep 2002;**25**(6):606−14.
35. Snell EK, Adam EK, Duncan GJ. Sleep and the body mass index and overweight status of children and adolescents. Child Dev 2007;**78**(1):309−23.
36. Carskadon MA, Acebo C, Seifer R. Extended nights, sleep loss, and recovery sleep in adolescents. Archives Italiennes de Biologie 2001;**139**(3):301−12.
37. Chervin RD, et al. Conduct problems and symptoms of sleep disorders in children. J Am Acad Child Adolesc Psychiatry 2003;**42**(2):201−8.
38. Chervin RD, et al. Symptoms of sleep disorders, inattention, and hyperactivity in children. Sleep 1997;**20**(12):1185−92.
39. Owens JA, et al. Effect of weight, sleep duration, and comorbid sleep disorders on behavioral outcomes in children with sleep-disordered breathing. Arch Pediatr Adolesc Med 2008;**162**(4):313−21.
40. Pilcher JJ, Ginter DR, Sadowsky B. Sleep quality versus sleep quantity: relationships between sleep and measures of health, well-being and sleepiness in college students. J Psychosom Res 1997;**42**(6):583−96.
41. Gangwisch JE, et al. Inadequate sleep as a risk factor for obesity: analyses of the NHANES I. Sleep 2005;**28**(10):1289−96.
42. Vorona RD, et al. Overweight and obese patients in a primary care population report less sleep than patients with a normal body mass index. Arch Intern Med 2005;**165**(1):25−30.
43. Patel SR, Hu FB. Short sleep duration and weight gain: a systematic review. Obesity (Silver Spring) 2008;**16**(3):643−53.
44. Locard E, et al. Risk factors of obesity in a five year old population. Parental versus environmental factors. Int J Obes Relat Metab Disord 1992;**16**(10):721−9.
45. von Kries R, et al. Reduced risk for overweight and obesity in 5- and 6-y-old children by duration of sleep—a cross-sectional study. Int J Obes Relat Metab Disord 2002;**26**(5):710−16.
46. Sekine M, et al. A dose-response relationship between short sleeping hours and childhood obesity: results of the Toyama Birth Cohort Study. Child Care Health Dev 2002;**28**(2):163−70.
47. Gnavi R, et al. Socioeconomic status, overweight and obesity in prepuberal children: a study in an area of Northern Italy. Eur J Epidemiol 2000;**16**(9):797−803.
48. Padez C, et al. Prevalence and risk factors for overweight and obesity in Portuguese children. Acta Paediatr 2005;**94**(11):1550−7.
49. Chaput JP, Brunet M, Tremblay A. Relationship between short sleeping hours and childhood overweight/obesity: results from the 'Quebec en Forme' Project. Int J Obes (Lond) 2006;**30**(7):1080−5.
50. Ben Slama F, et al. [Obesity and life style in a population of male school children aged 6 to 10 years in Ariana (Tunisia)]. Tunis Med 2002;**80**(9):542−7.
51. Hui LL, et al. Risk factors for childhood overweight in 6- to 7-y-old Hong Kong children. Int J Obes Relat Metab Disord 2003;**27**(11):1411−18.
52. Giugliano R, Carneiro EC. [Factors associated with obesity in school children]. J Pediatr (Rio J) 2004;**80**(1):17−22.
53. Eisenmann JC, Ekkekakis P, Holmes M. Sleep duration and overweight among Australian children and adolescents. Acta Paediatr 2006;**95**(8):956−63.
54. Dieu HT, et al. Prevalence of overweight and obesity in preschool children and associated socio-demographic factors in Ho Chi Minh City, Vietnam. Int J Pediatr Obes 2007;**2**(1):40−50.
55. Golding J. The Avon Longitudinal Study of Parents and Children (ALSPAC)—study design and collaborative opportunities. Eur J Endocrinol 2004;**151**(Suppl. 3):U119−23.
56. Agras WS, et al. Risk factors for childhood overweight: a prospective study from birth to 9.5 years. J Pediatr 2004;**145**(1):20−5.
57. Wolfson AR, Carskadon MA. Sleep schedules and daytime functioning in adolescents. Child Dev 1998;**69**(4):875−87.
58. Gupta NK, et al. Is obesity associated with poor sleep quality in adolescents? Am J Hum Biol 2002;**14**(6):762−8.
59. Benefice E, Garnier D, Ndiaye G. Nutritional status, growth and sleep habits among Senegalese adolescent girls. Eur J Clin Nutr 2004;**58**(2):292−301.
60. Knutson KL. Sex differences in the association between sleep and body mass index in adolescents. J Pediatr 2005;**147**(6):830−4.
61. Yu Y, et al. Short sleep duration and adiposity in Chinese adolescents. Sleep 2007;**30**(12):1688−97.
62. Chen MY, Wang EK, Jeng YJ. Adequate sleep among adolescents is positively associated with health status and health-related behaviors. BMC Public Health 2006;**6**:59.
63. Seicean A, et al. Association between short sleeping hours and overweight in adolescents: results from a US Suburban High School survey. Sleep Breath 2007;**11**(4):285−93.
64. Kripke DF, et al. Mortality associated with sleep duration and insomnia. Arch Gen Psychiatry 2002;**59**(2):131−6.
65. Taheri S, et al. Short sleep duration is associated with reduced leptin, elevated ghrelin, and increased body mass index. PLoS Med 2004;**1**(3):e62.
66. Patel SR, et al. A prospective study of sleep duration and mortality risk in women. Sleep 2004;**27**(3):440−4.
67. Bjorvatn B, et al. The association between sleep duration, body mass index and metabolic measures in the Hordaland Health Study. J Sleep Res 2007;**16**(1):66−76.
68. Pannain S, Cauter EV. Modulation of endocrine function by sleep-wake homeostasis and circadian rhythmicity. Sleep, Sleep Disorder and Hormones, Sleep Medicine Clinic 2007 2007;**2**(2):147−59.
69. Sakurai T, et al. Orexins and orexin receptors: a family of hypothalamic neuropeptides and G protein-coupled receptors that regulate feeding behavior. Cell 1998;**92**(5):1. page following 696.
70. Chemelli RM, et al. Narcolepsy in orexin knockout mice: molecular genetics of sleep regulation. Cell 1999;**98**(4):437−51.
71. de Lecea L, Sutcliffe JG. The hypocretins and sleep. FEBS J 2005;**272**(22):5675−88.
72. Currie A, Cappuccio FP. Sleep in children and adolescents: a worrying scenario: can we understand the sleep deprivation-obesity epidemic? Nutr Metab Cardiovasc Dis 2007;**17**(3):230−2.
73. Spiegel K, et al. Leptin levels are dependent on sleep duration: relationships with sympathovagal balance, carbohydrate regulation, cortisol, and thyrotropin. J Clin Endocrinol Metab 2004;**89**(11):5762−71.
74. Spiegel K, et al. Brief communication: Sleep curtailment in healthy young men is associated with decreased leptin levels, elevated ghrelin levels, and increased hunger and appetite. Ann Intern Med 2004;**141**(11):846−50.

REFERENCES

75. Tasali E, et al. *Sleep curtailment in healthy young adults is associated with increased ad lib food intake* Sleep 2009;**32**(Suppl):0394.
76. Nedeltcheva AV, et al. Sleep curtailment is accompanied by increased intake of calories from snacks. *Am J Clin Nutr* 2009;**89**(1):126–33.
77. Guilleminault C, et al. Preliminary observations on the effects of sleep time in a sleep restriction paradigm. *Sleep Med* 2003;**4**(3):177–84.
78. Schmid SM, et al. A single night of sleep deprivation increases ghrelin levels and feelings of hunger in normal-weight healthy men. *J Sleep Res* 2008;**17**(3):331–4.
79. Mullington JM, et al. Sleep loss reduces diurnal rhythm amplitude of leptin in healthy men. *J Neuroendocrinol* 2003;**15**(9):851–4.
80. Taheri S, et al. Short sleep duration is associated with reduced leptin, elevated ghrelin and increased body mass index. *PLoS Medicine* 2004;**1**(3):1–8.
81. Chaput JP, et al. Short sleep duration is associated with reduced leptin levels and increased adiposity: Results from the Quebec family study. *Obesity (Silver Spring)* 2007;**15**(1):253–61.
82. Saper CB, Scammell TE, Lu J. Hypothalamic regulation of sleep and circadian rhythms. *Nature* 2005;**437**(7063):1257–63.
83. Nunez A, et al. Hypocretin/Orexin neuropeptides: participation in the control of sleep-wakefulness cycle and energy homeostasis. *Curr Neuropharmacol* 2009;**7**(1):50–9.
84. Saper CB, Chou TC, Elmquist JK. The need to feed: homeostatic and hedonic control of eating. *Neuron* 2002;**36**(2):199–211.
85. Yamanaka A, et al. Hypothalamic orexin neurons regulate arousal according to energy balance in mice. *Neuron* 2003;**38**(5):701–13.
86. Badman MK, Flier JS. The gut and energy balance: visceral allies in the obesity wars. *Science* 2005;**307**(5717):1909–14.
87. Samson WK, Taylor MM, Ferguson AV. Non-sleep effects of hypocretin/orexin. *Sleep Med Rev* 2005;**9**(4):243–52.
88. Willie JT, et al. To eat or to sleep? Orexin in the regulation of feeding and wakefulness. *Annu Rev Neurosci* 2001;**24**:429–58.
89. Spiegel K, Leproult R, Van Cauter E. Impact of sleep debt on metabolic and endocrine function. *Lancet* 1999;**354**:1435–9.
90. Harris GC, Aston-Jones G. Arousal and reward: a dichotomy in orexin function. *Trends Neurosci* 2006;**29**(10):571–7.
91. Harris GC, Wimmer M, Aston-Jones G. A role for lateral hypothalamic orexin neurons in reward seeking. *Nature* 2005;**437**(7058):556–9.
92. Irwin M, et al. Effects of sleep and sleep deprivation on catecholamine and interleukin-2 levels in humans: clinical implications. *Journal of Clinical Endocrinology & Metabolism* 1999;**84**(6):1979–85.
93. Meier-Ewert HK, et al. Effect of sleep loss on C-reactive protein, an inflammatory marker of cardiovascular risk. *J Am Coll Cardiol* 2004;**43**(4):678–83.
94. Chen K, et al. Induction of leptin resistance through direct interaction of C-reactive protein with leptin. *Nat Med* 2006;**12**(4):425–32.
95. Rising R. Total daily energy expenditure. *J Am Coll Nutr* 1994;**13**(4):309–10.
96. Weaver T, et al. An instrument to measure functional status outcomes for disorders of excessive sleepiness. *Sleep* 1997;**20**(10):835–43.
97. Briones B, et al. Sleepiness and Health: Relationship between sleepiness and general health status. *Sleep* 1996;**19**(7):583–8.
98. Dinges D, et al. Cumulative sleepiness, mood disturbance, and psychomotor vigilance performance decrements during a week of sleep restricted to 4–5 hours per night. *Sleep* 1997;**20**:267–77.
99. Patel SR, et al. Association between reduced sleep and weight gain in women. *Am J Epidemiol* 2006;**164**(10):947–54.
100. Lauderdale DS, et al. Objectively measured sleep characteristics among early-middle-aged adults: the CARDIA study. *Am J Epidemiol* 2006;**164**(1):5–16.
101. Resnick HE, et al. Cross-sectional relationship of reported fatigue to obesity, diet, and physical activity: results from the third national health and nutrition examination survey. *J Clin Sleep Med* 2006;**2**(2):163–9.
102. Hitze B, et al. Determinants and impact of sleep duration in children and adolescents: data of the Kiel Obesity Prevention Study. *Eur J Clin Nutr* 2009;**63**(6):739–46.
103. Vaara J, et al. The effect of 60-h sleep deprivation on cardiovascular regulation and body temperature. *Eur J Appl Physiol* 2009;**105**(3):439–44.
104. Touchette E, et al. Associations between sleep duration patterns and behavioral/cognitive functioning at school entry. *Sleep* 2007;**30**(9):1213–19.
105. Dahl RE. The impact of inadequate sleep on children's daytime cognitive function. *Semin Pediatr Neurol* 1996;**3**(1):44–50.
106. O'Brien LM. The neurocognitive effects of sleep disruption in children and adolescents. *Child Adolesc Psychiatr Clin N Am* 2009;**18**(4):813–23.
107. Gislason T, Benediktsdottir B. Snoring, apneic episodes, and nocturnal hypoxemia among children 6 months to 6 years old. An epidemiologic study of lower limit of prevalence. *Chest* 1995;**107**(4):963–6.
108. Wing YK, et al. A controlled study of sleep related disordered breathing in obese children. *Arch Dis Child* 2003;**88**(12):1043–7.
109. Ievers-Landis CE, Redline S. Pediatric sleep apnea: implications of the epidemic of childhood overweight. *Am J Respir Crit Care Med* 2007;**175**(5):436–41.
110. Greene MG, Carroll JL. Consequences of sleep-disordered breathing in childhood. *Curr Opin Pulm Med* 1997;**3**(6):456–63.
111. Chervin RD, et al. Inattention, hyperactivity, and symptoms of sleep-disordered breathing. *Pediatrics* 2002;**109**(3):449–56.
112. Rosen CL, et al. Increased behavioral morbidity in school-aged children with sleep-disordered breathing. *Pediatrics* 2004;**114**(6):1640–8.
113. Gozal D. Sleep-disordered breathing and school performance in children. *Pediatrics* 1998;**102**(3 Pt 1):616–20.
114. Friedman BC, et al. Adenotonsillectomy improves neurocognitive function in children with obstructive sleep apnea syndrome. *Sleep* 2003;**26**(8):999–1005.
115. Montgomery-Downs HE, Crabtree VM, Gozal D. Cognition, sleep and respiration in at-risk children treated for obstructive sleep apnoea. *Eur Respir J* 2005;**25**(2):336–42.
116. Tauman R, Gozal D. Obesity and obstructive sleep apnea in children. *Paediatr Respir Rev* 2006;**7**(4):247–59.
117. Horner RL, et al. Sites and sizes of fat deposits around the pharynx in obese patients with obstructive sleep apnoea and weight matched controls. *Eur Respir J* 1989;**2**(7):613–22.
118. Naimark A, Cherniack RM. Compliance of the respiratory system and its components in health and obesity. *J Appl Physiol* 1960;**15**:377–82.
119. Lumeng JC, et al. Association between clinically meaningful behavior problems and overweight in children. *Pediatrics* 2003;**112**(5):1138–45.
120. Peppard PE, Young T. Exercise and sleep-disordered breathing: an association independent of body habitus. *Sleep* 2004;**27**(3):480–4.
121. Phillips BG, et al. Recent weight gain in patients with newly diagnosed obstructive sleep apnea. *J Hypertens* 1999;**17**(9):1297–300.
122. Ip MS, et al. Serum leptin and vascular risk factors in obstructive sleep apnea. *Chest* 2000;**118**(3):580–6.
123. Ozturk L, et al. The association of the severity of obstructive sleep apnea with plasma leptin levels. *Arch Otolaryngol Head Neck Surg* 2003;**129**(5):538–40.

124. Ulukavak Ciftci T, et al. Leptin and ghrelin levels in patients with obstructive sleep apnea syndrome. *Respiration* 2005;**72**(4): 395—401.
125. Tschop M, et al. Influence of hypobaric hypoxia on leptin levels in men. *Int J Obes Relat Metab Disord* 2000;**24**(Suppl. 2):S151.
126. Aygun AD, et al. Proinflammatory cytokines and leptin are increased in serum of prepubertal obese children. *Mediators Inflamm* 2005;**2005**(3):180—3.
127. Reinehr T, et al. Circulating soluble leptin receptor, leptin, and insulin resistance before and after weight loss in obese children. *Int J Obes (Lond)* 2005;**29**(10):1230—5.
128. Somers VK, et al. Sympathetic neural mechanisms in obstructive sleep apnea. *J Clin Invest* 1995;**96**(4):1897—904.
129. Saarelainen S, Lahtela J, Kallonen E. Effect of nasal CPAP treatment on insulin sensitivity and plasma leptin. *J Sleep Res* 1997;**6**(2):146—7.
130. Chin K, et al. Changes in intra-abdominal visceral fat and serum leptin levels in patients with obstructive sleep apnea syndrome following nasal continuous positive airway pressure therapy. *Circulation* 1999;**100**(7):706—12.
131. Ip S, et al. Serum leptin and vascular risk factors in obstructive sleep apnea. *Chest* 2000;**118**(3):580—6.
132. Shimizu K, et al. Plasma leptin levels and cardiac sympathetic function in patients with obstructive sleep apnoea-hypopnoea syndrome. *Thorax* 2002;**57**(5):429—34.
133. Sanner BM, et al. Influence of treatment on leptin levels in patients with obstructive sleep apnoea. *Eur Respir J* 2004;**23**(4):601—4.
134. Harsch IA, et al. Leptin and ghrelin levels in patients with obstructive sleep apnoea: effect of CPAP treatment. *Eur Respir J* 2003;**22**(2):251—7.
135. Nakra N, et al. Sleep-disordered breathing in children with metabolic syndrome: the role of leptin and sympathetic nervous system activity and the effect of continuous positive airway pressure. *Pediatrics* 2008;**122**(3):e634—42.
136. Broussard J, Tasali E, Van Cauter E. *Experimental suppression of slow wave sleep in healthy young men is associated with increased hunger and decreased vigor and mood Sleep* 2008;**31**:A110.
137. Spruyt K, et al. Dietary and physical activity patterns in children with obstructive sleep apnea. *J Pediatr*; 2009. in press.
138. Pediatrics AAO. Clinical practice guideline: diagnosis and management of childhood obstructive sleep apnea syndrome. *Pediatrics* 2002;**109**(4):704—12.
139. Mokhlesi B, Kryger MH, Grunstein RR. Assessment and management of patients with obesity hypoventilation syndrome. *Proc Am Thorac Soc* 2008;**5**(2):218—25.
140. Mokhlesi B, Tulaimat A. Recent advances in obesity hypoventilation syndrome. *Chest* 2007;**132**(4):1322—36.
141. O'Donnell C P, et al. Leptin prevents respiratory depression in obesity. *Am J Respir Crit Care Med* 1999;**159**(5 Pt 1):1477—84.
142. Tankersley CG, et al. Leptin attenuates respiratory complications associated with the obese phenotype. *J Appl Physiol* 1998;**85**(6):2261—9.
143. Verhulst SL, et al. The effect of weight loss on sleep-disordered breathing in obese teenagers. *Obesity (Silver Spring)* 2009;**17**(6): 1178—83.
144. Kalra M, et al. Obstructive sleep apnea in extremely overweight adolescents undergoing bariatric surgery. *Obes Res* 2005;**13**(7): 1175—9.
145. Epstein R, Chillag N, Lavie P. Starting Times of School: Effects on Daytime Functioning of Fifth-grade Children in Israel. *Sleep* 1998;**21**(3):250—6.
146. Foundation NS. 2004: Sleep in America Poll: Summary of findings; http://www.sleepfoundation.org/article/sleep-america-polls/2004-children-and-sleep.

CHAPTER 17

Cellular Remodeling during the Growth of the Adipose Tissue

Coralie Sengenès, Virginie Bourlier, Jean Galitzky, Alexia Zakaroff-Girard, Max Lafontan, Anne Bouloumié

Institut National de la Santé et de la Recherche Médicale (INSERM), U858, Toulouse, France, Université Toulouse III Paul Sabatier, Institut de Médecine Moléculaire de Rangueil, Equipe n°1 AVENIR

By the 1960s, the research of Tedeschi [1], Wasserman [2], and Liebelt [3] had pointed out that adipose tissue (AT) is not solely composed by fat cells or adipocytes but also by various stromal cells, resident and infiltrating immune cells, and an extensive endothelial network. Collectively, these cells are referred to as the stroma-vascular fraction of AT (AT-SVF). The physiological growth of AT, which occurs throughout normal development but also as a result of fat mass excessive enlargement associated with obesity, involves the remodeling of AT cell compartments, the adipocytes, and the SVF. Indeed, although it is well described that adipocytes, which are the site of AT metabolic activity, are able to adapt their size but also their number to maintain energy homeostasis, the cells from the SVF also appear to play an important role in the growth of AT. This review focuses on the changes occurring in AT during normal and excessive fat mass growth, including changes in adipocyte number and size and SVF cellular remodeling.

MATURE ADIPOCYTES

Research conducted before 1900 still provides the primary foundation upon which many histology texts rely for description of the growth of AT. The developmental history of AT starts in human embryo in sites called "primitive organs" [2]. These primitive organs are clearly delineated from surrounding connective tissue and possess a well-defined vascular network in the interstices of which cellular organization takes place. They contain fat cell clusters that possess at least several lipid droplets [2]. Then, in the second half of intrauterine growth, fetal mass enlargement is thought to exclusively depend on the appearance of new adipocytes leading to an increase of adipocyte number [4, 5]. At birth and from 1 to 18 months of age, fat depots appear to grow by virtue of adipocyte cell size alone because of the hypertrophy of the preexisting adipocytes, followed by increases in adipocyte cell number detected from 12 to 18 months of age. Then, adipocytes have been reported to enlarge slowly after 2 years of age in normal children and may reach adult levels by year 10 to 12. Subsequently, fat cell number may increase and be definitively set during adolescence [6—11].

During the onset and maintenance of obesity, extensive literature has described the changes in adipocyte mean size and number starting from Hirsch's study [6, 11—14]. Indeed, AT excessive development is thought to be the result of both adipocyte hypertrophy and hyperplasia [13—17]. Adipocyte hypertrophy would occur before hyperplasia to meet the need for additional fat storage capacity during the progression of obesity [13, 18]. Although rare "in vitro" data reported that adipocytes may exhibit proliferation potential through a dedifferentiation process [19], mature adipocytes are thought of as being terminally differentiated cells, incapable of division. Therefore, the appearance of new adipocytes is thought to be the result of adipocyte precursor cell (preadipocytes) differentiation into adipocytes.

ADIPOCYTE PRECURSOR CELLS

AT like muscle and bone is generally considered as having mesoderm origin. However, this may be an oversimplification, because precise lineage tracing studies are missing [20–22]. Indeed, recent data showed that a subset of adipocytes originates from the neural crest during normal mouse AT development, suggesting that the developmental origin of the adipocyte lineage might be more complex and heterogeneous than expected [21, 23].

Adipogenesis—that is, the appearance of new adipocyte from an undifferentiated immature cell—is generally described as a two-step process [24]. The first step constitutes the generation of committed adipocyte precursors (or preadipocytes) from mesenchymal stem cells (MSCs). The second step involves the terminal differentiation of these preadipocytes into mature functional adipocytes. By definition, MSCs are endowed with self-renewal properties and a differentiation potential toward all mesenchymal cell types, whereas preadipocytes have lost the ability to differentiate into mesenchymal derivatives other than adipocytes [21, 25]. To determine the phenotype of adipocyte progenitor cells in human AT, we demonstrated by flow cytometry and cell sorting approaches that among the cell populations present in human AT-SVF, a cell fraction characterized as positive for CD34 and negative for CD31 markers ($CD34^+/CD31^-$) was the only one able to differentiate into adipocytes [26]. We also showed that they exhibited, in situ, a proliferative activity, which was positively correlated to the adiposity degree [27]. Using similar strategies, mouse adipose progenitor cells were also characterized as $Lin^-/CD29^+/CD34^+/Sca-1^+/CD24^+$ and would reside in AT vasculature [28, 29]. Because adipocyte progenitors express in human as well as in mouse adult AT membrane markers known as hematopoietic stem cells markers, CD34 and Sca-1, respectively [30], it raises the question of the origin of such a cell type. Moreover, although most of the studies have focused on the resident adipocyte precursor cells from AT-SVF, several studies have suggested that non-AT resident source of cells could also serve as a source of new adipocytes. In support of the latter concept, Crossno et al. [31] reported that bone marrow-derived progenitor cells may contribute to new adipocytes formation in adult mouse AT. The authors exposed Green Fluorescent Protein (GFP)-labeled bone marrow-transplanted mice to two known inducers of new fat cell formation, either a high-fat diet or treatment with the thiazolidinedione (TZD) rosiglitazone. Subsequent examination demonstrated the presence of GFP^+ multilocular adipocytes within AT that were significantly increased in number by both high-fat feeding and TZD treatment. To note, controversial results have been reported [32].

ADIPOSE TISSUE-DERIVED STROMAL CELLS (ASCs)

As mentioned previously, AT is thought to originate from mesoderm. MSCs were initially identified in postnatal human bone marrow and have been used to model differentiating mesoderm. MSCs are defined as plastic adherent cells able to differentiate into adipocytes, osteoblasts, and chondrocytes [33] and would reside or originate from tissue vasculature [34]. AT-derived SVF cells isolated and maintained in MSC-related conditions have been shown to exhibit MSC-like activity and were named "adipose tissue-derived stromal cells" (ASCs). Indeed, they differentiate along multiple cell lineages, including adipocytes, cartilage, bone, skeletal muscle, neuronal cells, endothelial cells [35], cardiomyocytes and smooth muscle cells [34–39]. The surface immunophenotype of ASCs resembles that of bone marrow-derived MSCs [40], as direct comparisons between ASCs and MSC immunophenotypes reveal that they are >90% identical [36]. In vitro, ASCs have been shown to display a cell doubling time of 2 to 4 days depending on donor age and AT location (subcutaneous or visceral), culturing conditions, plating density, and culture media formulations [41, 42]. A cell population exhibiting similar properties has been isolated and characterized from AT of young donors and was named multipotent adipose-derived stem (MADS) cells. Human MADS (hMADS) cells display extensive self-renewal capacity in vitro, exhibit a normal diploid karyotype, and maintain the capacity to undergo differentiation into many mesenchymal cell types, and even brown adipocytes, at the single-cell level, even after extensive expansion [43–45].

AT MICROCIRCULATION AND AT-DERIVED ENDOTHELIAL CELLS

AT possesses a relatively dense network of blood capillaries, with almost every adipocyte surrounded by one capillary, ensuring adequate exposure to nutrients and oxygen. Moreover, the microvasculature within AT is rather unique. As AT has enormous growth potential given the appropriate metabolic challenge, it displays a high degree of plasticity with respect to its vascularization. During normal embryonic development, primitive fat organs are known to be associated with vascular structures [2, 46, 47]. Moreover, fetal adipocyte development is spatially and temporally related to capillary development [47], and arteriolar development has been shown to precede adipocyte differentiation in fat depots in the fetus [47]. During postnatal AT normal growth, AT requires continuous remodeling of the vascular network [47, 48] and the extracellular matrix (ECM) [47, 49, 50]. Different groups have repeatedly observed a close spatial and temporal relationship between adipocyte formation and blood vessel formation whatever the species studied [2, 51]. Indeed, in vitro studies revealed that differentiating adipocytes and AT explants trigger blood vessel formation [52, 53] and that, in turn, AT endothelial cells (ECs) promote preadipocyte differentiation [54].

We have studied the effects of human adult AT excessive development on AT-derived endothelial network. First, we characterized human AT-ECs as double positive for the membrane markers CD34 and CD31 [55]. Then, using the flow cytometry approach on freshly harvested human AT-SVF, we reported that AT-ECs percentage remained constant whatever the degree of obesity. Therefore, the excessive growth of human adult AT is associated with an extension of its vasculature. Moreover, several groups reported that AT growth in adult mice could be impaired with angiogenesis inhibitors [56–59]. In addition to angiogenesis, other processes such as endothelial progenitor cell (EPC) recruitment may contribute to the extension of the AT vascularization [60, 61]. EPCs circulate in the peripheral blood of adult mammals, including humans, and can be recruited to target organs where they differentiate into mature ECs and are incorporated into the developing vessels. Different groups have reported that AT-SVF and more precisely the $CD34^+CD31^-$ progenitor cell population exhibited in vitro angiogenic abilities, promoted angiogenesis, and participated in the revascularization of ischemic hind limbs of nude mice [35, 55, 62–65]. Thus, EC progenitors may reside in AT and could participate to postnatal neovascularization to support its excessive growth. It is also interesting to note that the expansion of AT results in hypoxia and increased levels of hypoxia-inducible factor 1α (HIF-1α) that, in turn leads to an up-regulation of various inflammatory adipokines [27, 66–70]. Moreover, hypoxia would also provoke AT fibrosis that may lead to further adipose dysfunction [70–72]. Hence, it is tempting to propose that angiogenesis within AT would be necessary to counteract hypoxia. To note, AT is rich in angiogenic factors as well as endothelial cells, progenitors, and immune cells, which could contribute to the capillary extension.

IMMUNE CELLS

A significant number of adipocyte-derived factors play an intricate role in various aspects of the innate and adaptive immune response [73]. It is therefore not surprising that local, obesity-driven changes in adipokine secretion have a systemic impact on a number of branches of the immune system [74]. The best-described phenomenon relates to changes in the inflammatory status. Indeed, the excessive growth of AT has been associated with changes in number of circulating leukocytes in children and adults together with an increase in many proinflammatory cytokine levels, suggesting that obesity should be considered as a low-level inflammatory condition [75–79]. In 2003, AT from obese mice and humans was shown to be infiltrated with macrophages; this information provided a major mechanistic advance into understanding how obesity propagates inflammation, which could explain some of the complications of the condition, particularly insulin resistance [80–82]. Evidence for a connection between obesity and inflammation has also been found in the context of clinical weight-loss studies. Weight loss achieved through dietary intervention alone or diet and exercise resulted in decreased circulating inflammatory factors in men and women of various age groups and degrees of obesity [83–85]. Not only do these findings strengthen the evidence for the direct contribution of obese AT to systemic inflammation, they also imply that many of the health benefits of weight loss are attributable to these decreases in inflammatory signals.

AT Macrophages

Macrophages are released from the bone marrow as immature monocytes and circulate in the blood before extravasation into their target tissues, where they differentiate into resident macrophages [86]. The increased number of macrophages in AT associated with excessive fat mass growth is a likely source of secreted proinflammatory factors, which might be responsible for inducing features of metabolic syndrome [87, 88]. Using an immunoselection approach, we isolated macrophages (i.e., $CD34^-/CD14^+$ cells) from freshly harvested human AT SVF and showed that they display monocyte/macrophage functions [89]. Moreover we demonstrated that they express higher levels of chemokines (Monocyte Chemotactic Protein-1 (MCP-1), Macrophage Inflammatory Protein-1α (MIP-1α), and Interleukin 8 (IL 8)) as well as resistin and visfatin when compared to mature adipocytes [90], suggesting that among the nonfat cells able to release proinflammatory products [91], the main source of inflammatory mediators within human AT are macrophages. Macrophages have remarkable plasticity that allows them to respond to environmental signals and changes, and their phenotype and physiology can be markedly altered by both innate and adaptive immune responses. Mirroring the type 1 T-helper (Th1)/ type 2 T-helper (Th2) concept of T-cell activation, a concept of M1/M2 polarization has recently been developed, where M1 or "classically" activated macrophage exhibit high inflammatory and bactericidal potential and M2 or "alternatively" activated macrophages have antiparasitic functions and ill-defined functions in tissue repair and remodeling [87–89].

We investigated human AT macrophage phenotypes and found that they were positive for a combination of common monocyte/macrophage markers (i.e., CD45, CD44, CD31, and HLA-DR) and for CD206 (or mannose receptor), usually described on M2-activated/resident macrophages [90]. Macrophages are found in every tissue of the body, and depending on the local microenvironment, they acquire specialized functions including phagocytosis, antigen presentation, tissue remodeling, and the secretion of a wide range of growth factors and cytokines [86]. Unexpectedly, human AT macrophages expressed both M1 and M2 activation cytokines and chemokines. Furthermore we showed that a subpopulation of these macrophages (i.e., $CD14^+/CD206^+/CD16^-$) increased with respect to AT excessive growth [90]. Surprisingly and conversely to data obtained in mice models [91, 92], human AT macrophages exhibited a more M2 phenotype with fat mass excessive enlargement [90]. AT macrophages may serve multiple functions, including the removal of necrotic adipocytes leading to lipid-engulfed foam cells, acting as proinflammatory mediators, and serving as angiogenic precursors [93, 94]. We and others have reported that AT macrophage-secreted factors stimulated angiogenesis and impaired adipogenesis in vitro [90, 95, 96]. In addition, we showed that secretions from AT macrophages reduced the proliferation of human AT $CD34^+/CD31^-$ progenitor cells in culture by oxidative stress generation [27]. Thus and paradoxically to their effect on angiogenesis, ATMs may affect fat mass development by reducing proliferation and differentiation of adipocyte progenitor cells.

AT Lymphocytes

The parallel development of adipose and lymphoid tissues in fetal and neonatal mammals was reported in the late 1950s. However, except during inflammatory processes, lymphocytes are not usually found within nonspecific immune organs apart from epithelial tissues, where they are involved in maintaining tissue integrity, defending against pathogens, and regulating inflammation [97, 98]. Interestingly, different studies have reported that AT from normal mice contains lymphocytes [99, 100]. Moreover, we and others have shown an increase in the ratio of $CD8^+$ to $CD4^+$ AT T cells during the excessive development of AT in the mouse as well as in the human [67, 99, 101–104]. Interestingly, the obesity-associated T-cell infiltration occurred weeks before AT macrophages typically infiltrate fat [105, 106]. The function of these fat-associated T cells and their conceivable roles in obesity, glucose homeostasis, or both are not understood, nor are their antigen specificities, activation history, or T sublineage profiles known [100]. However, very recently, a possible

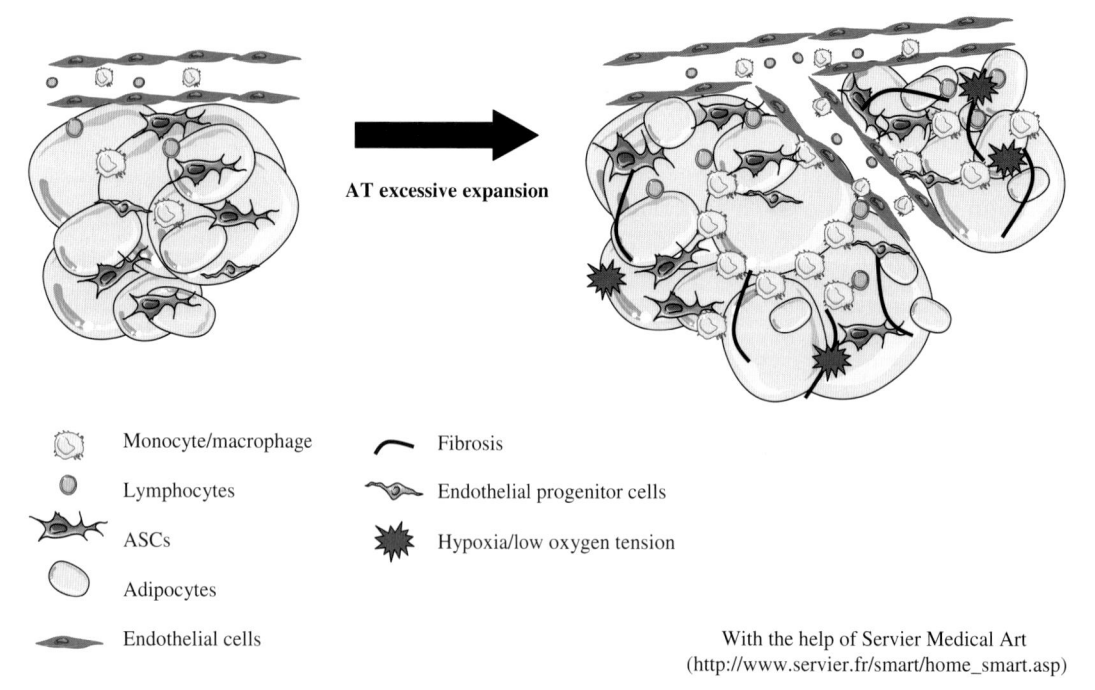

FIGURE 17.1 Cellular remodeling during the growth of AT. AT is composed of adipocytes as well as many additional cell types the proportion of which varies during AT normal or excessive growth. Indeed, AT expansion is the result of both adipocyte hypertrophy (increase in size) and hyperplasia (increase in number) and is associated with an increase in immune cell content (macrophages and lymphocytes) and an activation of the angiogenesis process.

fundamental role for T lymphocytes in the regulation of body weight, adipocyte hypertrophy, insulin resistance, and glucose tolerance was suggested [102].

CONCLUSION

The adipocyte is unique among cells in that one organelle, the lipid droplet, encompasses greater than 95% of the entire cell body. Hence, the adipocyte is traditionally viewed as a cell that is primarily involved in energy storage. However, it is now clear that the adipocyte has additional roles with the remaining 5% of its cellular mass. It has an exceptionally active secretory pathway whose function is not only to release products of conventional housekeeping genes but also to release many factors, the adipokines. The paracrine effects of adipokines have an impact on neighboring adipocytes as well as other local cell types within AT. Indeed and as discussed in the present chapter, AT is composed of adipocytes as well as many additional cell types, the proportion of which varies during AT normal or excessive growth. Since the late 1990s, increased focus has been placed on the cellular composition of AT depots and the factors influencing changes in AT composition in pathological states (Fig. 17.1). Studying AT cellular dynamics has provided great insight into AT biology, plasticity, and self-regenerative capacity as well as its central role toward the metabolic syndrome. Although we are in the midst of a dire and intertwined epidemic of diabesity, the recently described discoveries provide a hopeful light within this roiling tempest.

References

1. Tedeschi CG. "The fat cell; origin and structure". *Conn Med* 1960;**24**:33–40.
2. Wassermann F. The development of adipose tissue. In: Renold AE, Cahill GF, editors. *Handbook of physiology*, vol. 5. Washington: The Williams and Wilkins Company; 1965. pp. 87–100.
3. Liebelt RA, Vismara L, Liebelt AG. Autoregulation of adipose tissue mass in the mouse. *Proc Soc Exp Biol Med* 1968;**127**(2):458–62.
4. Enzi G, Inelmen EM, Caretta F, Rubaltelli F, Grella P, Baritussio A. Adipose tissue development "in utero." Relationships between some nutritional and hormonal factors and body fat mass enlargement in newborns. *Diabetologia* 1980;**18**(2):135–40.
5. Enzi G, Zanardo V, Caretta F, Inelmen EM, Rubaltelli F. Intrauterine growth and adipose tissue development. *Am J Clin Nutr* 1981;**34**(9):1785–90.
6. Hirsch J, Knittle JL. Cellularity of obese and nonobese human adipose tissue. *Fed Proc* 1970;**29**(4):1516–21.
7. Brook CG. Evidence for a sensitive period in adipose-cell replication in man. *Lancet* 1972;**2**(7778):624–7.
8. Knittle JL, Timmers K, Ginsberg-Fellner F, Brown RE, Katz DP. The growth of adipose tissue in children and adolescents. Cross-sectional and longitudinal studies of adipose cell number and size. *J Clin Invest* 1979;**63**(2):239–46.
9. Chumlea WC, Knittle JL, Roche AF, Siervogel RM, Webb P. Size and number of adipocytes and measures of body fat in boys and girls 10 to 18 years of age. *Am J Clin Nutr* 1981;**34**(9):1791–7.
10. Siervogel RM, Roche AF, Himes JH, Chumlea WC, McCammon R. Subcutaneous fat distribution in males and females from 1 to 39 years of age. *Am J Clin Nutr* 1982;**36**(1):162–71.
11. Spalding KL, Arner E, Westermark PO, Bernard S, Buchholz BA, Bergmann O, Blomqvist L, Hoffstedt J, Naslund E, Britton T, et al. Dynamics of fat cell turnover in humans. *Nature* 2008;**453**(7196):783–7.
12. Bjorntorp P, Sjostrom L. Adipose tissue cellularity. *Int J Obes* 1979;**3**(2):181–7.
13. van Harmelen V, Skurk T, Rohrig K, Lee YM, Halbleib M, Aprath-Husmann I, Hauner H. Effect of BMI and age on adipose tissue cellularity and differentiation capacity in women. *Int J Obes Relat Metab Disord* 2003;**27**(8):889–95.
14. Jo J, Gavrilova O, Pack S, Jou W, Mullen S, Sumner AE, Cushman SW, Periwal V. Hypertrophy and/or Hyperplasia: Dynamics of Adipose Tissue Growth. *PLoS Comput Biol* 2009;**5**(3):e1000324.
15. Bjorntorp P, Gustafson A, Persson B. Adipose tissue fat cell size and number in relation to metabolism in endogenous hypertriglyceridemia. *Acta Med Scand* 1971;**190**(5):363–7.
16. Hirsch J, Batchelor B. Adipose tissue cellularity in human obesity. *Clin Endocrinol Metab* 1976;**5**(2):299–311.
17. Arner E, Westermark PO, Spalding KL, Britton T, Ryden M, Frisen J, Bernard S, Arner P. Adipocyte Turnover: Relevance to Human Adipose Tissue Morphology. *Diabetes*; 2009.
18. Faust IM, Johnson PR, Stern JS, Hirsch J. Diet-induced adipocyte number increase in adult rats: a new model of obesity. *Am J Physiol* 1978;**235**(3):E279–86.
19. Fernyhough ME, Bucci LR, Hausman GJ, Antonio J, Vierck JL, Dodson MV. Gaining a solid grip on adipogenesis. *Tissue Cell* 2005;**37**(4):335–8.
20. Gesta S, Tseng YH, Kahn CR. Developmental origin of fat: tracking obesity to its source. *Cell* 2007;**131**(2):242–56.
21. Billon N, Monteiro MC, Dani C. Developmental origin of adipocytes: new insights into a pending question. *Biol Cell* 2008;**100**(10):563–75.
22. Hausman GJ, Dodson MV, Ajuwon K, Azain M, Barnes KM, Guan LL, Jiang Z, Poulos SP, Sainz RD, Smith S, et al. Board-invited review: the biology and regulation of preadipocytes and adipocytes in meat animals. *J Anim Sci* 2009;**87**(4):1218–46.
23. Billon N, Iannarelli P, Monteiro MC, Glavieux-Pardanaud C, Richardson WD, Kessaris N, Dani C, Dupin E. The generation of adipocytes by the neural crest. *Development* 2007;**134**(12):2283–92.
24. Lefterova MI, Lazar MA. New developments in adipogenesis. *Trends Endocrinol Metab* 2009;**20**(3):107–14.
25. Gregoire FM, Smas CM, Sul HS. Understanding adipocyte differentiation. *Physiol Rev* 1998;**78**(3):783–809.
26. Sengenes C, Lolmede K, Zakaroff-Girard A, Busse R, Bouloumie A. Preadipocytes in the human subcutaneous adipose tissue display distinct features from the adult mesenchymal and hematopoietic stem cells. *J Cell Physiol* 2005;**205**(1):114–22.
27. Maumus M, Sengenes C, Decaunes P, Zakaroff-Girard A, Bourlier V, Lafontan M, Galitzky J, Bouloumie A. Evidence of in situ proliferation of adult adipose tissue-derived progenitor cells: influence of fat mass microenvironment and growth. *J Clin Endocrinol Metab* 2008;**93**(10):4098–106.
28. Rodeheffer MS, Birsoy K, Friedman JM. Identification of white adipocyte progenitor cells in vivo. *Cell* 2008;**135**(2):240–9.

29. Tang W, Zeve D, Suh JM, Bosnakovski D, Kyba M, Hammer RE, Tallquist MD, Graff JM. White fat progenitor cells reside in the adipose vasculature. *Science* 2008;**322**(5901):583—6.
30. Weissman IL, Shizuru JA. The origins of the identification and isolation of hematopoietic stem cells, and their capability to induce donor-specific transplantation tolerance and treat autoimmune diseases. *Blood* 2008;**112**(9):3543—53.
31. Crossno Jr JT, Majka SM, Grazia T, Gill RG, Klemm DJ. Rosiglitazone promotes development of a novel adipocyte population from bone marrow-derived circulating progenitor cells. *J Clin Invest* 2006;**116**(12):3220—8.
32. Koh YJ, Kang S, Lee HJ, Choi TS, Lee HS, Cho CH, Koh GY. Bone marrow-derived circulating progenitor cells fail to transdifferentiate into adipocytes in adult adipose tissues in mice. *J Clin Invest* 2007;**117**(12):3684—95.
33. Phinney DG, Prockop DJ. Concise review: mesenchymal stem/multipotent stromal cells: the state of transdifferentiation and modes of tissue repair—current views. *Stem Cells* 2007;**25**(11): 2896—902.
34. Crisan M, Yap S, Casteilla L, Chen CW, Corselli M, Park TS, Andriolo G, Sun B, Zheng B, Zhang L, et al. A perivascular origin for mesenchymal stem cells in multiple human organs. *Cell Stem Cell* 2008;**3**(3):301—13.
35. Planat-Benard V, Silvestre JS, Cousin B, Andre M, Nibbelink M, Tamarat R, Clergue M, Manneville C, Saillan-Barreau C, Duriez M, et al. Plasticity of human adipose lineage cells toward endothelial cells: physiological and therapeutic perspectives. *Circulation* 2004;**109**(5):656—63.
36. Zuk PA, Zhu M, Ashjian P, De Ugarte DA, Huang JI, Mizuno H, Alfonso ZC, Fraser JK, Benhaim P, Hedrick MH. Human adipose tissue is a source of multipotent stem cells. *Mol Biol Cell* 2002;**13**(12):4279—95.
37. Gimble JM, Guilak F. Differentiation potential of adipose derived adult stem (ADAS) cells. *Curr Top Dev Biol* 2003;**58**: 137—60.
38. Yamamoto N, Akamatsu H, Hasegawa S, Yamada T, Nakata S, Ohkuma M, Miyachi E, Marunouchi T, Matsunaga K. Isolation of multipotent stem cells from mouse adipose tissue. *J Dermatol Sci* 2007;**48**(1):43—52.
39. Tholpady SS, Ogle RC, Katz AJ. Adipose stem cells and solid organ transplantation. *Curr Opin Organ Transplant* 2009;**14**(1): 51—5.
40. Pittenger MF, Mackay AM, Beck SC, Jaiswal RK, Douglas R, Mosca JD, Moorman MA, Simonetti DW, Craig S, Marshak DR. Multilineage potential of adult human mesenchymal stem cells. *Science* 1999;**284**(5411):143—7.
41. Mitchell JB, McIntosh K, Zvonic S, Garrett S, Floyd ZE, Kloster A, Di Halvorsen Y, Storms RW, Goh B, Kilroy G, et al. Immunophenotype of human adipose-derived cells: temporal changes in stromal-associated and stem cell-associated markers. *Stem Cells* 2006;**24**(2):376—85.
42. Izadpanah R, Trygg C, Patel B, Kriedt C, Dufour J, Gimble JM, Bunnell BA. Biologic properties of mesenchymal stem cells derived from bone marrow and adipose tissue. *J Cell Biochem* 2006;**99**(5):1285—97.
43. Rodriguez AM, Elabd C, Delteil F, Astier J, Vernochet C, Saint-Marc P, Guesnet J, Guezennec A, Amri EZ, Dani C, et al. Adipocyte differentiation of multipotent cells established from human adipose tissue. *Biochem Biophys Res Commun* 2004;**315**(2): 255—63.
44. Rodriguez AM, Pisani D, Dechesne CA, Turc-Carel C, Kurzenne JY, Wdziekonski B, Villageois A, Bagnis C, Breittmayer JP, Groux H, et al. Transplantation of a multipotent cell population from human adipose tissue induces dystrophin expression in the immunocompetent mdx mouse. *J Exp Med* 2005;**201**(9):1397—405.
45. Elabd C, Chiellini C, Carmona M, Galitzky J, Cochet O, Petersen R, Penicaud L, Kristiansen K, Bouloumie A, Casteilla L, et al. Human multipotent adipose-derived stem cells differentiate into functional brown adipocytes. *Stem Cells* 2009;**27**(11):2753—60.
46. Hausman GJ, Wright JT, Jewell DE, Ramsay TG. Fetal adipose tissue development. *Int J Obes* 1990;**14**(Suppl. 3):177—85.
47. Crandall DL, Hausman GJ, Kral JG. A review of the microcirculation of adipose tissue: anatomic, metabolic, and angiogenic perspectives. *Microcirculation* 1997;**4**(2):211—32.
48. Bouloumie A, Lolmede K, Sengenes C, Galitzky J, Lafontan M. Angiogenesis in adipose tissue. *Ann Endocrinol (Paris)* 2002; **63**(2):91—5.
49. Bouloumie A, Sengenes C, Portolan G, Galitzky J, Lafontan M. Adipocyte produces matrix metalloproteinase 2 and 9: involvement on adipose differentiation. *Diabetes* 2001 Sep;**50**(9): 2080—6.
50. Lijnen HR. Angiogenesis and obesity. *Cardiovasc Res* 2008;**78**(2): 286—93.
51. Hausman GJ, Campion DR, Martin RJ. Search for the adipocyte precursor cell and factors that promote its differentiation. *J Lipid Res* 1980;**21**(6):657—70.
52. Castellot Jr JJ, Karnovsky MJ, Spiegelman BM. Differentiation-dependent stimulation of neovascularization and endothelial cell chemotaxis by 3T3 adipocytes. *Proc Natl Acad Sci U S A* 1982;**79**(18):5597—601.
53. Montesano R, Mouron P, Orci L. Vascular outgrowths from tissue explants embedded in fibrin or collagen gels: a simple in vitro model of angiogenesis. *Cell Biol Int Rep* 1985;**9**(10):869—75.
54. Varzaneh FE, Shillabeer G, Wong KL, Lau DC. Extracellular matrix components secreted by microvascular endothelial cells stimulate preadipocyte differentiation in vitro. *Metabolism* 1994;**43**(7):906—12.
55. Miranville A, Heeschen C, Sengenes C, Curat CA, Busse R, Bouloumie A. Improvement of postnatal neovascularization by human adipose tissue-derived stem cells. *Circulation* 2004; **110**(3):349—55.
56. Rupnick MA, Panigrahy D, Zhang CY, Dallabrida SM, Lowell BB, Langer R, Folkman MJ. Adipose tissue mass can be regulated through the vasculature. *Proc Natl Acad Sci U S A* 2002;**99**(16):10730—5.
57. Liu JJ, Huang TS, Cheng WF, Lu FJ. Baicalein and baicalin are potent inhibitors of angiogenesis: Inhibition of endothelial cell proliferation, migration and differentiation. *Int J Cancer* 2003;**106** (4):559—65.
58. Kolonin MG, Saha PK, Chan L, Pasqualini R, Arap W. Reversal of obesity by targeted ablation of adipose tissue. *Nat Med* 2004;**10**(6):625—32.
59. Fukumura D, Ushiyama A, Duda DG, Xu L, Tam J, Krishna V, Chatterjee K, Garkavtsev I, Jain RK. Paracrine regulation of angiogenesis and adipocyte differentiation during in vivo adipogenesis. *Circ Res* 2003;**93**(9):e88—97.
60. Rossig L, Urbich C, Dimmeler S. Endothelial progenitor cells at work: not mature yet, but already stress-resistant. *Arterioscler Thromb Vasc Biol* 2004;**24**(11):1977—9.
61. Murasawa S, Asahara T. Endothelial progenitor cells for vasculogenesis. *Physiology (Bethesda)* 2005;**20**:36—42.
62. Moon MH, Kim SY, Kim YJ, Kim SJ, Lee JB, Bae YC, Sung SM, Jung JS. Human adipose tissue-derived mesenchymal stem cells improve postnatal neovascularization in a mouse model of hindlimb ischemia. *Cell Physiol Biochem* 2006;**17**(5-6): 279—90.
63. Grenier G, Scime A, Le Grand F, Asakura A, Perez-Iratxeta C, Andrade-Navarro MA, Labosky PA, Rudnicki MA. Resident endothelial precursors in muscle, adipose, and dermis

contribute to postnatal vasculogenesis. *Stem Cells* 2007;**25**(12): 3101—10.
64. Wosnitza M, Hemmrich K, Groger A, Graber S, Pallua N. Plasticity of human adipose stem cells to perform adipogenic and endothelial differentiation. *Differentiation* 2007;**75**(1):12—23.
65. Zimmerlin L, Donnenberg VS, Pfeifer ME, Meyer EM, Peault B, Rubin JP, Donnenberg AD. Stromal vascular progenitors in adult human adipose tissue. *Cytometry A* 2010 Jan;**77**(1):22—30. Erratum in: *Cytometry A*. 2010 Apr;**77**(4):406.
66. Hosogai N, Fukuhara A, Oshima K, Miyata Y, Tanaka S, Segawa K, Furukawa S, Tochino Y, Komuro R, Matsuda M, et al. Adipose tissue hypoxia in obesity and its impact on adipocytokine dysregulation. *Diabetes* 2007;**56**(4):901—11.
67. Rausch ME, Weisberg S, Vardhana P, Tortoriello DV. Obesity in C57BL/6J mice is characterized by adipose tissue hypoxia and cytotoxic T-cell infiltration. *Int J Obes (Lond)*; 2007.
68. Trayhurn P, Wang B, Wood IS. Hypoxia in adipose tissue: a basis for the dysregulation of tissue function in obesity? *Br J Nutr* 2008;**100**(2):227—35.
69. Pasarica M, Sereda OR, Redman LM, Albarado DC, Hymel DT, Roan LE, Rood JC, Burk DH, Smith SR. Reduced adipose tissue oxygenation in human obesity: evidence for rarefaction, macrophage chemotaxis, and inflammation without an angiogenic response. *Diabetes* 2009;**58**(3):718—25.
70. Halberg N, Khan T, Trujillo ME, Wernstedt-Asterholm I, Attie AD, Sherwani S, Wang ZV, Landskroner-Eiger S, Dineen S, Magalang UJ, et al. Hypoxia-inducible factor 1alpha induces fibrosis and insulin resistance in white adipose tissue. *Mol Cell Biol* 2009;**29**(16):4467—83.
71. Khan T, Muise ES, Iyengar P, Wang ZV, Chandalia M, Abate N, Zhang BB, Bonaldo P, Chua S, Scherer PE. Metabolic dysregulation and adipose tissue fibrosis: role of collagen VI. *Mol Cell Biol* 2009;**29**(6):1575—91.
72. Keophiphath M, Achard V, Henegar C, Rouault C, Clement K, Lacasa D. Macrophage-secreted factors promote a profibrotic phenotype in human preadipocytes. *Mol Endocrinol* 2009;**23**(1): 11—24.
73. Desruisseaux MS, Nagajyothi, Trujillo ME, Tanowitz HB, Scherer PE. Adipocyte, adipose tissue, and infectious disease. *Infect Immun* 2007;**75**(3):1066—78.
74. Tataranni PA, Ortega E. A burning question: does an adipokine-induced activation of the immune system mediate the effect of overnutrition on type 2 diabetes? *Diabetes* 2005;**54**(4):917—27.
75. Schwartz J, Weiss ST. Host and environmental factors influencing the peripheral blood leukocyte count. *Am J Epidemiol* 1991;**134**(12):1402—9.
76. Nieto FJ, Szklo M, Folsom AR, Rock R, Mercuri M. Leukocyte count correlates in middle-aged adults: the Atherosclerosis Risk in Communities (ARIC) Study. *Am J Epidemiol* 1992;**136**(5):525—37.
77. Visser M, Bouter LM, McQuillan GM, Wener MH, Harris TB. Elevated C-reactive protein levels in overweight and obese adults. *Jama* 1999;**282**(22):2131—5.
78. Visser M, Bouter LM, McQuillan GM, Wener MH, Harris TB. Low-grade systemic inflammation in overweight children. *Pediatrics* 2001;**107**(1):E13.
79. Zaldivar F, McMurray RG, Nemet D, Galassetti P, Mills PJ, Cooper DM. Body fat and circulating leukocytes in children. *Int J Obes (Lond)* 2006;**30**(6):906—11.
80. Weisberg SP, McCann D, Desai M, Rosenbaum M, Leibel RL, Ferrante Jr AW. Obesity is associated with macrophage accumulation in adipose tissue. *J Clin Invest* 2003;**112**(12):1796—808.
81. Xu H, Barnes GT, Yang Q, Tan G, Yang D, Chou CJ, Sole J, Nichols A, Ross JS, Tartaglia LA, et al. Chronic inflammation in fat plays a crucial role in the development of obesity-related insulin resistance. *J Clin Invest* 2003;**112**(12):1821—30.
82. Hotamisligil GS. Inflammation and metabolic disorders. *Nature* 2006;**444**(7121):860—7.
83. Heilbronn LK, Noakes M, Clifton PM. Energy restriction and weight loss on very-low-fat diets reduce C-reactive protein concentrations in obese, healthy women. *Arterioscler Thromb Vasc Biol* 2001;**21**(6):968—70.
84. Nicoletti G, Giugliano G, Pontillo A, Cioffi M, D'Andrea F, Giugliano D, Esposito K. Effect of a multidisciplinary program of weight reduction on endothelial functions in obese women. *J Endocrinol Invest* 2003;**26**(3):RC5—8.
85. Giugliano G, Nicoletti G, Grella E, Giugliano F, Esposito K, Scuderi N, D'Andrea F. Effect of liposuction on insulin resistance and vascular inflammatory markers in obese women. *Br J Plast Surg* 2004;**57**(3):190—94.
86. Murdoch C, Giannoudis A, Lewis CE. Mechanisms regulating the recruitment of macrophages into hypoxic areas of tumors and other ischemic tissues. *Blood* 2004;**104**(8): 2224—34.
87. Mosser DM. The many faces of macrophage activation. *J Leukoc Biol* 2003;**73**(2):209—12.
88. Martinez FO, Sica A, Mantovani A, Locati M. Macrophage activation and polarization. *Front Biosci* 2008;**13**:453—61.
89. Mantovani A, Garlanda C, Locati M. Macrophage diversity and polarization in atherosclerosis: a question of balance. *Arterioscler Thromb Vasc Biol* 2009;**29**(10):1419—23.
90. Bourlier V, Zakaroff-Girard A, Miranville A, De Barros S, Maumus M, Sengenes C, Galitzky J, Lafontan M, Karpe F, Frayn KN, et al. Remodeling phenotype of human subcutaneous adipose tissue macrophages. *Circulation* 2008;**117**(6): 806—15.
91. Lumeng CN, Bodzin JL, Saltiel AR. Obesity induces a phenotypic switch in adipose tissue macrophage polarization. *J Clin Invest* 2007;**117**(1):175—84.
92. de Luca C, Olefsky JM. Inflammation and insulin resistance. *FEBS Lett* 2008;**582**(1):97—105.
93. Cho CH, Koh YJ, Han J, Sung HK, Jong Lee H, Morisada T, Schwendener RA, Brekken RA, Kang G, Oike Y, et al. Angiogenic role of LYVE-1-positive macrophages in adipose tissue. *Circ Res* 2007;**100**(4):e47—57.
94. Heilbronn LK, Campbell LV. Adipose tissue macrophages, low grade inflammation and insulin resistance in human obesity. *Curr Pharm Des* 2008;**14**(12):1225—30.
95. Constant VA, Gagnon A, Landry A, Sorisky A. Macrophage-conditioned medium inhibits the differentiation of 3T3-L1 and human abdominal preadipocytes. *Diabetologia* 2006;**49**(6): 1402—11.
96. Lacasa D, Taleb S, Keophiphath M, Miranville A, Clement K. Macrophage-secreted factors impair human adipogenesis: involvement of proinflammatory state in preadipocytes. *Endocrinology* 2007;**148**(2):868—77.
97. Keller M, Spanou Z, Schaerli P, Britschgi M, Yawalkar N, Seitz M, Villiger PM, Pichler WJ. T cell-regulated neutrophilic inflammation in autoinflammatory diseases. *J Immunol* 2005; **175**(11):7678—86.
98. Batista FD, Harwood NE. The who, how and where of antigen presentation to B cells. *Nat Rev Immunol* 2009;**9**(1):15—27.
99. Caspar-Bauguil S, Cousin B, Galinier A, Segafredo C, Nibbelink M, Andre M, Casteilla L, Penicaud L. Adipose tissues as an ancestral immune organ: site-specific change in obesity. *FEBS Lett* 2005;**579**(17):3487—92.
100. Wu H, Ghosh S, Perrard XD, Feng L, Garcia GE, Perrard JL, Sweeney JF, Peterson LE, Chan L, Smith CW, et al. T-cell accumulation and regulated on activation, normal T cell expressed and secreted upregulation in adipose tissue in obesity. *Circulation* 2007;**115**(8):1029—38.

101. Kintscher U, Hartge M, Hess K, Foryst-Ludwig A, Clemenz M, Wabitsch M, Fischer-Posovszky P, Barth TF, Dragun D, Skurk T, et al. T-lymphocyte infiltration in visceral adipose tissue: a primary event in adipose tissue inflammation and the development of obesity-mediated insulin resistance. *Arterioscler Thromb Vasc Biol* 2008;**28**(7):1304—10.

102. Winer S, Chan Y, Paltser G, Truong D, Tsui H, Bahrami J, Dorfman R, Wang Y, Zielenski J, Mastronardi F, et al. Normalization of obesity-associated insulin resistance through immunotherapy. *Nat Med* 2009;**15**(8):921—9.

103. Feuerer M, Herrero L, Cipolletta D, Naaz A, Wong J, Nayer A, Lee J, Goldfine AB, Benoist C, Shoelson S, et al. Lean, but not obese, fat is enriched for a unique population of regulatory T cells that affect metabolic parameters. *Nat Med* 2009;**15**(8):930—9.

104. Duffaut C, Zakaroff-Girard A, Bourlier V, Decaunes P, Maumus M, Chiotasso P, Sengenes C, Lafontan M, Galitzky J, Bouloumie A. Interplay between human adipocytes and T lymphocytes in obesity: CCL20 as an adipochemokine and T lymphocytes as lipogenic modulators. *Arterioscler Thromb Vasc Biol* 2009;**29**(10):1608—14.

105. Duffaut C, Galitzky J, Lafontan M, Bouloumie A. Unexpected trafficking of immune cells within the adipose tissue during the onset of obesity. *Biochem Biophys Res Commun* 2009;**384**(4):482—5.

106. Nishimura S, Manabe I, Nagasaki M, Eto K, Yamashita H, Ohsugi M, Otsu M, Hara K, Ueki K, Sugiura S, et al. CD8+ effector T cells contribute to macrophage recruitment and adipose tissue inflammation in obesity. *Nat Med* 2009;**15**(8):914—20.

CHAPTER

18

Children Obesity, Glucose Tolerance, Ghrelin, and Prader-Willi Syndrome

Simonetta Bellone[*], Arianna Busti[*,†], Sara Belcastro[*,†], Gianluca Aimaretti[†], Gianni Bona[*], Flavia Prodam[*,†]

[*]Division of Paediatrics, Department of Medical Science, University of Piemonte Orientale, Novara, Italy and
[†]Endocrinology, Department of Clinical and Experimental Medicine, University of Piemonte Orientale, Novara, Italy

INTRODUCTION

Prader-Willi syndrome (PWS) is a complex multisystemic genetic disorder caused by the lack of expression of paternally inherited genes known to be imprinted and located in the chromosome 15q11-q13 region, named PWS region [1, 2]. Genomic imprinting is an epigenetic phenomenon whereby phenotype is modified by gender of the parent contributing that allele, and PWS was the first example described in humans [3]. It is known that 70% of PWS subjects presents a non-inherited deletion in the paternally PWS region. However, 25% of cases are due to a maternally disomy 15 (Uniparental disomy (UPD): maternal uniparental disomy) and the remaining cases to genomic imprinting defects such as microdeletion or epimutation or balanced chromosome translocations [4, 5]. It has been estimated that PWS occurs at a birth incidence at 1 in 30,000 individuals and has a population prevalence of around 1 in 50,000 in Caucasians [6, 7].

Although genotype-phenotype correlations have been widely described, it can be summarized that PWS is characterized by typical phenotypes including neonatal hypotonia, uncontrolled and precocious hyperphagia, morbid obesity, short stature, hypogonadism, and other somatic, endocrine, and psychological problems [2, 8]. Indeed, PWS is considered the most common genetic syndrome leading to life-threatening obesity. Notably, the loss of several paternally expressed genes in the PWS region is thought to contribute to the abnormalities of this syndrome, and *MKRN3, MAGEL2, NDN,* *SNURF-SNRPN,* and the sno-RNA genes like *Snord116* and *HBII-85* are all expressed in the brain, including the hypothalamus, to suggest that many features depend on hypothalamus-pituitary and brain signaling derangements [4, 8, 10].

Surveys have highlighted the high rates and varied causes of morbidity and mortality throughout the natural history of the disease, mostly because of disorders related to severe obesity and endocrine and metabolic impairment [11]. It has to be underlined that the PWS neuroendocrine and metabolic phenotype is partly different to what occurs in simple obesity, being an interesting model to investigate the complex and redundant regulation of fat distribution, energy balance, feeding, and central and peripheral signaling.

As the outcome of the studies on the investigation of PWS, like a model of morbid obesity with special characteristics partly different from those of primary obesity, the aim of this chapter is to review the knowledge about obesity in PWS children and adults paying particular attention to glucose metabolism and the ghrelin system, both of which seem to have a typical regulation in this syndrome.

CLINICAL FEATURES OF PWS: CHILDHOOD-ONSET OBESITY, BODY COMPOSITION, AND HYPERPHAGIA

PWS is the most commonly recognized genetic cause of early onset obesity. The most prominent feature of

PWS is childhood onset hyperphagia that can lead to morbid obesity. However, PWS can be divided in two distinct clinical phases. The second phase has been divided in two subphases to well describe childhood, adolescence, and adulthood [2].

Stage 1 occurs from birth to early infancy at around 2 years old. It is not characterized by obesity; on the contrary, PWS neonates and infants present mild prenatal growth retardation, severe hypotonia with poor suck, and feeding with or without failure to thrive [2, 4, 8, 12].

Stage 2 starts between 18 and 36 months of life and is characterized by a progressive weight increase. First, weight presents a hyperbolic trend to increase without significant higher caloric intake or interest in food. Afterward, children increase their weight with the onset of higher interest in food and mild hyperphagia [2, 4]. This stage is also characterized by low growth velocity and, as a consequence, short stature. Growth features seem to be mostly due to growth hormone deficiency (GHD) [2, 8, 13–15].

Stage 3 start ranges from 4 to 15 years of age. During this stage, the features are classically associated to PWS with uncontrollable hyperphagia and aggressive behavior in food seeking. PWS subjects present not only further weight gain but also delayed meal termination and gastric emptying and early meal initiation after previous food ingestion [16–18]. Consequences of unattended hyperphagia lead to maintenance of over 200% ideal body weight in at least 33% of the PWS population and occasionally death as a result of choking or stomach rapture [19–21]. All these aspects suggest a derangement in hormonal and metabolic satiety responses to food intake, and most of the recent studies have focused on endocrine and functional neuroimaging abnormalities.

Stage 4 occurs in a subset of individuals after 30 years of age. It is still characterized by increased appetite but without uncontrolled hyperphagia [2] and does not seem to present abnormal gastric emptying [22].

Childhood-onset PWS obesity shows a specific body composition. In fact, PWS subjects present in both prenatal and postnatal first months of life hypotonia because of persistent poor muscle tone. This feature proceeds with age, and reduced lean muscle mass as well as bone mineral content and density are associated with increased body fat from infancy to adulthood characterized by increased fat-to-lean mass ratios [23–25]. Total lean mass is significantly lower for arms, trunk, and especially legs; therefore, PWS differs from simple obesity in which an increase in lean tissue accompanies an increase in adipose tissue [26]. Notably, subjects with PWS have a reduced energy expenditure not only from reduced physical activity but also from lower energy utilization caused by their reduced lean body mass, which consists primarily of muscle in all ages [27, 28].

Accordingly, a low resting metabolic rate is normal when corrected for reduced lower free-fat mass and higher fat mass [29, 30]. During the life span, the percentage of body fat is significantly greater in the PWS population than in control individuals with a comparable degree of obesity [23, 24, 25, 31] and most of the fat accumulation tends to be in extraabdominal areas [26, 32]. In fact, PWS subjects present less trunk and, as a consequence, fat mass with respect to controls matched for obesity [26, 31]. This is evident as lower absolute visceral adipose tissue volume, percentage of total adipose tissue, or body mass. In contrast, no significant decrease in the amount of total or abdominal subcutaneous and nonvisceral internal adipose tissue is detected in respect to simple obesity [30, 33]. Fat distribution is similar between sexes, with a mean percentage body fat of 53% and 44% in adult PWS females and males, respectively, with similar results in children and adolescents [23, 29, 34].

Hence, it becomes clear that morbid obesity in PWS population resembles much more body composition of sedentary elderly and patients suffering of GHD than that of essential obesity. Consistent with this hypothesis, the GH/IGF-I axis has been widely explored in PWS individuals. GHD may be one of the candidate factors contributing to increased fat mass and, especially, to decreased muscle mass. Low spontaneous secretion and reduced GH peak to standard provocative tests as well as decreased circulating IGF-I levels have been demonstrated in PWS children and adults [2, 35, 36]. However, the etiology of impaired GH secretion is still controversial because it can be a functional effect of obesity alone and references cut off of normal responses to pharmacological stimuli are unavailable in such severe obesity [2, 8, 13, 14]. In addiction, because of different body composition in respect to simple obesity cut-off values that are simply stratified for body mass index (BMI) could be not really useful in PWS individuals. However, it has been shown that PWS adults present a lower GH response to growth hormone releasing hormone (GHRH) + arginine stimulus in respect to controls matched not only for BMI but also for percentage of fat mass. A severely impaired GH response is also associated with low IGF-I levels. These data support the hypothesis that GHD may be present in a significant subset of PWS patients and could influence their body composition, including low fat-free mass and other features like short stature, cardiovascular risk, osteoporosis, and psychological impairment [36]. The replacement with rhGH in PWS children is approved worldwide for some well-documented benefits, in particular the achievement of final adult height and an improvement in body composition, although without complete normalization [15]. A life-span replacement in PWS adults with well documented

GHD status could be useful basing on a recent multicenter trial [35, 36].

GHD and other dysfunctions like hypogenitalism as well as temperature and sleep disorders described in PWS subjects suggest hypothalamus-pituitary abnormalities. Accordingly, defects in the hypothalamus have been reported in studies using functional MRI or in post-mortem quantification of hypothalamic neuropeptides [30, 37, 38]. Pituitary MRI abnormalities including empty sella as well as anterior and posterior pituitary hypoplasia have been also reported [39].

Neuroanatomical and functional hypothalamic abnormalities may contribute to hyperphagia and behavioral PWS problems. Interestingly, the PWS hypothalamus presents a low oxytocin cell number otherwise orexin, GHRH, neuropeptide γ (NPγ), and agouti related protein (AgRP) neurons [30, 37, 39]. Given the effect of hyperphagia on health and quality of life of PWS subjects delineation of gene dysregulation, brain development and function is a challenge. It has already been shown that glucose administration is followed by a delayed signal reduction in hypothalamus, ventromedial prefrontal cortex, insula, and nucleo accumbens in these patients [38]. This effect is associated with a hyperresponsive neural network related to food process and a disruption of reward circuitry relating to food motivation in MRI functional studies [40–42]. Divergent neural mechanisms seem to be associated with behavioral phenotypes in genetic subtypes of PWS, suggesting that hyperphagia is a complex phenomenon and mechanisms linked to it are differently regulated by maternally imprinted or paternally expressed genes [18]. Position Emission Tomography (PET) protocols also demonstrated higher metabolism in the prefrontal and temporal lobe during fasting and reduced tracer binding to GABA-A receptors in the same regions [43, 44].

Hormonal abnormalities associated with neural derangement and hyperphagia are still unknown. Fasting and postprandial ghrelin levels are elevated in PWS subjects also before the onset of obesity [45], although peptide levels fall in normal extend after meal ingestion [46]. Acute somatostatin infusion also inhibits ghrelin secretion in PWS subjects but without modulating appetite [47]. Peptide YY (PYY) secretion is also modified in PWS with fasting lower levels and a blunted postprandial response, which present a similar altered profile to that observed for pancreatic polypeptide [48, 49].

It appears clear that morbid obesity and hyperphagia are the major problems of PWS, and obesity management requires environmental control with a low-caloric balanced diet and physical activity until pathogenetic mechanisms will not be clearly explained. As long as this remains a challenge, supervision, restriction to access to food, and money are needed.

GLUCOSE METABOLISM AND INSULIN SENSITIVITY

Type 2 diabetes has been reported in about 25% of adults with PWS with a mean age of 20 years [50]. Obesity is a common component of type 2 diabetes and plays an important role in the development of hyperinsulinemia and insulin resistance. The increase of visceral fat plays an integral role in the development of insulin resistance, glucose intolerance, and hyperlipidemia in obesity [51]. However, glucoregulatory mechanisms are different in obese PWS with respect to obese non-PWS subjects according to unusual fat patterning of the syndrome [34, 52, 53]. Euglycemic PWS patients have a reduced beta-cell response to glucose stimulation associated with an increased hepatic insulin extraction and a dissociation between obesity and insulin-resistance in respect to healthy obese subjects in both pediatric and adult ages after intravenous and oral glucose tolerance tests [52]. In particular, the first- and the second-phase insulin secretion responses are both lower in PWS with respect to matched obese subjects [52]. A state of relative hypoinsulinemia occurs in PWS individuals also after mixed meals [52, 54]. Therefore, nondiabetic PWS patients present normal or increased insulin sensitivity, suggesting that they may be protected from obesity-associated insulin resistance and metabolic syndrome [55–57]. Accordingly, insulin and insulin-resistance indexes in PWS are not associated with adipokines otherwise widely shown in simple obesity. Then, adipokines like adiponectin and resistin are differently modulated in PWS [58, 59]. In particular, high molecular weight (HMW) isoform of adiponectin and HMW/total adiponectin ratios are increased in PWS children, and these data are of particular interest because this isoform and the ratios better correlate with insulin sensitivity [57]. However, high levels of adiponectin may be a consequence, rather than a cause, of increased insulin sensitivity and hypoinsulinemia in PWS.

Many mechanisms could be linked to these metabolic PWS features, in particular GH and IGF/I deficiency. Glucose abnormalities and insulin resistance have been reported by some [52] but not all studies [35, 60, 61]. However, it has to be pointed out that GH treatment is followed by a modest increase in insulin, glucose, glycosylated hemoglobin (HbA1c), the homeostatic model assessment (HOMA) index, and the prevalence of metabolic syndrome in both pediatric and adult populations [35, 62], suggesting that the GH/IGF-I axis and fat distribution, which is influenced by hormone replacement, could have a role.

Despite a state of better insulin sensitivity in PWS, some individuals develop type 2 diabetes. Following the visceral fat area stratification reported by Despres,

PWS subjects with a visceral fat area higher than 130 cm² were found to have insulin sensitivity and resistance similar to obese-matched controls, suggesting that this population could be at higher risk of obesity-related disorders [53]. Moreover, diabetic PWS patients continue to have higher glucose levels with decreased precocious insulin levels during oral glucose tolerance test (OGTT), which are secondary to the pronounced reduced beta-cell response to glucose stimulation [33, 52, 56].

GHRELIN AND OBESTATIN REGULATION

PWS subjects typically present higher ghrelin levels [8, 63, 64]. Ghrelin is a 28–amino acid peptide, isolated from the stomach but also shown to be expressed in other tissues such as the pancreas, testes, placenta, pituitary, and hypothalamus [65]. Ghrelin has been identified as an endogenous ligand of the orphan GH secretagogue (GHS)-receptor type 1a [65, 66]. It circulates in blood in two forms: acylated (AG) and unacylated ghrelin (UAG). The acyl group, which binds ghrelin at the serine-3 residue, seems to be essential for the binding to GHS-receptor type 1a and the resulting neuroendocrine functions, namely GH secretion [65, 66]. UAG, which is devoid of the acyl group, represents the most abundant circulating form [67, 68]. UAG is biologically active, although it does not have direct neuroendocrine actions, suggesting the existence of some GHS-receptor subtypes [65, 66, 68–70]. The mechanism of acylation of the preproghrelin or UAG is largely unknown. Recently, it has been identified as the acyltransferase that octanoylates ghrelin [71].

Moreover, since its discovery (AG was identified first, followed by UAG), ghrelin emerged as a player in the regulation of food intake and energy expenditure, with AG the most potent peripheral orexigenic hormone known to date [65, 68, 70]. In animals and humans, AG, after both central and peripheral administration, has been shown to induce appetite and food intake [68]. Despite the clear orexigenic effects of AG, the actual physiological role of UAG in the regulation of appetite is still a matter of debate [68, 72].

It has also been clearly shown that both forms of ghrelin also influence energy metabolism at the peripheral level, most likely influencing fat oxidation [73, 74]. Reduced cellular fat oxidation and the promotion of adipogenesis each contributes to an increase in fat mass induced by AG but also UAG [68, 73, 75].

Consistent with its effects on food intake and its involvement in energy balance, circulating ghrelin levels are negatively associated with BMI in humans [68, 76, 77]. Several studies indicate that ghrelin hyposecretion in essential obesity is a functional impairment in response to body weight alteration [78]. Furthermore, most the data come from studies that have analyzed exclusively total ghrelin levels. Findings have also shown that UAG is decreased in obesity, whereas there are no concordant results for AG [68, 79, 80]. Ghrelin is implicated in the regulation of glucose homeostasis by modulating insulin secretion and action. It has also been demonstrated that insulin modulates ghrelin levels through inhibition [65, 68, 70, 81]. Ghrelin secretion is also modulated by nutrients, namely carbohydrates, whereas the role of fats and proteins is not completely understood because of discordant results [65, 68, 70, 81, 82].

In 2005, Zhang and coworkers, from a conserved region of preproghrelin sequence, identified a 23 amino acid peptide, which was named obestatin based on previous reported activities in animal models. It was initially characterized as the active ligand of the orphan receptor GPR39, but more recently this result is being discussed [75, 83–85].

Obestatin, like ghrelin, is expressed in several tissues, which include the stomach, duodenum, pancreas, and brain [75].

Obestatin initially appeared to be a new regulator of appetite and body weight [83]. Following studies, however, failed to reproduce obestatin's anorectic and antiobesity effects and questioned its existence as just a ghrelin-associated peptide [83].

Furthermore, previous data regarding the modulation of insulin secretion are limited and controversial [86, 87]. On the other hand, preliminary studies in vivo recently observed that obestatin is reduced in subjects with type 2 diabetes and impaired glucose tolerance as well as in obesity, whereas it is increased in anorexia [86].

As previously introduced, PWS individuals present higher ghrelin levels (from 3.0- to 3.6-fold) despite morbid obesity [63, 64, 88, 89]. This feature is typical of the syndrome unlike those with simple obesity, hypothalamic obesity due to craniopharyngioma, or other forms of genetic obesity [88, 89]. Hyperghrelinemia is also present in PWS infants, precedes morbid obesity, and maintains the age-dependent decrease [64, 90]. These results are in agreement with observations in a transgenic mouse model for the region equivalent to the human PWS region in which high ghrelin levels were observed from the third day after birth [91]. Some studies do not confirm higher ghrelin concentration in very young children, in particular children aged 17 to 60 months [45, 92], but these results could be influenced by rhGH therapy in the population [93]. Accordingly, high fasting total ghrelin levels in GH untreated PWS children were found to be decreased in the GH-treated group, although AG levels were not modified [64, 93, 94]. Indeed, total ghrelin could not be considered a surrogate for the acylated form, and the

GH replacement, at least in the PWS population, modulates ghrelin secretion in terms of AG: total ghrelin ratios [93]. Notably, gastric ghrelin-expressing cell density and quantity are both increased in the fundus and body of the stomach of PWS patients. This increase is not related to the IGF-I levels. In fact, gastric ghrelin-expressing cells are similar in both GH sufficient and GHD PWS subjects [17]. The increased density and quantity of ghrelin-expressing cells could also explain higher AG levels in PWS, according to the ghrelin O-acyltransferase (GOAT) expression in stomach and its mainly intracellular activity [71, 93–95].

Although many authors have reported higher AG levels, only one study evaluated UAG secretion in PWS without differences with respect to obese matched controls [95]. Preliminary conflicting data show obestatin not increased and elevated in PWS children [28, 96]. Although Park and coworkers failed to find a different regulation of obestatin secretion, this peptide positively correlated with the BMI standard deviation score in this population, similar to what was observed in some but not all studies performed to examine simple obesity [96–99]. Indeed, hyperghrelinemia in PWS seems to be a typical feature that involves the specific process of acylation without modulating the other forms derived from the prepropeptide.

Besides these results, many hypotheses on increased AG and total ghrelin secretion have been widely discussed. According to very early hyperghrelinemia in PWS infants, this hormonal derangement could play a role in early-onset obesity [64]. Moreover, it could explain at least two other major endocrine dysfunctions of the syndrome: obesity with reduced and delayed satiety and GHD [2, 63, 64, 89].

However, the role of elevated AG and total ghrelin levels in PWS hyperphagia has been questioned. Long-acting octreotide treatment successfully blunted fasting and postprandial AG and UAG levels without being followed by changes in body weight and composition, appetite, or behavior toward food in PWS children and adolescents [90, 100]. Similar data were obtained in PWS adults after an acute somatostatin infusion [47]. It has been suggested that the lack of reduction of appetite could be due to a consensual reduction of PYY, but this effect was obtained in an acute study on adults rather than in that with chronic administration in children [46, 47, 100]. Alternatively, the plasmatic inhibition of the peptide could not be associated with a consensual inhibition of its expression or activity. Indeed, increased appetite may be secondary to abnormal expression of nonghrelin genes, in particular serotoninergic pathways [101, 102]. Notably, similar falls in ghrelin levels after somatostatin infusion or octreotide therapy in PWS as in other studies of non-PWS individuals suggest that the cause of hyperghrelinemia probably is not an intrinsic primary abnormality of ghrelin expressing cells but, more likely, a loss of inhibitory, or excess of stimulatory, neural or hormonal inputs [46, 47, 90, 103, 104]. As vagotomy increases plasma ghrelin in rodents, the elevated AG and total ghrelin concentration in PWS subjects might result from reduced parasympathetic vagal efferent tone in PWS in agreement with similar data on disturbed parasympathetic cardiac autonomic function tests [89, 105].

Furthermore, a role in the development of GHD in PWS has been questioned. Goldstone and coworkers failed to demonstrate an association between plasma ghrelin and IGF-I levels even when adjusting for adiposity and insulin levels in PWS adults [89]. Similarly, GHRH neurons do not present abnormalities in postmortem PWS hypothalamus [106]. However, as previously discussed, GH replacement blunts ghrelin secretion, suggesting at least a functional role between these systems [93, 94].

It is clear that hyperghrelinemia is a new hormonal feature of PWS, but its pathophysiological role is still widely unclear at least with respect to hyperphagia, obesity, and GH status. The lack of modulation of UAG and obestatin remains to be investigated and could offer new hypotheses.

PRADER-WILLI SYNDROME (PWS), GLUCOSE METABOLISM, AND GHRELIN SYSTEM: WHAT IS THE LINK?

Insulin is a physiological modulator of glucose and ghrelin levels, as previously introduced. Insulin possesses an inhibitory effect on ghrelin secretion that is independent of plasma glucose concentration, although an additional effect cannot be excluded [68]. Insulin levels and insulin resistance have been shown to be major predictors of reduction of UAG and total ghrelin levels in obesity and metabolic syndrome [68, 79, 80].

PWS individuals present morbid obesity with typical fat distribution, relative hypoinsulinemia, higher insulin sensitivity, and grossly elevated ghrelin levels. As a consequence, the contribution of the ghrelin system on the PWS metabolic phenotype has been widely explored, with a contribution from studies in animal models. It has been reported that deficits of insulin and glucagon during fetal and postnatal life are prominent features in the transgenic PWS deletion mouse models, which also present hyperghrelinemia in the postnatal period at the onset of severe hypoglycemia. These findings suggest that higher ghrelin levels could be an adaptive response to restore normal glucose levels or glucose sensing. The same mechanism could also increase eating in this condition [91, 107]. Furthermore, insulin alone, which is reduced in PWS, is insufficient to lower basal ghrelin levels [107, 108]. Accordingly, Goldstone and coworkers have shown how higher ghrelin concentration in PWS adults may be partially contributed, but are not solely explained, by their abnormal fat distribution, relative hypoinsulinemia, or reduced insulin resistance in both fasting and fed conditions [46, 89]. These data are in agreement with similar results in studies of type 1 diabetes in which it has been shown that basal insulin is sufficient to suppress postprandial ghrelin in this population, whereas the lack of meal-induced ghrelin suppression could be caused by a severe insulin deficiency and might explain hyperphagia in individuals with uncontrolled type 1 diabetes [109]. However, regulatory influences in PWS secretion seem to be intact. Ghrelin levels maintain a normal postprandial fall by 32% in euglycemic PWS adults [46, 96] and are inhibited by somatostatin or its long-acting analogs in the same extent of non-PWS individuals [90, 100]. Moreover, the insulin-induced ghrelin suppression is more pronounced in PWS children during a euglycemic hyperinsulinemic clamp [107, 108]. Also AG levels are inhibited by carbohydrate administration in euglycemic PWS children with more sensitivity suppression by insulin [94, 95, 96, 107] but, unlike total ghrelin, are not modulated by GH replacement [94]. This variation of AG levels after a glucose challenge showed a significant correlation with the whole-body insulin sensitivity index (WBISI), and the decrease promptly starts with the delayed insulin surge [96].

A preliminary study evaluated fasting and postprandial AG and total ghrelin levels in PWS individuals with respect to their glucose tolerance. Notably, total ghrelin levels were similar, whereas AG levels and the AG: total ghrelin ratios were decreased in dysglycemic PWS with respect to euglycemic PWS adults. Fasting AG and ratio decreases have been hypothetically linked to higher insulin resistance in dysglycemic PWS despite similar adiposity. Moreover, AG levels increased after meals only in glucose-intolerant individuals and were predicted by glycemia during the oral glucose load, in particular in the first 60 minutes, suggesting that a fast increase of AG could modulate the relative hypoinsulinemia and hyperglycemic response to meals in PWS [110]. Alternatively, more pronounced low insulin levels are insufficient to inhibit postprandial AG levels with an inversion of the reciprocal pattern between insulin and ghrelin with respect to fasting and feeding conditions [109, 110, 111].

Paik and coworkers conducted the sole study on directly measured UAG levels in PWS. The findings suggested that UAG concentration was similar between PWS and healthy obese controls. Furthermore, AG and UAG secretions seem to be differently modulated by carbohydrates ingestion. Both peptides at fasting are correlated with WBISI, but this relationship is lost after the glucose challenge for UAG, unlike AG. Moreover, as previously discussed, AG promptly decreases with insulin surge, whereas UAG response is delayed for up to 90 minutes after glucose administration [95]. Because of different patterns of response, it has been hypothesized that insulin better inhibits AG in PWS or, conversely, a larger decrease in AG should induce greater insulin responses in PWS to preserve glucose tolerance [95, 110].

Obestatin levels have been shown to be elevated or unchanged in PWS with respect to healthy children [28, 96]. The authors also failed to find an association between obestatin and insulin levels in the syndrome, suggesting a different regulation among the two circulating forms of ghrelin and obestatin, at least in glucose metabolism in PWS [96].

All these data suggest that the ghrelin system is deeply involved in the regulation of glucose metabolism in PWS. It is also clear that AG, UAG, and obestatin are differently modulated. More data are needed to better clarify the pathophysiology of hyperghrelinemia in PWS, which until now has been based on the gross evaluation of total ghrelin. Relative hypoinsulinemia has a key role in fasting and postprandial regulation of these peptides, probably acting on many molecular pathways. The evaluation of PWS individuals with respect to their metabolic assessment in terms of glucose tolerance despite only total fat mass and fat distribution could offer new findings and potential therapeutic options.

CONCLUSION

PWS presents complex genetic and multiple phenotypes that mean a need for multidisciplinary and environmental approaches to reduce morbidity and mortality. Clinical features evolve from the neonatal period to adulthood with hyperphagia, typical fat distribution, and preserved insulin sensitivity. Alterations in the ghrelin system have been advocated to have a key role in this phenotype. Growing data suggest that hyperghrelinemia in PWS could be more likely a compensatory mechanism to other biochemical and hormonal alterations, in particular neonatal hypoglycemia and relative hypoinsulinemia. However, clear results are still scant because major investigations on total ghrelin levels have not included data on AG, UAG, and obestatin. Studies better focused on the complex evolution of the syndrome, paying particular attention to whom develops glucose intolerance, could offer new hypotheses on the role of the ghrelin system in PWS phenotypes as well as in features of simple obesity.

References

1. Nicholls RD, Knoll JH, Butler MG, Karam S, Lalande M. Genetic imprinting suggested by maternal heterodisomy in nondeletion Prader-Willi syndrome. *Nature* 1989;**342**:281–5.
2. Goldstone AP, Holland AJ, Hauffa BP, Hokken-Koelega AC, Tauber M. Recommendations for the diagnosis and management of Prader-Willi syndrome. *J. Clin. Endocrinol. Metab* 2008;**93**:4183–97.
3. Hanel ML, Wevrick R. The role of genomic imprinting in human developmental disorders: lessons from Prader-Willi syndrome. *Clin. Genet.* 2001;**59**:156–64.
4. Bittel DC, Butler MG. Prader-Willi syndrome: clinical genetics, cytogenetics and molecular biology. *Expert. Rev. Mol. Med.* 2005;**7**:1–20.
5. Buiting K, Gross S, Lich C, Gillessen-Kaesbach G, el-Maarri O, Horsthemke B. Epimutations in Prader-Willi and Angelman syndromes: a molecular study of 136 patients with an imprinting defect. *Am. J. Hum. Genet.* 2003;**72**:571–7.
6. Thomson AK, Glasson EJ, Bittles AH. A long-term population-based clinical and morbidity review of Prader-Willi syndrome in Western Australia. *J. Intellect. Disabil. Res.* 2006;**50**:69–78.
7. Vogels A, Van Den EJ, Keymolen K, Mortier G, Devriendt K, Legius E, Fryns JP. Minimum prevalence, birth incidence and cause of death for Prader-Willi syndrome in Flanders. *Eur. J. Hum. Genet.* 2004;**12**:238–40.
8. Goldstone AP. Prader-Willi syndrome: advances in genetics, pathophysiology and treatment. *Trends Endocrinol. Metab* 2004;**15**:12–20.
9. Ding F, Li HH, Zhang S, Solomon NM, Camper SA, Cohen P, Francke U. SnoRNA Snord116 (Pwcr1/MBII-85) deletion causes growth deficiency and hyperphagia in mice. *PLoS. One* 2008;**3**: e1709 (1–17).
10. de Smith AJ, Purmann C, Walters RG, Ellis RJ, Holder SE, Van Haelst MM, Brady AF, Fairbrother UL, Dattani M, Keogh JM, Henning E, Yeo GS, O'Rahilly S, Froguel P, Farooqi IS, Blakemore AI. A deletion of the HBII-85 class of small nucleolar RNAs (snoRNAs) is associated with hyperphagia, obesity and hypogonadism. *Hum. Mol. Genet.* 2009;**18**:3257–65.
11. Tauber M, Diene G, Molinas C, Hebert M. Review of 64 cases of death in children with Prader-Willi syndrome (PWS). *Am. J. Med. Genet. A* 2008;**146**:881–7.
12. Whittington JE, Butler JV, Holland AJ. Pre-, peri- and postnatal complications in Prader-Willi syndrome in a UK sample. *Early Hum. Dev.* 2008;**84**:331–6.
13. Burman P, Ritzen EM, Lindgren AC. Endocrine dysfunction in Prader-Willi syndrome: a review with special reference to GH. *Endocr. Rev.* 2001;**22**:787–99.
14. Hoybye C, Frystyk J, Thoren M. The growth hormone-insulin-like growth factor axis in adult patients with Prader Willi syndrome. *Growth Horm. IGF. Res.* 2003;**13**:269–74.
15. Lindgren AC, Lindberg A. Growth hormone treatment completely normalizes adult height and improves body composition in Prader-Willi syndrome: experience from KIGS (Pfizer International Growth Database). *Horm. Res.* 2008;**70**:182–7.
16. Holland AJ, Treasure J, Coskeran P, Dallow J, Milton N, Hillhouse E. Measurement of excessive appetite and metabolic changes in Prader-Willi syndrome. *Int. J. Obes. Relat Metab Disord.* 1993;**17**:527–32.
17. Choe YH, Jin DK, Kim SE, Song SY, Paik KH, Park HY, Oh YJ, Kim AH, Kim JS, Kim CW, Chu SH, Kwon EK, Lee KH. Hyperghrelinemia does not accelerate gastric emptying in Prader-Willi syndrome patients. *J. Clin. Endocrinol. Metab* 2005;**90**:3367–70.
18. Holsen LM, Zarcone JR, Chambers R, Butler MG, Bittel DC, Brooks WM, Thompson TI, Savage CR. Genetic subtype differences in neural circuitry of food motivation in Prader-Willi syndrome. *Int. J. Obes. (Lond)* 2009;**33**:273–83.
19. Butler MG. Management of obesity in Prader-Willi syndrome. *Nat. Clin. Pract. Endocrinol. Metab* 2006;**2**:592–3.
20. Stevenson DA, Heinemann J, Angulo M, Butler MG, Loker J, Rupe N, Kendell P, Cassidy SB, Scheimann A. Gastric rupture and necrosis in Prader-Willi syndrome. *J. Pediatr. Gastroenterol. Nutr.* 2007;**45**:272–4.
21. Stevenson DA, Heinemann J, Angulo M, Butler MG, Loker J, Rupe N, Kendell P, Clericuzio CL, Scheimann AO. Deaths due to choking in Prader-Willi syndrome. *Am. J. Med. Genet. A* 2007;**143**:484–7.
22. Hoybye C, Barkeling B, Naslund E, Thoren M, Hellstrom PM. Eating behavior and gastric emptying in adults with Prader-Willi syndrome. *Ann. Nutr. Metab* 2007;**51**:264–9.
23. Brambilla P, Bosio L, Manzoni P, Pietrobelli A, Beccaria L, Chiumello G. Peculiar body composition in patients with Prader-Labhart-Willi syndrome. *Am. J. Clin. Nutr.* 1997;**65**:1369–74.
24. Eiholzer, U., L'allemand, D., van, d. S., I, Steinert, H., Gasser, T. & Ellis, K. (2000). Body composition abnormalities in children with Prader-Willi syndrome and long-term effects of growth hormone therapy. *Horm. Res.* **53**, 200–206.
25. Eiholzer U, L'allemand D, Schlumpf M, Rousson V, Gasser T, Fusch C. Growth hormone and body composition in children younger than 2 years with Prader-Willi syndrome. *J. Pediatr.* 2004;**144**:753–8.
26. Theodoro MF, Talebizadeh Z, Butler MG. Body composition and fatness patterns in Prader-Willi syndrome: comparison with simple obesity. *Obesity. (Silver. Spring)* 2006;**14**:1685–90.
27. Bekx MT, Carrel AL, Shriver TC, Li Z, Allen DB. Decreased energy expenditure is caused by abnormal body composition in infants with Prader-Willi Syndrome. *J. Pediatr.* 2003;**143**: 372–6.
28. Butler MG, Theodoro MF, Bittel DC, Donnelly JE. Energy expenditure and physical activity in Prader-Willi syndrome: comparison with obese subjects. *Am. J. Med. Genet. A* 2007;**143**:449–59.
29. van Mil EA, Westerterp KR, Gerver WJ, Curfs LM, Schrander-Stumpel CT, Kester AD, Saris WH. Energy expenditure at rest and during sleep in children with Prader-Willi syndrome is explained by body composition. *Am. J. Clin. Nutr.* 2000;**71**:752–6.
30. Goldstone AP, Brynes AE, Thomas EL, Bell JD, Frost G, Holland A, Ghatei MA, Bloom SR. Resting metabolic rate, plasma leptin concentrations, leptin receptor expression, and adipose tissue measured by whole-body magnetic resonance imaging in women with Prader-Willi syndrome. *Am. J. Clin. Nutr* 2002;**75**:468–75.
31. Kennedy L, Bittel DC, Kibiryeva N, Kalra SP, Torto R, Butler MG. Circulating adiponectin levels, body composition and obesity-related variables in Prader-Willi syndrome: comparison with obese subjects. *Int. J. Obes. (Lond)* 2006;**30**:382–7.
32. Marzullo P, Marcassa C, Campini R, Eleuteri E, Minocci A, Priano L, Temporelli P, Sartorio A, Vettor R, Liuzzi A, Grugni G. The impact of growth hormone/insulin-like growth factor-I axis and nocturnal breathing disorders on cardiovascular features of adult patients with Prader-Willi syndrome. *J. Clin. Endocrinol. Metab* 2005;**90**:5639–46.
33. Goldstone AP, Thomas EL, Brynes AE, Bell JD, Frost G, Saeed N, Hajnal JV, Howard JK, Holland A, Bloom SR. Visceral adipose tissue and metabolic complications of obesity are reduced in

Prader-Willi syndrome female adults: evidence for novel influences on body fat distribution. *J. Clin. Endocrinol. Metab* 2001;**86**:4330–8.
34. Hoybye C, Hilding A, Jacobsson H, Thoren M. Metabolic profile and body composition in adults with Prader-Willi syndrome and severe obesity. *J. Clin. Endocrinol. Metab* 2002;**87**:3590–7.
35. Mogul HR, Lee PD, Whitman BY, Zipf WB, Frey M, Myers S, Cahan M, Pinyerd B, Southren AL. Growth hormone treatment of adults with Prader-Willi syndrome and growth hormone deficiency improves lean body mass, fractional body fat, and serum triiodothyronine without glucose impairment: results from the United States multicenter trial. *J. Clin. Endocrinol. Metab* 2008;**93**:1238–45.
36. Grugni G, Crino A, Bertocco P, Marzullo P. Body fat excess and stimulated growth hormone levels in adult patients with Prader-Willi syndrome. *Am. J. Med. Genet. A* 2009;**149A**:726–31.
37. Fronczek R, Lammers GJ, Balesar R, Unmehopa UA, Swaab DF. The number of hypothalamic hypocretin (orexin) neurons is not affected in Prader-Willi syndrome. *J. Clin. Endocrinol. Metab* 2005;**90**:5466–70.
38. Shapira NA, Lessig MC, He AG, James GA, Driscoll DJ, Liu Y. Satiety dysfunction in Prader-Willi syndrome demonstrated by fMRI. *J. Neurol. Neurosurg. Psychiatry* 2005;**76**:260–2.
39. Miller JL, Goldstone AP, Couch JA, Shuster J, He G, Driscoll DJ, Liu Y, Schmalfuss IM. Pituitary abnormalities in Prader-Willi syndrome and early onset morbid obesity. *Am. J. Med. Genet. A* 2008;**146A**:570–7.
40. Holsen LM, Zarcone JR, Brooks WM, Butler MG, Thompson TI, Ahluwalia JS, Nollen NL, Savage CR. Neural mechanisms underlying hyperphagia in Prader-Willi syndrome. *Obesity. (Silver. Spring)* 2006;**14**:1028–37.
41. Hinton EC, Holland AJ, Gellatly MS, Soni S, Patterson M, Ghatei MA, Owen AM. Neural representations of hunger and satiety in Prader-Willi syndrome. *Int. J. Obes. (Lond)* 2006;**30**:313–21.
42. Miller JL, James GA, Goldstone AP, Couch JA, He G, Driscoll DJ, Liu Y. Enhanced activation of reward mediating prefrontal regions in response to food stimuli in Prader-Willi syndrome. *J. Neurol. Neurosurg. Psychiatry* 2007;**78**:615–19.
43. Lucignani G, Panzacchi A, Bosio L, Moresco RM, Ravasi L, Coppa I, Chiumello G, Frey K, Koeppe R, Fazio F. GABA A receptor abnormalities in Prader-Willi syndrome assessed with positron emission tomography and [11C]flumazenil. *Neuroimage.* 2004;**22**:22–8.
44. Kim SE, Jin DK, Cho SS, Kim JH, Hong SD, Paik KH, Oh YJ, Kim AH, Kwon EK, Choe YH. Regional cerebral glucose metabolic abnormality in Prader-Willi syndrome: A 18F-FDG PET study under sedation. *J. Nucl. Med.* 2006;**47**:1088–92.
45. Haqq AM, Grambow SC, Muehlbauer M, Newgard CB, Svetkey LP, Carrel AL, Yanovski JA, Purnell JQ, Freemark M. Ghrelin concentrations in Prader-Willi syndrome (PWS) infants and children: changes during development. *Clin. Endocrinol. (Oxf)* 2008;**69**:911–20.
46. Goldstone AP, Patterson M, Kalingag N, Ghatei MA, Brynes AE, Bloom SR, Grossman AB, Korbonits M. Fasting and postprandial hyperghrelinemia in Prader-Willi syndrome is partially explained by hypoinsulinemia, and is not due to peptide YY3-36 deficiency or seen in hypothalamic obesity due to craniopharyngioma. *J. Clin. Endocrinol. Metab* 2005;**90**:2681–90.
47. Tan TM, Vanderpump M, Khoo B, Patterson M, Ghatei MA, Goldstone AP. Somatostatin infusion lowers plasma ghrelin without reducing appetite in adults with Prader-Willi syndrome. *J. Clin. Endocrinol. Metab* 2004;**89**:4162–5.
48. Zipf WB, O'Dorisio TM, Cataland S, Sotos J. Blunted pancreatic polypeptide responses in children with obesity of Prader-Willi syndrome. *J. Clin. Endocrinol. Metab* 1981;**52**:1264–6.
49. Gimenez-Palop O, Gimenez-Perez G, Mauricio D, Gonzalez-Clemente JM, Potau N, Berlanga E, Trallero R, Laferrere B, Caixas A. A lesser postprandial suppression of plasma ghrelin in Prader-Willi syndrome is associated with low fasting and a blunted postprandial PYY response. *Clin. Endocrinol. (Oxf)* 2007;**66**:198–204.
50. Butler JV, Whittington JE, Holland AJ, Boer H, Clarke D, Webb T. Prevalence of, and risk factors for, physical ill-health in people with Prader-Willi syndrome: a population-based study. *Dev. Med. Child Neurol.* 2002;**44**:248–55.
51. Bonora E, Kiechl S, Willeit J, Oberhollenzer F, Egger G, Targher G, Alberiche M, Bonadonna RC, Muggeo M. Prevalence of insulin resistance in metabolic disorders: the Bruneck Study. *Diabetes* 1998;**47**:1643–9.
52. Schuster DP, Osei K, Zipf WB. Characterization of alterations in glucose and insulin metabolism in Prader-Willi subjects. *Metabolism* 1996;**45**:1514–20.
53. Talebizadeh Z, Butler MG. Insulin resistance and obesity-related factors in Prader-Willi syndrome: comparison with obese subjects. *Clin. Genet.* 2005;**67**:230–9.
54. Eiholzer U, Gisin R, Weinmann C, Kriemler S, Steinert H, Torresani T, Zachmann M, Prader A. Treatment with human growth hormone in patients with Prader-Labhart-Willi syndrome reduces body fat and increases muscle mass and physical performance. *Eur. J. Pediatr.* 1998;**157**:368–77.
55. Zipf WB. Glucose homeostasis in Prader-Willi syndrome and potential implications of growth hormone therapy. *Acta Paediatr. Suppl* 1999;**88**:115–17.
56. Krochik AG, Ozuna B, Torrado M, Chertkoff L, Mazza C. Characterization of alterations in carbohydrate metabolism in children with Prader-Willi syndrome. *J. Pediatr. Endocrinol. Metab* 2006;**19**:911–18.
57. Haqq AM, Muehlbauer M, Svetkey LP, Newgard CB, Purnell JQ, Grambow SC, Freemark MS. Altered distribution of adiponectin isoforms in children with Prader-Willi syndrome (PWS): association with insulin sensitivity and circulating satiety peptide hormones. *Clin. Endocrinol. (Oxf)* 2007;**67**:944–51.
58. Hoybye C, Bruun JM, Richelsen B, Flyvbjerg A, Frystyk J. Serum adiponectin levels in adults with Prader-Willi syndrome are independent of anthropometrical parameters and do not change with GH treatment. *Eur. J. Endocrinol.* 2004;**151**:457–61.
59. Pagano C, Marin O, Calcagno A, Schiappelli P, Pilon C, Milan G, Bertelli M, Fanin E, Andrighetto G, Federspil G, Vettor R. Increased serum resistin in adults with Prader-Willi syndrome is related to obesity and not to insulin resistance. *J. Clin. Endocrinol. Metab* 2005;**90**:4335–40.
60. Greenswag LR. Adults with Prader-Willi syndrome: a survey of 232 cases. *Dev. Med. Child Neurol.* 1987;**29**:145–52.
61. de Lind van Wijngaarden RF, de Klerk LW, Festen DA, Duivenvoorden HJ, Otten BJ, Hokken-Koelega AC. Randomized controlled trial to investigate the effects of growth hormone treatment on scoliosis in children with Prader-Willi syndrome. *J. Clin. Endocrinol. Metab* 2009;**94**:1274–80.
62. Lammer C, Weimann E. [Changes in carbohydrate metabolism and insulin resistance in patients with Prader-Willi Syndrome (PWS) under growth hormone therapy]. *Wien. Med. Wochenschr.* 2007;**157**:82–8.
63. DelParigi A, Tschop M, Heiman ML, Salbe AD, Vozarova B, Sell SM, Bunt JC, Tataranni PA. High circulating ghrelin: a potential cause for hyperphagia and obesity in Prader Willi syndrome. *J. Clin. Endocrinol. Metab* 2002;**87**:5461–4.

64. Feigerlova E, Diene G, Conte-Auriol F, Molinas C, Gennero I, Salles JP, Arnaud C, Tauber M. Hyperghrelinemia precedes obesity in Prader-Willi syndrome. *J. Clin. Endocrinol. Metab* 2008;**93**:2800–5.
65. van der Lely AJ, Tschop M, Heiman ML, Ghigo E. Biological, physiological, pathophysiological, and pharmacological aspects of ghrelin. *Endocr. Rev.* 2004;**25**:426–57.
66. Kojima M, Kangawa K. Ghrelin: structure and function. *Physiol Rev.* 2005;**85**:495–522.
67. Gauna C, Delhanty PJ, Hofland LJ, Janssen JA, Broglio F, Ross RJ, Ghigo E, van der Lely AJ. Ghrelin stimulates, whereas des-octanoyl ghrelin inhibits, glucose output by primary hepatocytes. *J. Clin. Endocrinol. Metab* 2005;**90**:1055–60.
68. Wiedmer P, Nogueiras R, Broglio F, D'Alessio D, Tschop MH. Ghrelin, obesity and diabetes. *Nat. Clin. Pract. Endocrinol. Metab* 2007;**3**:705–12.
69. Broglio F, Gottero C, Prodam F, Gauna C, Muccioli G, Papotti M, Abribat T, van der Lely AJ, Ghigo E. Non-acylated ghrelin counteracts the metabolic but not the neuroendocrine response to acylated ghrelin in humans. *J. Clin. Endocrinol. Metab* 2004;**89**:3062–5.
70. Gil-Campos M, Aguilera CM, Canete R, Gil A. Ghrelin: a hormone regulating food intake and energy homeostasis. *Br. J. Nutr.* 2006;**96**:201–26.
71. Yang J, Brown MS, Liang G, Grishin NV, Goldstein JL. Identification of the acyltransferase that octanoylates ghrelin, an appetite-stimulating peptide hormone. *Cell* 2008;**132**:387–96.
72. Choi K, Roh SG, Hong YH, Shrestha YB, Hishikawa D, Chen C, Kojima M, Kangawa K, Sasaki S. The role of ghrelin and growth hormone secretagogues receptor on rat adipogenesis. *Endocrinology* 2003;**144**:754–9.
73. Thompson NM, Gill DA, Davies R, Loveridge N, Houston PA, Robinson IC, Wells T. Ghrelin and des-octanoyl ghrelin promote adipogenesis directly in vivo by a mechanism independent of the type 1a growth hormone secretagogue receptor. *Endocrinology* 2004;**145**:234–42.
74. Wortley KE, del Rincon JP, Murray JD, Garcia K, Iida K, Thorner MO, Sleeman MW. Absence of ghrelin protects against early-onset obesity. *J. Clin. Invest* 2005;**115**:3573–8.
75. Zhang JV, Ren PG, vsian-Kretchmer O, Luo CW, Rauch R, Klein C, Hsueh AJ. Obestatin, a peptide encoded by the ghrelin gene, opposes ghrelin's effects on food intake. *Science* 2005;**310**:996–9.
76. Tschop M, Weyer C, Tataranni PA, Devanarayan V, Ravussin E, Heiman ML. Circulating ghrelin levels are decreased in human obesity. *Diabetes* 2001;**50**:707–9.
77. Leite-Moreira AF, Soares JB. Physiological, pathological and potential therapeutic roles of ghrelin. *Drug Discov. Today* 2007;**12**:276–88.
78. Cummings DE, Weigle DS, Frayo RS, Breen PA, Ma MK, Dellinger EP, Purnell JQ. Plasma ghrelin levels after diet-induced weight loss or gastric bypass surgery. *N. Engl. J. Med.* 2002;**346**:1623–30.
79. Barazzoni R, Zanetti M, Ferreira C, Vinci P, Pirulli A, Mucci M, Dore F, Fonda M, Ciocchi B, Cattin L, Guarnieri G. Relationships between desacylated and acylated ghrelin and insulin sensitivity in the metabolic syndrome. *J. Clin. Endocrinol. Metab* 2007;**92**:3935–40.
80. Zwirska-Korczala K, mczyk-Sowa M, Sowa P, Pilc K, Suchanek R, Pierzchala K, Namyslowski G, Misiolek M, Sodowski K, Kato I, Kuwahara A, Zabielski R. Role of leptin, ghrelin, angiotensin II and orexins in 3T3 L1 preadipocyte cells proliferation and oxidative metabolism. *J. Physiol Pharmacol* 2007;**58**(Suppl. 1):53–64.
81. Baldelli R, Bellone S, Castellino N, Petri A, Rapa A, Vivenza D, Bellone J, Broglio F, Ghigo E, Bona G. Oral glucose load inhibits circulating ghrelin levels to the same extent in normal and obese children. *Clin. Endocrinol. (Oxf)* 2006;**64**:255–9.
82. Prodam F, Me E, Riganti F, Gramaglia E, Bellone S, Baldelli R, Rapa A, van der Lely AJ, Bona G, Ghigo E, Broglio F. The nutritional control of ghrelin secretion in humans: the effects of enteral vs. parenteral nutrition. *Eur. J. Nutr.* 2006;**45**:399–405.
83. Gourcerol G, St-Pierre DH, Tache Y. Lack of obestatin effects on food intake: should obestatin be renamed ghrelin-associated peptide (GAP)? *Regul. Pept.* 2007;**141**:1–7.
84. Holst B, Egerod KL, Schild E, Vickers SP, Cheetham S, Gerlach LO, Storjohann L, Stidsen CE, Jones R, Beck-Sickinger AG, Schwartz TW. GPR39 signaling is stimulated by zinc ions but not by obestatin. *Endocrinology* 2007;**148**:13–20.
85. Tang SQ, Jiang QY, Zhang YL, Zhu XT, Shu G, Gao P, Feng DY, Wang XQ, Dong XY. Obestatin: its physicochemical characteristics and physiological functions. *Peptides* 2008;**29**:639–45.
86. Harada T, Nakahara T, Yasuhara D, Kojima S, Sagiyama K, Amitani H, Laviano A, Naruo T, Inui A. Obestatin, acyl ghrelin, and des-acyl ghrelin responses to an oral glucose tolerance test in the restricting type of anorexia nervosa. *Biol. Psychiatry* 2008;**63**:245–7.
87. Qader SS, Hakanson R, Rehfeld JF, Lundquist I, Salehi A. Proghrelin-derived peptides influence the secretion of insulin, glucagon, pancreatic polypeptide and somatostatin: a study on isolated islets from mouse and rat pancreas. *Regul. Pept.* 2008;**146**:230–7.
88. Cummings DE, Clement K, Purnell JQ, Vaisse C, Foster KE, Frayo RS, Schwartz MW, Basdevant A, Weigle DS. Elevated plasma ghrelin levels in Prader Willi syndrome. *Nat. Med.* 2002;**8**:643–4.
89. Goldstone AP, Thomas EL, Brynes AE, Castroman G, Edwards R, Ghatei MA, Frost G, Holland AJ, Grossman AB, Korbonits M, Bloom SR, Bell JD. Elevated fasting plasma ghrelin in Prader-Willi syndrome adults is not solely explained by their reduced visceral adiposity and insulin resistance. *J. Clin. Endocrinol. Metab* 2004;**89**:1718–26.
90. Haqq AM, Farooqi IS, O'Rahilly S, Stadler DD, Rosenfeld RG, Pratt KL, LaFranchi SH, Purnell JQ. Serum ghrelin levels are inversely correlated with body mass index, age, and insulin concentrations in normal children and are markedly increased in Prader-Willi syndrome. *J. Clin. Endocrinol. Metab* 2003;**88**:174–8.
91. Stefan M, Ji H, Simmons RA, Cummings DE, Ahima RS, Friedman MI, Nicholls RD. Hormonal and metabolic defects in a Prader-Willi syndrome mouse model with neonatal failure to thrive. *Endocrinology* 2005;**146**:4377–85.
92. Erdie-Lalena CR, Holm VA, Kelly PC, Frayo RS, Cummings DE. Ghrelin levels in young children with Prader-Willi syndrome. *J. Pediatr.* 2006;**149**:199–204.
93. Hauffa BP, Petersenn S. GH treatment reduces total ghrelin in Prader-Willi syndrome (PWS) and may confound ghrelin studies in young PWS children. *Clin. Endocrinol. (Oxf)* 2009;**71**:155–6.
94. Hauffa BP, Haase K, Range IM, Unger N, Mann K, Petersenn S. The effect of growth hormone on the response of total and acylated ghrelin to a standardized oral glucose load and insulin resistance in children with Prader-Willi syndrome. *J. Clin. Endocrinol. Metab* 2007;**92**:834–40.
95. Paik KH, Choe YH, Park WH, Oh YJ, Kim AH, Chu SH, Kim SW, Kwon EK, Han SJ, Shon WY, Jin DK. Suppression of acylated ghrelin during oral glucose tolerance test is correlated with whole-body insulin sensitivity in children with Prader-Willi syndrome. *J. Clin. Endocrinol. Metab* 2006;**91**:1876–81.

96. Park WH, Oh YJ, Kim GY, Kim SE, Paik KH, Han SJ, Kim AH, Chu SH, Kwon EK, Kim SW, Jin DK. Obestatin is not elevated or correlated with insulin in children with Prader-Willi syndrome. *J. Clin. Endocrinol. Metab* 2007;**92**:229—34.
97. Lippl F, Erdmann J, Lichter N, Tholl S, Wagenpfeil S, Adam O, Schusdziarra V. Relation of plasma obestatin levels to bmi, gender, age and insulin. *Horm. Metab Res.* 2008;**40**:806—12.
98. Reinehr T, de SG, Roth CL. Obestatin and ghrelin levels in obese children and adolescents before and after reduction of overweight. *Clin. Endocrinol. (Oxf)* 2008;**68**:304—10.
99. Zou CC, Liang L, Wang CL, Fu JF, Zhao ZY. The change in ghrelin and obestatin levels in obese children after weight reduction. *Acta Paediatr.* 2009;**98**:159—65.
100. De Waele K, Ishkanian SL, Bogarin R, Miranda CA, Ghatei MA, Bloom SR, Pacaud D, Chanoine JP. Long-acting octreotide treatment causes a sustained decrease in ghrelin concentrations but does not affect weight, behaviour and appetite in subjects with Prader-Willi syndrome. *Eur. J. Endocrinol.* 2008;**159**:381—8.
101. Tauber M, Conte AF, Moulin P, Molinas C, Delagnes V, Salles JP. Hyperghrelinemia is a common feature of Prader-Willi syndrome and pituitary stalk interruption: a pathophysiological hypothesis. *Horm. Res.* 2004;**62**:49—54.
102. Zanella S, Watrin F, Mebarek S, Marly F, Roussel M, Gire C, Diene G, Tauber M, Muscatelli F, Hilaire G. Necdin plays a role in the serotonergic modulation of the mouse respiratory network: implication for Prader-Willi syndrome. *J. Neurosci.* 2008;**28**:1745—55.
103. Broglio F, Koetsveld PP, Benso A, Gottero C, Prodam F, Papotti M, Muccioli G, Gauna C, Hofland L, Deghenghi R, Arvat E, van der Lely AJ, Ghigo E. Ghrelin secretion is inhibited by either somatostatin or cortistatin in humans. *J. Clin. Endocrinol. Metab* 2002;**87**:4829—32.
104. Norrelund H, Hansen TK, Orskov H, Hosoda H, Kojima M, Kangawa K, Weeke J, Moller N, Christiansen JS, Jorgensen JO. Ghrelin immunoreactivity in human plasma is suppressed by somatostatin. *Clin. Endocrinol. (Oxf)* 2002;**57**:539—46.
105. Lee HM, Wang G, Englander EW, Kojima M, Greeley Jr GH. Ghrelin, a new gastrointestinal endocrine peptide that stimulates insulin secretion: enteric distribution, ontogeny, influence of endocrine, and dietary manipulations. *Endocrinology* 2002;**143**:185—90.
106. Goldstone AP, Unmehopa UA, Swaab DF. Hypothalamic growth hormone-releasing hormone (GHRH) cell number is increased in human illness, but is not reduced in Prader-Willi syndrome or obesity. *Clin. Endocrinol. (Oxf)* 2003;**58**:743—55.
107. Paik KH, Jin DK, Lee KH, Armstrong L, Lee JE, Oh YJ, Kim S, Kwon EK, Choe YH. Peptide YY, cholecystokinin, insulin and ghrelin response to meal did not change, but mean serum levels of insulin is reduced in children with Prader-Willi syndrome. *J. Korean Med. Sci.* 2007;**22**:436—41.
108. Paik KH, Lee MK, Jin DK, Kang HW, Lee KH, Kim AH, Kim C, Lee JE, Oh YJ, Kim S, Han SJ, Kwon EK, Choe YH. Marked suppression of ghrelin concentration by insulin in Prader-willi syndrome. *J. Korean Med. Sci.* 2007;**22**:177—82.
109. Murdolo G, Lucidi P, Di, Loreto. C, Parlanti N, De CA, Fatone C, Fanelli CG, Bolli GB, Santeusanio F, De FP. Insulin is required for prandial ghrelin suppression in humans. *Diabetes* 2003;**52**:2923—7.
110. Prodam F, Bellone S, Grugni G, Crino A, Ragusa L, Franzese A, Di BE, Corrias A, Walker G, Rapa A, Aimaretti G, Bona G. Influence of age, gender, and glucose tolerance on fasting and fed acylated ghrelin in Prader Willi syndrome. *Clin. Nutr.* 2009;**28**:94—9.
111. Cummings DE, Purnell JQ, Frayo RS, Schmidova K, Wisse BE, Weigle DS. A preprandial rise in plasma ghrelin levels suggests a role in meal initiation in humans. *Diabetes* 2001;**50**:1714—19.

CHAPTER
19

Insulin Resistance and Glucose Metabolism in Childhood Obesity

Subhashini Yaturu*, Sushil K. Jain[†]

*Department of Endocrinology, Stratton VA Medical Center, Albany, New York; Albany Medical College, Albany, NY, USA and [†]Department of Pediatrics, Louisiana State University Health Sciences Center, Shreveport, LA, USA

INTRODUCTION

The obesity epidemic is driving a large increase in type 2 diabetes mellitus (T2DM) and consequently setting the scene for an impending wave of cardiovascular morbidity and mortality. Obese adolescents demonstrate increased rates of early maturation, growth abnormalities, diabetes mellitus, obstructive sleep apnea, hypertension, steatosis, and polycystic ovarian syndrome, placing this group of children at risk for long-term health problems and reduced quality of life. A primary biochemical abnormality in most cases of T2DM is insulin resistance. The onset of insulin resistance commonly leads to relative insulin deficiency, with a slow decline in the regulation of blood glucose accompanied by hyperinsulinemia and elevated circulating free fatty acid (FFA) levels. This is followed later by a decrease in the ability to control plasma glucose, which manifests as rising fasting plasma glucose or rising peak plasma glucose levels in response to an oral glucose challenge with intermittent and persistent hyperglycemia, leading to a diagnosis of T2DM. Data from the Bogalusa Heart Study clearly show that almost 20% of obese children have adverse levels of at least one cardiovascular risk factor (hypercholesterolemia, hyperinsulinemia, hypertriglyceridemia, or hypertension) and that the presence of multiple risk factors is strongly associated with early stages of atherosclerosis [1].

INSULIN RESISTANCE

Insulin resistance is a fundamental aspect of the etiology of T2DM and is also linked to a wide array of other pathophysiological sequelae including hypertension, hyperlipidemia, atherosclerosis (i.e., the metabolic syndrome, or syndrome X), and polycystic ovarian disease [2]. Alterations related to diet-induced obesity have been found in insulin-resistant adipose tissue and muscle [3]. Several factors are implicated in the pathogenesis of obesity-related insulin resistance, such as increased free fatty acids and many hormones and cytokines released by adipose tissue.

INSULIN AND NORMAL INSULIN SIGNALING

Insulin is a key hormone whose actions play an important role in the growth and development of tissues and the control of glucose homeostasis [4]. Insulin is secreted by pancreatic beta cells as an inactive single-chain precursor, preproinsulin, with a signal sequence directing its passage into secretory vesicles. Proteolytic removal of the signal sequence results in the formation of proinsulin. In response to an increase in blood glucose or amino acid concentration, proinsulin is secreted and converted into active insulin by special proteases. The active insulin molecule is a small protein that consists of A and B chains held together by two disulfide bonds [5]. The primary role of insulin is to control glucose homeostasis by stimulating glucose transport into muscle and adipose cells while reducing hepatic glucose produced via gluconeogenesis and glycogenolysis. Insulin regulates lipid metabolism by increasing lipid synthesis in liver and fat cells while inhibiting lipolysis. Insulin is also a necessary hormone involved in the uptake of amino acids and protein synthesis [6]. The pleotrophic actions of insulin are all crucial for a cell to maintain normal homeostasis for cellular proliferation and differentiation.

Normal insulin signaling occurs through activation of a specific insulin receptor, which belongs to a subfamily of receptor tyrosine kinases [7]. The insulin molecule binds to the α subunit of the receptor, releasing the inhibition of tyrosine autophosphorylation by the β subunit [8, 9]. The receptor is autophosphorylated at distinct tyrosine residues. In contrast to most tyrosine kinase receptors, the activated insulin receptor directly phosphorylates insulin receptor substrates (IRS-1-4) on multiple tyrosine residues. Currently only four members of the IRS family are involved in insulin signaling, with IRS-1/2 being the most important for glucose transport [9, 10]. The subcellular distribution of these proteins between the cytoplasm and low-density membrane compartments of the cell have been shown to play a vital role in transmitting the proper insulin response [10, 11]. Tyrosine phosphorylated IRS proteins then act as a binding site for signaling molecules containing SH-2 (Src-homology-2) domains such as phosphatidylinositol 3'-kinase (PI3'-kinase), GRB-2/mSos, and SHP-2. These molecules bind the phosphorylated tyrosine residues of IRS proteins, forming a signaling complex to mediate the downstream signaling. PI3K is the main signal mediator of the metabolic and mitogenic actions of insulin. PI3K is composed of a p85 regulatory subunit that binds to IRS proteins and a p110 catalytic subunit. Following association of p85 with IRS-1/2, the p110 subunit has increased catalytic activity. This allows phosphorylation of its substrate-PtdIns(4,5)P$_2$- on the 3' position of the inositol ring to generate PtdIns [4, 12, 13] P$_3$ [9]. The second messenger, PtdIns [4, 12, 13] P$_3$, recruits the serine kinases PDK-1, PKB/Akt, and PKC to the plasma membrane via their PH domains. The activation of these kinases results in several of insulin's responses such as GLUT-4 translocation to the membrane, glycogen synthesis by phosphorylation of GSK-3, and lipogenesis by up-regulating synthesis of the fatty acid synthase gene.

In addition to insulin signaling via PI3K, insulin can activate the mitogen-activated protein (MAP) kinase, ERK, which leads to gene expression for various cellular proliferation or differentiation components. After phosphorylation of IRS-1/2, the adaptor proteins, Grb-2 and SOS are recruited and work together with a stimulated tyrosine phosphatase, SHP2, to activate membrane bound Ras. Activated Ras leads to a kinase cascade, allowing ERK to translocate to the nucleus for gene expression [9].

Insulin's main action of glucose uptake also requires activation of another signaling pathway involving tyrosine phosphorylation of the Cbl proto-oncogene. Cbl is associated with the adaptor protein CAP, which contains three SH3 domains and a sorbin homology (SoHo) domain. The SoHo domain of the phosphorylated Cbl-CAP complex allows translocation to lipid rafts and association with the protein flotillin. A signaling complex is formed at the site of the lipid raft resulting in the activation of a small G protein, TC10. TC10 is thought to act as a second signal in recruitment of the GLUT-4 protein to the membrane [4, 9].

EFFECTS OF INSULIN IN ADIPOSE STORAGE

Understanding the effects of insulin in adipose tissue makes it easier to understand the role of insulin resistance in obesity. The effects of insulin in adipose tissue include the following: (1) insulin stimulates the differentiation of preadipocytes to adipocytes; (2) in adipocytes, insulin promotes lipogenesis by stimulating the uptake of glucose and lipoprotein derived fatty acids; (3) insulin also causes transcriptional regulation in the hepatocyte; and (4) insulin diminishes triglyceride breakdown by inhibiting lipolysis.

ADIPOSE TISSUE AND INSULIN RESISTANCE

Obesity is associated with insulin resistance and is characterized by excess circulating lipid metabolites that would normally be "absorbed" by adipose tissue. In obesity, adipose tissue becomes refractory to suppression of fat mobilization by insulin and also to the normal acute stimulatory effect of insulin on activation of lipoprotein lipase (involved in fat storage). The net effect is that adipocytes become "full up" and resist further fat storage. Thus, in the postprandial period, there is an excess of circulating lipid metabolites that would normally have been "absorbed" by adipose tissue. This situation leads to fat deposition in other tissues. Accumulation of triacylglycerol in skeletal muscles and in liver is associated with insulin resistance.

VISCERAL FAT AND INSULIN RESISTANCE

When caloric intake exceeds caloric expenditure, the positive caloric balance and storage of energy in adipose tissue often causes adipocyte hypertrophy and visceral adipose tissue accumulation. These pathogenic anatomical abnormalities may incite metabolic and immune responses that promote T2DM, hypertension, and dyslipidemia. A study of Hispanic children with persistent prediabetes found them to have lower beta-cell function, resulting from a lower acute insulin response to glucose, and increasing visceral fat over time [14]. A study of 32 overweight or obese Hispanic children without diabetes but with a family history of T2DM indicated that increased visceral fat was independently related to both increased insulin resistance and decreased insulin secretion [15]. This study indicates that specific accumulation of visceral fat in addition to overall adiposity in Hispanic children increases the risk of T2DM [15]. Visceral fat is metabolically unique in children, being associated with elevated triglycerides and fasting insulin independent of total fat [16]. Insulin sensitivity and visceral fat were the only independent variables to emerge as significantly related to fasting insulin [16]. Similarly, in a Japanese study, both lower birth weight and visceral fat accumulation may be independently related to hyperinsulinemia and insulin resistance in obese Japanese children [17]. In a comparison of visceral adiposity and abdominal aortic elasticity, abdominal adipose tissue accumulation was noted to be closely associated with cardiovascular risk factors in obese children. Among abdominal adipose tissue compartments, visceral fat thickness was strongly correlated with the elastic properties of the abdominal aorta [18].

PATHOPHYSIOLOGY OF INSULIN RESISTANCE

The defects at the cellular level can be grouped into prereceptor, receptor, and postreceptor defects. The prereceptor defects may be related to abnormal insulin and insulin antibodies. The receptor defects may be due to decreased insulin receptors or decreased affinity. The postreceptor defects may be due to abnormal signal transduction or abnormal phosphorylation reactions. Note that when discussing insulin resistance, we generally refer to postreceptor defects.

METABOLIC SYNDROME IN CHILDHOOD OBESITY

Childhood obesity is increasingly common and is associated with health problems. The epidemic of childhood obesity has increased interest in the metabolic syndrome (MS) because of its potential projection into adulthood. The relationship between MS and T2DM and cardiovascular disease is well established in adults. This association can be suggested in children as well, although the syndrome in childhood urgently needs to be clearly defined. The most widely accepted hypothesis links the syndrome to obesity, because obesity plays a central role in the MS. Prevalence of the MS in adolescents has been estimated to be 6.7% in young adults and 4.2% in adolescents [19]. Figures rise from 0.9% for obesity and 12.4% for overweight [20] up to 31.1% in overweight and obese adolescents [21]. The rate of the MS increased progressively with increasing body mass index (BMI) categories ($P < 0.001$). Severely obese patients had a threefold increased risk with respect to moderately obese patients [22]. In the Bogalusa study, the four criterion risk variables considered were the highest quartile (specific for age, race, sex, and study year) of (1) BMI, (2) fasting insulin, (3) systolic or mean arterial blood pressure, and (4) total cholesterol to High-density lipoprotein (HDL) cholesterol ratio or triglycerides to HDL cholesterol ratio [23]. In this study, the best predictors were obesity and being in the upper quartile of basal insulin levels. Ethnic and genetic factors help to explain occurrence of the syndrome in the non-obese population and the differences of interobesity [23]. The constellation of metabolic syndrome variables at low levels in childhood is associated with lower measures of cardiovascular risk in adulthood [24].

INFLAMMATION AND CARDIOVASCULAR RISK IN OBESITY

Inflammatory stress conditions associated with childhood obesity, notably with abdominal fat deposition, may play a role in the development of the earliest stages of proatherosclerotic inflammatory processes and subsequent vascular dysfunction. These changes might be partially reversible by short-term diet and exercise intervention, even if patients do not reach ideal body weight [25].

Adolescent girls with menstrual disturbances within the spectrum of Polycystic ovary syndrome (PCOS) share several anthropometric, hormonal, and metabolic features of the metabolic syndrome [26–28]. The increasing rates of obesity, particularly abdominal obesity, with the resulting insulin resistance/hyperinsulinemia may trigger and permit the clinical expression of PCOS in genetically predisposed individuals through enhanced hyperinsulinemia-mediated metabolic pathways conducive to hyperandrogenemia [29]. Insulin resistance is the vital connection between PCOS and the metabolic syndrome [29]. Among children and adolescents, insulin resistance should be targeted for treatment, and lifestyle modification should always serve as the frontline strategy through exercise and dietary intervention. The role of pharmacotherapeutic agents remains unclear. A uniform definition of the metabolic syndrome for pediatric patients needs to be created. Early intervention should be instituted because many of the features of the syndrome continue from childhood into adulthood. Dietary fiber intake improves insulin sensitivity.

Obesity represents an increase in fat mass in which multiple metabolic pathways are deranged. The consequences of these metabolic derangements, including insulin resistance and inflammation, are reflected in obesity-related comorbidities and can be seen in the setting of pediatric obesity. Previously seen only rarely in the pediatric population, T2DM has now become increasingly common among obese adolescents, particularly among African American and Hispanic children. The early clinical manifestations of abnormalities related to childhood obesity, attributed to obesity-driven insulin resistance, are impaired glucose metabolism and nonalcoholic fatty liver disease. Both have no symptoms and demand a high index of suspicion and the proper choice of tests for establishing the diagnosis. The prevalence of impaired glucose tolerance is about 20% in American children and adolescents with a marked degree of obesity [30]. The most important risk factor for the rise of insulin resistance among young people is being overweight. The increased prevalence of T2DM parallels an increased prevalence of obesity in children and youth. Children have hyperinsulinism as a result of obesity, as do adults, and childhood obesity is commonly associated with impaired glucose metabolism [31]. The diagnostic criteria for diabetes mellitus in young people are (1) symptoms of diabetes mellitus and a random plasma-glucose concentration of ≥ 11.1 mmol/l, or (2) fasting plasma-glucose concentration of ≥ 7.0 mmol/l, or (3) 2-hour plasma-glucose levels following an oral glucose-tolerance test ≥ 11.1 mmol/l. The stress of obesity and the increased demand for insulin during adolescence explain the largely pubertal and postpubertal onset of T2DM in children. Another factor that has to be taken into consideration when assessing children and adolescents is their stage of pubertal development. Midpuberty is characterized by a reduction of peripheral insulin sensitivity by $\sim 30\%$ [32], thus placing further demands on the beta cells. The increasing incidence of type 2 diabetes is considered to be due in part to changing food patterns [33] and diets in South East Asia [34]. In contrast to adults, progression to full-blown T2DM seems to occur at a rapid rate in obese youth, especially African American children, pointing to an urgent need to alter the disease course in this population [35]. The first step is to determine which children should be screened for this condition. As overweight and obese children and adolescents are so commonly seen, the clinician is faced with the challenge of identifying individuals at greatest risk for morbidity. Interventions to halt weight gain and promote weight loss in children are of limited success and demand significant resources and continuous follow-up and monitoring [36]. The risk of developing T2DM in youth is markedly affected by the degree of obesity (particularly central obesity) and associated metabolic complications, such as insulin resistance, hyperinsulinemia, and dyslipidemia. A family history of T2DM in white children is associated with decreased insulin sensitivity and clearance, decreased IGFBP-1, and an impaired relationship between insulin action and beta-cell compensation [37]. Youth with T2DM have been reported to have a first- or second-degree relative with diabetes 75% to 100% of the time [38]. In the National Heart, Lung and Blood Institute Family Heart Study of 445 families, genetic correlations between BMI, waist circumference, HDL cholesterol, triglycerides, insulin, and plasminogen activator-1 antigen were found [39] and suggest that pleiotropic effects of genes or shared family environment contribute to the familial clustering of MS-related traits.

A positive family history of cardiovascular disease at an early age, T2DM, hypertension, or dyslipidemia, specifically in a parent who is not necessarily obese, may suggest that the child is already at risk for the development of adverse outcomes and that the addition of obesity may add a major metabolic burden, thus promoting and accelerating pathological processes even more. Insulin resistance seems to be the key element driving the development of the pathophysiological processes leading to the development of altered glucose metabolism, dyslipidemia, and hypertension. A history of being born small for gestational age has been shown to be an independent risk factor for the development of insulin resistance and the metabolic syndrome in adulthood [40]. A history of maternal gestational diabetes also has significant implications for the offspring. Maternal gestational diabetes is associated with adiposity and higher glucose and insulin concentrations in female offspring, at ages as early as 5 years [41]. Any child with a family history of T2DM or maternal gestational diabetes is a candidate for screening [42]. Peripubertal children and adolescents with obesity and signs of insulin resistance—such as acanthosis nigricans, the presence of hepatic steatosis, or ovarian hyperandrogenism—should be screened with an oral glucose tolerance test [43].

Increased visceral adiposity has also been shown to be related to a greater atherogenic metabolic profile in childhood [5]. Visceral fat has been shown to be related to greater insulin resistance and lower insulin secretory response in obese children and adolescents [5]. Adiponectin levels are lower in obese children with increased visceral fat deposition [44], even when the comparison is made between individuals with similar overall adiposity. Visceral adiposity appears to be more correlated with basal and stimulated insulin levels and inversely with insulin sensitivity [44]. An estimation of visceral fat can be performed using measurement of waist circumference. Although pediatric waist circumference reference charts are not readily available, data derived from the National Health and Nutrition Examination Survey (NHANES) have been shown to be clinically useful in identifying youth at risk for the metabolic syndrome. The assessment of waist circumference as well as BMI should both be performed in obese children and adolescents, as the cumulative data may provide a better tool for risk assessment.

INSULIN SENSITIVITY AND NUTRIENT AVAILABILITY

Obesity and excessive intake of nutrients has long been a risk factor for a variety of adverse health outcomes such as high blood pressure, insulin resistance, oxidative stress, and T2DM. Furthermore, studies have shown that calorie overload in rodents results in rapidly induced skeletal muscle and liver insulin resistance, whereas calorie restriction enhances skeletal muscle, liver, and insulin sensitivity [45]. Several key modulators are thought to act as sensors to the excessive intake of nutrients, including the regulatory subunits of PI3K, the protein deacetylase sirtuin 1 (SIRT1), and mTOR, a serine/threonine protein kinase [45], all of which also play key roles in modulating insulin action. Excess regulatory subunits of PI3K can have a negative effect on insulin signaling by binding to IRS-1 and inhibiting normal insulin signals. It has been reported that in insulin-resistant subjects, there is an excess of regulatory subunits of PI3K [46] and that calorie restriction increases the ratio of PI3K catalytic to regulatory subunits in rat skeletal muscle [47]. mTOR is also a nutrient-sensing pathway, and overactivation in rodent and human systems is associated with insulin resistance [45]. SIRT1 plays a key role in sensing calorie restriction and resulting in positive insulin sensitivity. Calorie restriction increases expression of SIRT1 through eNOS expression. Activation of SIRT1 results in activation of PGC-1α, one of the components of mitochondrial biogenesis [48]. Thus, it is safe to say that calorie restriction may be a positive mechanism by which to increase mitochondrial biogenesis and insulin sensitivity. Two approaches have been proposed to attenuate the causes of excessive nutrients leading to insulin resistance, one being weight loss to enhance insulin sensitivity and the other being alterations in the macronutrient content of diets to avoid stimulating compensatory insulin mechanisms [49]. These forms of therapeutic intervention may be a good way to improve insulin sensitivity and delay or stop the onset of insulin resistance.

PREVENTION

Given the strong association between obesity and insulin resistance and the development of metabolic syndrome and cardiovascular disease, prevention and treatment of childhood obesity appear to be essential to prevent the development of insulin resistance and its associated complications. Valid and reliable methods are essential to assess the presence and the extent of insulin resistance, the associated risk factors, and the effect of pharmacological and lifestyle interventions. The two most common tests to assess insulin resistance are the hyperinsulinemic euglycemic clamp and the frequently sampled intravenous glucose tolerance test utilizing the minimal model. However, neither of these tests is easily accomplished, and they are time consuming, expensive, and invasive. Simpler methods to assess insulin resistance based on surrogate markers derived from an oral glucose tolerance test or from fasting insulin and glucose levels have been validated in children and adolescents and are widely used. Early detection is very useful in obese children with three additional risk factors: diabetes type 2 in first- and second-degree relatives, members of certain ethnic groups, or indications of insulin resistance. Physical inactivity promotes obesity, insulin resistance, and diabetes, whereas physical activity and exercise reduce these risks. Studies performed in the school setting have shown the beneficial effects of exercise in children and youth. Weight loss in obese adolescents was shown to improve insulin sensitivity and lower glucose values [50]. Adiposity has the most significant influence on fasting insulin levels; however, increasing VO(2max) via exercise can lower insulin levels in those children with initially high levels of the hormone [50]. Because the beneficial effects of both aerobic exercise and resistance training can be short lived, exercise and physical activity must be sustained to optimize health and maintain weight loss.

CONCLUSION

The prevalence of obesity in children is increasing in epidemic proportions. The adverse metabolic consequences that accompany fat cell hypertrophy and visceral adiposity are best viewed as a pathological partnership between the pathogenic potential adipose tissue and the inherited or acquired limitations or impairments of other body organs. Early identification of children at risk for these complications, such as ethnicity and family history of diabetes or premature coronary artery disease, is a must. Lifestyle changes and exercise should be advocated.

Acknowledgments

Subhashini Yaturu is supported by the Merit Award of the Veterans Health Administration. Sushil K. Jain is supported by grants from National Institute of Diabetes and Digestive and Kidney Diseases (NIDDK) and the Office of Dietary Supplements of the National Institutes of Health (RO1 DK064797) and RO1 DK072433. The authors thank Georgia Morgan for the excellent editing of this manuscript.

References

1. Berenson GS, Srinivasan SR, Bao W, Newman 3rd WP, Tracy RE, Wattigney WA. Association between multiple cardiovascular risk factors and atherosclerosis in children and young adults. The Bogalusa Heart Study. *N Engl J Med* 1998;**338**:1650—6.
2. Reaven GM. Pathophysiology of insulin resistance in human disease. *Physiol Rev* 1995;**75**:473—86.
3. Bays HE, Gonzalez-Campoy JM, Bray GA, et al. Pathogenic potential of adipose tissue and metabolic consequences of adipocyte hypertrophy and increased visceral adiposity. *Expert Rev Cardiovasc Ther* 2008;**6**:343—68.
4. Pirola L, Johnston AM, Obberghen E. Modulation of insulin action. *Diabetologia* 2004;**47**:170—84.
5. Melloul D, Marshak S, Cerasi E. Regulation of insulin gene transcription. *Diabetologia* 2002;**45**:309—26.
6. Sesti G. Pathophysiology of insulin resistance. *Best Practice & Research Clinical Endocrinology & Metabolism* 2006;**20**:665—79.
7. Ogawa W, Matozaki T, Kasuga M. Role of binding proteins to IRS-1 in insulin signalling. *Molecular and Cellular Biochemistry* 1998;**182**:13—22.
8. Bloch-Damti A, Bashan N. Proposed Mechanisms for the Induction of Insulin Resistance by Oxidative Stress. *Antioxidants & Redox Signaling* 2005;**7**:1553—67.
9. Saltiel AR, Kahn CR. Insulin signalling and the regulation of glucose and lipid metabolism. *Nature* 2001;**414**:799—806.
10. Kriauciunas KM, Myers Jr MG, Kahn CR. Cellular Compartmentalization in Insulin Action: Altered Signaling by a Lipid-Modified IRS-1. *Mol. Cell. Biol* 2000;**20**:6849—59.
11. Anai M, et al. Different Subcellular Distribution and Regulation of Expression of Insulin Receptor Substrate (IRS)-3 from Those of IRS-1 and IRS-2. *J. Biol. Chem* 1998;**273**:29686—92.
12. Lasker RD. The Diabetes Control and Complications Trial: Implications for Policy and Practice. *N Engl J Med* 1993;**329**:1035—6.
13. Ahmad FK, Zhiheng H, King GL. Molecular Targets of Diabetic Cardiovascular Complications. *Current Drug Targets* 2005;**6**:487—94.
14. Goran MI, Lane C, Toledo-Corral C, Weigensberg MJ. Persistence of pre-diabetes in overweight and obese Hispanic children: association with progressive insulin resistance, poor beta-cell function, and increasing visceral fat. *Diabetes* 2008;**57**:3007—12.
15. Cruz ML, Bergman RN, Goran MI. Unique effect of visceral fat on insulin sensitivity in obese Hispanic children with a family history of type 2 diabetes. *Diabetes Care* 2002;**25**:1631—6.
16. Gower BA, Nagy TR, Goran MI. Visceral fat, insulin sensitivity, and lipids in prepubertal children. *Diabetes* 1999;**48**:1515—21.
17. Tanaka Y, Kikuchi T, Nagasaki K, Hiura M, Ogawa Y, Uchiyama M. Lower birth weight and visceral fat accumulation are related to hyperinsulinemia and insulin resistance in obese Japanese children. *Hypertens Res* 2005;**28**:529—36.
18. Polat TB, Urganci N, Caliskan KC, Akyildiz B. Correlation of abdominal fat accumulation and stiffness of the abdominal aorta in obese children. *J Pediatr Endocrinol Metab* 2008;**21**:1031—40.
19. Crespo PS, Prieto Perera JA, Lodeiro FA, Azuara LA. Metabolic syndrome in childhood. *Public Health Nutr* 2007;**10**:1121—5.
20. Tapia Ceballos L. [Metabolic syndrome in childhood]. *An Pediatr (Barc)* 2007;**66**:159—66.
21. Calcaterra V, Klersy C, Muratori T, et al. Prevalence of metabolic syndrome (MS) in children and adolescents with varying degrees of obesity. *Clin Endocrinol (Oxf)* 2008;**68**:868—72.
22. Calcaterra V, Klersy C, Muratori T, et al. *Clin Endocrinol (Oxf)* 2008;**68**:868—72.
23. Srinivasan SR, Myers L, Berenson GS. Predictability of childhood adiposity and insulin for developing insulin resistance syndrome (syndrome X) in young adulthood: the Bogalusa Heart Study. *Diabetes* 2002;**51**:204—9.
24. Chen W, Srinivasan SR, Li S, Xu J, Berenson GS. Metabolic syndrome variables at low levels in childhood are beneficially associated with adulthood cardiovascular risk: the Bogalusa Heart Study. *Diabetes Care* 2005;**28**:126—31.
25. Kelishadi R, Hashemi M, Mohammadifard N, Asgary S, Khavarian N. Association of changes in oxidative and proinflammatory states with changes in vascular function after a lifestyle modification trial among obese children. *Clin Chem* 2008;**54**:147—53.
26. Coviello AD, Legro RS, Dunaif A. Adolescent girls with polycystic ovary syndrome have an increased risk of the metabolic syndrome associated with increasing androgen levels independent of obesity and insulin resistance. *J Clin Endocrinol Metab* 2006;**91**:492—7.
27. de Ferranti SD, Gauvreau K, Ludwig DS, Neufeld EJ, Newburger JW, Rifai N. Prevalence of the metabolic syndrome in American adolescents: findings from the Third National Health and Nutrition Examination Survey. *Circulation* 2004;**110**:2494—7.
28. Ford ES. Prevalence of the metabolic syndrome defined by the International Diabetes Federation among adults in the U.S. *Diabetes Care* 2005;**28**:2745—9.
29. Tfayli H, Arslanian S. Menstrual health and the metabolic syndrome in adolescents. *Ann N Y Acad Sci* 2008;**1135**:85—94.
30. Sinha R, Fisch G, Teague B, et al. Prevalence of impaired glucose tolerance among children and adolescents with marked obesity. *N Engl J Med* 2002;**346**:802—10.
31. Martin MM, Martin AL. Obesity, hyperinsulinism, and diabetes mellitus in childhood. *J Pediatr* 1973;**82**:192—201.
32. Goran MI, Gower BA. Longitudinal study on pubertal insulin resistance. *Diabetes* 2001;**50**:2444—50.
33. Kitagawa T, Owada M, Urakami T, Tajima N. Epidemiology of type 1 (insulin-dependent) and type 2 (non-insulin-dependent) diabetes mellitus in Japanese children. *Diabetes Res Clin Pract* 1994;**24**(Suppl):S7—13.
34. Misra A, Khurana L, Isharwal S, Bhardwaj S. South Asian diets and insulin resistance. *Br J Nutr* 2009;**101**:465—73.
35. Weiss R, Taksali SE, Tamborlane WV, Burgert TS, Savoye M, Caprio S. Predictors of changes in glucose tolerance status in obese youth. *Diabetes Care* 2005;**28**:902—9.
36. Summerbell CD, Waters E, Edmunds LD, Kelly S, Brown T, Campbell KJ. Interventions for preventing obesity in children. *Cochrane Database Syst Rev*; 2005:CD001871.
37. Arslanian SA, Bacha F, Saad R, Gungor N. Family history of type 2 diabetes is associated with decreased insulin sensitivity and an impaired balance between insulin sensitivity and insulin secretion in white youth. *Diabetes Care* 2005;**28**:115—19.
38. Silverstein JH, Rosenbloom AL. Type 2 diabetes in children. *Curr Diab Rep* 2001;**1**:19—27.
39. Tang W, Hong Y, Province MA, et al. Familial clustering for features of the metabolic syndrome: the National Heart, Lung, and Blood Institute (NHLBI) Family Heart Study. *Diabetes Care* 2006;**29**:631—6.

40. Levy-Marchal C, Jaquet D. Long-term metabolic consequences of being born small for gestational age. *Pediatr Diabetes* 2004;**5**: 147–53.
41. Krishnaveni GV, Hill JC, Leary SD, et al. Anthropometry, glucose tolerance, and insulin concentrations in Indian children: relationships to maternal glucose and insulin concentrations during pregnancy. *Diabetes Care* 2005;**28**:2919–25.
42. Caprio S. Treatment of impaired glucose tolerance in childhood. *Nat Clin Pract Endocrinol Metab* 2008;**4**:320–1.
43. Lee S, Bacha F, Gungor N, Arslanian SA. Racial differences in adiponectin in youth: relationship to visceral fat and insulin sensitivity. *Diabetes Care* 2006;**29**:51–6.
44. Caprio S. Insulin resistance in childhood obesity. *J Pediatr Endocrinol Metab* 2002;**15**(Suppl. 1):487–92.
45. Schenk S, Saberi Maziyar, Jerrold M. Olefsky Insulin sensitivity: modulation by nutrients and inflammation. *J. Clin. Invest* 2008;**118**:2992–3002.
46. Bandyopadhyay GK, et al. Increased p85/55/50 Expression and Decreased Phosphotidylinositol 3-Kinase Activity in Insulin-Resistant Human Skeletal Muscle. *Diabetes* 2005;**54**: 2351–9.
47. McCurdy CE, Davidson RT, Cartee GD. Calorie restriction increases the ratio of phosphatidylinositol 3-kinase catalytic to regulatory subunits in rat skeletal muscle. *Am J Physiol Endocrinol Metab* 2005;**288**:E996–1001.
48. Kim J-a, Wei Y, Sowers JR. Role of Mitochondrial Dysfunction in Insulin Resistance. *Circ Res* 2008;**102**:401–14.
49. Reaven GM. The insulin resistance syndrome: definition and dietary approaches to treatment. *Annual Review of Nutrition* 2005;**25**:391–406.
50. McMurray RG, Bauman MJ, Harrell JS, Brown S, Bangdiwala SI. Effects of improvement in aerobic power on resting insulin and glucose concentrations in children. *Eur J Appl Physiol* 2000;**81**: 132–9.

CHAPTER 20

Insulin Resistance in Pediatric Obesity
Physiological Effects and Possible Diet Treatment

Ulf Holmbäck
Department of Public Health and Caring Sciences, Clinical Nutrition and Metabolism,
Uppsala University, Uppsala, Sweden

INTRODUCTION

The prevalence of obesity has increased in both affluent and nonaffluent countries. For example, in Sweden several studies show that since the 1990s, the prevalence of obesity has more doubled in children [1–4]. Similar prevalence figures have been found in the United States and elsewhere [5]. The suggested reasons for this increase are many: lack of physical activity, increased television viewing, and greater access to energy-dense foods and snacks (reviewed in [6]). As overweight and obese children commonly become overweight and obese adults [7], with increased risk of developing cardiovascular disease [8] and type 2 diabetes [9], it is important to find ways of treating childhood obesity. Even though the children of today have a changed environment with immediate access to easily digestible food and nonphysical activity entertainment, the majority of children do not become overweight or obese. It is thus apparent that individual differences have a big part to play when deciding who will become obese and who will stay slim. This chapter shows how individual metabolism affects how food is metabolized with special emphasis on insulin and argues that it is important to know the obese pediatric patient's insulin sensitivity before any macronutrient recommendation is given. One possible explanation for the rather poor result of dietary interventions [10] may be that differences in metabolism have not been taken into consideration. Starting with fat storage and fat metabolism, and how insulin plays a big part in these processes, this chapter then discusses insulin function and effects on obesity, followed by diet intervention studies in children. Lastly, this chapter tries to sum up and suggest one way to consider individual metabolism.

FAT STORAGE AND FAT METABOLISM: THE ROLE OF INSULIN

A brief and simplistic overview of the major catabolic and anabolic hormones is presented in Figure 20.1. The figure shows how crucial insulin is for energy storage and, by extension, growth. All macronutrients are under the metabolic control of insulin, and it can perhaps be said that insulin is the most important anabolic hormone. This section discusses in some detail the effects of insulin on fat turnover, as some knowledge about fat turnover is essential to understand the impact of the various macronutrients on fat storage.

Fat from the diet is transported as triglycerides in chylomicrons from enterocytes. During circulation, triglycerides can be picked up by various cell types after being hydrolyzed by lipoprotein lipase (LPL). Chylomicrons will end up in the liver and then be "rearranged" into VLDL-particles for another round in the circulatory system. Figure 20.2 shows the uptake and storage of fatty acids in the adipocyte and Figure 20.3 depicts the transportation of fat inside the muscle cell. Insulin stimulates the LPL to hydrolyze the triglycerides from triglycerides in the blood vessels and inhibit hormone-sensitive lipase (HSL), thereby limiting the release of fatty acids from the adipocyte to the circulation. An important factor not mentioned in figure 20.2 is the perilipin, adipophilin, and TIP47 protein system [11], where perilipin is that major component [11]. When stimulated by catecholamines, perilipin interacts with hormone-sensitive lipase and increases its activity [11]. Insulin, via decreased phosphoenol kinase A activity, inhibits the activity of both perilipin and HSL (see [12] for a more detailed description of the storage and release of TG).

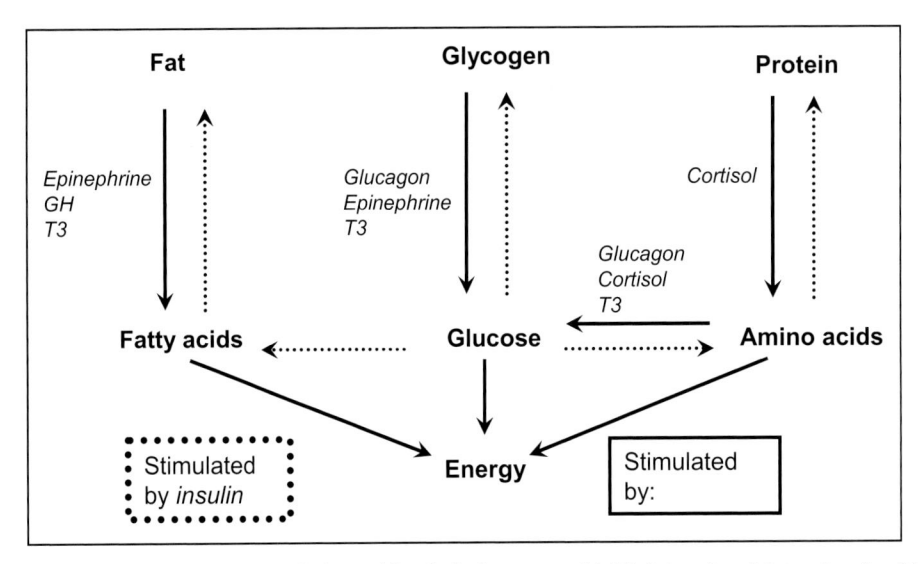

FIGURE 20.1 Simplified scheme of the major anabolic and katabolic hormones, highlighting the pleiotropic role of insulin

REGULATION OF ENTRANCE OF FATTY ACIDS INTO MITOCHONDRIA

The key regulatory step in the fat oxidation process is the entrance of fatty acids into the mitochondria [13]. This is an active transportation process that requires the assistance of the carnitine-shuttle enzyme complex (Figure 20.4). The rate-limiting step is the first part where carnitine-palmitoyl-transferase-1 (CPT1) transports the fatty acyl-CoA over the outer mitochondrial membrane. We have previously shown that human skeletal muscle CPT-1 activity is decreased by physiological hyperglycemia with hyperinsulinemia [14]. It important to note that the uptake into the muscle cell is not decreased [14], which leads to an accumulation of fatty acids in the skeletal muscle cell. This accumulation of fatty acids within the skeletal muscle cell has deleterious effects; among others, intramuscular triglyceride content is associated with decreased insulin sensitivity [15]. Studies comparing obese children with normal insulin sensitivity with obese children with decreased insulin sensitivity usually find more intramuscular fat in the insulin-resistant children [16]. This will be briefly discussed next.

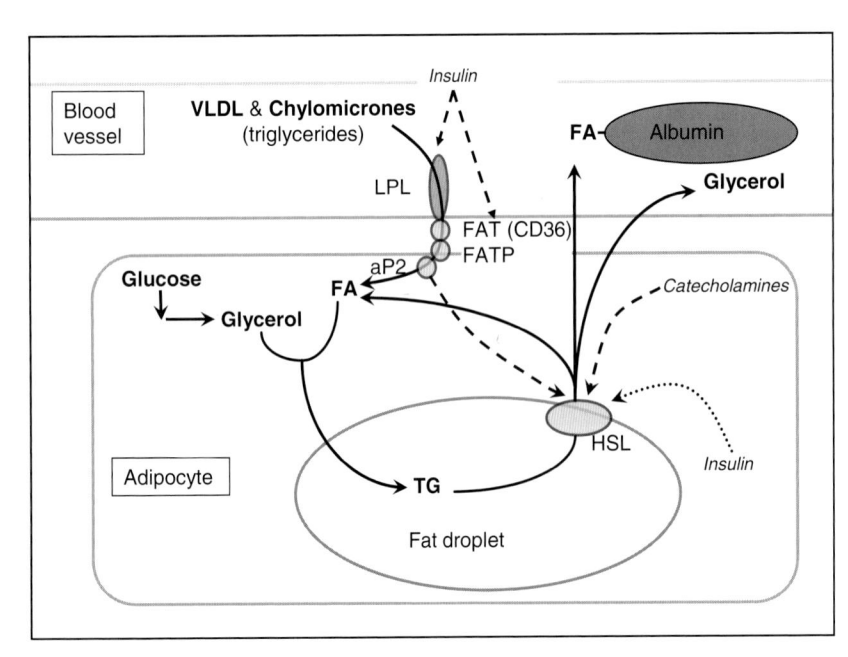

FIGURE 20.2 Fat turnover in the adipocyte. LPL, lipoprotein lipase; HSL, hormone sensitive lipase; FA, fatty acids; TG, triglycerides. Dashed arrows depict stimulation and dotted arrow depicts inhibition.

II. PATHOPHYSIOLOGY

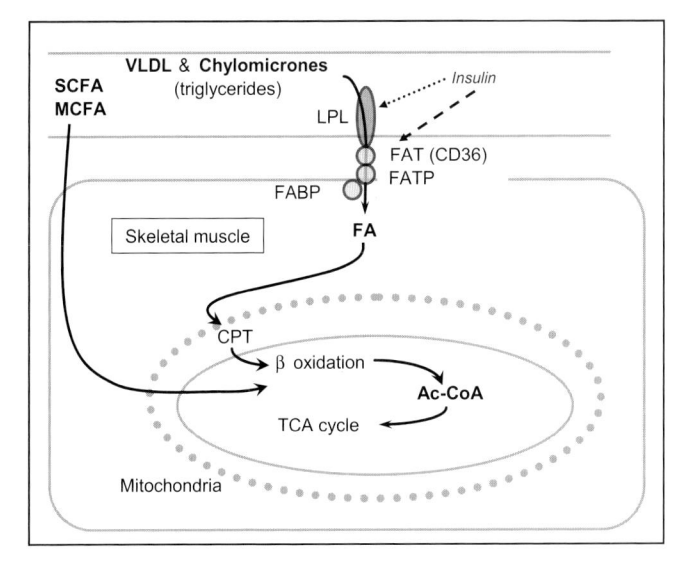

FIGURE 20.3 Fat transportation in the skeletal muscle cell. LPL, lipoprotein lipase; FA, fatty acids; TG, triglycerides; SCFA, short chained fatty acids; MCFA, medium chained fatty acids; FAT, fatty acid translocase (also known as CD36); FATP, fatty acids transporting protein; FABP, fatty acid binding protein; CPT, carnitine palmitoyl-enzyme complex (see Figure 20.4). Dashed arrows depict stimulation and dotted arrow depicts inhibition.

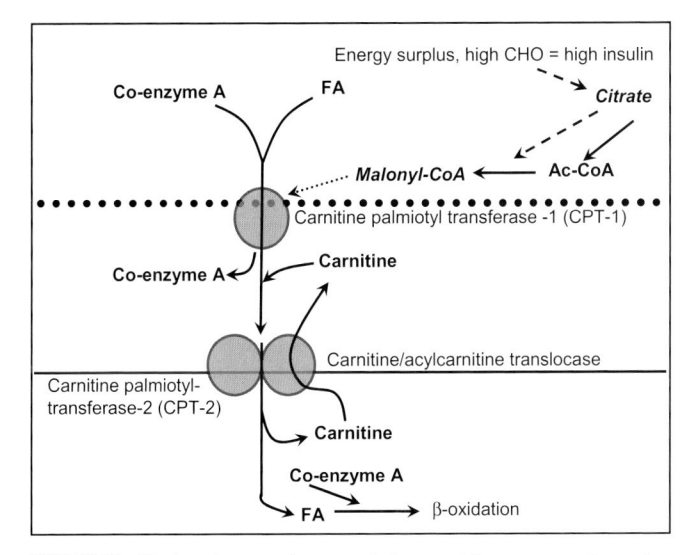

FIGURE 20.4 The regulation of fatty acid transport into the mitochondria. Dashed arrows depict stimulation and dotted arrow depicts inhibition.

MEASURING INSULIN FUNCTION

Before going into methods, a few words about the various components of insulin function. Insulin sensitivity is usually equal to insulin responsiveness, where a low insulin responsiveness (longer insulin half-life) is considered decreased insulin sensitivity [17]. Thus, insulin resistance is usually defined as decreased sensitivity or responsiveness to metabolic actions of insulin [17]. The most common way of looking at the insulin regulatory system is measuring fasting glucose and fasting insulin. However, these values are not sensitive enough to smaller changes in insulin functioning. Various formulas have evolved, such as HOMA and QUICKI, which from fasting values calculate insulin sensitivity. The main benefit with these methods is that they require only one blood sample and can be used in large studies. The problem with these calculations is that the data come from fasting values; it can be argued that it is the handling of glucose (i.e., meals) that is the problem. Therefore, the standard method for diagnosing impaired glucose tolerance or diabetes is the oral glucose tolerance test (OGTT), where the subject consumes 75 g of glucose and blood is sampled regularly for ~120 minutes. This test works to sort out "healthy" from "nonhealthy" and gives an estimate of glucose tolerance, but it will not give a clear answer about insulin sensitivity. The more invasive and much more laborious methods are the intravenous glucose tolerance test (IVGTT) and the hyperinsulinemic euglycemic clamp. In the IVGTT, glucose is first injected, followed by an insulin bolus, and blood is sampled frequently. The IVGTT will not only give values for insulin sensitivity (SI), it will also measure the acute insulin response (AIR) and the disposition index (DI). A high AIR indicates that body reacts strongly to the challenge, which is often seen together with low insulin sensitivity. The DI, which is a product of SI and AIR, gives an indication of β-cell function. A normal DI together with a low SI means that the pancreas is responsive and still able to produce insulin in large amounts. A fall or low DI indicates that the β-cells are less responsive or that insulin production is decreased (see [18] for a more detailed explanation of the IVGTT). The hyperinsulinemic euglycemic clamp is considered the golden standard for measuring insulin function [17]. First insulin is infused at a constant rate and glucose levels are then "clamped" at a certain level by a dextrose infusion [17]. When steady-state conditions have been achieved for plasma insulin, blood glucose, and the glucose infusion rate (GIR), the glucose disposal rate (M) can be calculated as an estimate of insulin sensitivity. An alternative insulin sensitivity index (SI) can be derived by normalizing M for steady-state blood glucose concentration and difference between fasting and steady-state plasma insulin [17]. IVGTT and the clamp will not always give the same result, so a fair understanding is required of the subject population when interpreting the results [17, 19].

INSULIN RESISTANCE AND WEIGHT GAIN

As children enter puberty, there is a natural decrease in insulin sensitivity [20]. As children progress from

Tanner stage I to Tanner stage III, their insulin sensitivity falls with ~30%, and this natural fall is independent of age, ethnicity, and body fat [20]. This means that obese children that already have a low insulin sensitivity will decrease their insulin sensitivity even more [20]. Also the disposition index falls, and this fall is greater in the highest body fat tertile [20]. The precise agent for this decrease in insulin sensitivity is yet to be fully determined, although GH/IGF-1 seems like likely factors [21]. The natural decline in insulin sensitivity during puberty means that any pharmacological intervention to increase insulin sensitivity has to be carefully planned. However, one could hypothesize that for children in the highest fat mass tertile, a pharmacological agent that maintains insulin sensitivity might not be all bad as it has been shown that their prepubertal insulin sensitivity was less than the Tanner stage III values in the low and medium body fat mass tertile [20].

Several longitudinal studies have looked at insulin funtion and subsequent weight gain. Adam et al. [22] studied 96 overweight Hispanic children and observed that decreased insulin sensitivity (over 1 year) was strongly associated with subsequent weight gain, also when controlling for fat free mass, age, Tanner stage, and gender. Odeleye et al. [23] measured fasting insulin in 328 5- to 9-year-old Pima Indian children and did a follow-up ~10 years later. The yearly rate of weight gain was moderately but significantly associated with fasting insulin, independently from age, gender, changes in height, and initial relative weight [23]. Johnson et al. [24] measured 8-year-old children with DEXA and IVGTT and remeasured them annually for 3 to 6 years. The fat mass rate of increase was significantly associated with fasting insulin (positive), SI (negative), and AIR (positive) [24]. Furthermore, lower SI or higher AIR at the start and greater decreases in SI or increases in AIR were associated with greater increases in fat mass [24]. Interestingly, this effect was larger in Caucasians than in African Americans. The authors speculate that the decreased SI is mainly an effect on muscle tissues, whereas the adipose tissue remains insulin sensitive, thereby being even more prone to accumulate fat [24]. Also other endocrine differences are observed in insulin-resistant children. Weight loss typically increases ghrelin concentration, but in obese children with decreased insulin sensitivity, this increase does not occur [25].

Srinivasas et al. [26] followed 745 8- to 17-year-old children for a mean of ~12 years. The possibility of developing metabolic syndrome (in this case, high body mass index [BMI], high fasting insulin, high blood pressure, and high blood lipids) was strongly associated with BMI and fasting insulin. The lowest quartile of insulin had a ~3% incidence of the metabolic syndrome, whereas the highest quartile had a ~12% incidence [26]. The insulin association was not significant when corrected for BMI (CI 0.7 to 4.7), whereas the BMI association remained after adjusting for insulin [26]. Li et al. [27], compared low-birth-weight (LBW) children with normal-weight children and found that ethnicity played a much more dominating role than birth weight. In the Caucasian children, birth weight was not associated with various markers of insulin sensitivity [27]. However, the African American LBW children had higher fasting insulin and lower AIR compared to normal-weight children [27]. Overall, the African American children were more insulin resistant than the Caucasian children [27].

INSULIN SENSITIVITY IN OBESE CHILDREN

Certain subgroups seem to have an increased frequency of altered insulin sensitivity (e.g., Pima Indians and Hispanics in the United States). But studies on other populations reveal that a substantial part of the obese population might be at risk. Wiegand et al. [28] examined 491 obese children and after excluding patients with obesity syndromes and other illnesses. In all, 102 boys and girls fulfilled the American Diabetes Association (ADA) screening criteria (obese and at least another risk factor) for diabetes type 2 [28]. An OGTT was performed; 37 children had impaired glucose tolerance, and 6 had diabetes type 2 [28]. Taksali et al. [29] studied 118 obese children and divided them into tertiles of visceral fat. The tertile with the highest amount of visceral fat was more insulin resistant than the other tertiles, despite having a lower BMI [29].

WHY INSULIN SENSITIZING INCREASES WEIGHT

If decreased insulin sensitivity is the problem, then increasing insulin sensitivity with pharmaceutical agents would ameliorate this problem. The problem is the pleiotropic activity of insulin. The thiazolidinediones are PPAR-γ-agonists and among other things they increase insulin sensitivity. However, this increase seems to be fat depot-specific, and they lead to weight gain [30, 31] and rosiglitazone increases triglyceride-rich lipoprotein particle production and reduces particle clearance [32]. As pathological lipid profile is part of insulin-resistant obese patients, this effect is far from desirable. Metformin, on the other hand, seems to be less effective at increasing insulin sensitivity but more effective in decreasing body weight. In studies on children and adolescents, metformin has been shown to decrease weight and body composition without significantly affecting insulin sensitivity [26], although fasting insulin was decreased [26]. In this study [26] there was considerable individual variation, and only 50% of the studied children displayed any weight loss. As always, compliance makes it hard to see if this variation is physiological or psychological as adherence varied between 15% and 99% [26]. In one meta-analysis (five trials encompassing 320 insulin-resistant obese children), metformin was shown to decrease BMI and HOMA-IR after 6 months [33]. The effect was similar to that of orlistat and sibutramin [33]. However, no long-term data exist but perhaps metformin may be warranted in patients where other interventions will not work.

DIET STUDIES ON CHILDREN

Despite the fact that pediatric obesity has been a problem for quite some time, there are few diet intervention studies. In a systematic review by Gibson et al. [34], only nine intervention studies fulfilled their criteria. Major reasons for exclusion were inappropriate intervention (e.g., behavioral interventions, very short term dietary interventions), ineligible study population (e.g., only adults, a mixture of obese and nonobese children), and inappropriate study design (e.g., observational study, lack of comparison group). There was a considerable spread in results, with interventions performing slightly better in shorter studies, but few differences were seen ≥1 year studies [34]. The authors concluded, "Ad libitum diets are of particular interest in view of the ineffectiveness of energy-restricted diets" (p. 1551) [34]. In a similar, later meta-analysis, McGovern et al. [35] included six studies and found no significant difference between interventions and control (confidence interval for standard mean difference was −0.56 to 0.11). However, these two articles have only focused on weight, which may be a somewhat reductionistic way of looking at the effect of diets. Here are some studies where carbohydrate quality or quantity has been the main focus.

Low GI-Diet Studies in Children

Spieth et al. [36] divided 107 obese children into a standard low-fat, low-calorie group and a group following a low-glycemic index diet without energy restriction. During the ~4 month intervention, more weight was lost in the low glycemic index group, and this weight loss was not dependent on age, sex, ethnicity, BMI or baseline weight [36]. Ebbeling et al. [37] randomized 16 obese adolescents (13 to 21 years) to a standard low-fat diet or a low-glycemic load diet (slightly higher allowance for fat); both were ad libitum diets. Fat mass was lower in the low-glycemic load group at the end of the 6-month intervention as well as at 6-month follow-up; and HOMA index increased less in this group. In a bivariate linear regression analysis glycemic load (GL) explained 51% of the variance in body fat, whereas dietary fat content was not associated with body fat [37].

In a pilot study, Fajcsak et al. [38] followed eight obese children that consumed a low-glycemic index diet during 6 weeks. Weight did not decrease, but fat mass, hunger, and various risk markers decreased [38]. Ventura et al. [39] observed decreased glucose and insulin response after IVGTT in Latino children advised to eat less sugar. In a similar study by Cummings et al. [40], children were instructed to eat healthier and especially limit consumption of sugar-containing beverages. Those with a decrease or no change in BMI z-score had greater insulin resistance than those whose BMI z-score increased. In other words, the benefit of removing sugar-containing beverages was much greater in insulin-resistant children [40].

Low-Carbohydrate Diet Studies in Children

In a relative large study, 104 overweight children (6 to 14 years old) were randomized to an ad lib low-carbohydrate (CHO) diet (max. 20 g CHO/day) or a 1000 kcal/day (4.2 MJ/day) standard diet (50 E% CHO, 30 E% fat, and 20 E% protein) [41]. The diets were consumed for 8 weeks and weight loss was similar between the two diets. Fasting insulin decreased from almost 29 μU/ml to 7 μU/L in the low-carbohydrate diet group, whereas no significant change was observed in the standard diet group [41]. Noteworthy is perhaps that the patients reported that the ad lib component of the low-carbohydrate diet was appreciated [41]. Of note is, of course, that ad lib gets quite restricted when only 20 g of CHO is allowed per day.

In a pilot study, Bailes et al. [42] studied 55 5- to 18-year-old obese children who chose either a low-carbohydrate diet (max 30 g CHO/day) or a standard low-calorie diet (max. 30 E% fat, 15 to 20 E% protein, and 55 E% CHO; 80% of calculated energy need). Participants were instructed to choose the diet that they thought would be easiest to follow based on their own food preferences; 36 children chose low CHO and 16 chose low calorie. Children (27 at 2-month follow-up) in the low-CHO diet group lost 5.21± 3.44 kg, whereas subjects in the low-calorie diet group (10 at 2-month follow-up) gained 2.36 ± 2.54 kg. No biochemical or other supplemental data were given, so the results are somewhat difficult to interpret. This is more of a proof-of-principle study (i.e., a self-selected diet can give rise to good treatment results). However, whether long-term success is also helped by self-selection was not addressed in this study. In another pilot study, Siegel et al. [43] studied children between 12 and 18 years. Subjects with a BMI above the 95th percentile were instructed to eat less than 50 grams of carbohydrate daily but were not restricted on fat and protein intake. There was a major dropout, as 6 months results are only available for 38 of 63 children who started the study. Of these 38 children, 32 lost weight and 5 gained weight. The children reported decreasing their CHO intake substantially, but they did not increase fat and protein, which meant that the reported caloric intake was halved compared to baseline. Underreporting must have been substantial as 5 subjects managed to increase their weight [43].

In a similar but more controlled study, Sondike et al. [44] randomized 30 obese adolescents to either low carbohydrate (LC) (<20 g CHO for 2 weeks, followed by <40 g CHO for 8 weeks) or HC (standard low-calorie protocol). The LC group reported eating 1830 kcal/day and the HC 1100 kcal/day. Despite these reported calorie intakes, the LC group lost on average ~10 kg, and the HC group lost ~ 4 kg. Eight of the 16 subjects in the LC group lost more than 5 kg, whereas 4 out of 14 in the HC group lost more than 5 kilos [44]. In these three studies, groups or individuals gain weight despite reporting eating low-calorie diets. In adults it is frequently reported that despite that the low-calorie groups report eating fewer calories than the low-carbohydrate groups, the weight loss is usually less in the low-calorie group [45]. Underreporting is always of concern in diet studies, as it is laborious to correctly report all food items. But it is not readily apparent why it should be harder to correctly report low-calorie/low-fat diets than low-carbohydrate diets.

Treuth et al. [46] randomized 24 normal-weight children aged 6 to 16 years to a low-fat group (25 E% fat and 60 E% CHO) and a high-fat group (55 E% fat, 30 E% CHO). Each diet period was 7 days with a 2- to 8-week washout. The children were able to adjust to the two diets as respiratory quotient (RQ) reflected the diet composition. An IVGTT was also performed and higher SI was observed in the adolescents after the low-fat diet [47], although fasting insulin and c-peptide were lower after the high-fat diet [46, 47]. In a follow-up study [48], obese adolescents followed the same protocol. In contrast to the lean adolescents, no diet difference in SI was seen, but the obese adolescents were much more insulin resistant [48]. More insulin (a two-fold increase) was secreted during the IVGTT in the obese adolescents after the low-fat diet than after the high-fat diet [48]. Altering the contribution from glucose and fructose did not affect insulin secretion [49].

Demol et al. [50] randomized 55 obese adolescents to three groups: low-carbohydrate, low-fat diet (max. 20 E% CHO, 30 E% fat, and 50 E% protein); low-carbohydrate, high-fat diet (max. 20 E% CHO, 60 E% fat, and 20 E% protein); and high-carbohydrate diet (50 to 60 E% CH, 30 E% fat, and 20 E% proteins). All diets were energy-restricted to 1200 to 1500 kcal/day and were consumed for 12 weeks. No differences were seen in weight changes at the end of the study and at the 9-month follow-up [50]. The dropout rate was 17% in the low-carbohydrate, low-fat group, 29% in the low-carbohydrate, high-fat group, and 31% in the high-carbohydrate, low-fat group (p = ns) [51]. However, decreased fasting insulin and HOMA levels were observed in the two low-carbohydrate diet groups at the end of the study and at the 9-month follow-up [50]. Psychological functioning was assessed with a health-related quality-of-life questionnaire [51]. Despite similar weight changes, improvements in psychological functioning were seen in low CHO, low-fat, and high CHO group but not in low CHO, high-fat diet group [51], although the lack of change in the low CHO, high-fat group might have been a power issue as there was only 12 subjects in this group (see Table 2 in [51]).

More Draconian diets have been used. For example, Sothern et al. [52] used a virtually fat and carbohydrate free ketogenic diet in obese adolescents for 10 weeks and noted a ~10% decrease in weight and very little attrition. However, these kinds of ketogenic diets are more for the dietary treatment of epilepsy and not within the scope of this chapter.

HEALTH ASPECTS OF A LOW-CARBOHYDRATE DIET

Many countries have food guidelines that recommend keeping saturated fat intake low [53] [54], the rational being that saturated fat directly or indirectly causes cardiovascular disease. As low-carbohydrate diets often are high in saturated fat (though that is not always the case [55]), the impact of saturated fat on health has to be addressed, especially if children end up eating a low-carbohydrate diet for a long time. Currently few studies have been done to examine saturated fat and health in children. In the STRIP study [56], families with infants were randomized to intervention (low saturated and cholesterol intake) and control. The children were measured annually; interestingly, despite the fact that both boys and girls reported eating less saturated fat and cholesterol, only boys showed a significant decrease in LDL-cholesterol [56].

Samuelsson et al. [57] observed that the estimated dietary intake of saturated short chain fatty acids was inversely related to the serum cholesterol in adolescents. In short, it is not clear-cut that low saturated fat intake equals low total or LDL cholesterol concentration. When looking at studies in adults, decreasing saturated fat commonly decreases HDL cholesterol concentration [58]. Moreover, it has become increasingly apparent that the concentration of LDL may not be a major prognostic factor in cardiovascular disease, but rather the different subclasses of the LDL particle are important. Of the different LDL subclasses, the small dense LDL-III (or LDL-C<255Å) particle is the most atherogenic [59–62]. Some have found a relationship between LDL concentration and LDL size [63], whereas others found no relationship [64]. It has been shown that as saturated fat content in the diet decreases, the size of the LDL particle decreases [63, 65–67], although some find no change in LDL particle size when changing diet [58, 68], and others find increased concentrations of small dense LDL with increased saturated fat intake [69]. The same group had previously found that a very low carbohydrate diet with ~25% of the energy from saturated fat increased the size of the LDL particles in men [70] but not in women [71].

Nielsen et al. [72] found that VLDL particles were more resistant to oxidative modifications after palm oil, olive oil, or butter meals compared to sunflower and rapeseed oil meals. Korpela et al. [73] found that LDL from "high fish" eaters were more susceptible to oxidation than that from "high milk" eaters. Decreasing the saturated fat content of the diet has been shown to decrease the primary cardioprotective HDL2 [74]. Moreover, some of the associations between saturated fat intake and risk markers for cardiovascular disease seem to be different when CHO intake is low. Warensjö et al. [75] have shown that high saturated fat intake was associated with increased stearoyl-Coenzyme A desaturase 1 (SCD-1) activity (measured as ratio between unsaturated product and saturated precursor). SCD-1 is an enzyme that converts 16:0 and 18:0 to 16:1 and 18:1, and its activity has been shown to be associated with increased risk of cardiovascular disease [76]. However, Mangravite et al. [77] studied transcriptional expression after diets with varying amounts of CHO and saturated fat and observed an inverse relationship between SCD-1 expression and saturated fat intake. The association was strongest between CHO intake and SCD-1 [77]. In another diet comparison study, Forsythe et al. [78] compared a very low carbohydrate diet (12 E% CHO) with a low-fat diet and observed a lower 16:1/16:0 ratio after 12 weeks on very low carbohydrate diet.

In short-term and long-term low-carbohydrate, high-saturated fat diet trials, the fasting triglyceride concentration is typically decreased compared to habitual or control diets [45], even when there is no difference in body weight [79]. Also, in short-term low-carbohydrate diet trials, the postprandial triglyceride concentration after a test meal is typically decreased compared to low-fat diets [71, 80]. Moreover, total as well as LDL cholesterol is higher after low-carbohydrate diets than after low-fat diets [45]. There has been a fear that low-carbohydrate diets will lead to high-protein diets, which will increase the risk of kidney stones and affect bone mineralization. For example, Reddy et al. [81] observed lower urine pH and higher urinary calcium in subjects eating a ketogenic high-protein, low-carbohydrate diet. This would indicate that long-term intake of this diet could increase the risk of kidney stones and affect the integrity of the skeleton [81]. One should note that in that study, the subjects consumed almost 35 E% protein [81]. In one epidemiological study in elderly women, Dargent-Molina et al. [82] observed that although no overall association between total protein or net acid excretion and fracture risk was found, high-protein diets were associated with an increased risk of fracture when calcium intake was low. On the other hand, Munger et al. [83] also studied elderly women and observed an inverse relationship between hip fracture and the intake of animal protein. Furthermore, a recent meta-analysis could not find any association between a marker of bone metabolism (N-telopeptides), and net acid excretion or urine calcium [84]. All in all it seems that protein intake (at least between 15 E% to 30 E%) does not have any significant negative effect on bone metabolism.

The above-mentioned relationships between diet and various risk markers/risk factors have to be seen in the light of potential weight loss. A diet that normalizes a child's weight will most probably decrease the risk of future disease. Thus, the potential problem of an increased LDL concentration must be seen in light of decreased weight and triglycerides.

Gastrointestinal problems, such as constipation, have been mentioned has possible side effects of a low-carbohydrate diet. In the study by Demol et al. [50], mentioned previously, side effects as well as attrition were similar between low-carbohydrate and high-carbohydrate groups. Brinkworth et al. [85] studied adults and did not find any difference in gastrointestinal complaints between a low-carbohydrate, high-protein diet and a high-carbohydrate, low-fat diet. Also cognitive function is of concern, as glucose is the main fuel for the brain. A low intake of carbohydrate could then hypothetically affect learning. However, studies looking at the effect of breakfast versus no breakfast on mental performance show that significant effects are only seen in malnourished children [86]. Thus, as long as adequate energy intake is observed, there are no current indications that a low-carbohydrate diet should affect learning significantly.

THE INSULIN SYSTEM IN AN EVOLUTIONARY PERSPECTIVE

In 1962 Neel [87] put forward the "thrifty gene hypothesis," which stated that individuals that easily could store extra energy would have had an evolutionary advantage during famines. Obese and overweight individuals accordingly have this "thrifty gene." Some researchers have discussed the thrifty gene hypothesis and why it is not valid [88, 89]. In short, where feast and famine would possibly occur (far away from the equator), the presence of overweight and type 2 diabetes is lower [88, 89]. Moreover, any species that cannot plan and cannot adapt to new circumstances will become extinct, and the presence of a thrifty gene will not compensate the lack of planning. The individual variation we see is more a sign that nature did not bother to regulate tightly a possible positive energy balance, as it would resolve itself without direct body interference. The human body has many appetite-increasing systems but fewer satiating systems. Evolutionary there has been less of a need for satiating systems. In the preagrarian society, food was collected via physical activity; therefore, any excess weight from an overfeeding episode (e.g., a successful hunt) would increase caloric demand and require even more activity to maintain the excess weight, otherwise weight would decrease to the level of every day's caloric intake. However, the cost of activity decreases as body weight decreases, so other processes have to ensure that proper caloric intake is maintained. Thus, the ghrelin and other satiating systems are weak in comparison to the appetite-promoting power of palatable foods of today, with the concomitant rise of insulin. Moreover, insulin-counteracting hormones, such as glucagon, were most probably set to fight insulin extensively. Nowadays, there is little cost of excess weight with escalators, cars, moving sidewalks, drive-in ATMs, home delivery, and remote controls. Weight has to increase to levels never before seen before the costs appear. As can be seen in the United States, where the majority of the population is overweight or obese, actually a minority of the population can withstand a truly obesogenic environment, as there was no need for nature to factor in caloric surplus until, say, the 1950s.

AMALGAMATION

This chapter has described how important insulin is for the fat metabolism and explained that altered insulin functioning is strongly associated with obesity. Although obesity is a complex and multifaceted disease, with strong behavioral and psychosocial components, it is vital to characterize correctly the pediatric obesity patient before dietary recommendations are given. Although the

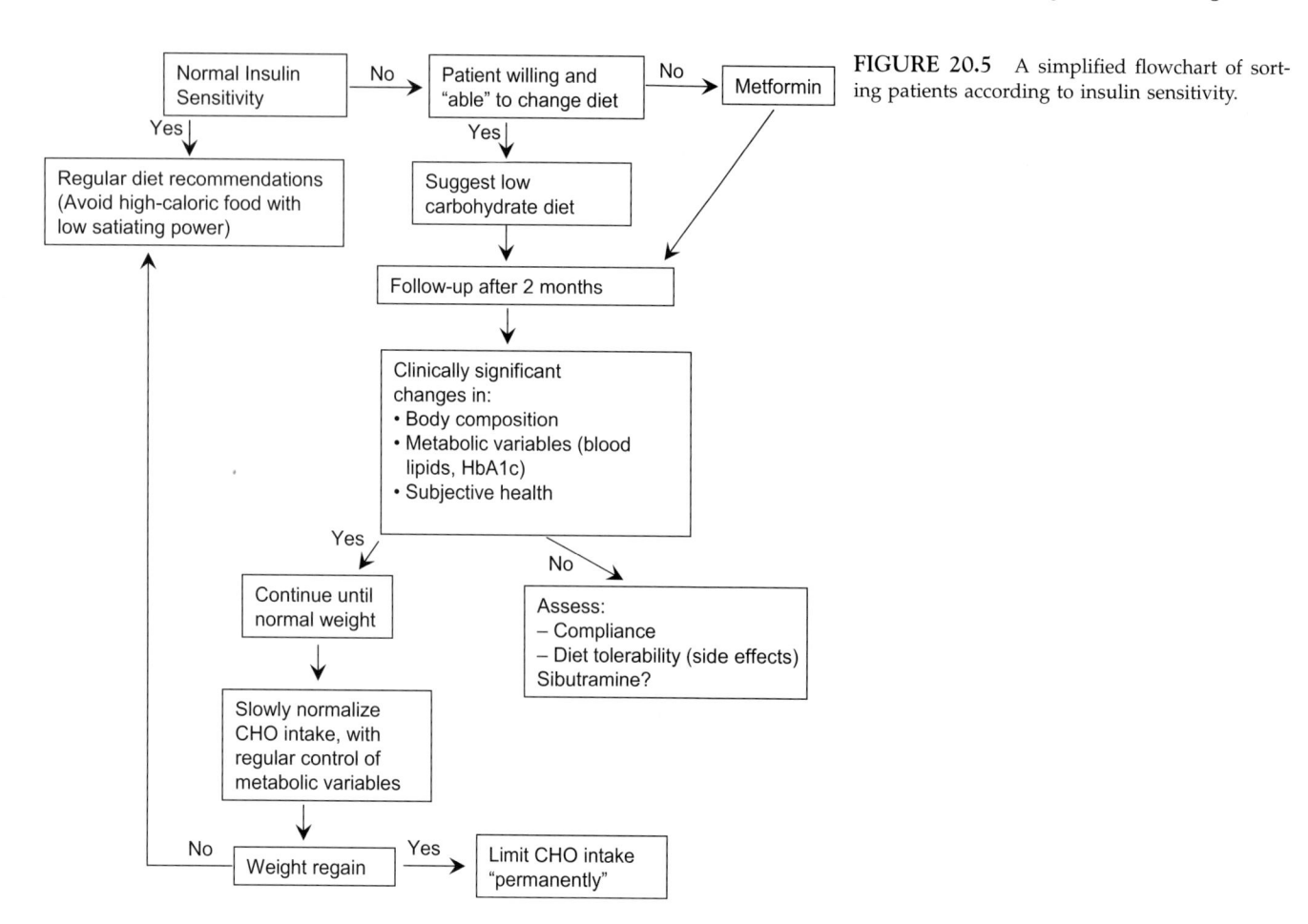

FIGURE 20.5 A simplified flowchart of sorting patients according to insulin sensitivity.

evidence still is quite weak, most studies indicate that for obese subjects with decreased insulin sensitivity, a diet with a large proportion of carbohydrate will not assist in weight loss or weight maintenance. It is important to differentiate between the dietary advice given to healthy or mildly overweight children and the more individual approach one has to take to treat the obese child. Just as proper nutrition cannot by itself make all children lean, even the most rigorous behavior program will most probably fail if the diet component is not suited to the metabolism of the patient. Although there may be hesitation within the nutrition community to recommend low-carbohydrate diets, it is important to recognize the risk of future disease if the obese pediatric patient is not treated. As argued earlier, the potential health risks of eating a well-balanced low-carbohydrate diet are small compared to the health benefits.

Again, it is important to characterize the patient, as obese subjects with high insulin sensitivity most probably will not benefit from a low-carbohydrate diet. It is also important that professionals help patients to learn how to eat in a new way; otherwise, nonprofessionals (such as vocal groups on the Internet) will provide dietary guidance. These groups might not have the required skills to construct an adequate diet for a growing child. This chapter focuses more or less completely on insulin action and not on genetic makeup. The genetic studies have so far not given enough information to help in determining which patient should be given what advice, with perhaps the possible exception of FTO. Sonestedt et al. [90] have shown that BMI was somewhat higher in subjects with the AA allele compared to subjects with the TT allele; and this relationship was dependent on dietary fat intake. However, the differences were small, and so far no intervention study has addressed the impact of FTO on response to various macronutrients.

To conclude, there is currently a tidal wave of untreated obese children and it is important to find ways of using the resources as efficiently as possible. Included is a simple flow sheet (Figure 20.5) that can be used to sort patients according to insulin sensitivity. The better the patient is characterized, the easier it will be to find the proper individual treatment plan. If some patients can be treated with a diet that fits their metabolism, possibly more resources can be used for the more laborious patients where psychosocial environment and behavior need to be changed.

References

1. Holmback U, Fridman J, Gustafsson J, Proos L, Sundelin C, Forslund A. Overweight more prevalent among children than among adolescents. *Acta Paediatr* 2007;**96**:577−81.
2. Mårild S, Bondestam M, Bergstrom R, Ehnberg S, Hollsing A, Albertsson-Wikland K. Prevalence trends of obesity and overweight among 10-year-old children in western Sweden and relationship with parental body mass index 1. *Acta Paediatr* 2004;**93**:1588−95.
3. Ekblom O, Oddsson K, Ekblom B. Prevalence and regional differences in overweight in 2001 and trends in BMI distribution in Swedish children from 1987 to 2001 1. *Scand J Public Health* 2004;**32**:257−63.
4. Petersen S, Brulin C, Bergstrom E. Increasing prevalence of overweight in young schoolchildren in Umea, Sweden, from 1986 to 2001 1. *Acta Paediatr* 2003;**92**:848−53.
5. Cali AM, Caprio S. Obesity in children and adolescents. *The Journal of Clinical Endocrinology and Metabolism* 2008;**93**:S31−6.
6. Hardy LR, Harrell JS, Bell RA. Overweight in children: definitions, measurements, confounding factors, and health consequences 1. *J Pediatr Nurs* 2004;**19**:376−84.
7. Serdula MK, Ivery D, Coates RJ, Freedman DS, Williamson DF, Byers T. Do obese children become obese adults? A review of the literature 1. *Prev Med* 1993;**22**:167−77.
8. Singhal A. Endothelial dysfunction: role in obesity-related disorders and the early origins of CVD 1. *Proc Nutr Soc* 2005;**64**:15−22.
9. Field AE, Cook NR, Gillman MW. Weight status in childhood as a predictor of becoming overweight or hypertensive in early adulthood 1. *Obes Res* 2005;**13**:163−9.
10. Collins CE, Warren J, Neve M, McCoy P, Stokes BJ. Measuring effectiveness of dietetic interventions in child obesity: a systematic review of randomized trials. *Archives of Pediatrics & Adolescent Medicine* 2006;**160**:906−22.
11. Tai ES, Ordovas JM. The role of perilipin in human obesity and insulin resistance. *Current opinion in lipidology* 2007;**18**:152−6.
12. Wang S, Soni KG, Semache M, Casavant S, Fortier M, Pan L, Mitchell GA. Lipolysis and the integrated physiology of lipid energy metabolism. *Molecular Genetics and Metabolism* 2008;**95**: 117−26.
13. Rasmussen BB, Wolfe RR. Regulation of fatty acid oxidation in skeletal muscle. *Annual Review of Nutrition* 1999;**19**:463−84.
14. Rasmussen BB, Holmback UC, Volpi E, Morio-Liondore B, Paddon-Jones D, Wolfe RR. Malonyl coenzyme A and the regulation of functional carnitine palmitoyltransferase-1 activity and fat oxidation in human skeletal muscle. *The Journal of Clinical Investigation* 2002;**110**:1687−93.
15. Perseghin G, Scifo P, De Cobelli F, Pagliato E, Battezzati A, Arcelloni C, Vanzulli A, Testolin G, Pozza G, Del Maschio A, Luzi L. Intramyocellular triglyceride content is a determinant of in vivo insulin resistance in humans: a 1H-13C nuclear magnetic resonance spectroscopy assessment in offspring of type 2 diabetic parents. *Diabetes* 1999;**48**:1600−6.
16. Weiss R, Dufour S, Taksali SE, Tamborlane WV, Petersen KF, Bonadonna RC, Boselli L, Barbetta G, Allen K, Rife F, Savoye M, Dziura J, Sherwin R, Shulman GI, Caprio S. Prediabetes in obese youth: a syndrome of impaired glucose tolerance, severe insulin resistance, and altered myocellular and abdominal fat partitioning. *Lancet* 2003;**362**:951−7.
17. Muniyappa R, Lee S, Chen H, Quon MJ. Current approaches for assessing insulin sensitivity and resistance in vivo: advantages, limitations, and appropriate usage. *Am J Physiol Endocrinol Metab* 2008;**294**:E15−26.
18. Bergman RN. Toward physiological understanding of glucose tolerance. Minimal model approach. *Diabetes* 1989;**38**:1512−27.
19. Gordillo-Moscoso A, Valadez-Castillo JF, Mandeville PB, Hernandez-Sierra JF. Comparison of equivalence and determination of diagnostic utility of min-mod and clamp methods for insulin resistance in diabetes free subjects: a meta-analysis. *Endocrine* 2004;**25**:259−63.
20. Goran MI, Gower BA. Longitudinal study on pubertal insulin resistance. *Diabetes* 2001;**50**:2444−50.

21. Moran A, Jacobs Jr DR, Steinberger J, Cohen P, Hong CP, Prineas R, Sinaiko AR. Association between the insulin resistance of puberty and the insulin-like growth factor-I/growth hormone axis. *The Journal of Clinical Endocrinology and Metabolism* 2002;**87**: 4817–20.
22. Adam TC, Toledo-Corral C, Lane CJ, Weigensberg MJ, Spruijt-Metz D, Davies JN, Goran MI. *Insulin Sensitivity as an Independent Predictor of Fat Mass Gain in Hispanic Adolescents*. Diabetes care; 2009.
23. Odeleye OE, de Courten M, Pettitt DJ, Ravussin E. Fasting hyperinsulinemia is a predictor of increased body weight gain and obesity in Pima Indian children. *Diabetes* 1997;**46**:1341–5.
24. Johnson MS, Figueroa-Colon R, Huang TT, Dwyer JH, Goran MI. Longitudinal changes in body fat in African American and Caucasian children: influence of fasting insulin and insulin sensitivity. *The Journal of Clinical Endocrinology and Metabolism* 2001;**86**:3182–7.
25. Krohn K, Boczan C, Otto B, Heldwein W, Landgraf R, Bauer CP, Koletzko B. Regulation of ghrelin is related to estimated insulin sensitivity in obese children. *International Journal of Obesity* 2006;**30**:1482–7. 2005.
26. Srinivasan S, Ambler GR, Baur LA, Garnett SP, Tepsa M, Yap F, Ward GM, Cowell CT. Randomized, controlled trial of metformin for obesity and insulin resistance in children and adolescents: improvement in body composition and fasting insulin. *The Journal of Clinical Endocrinology and Metabolism* 2006;**91**:2074–80.
27. Li C, Johnson MS, Goran MI. Effects of low birth weight on insulin resistance syndrome in Caucasian and African-American children. *Diabetes care* 2001;**24**:2035–42.
28. Wiegand S, Maikowski U, Blankenstein O, Biebermann H, Tarnow P, Gruters A. Type 2 diabetes and impaired glucose tolerance in European children and adolescents with obesity — a problem that is no longer restricted to minority groups. *European journal of endocrinology / European Federation of Endocrine Societies* 2004;**151**:199–206.
29. Taksali SE, Caprio S, Dziura J, Dufour S, Cali AM, Goodman TR, Papademetris X, Burgert TS, Pierpont BM, Savoye M, Shaw M, Seyal AA, Weiss R. High visceral and low abdominal subcutaneous fat stores in the obese adolescent: a determinant of an adverse metabolic phenotype. *Diabetes* 2008;**57**:367–71.
30. Virtanen KA, Hallsten K, Parkkola R, Janatuinen T, Lonnqvist F, Viljanen T, Ronnemaa T, Knuuti J, Huupponen R, Lonnroth P, Nuutila P. Differential effects of rosiglitazone and metformin on adipose tissue distribution and glucose uptake in type 2 diabetic subjects. *Diabetes* 2003;**52**:283–90.
31. Kang JG, Park CY, Ihm SH, Yoo HJ, Park H, Rhee EJ, Won JC, Lee WY, Oh KW, Park SW, Kim SW. Mechanisms of adipose tissue redistribution with rosiglitazone treatment in various adipose depots. *Metabolism: Clinical and Experimental* 2009;**48**(7): 745–9.
32. Duez H, Lamarche B, Uffelman KD, Valero R, Szeto L, Lemieux S, Cohn JS, Lewis GF. Dissociation between the insulin-sensitizing effect of rosiglitazone and its effect on hepatic and intestinal lipoprotein production. *The Journal of Clinical Endocrinology and Metabolism* 2008;**93**:1722–9.
33. Park MH, Kinra S, Ward KJ, White B, Viner RM. Metformin for obesity in children and adolescents: a systematic review. *Diabetes Care* 2009;**32**:1743–5.
34. Gibson LJ, Peto J, Warren JM, dos Santos Silva I. Lack of evidence on diets for obesity for children: a systematic review. *International Journal of Epidemiology* 2006;**35**:1544–52.
35. McGovern L, Johnson JN, Paulo R, Hettinger A, Singhal V, Kamath C, Erwin PJ, Montori VM. Clinical review: treatment of pediatric obesity: a systematic review and meta-analysis of randomized trials. *The Journal of Clinical Endocrinology and Metabolism* 2008;**93**:4600–5.
36. Spieth LE, Harnish JD, Lenders CM, Raezer LB, Pereira MA, Hangen SJ, Ludwig DS. A low-glycemic index diet in the treatment of pediatric obesity. *Archives of Pediatrics & Adolescent Medicine* 2000;**154**:947–51.
37. Ebbeling CB, Leidig MM, Sinclair KB, Hangen JP, Ludwig DS. A reduced-glycemic load diet in the treatment of adolescent obesity. *Archives of Pediatrics & Adolescent Medicine* 2003;**157**: 773–9.
38. Fajcsak Z, Gabor A, Kovacs V, Martos E. The effects of 6-week low glycemic load diet based on low glycemic index foods in overweight/obese children—pilot study. *Journal of the American College of Nutrition* 2008;**27**:12–21.
39. Ventura E, Davis J, Byrd-Williams C, Alexander K, McClain A, Lane CJ, Spruijt-Metz D, Weigensberg M, Goran M. Reduction in risk factors for type 2 diabetes mellitus in response to a low-sugar, high-fiber dietary intervention in overweight Latino adolescents. *Archives of Pediatrics & Adolescent Medicine* 2009;**163**: 320–7.
40. Cummings DM, Henes S, Kolasa KM, Olsson J, Collier D. Insulin resistance status: predicting weight response in overweight children. *Archives of Pediatrics & Adolescent Medicine* 2008;**162**: 764–8.
41. Pena L, Pena M, Gonzalez J, Claro A. A comparative study of two diets in the treatment of primary exogenous obesity in children. *Acta Paediatrica Academiae Scientiarum Hungaricae* 1979;**20**:99–103.
42. Bailes JR, Strow MT, Werthammer J, McGinnis RA, Elitsur Y. Effect of low-carbohydrate, unlimited calorie diet on the treatment of childhood obesity: a prospective controlled study. *Metabolic Syndrome and Related Disorders* 2003;**1**:221–5.
43. Siegel RM, Rich W, Joseph EC, Linhardt J, Knight J, Khoury J, Daniels SR. A 6-Month, Office-Based, Low-Carbohydrate Diet Intervention in Obese Teens. *Clinical Pediatrics*; 2009;.
44. Sondike SB, Copperman N, Jacobson MS. Effects of a low-carbohydrate diet on weight loss and cardiovascular risk factor in overweight adolescents. *The Journal of Pediatrics* 2003;**142**: 253–8.
45. Nordmann AJ, Nordmann A, Briel M, Keller U, Yancy Jr WS, Brehm BJ, Bucher HC. Effects of low-carbohydrate vs low-fat diets on weight loss and cardiovascular risk factors: a meta-analysis of randomized controlled trials. *Archives of Internal Medicine* 2006;**166**:285–93.
46. Treuth MS, Sunehag AL, Trautwein LM, Bier DM, Haymond MW, Butte NF. Metabolic adaptation to high-fat and high-carbohydrate diets in children and adolescents. *The American Journal of Clinical Nutrition* 2003;**77**:479–89.
47. Sunehag AL, Toffolo G, Treuth MS, Butte NF, Cobelli C, Bier DM, Haymond MW. Effects of dietary macronutrient content on glucose metabolism in children. *The Journal of Clinical Endocrinology and Metabolism* 2002;**87**:5168–78.
48. Sunehag AL, Toffolo G, Campioni M, Bier DM, Haymond MW. Effects of dietary macronutrient intake on insulin sensitivity and secretion and glucose and lipid metabolism in healthy, obese adolescents. *The Journal of Clinical Endocrinology and Metabolism* 2005;**90**:4496–502.
49. Sunehag AL, Toffolo G, Campioni M, Bier DM, Haymond MW. Short-term high dietary fructose intake had no effects on insulin sensitivity and secretion or glucose and lipid metabolism in healthy, obese adolescents. *J Pediatr Endocrinol Metab* 2008;**21**: 225–35.
50. Demol S, Yackobovitch-Gavan M, Shalitin S, Nagelberg N, Gillon-Keren M, Phillip M. Low-carbohydrate (low & high-fat) versus high-carbohydrate low-fat diets in the treatment of obesity in adolescents. *Acta Paediatr* 2009;**98**:346–51.
51. Yackobovitch-Gavan M, Nagelberg N, Demol S, Phillip M, Shalitin S. Influence of weight-loss diets with different

macronutrient compositions on health-related quality of life in obese youth. *Appetite* 2008;**51**:697−703.
52. Sothern MS, Despinasse B, Brown R, Suskind RM, Udall Jr JN, Blecker U. Lipid profiles of obese children and adolescents before and after significant weight loss: differences according to sex. *Southern Medical Journal* 2000;**93**:278−82.
53. Becker W, Lyhne N, Pedersen AN, Aro A, Fogelholm M, Thorsdottir I, Alexander JT, Anderssen SA, Meltzer HM, Pedersen JI. Nordic Nutrition Recommendations 2004-integrating nutrition and physical activity. *Scandinavian Journal of Nutrition* 2004;**48**:178−87.
54. Gifford KD. Dietary fats, eating guides, and public policy: history, critique, and recommendations. *The American Journal of Medicine* 2002;**113**(Suppl. 9B):89S−106S.
55. Jenkins DJ, Wong JM, Kendall CW, Esfahani A, Ng VW, Leong TC, Faulkner DA, Vidgen E, Greaves KA, Paul G, Singer W. The effect of a plant-based low-carbohydrate ("Eco-Atkins") diet on body weight and blood lipid concentrations in hyperlipidemic subjects. *Archives of Internal Medicine* 2009;**169**:1046−54.
56. Rask-Nissila L, Jokinen E, Ronnemaa T, Viikari J, Tammi A, Niinikoski H, Seppanen R, Tuominen J, Simell O. Prospective, randomized, infancy-onset trial of the effects of a low-saturated-fat, low-cholesterol diet on serum lipids and lipoproteins before school age: The Special Turku Coronary Risk Factor Intervention Project (STRIP). *Circulation* 2000;**102**:1477−83.
57. Samuelson G, Bratteby LE, Mohsen R, Vessby B. Dietary fat intake in healthy adolescents: inverse relationships between the estimated intake of saturated fatty acids and serum cholesterol. *Br J Nutr* 2001;**85**:333−41.
58. Li Z, Otvos JD, Lamon-Fava S, Carrasco WV, Lichtenstein AH, McNamara JR, Ordovas JM, Schaefer EJ. Men and women differ in lipoprotein response to dietary saturated fat and cholesterol restriction. *The Journal of Nutrition* 2003;**133**:3428−33.
59. Chait A, Brazg RL, Tribble DL, Krauss RM. Susceptibility of small, dense, low-density lipoproteins to oxidative modification in subjects with the atherogenic lipoprotein phenotype, pattern B. *Am J Med* 1993;**94**:350−6.
60. Watts GF, Mandalia S, Brunt JN, Slavin BM, Coltart DJ, Lewis B. Independent associations between plasma lipoprotein subfraction levels and the course of coronary artery disease in the . *St Thomas' Atherosclerosis Regression Study (STARS) 1. Metabolism: Clinical and Experimental* 1993;**42**:1461−7.
61. Williams PT, Superko HR, Haskell WL, Alderman EL, Blanche PJ, Holl LG, Krauss RM. Smallest LDL particles are most strongly related to coronary disease progression in men 1. *Arterioscler Thromb Vasc Biol* 2003;**23**:314−21.
62. St-Pierre AC, Cantin B, Dagenais GR, Mauriege P, Bernard PM, Despres JP, Lamarche B. Low-density lipoprotein subfractions and the long-term risk of ischemic heart disease in men: 13-year follow-up data from the Quebec Cardiovascular Study. *Arterioscler Thromb Vasc Biol* 2005;**25**:553−9.
63. Campos H, Blijlevens E, McNamara JR, Ordovas JM, Posner BM, Wilson PW, Castelli WP, Schaefer EJ. LDL particle size distribution. Results from the Framingham Offspring Study. *Arterioscler Thromb* 1992;**12**:1410−19.
64. Lamarche B, Moorjani S, Cantin B, Dagenais GR, Lupien PJ, Despres JP. Associations of HDL2 and HDL3 subfractions with ischemic heart disease in men. Prospective results from the Quebec Cardiovascular Study. *Arterioscler Thromb Vasc Biol* 1997;**17**:1098−105.
65. Dreon DM, Fernstrom HA, Campos H, Blanche P, Williams PT, Krauss RM. Change in dietary saturated fat intake is correlated with change in mass of large low-density-lipoprotein particles in men. *Am J Clin Nutr* 1998;**67**:828−36.
66. Dreon DM, Fernstrom HA, Williams PT, Krauss RM. A very low-fat diet is not associated with improved lipoprotein profiles in men with a predominance of large, low-density lipoproteins. *Am J Clin Nutr* 1999;**69**:411−18.
67. Kratz M, Gulbahce E, von Eckardstein A, Cullen P, Cignarella A, Assmann G, Wahrburg U. Dietary mono- and polyunsaturated fatty acids similarly affect LDL size in healthy men and women. *The Journal of Nutrition* 2002;**132**:715−18.
68. Rivellese AA, Maffettone A, Vessby B, Uusitupa M, Hermansen K, Berglund L, Louheranta A, Meyer BJ, Riccardi G. Effects of dietary saturated, monounsaturated and n-3 fatty acids on fasting lipoproteins, LDL size and post-prandial lipid metabolism in healthy subjects. *Atherosclerosis* 2003;**167**:149−58.
69. Wallace AJ, Humphries SE, Fisher RM, Mann JI, Chisholm A, Sutherland WH. Genetic factors associated with response of LDL subfractions to change in the nature of dietary fat. *Atherosclerosis* 2000;**149**:387−94.
70. Sharman MJ, Kraemer WJ, Love DM, Avery NG, Gomez AL, Scheett TP, Volek JS. A ketogenic diet favorably affects serum biomarkers for cardiovascular disease in normal-weight men 1. *J Nutr* 2002;**132**:1879−85.
71. Volek JS, Sharman MJ, Gomez AL, Scheett TP, Kraemer WJ. An isoenergetic very low carbohydrate diet improves serum HDL cholesterol and triacylglycerol concentrations, the total cholesterol to HDL cholesterol ratio and postprandial pipemic responses compared with a low fat diet in normal weight, normolipidemic women 1. *J Nutr* 2003;**133**:2756−61.
72. Nielsen NS, Marckmann P, Hoy C. Effect of meal fat quality on oxidation resistance of postprandial VLDL and LDL particles and plasma triacylglycerol level 1. *Br J Nutr* 2000;**84**:855−63.
73. Korpela R, Seppo L, Laakso J, Lilja J, Karjala K, Lahteenmaki T, Solatunturi E, Vapaatalo H, Tikkanen MJ. Dietary habits affect the susceptibility of low-density lipoprotein to oxidation. *Eur J Clin Nutr* 1999;**53**:802−7.
74. Berglund L, Oliver EH, Fontanez N, Holleran S, Matthews K, Roheim PS, Ginsberg HN, Ramakrishnan R, Lefevre M. HDL-subpopulation patterns in response to reductions in dietary total and saturated fat intakes in healthy subjects 1. *Am J Clin Nutr* 1999;**70**:992−1000.
75. Warensjo E, Riserus U, Gustafsson IB, Mohsen R, Cederholm T, Vessby B. Effects of saturated and unsaturated fatty acids on estimated desaturase activities during a controlled dietary intervention. *Nutr Metab Cardiovasc Dis* 2008;**18**:683−90.
76. Warensjo E, Sundstrom J, Vessby B, Cederholm T, Riserus U. Markers of dietary fat quality and fatty acid desaturation as predictors of total and cardiovascular mortality: a population-based prospective study. *The American Journal of Clinical Nutrition* 2008;**88**:203−9.
77. Mangravite LM, Dawson K, Davis RR, Gregg JP, Krauss RM. Fatty acid desaturase regulation in adipose tissue by dietary composition is independent of weight loss and is correlated with the plasma triacylglycerol response. *The American Journal of Clinical Nutrition* 2007;**86**:759−67.
78. Forsythe CE, Phinney SD, Fernandez ML, Quann EE, Wood RJ, Bibus DM, Kraemer WJ, Feinman RD, Volek JS. Comparison of low fat and low carbohydrate diets on circulating fatty acid composition and markers of inflammation. *Lipids* 2008;**43**:65−77.
79. Foster GD, Wyatt HR, Hill JO, McGuckin BG, Brill C, Mohammed BS, Szapary PO, Rader DJ, Edman JS, Klein S. A randomized trial of a low-carbohydrate diet for obesity 1. *N Engl J Med* 2003;**348**:2082−90.
80. Sharman MJ, Volek JS. Weight loss leads to reductions in inflammatory biomarkers after a very-low-carbohydrate diet and a low-fat diet in overweight men 1. *Clin Sci (Lond)* 2004;**107**:365−9.

81. Reddy ST, Wang CY, Sakhaee K, Brinkley L, Pak CY. Effect of low-carbohydrate high-protein diets on acid-base balance, stone-forming propensity, and calcium metabolism. *Am J Kidney Dis* 2002;**40**:265–74.
82. Dargent-Molina P, Sabia S, Touvier M, Kesse E, Breart G, Clavel-Chapelon F, Boutron-Ruault MC. Proteins, dietary acid load, and calcium and risk of postmenopausal fractures in the E3N French women prospective study. *J Bone Miner Res* 2008;**23**:1915–22.
83. Munger RG, Cerhan JR, Chiu BC. Prospective study of dietary protein intake and risk of hip fracture in postmenopausal women. *The American Journal of Clinical Nutrition* 1999;**69**:147–52.
84. Fenton TR, Lyon AW, Eliasziw M, Tough SC, Hanley DA. Meta-analysis of the effect of the acid-ash hypothesis of osteoporosis on calcium balance. *J Bone Miner Res* 2009;**24**:1835–40.
85. Brinkworth GD, Noakes M, Clifton PM, Bird AR. Comparative effects of very low-carbohydrate, high-fat and high-carbohydrate, low-fat weight-loss diets on bowel habit and faecal short-chain fatty acids and bacterial populations. *The British Journal of Nutrition* 2009;**101**:1493–502.
86. Bellisle F. *Effects of diet on behaviour and cognition in children*. The British Journal of Nutrition 2004;**92**(Suppl. 2):S227–32.
87. Neel JV. Diabetes mellitus: a "thrifty" genotype rendered detrimental by "progress"? *American Journal of Human Genetics* 1962;**14**:353–62.
88. Paradies YC, Montoya MJ, Fullerton SM. Racialized genetics and the study of complex diseases: the thrifty genotype revisited. *Perspectives in Biology and Medicine* 2007;**50**:203–27.
89. Watve MG, Yajnik CS. Evolutionary origins of insulin resistance: a behavioral switch hypothesis. *BMC Evolutionary Biology* 2007;**7**:61.
90. Sonestedt E, Roos C, Gullberg B, Ericson U, Wirfalt E, Orho-Melander M. Fat and carbohydrate intake modify the association between genetic variation in the FTO genotype and obesity. *The American Journal of Clinical Nutrition* 2009;**90**:1418–25.

CHAPTER 21

Role of Fatty Liver Disease in Childhood Obesity

Valerio Nobili, Anna Alisi, Melania Manco
Scientific Directorate, Bambino Gesù Children's Hospital and Research Institute, Rome, Italy

INTRODUCTION

In the context of the obesity epidemic, fatty liver disease has become one of the most common complications of weight gain in obese children and adolescents. Nowadays it also represents the most frequent hepatic disease among youngsters in the United States [1] and probably worldwide [2]. Data from National Health and Nutrition Examination Survey 1999—2004 (N = 2450 children; age range 12 to 18 years) found elevated levels of alanine aminotransferases (ALT), a poor index of fatty liver, in 75 (3%) of adolescents. The prevalence of increased ALT rose to 6% in overweight and to 10% in obese adolescents [3]. In a case series of autopsies performed on more than 800 U.S. children of various body weight and ethnicity aged 2 to 19 years who died of unnatural causes, the prevalence of histologically proven fatty liver was 9.6% [4]. The Child and Adolescent Trial for Cardiovascular Health (CATCH), a school-based trial, recruited third-graders from public elementary schools in California, Louisiana, Minnesota, and Texas (N = 2575) and followed them through the 12th grade. This survey found a prevalence of unexplained elevated ALT of 23% among obese adolescents (N = 127) [5]. Of note, the highest rate of elevated ALT occurred in Hispanic adolescents (36%), followed by non-Hispanic whites (22%) and black individuals (14%). In some reports, prevalence of disease becomes much higher depending on diagnostic criteria and selection of the population. One study has suggested a prevalence of fatty liver as high as 53% in overweight and obese children [6].

The prevalence of the disease has been rapidly growing since the late 1990s, probably paralleling the rise of both epidemic overweight and obesity in youth and of consciousness of the disease among healthcare providers. One study investigated the rate of hospitalization and discharge for nonalcoholic fatty liver disease (NAFLD), obesity, and type 2 diabetes (T2DM) in youngsters [7]. The study found that between 1986 to 1988 and 2004 to 2006, hospitalizations with NAFLD diagnosis increased from 0.9 to 4.3/100,000 young individuals. Diabetes was reported in 32% of discharges with NAFLD [7].

Nonalcoholic fatty liver disease consists of the fatty infiltration of the liver without excessive or with no consumption of alcohol. NAFLD encompasses a spectrum of disease, which ranges from fatty infiltration with no inflammation, termed simple steatosis, to necro-inflammation (nonalcoholic steatohepatitis, otherwise termed NASH), to fibrosis and, either, cirrhosis.

Simple steatosis has for a long time been considered a benign entity as compared with NASH, which, conversely, may progress up to fibrosis, cirrhosis, and liver failure [8, 9]. Nonetheless, one report contradicts this assumption, suggesting a pivotal role of fatty liver in the development of cardiovascular disease and type 2 diabetes [10]. As high is the intrahepatic fat content as worst is the lipid profile of the young patients and higher are values of 2-hour plasma glucose [10]. Thus, fatty liver is associated with proatherogenic [11] and proinflammatory [10] profiles that make fatty liver not just a marker of cardiovascular disease [12—15] but a strong determinant. This is not only the result of the clustering of fatty liver with insulin resistance and components of the metabolic syndrome. Fatty liver seems able to promote *per se* and anticipate the onset of the cardiovascular disease at unexpected ages in obese children.

PATHOGENESIS

Pathogenetic mechanisms causing NAFLD and determining the progression to NASH and fibrosis have not yet been fully elucidated. It is likely that fat accumulation and insulin resistance are the first hit. Then, multiple subsequent hits ("two-hit hypothesis") cause fatty liver to progress to necro-inflammation and fibrosis [16]. Fatty acids deriving from excessive dietary consumption of fats or enhanced lipolysis from adipocytes overflow to the liver ("overflow hypothesis"), where they accumulate. Deposition of fat within the liver (hepatic steatosis) is unavoidably associated with local insulin resistance. The relationship between fat deposition and insulin resistance is one of the chicken-egg questions that characterize our knowledge on the pathogenesis of NAFLD. In fact, insulin resistance promotes fat deposition and intrahepatic fat accumulation causes insulin resistance. The temporal sequence between fatty liver and insulin resistance is not yet determined. Recent studies provide evidence that fatty liver may develop independent of insulin resistance and that liver-secreted cytokines may affect insulin signaling in muscle and adipose tissue [17]. Steatotic liver is more vulnerable to secondary hits, which may promote progression to NASH and predispose liver to advanced fibrosis, cirrhosis, and hepatocellular carcinoma [18]. Secondary hits would include mitochondrial dysfunction, oxidative stress, lipid peroxidation, inflammation, and a number of cytokines largely secreted from the abundant adipose tissue (adipocytokines) [18, 19]. In the progression to NASH and fibrosis, gut-derived bacterial endotoxin can play a pivotal role [20]. This is at present the most accredited pathogenetic model (Fig. 21.1). The notion of the metabolic endotoxemia, first hypothesized by Cani and colleagues [21, 22], supports the concept that endotoxin can promote insulin resistance, weight gain, fatty liver, and hepatic inflammation as well as cardiovascular disease. In this context, endotoxin may represent a strong link between fatty liver and cardiovascular disease [23].

Enhanced accumulation of fat within the hepatic parenchyma is due to several factors: mainly increased uptake of fat from the bloodstream in front of excessive dietary consumption or increased release of fatty acids from the adipocytes (lipolysis), reduced beta-oxidation [24–26], reduced export via lipoproteins, and increased synthesis (*de novo* lipogenesis). The fate of fatty acids within the liver is to enter a slow or a rapid turnover pool of fats. Fatty acids can be either oxidized or rapidly incorporated into complex lipids (i.e., triglycerides, phospholipids, and glycolipids), which can serve as structural lipids or bind apolipoproteins to be secreted into plasma. Systemic insulin resistance can precede fat infiltration of the liver, causing hepatic insulin resistance or, vice versa, fatty liver can lead to local and then systemic reduced insulin sensitivity [27, 28]. Increased *de novo* lipogenesis and unsuppressed gluconeogenesis are both the results of hepatic insulin resistance. Stable isotopes techniques demonstrated that 59% of hepatic triglycerides derive from adipose tissue spillover, 26% from *de novo* lipogenesis (versus 5% in control subjects), and 15% from dietary sources in adults with fatty liver [26]. Insulin resistance translates also into reduced beta fatty acid oxidation and export [27, 29]. In the dysregulation of hepatic fatty acid metabolism, proteins such as the protein-binding elements in response to sterols (SREBs), the liver nuclear receptor LXR-alpha, the carbohydrate response element binding protein (ChREBP), and the peroxisome proliferator receptor (PPAR) are pivotal [30–34]. Moreover, fatty acids interact also with Toll-like receptors (TLRs), activate cellular apoptosis, induce oxidative stress, and interfere with cytokine secretion [35]. Hyperinsulinemia and hyperglycemia can contribute to enhanced oxidative stress, necro-inflammatory response, and apoptosis in a vicious

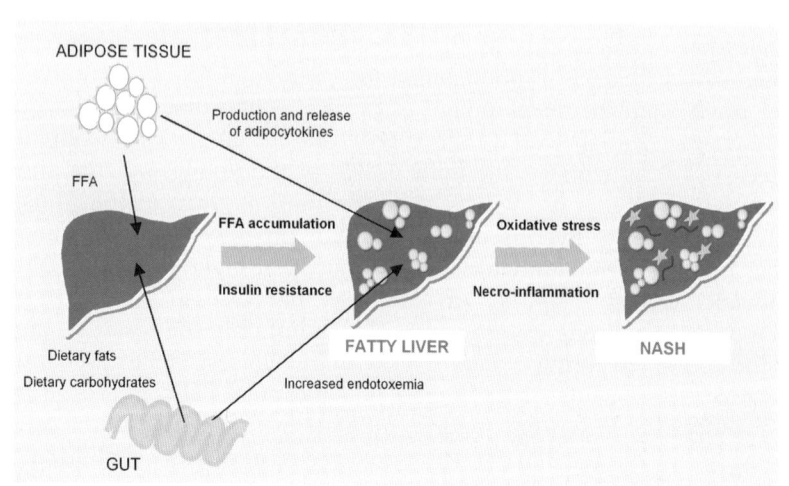

FIGURE 21.1 *Metabolic endotoxemia in the progression from NAFLD to NASH.* Nutritional factors influence the gut microbiota and the intestinal permeability. The leaky intestine permits the passage of endotoxin across the gut barrier, thus causing "metabolic endotoxemia." Endotoxin is the most powerful trigger for the Toll-like receptor 4 (TLR4), which initiates within hepatocytes and Kupffer cells a cascade of proinflammatory, prooxidative, and profibrotic signals. All these signals result in the progression from simple fatty liver to NASH and fibrosis. TLR4s are ubiquitously located. On adipocytes and endothelium cells, the binding of LPS with TLRs favors local and systemic low-grade inflammation.

cycle of cellular dysfunction [18] via chemical alterations of biological macromolecules (i.e., DNA, lipids and proteins) [36–38]. Of note, fatty liver is particularly susceptible to oxidative damage and fibrogenic process [37, 39]. Intrahepatic accumulation of fats leads to the saturation of the mitochondrial extramitochondrial oxidation processes (peroxisome β-oxidation and microsomal ω-oxidation), both determining the release of hydrogen peroxide and other reactive oxygen species (ROS). When ROS exceed the defensive capacity of antioxidant systems, they cause release of proinflammatory and profibrotic cytokines, lipid peroxidation and, finally, steatohepatitis and fibrosis [37, 39]. Lipid peroxidation of cellular membranes causes cell necrosis, formation of Mallory hyaline substance, and activation of hepatic stellate cells (HSC) that, in turn, synthesize collagen. Oxidative stress boosts the further release of proinflammatory and prooxidative cytokines such as tumor necrosis factor-alpha (TNF-α), transforming growth factor (TGF)-β; interleukin (IL)-6, and leptin by hepatocytes, Kupffer cells, and adipocytes [39–41]. These cytokines cause apoptosis, leukocyte chemotaxis, and phenomena of inflammation locally with further damage of the mitochondrial respiratory chain [42, 43].

TNF-α, interferes mainly with the mechanisms of insulin signaling, which results in decreased cell glucose uptake [18, 41, 44]. However, increased TNF-α may also alter the activity of mitochondrial enzymes, thereby contributing to apoptotic and profibrotic processes [44–46]. IL-6 exerts several biological effects on hepatocytes [47], favoring inflammation and fibrosis [41, 48]. IL-6 derives from the adipose tissue and reaches the liver via the portal route. Here, it binds its specific receptor and causes the activation of the suppressors of cytokine signaling 3 (SOCS-3), which, in turn, causes the inhibition of tyrosine phosphorylation of insulin receptor substrates (IRS), further causing insulin resistance [41, 47]. Differently from TNF-α and IL-6, adiponectin has anti-inflammatory properties and may play a role in the protection from necro-inflammation [48, 49]. Adiponectin binds two specific receptors, one located on the surface of hepatocytes [49] and the other one sited on muscle cells [50, 51]. In both cases, by binding the receptor, adiponectin can ameliorate insulin sensitivity, inflammation, and energy metabolism. It is worth mentioning that children with NAFLD have reduced levels of adiponectin as compared with obese controls without fatty liver [52, 53]. Leptin, the product of the ob gene, modulates lipid accumulation in adipose tissues, myocardium, skeletal muscle, liver, and pancreas through the modulation of β-oxidation. Its circulating concentrations are positively correlated with the degree of visceral obesity [54, 55]. High levels of leptin modulate the production of TNF-α and activation of macrophages, thus promoting inflammation and insulin resistance [41, 48, 56]. Leptin also contributes to activation of the stellate cells. In our series, high values of leptin alone or in combination with TNF-α are able to discriminate children and adolescents with hepatic necro-inflammation [57]. Other molecules are likely to play a role in the inflammatory process that is aroused in young individuals with fatty liver. They include resistin [58], retinol binding protein 4 (RBP4), plasminogen activator inhibitor type 1 (PAI-1), and visfatin [59–61].

Measurement of some cytokines can be of interest with the aim at identified children and adolescents with more severe histological derangement. We have observed that levels of leptin correlated significantly with grade of steatosis and necro-inflammation [62]. TNF-α also is a good predictor of necro-inflammation [24] as well as levels of endotoxin and PAI-1 [63]. Children with fatty liver, particularly those with fibrosis, have higher levels of RBP4 [60].

DIAGNOSIS

The revised 2007 Expert Committee recommendations on the assessment, prevention, and treatment of child and adolescent overweight and obesity now include screening and recommendations for NAFLD, a condition that was not included previously [64]. It is highly advisable that overweight and obese children and adolescents are routinely screened for increased aminotransferases and, at least once, evaluated for fatty liver. The risk to have fatty liver will be higher in male pubertal individuals, particularly of ethnic minorities, and in presence of visceral adiposity. The course of the disease may be completely asymptomatic and be discovered with an accidental report of abnormal ALT or echogenic liver. Children seldom complain of fatigue, malaise, or vague and aching right upper quadrant discomfort. Hepatomegaly is a frequent report. Acanthosis nigricans may be noted.

Liver enzyme may be within normal range, mildly or severely elevated, or fluctuating over time. Normal ALT does not exclude, in presence of echogenic liver, the occurrence of either simple fatty liver or nonalcoholic steatohepatitis. At the time of liver biopsy, up to 20% of children and adolescents with liver necro-inflammation and even fibrosis have normal ALT [65].

Simple fatty liver is defined as the accumulation of fat inside the hepatic tissue exceeding 5% of the normal amount. Fatty liver is usually diagnosed in presence of hyperechogenic liver tissue with fine, tightly packed echoes, posterior darkness and loss of definition of the diaphragm (posterior beam attenuation), or increased liver/kidney echo pattern at ultrasound [66]. Limits of the ultrasonography are the inability to discriminate between simple steatosis and steatohepatitis; to be operator and machine dependent technique; and to be not reproducible and affected by several variables including degree of adiposity [67], coexisting fibrosis, or inflammation [68]. Studies in adults with NAFLD demonstrate that the sensitivity of ultrasonography falls when evaluating patients with less than 30% to 43% steatosis on biopsy [69], whereas sensitivity for liver fat detection in children has not been established yet.

Computed tomography, nuclear magnetic resonance, and spectroscopy are more fine techniques that permit quantification of fat content, but both are costly. Computed tomography uses ionizing radiation and therefore is not favored for evaluation of liver fat in the absence of another clinical indication. Nuclear magnetic resonance (NMR) and spectroscopy can decompose the signal coming from the liver into its water and fat components, thereby permitting estimation of the fractional fat content of the liver as a measure of hepatic triglyceride concentration. Spectroscopy is currently considered the most accurate for measurement of liver triglyceride concentration. However, the techniques is time consuming, restricted in spatial coverage, and requires off-scan analysis by an expert. Because of these limitations, it is best suited for research studies at specialized centers and is not appropriate for widespread use. Unlike spectroscopy, which provides exquisite biochemical information from small regions of interest in the liver, NMR can assess fat in the entire liver. It is easy to perform and interpret and, therefore, may be more suitable for widespread use.

The gold standard for the diagnosis of fatty liver or NASH remains the liver biopsy. The procedure is, however, biased from sampling variability, high cost, and risks. The histological appearance of fatty liver is characterized by macrovesicular steatosis (the fat globules vary in size from very small to nearly filling the hepatocytes). Ballooning degeneration with or without Mallory bodies, and lobular or portal inflammation, with or without fibrosis, are characteristics of NASH [70]. In youngsters, diagnosis of NASH can be challenging because the ballooning degeneration, classic zone 3 fibrosis, and parenchymal inflammation that are commonly seen in adult NASH are less common in children [71]. The histological adult-type pattern of NASH, which is termed type 1 and characterized by steatosis with ballooning degeneration and lobular inflammation, with or without perisinusoidal fibrosis, and without portal inflammation, occurs in only 17% of U.S. children. Type 2 NASH, which is defined by macrovesicular hepatocellular steatosis with portal inflammation, with or without portal fibrosis, and no or minimal ballooning degeneration, is the predominant histological injury pattern seen in 51% of children [72]. The remaining 32% of patients had a pattern of overlap with features common to both the type 1 and type 2 NASH patterns. Children with type 2 NASH are more likely to be male, younger, heavier, and non-white [33]. Isolated portal fibrosis is four times more likely to occur in children than adults [70].

In the clinical care of obese children and adolescents with fatty liver, the question is who should be biopsied and when. We have recently proposed a diagnostic algorithm [73], which can be simplified as in Figure 21.2. Accordingly, obese children and adolescents with ultrasonographic evidence of fatty liver who are pubertal, male, and from ethnic minorities deserve liver biopsy, particularly if they have increased or fluctuating levels of liver enzymes, visceral obesity (as determined using the waist circumference centile for age, sex, and ethnicity), severe insulin resistance, and disordered carbohydrate metabolism (prediabetes and type 2 diabetes), dyslipidemia, and hypertension. It is worth mentioning that clustering metabolic abnormalities (i.e., visceral adiposity, impaired glucose tolerance, dyslipidemia, and hypertension) augments all the chances to have complicated fatty liver disease [74]. The causal relationship between visceral adiposity and fatty liver has not been fully elucidated. Visceral adiposity may result causative of fatty liver as it favors increased splanchnic lipolysis [75]; or increased portal efflux of proinflammatory cytokines; or probably it occurs simultaneously to fatty liver, both conditions being the net result of a systemic disorder of lipid storage [76].

Factors potentially explaining the higher rate of fatty liver in male adolescents include hormonal changes surrounding puberty or their increased control over unhealthy food choices and sedentary physical activity with age. At puberty, an increase in mean serum insulin levels is observed as well as consistent changes in the hormonal milieu. The rise in serum insulin levels coincides with Tanner stage 2, and these levels are sustained throughout adolescence [77]. Estrogens may be potentially protective, or, conversely, androgens may aggravate necro-inflammation [5].

FATTY LIVER, CARDIOVASCULAR DISEASE, AND TYPE 2 DIABETES

Suspected fatty liver disease as based on elevated serum ALT is associated with increased risk of cardiovascular and all-cause mortality (in addition to liver mortality) in adults [78]. Increased cardiovascular risk in individuals with fatty liver can be due to different factors, which include insulin resistance per se, proatherogenic profile, and exposure to higher levels of insulin, glucose, and prooxidative and proinflammatory milieu.

As a consequence of the impaired lipid metabolism and, particularly of the reduced rate of hepatic lipid

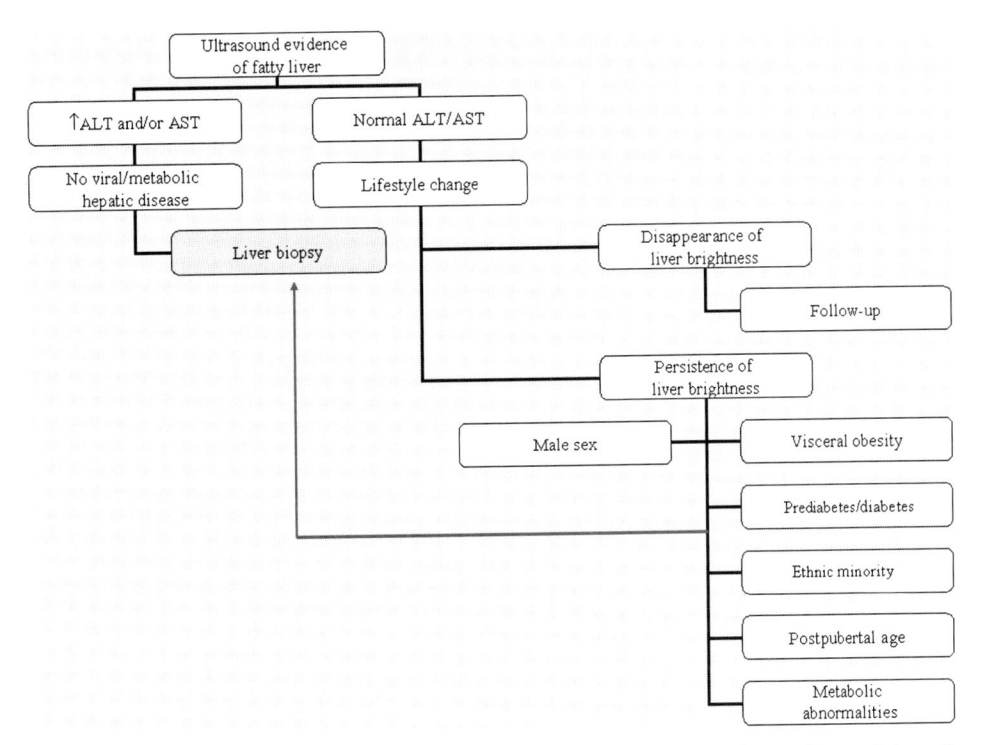

FIGURE 21.2 *Algorithm for liver biopsy.* Obese children and adolescents with ultrasonographic evidence of fatty liver have to undergo periodically biochemical screening for increased levels of aminotransferases. Those individuals who present increased levels of aminotransferases may deserve liver biopsy if they are pubertal males and from ethnic minorities; if they have abnormalities of the metabolic syndrome, and particularly if they have prediabetes or overt type 2 diabetes. In the present flowchart, there is no mention of measurement of serum biomarkers and novels imagine techniques, which have been used so far only for research purposes.

export, abnormalities in blood lipids, namely hypertriglyceridemia, low High Density Lipoprotein (HDL) concentrations, and small, dense low-density lipoprotein particles are commonly observed in these patients. Elevated triglycerides have been found to be associated with hepatic steatosis in a series of children [10, 74]. Hepatic fat content as measured by using fast Pre-magnetic resonance imaging (MRI) in 49 obese adolescents with normal glucose tolerance was associated with a pronounced dyslipidemic profile characterized by large Very Low Density Lipoprotein (VLDL), small dense Low Density Lipoprotein (LDL), and decreased large HDL concentrations [10]. Also the prevalence of the metabolic syndrome was the highest in the tertile with the highest content of hepatic fat. Studies have demonstrated that children with biopsy-proven NAFLD are more likely to have dyslipidemia, hypertension, insulin resistance, and more components of metabolic syndrome than age/sex/body mass index (BMI)—matched controls without NAFLD [79] and that to have more components of the metabolic syndrome augments the risk for more severe derangement of the hepatic parenchyma [74]. Because fatty liver is constantly characterized by impaired insulin sensitivity and clusters with all the metabolic abnormalities of the metabolic syndrome, it is widely considered the hepatic component of the syndrome [15, 59, 74]. A recent study revised retrospectively data from a hospital-based cohort study. Sixty-six children with NAFLD were followed for up to 20 years. The metabolic syndrome was present in 29% of the children at the time of NAFLD diagnosis, with 83% presenting with at least one feature of the metabolic syndrome including obesity, hypertension, dyslipidemia, or hyperglycemia. Four children with baseline normal fasting glucose developed type 2 diabetes 4 to 11 years after NAFLD diagnosis [9].

In the absence of a larger longitudinal study, it is hard to investigate the relationship between pediatric fatty liver and increased morbidity and mortality from cardiovascular disease. Thus, in a pediatric setting, cardiovascular risk can be predicted indirectly and, for instance, by evaluating vascular reactivity through the measurement of circulating molecules, which can be involved in the disruption of the plaque, or in the monocytes recruitment at the endothelium site, the evaluation of the carotid intima media thickness, the Ankle Brachial Pressure Index (ABPI), or by estimating microalbuminuria.

A couple of studies have observed higher levels of intima media thickness in children with fatty liver as compared with obese children without fatty liver or normal-weight controls [80, 81]. In our series, carotid intima media thickness did not differ between obese children with and without fatty liver [82]. Furthermore, in a regression model, we tried, but unsuccessfully, to rule out if the relationship between cardiovascular disease and fatty liver could be mediated by reduced levels of adiponectin. Measurement of 24 urinary excretions of albumin also failed to differentiate obese children with fatty liver from those without [83].

The association between fatty liver, prediabetes, or overt diabetes seems more evident. Moderate elevation in alanine aminotransferase levels was found to be associated with high-normal glucose levels [84], whereas abnormal ALT levels were reported in youngsters with type 2 diabetes [85], raising the question of a potential role of fatty liver in the onset of T2DM in obese youth. One study [10] demonstrated that independent of overall obesity, the severity of hepatic steatosis strongly affects the presence of prediabetes and diabetes in obese adolescents. The hepatic content of fat has been estimated by using nuclear magnetic spectroscopy, and patients with a content of fat in the highest tertile of the sample had significantly higher values of 2h plasma glucose. In a large sample of children and adolescents with ultrasonographic evidence of fatty liver, we have observed that subjects with fatty liver have 2h plasma glucose higher than those without and that the mean difference between values in the two groups is 13 mg/dl [86]. Children with fatty liver seem able to compensate with increased beta cell function for reduced insulin sensitivity [10, 86]. In fact, although insulin sensitivity decreases across tertiles of hepatic liver content, beta cell function increases [10].

TREATMENT

The only proven therapeutic strategy for the treatment of fatty liver in overweight and obese children consists of stable lifestyle changes. So far, the prescription of medications, including insulin sensitizers and antioxidants, did not provide better results than lifestyle changes in terms of both biochemical parameters and liver histology. Other medications (i.e., orlistat or lipid-lowering drugs) or medical and surgical procedures (i.e., the Roux-en-Y gastric bypass [RYGB]) may be prescribed in the presence of poor compliance to the prescription of lifestyle changes or severe metabolic abnormalities associated with overweight and obesity.

Trials have demonstrated the efficacy of lifestyle changes (achieved by a hypocaloric diet and physical exercise) in reducing levels of transaminases and liver brightness [87], or grade of steatosis and inflammation [88, 89]. On the contrary, no study has proved the efficacy of lifestyle changes to revert or, at least, ameliorate fibrosis [88, 89].

In these trials, nutritional advices consisted of a balanced hypocalorie diet, tailored for the individual's needs. A multidisciplinary team took care of children and their families in order to achieve durable results [88, 90]. No controlled trial has compared the efficacy of different dietary regimens (i.e., low-carbohydrate versus normal carbohydrate diet). It is conceivable that saturated fats and high glycemic foods, including simple sugars, refined grains, rice, and potatoes, should be limited or avoided in favor of whole grains, legumes, and low glycemic index fruits and vegetables. Consumption of low-glycemic meals can reduce glucose stimulated insulin secretion, thereby promoting nutrient oxidation and reducing hepatic lipid synthesis and storage. Conversely, simple sugars can enhance insulin secretion. Fructose, which is particularly present in sweetened beverages, leads to increased *de novo* lipogenesis and subsequent hypertriglyceridemia. Fructose consumption causes fat to accumulate viscerally [91]. Furthermore, high fructose consumption affects gut microflora and intestinal permeability and thus promotes metabolic endotoxemia [92].

Pharmacological therapies, so far, evaluated for the treatment of fatty liver in youngsters have included antioxidant agents and insulin sensitizers. This form of therapy is undergoing a placebo-controlled trial for comparing simultaneously the effect of vitamin E and metformin on liver histology [89, 90].

After short pilot studies, however, both medications have been evaluated in two separate placebo-controlled studied [89, 90] and compared with lifestyle change. Metformin (1.5 g/d) was prescribed for 1 year in 27 overweight/obese young patients with biopsy-proven NAFLD with the aim of estimating the effect of metformin on liver enzymes. At the end of first year, the code was opened and the patients asked to continue the treatment in an open fashion to estimate outcomes on liver histology. The control group (N = 30) was obtained from a separate but parallel ongoing study that had identical inclusion criteria on the use of antioxidants in NAFLD. ALT significantly improved from baseline with decreasing body weight in both groups. Steatosis was reduced in the two groups as well as ballooning and necro-inflammation. No significant changes in fibrosis were detected [89]. Among insulin sensitizers, the PPAR-gamma agonists, the thiazolidinediones (TZD) can be promising as they have important anti-inflammatory and antiatherogenic properties [93], but this class of drugs has not been approved by the Food and Drug Administration for use in children and adolescents. Fifty-five patients with disordered carbohydrate metabolism and liver biopsy-confirmed nonalcoholic steatohepatitis underwent a 6-month treatment with a hypocalorie diet and pioglitazone (45 mg daily) or placebo. Diet plus pioglitazone, as compared with diet plus placebo, improved significantly glycemic metabolism and glucose tolerance, normalized liver aminotransferase levels, decreased hepatic fat content, and increased hepatic insulin sensitivity. Treatment with pioglitazone, as compared with placebo, was associated with improvement in histological findings with regard to steatosis, ballooning necrosis, and inflammation. No significant amelioration in degree of fibrosis was observed as compared with placebo [94]. Of note, treatment with pioglitazone is able to ameliorate adipocyte insulin resistance in adult patients with NASH [95].

In the controlled trial with the use of vitamin E, 53 young patients (age 5.7 to 18.8 years) were enrolled and randomized to alpha-tocopherol 600 IU/day plus ascorbic acid 500 mg/day (N = 25) or placebo (N = 28). The study lasted 24 months. The primary end point of this study was the change in liver histology on repeated biopsy at 24 months. The amelioration of steatosis, lobular inflammation, hepatocyte ballooning, and NAFLD activity score was seen in both groups, and it was likely the result of the lifestyle change. Levels of aminotransferases, triglycerides, cholesterol, fasting glucose, and insulin and insulin sensitivity indices improved significantly as well in both arms [90].

Ursodeoxycholic acid (UDCA) is a cytoprotective agent that has been studied as potential therapy for NAFLD in pediatric settings. In an open controlled study [96], obese children (N = 31) were assigned to the treatment according to their anticipated success with lifestyle modification with UDCA (10 to 12.5 mg/kg/day) with or without a weight-reduction diet. Control groups consisted of children treated with diet alone or no intervention. The study was quite unusual in its design, and underpowered. At 6 months, the addition of UDCA to the diet was no more effective than diet alone in reducing serum aminotransferases or the appearance of steatosis, as revealed by ultrasonography. No difference was observed between children treated with UDCA and those receiving no intervention; however, the children assigned to these treatment arms were those who were judged unlikely to comply with lifestyle advice.

The RYGB is the only bariatric technique whose use is approved by the Food and Drug Administration for treatment of morbidly obese adolescents (BMI > 40 kg/m^2 or BMI>35 kg/m^2 plus two comorbidities). RYGB can reverse disordered carbohydrate metabolism, features of the metabolic syndrome, and ameliorate fatty liver [97]. A multicenter study for the Follow-up of Adolescent Bariatric Surgery (FABS) concluded in April 2010.

CONCLUSION

Nonalcoholic fatty liver disease can no longer be considered a benign entity, as the fat infiltration of the hepatic parenchyma is significantly associated with visceral adiposity, features of the metabolic risk (mainly increased risk for prediabetes and type 2 diabetes and anticipated cardiovascular disease). No matter what the mechanisms of the progression from NAFLD to NASH are, it seems that even fatty liver can be a worrisome condition, able to significantly impact health costs. It is also likely that by counteracting NAFLD, the onset of the cardiovascular disease can be delayed or reduced.

References

1. Shneider BL, Gonzalez-Peralta R, Roberts EA. Controversies In The Management Of Pediatric Liver Disease: Hepatitis B, C And Nafld: Summary Of A Single Topic Conference. *Hepatology* 2006;44:1344—54.
2. Manco M, Bottazzo G, Devito R, Marcellini M, Mingrone G, Nobili V. Nonalcoholic Fatty Liver Disease In Children. *J Am Coll Nutr* 2008;27:667—76.
3. Strauss RS, Barlow SE, Dietz WH. Prevalence Of Abnormal Serum Aminotransferase Values In Overweight And Obese Adolescents. *J Pediatr* 2000;136:727—33.
4. Schwimmer JB, Deutsch R, Kahen T, Lavine JE, Stanley C, Behling C. Prevalence Of Fatty Liver In Children And Adolescents. *Pediatrics* 2006;118:1388—93.
5. Schwimmer JB, Mcgreal N, Deutsch R, Finegold MJ, Lavine JE. Influence Of Gender, Race, And Ethnicity On Suspected Fatty Liver In Obese Adolescents. *Pediatrics* 2005;115:E561—5.
6. Dunn W, Schwimmer JB. The Obesity Epidemic And Nonalcoholic Fatty Liver Disease In Children. *Curr Gastroenterol Rep* 2008;10:67—72.
7. Koebnick C, Getahun D, Reynolds K, Coleman KJ, Porter AH, Lawrence JM, Punyanitya M, Quinn VP, Jacobsen SJ. Trends In Nonalcoholic Fatty Liver Disease-Related Hospitalizations In Us Children, Adolescents, And Young Adults. *J Pediatr Gastroenterol Nutr* 2009;48:597—603.
8. Caldwell SH, De Freitas LA, Park SH, Moreno ML, Redick JA, Davis CA, Sisson BJ, Patrie JT, Cotrim H, Argo CK, Al-Osaimi A. Intramitochondrial Crystalline Inclusions In Nonalcoholic Steatohepatitis. *Hepatology* 2009;49:1888—95.
9. Feldstein AE, Charatcharoenwitthaya P, Treeprasertsuk S, Benson JT, Enders FB, Angulo P. The Natural History Of Non-Alcoholic Fatty Liver Disease In Children: A Follow-Up Study For Up To 20 Years. *Gut* 2009;58:1538—44.
10. Cali AM, De Oliveira AM, Kim H, Chen S, Reyes-Mugica M, Escalera S, Dziura J, Taksali SE, Kursawe R, Shaw M, Savoye M, Pierpont B, Constable RT, Caprio S. Glucose Dysregulation And Hepatic Steatosis In Obese Adolescents: Is There A Link? *Hepatology* 2009;49:1896—903.
11. Targher G, Chonchol M, Miele L, Zoppini G, Pichiri I, Muggeo M. Nonalcoholic Fatty Liver Disease As A Contributor To Hypercoagulation And Thrombophilia In The Metabolic Syndrome. *Semin Thromb Hemost* 2009;35:277—87.
12. Loria P, Lonardo A, Targher G. Is Liver Fat Detrimental To Vessels?: Intersections In The Pathogenesis Of Nafld And Atherosclerosis. *Clin Sci (Lond)* 2008;115:1—12.

13. Targher G, Chonchol M, Miele L, Zoppini G, Pichiri I, Muggeo M. Nonalcoholic Fatty Liver Disease As A Contributor To Hypercoagulation And Thrombophilia In The Metabolic Syndrome. *Semin Thromb Hemost* 2009;**35**:277–87.
14. Targher G, Bertolini L, Padovani R, Rodella S, Tessari R, Zenari L, Day C, Arcaro G. Prevalence Of Nonalcoholic Fatty Liver Disease And Its Association With Cardiovascular Disease Among Type 2 Diabetic Patients. *Diabetes Care* 2007;**30**:1212–8.
15. Targher G, Marra F, Marchesini G. Increased Risk Of Cardiovascular Disease. In Non-Alcoholic Fatty Liver Disease: Causal Effect Or Epiphenomenon? *Diabetologia* 2008;**51**:1947–53.
16. Day CP, James OF. Steatohepatitis: A Tale Of Two "Hits"? *Gastroenterology* 1998;**114**:842–5.
17. Stefan N, Kantartzis K, Haring HU. Causes And Metabolic Consequences Of Fatty Liver. *Endocr Rev* 2008;**29**:939–60.
18. Tilg H, Moschen AR. Insulin Resistance, Inflammation, And Non-Alcoholic Fatty Liver Disease. *Trends Endocrinol Metab* 2008;**19**:371–9.
19. Cave M, Deaciuc I, Mendez C, Song Z, Joshi-Barve S, Barve S, Mcclain C. Nonalcoholic Fatty Liver Disease: Predisposing Factors And The Role Of Nutrition. *J Nutr Biochem* 2007;**18**:184–95.
20. Baffy G. Kupffer Cells In Non-Alcoholic Fatty Liver Disease: The Emerging View. *J Hepatol* 2009;**51**:212–23.
21. Cani PD, Amar J, Iglesias MA, Poggi M, Knauf C, Bastelica D, Neyrinck AM, Fava F, Tuohy KM, Chabo C, Waget A, Delmee E, Cousin B, Sulpice T, Chamontin B, Ferrieres J, Tanti JF, Gibson GR, Casteilla L, Delzenne NM, Alessi MC, Burcelin R. Metabolic Endotoxemia Initiates Obesity And Insulin Resistance. *Diabetes* 2007;**56**:1761–72.
22. Cani PD, Bibiloni R, Knauf C, Waget A, Neyrinck AM, Delzenne NM, Burcelin R. Changes In Gut Microbiota Control Metabolic Endotoxemia-Induced Inflammation In High-Fat Diet-Induced Obesity And Diabetes In Mice. *Diabetes* 2008;**57**:1470–81.
23. Manco M. Endotoxin As A Missed Link Among All The Metabolic Abnormalities In The Metabolic Syndrome. *Atherosclerosis* 2009;**206**:36.
24. Tessari P, Coracina A, Cosma A, Tiengo A. Hepatic Lipid Metabolism And Non-Alcoholic Fatty Liver Disease. *Nutr Metab Cardiovasc Dis* 2009;**19**:291–302.
25. Cheung O, Sanyal AJ. Abnormalities Of Lipid Metabolism In Nonalcoholic Fatty Liver Disease. *Semin Liver Dis* 2008;**28**:351–9.
26. Donnelly KL, Smith CI, Schwarzenberg SJ, Jessurun J, Boldt MD, Parks EJ. Sources Of Fatty Acids Stored In Liver And Secreted Via Lipoproteins In Patients With Nonalcoholic Fatty Liver Disease. *J Clin Invest* 2005;**115**:1343–51.
27. Musso G, Gambino R, Cassader M. Recent Insights Into Hepatic Lipid Metabolism In Non-Alcoholic Fatty Liver Disease (Nafld). *Prog Lipid Res* 2009;**48**:1–26.
28. Marra F, Gastaldelli A, Svegliati Baroni G, Tell G, Tiribelli C. Molecular Basis And Mechanisms Of Progression Of Non-Alcoholic Steatohepatitis. *Trends Mol Med* 2008;**14**:72–81.
29. Tsochatzis EA, Manolakopoulos S, Papatheodoridis GV, Archimandritis AJ. Insulin Resistance And Metabolic Syndrome In Chronic Liver Diseases: Old Entities With New Implications. *Scand J Gastroenterol* 2009;**44**:6–14.
30. Qi L, Saberi M, Zmuda E, Wang Y, Altarejos J, Zhang X, Dentin R, Hedrick S, Bandyopadhyay G, Hai T, Olefsky J, Montminy M. Adipocyte Creb Promotes Insulin Resistance In Obesity. *Cell Metab* 2009;**9**:2772–86.
31. Jh Lee, Zhou J, Xie W. Pxr And Lxr In Hepatic Steatosis: A New Dog And An Old Dog With New Tricks. *Mol Pharm* 2008;**5**:60–6.
32. Ferré P, Foufelle F. Srebp-1c Transcription Factor And Lipid Homeostasis: Clinical Perspective. *Horm Res* 2007;**68**:72–82.
33. George J, Liddle C. Nonalcoholic Fatty Liver Disease: Pathogenesis And Potential For Nuclear Receptors As Therapeutic Targets. *Mol Pharm* 2008;**5**:49–59.
34. Reddy JK, Rao MS. Lipid Metabolism And Liver Inflammation. II. Fatty Liver Disease And Fatty Acid Oxidation. *Am J Physiol Gastrointest Liver Physiol* 2006;**290**:G852–8.
35. Gentile CL, Pagliassotti MJ. The Role Of Fatty Acids In The Development And Progression Of Nonalcoholic Fatty Liver Disease. *J Nutr Biochem* 2008;**19**:567–76.
36. Djordjević VB. Free Radicals In Cell Biology. *Int Rev Cytol* 2004;**237**:57–89.
37. Malaguarnera M, Di Rosa M, Nicoletti F, Malaguarnera L. Molecular Mechanisms Involved In Nafld Progression. *J Mol Med.* 2009;**87**:679–95. Epub 2009 Apr 8.
38. Duvnjak M, Lerotić I, Barsić N, Tomasić V, Virović Jukić L, Velagić V. Pathogenesis And Management Issues For Non-Alcoholic Fatty Liver Disease. *World J Gastroenterol* 2007;**13**:4539–50.
39. Jou J, Choi SS, Diehl AM. Mechanisms Of Disease Progression In Nonalcoholic Fatty Liver Disease. *Semin Liver Dis* 2008;**28**:370–9.
40. Kamada Y, Takehara T, Hayashi N. Adipocytokines And Liver Disease. *J Gastroenterol* 2008;**43**:811–22.
41. Polyzos SA, Kountouras J, Zavos C. Nonalcoholic Fatty Liver Disease: The Pathogenetic Roles Of Insulin Resistance And Adipocytokines. *Curr Mol Med* 2009;**9**:299–314.
42. Browning JD, Horton JD. Molecular Mediators Of Hepatic Steatosis And Liver Injury. *J Clin Invest* 2004;**114**:147–52.
43. Wei Y, Rector RS, Thyfault JP, Ibdah JA. Nonalcoholic Fatty Liver Disease And Mitochondrial Dysfunction. *World J Gastroenterol* 2008;**14**:193–9.
44. Tilg H, Moschen AR. Inflammatory Mechanisms, In The Regulation Of Insulin Resistance. *Mol Med* 2008;**14**:222–31.
45. Fromenty B, Robin MA, Igoudjil A, Mansouri A, Pessayre D. The Ins And Outs Of Mitochondrial Dysfunction In Nash. *Diabetes Metab* 2004;**30**:121–38.
46. Begriche K, Igoudjil A, Pessayre D, Fromenty B. Mitochondrial Dysfunction In Nash: Causes, Consequences And Possible Means To Prevent It. *Mitochondrion* 2006;**6**:1–28.
47. Kim JH, Bachmann RA, Chen J. Interleukin-6 And Insulin Resistance. *Vitam Horm* 2009;**80**:613–33.
48. Marra F, Bertolani C. Adipokines, In Liver Diseases. *Hepatology* 2009;**50**:957–69.
49. Lu JY, Huang KC, Chang LC, Huang YS, Chi YC, Su TC, Chen CL, Yang WS. Adiponectin: A Biomarker Of Obesity-Induced Insulin Resistance In Adipose Tissue And Beyond. *J Biomed Sci* 2008;**15**:565–76.
50. Kadowaki T, Yamauchi T. Adiponectin And Adiponectin Receptors. *Endocr Rev* 2005;**26**:439–51.
51. Whitehead JP, Richards AA, Hickman IJ, Macdonald GA, Prins JB. Adiponectin—A Key Adipokine In The Metabolic Syndrome. *Diabetes Obes Metab* 2006;**8**:264–80.
52. Denzer C, Thiere D, Muche R, Koenig W, Mayer H, Kratzer W, Wabitsch M. Gender-Specific Prevalences Of Fatty Liver In Obese Children And Adolescents: Roles Of Body Fat Distribution, Sex Steroids, And Insulin Resistance. *J Clin Endocrinol Metab* 2009;**94**:3872–81.
53. Louthan MV, Barve S, Mcclain CJ, Joshi-Barve S. Decreased Serum Adiponectin: An Early Event In Pediatric Nonalcoholic Fatty Liver Disease. *J Pediatr* 2005;**147**:835–8.
54. Anubhuti, Arora S. Leptin And Its Metabolic Interactions: An Update. *Diabetes Obes Metab* 2008;**10**:973–93.
55. Jéquier E. Leptin Signaling, Adiposity, And Energy Balance. *Ann N Y Acad Sci* 2002;**967**:379–88.
56. Rabe K, Lehrke M, Parhofer KG, Broedl UC. Adipokines And Insulin Resistance. *Mol Med* 2008;**14**:741–51.

57. Manco M, Marcellini M, Giannone G, Nobili V. Correlation Of Serum TNF-α Levels And Histologic Liver Injury Scores In Pediatric Nonalcoholic Fatty Liver Disease. *Am J Clin Pathol* 2007;**127**:954—60.

58. Tsochatzis E, Papatheodoridis GV, Hadziyannis E, Georgiou A, Kafiri G, Tiniakos DG, Manesis EK, Archimandritis AJ. Serum Adipokine Levels In Chronic Liver Diseases: Association Of Resistin Levels With Fibrosis Severity. *Scand J Gastroenterol* 2008;**43**:1128—36.

59. Thuy S, Ladurner R, Volynets V, Wagner S, Strahl S, Königsrainer A, Maier KP, Bischoff SC, Bergheim I. Nonalcoholic Fatty Liver Disease, In Humans Is Associated With Increased Plasma Endotoxin And Plasminogen Activator Inhibitor 1 Concentrations And With Fructose Intake. *J Nutr* 2008;**138**:1452—5.

60. Nobili V, Alkhouri N, Alisi A, Ottino S, Lopez R, Manco M, Feldstein AE. Retinol-Binding Protein 4: A Promising Circulating Marker Of Liver Damage, In Pediatric Nonalcoholic Fatty Liver Disease. *Clin Gastroenterol Hepatol* 2009;**7**:575—9.

61. Aller R, De Luis DA, Izaola O, Sagrado MG, Conde R, Velasco MC, Alvarez T, Pacheco D, González JM. Influence Of Visfatin On Histopathological Changes Of Non-Alcoholic Fatty Liver Disease. *Dig Dis Sci* 2009;**54**:1772—7.

62. Nobili V, Manco M, Ciampalini P, Diciommo V, Devito R, Piemonte F, Comparcola D, Guidi R, Marcellini M. Leptin, Free Leptin Index, Insulin Resistance And Liver Fibrosis In Children With Non-Alcoholic Fatty Liver Disease. *Eur J Endocrinol* 2006;**155**:735—43.

63. Alisi A, Manco M, Devito R, Piemonte F, Nobili V. Endotoxin And Plasminogen Activator Inihibitor-1 Serum Levels Associate With Non Alcholic Steatohepatitis In Children. *J Ped Gastroenterol Nutr* 2010;**50**(6):645—9.

64. Barlow SE, Expert Committee. Expert Committee Recommendations Regarding The Prevention, Assessment, And Treatment Of Child And Adolescent Overweight And Obesity: Summary Report. *Pediatrics* 2007;**120**(Suppl 4):S164—92.

65. Manco M, Alisi A, Nobili V. Risk Of Severe Liver Disease, In Nafld With Normal Alt Levels: A Pediatric Report. *Hepatology* 2008;**48**:2087—8.

66. Charatcharoenwitthaya P, Lindor KD. Role Of Radiologic Modalities In The Management Of Non-Alcoholic Steatohepatitis. *Clin Liver Dis* 2007;**11**:37—54.

67. Taylor KJ, Gorelick FS, Rosenfield AT, Riely CA. Ultrasonography Of Alcoholic Liver Disease With Histological Correlation. *Radiology* 1981;**141**:157—61.

68. Hepburn MJ, Vos JA, Fillman EP, Lawitz EJ. The Accuracy Of The Report Of Hepatic Steatosis On Ultrasonography, In Patients Infected With Hepatitis C In A Clinical Setting: A Retrospective Observational Study. *Bmc Gastroenterol* 2005;**5**:14.

69. Saadeh S, Younossi ZM, Remer EM, Gramlich T, Ong JP, Hurley M, Mullen KD, Cooper JN, Sheridan MJ. The Utility Of Radiological Imaging, In Nonalcoholic Fatty Liver Disease. *Gastroenterology* 2002;**123**:745—50.

70. Kleiner DE, Brunt EM, Van Natta M, Behling C, Contos MJ, Cummings OW, Ferrell LD, Liu YC, Torbenson MS, Unalp-Arida A, Yeh M, Mccullough AJ, Sanyal AJ, Nonalcoholic Steatohepatitis Clinical Research Network. Design And Validation Of A Histological Scoring System For Nonalcoholic Fatty Liver Disease. *Hepatology* 2005;**41**:1313—21.

71. Carter-Kent C, Yerian LM, Brunt EM, Angulo P, Kohli R, Ling SC, Xanthakos SA, Whitington PF, Charatcharoenwitthaya P, Yap J, Lopez R, Mccullough AJ, Feldstein AE. Nonalcoholic Steatohepatitis, In Children: A Multicenter Clinicopathological Study. *Hepatology* 2009;**50**:1113—20.

72. Schwimmer JB, Behling C, Newbury R, Deutsch R, Nievergelt C, Schork NJ, Lavine JE. Histopathology Of Pediatric Nonalcoholic Fatty Liver Disease. *Hepatology* 2005;**42**:641—9.

73. Manco M, Bottazzo G, Devito R, Marcellini M, Mingrone G, Nobili V. Nonalcoholic Fatty Liver Disease In Children. *J Am Coll Nutr* 2008;**27**:667—76.

74. Manco M, Marcellini M, Devito R, Comparcola D, Sartorelli MR, Nobili V. Metabolic Syndrome And Liver Histology In Paediatric Non-Alcoholic Steatohepatitis. *Int J Obes (Lond)* 2008;**32**:381—7.

75. Nielsen S, Guo Z, Johnson CM, Hensrud DD, Jensen MD. Splanchnic Lipolysis In Human Obesity. *J Clin Invest* 2004;**113**:1582—8.

76. Despres JP, Lemieux I. Abdominal Obesity And Metabolic Syndrome. *Nature* 2006;**444**:881—7. Doi:10.1038/Nature05488.

77. Potau N, Ibanez L, Rique S, Carrascosa A. Pubertal Changes In Insulin Secretion And Peripheral Insulin Sensitivity. *Horm Res* 1997;**48**:219—26.

78. Lee TH, Kim WR, Benson JT, Therneau TM, Melton 3rd LJ. Serum Aminotransferase Activity And Mortality Risk In A United States Community. *Hepatology* 2008;**47**:880—7.

79. Schwimmer JB, Pardee PE, Lavine JE, Blumkin AK, Cook S. Cardiovascular Risk Factors And The Metabolic Syndrome In Pediatric Nonalcoholic Fatty Liver Disease. *Circulation* 2008;**118**:277—83.

80. Demircioglu F, Kocyigit A, Arslan N, Cakmakci H, Hizli S, Sedat AT. Intima-Media Thickness Of Carotid Artery And Susceptibility To Atherosclerosis In Obese Children With Nonalcoholic Fatty Liver Disease. *J Pediatr Gastroenterol Nutr* 2008;**47**:68—75.

81. Pacifico L, Cantisani V, Ricci P, Osborn JF, Schiavo E, Anania C, Ferrara E, Dvisic G, Chiesa C. Nonalcoholic Fatty Liver Disease And Carotid Atherosclerosis, In Children. *Pediatr Res* 2008;**63**:423—7.

82. Manco M, Bedogni G, Monti L, Morino G, Natali G, Nobili V. Intima-Media Thickness And Liver Histology In Obese Children And Adolescents with Non-Alcoholic Fatty Liver Disease. *Atherosclerosis* 2010;**209**(2):463—8.

83. Manco M, Ciampalini P, Devito R, Vania A, Cappa M, Nobili V. Albuminuria And Insulin Resistance, In Children With Biopsy Proven Non-Alcoholic Fatty Liver Disease. *Pediatr Nephrol* 2009;**24**:1211—17.

84. Burgert TS, Taksali SE, Dziura J, Goodman TR, Yeckel CW, Papademetris X, Constable RT, Weiss R, Tamborlane WV, Savoye M, Seyal AA, Caprio S. Alanine Aminotransferase Levels And Fatty Liver, In Childhood Obesity: Associations With Insulin Resistance, Adiponectin, And Visceral Fat. *J Clin Endocrinol Metab* 2006;**91**:4287—94.

85. Nadeau KJ, Klingensmith G, Zeitler P. Type 2 Diabetes In Children Is Frequently Associated With Elevated Alanine Aminotransferase. *J Pediatr Gastroenterol Nutr* 2005;**41**:94—8.

86. Manco M, Gastaldelli A, Bedogni G, Grugni G, Sartorio A. Phenotypes Of Prediabetes And Non Alcoholic Fatty Liver Disease, In Obese Children And Adolescents. *Diabetologia* 2009;**52**:S347.

87. Vajro P, Fontanella A, Perna C, et al. Persistent Hyperaminotransferasemia Resolving After Weight Reduction, In Obese Children. *J Pediatr* 1994;**125**:239—41.

88. Nobili V, Marcellini M, Devito R, Ciampalini P, Piemonte F, Comparcola D, Sartorelli MR, Angulo P. Nafld, In Children: A Prospective Clinical-Pathological Study And Effect Of Lifestyle Advice. *Hepatology* 2006;**44**:458—65.

89. Nobili V, Manco M, Ciampalini P, Alisi A, Devito R, Bugianesi E, Marcellini M, Marchesini G. Metformin Use, In Children With Nonalcoholic Fatty Liver Disease: An Open-Label, 24-Month, Observational Pilot Study. *Clin Ther* 2008;**30**:1168—76.

90. Nobili V, Manco M, Devito R, Di Ciommo V, Comparcola D, Sartorelli MR, Piemonte F, Marcellini M, Angulo P. Lifestyle Intervention And Antioxidant Therapy, In Children With Nonalcoholic Fatty Liver Disease: A Randomized, Controlled Trial. *Hepatology* 2008;**48**:119–28.
91. Stanhope KL, Schwarz JM, Keim NL, Griffen SC, Bremer AA, Graham JL, Hatcher B, Cox CL, Dyachenko A, Zhang W, Mcgahan JP, Seibert A, Krauss RM, Chiu S, Schaefer EJ, Ai M, Otokozawa S, Nakajima K, Nakano T, Beysen C, Hellerstein MK, Berglund L, Havel PJ. Consuming Fructose-Sweetened, Not Glucose-Sweetened, Beverages Increases Visceral Adiposity And Lipids And Decreases Insulin Sensitivity, In Overweight/Obese Humans. *J Clin Invest* 2009;**119**:1322–34. Doi:10.1172/Jci37385.
92. Spruss A, Bergheim I. Dietary Fructose And Intestinal Barrier: Potential Risk Factor, In The Pathogenesis Of Nonalcoholic Fatty Liver Disease. *J Nutr Biochem* 2009;**20**:657–62. Doi:10.1016/J.Jnutbio.2009.05.006.
93. Chiquette E, Ramirez G, Defronzo RA. A Meta-Analysis Comparing The Effect Of Thiazolidinediones On Cardiovascular Risk Factors. *Arch Inter Med* 2004;**164**:2097–104.
94. Belfort R, Harrison SA, Brown K, Darland C, Finch J, Hardies J, Balas B, Gastaldelli A, Tio F, Pulcini J, Berria R, Ma JZ, Dwivedi S, Havranek R, Fincke C, Defronzo R, Bannayan GA, Schenker S, Cusi K. A Placebo-Controlled Trial Of Pioglitazone, In Subjects With Nonalcoholic Steatohepatitis. *N Engl J Med* 2006;**355**: 2297–307. Doi:10.1056/Nejmoa060326.
95. Gastaldelli A, Harrison SA, Belfort-Aguilar R, Hardies LJ, Balas B, Schenker S, Cusi K. Importance Of Changes In Adipose Tissue Insulin Resistance To Histological Response During Thiazolidinedione Treatment Of Patients With Nonalcoholic Steatohepatitis. *Hepatology* 2009;**50**:1087–93. Doi:10.1002/Hep.23116.
96. Vajro P, Franzese A, Valerio G, Iannucci MP, Aragione N. Lack Of Efficacy Of Ursodeoxycholic Acid For The Treatment Of Liver Abnormalities, In Obese Children. *J Pediatr* 2000;**136**: 739–43.
97. Pratt JS, Lenders CM, Dionee EA, Hoppin AG, Hsu GL, Inge TH, Lawlor DF, Marino MF, Meyers AF, Rosenblum JL, Sanchez VM. Best Practice Updates For Pediatric/Adolescent Weight Loss Surgery. *Obesity* 2009;**17**:901–10.

SECTION III

PSYCHOLOGICAL AND BEHAVIORAL FACTORS

CHAPTER 22

An Overview of Psychosocial Symptoms in Obese Children

Lisa Y. Gibson

Telethon Institute for Child Health Research, Centre for Child Health Research, The University of Western Australia, Perth, Western Australia

BACKGROUND

Considering the pervasive nature of childhood obesity, there is an increased need to investigate the effects of obesity on a child's physical and psychosocial health. Although the physical health effects of obesity have been widely documented (e.g., [1, 2, 3]), much less is known about the psychosocial consequences of excess weight in children. Despite this lack, there is recent speculation that the psychosocial consequences of excess weight are more prevalent than the physical health consequences [4].

A number of psychosocial constructs are examined in relation to obesity. These include self-esteem, depression, social functioning, eating disorder psychopathology, quality of life, body dissatisfaction, and bias and discrimination. Each of these issues is discussed in detail in this chapter.

BIAS AND DISCRIMINATION

There is considerable evidence to suggest that overweight and obese individuals are discriminated against across multiple domains of living, including education, employment, income, healthcare, and interpersonal relationships [5]. There is evidence to suggest that bias against people who are overweight or obese (which leads to discrimination) is also found among young children.

A landmark study in this area was conducted in 1961 by Richardson and colleagues [6]. Children aged 10 and 11 years were shown six line drawings and asked to rank them according to which of the people depicted they would most prefer to be friends with. Four of the drawings showed children with various disabilities, such as in a wheelchair, on crutches, with an amputated hand, and with a facial disfigurement. Of the other two drawings, one picture showed an overweight child and the other showed a child of average weight with no disability. Consistently, the children rated the overweight child as being the least liked of the six pictures and that drawing was ranked last, whereas the image of the average weight child was ranked at the top. These findings have been replicated in a more recent study using the same methodology [7].

Whereas Puhl and Brownell [5] reported the existence of this bias in children 8 years of age, other studies have found negative attitudes toward overweight and obese children as young as 3 years [8]. In Cramer and Steinwert's research [8], preschool children aged 3 to 5 years were told a simple story that described the behavior of two children. The behavior of one child was "mean," and the behavior of the other child was "nice." Two target figures that differed only in size—one figure was chubby and one was thin—were presented to the children. The children were asked to identify which picture represented the mean child and which picture represented the nice child. For both boys and girls, the figure of the chubby child was selected significantly more often as the mean child. Other studies have assessed the bias against overweight and obese children by presenting children with images of different body types and asking them to assign attributes to the pictures from a list (e.g., [9, 10]). Hill and Silver [10] presented 9-year-old children with two images of body types, one thin and one overweight. The overweight figures were rated as having significantly fewer friends, doing less well at school, and being unhealthy. Wardle, Volz, and Golding [11] reported similar findings, with obese children being rated as less popular, friendly, intelligent, and attractive, and more mean, lazy, argumentative, sad, and dirty than nonobese children.

In addition, some studies have examined the influence of children's own weight or build on their judgments of stereotypical figures [10, 12, 13]. These studies have found that even overweight children hold negative attitudes toward overweight people. However, overweight children do not regard themselves as sharing those same negative attributes [10, 13]. Cramer and Steinwert [8] found that, in some cases, overweight preschoolers actually held stronger negative stereotypes than their healthy-weight peers. This research suggests that overweight and obese children are just as likely to support stigmatizing attitudes toward overweight and obesity as their healthy-weight counterparts.

Generally, the literature provides evidence for a negative attitude toward not only obese adults but also obese children. The stigma attached to obesity is pervasive and can have detrimental effects across a variety of life areas such as interpersonal difficulties, being the target of bullying and victimization, psychological problems, and a decreased quality of life [14].

SELF-ESTEEM

One of the most frequently researched psychosocial consequences of obesity in children is self-esteem. Self-esteem refers to an individual's feelings of his or her self-worth and competence and is considered an important marker of a child's well-being and mental health. Although the relationship between obesity and self-esteem in children has been widely examined, the findings tend to be inconsistent. A number of studies have found lower levels of self-esteem among obese children compared with nonobese children [15–20]. On the other hand, some studies have reported levels of self-esteem within the normal range for obese children [21–23].

The inconsistent findings may be due, in part, to important developmental differences in self-esteem among overweight and obese participants. In a review of the literature on self-esteem and obesity, French, Story, and Perry [24] reported that of the 25 cross-sectional studies included in the review, only 13 studies had found significantly lower self-esteem among obese participants. The studies among 7- to 12-year-old children generally found little or no significant differences between obese and healthy-weight children on the measure of self-esteem. However, the cross-sectional studies among 13- to 18-year-olds were consistent in finding lower levels of self-esteem in obese participants when compared with healthy-weight participants. This suggests that the association between obesity and self-esteem may strengthen with age, so that obese adolescents are more likely to experience low self-esteem than preadolescent obese children.

The results of longitudinal studies also support this suggestion [17, 25]. Among a sample of 1520 children aged 9 to 10 years at baseline, Strauss [17] found no significant differences in global self-esteem between the obese and nonobese children. At the follow-up assessment conducted 4 years later (aged 13 to 14 years), there was a significant decrease in the self-esteem of obese females and a mild decrease in the self-esteem of obese males. The lower levels of self-esteem at follow-up among the obese children were found to be associated with higher levels of sadness, loneliness, nervousness, and smoking and drinking. Hesketh, Wake, and Waters [25] also examined the temporal relationship between self-esteem and obesity among a sample of children tracked for 3 years during primary school. At baseline (5 to 10 years old), there was a significant inverse association between body mass index (BMI) and self-esteem so that, as BMI increased, scores on the measure of self-esteem decreased. At follow-up, there was a stronger relationship between BMI and self-esteem with almost 50% of the obese children scoring in the lowest 15% of the self-esteem measure.

A number of other factors are purported to account for the inconsistent findings in the research on self-esteem and obesity. These include gender, ethnicity, whether the obese sample was recruited from the community (nontreatment seeking) or clinical (treatment seeking) sample, and the particular aspect of self-esteem measured [15, 24, 26].

Self-esteem is a multidimensional construct conceptualized in terms of global self-evaluation as well as several distinct behavioral domains. For example, physical appearance, social competence, scholastic competence, athletic competence, and behavioral conduct are the five domains assessed in the Self-perception Profile for Children, one of the most frequently used measures of self-esteem [27]. Typically, studies have measured only global or overall self-esteem, ignoring the various aspects of self-concept that contribute to the general self-concept. Of the studies that have measured the individual components of self-esteem, weight status has been more consistently associated with the physical appearance (i.e., body esteem) and athletic competence subscales, such that obese children report lower levels of these aspects of self-esteem in comparison to healthy-weight children [15, 23, 26, 28–30]. In addition, some studies have found impaired body esteem among overweight and obese children but preserved global self-esteem (e.g., [22, 26]). Body esteem is the component of self-esteem that refers to an individual's attitudes, evaluations, and feelings about his or her body [31]. Hence, it is not surprising that studies have found this aspect of self-esteem to be lower in overweight and obese samples than in healthy-weight samples.

DEPRESSION

Overweight and obese children are perceived to be unhappy with their weight and at risk of experiencing depression. Generally, studies among treatment seeking samples of obese children have found a positive relationship between depressive symptoms and obesity [32–36]. These studies suggest that obese children report higher levels of depression compared with healthy-weight children.

Population-based studies examining the relationship between BMI and depressive symptoms among children and adolescents have been inconclusive. In a population sample of 4703 15- to 17-year-olds, Sjoberg, Nilsson, and Leppart [37] found higher levels of depressive symptoms among the obese adolescents compared with overweight and healthy-weight peers. More specifically, those adolescents with the highest BMIs were significantly more likely to experience major depression in accordance with the DSM-IV criteria. Studies demonstrating a positive association between obesity and depression tend be limited to adolescent samples. However, community-based samples show that overweight children do not differ in levels of depression compared with those of average-weight peers, suggesting that overweight and obese children are no more likely to suffer from depression than healthy-weight children [38–40]. Furthermore, studies that included a clinical obese sample, a nonclinical obese sample, and a normal-weight control group have found higher levels of depression in their clinical group but no differences in depression between the nonclinical obese group and the normal-weight controls in Diagnostic and Statistical Manual of Mental Disorders (DSM) diagnoses of depression [33, 34].

Studies using population samples indicate that gender may impact on the relationship between BMI and depression. Erickson, Robinson, Haydel, and Killen [41] examined whether body fat and depressive symptoms were associated in a sample of third-grade children (N = 868, mean age = 8.4 years). A modest but significant association was found between depressive symptoms (as assessed by the Children's Depression Inventory) and BMI for girls. However, BMI and depressive symptoms were not correlated in boys. Gibson et al. [42] also reported gender differences on the Children's Depression Inventory among a sample of 8- to 12-year-old children. A significant interaction was found between BMI z-score and gender on the measure of depression, with girls having a significantly greater increase in depression than boys as the BMI z-score increased.

The cross-sectional research on the association between obesity and depression in children and adolescents seems clearly divided. Studies with treatment-seeking samples consistently report a moderate positive relationship, whereas studies involving population-based samples tend to report either no relationship or a weak positive relationship between obesity and depression.

Longitudinal studies have been able to examine the temporal relationship between obesity and depression. Several prospective studies of adolescent girls found that obesity at baseline did not predict depression at follow-up [43, 44]. Two prospective studies from the United States supported the notion that depression may predispose individuals to the development of obesity. Pine and colleagues studied more than 700 adolescents in 1983 and again 9 years later and found that depression in adolescence predicted significantly elevated BMIs in adulthood [45]. A subsequent prospective study by the same research group compared adult BMIs of children who had or had not experienced major depression between the ages of 6 to 17 years [46]. Those who had experienced depression during childhood or adolescence had significantly higher BMIs in adulthood.

In the Pine, Goldstein, Wolk, and Weissman [45] study, the duration of depressive symptoms in adolescence was found to be an independent predictor of obesity severity, suggesting that the risk of adult obesity may increase with reoccurrence or persistence of depression. Hence, it is possible that the duration of depression is the key risk factor for the development of obesity in adulthood. Richardson et al. [47] found a similar dose-response relationship between depression in adolescents and risk of adult obesity in a community cohort. In girls, there was an increased risk for obesity in adulthood with increasing number of times the study member had met the criteria for major depression in late adolescence. The longitudinal study by Richardson et al. [47] is the first to report that the relationship between depression and obesity differs significantly by gender. This finding is consistent with prior cross-sectional studies (e.g., [41]), which have observed a positive association between depression and obesity in female participants.

The longitudinal studies examining the relationship between obesity and depression suggest that depression at baseline predicts obesity at follow-up, rather than obesity predicting depression. These studies provide evidence for the notion that depression is not just a consequence of obesity but it perhaps plays a causal role. Although depression in childhood is a risk factor for the development of obesity, the exact causal pathway remains to be established.

BODY DISSATISFACTION

Body image refers to the subjective image an individual has of his or her own body and is typically measured using body figure rating scales. These rating scales are usually figure drawings of increasing size from which respondents must select their actual and ideal body sizes. The discrepancy between actual and ideal body size is used as an index of body dissatisfaction. Although body dissatisfaction is prevalent in normal-weight groups (especially adolescent girls), it has also been found to be widespread in adult obese populations. An association between BMI and body dissatisfaction has also been found in children, in particular girls [48].

Although few studies have measured body dissatisfaction in treatment-seeking samples of obese youths [49] there are numerous community-based studies that consistently report higher levels of body dissatisfaction among overweight and obese children and adolescents (e.g., [23, 24, 50]). For example, Truby and Paxton [51] confirmed the finding that body dissatisfaction is frequently observed in children, especially girls. Furthermore, perceptions of body size (as assessed using the Children's Body Image Scale) were found to be related to BMI in the sample of 254 Australian children aged 8 to 12 years.

Establishing a developmental pattern of body dissatisfaction has been made difficult by the few studies that have included a sample of both preadolescents and adolescents. Davison and colleagues [52, 53] documented the development of weight concerns and body dissatisfaction in a cohort of 197 girls assessed at ages 5, 7, and 9. Across all time points, body esteem was lower in the girls with higher BMI. In addition, the associations between weight concern, body dissatisfaction, and weight status increased with age [52, 53]. This suggests body concerns emerge early, at least in girls, and continue to increase throughout a child's development.

Body dissatisfaction is thought to be of concern primarily in females, but it appears that body dissatisfaction may have a markedly different effect in boys and girls. Kostanski, Fisher, and Gullone [54] found girls were more dissatisfied with their bodies with increasing weight; however, both overweight and underweight boys expressed increased levels of body dissatisfaction. Ricciardelli and McCabe [48] conducted a review of studies of body image in males and argued that the relationship between weight and body dissatisfaction in males was not as clear-cut as those for females. The review indicated that girls generally want to be thinner whereas boys generally want to be bigger. Identifying these gender differences is difficult because current measures of body image often do not differentiate between "bigger" as a result of more muscle and "bigger" because of more fat. These gender differences with respect to body dissatisfaction may reflect the different sociocultural pressures on girls and boys to conform to an idealized physique, girls to the thin ideal and boys to a muscular body type [55].

DISORDERED EATING

Childhood obesity has been shown to be associated with the cognitive and behavioral symptoms of eating disorders, such as increased weight and shape concern and binge eating [56, 57]. This is of concern as these behaviors have been identified as important causal factors for the development of eating disorders such as bulimia nervosa and binge eating disorder [58, 59].

Although obesity is purported to be a risk factor for binge eating in adulthood [60], it is unclear whether BMI predicts binge eating behaviors in adolescents. The relationship between increased BMI and binge eating in adolescents has been demonstrated in some cases, although other studies did not find body mass predicted binge eating. In a sample of primary school children, Neumark-Sztainer et al. [61] found that overweight participants reported more binge eating episodes than healthy-weight children. Furthermore, evidence from longitudinal studies among adolescents suggests that dieting is a risk factor for binge eating. Overweight and obese adolescents are more likely to diet, possibly in an attempt to conform sociocultural pressures to adhere to the thin ideal, putting themselves at increased risk for binge eating.

Tanofky-Kraff et al. [57] measured binge eating behaviors and eating disorder cognitions using the Child Eating Disorder Examination (ChEDE) in a community sample of children aged 6 to 13 years. The researchers found that overweight children scored significantly higher on the restraint, shape, and weight concern, and eating concern subscales of the ChEDE than the healthy-weight children. The sample of overweight children also reported more subjective binge eating with loss-of-control episodes than their healthy-weight counterparts. The finding that overweight participants with BMIs at or above the 95th percentile, in comparison to those from 85th up to the 95th percentile, had higher ChEDE scores suggests that as BMI increases, so does eating disorder psychopathology.

Several studies have shown a link between weight status and weight and shape concern in children. Weight and shape concern refers to a preoccupation with, or overconcern about, issues relating to weight and shape and to the evaluation of self-worth largely in terms of weight and shape [62]. In an interview-based study, overweight girls were found to have higher concerns about shape, weight, and eating and higher levels of dietary restraint than normal-weight peers [56]. Allen, Byrne, Blair, and Davis [63] used the ChEDE to assess eating disorder psychopathology in a sample of primary school-aged children (8 to 12 years). Overweight children were found to be more concerned about their weight and shape than healthy-weight children. A large-scale questionnaire study of elementary school children also revealed obese children, particularly girls, were significantly more likely to report concerns about their weight and to report restraining their eating than average-weight children [64]. The association between weight status and weight and shape concern may explain why childhood obesity is a risk factor for eating disorders such as bulimia nervosa and binge eating disorder, as previous research has found high weight and shape concern predicts the development and maintenance of disordered eating [65, 66].

Body dissatisfaction is also thought to be an important precursor to the development of disordered eating. Cross-sectional studies have found associations between body dissatisfaction and symptoms of eating disorders in children. Vander Wal and Thelen [64] reported an association between obesity and four characteristics of disordered eating: dieting, restrained eating, fear of overweight, and body dissatisfaction among a sample of 9- to 12-year-old children. Although both healthy-weight and obese children reported body dissatisfaction and weight control behaviors, these behaviors were more frequent among the sample of obese children. In addition, longitudinal studies demonstrate that body dissatisfaction is a risk factor for the development of disordered eating. Girls with the greatest weight and shape concerns at baseline were more likely to develop eating disorder symptomatology over a 4-year period than girls with the fewest concerns [65].

This research demonstrates higher eating disorder cognitions and behaviors among overweight and obese children and adolescents. Furthermore, it is suggested that overweight children may be at greater risk of developing full-syndrome eating disorder diagnoses in the future compared with their normal-weight peers.

QUALITY OF LIFE

Health related quality of life (QoL) is a multidimensional construct that includes physical health, school functioning, and emotional and social well-being. Health-related QoL reflects an individual's own judgment of his or her well-being and functioning within the context of day-to-day life. QoL has been examined in relation to a number of childhood disorders, including cancer, asthma, and cystic fibrosis. Although studies have consistently demonstrated lower QoL among obese adults (e.g., [67, 68]), there is limited information about QoL in obese children.

Schwimmer, Burwinkle, and Varni [69] compared QoL among three groups of children and adolescents—a treatment-seeking sample of obese children, a sample receiving treatment for cancer, and a healthy-weight sample—aged 5 to 18 years. Obese children and adolescents reported significantly lower QoL than the healthy-weight sample across all domains measured (i.e., physical, social, emotional, school, and global functioning). Furthermore, the level of QoL reported by obese children and adolescents was similar to children diagnosed with cancer. A number of other studies have examined QoL in a clinical or treatment-seeking sample of obese children and adolescents and have also shown impairments in QoL in all domains relative to norms for healthy-weight youths (e.g., [70–72]). These studies suggest the everyday life of treatment-seeking obese children is globally impacted by this condition.

However, Hughes, Farewell, Harris, and Reilly [73] found that only the physical domain scores were significantly lower for a clinical obese sample than the control group using a self-report QoL measure. This is in contrast to studies such as Schwimmer et al. [69], which found psychosocial health and emotional and social functioning were the most severely impaired in the clinical sample of obese children. In Hughes et al. these aspects of QoL were relatively unaffected in the clinical sample of obese children. A possible reason may be that Schwimmer et al.'s sample included adolescents and young adults, and perhaps psychosocial rather than physical issues predominate in adolescents and adults.

What is not clear from the majority of studies is whether increasing weight is associated with increasing impairment in QoL (i.e., a negative linear relationship), or whether there is a threshold effect, such that a child's weight may need to reach a certain level for QoL deficits to emerge. Data from Williams, Wake, Hesketh, Maher, and Waters [74] and Shoup, Gattshall, Dandamudi, and Estabooks [75] suggest that there are weight-related differences. Williams et al. [74] examined QoL in a community sample of Australia primary school-aged children, aged 9 to 12 years. Both parent proxy and child-reported QoL was found to decrease with increasing child weight. In particular, obese children were found to have lower physical and social functioning compared to healthy-weight children, suggesting that some dimensions of QoL may be more affected by excess weight than others. A U.S. population-based study also found that increasing weight was associated with lower QoL scores [75]. In comparison with the overweight participants, obese children reported lower psychosocial, physical, and total QoL scores. These findings suggest that the severity of QoL impairments and the domains affected vary with degree of adiposity.

Some of the research on QoL in overweight and obese children and adolescents also suggests that gender may impact on the relationship between weight and QoL. Swallen, Reither, Hass, and Meier [76] found BMI more strongly associated with functional impairments in QoL for adolescent boys than girls, with overweight boys reporting significantly worse physical health than boys with normal BMIs. Similarly, Ingerski, Janicke, and Silverstein [71] found a relationship between gender and physical QoL in overweight youth, with adolescent males reporting better physical QoL than females. Whereas Swallen et al. [74] and Ingerski et al. [71] both reported that the relationship between BMI and QoL varies according to gender in their samples of adolescents, Schwimmer et al. did not find gender differences among their sample of youth aged 5 to 18 years. The discrepant findings may suggest that gender differences in self-reported QoL are slight in overweight and obese children but become apparent or increase in adolescence.

Although QoL measures, such as the PedsQL, include both a parent-proxy or child-report scale, few studies have utilized both to measure QoL in overweight children and adolescents. Of the few studies that have assessed child and parent report, the findings generally suggest that parents report worse QoL than their children [69–71]. Child- and parent-reported QoL tend not to concur. QoL impairments are found to be greater when assessed from the parent perspective in comparison with the child's perspective, with parents being much less optimistic about their child's health and well-being. In particular, some research suggests that parents tend to report much more severe deficits in the domain of emotional health [77, 78]. It is possible that parents have a limited awareness of their child's internal states, such as their psychosocial health, but a greater understanding of more observable behaviors. However, it is not clear whether parents are overestimating the impact of a child's weight on the child's QoL or whether children tend to downplay or underreport their impairments.

SOCIAL FUNCTIONING (PEER RELATIONS AND BULLYING-VICTIMIZATION)

The majority of the research on social functioning in overweight and obese children suggests that the bias and discrimination toward obese individuals has a negative impact on social relationships for overweight children [79]. Generally, the research has found that obese adolescents have fewer friends, are less liked, and are rejected more often than their healthy-weight counterparts [20, 50].

However, the impact of weight on an individual's social functioning may differ with respect to age. Using a peer-nomination method, Phillips and Hill [26] examined children's popularity with same-sex classmates. Children were asked to identify up to three children they would sit next to in class, play with at break time, or invite home for tea. There was no influence of weight on peer choices among this sample of primary school-aged children. Obese boys and girls were as likely to be chosen as their healthy-weight peers to socialize with both at school and at home. U.S. researchers Strauss and Pollack [50] analyzed data on social network mapping from the National Survey of Adolescent Health. This survey contained peer-report sociometric measures from 90,000 13- to 18-year-olds. Overweight and obese adolescents were significantly more likely than healthy-weight peers to have three or fewer nominations from other adolescents, whereas healthy-weight adolescents were significantly more likely to have six or more friendship nominations compared with overweight or obese children. Compared to healthy-weight adolescents, overweight and obese adolescents were more likely to be socially isolated and were less likely to be nominated as friends by their peers. Furthermore, although the majority of overweight and obese adolescents received at least one friendship nomination, they tended to receive less reciprocal nominations. In other words, overweight and obese children were less likely to be nominated as a friend by a peer they had chosen as a friend. This lack of reciprocity indicates that friendships for overweight and obese children are fewer and more fragile.

The bias and discrimination toward obese individuals is suggested to go beyond isolation or social marginalization, with overweight and obese youth experiencing bullying-victimization. Bullying-victimization refers to an individual being repeatedly exposed to the negative actions of others with the intention to hurt [80] and is frequent in school settings. The bullying can be overt (physical [e.g., hitting]), verbal (e.g., name calling), or relational (e.g., social exclusion). Being overweight or obese is thought to be a salient target for bullying and victimization.

Although research is yet to determine the exact prevalence of weight-related bullying-victimization, the evidence suggests that it is widespread and greater among overweight children [81–83]. Obese children report being the victims of all types of bullying—physical, verbal, and relational—although verbal and relational bullying are found to be more common [82]. A study of 10- to 14-year-olds (N = 156) found that weight-based teasing was more severe, frequent, and upsetting among overweight children compared with nonoverweight children [84]. Janssen et al. [83] examined bullying-victimization among 5749 youths aged 11 to 16 years. Overweight and obese adolescents in all age groups (with the exception of 15- to 16-year-old boys) were more likely to be victims of bullying behaviors than were average-weight peers. Janssen et al. [83] also found that as BMI increased, there was an increase in verbal, physical, and relational peer victimization, such that the likelihood of bully-victimization was lower in normal-weight youth by comparison to overweight youth, who in turn had a lower likelihood of bully-victimization than obese youth. This is consistent with the research of Neumark-Sztainer et al. [81], which suggests that bully-victimization experiences are more prevalent in children with higher levels of obesity.

Research on perpetrators of bullying-victimization and obesity generally suggest that obese preadolescent boys [82] and male and female obese adolescents [83] are also the perpetrators of bullying. This has been suggested to be due to their physical dominance over their peers or possibly due to confrontation as a result of the victimization [82]. Although both preadolescent and adolescents boys engage in bullying-perpetrating, bully-perpetrating is reported to increase in girls as they get older. Janssen et al. [83] reported a relationship between bullying-perpetrating and obesity in both adolescent boys and girls. Among 15- to 16-year-old boys, BMI was also positively associated with being the perpetrator of bullying behaviors, whereas among 15- to 16-year-old girls, BMI was positively associated with being both a perpetrator and a victim of bullying.

The specific type of bullying-victimization behavior experienced by overweight and obese children may differ according to gender. Overweight and obese boys are at risk of being verbally teased and victims of physical aggression by peers (e.g., punched, kicked). On the other hand, recent evidence indicates that girls are at risk of relational victimization. This research suggests that girls are more likely to use their friendship status as a way of inflicting social harm—for example, by purposefully excluding a peer from social activities or threatening to withdraw one's friendship [85].

Longitudinal research on weight-based teasing has highlighted possible pathways between obesity and bullying-victimization. Griffiths et al. [82] reported that weight-category was a significant predictor of future victimization among 8210 children. Specifically, obese boys and girls were more likely to be victims of overt bullying 1 year later, but this was not the case for overweight boys and girls. A prospective cohort study in the United Kingdom also examined whether weight category at age 7 predicted bullying-victimization behaviors 1 year later [86]. Compared to average-weight children, obese boys were more likely to be both victims and perpetrators of overt bullying, and obese girls were more likely to be victims of overt bullying a year later. Overt bullying includes behaviors such as having something stolen, being threatened or blackmailed, being hit or beaten up, being called nasty names, or having tricks played on them. Griffiths et al. [82, 86] found that obesity, but not overweight status, was a significant predictor of involvement in bullying-victimization, suggesting the actual level of adiposity is significant in predicting future bullying involvement.

Griffiths et al. [82] used qualitative research to understand the impact of weight-related victimization on peer relationships among obese adolescents. Those who had experienced weight-related victimization tended to report low self-confidence, body dissatisfaction, and depressive feelings, whereas some adolescents internalized attributes of social worthlessness. Neumark-Sztainer et al. [81] found that not only are overweight adolescent boys and girls at greatest risk of being teased about their weight, but they are also more likely to be bothered by it. Weight-based teasing was found to be associated with disordered eating behaviors, with adolescents who were teased about their weight more likely to use unhealthy-weight control methods and engage in binge eating. This is of concern as these disordered eating behaviors may place overweight and obese youth at further risk for future weight gain. The consequences of bullying in terms of self-confidence, isolation, and peer anxiety may in turn affect the social development of overweight and obese youth. As well as the immediate effect on an individual's psychosocial health and peer relationships, bullying-victimization is also thought to have a negative long-term impact. Research has shown that individuals bullied repeatedly throughout adolescence have lower self-esteem and more depressive symptoms as adults [80].

RELATIONSHIP BETWEEN PSYCHOSOCIAL SYMPTOMS

The majority of studies documenting the psychosocial burden of excess weight in children have been confined to isolated aspects of psychosocial functioning, rather than examining the relationship between excess weight and a broad range of psychosocial constructs measured concurrently. What is unclear from the research presented in this chapter is whether particular psychosocial problems coexist in overweight and obese children, whether the nature of such combinations varies with degree of adiposity, or whether increasing adiposity is associated in an increasing number of psychosocial problems.

Gibson, Byrne, Blair, Jacoby, and Zubrick [42] were able to examine these issues in a sample of 262 primary school children aged 8 to 13 years. Of the 262 children, 158 children were classified as healthy weight, 104 as overweight, and 27 as obese. Of the overweight and obese children, 19 were recruited from a pediatric hospital outpatient setting (clinical sample) and 85 were recruited from metropolitan primary schools in Western Australia (community sample). Measures of depression, self-esteem, health-related quality of life, body dissatisfaction, bullying, eating disorder psychopathology, and behavioral and emotional problems were administered to all children. Higher BMI z-scores were found to be associated with statistically significant increases in depression, body dissatisfaction, frequency of eating disorder symptoms, internalizing and externalizing problems on the Child Behavior Checklist (CBCL), and the frequency of being bullied, and with decreasing levels of quality of life and self-esteem.

In addition, a positive association was found between the number of psychosocial problems and child BMI z-score, indicating that as BMI increases, children are likely to experience an increasing number of psychosocial problems. These findings demonstrate that overweight and obese children report both higher levels of psychosocial distress and a greater number of psychosocial problems than healthy-weight children.

The inclusion of a range of measures of psychosocial functioning allowed the clustering of psychosocial problems to be examined for the overweight/obese children and the healthy-weight children using principal component analysis. One of the clustering profiles common in the overweight/obese group, but not the healthy-weight group, was the clustering of global self-worth with body dissatisfaction and eating disorder symptoms. This suggests that for overweight and obese children, their sense of self-worth is closely tied with issues regarding weight and shape concern and body image.

Even among young primary school-aged children the psychosocial burden of excess weight is significant and broad reaching. Overweight and obese children are likely to experience multiple psychosocial problems, in particular their self-worth is strongly associated with weight, shape, eating concern, and body dissatisfaction.

NOT ALL CHILDREN EXPERIENCE PSYCHOSOCIAL SYMPTOMS: WHY?

Although there is substantial evidence that overweight and obese children and adolescents suffer from impaired psychosocial functioning compared with healthy-weight children, it is clear that not all overweight and obese children experience psychosocial problems. Hence, it is suggested that individuals with obesity are a heterogeneous group with substantial variation in psychosocial functioning [87]. Recently there has been a move away from investigating if obese children and adolescents suffer from psychosocial problems to searching for risk factors that explain why some obese individuals suffer negative psychosocial consequences and others do not. Although the majority of this chapter has focused on how weight impacts on a child's psychosocial functioning, research has also begun to examine other factors that may protect some overweight and obese children and adolescents or make others more vulnerable to psychosocial problems.

It has been suggested that psychosocial problems, in particular depression and self-esteem, in obese children and adolescents, may in part be accounted for by concerns about being overweight, dissatisfaction with one's body size, or being teased about one's weight or shape.

One of the first studies to suggest that concerns about being overweight may have an impact on the relationship between BMI and psychosocial functioning was conducted by Erickson et al. [41]. Erickson and colleagues examined the relationship between BMI and depressive symptoms in a community sample of children aged 8.4 years. A modest association was found between BMI and depressive symptoms among girls, but not boys. However, the relationship between BMI and depressive symptoms was limited to girls who also reported overweight concerns. The sum of all endorsed attitudes and behaviors on the Kids Eating Disorder Survey was used as a measure of overweight concerns in the analysis. This questionnaire includes items such as desire to lose weight, fear of gaining weight, dieting to lose weight, and fasting to lose weight. Overweight concerns were found to be significantly and positively associated with depressive symptoms among girls. However, after controlling for overweight concerns, BMI was no longer significantly associated with depressive symptoms. On the other hand, after controlling for BMI, reported overweight concerns were still significantly associated with depressive symptoms. Therefore, the relationship between BMI and depressive symptoms was mostly limited to those girls who also reported overweight concerns. As a group, overweight girls who did not report overweight concerns also did not report significantly more depressive symptoms than their healthy-weight peers. In addition, healthy-weight girls who reported more overweight concerns also reported more depressive symptoms. The findings of this study suggest that overweight concerns play an important role in mediating the relationship between BMI and depressive symptoms.

Similarly, Allen et al. [63] found that weight and shape concern accounted for individual differences in the psychological consequences of obesity in primary school-aged children. Weight and shape concern refers to a preoccupation with, or overconcern about, issues relating to weight and shape, and the evaluation of self-worth largely in terms of weight and shape [62, 63]. Allen et al. [63] found that overweight children reported more concern about their weight and shape than healthy-weight children. In addition, after controlling for BMI, children with high weight and shape concern reported lower self-esteem, higher body dissatisfaction, and higher depression than children with low weight and shape concern. Weight and shape concern also mediated the link between weight status and self-esteem, body dissatisfaction, and depression. More specifically, in this sample of primary school children, it was only children with a high degree of weight and shape concern that experienced psychosocial problems. Hence, the results of this study suggest that it is an individual's level of weight and shape concern rather than the person's actual weight that is associated with psychosocial problems in children.

It has also been suggested that psychosocial functioning in overweight and obese children and adolescents may depend in part on their level of satisfaction with their body weight and appearance [88]. Although it is suggested that overweight and obese children may become vulnerable to psychosocial problems once they become dissatisfied with their body, few studies have examined this idea in children.

Watt, Byrne, Gibson, and Davis [89] examined whether an objective (BMI z-score) or subjective (body dissatisfaction) measure of adiposity best predicts the presence of adverse mental health outcomes, as measured by the Child Behavior Checklist (CBCL). Whereas anthropometric measures of adiposity give an actual indication of excess weight, subjective measures provide an attitudinal indication of an individual's perception of, and importance attached to, and dissatisfaction with his or her size and shape. It was predicted that the subjective measure (body dissatisfaction) would be a better predictor of psychosocial complication than an objective measure (BMI z-score). Multivariate analyses conducted on 292 healthy-weight, overweight, and obese children found that although both BMI z-score and body dissatisfaction were associated with mental health outcomes, it was the body dissatisfaction that was more strongly associated with the presence of adverse mental health outcomes in children and adolescents. More specifically, a greater level of body dissatisfaction was associated with higher scores on the Internalizing and Externalizing subscales of the CBCL, indicating more emotional and behavioral problems among children dissatisfied with their body. This study suggests that it is how individuals perceive themselves, rather than their actual adiposity, that is important in determining psychosocial functioning in children.

There is also evidence that weight-based teasing may mediate the relationship between obesity and psychosocial functioning in children. Eisenberg and colleagues examined weight-based teasing in a school sample of 4746 adolescents in the United States [39]. Teasing about weight (by either peers or family members) was associated with low body satisfaction, low self-esteem, high depressive symptoms and thinking about and attempting suicide. These associations were found for both males and females, across racial and ethnic groups, and across weight categories. In addition, weight was not significantly associated with the psychological functioning after teasing was entered into the multivariate models, suggesting that being teased about weight, rather than an individual's weight, is a key risk factor for low self-esteem, depressive symptoms, and suicidal ideation and attempts.

IMPLICATIONS FOR INTERVENTION AND PREVENTION

The sections within this chapter have demonstrated substantial evidence that overweight and obese children and adolescents are at risk of suffering from psychosocial problems, such as low self-esteem, depression, poor quality of life, impaired social relationships, and eating disorder psychopathology. However, traditionally psychosocial problems have received less attention in the majority of interventions for obesity than physical health problems. Considering both the immediate and long-term impact of obesity on an individual's psychosocial functioning, cognitive-behavioral strategies to improve social and peer relationships, body dissatisfaction, depression, and self-esteem are an essential component to obesity treatments for children and adolescents. In fact, some of the more successful treatments for obesity in children and adolescents are psychology-based treatments [90, 91].

Advances in identifying risk factors for the development of psychosocial problems in obese children and adolescents have highlighted the importance of factors such as weight and shape concern, body satisfaction, and teasing as possible mediators of the relationship between weight status and psychosocial problems. This research has important implications for prevention programs aimed at reducing psychosocial distress among overweight and obese children. For example, early detection of high weight and shape concern combined with appropriate interventions that aim to reduce this concern may prevent or reduce psychological distress in overweight individuals. Likewise, programs to develop healthy body image in children may decrease the risk of psychosocial problems in overweight and obese children and adolescents.

References

1. Burke VL. Predictors of body mass index and associations with cardiovascular risk factors in Australia children: a prospective cohort study. *International Journal of Obesity* 2005;**29**:15−23.
2. Oddy WH, Sherriff JL, de Klerk NH, Kendall GE, Sly PD, Beilin LJ, Blake KB, Landau LI, Stanley FJ. The relation of breastfeeding and body mass index to asthma and atopy in children: A prospective cohort study to age 6 years. *American Journal of Public Health* 2004;**94**:1531−7.
3. Must A, Strauss RS. Risks and consequences of childhood and adolescent obesity. *International Journal of Obesity* 1999;**23**:2−11.
4. Lee YS. Consequences of childhood obesity. Annuals. *Academy of Medicine Singapore* 2009;**38**:75−81.
5. Puhl RM, Brownell KD. Bias, discrimination, and obesity. *Obesity Research* 2001;**9**(12):788−805.
6. Richardson SA, Goodman N, Hastorf AH, Dornbusch SM. Cultural uniformity in reaction to physical disabilities. *American Sociological Review* 1961;**26**:241−7.
7. Latner J, Stunkard AJ. Getting worse: The stigmatization of obese children. *Obesity Research* 2003;**11**:452−6.
8. Cramer P, Steinwert T. Thin is Good, Fat is Bad: How Early Does it Begin? *Journal of Applied Developmental Psychology* 1998;**19**(3):429−51.
9. Brylinsky JA, Moore JC. The identification of body build stereotypes in young children. *Journal of Research in Personality* 1994;**28**:170−81.
10. Hill AJ, Silver EK. Fat, friendless and unhealthy: 9-year old children's perception of body shape stereotypes. *International Journal of Obesity* 1995;**19**:423−30.
11. Wardle J, Volz C, Golding C. Social variation in attitudes to obesity in children. *International Journal of Obesity* 1995;**19**:562−9.
12. Davidson KK, Birch LL. Predictors of fat stereotypes among 9-year-old girls and their parents. *Obesity Research* 2004;**12**:86−94.
13. Lerner RM, Korn SJ. The development of body-build stereotypes in males. *Child Development* 1972;**43**:908−20.
14. Latner J, Schawartz MB. Weight bias in the child's world. In: Brownell KD, Weight bias, editors. *Nature, Consequences, and Remedies*. London: Guildford Press; 2005.
15. Braet C, Mervielde I, Vandereycken W. Psychological aspects of childhood obesity: A controlled study in a clinical and non-clinical sample. *Journal of Pediatric Psychology* 1997;**22**:59−71.
16. Pierce JW, Wardle J. Cause and effect beliefs and self-esteem of overweight children. *Journal of Child Psychology and Psychiatry* 1997;**38**:645−50.
17. Strauss R. Childhood obesity and self-esteem. *Pediatrics* 2000;**105**:1−5.
18. Allon N. Self-perception of the stigma of overweight on relationship to weight-losing patterns. *American Journal of Clinical Nutrition* 1979;**32**:470−80.
19. Sallade J. A comparison of the psychological adjustment of obese vs. nonobese children. *Journal of Psychosomatic Research* 1973;**17**:89−96.
20. Strauss CC, Smith K, Frame C, Forehand R. Personal and interpersonal characteristics associated with childhood obesity. *Journal of Pediatric Psychiatry* 1985;**10**:337−43.
21. Wadden TA, Foster GD, Brownell KD, Finley E. Self-concept in obese and normal weight children. *Journal of Consulting & Clinical Psychology* 1984;**52**:1104−5.
22. Mendelson B, White DR. Relation between body-esteem and self-esteem of obese and normal children. *Perceptual Motor Skills* 1982;**54**:899−905.
23. Renman C, Engstrom I, Silverdal S-A, Aman J. Mental health and psychosocial characteristics in adolescent obesity: a population-based case control study. *Acta Pediatrics* 1999;**88**:998−1003.
24. French SA, Story M, Perry CL. Self-esteem and obesity in children and adolescents: A literature review. *Obesity research* 1995;**5**:479−90.
25. Hesketh K, Wake M, Waters E. Body mass index and parent-reported self-esteem in elementary school children: evidence for a causal relationship. *International Journal of Obesity* 2004;**28**:1233−7.
26. Phillips RG, Hill AJ. Fat, plain, but not friendless: self-esteem and peer acceptance of obese and pre-adolescent girls. *International Journal of Obesity* 1998;**22**:287−93.
27. Harter S. *Self-perception Profile for Children*. Denver, CO: University of Denver; 1985.
28. Franklin J, Denyer G, Steinbeck KS, Caterson ID, Hill AJ. Obesity and risk of low self-esteem: A statewide survey of Australian children. *Pediatrics* 2006;**118**:2481−7.
29. Stradmeijer M, Bosch J, Koops W, Seidell J. Family functioning and psychosocial adjustment in overweight youngsters. *International Journal of Eating Disorders* 2000;**27**:110−14.
30. French SA, Perry CL, Leon GR, Fulkerson JA. Self-esteem and changes in body mass index over 3 years in a cohort of adolescents. *Obesity Research* 1996;**4**:27−33.
31. Fisher S, Cleveland SE. *Body image and personality*. 2nd ed. New York: Dover Publications; 1968.
32. Banis HT, Varni JW, Wallander JL, Korsch BM, Jay. SM, Adler R, Garcia-Temple E, Negrete V. Psychological and social adjustment of obese children and their families. *Child Care Health and Development* 1988;**14**:157−73.
33. Britz B, Siegfried W, Ziegler A, Lamertz C, Herpertz-Dahlmann BM, Remschmidt H, Wittchen H-U, Hebebrand J. Rates of psychiatric disorders in a clinical study group of adolescents with extreme obesity and in obese adolescents ascertained via a population based study. *International Journal of Obesity* 2000;**24**:1707−14.
34. Erermis S, Cetin N, Tamar M, Bukusoglu N, Akdeniz F, Goksen D. Is obesity a risk factor for psychopathology among adolescents? *Pediatrics International* 2004;**46**:296−301.
35. Israel AC, Shapiro LS. Behavioral problems in obese children enrolling in a weight reduction program. *Journal of Pediatric Psychology* 1985;**10**:449−60.
36. Epstein LH, Wisniewski L, Weng R. Child and parent psychological problems influence children weight control. *International Journal of Eating Disorders* 1994;**15**:151−8.
37. Sjoberg RL, Nilsson KW, Leppart J. Obesity, shame and depression in school-aged children: A population based study. *Pediatrics* 2005;**116**:389−92.
38. Brewis A. Biocultural aspects of obesity in young Mexican schoolchildren. *American Journal of Human Biology* 2003;**15**:446−60.
39. Eisenberg ME, Neumark-Sztainer D, Story M. Associations of weight-based teasing and emotional well-being among adolescents. *Archives of Pediatrics and Adolescent Medicine* 2003;**157**:733−8.
40. Wardle J, Williamson S, Johnson F, Edwards C. Depression in adolescent obesity: Cultural moderators of the association between obesity and depressive symptoms. *International Journal of Obesity* 2006;**30**:634−43.
41. Erickson SJ, Robinson TN, Haydel KF, Killen JD. Are overweight children unhappy? Body mass index, depressive symptoms, and overweight concerns in elementary school children. *Archives of Pediatrics & Adolescent Medicine* 2000;**154**:931−6.

REFERENCES

42. Gibson LY, Byrne SM, Blair E, Davis EA, Jacoby P, Zubrick SR. Clustering of psychosocial symptoms in overweight children. *Australian and New Zealand Journal of Psychiatry* 2008;**42**:118–25.
43. Stice E, Bearman SK. Body-image and eating disturbances prospectively predicts increases in depressive symptoms in adolescent girls: A growth curve analysis. *Developmental Psychology* 2001;**37**:597–607.
44. Stice E, Hayward C, Cameron RP, Killen JD, Taylor CB. Body-image and eating disturbances predict onset of depression among female adolescents: A longitudinal study. *Journal of Abnormal Psychology* 2000;**109**:438–44.
45. Pine DS, Goldstein RB, Wolk S, Weissman MM. The association between childhood depression and adulthood body mass index. *Pediatrics* 2001;**107**:1049–56.
46. Goodman E, Whitaker RC. A prospective study of the role of depression in the development and persistence of adolescent obesity. *Pediatrics* 2002;**110**:497–504.
47. Richardson LP, Davis R, Poulton R, McCauley E, Moffitt TE, Caspi A, Connell F. A longitudinal evaluation of adolescent depression and adult obesity. *Archives of Pediatrics and Adolescent Medicine* 2003;**157**:739–45.
48. Ricciardelli LA, McCabe MP. Children's body image concerns and eating disturbance: A review of the literature. *Clinical Psychology Review* 2001;**21**:325–44.
49. Braet C, Tanghe A, Decaluwe V, Moens E, Rosseel Y. Inpatient treatment for children with obesity: Weight loss, psychological well-being, and eating behavior. *Journal of Pediatric Psychology* 2004;**29**:519–29.
50. Strauss RS, Pollack HA. Social marginalization of overweight children. *Archives of Pediatric & Adolescent Medicine* 2003;**157**:746–52.
51. Truby H, Paxton S. Development of the Children's Body Image Scale. *British Journal of Clinical Psychology* 2002;**41**:185–203.
52. Davidson KK, Birch LL. Weight status, parent reaction and self-concept in five-year-old girls. *Pediatrics* 2001;**107**:46–53.
53. Davidson KK, Markey CN, Birch LL. A longitudinal examination of patterns in girls' weight concerns and body satisfaction from ages 5 to 9 years. *International Journal of Eating Disorders* 2003;**33**:320–32.
54. Kostanski M, Fisher A, Gullone E. Current conceptualisation of body image dissatisfaction: have we got it wrong? *Journal of Child Psychology and Psychiatry* 2004;**45**:1317–25.
55. Wardle J, Cooke L. The impact of obesity on psychological well-being. *Best Practice & Research Clinical Endocrinology & Metabolism* 2005;**19**:421–40.
56. Burrows A, Cooper M. Possible risk factors in the development of eating disorders in overweight pre-adolescent girls. *International Journal of Obesity* 2002;**26**:1268–73.
57. Tanofsky-Kraff M, Yanovski SZ, Wilfley DE, Marmarosh C, Morgan CM, Yanovski JA. Eating-disordered behaviors, body fat, and psychopathology in overweight and normal-weight children. *Journal of Consulting and Clinical Psychology* 2004;**72**(1):53–61.
58. Johnson F, Wardle J. Dietary restraint, body dissatisfaction, and psychological distress: A prospective analysis. *Journal of Abnormal Psychology* 2005;**114**(1):119–25.
59. Neumark-Sztainer D, Story M, Falkner NH, Beuhring T, Resnick MD. Sociodemographic and personal characteristics of adolescents engaged in weight loss and weight/muscle gain behaviors: Who is doing what? *Preventive Medicine* 1999;**28**:40–50.
60. Vogeltanz-Holm ND, Wonderlich SA, Lewis BA, Wilsnack SC, Harris TR, Wilsnack RW, Kristjanson AF. Longitudinal predictors of binge eating, intense dieting, and weight concerns in a national sample of women. *Behavior Therapy* 2000;**31**:221–35.
61. Neumark-Sztainer D, Story M, French SA, Hannan PJ, Resnick MD, Blum RW. Psychosocial concerns and health compromising behaviours among overweight and nonoverweight adolescents. *Obesity Research* 1997;**5**:237–49.
62. Fairburn CG, Cooper Z, Shafran R. Cognitive-behaviour therapy for eating disorders: A "transdiagnostic" theory and treatment. *Behavior Research and Therapy* 2003;**41**:509–28.
63. Allen KL, Byrne SM, Blair EM, Davis EA. Why do some overweight children experience psychological problems? The role of weight and shape concern. *International Journal of Pediatric Obesity* 2006;**1**(4):239–47.
64. Vander Wal JS, Thelen MH. Eating and body image concerns among obese and average-weight children. *Addictive Behaviors* 2000;**25**(5):775–8.
65. Killen JD, Taylor CB, Hayward C, Wilson DM, Haydel KF, Hammer LD, et al. Weight concerns influence the development of eating disorders: A 4-year prospective study. *Journal of Clinical Child and Adolescent Psychology* 1996;**64**:936–40.
66. Fairburn CG, Harrison PJ. Eating Disorders. *The Lancet* 2003;**361**:407–16.
67. Kolotkin RL, Crosby RD, Williams GR. Health-related quality of life varies among obese subgroups. *Obesity Research* 2002;**10**:748–56.
68. Fontaine KB, Barofsky I. Obesity and health-related quality of life. *Obesity Review* 2001;**2**:173–82.
69. Schwimmer JB, Burwinkle TM, Varni JW. Health related quality of life among severely overweight, treatment-seeking adolescents. *JAMA* 2003;**289**:1813–19.
70. Zeller MH, Modi AC. Predictors of health-related quality of life in obese youth. *Obesity* 2006;**14**:122–30.
71. Ingerski LM, Janicke DM, Silverstein JH. Brief Report: Quality of Life in Overweight Youth – The role of multiple informants and perceived social support. *Journal of Pediatric Psychology* 2007;**32**:869–74.
72. Janicke DM, Marciel KK, Ingerski LM, Novoa W, Lowry KW, Sallinen BJ, et al. Impact of psychosocial factors on quality of life in overweight youth. *Obesity* 2007;**15**:869–74.
73. Hughes AR, Farewell K, Harris D, Reilly JJ. Quality of life in a clinical sample of obese children. *International Journal of Obesity* 2007;**31**:39–44.
74. Williams J, Wake M, Hesketh K, Maher E, Waters E. Health-related quality of life of overweight and obese children. *JAMA* 2005;**293**:70–6.
75. Shoup JA, Gattshall M, Dandamudi P, Estabrooks P. Physical activity, quality of life and weight status in overweight children. *Quality of Life Research* 2000;**17**:407–12.
76. Swallen KC, Reither EN, Haas SA, Meier AM. Overweight, obesity, and health-related quality of life among adolescents: The National Longitudinal Study of Adolescent Health. *Pediatrics* 2005;**115**(2):340–7.
77. Wake M, Salmon L, Waters E, Wright M, Hesketh K. Parent-reported health status of overweight and obese Australian primary school children: a cross sectional population survey. *International Journal of Obesity* 2002;**26**:717–24.
78. Pinhas-Hamiel O, Singer S, Pilpel N, Fradkin A, Modan D, Reichman B. Health-related quality of life among children and adolescents: association with obesity. *International Journal of Obesity* 2006;**30**:267–72.
79. Puhl R, Latner J. Obesity, stigma, and the health of the nation's children. *Psychological Bulletin* 2007;**133**:557–80.
80. Olweus D. Sweden. In: Smith PK, et al., editors. *The nature of school bullying: A cross-nation perspective*. London, UK: Routledge; 1999.
81. Neumark-Sztainer D, Falkner N, Story M, Perry C, Hannan PJ, Mulert S. Weight-teasing among adolescents: correlations with weight status and disordered eating behaviors. *International Journal of Obesity* 2002;**26**:123–31.

82. Griffiths LJ, Wolke D, Page AS, Horwood JP, ALSPAC Study Team. Obesity and bullying: different effects for boys and girls. *Archives of Disease in Childhood* 2006;**91**:121–5.
83. Janssen I, Craig WM, Boyce WF, Pickett W. Associations between overweight and obesity with bullying behaviors in school-aged children. *Pediatrics* 2004;**113**:1187–94.
84. Hayden-Wade H, Stein R, Ghaderi A, Saelens BE, Zabinski MF, Wilfley DE. Prevalence, characteristics, and correlates of teasing experiences among overweight children vs. non-overweight peers. *Obesity Research* 2005;**13**:1381–92.
85. Pearce MJ, Boergers J, Prinstein MJ. Adolescent obesity, overt and relational victimization, and romantic relationships. *Obesity Research* 2002;**10**:386–93.
86. Griffiths LJ, Wolke D, Page AS, Horwood JP. ALSPAC Study team. Obesity and bullying: different effects for boys and girls. *Archives of Disease in Childhood* 2006;**91**:121–5.
87. Friedman MA, Brownell KD. Psychological correlates of obesity: Moving to the next research generation. *Psychological Bulletin* 1995;**117**:3–20.
88. Shin NY, Shin MS. Body dissatisfaction, self-esteem, and depression in obese Korean children. *Journal of Pediatrics* 2008;**152**:502–6.
89. Watt F, Byrne S, Gibson L, Davis E. Measures of adiposity for predicting mental health outcomes in children and adolescent. *Obesity* 2007;**16**:S285.
90. Tsiros M, Sinn N, Brennan L, Coates AM, Walkey JW, Petkov J, Howe PRC, Buckley JD. Cognitive behavioral therapy improves diet and body composition in overweight and obese adolescents. *American Journal of Clinical Nutrition* 2008;**87**:1134–40.
91. Braet C, Van Winckel M. Long term follow-up of a cognitive behavioral treatment program for obese children. *Behavior Therapy* 2000;**31**:55–74.

CHAPTER 23

Childhood Obesity: Depression, Anxiety and Recommended Therapeutic Strategies

Dana L. Rofey,* Jessica J. Black,† Jennifer E. Phillips,* Ronette Blake,* KayLoni Olson*

*Children's Hospital of Pittsburgh, PA, USA and †University of Cincinnati, OH, USA

INTRODUCTION

Since the 1980s, childhood obesity rates have more than tripled for children 6 to 11 years old and more than doubled for preschool children 2 to 5 years old and adolescents 12 to 19 years old [1]. Based on the National Health and Nutrition Examination Survey (NHANES), 31% of children aged 6 to 19 are at risk for overweight and obesity and 16% of children aged 6 to 19 are already overweight [2]. This obesity epidemic highlights the need to increase prevention and intervention efforts, possibly by targeting younger and less overweight children. Thus, it is critical to identify factors that are associated with increased weight in childhood.

One approach to controlling the national obesity epidemic involves an increased understanding of, and attention to, the relationship between weight and mood disturbances [3, 4]. Given the strong correlations among clinically significant weight gain, depression, and anxiety [5, 6] in adult populations, a current area of focus is the connection between psychopathology and weight in childhood.[1] Affective disturbances commonly occur during development [7, 8], and recent studies suggest that increased weight is correlated with depressive and anxiety symptoms in childhood, as demonstrated by greater body mass index percentiles (BMI percentile, defined as height-to-weight ratio [kilograms/meters squared]), adjusted for sex and age [6, 9–11]. Given that adolescence is a significant period of emotional and physical maturation [12], it is fundamental to acknowledge and further explore the influence of depression/anxiety disorders on weight in order to more effectively understand, prevent, and treat pediatric obesity [3, 12–14]. This chapter describes current treatment practices for each condition separately and research studies examining treatment across behavioral (weight) and emotional (mood) processes. Given the brevity of this chapter, the purpose is to provide preliminary data, encourage additional research on inclusive treatments, and encourage the development and application of broad-based, enhanced interventions.

OBESITY AND DEPRESSION

Evidence against a Relationship between Childhood Depression and Obesity

The directional nature of the relationship between obesity and depression in children and adolescents remains unclear. Research has shown that community-based samples of obese children do not differ in levels of depression compared to average-weight peers [15–17]. These findings exist across cultures. For example, Brewis investigated an urban, high socioeconomic sample (N = 219) of Mexican schoolchildren (aged 6 to 12) and found that obese children did not experience more depressive symptoms than their non-obese peers. Data from two large demographically diverse English school-based studies (N = 4320,

---

[1]This chapter highlights the literature on depression and anxiety. For other psychiatric comorbidities, please see Chapter 19.

N = 1824; ages ~11 and ~14–15) show that even after controlling for gender, socioeconomic status, and ethnicity, depressive symptoms are not significantly higher in obese adolescents than in their non-obese peers [17]. Similarly, another secondary analysis of U.S. children (N = 4746; grades 7 to 12) from various public schools in a Midwest state supports these findings in Mexican and English youth populations—adolescent weight is not associated with depressive symptoms [15].

Evidence for a Relationship between Depression and Obesity in Children

In contrast to the aforementioned, clinical samples seem to indicate a different relationship than community-based samples. Treatment-seeking obese children appear to display higher levels of depression than normal-weight controls [18, 19]. In both a clinical sample of German (N = 1655) and Turkish (N = 90) adolescents, a comparison of means revealed that obese adolescents seeking weight-related treatment reported higher rates of depression than obese adolescents in the general population. Another study by Vlierberghe and colleagues [20] also found that overweight children referred for treatment are both heavier and have more reported depressive symptoms than overweight children not seeking treatment. The possible long-term negative sequelae of both obesity and depression reinforce the need for clarifying directional relationships.

Obesity Predicting Depression

Several prospective studies have provided evidence for obesity causing depression and vice versa. Using U.S. nationally representative data from the National Longitudinal Study of Adolescent Health (baseline 1995), Merten and colleagues reported that obesity in adolescence significantly predicted an increase in depressive symptoms 6 years later for young adult women but not men (aged 12 to 18 at baseline and 19 to 26 at follow-up) [21]. It is important to note that longitudinal research conducted by Mustillo et al. found a modest relationship between chronic obesity and higher levels of depression over an 8-year period in boys only [22]. Although existing research sheds some light on obesity as a predictor of depression in youth, results are contradictory and sample demographics are heterogeneous, making it difficult to compare across studies.

Depression Predicting Obesity

In contrast, other evidence indicates that it is childhood depression that predicts the development of obesity in both children [23] and adults [14, 24, 25]. For example, Rofey et al. [14] found that childhood depression ($\chi^2 = 4.6$, $p = 0.03$) was associated with increased BMI percentiles. Compared to controls, BMI percentiles of depressed females over the course of the study differed profoundly ($\chi^2 = 7.0$, $p = 0.01$). Moreover, Ternouth and colleagues [26] extracted weight and mood data from 6500 individuals from the 1970 Birth Cohort Study. After controlling for childhood BMI, parental BMI, and social class, the authors found that childhood emotional problems predicted weight gain in women only (least squares regression N = 3359; coefficient 0.004, p = .032).

In summary, looking at the association between depressive symptomology and weight among the general population does not appear to differ between obese children and adolescents and their non-obese peers. However, obese youth seeking weight-related treatment are more likely to experience higher rates of depression. Though existing data are mixed, accumulating evidence indicates that obesity may predict depression, and future longitudinal research may further clarify the casual relationship between depression and obesity. Research on depressive symptoms and emotional disturbances predicting increased weight appear to be clearer, drawing attention to a possible gender difference (i.e., evidence supports that young girls and women may be at higher risk than their male counterparts). Additional longitudinal research efforts that focus on treatment-seeking youth with an emphasis on gender differences would be helpful in developing a paradigm for childhood obesity and depression.

OBESITY AND ANXIETY

In contrast to depression and obesity, relatively few studies have examined the relationship between anxiety and obesity. Findings from community samples are mixed, whereas findings from clinical samples present a clearer relationship.

Evidence against a Relationship between Childhood Obesity and Anxiety

Evidence from community-based adolescent samples in both the U.S. [27] and Germany [28] demonstrate no differences in anxiety symptoms between overweight and non-overweight youth. This cross-sectional study, conducted by Lamertz et al., employed data from the Early Developmental Stages of Psychopathology (EDSP) collected in 1994 and compared survey data from 14- to 17-year-olds with survey data from 18- to 24-year-olds. It is interesting to note that when combined, gender and BMI significantly predicted anxiety disorders among 18- to 24-year-old women. Although both these studies on U.S. and German youth did not find a relationship between weight and increased anxiety, some researchers have found such a relationship among community based samples [24, 27, 28].

Evidence for a Relationship between Childhood Obesity and Anxiety

In a nonclinical sample of Swiss high school girls (N = 136; aged 15 to 20), Buddeburg-Fisher and colleagues [24] found higher rates of anxiety disorders among overweight girls. Utilizing a more diverse sample, Britz and colleagues [18] reported findings on a rich data set in that it encompassed obese adolescents seeking inpatient weight-related treatment (N = 47) and matched obese, community adolescents (N = 47) and non-obese, community adolescents (N = 1608) all between the ages of 15 and 21. Obese adolescents in the clinical condition reported higher lifetime prevalence of anxiety disorders as compared to community-based obese and nonobese controls [18]. The most common anxiety disorder was social phobia and anxiety not otherwise specified; a diagnosis of anxiety "not otherwise specified" was due to patients reporting that their obesity underlined their presenting social anxiety [18]. Similar to Britz's findings that clinical populations may exhibit higher rates of anxiety than community populations are findings from a study conducted by Vlierberghe and colleagues [20]. Vlierberghe et al. [20] investigated European youth who visited a weight-management treatment center (N = 155; mean age 13.76) and overweight youth from a nonclinical community sample (N = 73; mean age 13.74). Although Vlierberghe [20] reported overweight youth suffer from high rates of mental disorders, those referred for treatment suffered more so, particularly with anxiety disorders, than nonreferred youth. However, the difference was not significant [20]. Compounding evidence for a relationship between anxiety and obesity in clinical youth samples, Duffecy et al. [29] noted frequent reports of anxiety symptoms in a sample of adolescents pursuing laparoscopic surgery (N = 40; 12 to 18 years). Extant research indicates youth in clinical populations display more anxiety than nonclinical peers, whereas research among youth in community populations is mixed. Limited research suggests various findings in community youth may be due to gender differences.

Prospective Studies on Childhood Obesity and Anxiety

Unfortunately, prospectively there is an even greater dearth of research between obesity and psycho pathology. The one known longitudinal study of psychological factors and pediatric weight gain was conducted by Rofey and colleagues [14] and demonstrated more substantial increases in BMI over three time points in nonobese youth with anxiety as compared to nonanxious or depressed youth [14]. More specifically this longitudinal analysis found that childhood anxiety ($\chi^2 = 6.0$, $p = 0.01$) was associated with increased BMI percentiles. Compared to controls, BMI percentiles of anxious females approached significance ($\chi^2 = 3.7$, $p = 0.06$). Males with anxiety showed a greater trend toward being overweight ($\chi^2 = 3.3$, $p = 0.07$) in comparison to controls.

Additional Considerations

Considering the paucity and inconsistency of existing research on this topic, it may be helpful to examine studies that report important covariates between weight and anxiety. An epidemiological study conducted with German youth found that even when BMI was controlled, those with disordered eating have higher rates of anxiety than youth without disordered eating (N = 1895, 11 to 17 years of age) [30]. Similar findings were reported in a sample of overweight treatment-seeking youth (N = 122; aged 8 to 18) from a Northeastern U.S. state: adolescents with eating disorders not otherwise specified (EDNOS) reported more symptoms of anxiety and depression than other overweight treatment-seeking youth [31]. Social factors may also influence the association between anxiety and weight. Storch and colleagues [32] reported that peer victimization among U.S. children from a southern state was related to reports of general and social physique anxiety among overweight and at-risk-for-overweight youth (N = 92, aged 8 to 18; mean age 13). Unfortunately, this study involved overweight and at-risk-for-becoming-overweight children only, and the relationship of BMI was not explored [32]. Positive relationships between variables such as disordered eating and anxiety in overweight youth indicate more research on factors besides weight may be helpful in conceptualizing the relationship between childhood anxiety and weight.

Currently the data on childhood obesity and anxiety remains inconclusive. Community-based research findings are mixed, perhaps due in part to gender differences. However, research on clinical samples indicates that there is a relationship between overweight youth seeking treatment and higher rates of anxiety. To date, the one known longitudinal study reports that childhood anxiety is predictive of increased BMI. Additionally, the relationship between anxiety and obesity for treatment-seeking youth may be explained by the predisposition of these youth to worry more about health and weight issues, making them more likely to seek treatment than non-anxious obese individuals. Future research in this area could help to clarify the relationship between anxiety and obesity in childhood, as well as to enhance treatment strategies and identify which populations may benefit most from prevention efforts.

EMPIRICALLY SUPPORTED TREATMENTS

The following discussion is an attempt to highlight the empirically validated treatments for obesity, depression, and anxiety (see Table 23.1). Given the scope of this chapter, the focus will be on psychotherapeutic interventions. However, ample evidence exists that highlights pharmacotherapy and surgical options for obesity (see Chapters 33 and 35, respectively). This chapter is meant to serve as an introduction for examining these interregulatory processes. Further, the argument is made to provide an enhanced intervention that addresses co-occurring disturbances. More directly addressing the interactions among psychological (depression, anxiety) and behavioral (nutrition/physical activity) disturbances in adolescents with obesity is a critical component of understanding the disease process and developing effective interventions. The rationale for this interdisciplinary mindset is framed by (at least) three lines of evidence connecting these mind-body functions: (1) adolescents with obesity are more likely to exhibit depression or anxiety, (2) emotional problems can increase aberrant eating patterns as well as sedentary behavior and decrease physical activity, and (3) physical activity can assist in positive affect.

For adults, the current gold-standard intervention results in a 10% reduction in body weight, which is typically regained within a few years of treatment [33]. Obesity interventions for children have yielded similar results, though family-based interventions have produced more persistent weight loss over time [34–36]. As shown in detail later in this discussion, Epstein et al. [34] have shown significant decreases in percentage overweight and long-term improvements in fitness level and cardiovascular risk factors for children [37]. Research of family-based behavioral treatment has also found preliminary effects such as improvements in depressive symptoms and self-esteem [38]. Epstein and colleagues [39] revealed that after 25 years of family-based interventions, "Efficacy research is needed to guide effectiveness studies…on a broader base of participants…and consist of youth who may have psychological [or medical] problems." (p. 388). Epstein and colleagues also argued that effectiveness research may indicate that the treatments are ready for broad application or may reveal important facets that make certain patients less likely to succeed. This chapter begins to present a framework offering support for including children with mood disturbances. Refer to Chapter 36 for more information on psychotherapy as an intervention for obesity.

INTERVENTIONS FOR PEDIATRIC OBESITY

Fortunately, a number of strategies have been shown to help reduce childhood obesity, and research demonstrates the positive health impact of weight-loss interventions for pediatric populations [40–42]. Similarly, long-term improvements in psychological factors (e.g., anxiety, depression) have been noted in children who have completed a weight-loss program [43].

Empirically supported treatments for pediatric obesity typically include nutritional education [44–46] and the promotion of increased physical activity [47, 48]. In addition, findings suggest that the involvement of both children and parents in treatment [49–52] contributes significantly to pediatric weight-loss efforts. Ample evidence exists for the efficacy of behavioral strategies in the treatment of pediatric obesity [52]. Behavior-based therapies stress the development of new eating and physical activity habits, as well as providing specific strategies for changing the environment. The components used in behavioral weight management treatment generally include stimulus control, self-monitoring, reinforcement of behavior change, and modeling of healthier behaviors [52]. Additionally, parent training is a key element in behavioral pediatric weight management. Parents are asked to engage in several strategies to assist their children in meeting weight-loss goals, including *contingency contracting*—parents agree to make behavioral changes alongside those of their children; *functional analysis*—parents observe and quantify the frequency of a target behavior (i.e., overeating, sedentary behavior) and subsequently note the consequences of the target behavior; and *reinforcement* programs—parents use "alternate" behavioral consequences to affect the rate of a specific behavior (e.g., money, praise, tokens, clothing). Behavioral therapy programs also utilize stimulus control techniques such as teaching individuals to clear the house of high-fat/high-calorie foods, eat more slowly, delay gratification, eat in one designated area, and eat low-calorie snacks.

One such technique developed by Leonard Epstein in the 1970s teaches a "color-coded" food strategy: high-calorie foods (greater than 5 grams of fat per serving) are coded red and should only be eaten rarely; moderate-calorie foods (between 2 and 5 grams of fat) are coded yellow and can be eaten in moderation; and low-calorie foods (less than 2 grams of fat) are coded green and can be consumed freely. Self-monitoring behavior is also a central strategy of behavioral weight-loss programs. Using this technique, the

TABLE 23.1 Examples of Empirically-validated Psychotherapeutic Strategies for the Treatment of Pediatric Obesity, Depression, and Anxiety

Therapeutic orientation	Key components	Specific techniques		
		Obesity	Depression	Anxiety
Behavioral Therapy[a]	Education	Caloric value of dietary and physical activity	Depression as a medical condition	Physiological basis of anxiety
	Behavioral monitoring	Food/activity "logging"	Daily activity monitoring	Increase awareness of anxiety "triggers" through daily self-monitoring records
	Contingency contracting and reinforcement programs	Praise/tokens for maintaining healthy eating/exercise schedule	Behavioral activation—gradually increase rewarding activities	Rewarding each phase in gradual exposure to anxiety-provoking stimuli (i.e., rewarding consecutive days of school attendance for treatment of school avoidance)
	Stimulus control techniques	Removing certain foods from home, eating in designated area	Increase time spent in positive environments	
Cognitive/ Cognitive Behavioral Therapy[b] (CBT)	Recognize connections between thoughts, feelings, and behavior and identify faulty cognitions	Identify alterations in eating behavior related to mood changes	Counter distorted thoughts ("I'm a failure") with more realistic appraisals ("I'm better at some things than others")	Identify underlying physiology of anxiety-related sensations
	Positive self-statements	Write positive script (reminders) for reference during episodes of craving	Write positive script for reference during depressive episodes	Write positive thoughts when feeling anxious sensations
	Relaxation training	Distraction, imagery	Imagery, diaphragmatic breathing, muscle relaxation	Controlled breathing, progressive muscle relaxation
	Problem solving	Role-playing, delaying gratification in "tempting" situations	Identification of the triggers and high-risk hierarchies that lead to depressogenic thoughts	Discuss support seeking from family/friends
Interpersonal Psychotherapy[c]	Focus on specific interpersonal problem areas	Identification of problem areas that have contributed to the emergence of the disorder over time, regulate emotional states that maintain bingeing behavior	Focuses on functional role of depression (rather than on etiology), examine how problematic interactions develop in response to depression	
	Grief (complicated bereavement after death of a loved one)	Identify "emotional eating" as attempt to avoid painful feelings of grief	"Revisiting"—promote sense of connection to the deceased through letter writing and similar activities	
	Role disputes (conflict with a parent, sibling, friend, etc.)	Identify conflict avoidance as possible trigger for binge eating	Identify nature of dispute; determine plan of action; modify unsatisfying patterns or reassess expectations	
	Role transitions (change in "life status," i.e., parental divorce, changing schools, etc.)	Identify difficulties with role expectations	Express feelings of guilt, anger, loss, let go of previous role; acquire new skills; develop social network around new role	
	Interpersonal deficits (chronic difficulty in initiating/sustaining relationships)	Identify deficiencies in solving social problems	Reduce social isolation by focusing on therapeutic relationship and forming new relationships	

(Continued)

TABLE 23.1 Examples of Empirically-validated Psychotherapeutic Strategies for the Treatment of Pediatric Obesity, Depression, and Anxiety—cont'd

Therapeutic orientation	Key components	Specific techniques Obesity	Depression	Anxiety
Psychodynamic Therapy[d]				Use play therapy to identify conflict driving maladaptive coping behavior (i.e., chaotic family environment drives child to employ obsessive rituals) to understand current behavior
Motivational Interviewing[e]	Collaborative—focus on individual's goals and values	"How would your life change if you adopted a healthier lifestyle?"		
		Identify the behaviors that you would like to change		
	Directive—focus on function of ambivalence to elicit motivation	"What are the good things about eating healthier or being more physically active? What are some not-so-good things?"		
	Incorporates "change talk"	If ambivalent, listen for the desire/ability/reason/need talk		
	Rolling with resistance	Use simple and complex reflections to come alongside of the patient to acknowledge the negatives about change		

[a]Wadden, T.A., & Foster, G.D. (2000). Behavioral treatment of obesity. *The Medical Clinics of North America, 84,* 441-461.
[b]Beck A. (1997). The past and future of cognitive therapy. *Journal of Psychotherapy Practice and Research, 6,* 276-284.
[c]Weissman, M.M., Markowitz, J., & Klerman, G.L. (2000). *Comprehensive Guide to Interpersonal Psychotherapy.* New York: Basic Behavioral Science Books.
[d]Warren, C.S., & Messer, S.B. (1999). Brief psychodynamic therapy with anxious children. In S.W. Russ & T.H. Ollendick (Eds.), *Handbook of Psychotherapies with Children and Families.* New York: Springer.
[e]Miller, W., & Rollnick, S. (2002). *Motivational Interviewing (2nd ed.). Preparing People for Change.* New York: Guilford Press.

individuals maintain records of when and where they engage in behaviors that are either supportive of or detrimental to weight-loss efforts.

Early research from the 1970s and 1980s [36, 53–56], as well as more recent work from the 1990s [35, 42, 56], support the use of behavioral family-based interventions for pediatric weight loss. In particular, the work of Epstein and colleagues provides compelling evidence for using behavioral interventions in the treatment of pediatric obesity [42, 56]. The results of several of Epstein's randomized clinical trials, in which children aged 6 to 12 years (along with one supportive caregiver) received a 6-month behavioral weight-loss intervention, show that 30% of the children were no longer obese 10 years post intervention. Overall, behavioral-based family therapy and lifestyle modification appear to be effective in the treatment of obesity in children.

Though some evidence suggests that a behavioral approach to pediatric obesity may be superior to cognitive strategies [57], the inclusion of cognitive components in laboratory-based investigations of childhood and adult weight loss have shown favorable results [36, 56, 58, 59]. Cognitive behavioral therapy (CBT) attempts to address issues that may have been overlooked in early behavioral programs, including cognitive distortions regarding body image and eating, instruction in self-monitoring, problem-solving techniques, motivational issues, and focusing on specific weight-loss goals and barriers to healthy behavior. Similar to behavioral programs, cognitive components are typically used in conjunction with dietary and physical activity education. One early cognitive-behavioral treatment program for children aged 9 to 13 years utilized a 9-week program that included dietary and physical activity self-monitoring, cognitive strategies for managing negative self-statements, and assertiveness training [60]. Children in the cognitive treatment group lost significantly more weight than controls and retained their weight loss at 3-month follow-up. Duffy and Spence [61] randomly assigned 27 overweight children (aged 7 to 13 years) to eight sessions of either behavioral management or combined CBT. No differences between treatment groups were noted, and both groups of children demonstrated significant improvements in weight at 6- and 9-month follow-up. Thus, although additional research is needed to establish whether differences in outcomes may exist between behavioral treatment and cognitively based strategies, it appears that the two approaches to pediatric weight loss may be equally valuable.

Interpersonal psychotherapy (IPT) has been adapted for the treatment of binge eating disorder, which has been associated with obesity [62, 63]. Originally designed as a time-limited treatment for depression, IPT is based on the theory that interpersonal functioning is a key component of well-being and approaches treatment in the context of interpersonal difficulties in one or more problem areas [64]. In light of evidence linking binge eating behavior to difficulty in social interactions, feelings of loneliness, or other negative emotions [65, 66], IPT has been modified for treatment of patients with eating disturbances [67–69]. IPT has been successful in the treatment of bulimia nervosa [67] and has shown efficacy in reducing binge eating episodes in response to negative affect and disordered eating psychopathology in adults [68, 69]. It has been suggested that IPT may be useful in reducing excessive weight gain over time in adolescents at risk for overweight; to date, however, only one pilot study exists in this area [70].

Research on motivational interviewing (MI) for treatment of obesity in pediatric populations is limited, yet promising. MI is a therapeutic strategy aimed at helping individuals to explore ambivalence about making behavioral changes and has been suggested as a possible tool for helping achieve dietary and physical activity modifications [71]. Utilizing reflective listening and methods to elicit "change talk," MI seeks to resolve ambivalence and strengthen the client's reasons for engaging in positive behavior change consistent with one's goals and values [72]. Although behavioral modification is considered to be efficacious for weight loss in youth, compliance issues often lead the families of obese children and adolescents to seek alternate, though riskier, strategies (e.g., pharmacotherapy, bariatric surgery) [44]. Motivational interviewing techniques aimed toward enhancing adherence to dietary and exercise recommendations in children and families could play a key role in promoting weight management.

To date, however, little research has been done in the area of MI and pediatric weight loss. Some data suggest that MI assists in promoting healthier eating habits, increasing physical activity, and improving weight status in adults, but these findings are not consistent [73–75]. Thus far, only two pediatric weight-loss interventions have employed MI techniques: the Healthy Lifestyles Pilot Study [76] and Go Girls [77].

The Healthy Lifestyles Pilot Study, conducted from 2004 to 2005, was aimed at preventing obesity among children 3 to 7 years old [76]. Pediatric Research in Office Settings (PROS) clinicians were trained to provide motivational interviewing to patients during office visits. Patients in the control group received usual care, whereas those in the "Minimal" group received one MI session and those in the "Intensive" group received two MI sessions during office visits. At the 6-month follow-up, patients in the Minimal and Intensive groups showed a trend of decreasing BMI-for-age percentiles, though results were not statistically significant. Decreases in families' "eating out" behavior and high-calorie snacking were also noted. Thus, although children's weight changes failed to reach significance, this study demonstrated the feasibility of implementing a brief, physician office-based obesity prevention program using MI. Go Girls was a church-based nutrition and physical activity program designed for overweight African American adolescent females. In one of the treatment conditions, girls received four to six MI telephone counseling calls focused on the participants' progress. Unfortunately, both 6-month and 1-year post assessments indicated no significant BMI differences between the MI group and controls. Thus, at present, insufficient data exist to determine the efficacy of MI for the prevention or treatment of pediatric obesity in children [78].

Childhood Depression

Major depressive disorder is relatively common during childhood with an estimated prevalence of approximately 1% to 2% in school-aged children (6- to 12-year-olds) and 2% to 5% in adolescents (13- to 18-year-olds) [79]. Depression in adolescence interferes with normative social and emotional processes during a sensitive period of development and may have lasting negative consequences on future adult functioning [80, 81].

Although extensive clinical intervention research has been conducted on adult depression, clinical interventions for child and adolescent depression have been understudied. Both psychotherapeutic and pharmacological treatment studies of major depression through the lifespan are complicated by a relatively high placebo or nonspecific treatment response rate, approaching 30% [82]. CBT seems to be effective in treating child and adolescent depression [83, 84]. CBT for depression involves several essential features: identifying and correcting inaccurate thoughts associated with depressed feelings (cognitive restructuring), helping patients to engage more often in enjoyable activities (behavioral activation), and enhancing problem-solving skills. To date, there have been no large-scale efficacy studies comparing psychosocial treatments for preadolescent depression and, hence, no efficacious treatments have been identified for this high-risk group. The only study that compares treatment with non-waitlist controls is the study of Brent and colleagues [85] that showed superiority of CBT over family and supportive therapies with good control for treatment contact amount and treatment expectancy. In the Treatment for Adolescents with Depression Study (TADS)—the only controlled study comparing psychotherapeutic and pharmacological approaches—CBT alone (43% response rate) was not superior to placebo (35% response rate) in any analysis, fluoxetine alone (61% response rate) was superior to CBT alone in both preplanned analyses and was superior to placebo in one of the two analyses, and CBT plus a selective serotonin reuptake inhibitor (SSRI) (71% response rate) was superior to CBT alone and placebo alone in both analyses and slightly better than SSRI alone in one analysis. However, two emerging CBT treatment protocols, Taking Action [86] and Primary and Secondary Control Enhancement Training [87], have demonstrated promise in effectively treating childhood depression as compared to waitlist control groups. Interpersonal psychotherapy (IPT) has also been studied by two groups in open and controlled trials for adolescent depression [88, 89]. IPT was shown to be superior to a treatment-as-usual control [88], and in another study, both IPT and CBT were significantly better than a waitlist approach [89].

Childhood Anxiety

Anxiety disorders represent one of the most common forms of psychopathology among children and adolescents, but they often go undetected or untreated. Early identification and effective treatment may reduce the impact of anxiety on academic and social functioning in youth and may reduce the persistence of anxiety disorders into adulthood. Psychotherapy and medication treatment of childhood anxiety have emerged as evidence-supported treatment [90]. In the recent Cochran review of CBT for anxiety disorders in children and adolescents [91], 13 studies with a total of 498 subjects and 311 controls were included in the meta-analysis. Analyses for all children enrolled showed a 56% overall response rate for CBT versus 28.2% for controls (RR 0.58, 95% CI 0.50-0.67). The standardized mean difference in reduction in anxiety symptoms across the studies was −0.58 (superiority of treatment over control). Across studies, 87.3% of subjects in the CBT groups completed the treatment trial and only 12.4% were lost to follow-up. All subjects in these trials were outpatients. Post-hoc analyses found that individual, group, and family/parental formats of CBT produced similar outcomes. The improvement from therapy appears durable—in the 10 studies that reported follow-up data (mean follow-up = 13 months; range, 3 to 72 months), the proportion in remission at follow-up was 69%. These figures are compatible with an earlier meta-analysis [92]. These data suggest that CBT for child anxiety is efficacious and well tolerated by patients and their families.

Numerous case studies indicate that psychodynamic therapy is helpful for anxiety disorders [93–95]; however, there is limited research on the efficacy or effectiveness of psychodynamic therapy alone, in combined treatments, or compared with other modalities [96]. Psychodynamic therapists "understand anxiety as a signal of internal distress and conflict that motivates the individual to employ internalized, largely unconscious coping strategies, defense mechanisms, and compromise formations. Anxiety disorders result when the signals interfere with normal behavior and development" (p. 275). Thus, the goal of psychodynamic therapy is to bring the anxiety back to functional levels and for the child to regain a healthy developmental trajectory [90].

Last, research and clinical experience suggest that parents and families may play an important role in the development and maintenance of childhood anxiety. Parental anxiety, parenting anxiety, parenting styles, insecure attachment, and parent-child interactions are risk factors that may not be addressed by child-only interventions. Selective serotonin reuptake inhibitors (SSRIs) have also emerged as the medication of choice in the treatment of childhood anxiety disorders. When anxiety disorder symptoms are moderate or severe or impairment makes participation in psychotherapy challenging, pharmacology is recommended [97, 98].

ENHANCED TREATMENT

Considering that psychological and emotional disturbances are intertwined with obesity and that more than one-third of obese patients seeking treatment are depressed [99], it is important for interventionists and researchers to consider treatment of both disorders. Regardless of causality, treating depression/anxiety and obesity may enhance the treatment and show greater effects in both areas. Zametkin, Jacobs, and Parrish [100] have suggested that treating one disorder (obesity or mood disorders) may lead to improvements in the other disorder. Moreover, it should be noted that pervasive, genetically driven psychopathology may need to be treated before weight management based on the presenting circumstances (e.g., suicidality, more severe mental illness [bipolar disorder/psychotic presentations]). The notion that treating both disorders may increase the overall effectiveness of the treatment program may be a logical hypothesis.

Although there is a strong link between psychological disorders and obesity, and it seems obvious to theorize that treating both may lead to better treatment outcomes, current research often excludes participants with psychological diagnoses [100]. A direct result of this lack of research is that no evidence-based interventions currently exist for depressed, obese individuals [99]. Furthermore, even less research has been conducted on treatments for obese individuals diagnosed with an anxiety disorder, and no evidence-based interventions focusing on both facets are available. One reason for the lack of treatment designed for obese and anxious individuals may be due to the highly confounded nature of depression and anxiety. Some may argue that early childhood anxiety may eventually lead to depression given that two thirds of youth diagnosed with an anxiety disorder later develop depression [101–103]. Because of the lack of interventions focusing on anxiety and obesity and the comorbidity of depression and anxiety, this section primarily focuses on two enhanced treatments working to treat depression and obesity.

Pagoto et al. recognized the need for empirical evidence for treatment of psychopathologies in conjunction with treatment for obesity [99]. This study targeted weight reduction and depression in 14 adult participants through behavioral activation (BA) treatment, a treatment commonly used with depressed patients that "aims to increase exposure to the positive consequences of healthy behavior in order to increase the frequency of healthy behaviors and reduce the frequency of depressive behaviors" (p. 411). Using BA to treat overweight patients stems from Pagoto and colleagues' previous research that revealed that women with a high BMI tended to participate in less rewarding behaviors than women with a lower BMI [104]. Results from Pagoto, et al.'s [99] current study indicates that BA may be helpful in weight-loss treatment for depressed individuals as participants showed an overall decrease in weight and caloric intake as well as depressive symptoms following treatment.

Another study that targeted this scantily researched area focused on treatment of depression and obesity in adolescent girls with polycystic ovary syndrome (PCOS), an endocrine disorder that predisposes women to suffer from depressive symptoms and obesity [4]. This study involved 12 depressed and overweight adolescent girls diagnosed with PCOS. Treatment involved CBT sessions enhanced with nutrition and fitness goals, primary and secondary control enhancement training (PASCET-PI-2), and family psychoeducation. Participants met individually with a behavioral coach for eight sessions that focused on weight and depression, scheduling behaviorally activating events, and positive thinking and cognitive restructuring. Simultaneously, the family met with a behavioral coach for three sessions that focused on similar topics. Each individual session was followed with 15 to 20 minutes of physical activity. Following this intervention, participants in Rofey et al.'s study showed a significant decrease in weight and a significant decrease in depressive symptoms.

There is an overall lack of interventions for treating both emotional disturbances and obesity. Studies such as Pagoto et al.'s [99] and Rofey et al.'s [4] provide evidence that enhanced treatment focusing on psychopathologies in addition to obesity are feasible and may be useful for a subset of patients. Moreover, as Table 23.1 shows, many of the therapeutic interventions for the individual presenting symptoms (obesity, depression, and anxiety) target similar underlying processes. More research like this, that does not exclude patients based on psychological diagnoses, is needed. These studies will assist in assessing the effectiveness of broad-based interventions bridging interregulatory processes for a subset of patients.

CONCLUSION

Obesity in pediatric and adolescent populations has reached epidemic proportions in the United States. In addition to the increased risk of cardiovascular [105, 106], orthopedic [107], and pulmonary [108] complications faced by overweight youth, the accompanying psychosocial correlates of obesity may adversely affect overall quality of life [39, 109]. To complicate obesity treatment, many empirically validated interventions exclude participants who have comorbid psychiatric diagnoses. The complex, intertwined relationships between behavioral (nutrition/physical activity) and emotional (depression, anxiety) disturbances complicate treatment as the age-old questions arise—what comes first and how do we treat it? Some researchers argue that a patient must be stabilized psychiatrically before engaging in weight management [100]. However, few studies have examined low-level psychopathology and whether it is more effective to utilize empirically validated obesity treatment first, alongside, or simultaneous to treating the presenting psychopathology. As this discussion shows, few studies have methodically addressed these issues while providing treatment. Data are provided that show that the same techniques that are empirically validated for the treatment of childhood obesity—CBT, IPT, and MI therapies—may be efficacious in treating childhood mood disturbances (namely depression and anxiety). Even in more severe cases of obesity and mood disorders, when practitioners may consider additional approaches such as pharmacotherapy or bariatric surgery, these therapies can make a significant contribution to enhancing patients' quality of life and compliance with the interventions [110].

References

1. Institute of Medicine. *Preventing childhood obesity*. Washington, DC: National Academy of Science; 2004.
2. Center for Disease Control. *Prevalence of overweight and obesity among adults*. Hyattsville, MD: U.S. Department of Health and Human Services; 2003.
3. Anderson S, Cohen P, Naumova E, Must A. Association of depression and anxiety disorders with weight change in a prospective community-based study of children followed up into adulthood. *Archives of Pediatric and Adolescent Medicine* 2006;**160**:285–91.
4. Rofey DL, Szigethy E, Noll R, Dahl R, Iobst E, Arslanian S. Cognitive-behavioral therapy for physical and emotional disturbances in adolescents with Polycystic Ovary Syndrome: A pilot study. *Journal of Pediatric Psychology* 2009;**34**:156–63.
5. Faith M, Allison D, Geliebter A. Emotional eating and obesity: Theoretical considerations and practical recommendations. In: Dalton S, editor. *Obesity and weight control: The health professional's guide to understanding and practice*. Gaithersburg, MD: Aspen; 1997. pp. 439–65.
6. Franko D, Striegel-Moore R, Thompson D, Schreiber G, Daniels S. Does adolescent depression predict obesity in black and white young adult women? *Psychological Medicine* 2005;**35**: 1505–13.
7. Dahl R. Adolescent brain development: a period of vulnerabilities and opportunities. *Annals of the New York Academy of the Sciences* 2004;**1021**:1–22.
8. Lewinsohn P, Hops H, Roberts R, Seeley J, Andrews J. Adolescent psychopathology: I. Prevalence and incidence of depression and other DSM-III-R disorders in high school students. *Journal of Abnormal Psychology* 1993;**102**:133–44.
9. Goodman E, Whitaker R. A prospective study of the role of depression in the development and persistence of adolescent obesity. *Pediatrics* 2002;**110**:497–504.
10. Pine D, Goldstein R, Wolk S, Weissman M. The association between childhood depression and adulthood body mass index. *Pediatrics* 2001;**107**:1049–56.
11. Vila G, Zipper E, Dabbas M, Bertrand C, Robert J, Ricour C. Mental disorders in obese children and adolescents. *Psychosomatic Medicine* 2004;**66**:387–94.
12. Pietrobelli A, Flodmark C, Lissau I, Moreno L, Widhalm K. From birth to adolescence: Vienna 2005 European Childhood Obesity Group International Workshop. *International Journal of Obesity* 2005;**29**:1–6.
13. O'Dea J, Wilson R. Socio-cognitive and nutritional factors associated with body mass index in children and adolescents: Possibilities for childhood obesity prevention. *Health Education Research* 2006;**21**:796–805.
14. Rofey D, Kolko R, Iosif A, Silk J, Bost J, Feng W. A longitudinal study of childhood depression and anxiety in relation to weight gain. *Child Psychiatry and Human Development* 2009;**40**: 517–26.
15. Eisenberg M, Neumark-Sztainer D, Story M. Associations of weight-based teasing and emotional well-being among adolescents. *Archives of Pediatric and Adolescent Medicine* 2003;**157**:733–8.
16. Brewis A. Biocultural aspects of obesity in young Mexican schoolchildren. *American Journal of Human Biology* 2003;**15**: 446–60.
17. Wardle J, Williamson S, Johnson F, Edwards C. Depression in adolescent obesity: Cultural moderators of the association between obesity and depressive symptoms. *International Journal of Obesity* 2006;**30**:543–634.
18. Britz B, Siegfried W, Ziegler A, Lamertz C, Herpertz-Dahlmann B, Remschmidt H. Rates of psychiatric disorders in a clinical study group of adolescents with extreme obesity and in obese adolescents ascertained via a population based study. *International Journal of Obesity and Related Metabolic Disorders* 2000;**24**:1707–14.
19. Erermis S, Cetis N, Tamar M, Bukusoglu N, Akdeniz F, Goksen D. Is obesity a risk factor for psychopathology among adolescents? *Pediatrics International* 2004;**46**:296–301.
20. Vlierberghe L, Braet C, Goossens L, Mels S. Psychiatric disorders and symptom severity in referred versus non-referred overweight children and adolescents. *European Child and Adolescent Psychiatry* 2009;**18**:164–73.
21. Merten M, Wickrama K, Williams A. Adolescent obesity and young adult psychosocial outcomes: Gender and racial differences. *Journal of Youth and Adolescence* 2008;**37**:1111–12.
22. Mustillo S, Worthman C, Erkanli A, Keeler G, Angold A, Costello E. Obesity and psychiatric disorder: Developmental trajectories. *Pediatrics* 2003;**111**:851–9.
23. Goodman E, Whitaker R. A prospective study of the role of depression in the development and persistence of adolescent obesity. *Pediatrics* 2002;**110**:497–504.
24. Buddeburg-Fisher B, Klaghofer R, Reed V. Associations between body weight, psychiatric disorders and body image in female adolescents. *Psychotherapy and Psychosomatics* 1999;**68**:325–32.
25. Anderson S, Cohen P, Naumova E, Jacques P, Must A. Adolescent obesity and risk for subsequent major depressive disorder and anxiety disorder: Prospective evidence. *Psychosomatic Medicine* 2007;**69**:740–7.
26. Ternouth A, Collier D, Maughan B. Childhood emotional problems and self-perceptions predict weight gain in a longitudinal regression model. *BMC Medicine* 2009;**7**:46.
27. Tanofsky-Kraff M, Yanovski S, Wilfley D, Marmarosh C, Morgan C, Yanovski J. Eating-disordered behaviors, body fat, and psychopathology in overweight and normal-weight children. *Journal of Consulting and Clinical Psychology* 2004;**72**:53–61.
28. Lamertz C, Jacobi C, Yassouridis A, Arnold K, Henkel A. Are obese adolescents and young adults at risk for mental disorders? A community survey. *Obesity Research* 2002;**10**:1152–60.
29. Duffecy J, Bleil M, Labott S, Browne A, Galvani C. Psychopathology in adolescents presenting for laparoscopic banding. *Journal of Adolescent Health* 2008;**43**:623–5.
30. Herpertz-Dahlmann B, Wille N, Holling H, Vloet T, Ravens-Sieberer U. Disordered eating behaviour and attitudes, associated psychopathology and health-related quality of life: Results of the BELLA study. *European Child and Adolescent Psychiatry* 2008;**17**:82–91.
31. Eddy K, Tanofsky-Kraff M, Thompson-Brenner H, Herzog D, Brown T, Ludwig D. Eating disorder pathology among overweight treatment-seeking youth: Clinical correlates and cross-sectional risk modeling. *Behaviour Research and Therapy* 2007;**45**:2360–71.
32. Storch E, Milsom V, DeBraganza N, Lewin A, Geffken G, Silverstein J. Peer victimization, psychosocial adjustment, and physical activity in overweight and at-risk-for-overweight youth. *Journal of Pediatric Psychology* 2007;**32**:80–9.

REFERENCES

33. Jeffery R, Drewnowski A, Epstein L, Stunkard A, Wilson G, Wing R, et al. Long-term maintenance of weight loss: Current status. *Health Psychology* 2000;**19**:5—16.
34. Epstein L, Myers M, Raynor H, Saelens B. Treatment of pediatric obesity. *Pediatrics* 1998;**101**:554—70.
35. Epstein L, Valoski A, Wing R, McCurley J. Ten-year follow-up of behavioral, family-based treatment for obese children. *Journal of the American Medical Association* 1990;**264**:2519—23.
36. Flodmark C, Ohlsson T, Ryden O, Sveger T. Prevention of progression to severe obesity in a group of obese school children treated with family therapy. *Pediatrics* 1993;**91**:880—4.
37. Epstein L, Kuller L, Wing R, Valoski A, McCurley J. The effect of weight control on lipid changes in obese children. *American Journal of Diseases of Children* 1989;**143**:454—7.
38. Levine M, Ringham R, Kalarchian M, Wisniewski L, Marcus M. Is family-based behavioral weight control appropriate for severe pediatric obesity? *International Journal of Eating Disorders* 2001;**30**:318—28.
39. Epstein L, Paluch R, Roemmich J, Beecher M. Family-based obesity treatment, then and now: Twenty-five years of pediatric obesity treatment. *Health Psychology* 2007;**26**:381—91.
40. Schwimmer J, Burwinkle T, Varni J. Health-related quality of life of severely obese children and adolescents. *Journal of the American Medical Association* 2003;**289**:1813—19.
41. Becque M, Katch V, Rocchini A, Marks C, Moorehead C. Coronary risk incidence of obese adolescents: Reduction by exercise plus diet intervention. *Pediatrics* 1988;**81**:605—12.
42. Epstein L, Valoski A, Kalarchian M, McCurley J. Do children lose and maintain weight easier than adults: A comparison of child and parent weight changes from six months to ten years. *Obesity Research* 1995;**3**:411—17.
43. Katch V, Becque M, Marks C, Moorehead C, Rocchini A. Basal metabolism of obese adolescents: Inconsistent diet and exercise effects. *American Journal of Clinical Nutrition* 1988;**48**:565—9.
44. Epstein L, Wing R, Koeske R, Valoski A. Effects of diet plus exercise on weight change in parents and children. *Journal of Consulting and Clinical Psychology* 1984;**52**:429—37.
45. Epstein L, Wing R, Penner B, Kress M. The effect of diet and controlled exercise on weight loss in obese children. *Journal of Pediatrics* 1985;**107**:358—61.
46. Emes C, Velde B, Moreau M, Murdoch D, Trussell R. An activity based weight control program. *Adapted Physical Activity Quarterly* 1990;**7**:314—24.
47. Epstein L. Exercise in the treatment of childhood obesity. *International Journal of Obesity and Related Metabolic Disorders* 1995;**19**:S117—21.
48. Epstein L, Goldfield G. Physical activity in the treatment of childhood overweight and obesity: Current evidence and research issues. *Medicine and Science in Sports and Exercise* 1999;**31**:S553—9.
49. Brownell K, Kelman J, Stunkard A. Treatment of obese children with and without their mothers: Changes in weight and blood pressure. *Pediatrics* 1983;**71**:515—23.
50. Kingsley R, Shapiro J. A comparison of three behavioral programs for the control of obesity in children. *Behavior Therapy* 1977;**8**:30—6.
51. Renjilian D, Perri M, Nezu A, McKelvey W, Shermer R, Anton SD. Individual versus group therapy for obesity: Effects of matching participants to their treatment preferences. *Journal of Consulting and Clinical Psychology* 2001;**69**:717—21.
52. Epstein L, Paluch R, Kilanowski C, Raynor H. The effect of reinforcement or stimulus control to reduce sedentary behavior in the treatment of pediatric obesity. *Health Psychology* 2004;**23**:371—80.
53. Aragona J, Cassady J, Drabman R. Treating overweight children through parental training and contingency contracting. *Journal of Applied Behavioral Analysis* 1975;**8**:269—78.
54. Coates T, Killen J, Slinkard L. Parent participation in a treatment program for overweight adolescents. *International Journal of Eating Disorders* 1982;**1**:37—48.
55. Gross I, Wheeler M, Hess K. The treatment of obesity in adolescents using behavioral self-control. *Clinical Pediatrics* 1976;**15**:920—4.
56. Epstein L, Valoski A, Wing R, McCurley J. Ten year outcomes of behavioral family-based treatment for childhood obesity. *Health Psychology* 1994;**13**:373—83.
57. Herrera E, Johnston C, Steele R. Comparison of cognitive and behavioral treatments for pediatric obesity. *Children's Health Care* 2004;**33**:151—67.
58. Senediak C, Spence S. Rapid versus gradual scheduling of therapeutic contact in a family-based behavioral weight control program for children. *Behavioral Psychotherapy* 1985;**13**:265—87.
59. Williams C, Bollella M, Carter B. Treatment of childhood obesity in pediatric practice. *Annals of the New York Academy of Science* 1993;**699**:207—19.
60. Kirschenbaum D, Harris E, Tomarken A. Effects of parental involvement in behavioral weight loss therapy for preadolescents. *Behavior Therapy* 1984;**15**:485—500.
61. Duffy G, Spence S. The effectiveness of cognitive self-management as an adjunct to a behavioral intervention for childhood obesity: A research note. *Journal of Child Psychology and Psychiatry* 1993;**34**:1043—50.
62. de Zwaan M. Binge eating disorder and obesity. International journal of obesity and related metabolic disorders. *Journal of the International Association for the Study of Obesity* 2001;**25**:S51—5.
63. Yanovski S, Nelson J, Dubbert B, Spitzer R. Association of binge eating disorder and psychiatric comorbidity in obese subjects. *American Journal of Psychiatry* 1993;**150**:1472—9.
64. Weissman M, Markowitz J, Klerman G. *Comprehensive Guide to Interpersonal Psychotherapy*. New York: Basic Books; 2000.
65. Steiger H, Gauvin L, Jabalpurwala S, Seguin R, Stotland S. Hypersensitivity to social interactions in bulimic syndromes: Relationship to binge eating. *Journal of consulting and clinical psychology* 1999;**67**:765—75.
66. Wilfley D, Pike K, Streigel-Moore R. Toward an integrated model of risk for binge eating disorder. *Journal of Gender, Culture, and Health* 1997;**2**:1—3.
67. Fairburn C, Jones R, Peveler R. Three psychological treatments for bulimia nervosa. A comparative trial. *Archives of General Psychiatry* 1991;**48**:463—9.
68. Wilfley D, Agras W, Telch C, Rossiter E, Schneider J, Cole A, et al. Group cognitive behavioral therapy and group interpersonal psychotherapy for the nonpurging bulimic individual: A controlled comparison. *Journal of Consulting and Clinical Psychology* 1993;**61**:296—305.
69. Wilfley D, Welch R, Stein R, Spurrell E, Cohen L, Saelens B, et al. A randomized comparison of group cognitive-behavioral therapy and group interpersonal psychotherapy for the treatment of overweight individuals with binge-eating disorder. *Archives of general psychiatry* 2002;**59**:713—21.
70. Tanofsky-Kraff M, Wilfley D, Young J, Mufson L, Yanovski S, Glasofer D. Preventing excessive weight gain in adolescents: Interpersonal psychotherapy for binge eating. *Obesity* 2007;**15**:1345—55.
71. DiLillo V, Siegfried N, Smith W. Incorporating motivational interviewing into behavioral obesity treatment. *Cognitive and Behavioral Practice* 2004;**10**:120—30.
72. Miller W, Rollnick S. Preparing People for Change., *Motivational Interviewing*. 2nd ed. New York: Guilford Press; 2002.

73. Dunn C, Deroo L, Rivara F. The use of brief interventions adapted from motivational interviewing across behavioral domains: A systematic review. *Addiction* 2001;**12**:1725–42.
74. Berg-Smith S, Stevens V, Brown K, Van Horn L, Gernhofer N, Peters E. A brief motivational intervention to improve dietary adherence in adolescents. The Dietary Intervention Study in Children (DISC) Research Group. *Health Education Research* 1999;**14**:399–410.
75. Smith D, Heckemeyer C, Kratt P, Mason D. Motivational interviewing to improve adherence to a behavioral weight-control program for older obese women with NIDDM: A pilot study. *Diabetes Care* 1997;**20**:52–4.
76. Schwartz R, Hamre R, Dietz W, Wasseman R, Slora E, Myers E, et al. Office-based motivational interviewing to prevent childhood obesity: A feasibility study. *Archives of Pediatrics and Adolescent Medicine* 1997;**161**:495–501.
77. Resnicow K, Taylor R, Baskin M. Results of go girls: A nutrition and physical activity intervention for overweight African American adolescent females conducted through Black churches. *Obesity Research* 2005;**13**:1739–48.
78. Resnicow K, Davis R, Rollnick S. Motivational Interviewing for pediatric obesity: Conceptual issues and evidence review. *Journal of American Dietetic Association* 2006;**106**:2024–33.
79. Fleming J, Offord D. Epidemiology of childhood depressive disorders: A critical review. *Journal of the American Academy of Child and Adolescent Psychiatry* 1990;**29**:571–80.
80. Fergusson D, Horwood L, Ridder E, Beautrais A. Suicidal behavior in adolescence and subsequent mental health outcomes in young adulthood. *Psychological Medicine* 2005;**35**:983–93.
81. Lewinsohn P, Rohde P, Klein D, Seeley J. Natural course of adolescent major depressive disorder: I. Continuity into young adulthood. *Journal of the American Academy of Child and Adolescent Psychiatry* 1999;**38**:56–63.
82. Ryan N. Treatment of depression in children and adolescents. *The Lancet* 2005;**366**:933–40.
83. Harrington R, Campbell F, Shoebridge P, Whittaker J. Meta-analysis of CBT for depression in adolescents. *Journal of the American Academy of Child and Adolescent Psychiatry* 1998;**37**:1005–7.
84. Lewinsohn P, Clarke G. Psychosocial treatments for adolescent depression. *Clinical Psychology Review* 1999;**19**:329–42.
85. Brent D, Holder D, Kolko D, Birmaher B, Baugher M, Roth C, et al. A clinical psychotherapy trial for adolescent depression comparing cognitive, family, and supportive therapy. *Archives of General Psychiatry* 1997;**54**:877–85.
86. Stark K, Kendall P, McCarthy M, Stafford M, Barron R, Thomeer M. *Taking action: A workbook for overcoming depression.* Ardmore, PA: Workbook Publishing; 1996.
87. Weisz J, Thurber C, Sweeney L, Proffitt V, LeGagnoux G. Brief treatment of mild-to-moderate child depression using primary and secondary control enhancement training. *Journal of Consulting and Clinical Psychology* 1997;**65**:703–7.
88. Mufson L, Pollack Dorta K, Moreau D, Weissman M. *Interpersonal psychotherapy for depressed adolescents.* 2nd ed. New York: Guilford Publications, Inc; 2004.
89. Rossello J, Bernal G. The efficacy of cognitive-behavioural and interpersonal treatments for depression in Puerto Rican adolescents. *Journal of Consulting and Clinical Psychology* 1999;**67**:734–45.
90. Connolly S, Bernstein G, Bernet W, Bukstein O, Arnold V, Beitchman J, et al. Practice parameter for the assessment and treatment of children and adolescents with anxiety disorder. *Journal of the American Academy of Child and Adolescent Psychiatry* 2007;**46**:267–83.
91. James A, Soler A, Weatherall R. Cognitive behavioural therapy for anxiety disorders in children and adolescents. *Cochrane Database System Review, 4, CD004690*; 2005.
92. Weisz J, Thurber C, Sweeney L, Proffitt V, LeGagnoux G. Brief treatment of mild-to-moderate child depression using primary and secondary control enhancement training. *Journal of Consulting and Clinical Psychology* 1997;**65**:703–7.
93. Goldberger M. Enactment and play following medical trauma: An analytic case study. *Psychoanalytic Study of the Child* 1995;**50**:252–71.
94. McGehee R. Child psychoanalysis and obsessive-compulsive symptoms: The treatment of a ten-year-old boy. *Journal of the American Psychoanalytic Association* 2005;**53**:213–37.
95. Novick K. Issues in the analysis of a preschool girl. *Psychoanalytic Study of the Child* 1974;**29**:319–40.
96. Lis A, Zennaro A, Mazzeschi C. Child and adolescent empirical psychotherapy research: A review focused on cognitive-behavioral and psychodynamic-informed psychotherapy. *European Journal of Psychology* 2001;**6**:36–64.
97. Birmaher B, Yelovich K, Renaud J. Pharmacologic treatment for children and adolescents with anxiety disorders. *Pediatrics Clinic of North America* 1998;**45**:1187–204.
98. Labellarte M, Ginsburg G, Walkup J, Riddle M. The treatment of anxiety disorders in children and adolescents. *Biological Psychiatry* 1999;**46**:1567–78.
99. Pagoto S, Bodenlos J, Schneider K, Olendzki B, Spates C, Ma Y. Initial investigation of behavioral activation treatment for comorbid major depressive disorder and obesity. *Psychotherapy: Theory, Research and Practice* 2008;**45**:410–15.
100. Zametkin A, Jacobs A, Parrish J. Treatment of children and adolescents with obesity and comorbid psychiatric conditions. In: Jelalian E, Steele R, editors. *Handbook of Childhood and Adolescent Obesity: Treatment of children and adolescents with obesity and comorbid psychiatric conditions.* New York: Springer-Verlag; 2008. pp. 425–43.
101. Brady E, Kendall P. Comorbidity of anxiety and depression in children and adolescents. *Psychological Bulletin* 1992;**111**:244–55.
102. Kovacs M, Gatsonis C, Paulauskas S, Richards C. Depressive disorders in childhood. IV. A longitudinal study of comorbidity with and risk for anxiety disorders. *Archives of General Psychiatry* 1989;**46**:776–82.
103. Pine D, Cohen P, Gurley D, Brook J, Ma Y. The risk for early-adulthood anxiety and depressive disorders in adolescents with anxiety and depressive disorders. *Archives of General Psychiatry* 1998;**55**:56–64.
104. Pagoto S, Spring B, Cook J, McChargue D, Schneider K. High BMI and reduced frequency and enjoyment of pleasant events. *Personality and Individual Differences* 2006;**40**:1421–31.
105. Must A, Strauss R. Risks and consequences of childhood and adolescent obesity. *International Journal of Obesity and Related Metabolic Disorders* 1999;**23**:S2–11.
106. Reilly J, Methven E, McDowell Z, Hacking B, Alexander D, Stewart L, Kelnar C. Health consequences of obesity. *Archives of Disease in Childhood* 2003;**88**:748–52.
107. Dietz W. Health consequences of obesity in youth: Childhood predictors of adult disease. *Pediatrics* 1998;**101**:518–24.
108. Kolotkin R, Crosby R, Corey-Lisle P, Li H, Swanson J. Performance of a weight-related measure of quality of life in a psychiatric sample. *Quality of Life Research* 2006;**15**:587–96.
109. Lazarus R, Colditz G, Berkey C, Speizer F. Effects of body fat on ventilatory function in children and adolescents: Cross-sectional findings from a random population sample of school children. *Pediatric Pulmonology* 1997;**24**:187–94.
110. Kalarchian M, Marcus M. Management of the bariatric surgery patient: Is there a role for the cognitive behavior therapist? *Cognitive and Behavioral Practice* 2003;**10**:112–19.

CHAPTER 24

The Emotional Impact of Obesity on Children

Robert E. Cornette
Department of Nursing, Berea College, Berea, Kentucky

INTRODUCTION

"Fatty, Fatty, two by four, can't fit through the kitchen door." Most of us have heard either this taunt or similar ridicule directed toward a peer in school. Whether you were the perpetrator, the victim, or a bystander, you were acutely aware of the profound influence of these attacks. We really never knew why overweight children were the targets of such harassment. Possibly because they looked different (that may explain why children that were taller, shorter, thinner, etc. were also the targets of verbal derision), or was it because of the stereotypes associated with obese people? Stereotypical beliefs that obese people are: lazy, weak, dumb, helpless, spoiled, or just different. After all, when members of the baby-boomer generation were children during the 1950s and 1960s, overweight children accounted for only about 4% of the population as compared to about 35% today (12- to 19-year-olds) [1].

Certainly, as children we did not consider the consequences of the name calling or teasing these young children suffered beyond the immediate crying or fleeing by the victim. But what is the emotional toll suffered by these victims, and are the effects only short-lived or more enduring? Are the emotional consequences of being an obese child solely the result of taunting by others, or are there other, more intrinsic sequelae that manifest during adolescence or as an adult? With the declaration that obesity has become an epidemic in the United States as well as numerous other countries, much attention has been given to the physical consequences of obesity on children and even the fiscal cost for taxpayers. But little attention has been focused on the emotional, psychological, social, and spiritual effects of living as an obese child. This chapter focuses on the metaphysical consequences of obesity on children and adolescents. In addition, we will attempt to answer these questions: Do all obese children suffer some emotional consequence merely from being overweight? What are the immediate and long-term emotional tolls of being an obese child? Are current treatment modalities efficacious in addressing these emotional symptoms? Finally, whereas other chapters of this book will investigate possible solutions to prevent childhood obesity, this chapter examines some possible interventions to prevent or treat the emotional consequences of obesity during childhood.

OBESITY AND PSYCHOLOGICAL DISORDERS

Obesity itself is not a psychological disorder according to the Diagnostic and Statistical Manual IV (DSM). Some researchers are investigating the possibility of moving obesity out of the realm of the medical arena and into the science of the psychological. The possibility of considering obesity as a mental or behavioral problem has been explored. The moralistic view of obesity (i.e., people are obese because they choose to eat too much) does not take into account that appetite is influenced by genetic and environmental factors that may supersede conscious control [2]. One researcher concluded that if eating was controlled solely by homeostatic mechanisms we would be at our ideal body weight and eating would be a mundane and unexciting activity like breathing [3]. An association between nonhomeostatic eating (i.e., energy consumption in excess of energy expenditure) and factors that contribute to compulsive drug use explains research findings that an addiction to food is similar to an addiction to drugs and alcohol and shares the characteristics of tolerance, withdrawal, and substance-seeking behavior [4, 5]. Lastly, the behavior of nonhomeostatic eating as a coping mechanism in response to internal or external stressors should be recognized. Although not the result of physical influences, overeating as a coping mechanism to stressors could be considered as a manifestation of a psychological dysfunction and, in fact, treatment approaches that have focused on dialectical behavioral therapy rather than nutritional management have been promising [6].

Clearly, there are some psychological disorders that manifest with compulsive eating (e.g., pica, anorexia nervosa, and bulimia), but one study found that whereas binge-eating disorders only affect 2% to 3% of the general population, they are reported in 25% or more of obese people [7]. Nevertheless, obesity remains a physical or medical condition that results from nonhomeostatic eating. Although the excessive caloric intake may result from metabolic conditions such as Prader-Willi syndrome, a genetic disorder characterized by uncontrolled, compulsive eating, more often it is the result of the individual eating more calories than he or she expends. Possibly because obesity has been considered a medical rather than a psychological condition, little attention has been focused on the psychological ramifications of living as an obese individual. Often, healthcare professionals counsel obese patients on methods to lose weight and educate on the physical consequences of failing to do so. Rarely, this counseling includes surveillance of the patient's emotional state or assumes that any emotional trauma from being obese will be alleviated with weight loss.

THE PSYCHOLOGICAL HISTORY OF OBESITY

For most people, the issue of the rapidly rising number of overweight and obese children, adolescents, and adults is one that has just recently come into the public's consciousness. Although the current number of overweight and obese people is the highest our planet has seen, it is fair to say that overweight people have existed throughout history. And though the perception of these overweight individuals may have varied according to the predominate culture, these views may shed some insight into the origins of the development of current labels, stereotypes, or biases regarding the overweight and obese.

It may be impossible to determine when the first obese person existed in history, if he or she were a child, or what emotional consequences that individual experienced as a result. We do know that figurines, called the Venus of Willendorf, date back 30,000 years and depict an obese woman. It is uncertain if the figurines were fertility symbols or erotic tokens [8]. Obesity in early history most likely rarely occurred and may have been prized as a symbol of status and prosperity. But as early as 400 BC, Hippocrates, the father of medicine, wrote of the association between obesity, disease, and early death [9]. Early Egyptians were concerned with diet as a means of maintaining health [8] but utilized extreme measures to limit the quantity of food they digested such as purging, vomiting, and fasting [10].

Early writings regarding the stigmatization associated with being obese occurred in medieval Japan. Scrolls from the 12th century depict a wealthy woman who became obese. It explains that the woman could no longer walk easily, needed assistance with her activities of daily living, perspired profusely, and gasped for breath [11]. The culture in Japan at the time saw this woman's obesity as a result of her greed and selfishness [12]. In Europe, even during the culture of voluptuous women depicted in the paintings of Rubens and Renoir [13], society was being influenced by the Christian ideology that obesity was a characteristic of gluttony, which would eventually be categorized in the 5th century as one of the Seven Deadly Sins [14]. Obesity was not only seen as a moral failure but now it was a transgression against God [13].

THE METAPHYSICAL CONSEQUENCES FOR OBESE CHILDREN

For the first time in recent history, children today may be facing a shorter life span than their parents due, in large part, to the alarming rise in obesity [15]. Thirty states have rates of childhood overweight (body mass index [BMI] of or greater than 85th percentile for age and gender) and obesity (BMI of or greater than 95th percentile for age and gender) for children age 10 to 17 above 30%, with one state, Mississippi, obtaining a rate of 44% [16]. Overall, one in three children (10 to 17 years old) is overweight or obese [17]. A national survey found that obese adolescents had the following risks:

- A 60% higher risk of being diagnosed with anxiety or depression
- A 40% greater risk of having feelings of worthlessness
- A 40% greater risk of parental concerns about their child's self-esteem
- A 70% greater risk of being told by a healthcare provider that they have behavioral problems
- A 30% greater risk of being withdrawn
- A 40% greater risk of bullying others [18]

Given the increase in the rate of obesity in children, it could be assumed that there would be a reduction in the stigmatization of obese children; yet negative views of obese children are higher now than that of four decades ago [19]. Nonobese children have stated that they would prefer to befriend a child with a physical disability, such as a missing limb or blindness, than an obese child [20–23]. The consequences for obese children are varied and can be categorized as teasing and bullying, emotional problems, and school and daily functioning problems [24]. These categories will serve as an outline to examine the emotional consequences of obesity on children and adolescents.

TEASING AND BULLYING

At the beginning of this chapter, you read a poem used to taunt overweight and obese children. Although it may appear silly and inconsequential on initial inspection, these words, as well as those similar in nature, are capable of inflicting profound and enduring wounds on their victims. Obese children are the victims of teasing three times more often than their average weight peers [25]. Evidence is revealing that the consequences of such teasing may impact all areas of the child's development, including the child's psychological, social, emotional, academic, professional, and spiritual development, not only during growth into adulthood but possibly well into middle age and beyond. One study found that 98% of obese adults reported being the victim of harassment, criticism, or teasing from family members and friends. Seventy-five percent reported that they were criticized or teased at work, whereas 50% indicated that the criticism or teasing came from their supervisor, and 33% reported being called negative names by a heathcare professional [26]. Children are most frequently teased by unfamiliar children and classmates, then familiar classmates and siblings, and even parents, adults in their lives, and adult strangers [24, 25]. In a study examining the attitudes of high school teachers on obesity, the teachers indicated their belief that obese teens were unkempt, emotional, less likely to succeed, and had more family problems. Forty-three percent of the teachers believed that people felt uncomfortable around obese people, 55% believed that obesity stemmed from a lack of love or attention, and 28% believed that becoming obese was the worst thing that could happen to a person [27].

Although the frequency of teasing varies between boys and girls, girls indicate that the teasing is more stressful and results in greater incidents of emotional problems, such as anxiety and sadness, than that reported by boys, who exhibit greater behavioral problems and fighting [28, 29]. Although many obese children are the victims of teasing and bullying, it should be noted that obese children are also the perpetrators of bullying. Bullying behavior can manifest in various forms including name calling/teasing, threats, physical harm, social rejection, rumors, or sexual harassment [30, 31]. Physically aggressive behavior is more common in boys, with girls engaging in more relational aggressive behavior such as threatening to withdraw friendship or rumor spreading [32]. Often the verbal teasing/bullying by obese children is in the form of attacks on a peer's ethnic, religious, or sexual characteristics in order to divert attention from themselves and the focus on weight [33].

Evidence indicates that the negative stereotypes associated with obesity in childhood appear to decline with age, especially for boys [34]. However, the incidence of perpetrating bullying behavior by obese children appears to increase as these youth move into adolescence [35, 36], possibly as a means of initiating domination of their peer group during the time when peer group recognition is most important [33]. The following sections further examine the impacts of weight-based victimization (e.g., greater levels of loneliness, sadness, and nervousness [35]; poorer academic performance in high school and decreased college acceptance [36, 37]; and decreased likelihood of marrying as an adult and lower household incomes than their nonobese counterparts [38]).

EMOTIONAL CONSEQUENCES

With the growing public awareness regarding the epidemic of obesity plaguing our youth, we have been exposed to a plethora of information pertaining to the physical toll excess weight takes on our health. In contrast, far less attention has been focused on the psychological, social, emotional, and spiritual consequences of being an obese child or adolescent. As a result, little evidence is available regarding the nonphysical ramifications of obesity experienced by children during their childhood and adult lives. It is fair to argue that the nonphysical consequences of childhood obesity are as devastating as the physical consequences, if not more so, because of their ability to affect numerous aspects of a person's life.

Although there are a multitude of conditions that can affect the human psyche, this discussion focuses on the consequences of obesity pertaining to self-esteem/image, mood (e.g., depression), and anxiety disorders. Obese children are more likely to suffer from negative or decreased self-esteem or self-image, increased anxiety, sad affect, and symptoms of depression [24]. One study found that 42% of obese children met the DSM-IV criteria for a mood disorder and 40% for an anxiety disorder [39]. There is a direct correlation between the baseline body mass index (BMI) and lower self-esteem [40] in adolescents, but the inverse (i.e., lower self-esteem correlated with increased body weight) was not noted. Interestingly, whereas girls who are greatly overweight reported lower self-esteem than girls who were not as overweight, the same was not true with boys [41]. In fact, the overweight boys reported higher self-esteem, possibly because of the value placed on weight and strength in sports such as American football. The greater dissatisfaction with body image and self-esteem in girls may explain why girls are more likely to participate in dieting as a means to improve their self-worth [42].

Self-Esteem

Even though early studies indicated that there was no significant relationship between being obese and low self-esteem in children [43], subsequent studies revealed interesting correlations between self-esteem and obesity in children. Obesity has been found to be a determinate of future low self-esteem in children [35, 40, 44–46] and obese children whose self-esteem decreased over a period of a few years were at greater risk of engaging in unhealthy lifestyle behaviors, such as smoking tobacco and alcohol use [35]. It is speculated that the lower self-esteem observed in these children may result from lower self-perceptions of physical appearance and athletic competence [47], poorer body esteem, and perceived cognitive capacities [45]. Other contributing factors to lower self-esteem in obese children may come from the child's internalization of the responsibility for the additional weight. Children, especially girls, who experienced the perception that they were being blamed by their parents for their obesity reported negative self-perceptions [45], as did children who believed that they were responsible for their condition, rather than external causes beyond their control [48].

Depression

Like self-esteem, the relationship between depression and obesity in children is tenuous. Whereas some studies indicate that obese children are more inclined to suffer depressive symptoms, other studies fail to find these results. When weight-related teasing was examined regarding its influence on depression, a positive relationship was found but raised the question of whether the weight or the teasing contributed to the depressive condition [49]. Interestingly, research has focused on the inverse relationship by investigating whether children who suffer depressive symptoms are more likely to become obese in adolescence or adulthood. Although the research in this area is not conclusive, evidence indicates that children who experience depressive symptoms are more likely to experience higher weights in their youth or adulthood [50], and the findings are more characteristic of female rather than male youths [51].

Body Dissatisfaction

Body dissatisfaction is higher in overweight and obese children and adolescents, especially in obese girls [52]. Similar to depressive symptoms, research has found that weight-related teasing has a negative relationship to body image in both male and female youths and the development of eating disorders in females [53]. The greater the teasing as a child, the more likely the child will suffer body dissatisfaction as an adult and, subsequently, lower self-esteem [54]. Additional research has determined that the weight-related teasing rather than the child's weight was the stronger predictor of body dissatisfaction [53], and when body image was modified without weight change, self-esteem improved [55].

PROBLEMS WITH SCHOOL AND SOCIAL FUNCTIONING

In 1967, researchers first recognized that peers treated overweight and obese children differently [56]. They found that overweight boys were least likely to be nominated as a close friend by their peers. Other studies have found that normal-weight children characterize obese peers as mean and they are among the least liked and least desirable playmates [57]. Since that time, research has unveiled that overweight and obese youths are more likely to be isolated and spend less time with their friends, more likely to report that they felt their friends did not care about them, less likely to have ever dated, more dissatisfied with their dating status, and less likely to marry as an adult [38, 58–60]. Of normal-weight children, only 12% indicated that they ever dated an overweight peer (with girls more likely to date an overweight peer) and they were uncomfortable dating obese peers [61]. Not only do obese adolescents report experiencing more social rejection and isolation, but their normal-weight friends may also experience stigmatization as a result of socializing with the obese teens [62]. As much as 50% of obese boys and 58% of obese girls report experiencing significant problems with peer relationships [24].

Obese girls experience more social marginalization in the form of ostracizing, having rumors or lies spread regarding them, or being given the silent treatment [60, 63]. In all age ranges, girls experience more social victimization than boys and, interestingly, experience more stigmatization by their parents than boys [25, 61, 64]. Girls may also experience more social victimization as their social economic status rises [65]. The increased vulnerability obese girls experience to psychosocial victimization may contribute to their decreased academic and social competencies [66]. One study found that obese girls in the 7th, 9th, and 11th grades were more likely to have been held back a year in school [69]. One study found that 16-year-old girls in the top 10% of the BMI range earned 7.4% less income when they were 23 years of age [67]. Overweight girls tend to receive less financial support for education from their parents, are not as represented at prominent universities as obese men, and are less likely to finish college [68, 69].

For both sexes, researchers have found that obese children need twice as many learning aids as normal-weight children [70] and consider themselves below-average students, with obese boys being more likely to expect themselves to quit school [69]. In addition, they report that they often enjoy fewer sports and athletic activities, such as running or walking, and activities of daily living, such as buying clothes, dancing, or eating out with friends [71].

SUICIDAL BEHAVIOR

Without a doubt, the most disturbing consequence of obesity victimization is the development of suicidal ideation or behavior. After consideration of the numerous psychosocial consequences of being an obese child or adolescent, it is not difficult to conceive that obese adolescents are more likely to consider suicide as an escape from the torment they experience [59, 71]. Obese girls are 1.7 times more likely to attempt suicide than their normal-weight peers and research has demonstrated that BMI and self-perceptions of being overweight, even slightly, were positively associated with suicidal ideation in Caucasian, Hispanic, and African American girls [72]. Research into the effects of teasing on obese youths has revealed that obese teens who were teased about their weight were two to three times more likely to develop suicidal ideation than obese teens who were not teased [49]. More specifically, 51% of girls and 13% of boys who were teased about their weight reported suicidal ideation compared to 25% and 4%, respectively, of those who were not teased [25]. These numbers speak to the need to focus on the quality of life experienced by obese children. Although it may not be surprising than obese children report a lower quality of life than their normal-weight peers, it may be alarming that obese children report a quality of life similar to children suffering from cancer [73].

INTERVENTIONS

After considering the significant psychosocial and emotional impact associated with the stigmatization of obese children and adolescents, we can appreciate the need for interventions to address this issue. Interventions should not just focus on the reduction of weight, but rather interventions should be developed that reduce or eliminate the bias against obese individuals that is the source of the marginalizing of these youth. Research has demonstrated that bias against obesity can develop in children as young as 3 years of age [74], suggesting that the foundation of this bias may come from parents as well as from social and media sources. Research has determined that parents can convey weight bias in subtle forms such as portraying overweight characters in stories in negative manners or through their efforts to control their child's weight [75]. To the child, these messages communicate that fat is synonymous with undesirable characteristics. Teachers and school officials who perpetrate the stereotypes discussed previously, only serve to reinforce these messages. Even healthcare professionals may, in their zeal to improve children's health, convey a message that fat is bad and children should achieve and maintain a healthy weight. This illustrates that bias and victimization of obese youth is a socially sanctioned behavior among children and adults [76]. As a result, interventions to address the stigmatization of obese youth will need to challenge the sanctioning of these behaviors.

One theory states that negative stereotyping behavior will decrease if the perpetrator of the behavior believes that the obesity is not within the victim's control [77]. Studies conducted to examine this theory found that when obese children were identified as being overweight because of a medical condition, perpetrators of negative stereotypes were less likely to victimize them but they tended to avoid interacting with the obese child [78]. This suggested that the medical explanation may have also served to illustrate the differences between the two children. Clearly, interventions intending to explain the cause of obesity are not as effective as interventions designed to abate the social sanctioning of behavior intended to marginalize an obese person. Interventions to decrease the social sanctioning of negative stereotyping should include the following:

- Targeting parents by increasing their awareness of the intentional and unintentional messages they may convey to their children
- Challenging the negative beliefs teachers may have toward obese children while increasing their awareness of the impact negative biases have on children
- Instituting antiweight teasing rules in school to prevent portraying obese people in a negative manner in students' lessons and to begin portraying them in a more positive manner
- Targeting societal beliefs that fat is bad and changing media messages that promote weight bias [79]

In addition, interventions should be developed to help obese youth develop effective coping mechanisms to assist them in buffering the negative effects of weight bias, increasing supportive peer and family relationships, and providing obese children with supportive opportunities to participate in social and recreational activities [25, 58]. Finally, interventions should be framed in a manner that emphasizes positive behavioral changes such as monitoring television viewing time, sensible fast-food and sweets consumption, and physical activity, rather than motivating change through body-image modification [80].

CONCLUSION

Throughout the history of the human race people have been victimized for their beliefs, their practices, or their appearance. Children today are faced with a culture that deeply values physical appearance and views obesity as a symptom of laziness, weakness, and selfishness. Thus, it is easy to fathom the emotional sequela experienced by overweight and obese children and adolescents. While obesity is not classified as a psychiatric disorder it can manifest several psychological symptoms such as: anxiety; feelings of worthlessness; low self esteem; aggression; social withdrawal; depression; and even suicidal behavior. With the rapid increase in the number of obese children, it stands to reason that we will see an increase in the number of children suffering from mental health disorders. Interventions should be directed towards the psychological as well as the nutritional health of the child. Additionally, interventions should be crafted that: reduce social biases towards the obese; help develop effective coping mechanisms for obese children; increase supportive relationships; and emphasize positive lifestyle changes rather than modifying body image.

References

1. National Health and Nutrition Examination Survey (NHANES). (2006). Atlanta: Center for Disease Control and Prevention.
2. Devlin M. Is there a place for obesity in the DSM V? *International Journal of Eating Disorders* 2007;**40**:S83–8.
3. Saper C, Chou T, Elmquist J. The need to feed: Homeostatic and hedonic control of eating. *Neuron* 2002;**36**:199–211.
4. Colantuoni C, Rada P, McCarthy J, Patten C, Avena N, Chadeayne A, Hoebal B. Evidence that intermittent, excessive sugar intake causes endogenous opioid dependence. *Obesity Research* 2002;**10**:478–88.
5. Avena N, Hoebel B. A diet promoting sugar dependency causes behavioral cross sensitivity to a low dose of amphetamine. *Neuroscience* 2003;**122**:17–20.
6. Telch C, Agras W, Linehan M. Dialectical behavioral therapy for binge eating disorder. *Journal of Consulting Clinical Psychology* 2001;**69**:1061–5.
7. Pull C. Binge Eating Disorder. *Current Opinion in Psychiatry* 2004;**17**(1):43–8.
8. Haslam D. Obesity: A medical history. *Obesity Reviews* 2007;**8**(1): 31–6.
9. Hippocrates (400 BC). De Priscina Medicina.
10. Siculus (20 BC). "Bibliotheca historica."
11. Komatsu S. "Gaki-zoshi Jigoku-zoshi Yamai-zoshi Kusoshi-emaki," Vol. 7 Nihon no emaki. Tokyo: Chuo koronsha; 1990. pp. 102–47.
12. Lafleur W. "The Karma of words: Buddhism and the Literary Arts of Medieval Japan". Berkeley: University of California Press; 1983. pp. 35–7.
13. Stunkard A, LaFleur W, Wadden T. Stigmatization of obesity in medieval times: Asia and Europe. *International Journal of Obesity* 1998;**22**:1141–4.
14. Schwartz H. "Never Satisfied: A cultural history of diets, fantasies and fat". New York: Anchor Books; 1990.
15. Olshansky S, Passaro D, Hershow R. A potential decline in Life Expectancy in the Unites States in the 21st century. *The New England Journal of Medicine* 2005;**352**:1138–45.
16. Trust for America's Health, (2009). F as in fat: How obesity policies are failing in America. Washington, DC: Robert Wood Johnson Foundation.
17. National Survey of Children's Health. Portland: Oregon Health & Science University. (2007).
18. Belue R, Francis L, Colaco B. Mental health problems and overweight in a nationally representative sample of adolescents: Effects of race and ethnicity. *Pediatrics* 2009;**123**(2): 697–702.
19. Latner J, Stunkard A. Getting worse: The stigmatization of obese children. *Obesity Research* 2003;**11**:452–6.
20. Staffieri J. A study of stereotype of body image in children. *Journal of Personality and Social Psychology* 1967;**7**:101–4.
21. Goodman N, Dornbusch S, Richardson S, Hastorf A. Variant reactions to physical disabilities. *American Sociology Review* 1963;**28**:429–35.
22. Maddox G, Back K, Liederman V. Overweight as a social deviance and disability. *Journal of Health and Social Behavior* 1968;**9**: 287–98.
23. Richardson S, Goodman N, Hastorf A, Dornbusch S. Cultural uniformity in reaction to physical disabilities. *American Sociological Reviews* 1961;**26**:241–7.
24. Warschburger P. Unhappy obese child. *International Journal of Obesity* 2005;**29**:S127–9.
25. Neumark-Sztainer D, Falkner N, Story M, Perry C, Hannah P, Mulert S. Weight teasing among adolescents: Correlations with weight status and disordered eating behavior. *International Journal of Obesity* 2002;**26**:123–31.
26. Rothblum E, Brand P, Miller C, Oetjen H. Results of the NAAFA survey on employment discrimination: Part II. *NAAFA Newsletter* 1989;**17**:4–6.
27. Neumark-Sztainer D, Story M, Harris T. Beliefs and attitudes about obesity among teachers and school health care providers working with adolescents. *Journal of Nutritional Education* 1999;**31**: 3–9.
28. Kimm S, Sweeney C, Janosky J, MacMillian J. Self-concept measure and childhood obesity: A descriptive analysis. *Journal of Developmental Behavioral Pediatrics* 1991;**12**:19–24.
29. Manus H, Killeen M. Maintenance of self-esteem by obese children. *Journal of Child and Adolescent Psychiatric Nursing* 1995;**8**: 17–24.
30. Loeber R. Developmental and risk factors of juvenile antisocial behavior and delinquency. *Clinical Psychology Reviews* 1990;**10**: 1–41.
31. Crick N. Engagement in gender normative versus non-normative forms of aggression: Links to social psychological adjustment. *Developmental Psychology* 1997;**33**:610–17.

REFERENCES

32. Crick N, Grotpeter J. Relational aggression, gender, and social-psychological adjustment. *Child Development* 1995;**66**:710−22.
33. Janssen I, Craig W, Boyce W, Pickett W. Associations between overweigh and obesity with bullying behaviors in school aged children. *Pediatrics* 2004;**113**:1187−94.
34. Kirkpatrick S, Sanders D. Body image stereotypes: A developmental comparison. *Journal of Genetic Psychology* 1978;**132**:87−95.
35. Strauss R. Childhood obesity and self-esteem. *Pediatrics* 2000; **105**(1):1−5.
36. Canning H, Mayar J. Obesity: An influence on high school performance. *American Journal of Clinical Nutrition* 1967;**20**:352−4.
37. Canning H, Mayar J. Obesity: It's possible effect on college acceptance. *New England Journal of Medicine* 1967;**20**:352−4.
38. Gortmaker S, Must P, Perrin J, Sobol A, Dietz W. Social and economic consequences of overweight in adolescence and young adulthood. *New England Journal of Medicine* 1993;**329**: 1008−12.
39. Britz B, Siegfried W, Ziegler A, Lamertz C, Herpetz-Dahlmann B, Remschmidt H, Wittchen H, Hebebrand J. Rates of psychiatric disorders in a clinical study of adolescents with extreme obesity and in obese adolescents ascertaining via a population based study. *International Journal of Obesity* 2000;**24**:1707−14.
40. Hesketh K, Wake M, Waters E. Body mass index and parent reported self esteem in elementary school children: Evidence of a causal relationship. *International Journal of Obesity* 2004;**28**: 1233−7.
41. Israel A, Ivanova M. Global and dimensional self esteem in preadolescent children who are overweight: Age and gender differences. *International Journal of Eating Disorders* 2002;**31**: 424−9.
42. Hill A, Pallin V. Dieting awareness and low self-worth: Related issues in 8 year old girls. *International Journal of Obesity* 1998;**24**: 405−13.
43. French S, Story M, Perry C. Self esteem and obesity in children and adolescent: A literature review. *Obesity Research* 1995;**3**: 479−90.
44. Brown K, McMahon R, Biro F, Crawford P, Schreiber G, Similo S. Changes in self-esteem in black and white girls between the ages of 9 and 14 years. The NHLBI Growth and Heath Study. *Journal of Adolescent Health* 1998;**23**:7−19.
45. Davidson K, Birch L. Weight status, parents reaction, and self concepts in five year old girls. *Pediatrics* 2001;**107**:46−53.
46. Tiggemann M. Body dissatisfaction and adolescent self esteem: Prospective findings. *Body Image* 2005;**2**:129−35.
47. Phillips R, Hill A. Fat, plain, but not friendless: Self esteem and peer acceptance of obese preadolescent girls. *International Journal of Obesity* 1998;**22**:287−93.
48. Pierce J, Wardle J. Cause and effect beliefs and self esteem of overweight children. *Journal of Child Psychology & Psychiatry* 1997;**38**:645−50.
49. Eisenberg M, Neumark-Sztainer D, Story M. Associations of weight based teasing and emotional well-being among adolescents. *Archives of Pediatric and Adolescent Medicine* 2003;**157**:733−8.
50. Richardson L, Davis R, Poulton R, McCauley E, Moffit T, Caspi A, Connell F. A longitudinal evaluation of adolescent depression and adult obesity. *Archives of Pediatrics and Adolescent Medicine* 2003;**157**:739−45.
51. Anderson S, Cohen P, Naumova E, Must A. Associations of depression and anxiety disorders with weight change in a prospective community based study of children following into adulthood. *Archives of Pediatric and Adolescent Medicine* 2006;**160**: 285−91.
52. Ricciardelli L, McCabe M. Children's body image concerns and eating disturbances: A review of literature. *Clinical Psychology Review* 2001;**21**:325−44.
53. Thompson J, Coovert M, Richards K, Johnson S, Cattarin J. Development of body image, eating disturbance, and general psychological functioning in female adolescents: Covariance structure modeling and longitudinal investigations. *International Journal of Eating Disorders* 1995;**18**:221−36.
54. Grilo C, Wilfrey D, Brownwell K, Rodin J. Teasing, body image, and self esteem in a clinical sample of obese women. *Addictive Behaviors* 1994;**19**:443−50.
55. Pesa J, Syre T, Jones E. Psychosocial differences associated with body weight among female adolescents: The importance of body image. *Journal of Adolescent Health* 2000;**26**:330−7.
56. Staffieri J. A study of social stereotype of body image in children. *Journal of Personality and Social Psychology* 1967;**7**:101−4.
57. Kraig K, Keel P. Weight-based stigmatization in children. *International Journal of Obesity* 2001;**25**:1661−6.
58. Strauss R, Pollack H. Social marginalization of overweight children. *Archives of Pediatric and Adolescent Medicine* 2003;**157**:746−52.
59. Falkner N, Neumark-Sztainer D, Story M, Jeffery R, Beuhring T, Resnick M. Social, educational and psychological correlations of weight status in adolescents. *Obesity Research* 2001;**9**:32−42.
60. Pearce M, Boergers J, Prinstein M. Adolescent obesity, overt and relational peer victimization, and romantic relationships. *Obesity Research* 2002;**10**:386−93.
61. Sobal J, Nicolopoulos V, Lee L. Attitudes about overweight and dating among secondary students. *International Journal of Obesity* 1995;**19**:376−81.
62. Hebl M, Mannix L. The weight of obesity in evaluating others: A mere proximity effect. *Personality and Social Psychology Bulletin* 2003;**29**:28−38.
63. Janssen I, Craig W, Boyce W, Pickett W. Associations between overweight and obesity with bullying behaviors in school aged children. *Pediatrics* 2004;**113**:1187−94.
64. Pierce J, Wardle J. Self esteem, parental appraisal and body size in children. *Journal of Child Psychology and Psychiatry* 1993;**34**: 1125−36.
65. Turnbull J, Heaslip S, McLeod H. Pre-school children's attitudes to fat and normal male and female stimulus figures. *International Journal of Obesity Related Metabolic Disorders* 2000;**24**:1705−6.
66. Datar A, Sturm R. Childhood overweight and elementary school outcomes. *International Journal of Obesity* 2006;**30**:1449−60.
67. Sargent J, Blanchflower D. Obesity and stature in adolescence and earning in young adulthood. *Archives of Pediatric and Adolescent Medicine* 1994;**148**:681−7.
68. Canning H, Mayer J. Obesity: An influence in high school performance. *American Journal of Clinical Nutrition* 1967;**24**:352−4.
69. Tershakoves A, Weller S, Gallagher P. Obesity, school performance and behavior of black, urban elementary school children. *International Journal of Obesity Related Metabolic Disorders* 1994;**18**:323−7.
70. Warschburger P, Buchholtz H, Petermann F. Entwicklung eines krankheissoezifischen interviews zur Erfassung der Lebensquailtat adiposer Kinder und Jugendlicher. *Z Klinical Psychology, Psychiatry and Psychotherapy* 2001;**49**:247−61.
71. Ackard D, Neumark-Sztainer D, Story M, Perry C. Overeating among adolescents: Prevalence and associations with weight related characteristics and psychological health. *Pediatrics* 2003;**111**:67−74.
72. Eaton D, Lowry R, Brener N, Galuska D, Crosby A. Associations of body mass index and perceived weight with suicidal ideation and suicidal attempts among U.S. high school students. *Archives of Pediatrics and Adolescent Medicine* 2005;**159**:513−19.
73. Schwimmer J, Burwinkle T, Varni J. Health related quality of life of severely obese children and adolescents. *Journal of the American Medical Association* 2003;**289**:1813−19.
74. Brylinski J, Moore J. The identification of body build stereotypes in young children. *Journal of Res Pers* 1994;**28**:170−81.

75. Adams GR, Hicken M, Salehi M. Socialization of the physical attractiveness stereotype: Parent expectations and verbal behaviors. *International Journal of Psychology* 1988;**23**:137−49.
76. Hayden-Wade H, Stein R, Ghaderi A, Saelens B, Zabinski M, Wilfrey D. Prevalence, characteristics and correlations of teasing experiences among obese vs. non-obese peers. *Obesity Research* 2005;**13**:1381−92.
77. Weiner B, Graham S. An attributional approach to emotional development. In: Izard CE, Kagan J, Zojonc RB, editors. *"Emotions, cognitions, and behavior"*. Cambridge: Cambridge University Press; 1984. pp. 167−91.
78. Bell S, Morgan S. Children's attitudes and behavioral interventions towards a peer presented as obese: Does a medical explanation for the obesity make a difference? *Journal of Pediatric Psychology* 2000;**25**:137−45.
79. Gray W, Kahnan N, Janicke D. Peer victimization and pediatric obesity: A review of literature. *Psychology in the Schools* 2009;**46**(8):720−7.
80. Dolan M, Faith M. Prevention of overweight with young children and families. In: Latner J, Wilson G, editors. *"Self-help approach for obesity and eating disorders: Research and practice"*. New York: Guilford Press; 2007. pp. 265−88.

CHAPTER 25

Psychiatric Illness, Psychotropic Medication, and Childhood Obesity

Lawrence Maayan, Leslie Citrome

New York University School of Medicine, New York City, New York, and Nathan S. Kline Institute for Psychiatric Research, Orangeburg, New York

INTRODUCTION

Weight gain and obesity have become a critical issue for U.S. children. For those with psychiatric illness, obesity is an additional health burden with problematic sequelae. Although psychiatric illness and medication often have metabolic effects, it appears that the newer antipsychotic medications—used as primary treatments for pediatric autism, psychotic and bipolar disorders, and adjunctive treatments for others—are particularly likely to cause weight gain in some children. In this chapter we examine current research delineating the extent of psychotropic-associated weight gain in youth, with emphasis on second-generation antipsychotic medications as well as underlying mechanisms and pharmacogenetics. Also summarized are current data on pharmacological and behavioral treatments as well as future directions in research.

PEDIATRIC OBESITY

The prevalence of child and adolescent obesity in the United States has more than tripled since 1970 [1]. Although recent evidence suggests that the prevalence of obesity in children may have plateaued, the present rates predict a public health problem of considerable personal and societal costs in the coming decades as these individuals age and develop likely cardiovascular and endocrine illness [2–4]. Furthermore, pediatric obesity has disproportionately afflicted children in minority communities [1] who often have the least access to health services [5]. The severity of the consequences of obesity are becoming increasingly evident, with longitudinal data from large population-based studies showing carotid intimal media thickness in adults, a risk factor for stroke, related to low-density lipoprotein cholesterol levels [6] and body mass index (BMI)[7] in childhood. Some of these cardiometabolic effects of obesity are even becoming evident in childhood itself, with evidence showing an increased rate of metabolic syndrome [8] and carotid intimal media thickening [9]. Type 2 diabetes, once a disease almost exclusively found in adults, is increasingly prevalent in children both in the United States [10–12] and in the rest of the world. Studies looking at the rates of pediatric usage of antihypertensive, antidiabetic, and dyslipidemic medications have shown increases in these rates as well, suggesting an increase in hyperglycemia and cardiovascular disease in childhood [13].

PREVALENCE OF PSYCHIATRIC ILLNESS IN CHILDHOOD

In a separate but not entirely unrelated development the diagnosis and treatment of child psychiatric disorders has increased dramatically during the same period [14]. In a review paper, the authors of the Great Smoky Mountain Study, a large epidemiological study of pediatric mental health in the 1990s funded by the National Institutes of Health (NIH), found the current median prevalence of child and adolescent psychiatric disorders to be 27% [15]. This is parsed into major depressive disorder, anxiety disorders (including obsessive compulsive disorder (OCD)), conduct disorder (CD), oppositional defiant disorder (ODD), and attention deficit hyperactivity disorder (ADHD) as the five most common psychiatric illnesses in this population. Each of these disorders can be debilitating in its own right.

Major depression affects an estimated 2.5% of children and 8.3% of U.S. adolescents. These rates account for approximately 2.6 million youth aged 6 to 17 [16]. It frequently is associated with disabling anxiety and with thoughts of suicide experienced by 40% to 80% of youth with the illness [17–22], suicide attempts by up to 35% of depressed youth [17, 18, 21–25], and, much less commonly, completed suicides. In the United States, approximately 2000 young people die each year as a result of suicide. On an annual basis, 1.3 of every 100,000 children aged 10 to 14, 8.2 of every 100,000 15- to 19-year-olds, and 12.5 of every 100,000 20- to 24-year-olds die from suicide, making it the third leading cause of death for individuals aged 15 to 24 [26].

Since the mid-1990s, conclusive work has come out demonstrating the importance of pharmacological and psychotherapeutic treatment culminating with the National Institutes of Mental Health (NIMH)-sponsored treatment of adolescents with depression study (TADS) [27] and the Treatment of Adolescent Suicide Attempters study [28] showing the efficacy of fluoxetine in the treatment of pediatric depression. Fluoxetine and escitalopram are the only antidepressants of the serotonin-specific reuptake inhibitor (SSRI) class with a Food and Drug Administration (FDA) indication for the treatment of pediatric major depressive disorder.

Prevalence estimates for anxiety disorders range from 3% to 30% with a median of 8% [15]. It can be comorbid with major depressive disorder [29]. In 2008, the NIMH-funded Child and Adolescent Anxiety Multimodal Study (CAMS) supported SSRI (such as sertraline) alone or in combination with psychotherapy as effective treatment [30].

Attention deficit hyperactivity disorder has a prevalence of approximately 6.7% as estimated by the U.S. National Health Interview Survey for the period 1997–2000 [31]. Although stimulants such as methylphenidate and mixed amphetamine salts have been available for many years, the NIMH-supported Multimodal Treatment of ADHD (MTA) study solidly established the efficacy and safety of methylphenidate as treatment for ADHD in school-aged children [32] and the Preschool ADHD Treatment Study (PATS) in children down to age 3 [33]. Atomoxetine, a nonstimulant drug, is also FDA approved for ADHD with studies showing safety and efficacy down to age 5 [34].

Data from several other NIMH sponsored trials examining treatment of child psychiatric disorders have emerged since the late 1990s, including the pediatric Obsessive Compulsive Disorder Treatment Study (POTS) in OCD [35] and the treatment of Early Onset Schizophrenia Syndrome study of pediatric psychosis and schizophrenia (TEOSS) [36]. As the quality and quantity of evidence-based research regarding pharmacological treatment of mental illness in children has increased, the rate of prescription of medications has risen as well with a 2003 study showing rates of use in children approaching the same level as in adults [14].

OBESITY ASSOCIATED WITH PSYCHIATRIC ILLNESS

Psychiatric illness in children has its own independent relationship with weight abnormalities and obesity. Using data from the Great Smoky Mountain Study, Mustillo and colleagues found chronic obesity to be correlated with having a psychiatric disorder. In particular they noted higher rates of oppositional defiant disorder (in both sexes) and major depression (in boys only) in children with chronic obesity. They did not attribute causality but noted that the obesity in these children had been present from an early age, often preexisting the psychiatric diagnosis [37].

Although Mustillo's group did not find evidence of a correlation between obesity and ADHD, there is other research that has [38, 39]. The most thorough examination to date looked at a cross-sectional analysis of 62,887 children and adolescents aged 5 to 17 years from the 2003–2004 National Survey of Children's Health, a nationally representative sample of youth in the United States, and found that unmedicated children and adolescents with ADHD had 1.5 times the odds of being overweight. The authors hypothesized that this may be due to either untreated impulsivity resulting in poor dietary choices or increased time spent with video games or television [39].

Likewise there is evidence that children who are identified as having bipolar disorder are more likely to be overweight. Looking at a clinical sample of 348 youth, Goldstein and colleagues found a trending towards significant odds ratio of 1.25 (95% CI 0.99 – 1.57) of being overweight in youth with bipolar disorder as opposed to the general population. As in ADHD, they attributed impulsive eating, but also speculated as to the existence of neurobiological dysfunction underlying both behavior and the regulation of satiety and eating behaviors.

PSYCHOTROPIC MEDICATION UTILIZATION: SECOND-GENERATION ANTIPSYCHOTICS

The area of interaction between metabolic and psychiatric function merits its own extensive treatment; however, for the purpose of this chapter we will focus on the effects of medication and in particular on second-generation antipsychotics, which appear to be the most

TABLE 25.1 Relative Effect on Weight of Psychotropic Medications

Medication classes	Effect on weight[a]
Antipsychotics	+++ [36, 65]
Anticonvulsants	++ [100]
Lithium	++ [101, 102]
Antidepressants	+ [103, 104]
Amphetamines	− [105, 106]

[a] − = (weight loss), + = (little weight gain), ++ = (moderate weight gain), +++ = great weight gain.

likely of psychotropics indicated in children to cause weight gain (Table 25.1). Second-generation antipsychotics (SGAs) include aripiprazole, clozapine, olanzapine, paliperidone, quetiapine, risperidone, and ziprasidone [40]. Newer agents that received adult FDA approval in 2009 include iloperidone [41] and asenapine [42]. Although SGAs have a lower likelihood of causing extrapyramidal side effects, they have a higher propensity to cause increases in body weight. This in turn increases the risk for cardiometabolic problems. Over the past decade, usage of SGAs in child psychiatry has increased considerably up to six-fold by some estimates [40].

This increase in usage of SGAs is partly related to higher prevalence rates for diagnoses where SGAs are the first line treatment, as well as a concomitant rise in off-label usage. Currently, risperidone and aripiprazole have indications in pediatric schizophrenia, in bipolar disorder, and for irritability associated with autistic disorder. The other SGAs are also used under these circumstances, although this use is off label (Table 25.2).

In terms of these diagnoses, rates of pediatric schizophrenia have remained essentially stable. There is, however, a small but increasing percentage of children who have been diagnosed with pervasive developmental disorders (PDD) such as autism, Asperger's, and Rett's disorders [43] with prevalence rates rising from 3 to 6 per 10,000 before 1990 [44] to rates of 45 per 10,000 in the early 2000s and up to 110 per 10,000 in a recent study [43], mostly the result of knowledge of the disorder and increased sensitivity of assessment. Similarly rates of pediatric bipolar disorder have doubled since the mid-1990s [45, 46], in part because of the development of diagnostic tools designed to categorize the irritability and ultradian cycling (i.e., recurrent periods or cycles repeated throughout a 24-hour circadian day) sometimes observed in behaviorally disrupted youth under the rubric of possible mood symptoms. These nosologic and conceptual changes, combined with clinical research findings demonstrating benefit for children with PDD [47] and bipolar disorder [48], helped spur the growing usage of SGAs in this population.

In addition, the increase in the amount of off-label usage of antipsychotics has been driven in part by an evidence base showing some benefit for children with these treatments for common symptoms like aggression and irritability associated with disruptive behavior disorders such as ADHD, oppositional defiant disorder, and conduct disorder [49, 50] and a lack of other demonstrated beneficial alternatives for childhood disorders. On a population-based level, this has been described by research reviewing several state registries, as summarized in the following discussion.

A study examining records from children in Tennessee in the statewide public insurance program showed a doubling of antipsychotic usage rates between 1996 and 2001 with much of the increase attributable to increased usage in ADHD and affective disorders [51]. A study conducted in Central New York showed that 77% of children prescribed an antipsychotic did not have a psychotic disorder and that the most common medication combination was that of a stimulant and an antipsychotic [52]. A nationwide survey of outpatient visits showed a six-fold increase from 1993 to 2002 with again the most common diagnoses for which antipsychotics were prescribed being disruptive behavior disorders, including ADHD, ODD, and CD (37.8%) and mood disorders (31.8%) being the second most common followed by pervasive developmental or mental retardation (17.3%) and psychotic disorders (14.2%) [40]. A study examining Medicaid data in Florida from 2002 to 2005 demonstrated a higher utilization of antipsychotics than in the prior decade [53]. Although "prescription-based evidence" is not a substitute for clinical trials testing the utility of these treatments, they do make it clear that these psychotropic agents are widely used.

WEIGHT GAIN ON ANTIPSYCHOTICS

The data documenting antipsychotic associated weight gain in adults are conclusive. A landmark meta-analysis and review produced by David Allison and colleagues [54] showed SGA-associated weight gain of over 4 kg with olanzapine and clozapine and over 2 kg with risperidone in a 10-week period contrasted with a mean weight loss on placebo of 0.74 kg. This was followed up by multiple confirmatory studies. Medication-associated weight gain appeared even more pronounced in individuals early in treatment with findings from the yearlong European First Episode Schizophrenia Trial (EUFEST) showing 13.9 kg on olanzapine, 10.5 kg on quetiapine, 4.8 kg on ziprasidone, and 7.3 kg on the first-generation haloperidol in a year of treatment [55]. Even more relevant are the proportions of patients who gain a clinically meaningful greater than 7% of their initial body weight over the course of time. In the

TABLE 25.2 FDA-Approved Antipsychotic Medications for Use in Children (Table 2)

Generic name	Trade name	FDA indication
Aripiprazole	Abilify	1. Treatment of manic and mixed episodes associated with Bipolar I disorder in pediatric patients 10 to 17 years of age. 2. Treatment of Schizophrenia in adults and in adolescents 13 to 17 years of age. 3. Treatment of irritability associated with autistic disorder in children and adolescents aged 5 to 16 years [107].
Chlorpromazine	Thorazine	For the treatment of severe behavioral problems in children (1 to 12 years of age) marked by combativeness or explosive hyperexcitable behavior (out of proportion to immediate provocations) and as a short-term treatment for hyperactivity in children who are refractory to psychotherapy or other medications [108].
Chlorprothixene	Taractan, Truxal	1. Treatment of psychotic disorders in adults and children 6 and up. 2. Treatment of acute mania occurring as part of bipolar disorders in adults and children 6 and up [109].
Haloperidol	Haldol	1. Management of manifestation of psychotic disorders 3–12. 2. Control of tics and vocal utterances of Tourette's disorder in children and adults 3–12. 3. For severe behavior disorders or as a short-term treatment for hyperactivity in children over 12 who are refractory to psychotherapy or other medications [110].
Molindone	Moban	Treatment of schizophrenia in adults and children 12 and up [111].
Olanzapine	Zyprexa	1. Treatment of schizophrenia in adults and in adolescents 13–17 years of age. 2. Treatment of bipolar disorder in adults and in adolescents 13–17 years of age. [112] dailymed.nlm.nih.gov/dailymed/drugInfo.cfm?id=18711.
Risperidone	Risperdal	1. Treatment of schizophrenia in adults and adolescents aged 13 to 17 years. 2. Alone, or in combination with lithium or valproate, for the short-term treatment of acute manic or mixed episodes associated with Bipolar I disorder in adults, and alone in children and adolescents aged 10 to 17 years. 3. Treatment of irritability associated with autistic disorder in children and adolescents aged 5 to 16 years [112].
Perphenazine	Trilafon	Treatment of schizophrenia in adults and children 12 and up [113].
Pimozide	Orap	Suppression of motor and phonic tics in patients with treatment-resistant Tourette's disorder in adults and children 12 and up [114].
Quetiapine	Seroquel	1. Treatment of schizophrenia in adults and adolescents aged 13–17 years of age. 2. Treatment of bipolar disorder in adults and adolescents aged 10–17 years. [115] dailymed.nlm.nih.gov/dailymed/drugInfo.cfm?id=18562.
Thioridazine	Mellaril	For the management of treatment-resistant schizophrenia in children and adults [115].
Thiothixene	Navane	For the management of schizophrenia in adults and children 12 and up [116].
Trifluoperazine	Stelazine	1. For the management of schizophrenia and psychosis in children 6 and up. 2. For the short-term treatment of generalized nonpsychotic anxiety [117].

aforementioned EUFEST study, this occurred in 53% of those randomized to haloperidol, 63% of those randomized to amisulpride, 86% of those randomized to olanzapine, 65% of those randomized to quetiapine, and 37% of those randomized to ziprasidone.

The Consensus Development Conference on Antipsychotic Drugs and Obesity and Diabetes [56] supported the weight-gain correlation demonstrated in previous studies and indicated that clozapine and olanzapine were most likely to cause weight gain, followed closely by risperidone and quetiapine, with aripiprazole and ziprasidone being the least likely. Observational evidence in olanzapine suggests this weight gain to be most rapid in the first 6 weeks of treatment [57], particularly in those who eventually gain the most weight.

There have been fewer studies of the correlation between SGA use and weight gain in children and adolescents; however, those that exist show a larger and more rapid pattern of weight gain. A prospective study comparing adolescents 13 to 19 years old on olanzapine, risperidone, and haloperidol over a 12-week period showed 7.2 kg of increase on olanzapine with 90.5% gaining at least 7% of their baseline body weight and 3.9 kg on risperidone with 42.9% gaining 7% or more of their baseline body weight [58].

A more recent double-blind, randomized, comparative study, the Treatment of Early Onset Schizophrenia Spectrum disorders (TEOSS), showed a similar amount of increase over a shorter period—over 6.1 kilograms for olanzapine and 3.6 kilograms for risperidone in 8 weeks compared with a negligible 0.3 kg for the molindone/benztropine comparator [36]. In the TEOSS study, the findings for olanzapine were so dramatic that the data safety monitoring board reconsidered their risk-benefit assessment and recommended against enrolling additional participants after an interim analysis [59]. Even over a period as short as 6 weeks, children and adolescents 9 to 21 years old [60] showed a mean 4.6 kg weight gain on olanzapine, compared with 2.8 kg on risperidone. The authors, assuming comparability of the studies, pointed out that this is significantly more rapid than in adults. Categorical changes on weight were not reported, but the distribution of weight gain/loss was described graphically in the published report [36] with some patients gaining weight and others losing weight, no matter the medication assignment. Although these studies are not placebo controlled, the comparison with a more weight-neutral comparator in the TEOSS study supports that this weight gain is likely associated with medication and not with underlying illness.

In a systematic review conducted by Safer in 2004 [61] examining young children, adolescents, adults, and elderly, there was an inverse relationship between age and percentage of baseline body weight gained. Clinical research that has examined concomitant administration of SGAs along with stimulants [62] and mood stabilizers [63] has shown that the antipsychotics still confer increased metabolic risk, even as adjunctive medications. This weight gain persists over long-term treatment as well, with youth on risperidone for longer than 2 years showing greater than a half standard deviation increase in BMI z-score, a developmentally inappropriate increase in weight [64] (Table 25.3).

Findings of a higher rate and relative amount of weight gain in children have led to two divergent hypotheses. One posited that developmental effects of differential metabolism in children caused increased vulnerability to medication-associated weight gain, whereas another line of thought viewed the findings

TABLE 25.3 Selected Studies Demonstrating Antipsychotic Associated Weight Gain in Youth

Atypical antipsychotic	Age (n)	Design	Duration (weeks)	Weight gain (kg)	7% Weight gain (%)
Calarge et al., 2009 [64] Risperidone	11.6 (99)	Longitudinal	156	0.6^b	N/A^d
Correll et al., 2009 [65] Aripiprazole Olanzapine Quetiapine Risperidone Comparison Group	13.9 ± 3.6 (272) 13.4 ± 3.1 (41) 14.7 ± 3.2 (45) 14.0 ± 3.1 (36) 12.6 ± 4.0 (135) 15.5 ± 2.0 (15)	Naturalistic open label	12	4.44 (3.71–5.18)^a 8.54 (7.38–9.69)^a 6.06 (4.90–7.21)^a 5.34 (4.81–5.87)^a 0.19 (−1.04–1.43)^a	4–12.3 9.9–14.5 15–16 41.9–45.8
Hrdlicka et al., 2009 [118] Risperidone Olanzapine Haloperidol	15.8 ± 1.6 (109)	Chart review	6	4.9 ± 3.6 7.1 ± 4.1 3.5 ± 3.7	N/A^d
Verma et al., 2009 [119] Risperidone	29.8 ± 6.2 (56)	Naturalistic open label	26	6.2 ± 7.0	65
Sikich et al., 2008 [36] Olanzapine Risperidone Molindone	8–19 (116) (35) (41) (40)	Randomized, double-blind multisite trial	8	6.1 ± 3.6 3.6 ± 4.0 0.3 ± 2.9	N/A^d
Kumra et al., 2008 [120] Clozapine Olanzapine	10–18 (21) (18) (21)	Randomized, double-blind, controlled	12	0.7 ± 3.4^c 1.5 ± 9.1^c	16.7 9.5
Tohen et al., 2007 [121] Olanzapine	13–17 (107)	Randomized, double-blind, controlled	20.6	3.66 ± 2.18	41.9
Delbello et al., 2006 [122] Quetiapine	12–18 (25)	Randomized, double-blind, controlled	4	4.4 ± 5.0	N/A^d
Fleischhaker et al., 2006 [60] Olanzapine Risperidone Clozapine	17.2 ± 1.8 (16) 15.8 ± 1.4 (16) 15.6 ± 2.6 (19)	Naturalistic open label	6	4.6 ± 1.9 2.8 ± 1.3 2.5 ± 2.9	N/A^d
Shaw et al., 2006 [123] Clozapine Olanzapine	7–16 (25) (12) (13)	Randomized, double-blind, controlled	8	3.8 ± 6.0 3.6 ± 4.0	N/A^d

(Continued)

TABLE 25.3 Selected Studies Demonstrating Antipsychotic Associated Weight Gain in Youth—cont'd

Atypical antipsychotic	Age (n)	Design	Duration (weeks)	Weight gain (kg)	7% Weight gain (%)
Biederman et al., 2005 [124] Olanzapine Risperidone	4–6 (31) (15) (16)	Open label	8	3.2 ± 0.7 2.2 ± 0.4	N/A[d]
Biederman et al., 2005 [125] Risperidone	6–17 (30)	Open label	8	2.1 ± 2.0	N/A[d]
Marchand et al., 2004 [126] Quetiapine	4–17 (19)	Randomized, controlled	10	0.8[c]	N/A[d]
Sikich et al., 2004 [72] Olanzapine Risperidone	6 (36) (16) (20)	Randomized, double-blind, controlled	8	7.2 ± 0.1 4.9 ± 0.4	N/A[d]
Masi et al., 2002 [127] Clozapine	12–17 (10)	Randomized, controlled	14.8	7.0 ± 3.1	N/A[d]
Ratzoni et al., 2002 [58] Olanzapine Risperidone Haloperidol	17.0 ± 1.6 (21) 17.1 ± 2.1 (21) 17.3 ± 1.3 (8)	Naturalistic open label	12	7.2 ± 6.3 3.9 ± 4.8 1.1 ± 3.3	90.5 42.9 12.5
Frazier et al., 2001 [128] Clozapine	5–14 (23)	Open label	8	5.0 ± 2.3	N/A[d]

[a]Standard deviation values were not available, but 95% confidence interval is provided.
[b]Mean BMI z-score, utilized instead of mean weight gained in order to control for developmentally appropriate weight gain.
[c]Mean BMI.
[d]Information was not provided.

simply an artifact caused by the fact that younger individuals were less likely to be exposed to medication than adults and that the increased weight gain seen in studies of youth was similar to that shown in first-episode adults [65]. The findings of the 6-year Second-Generation Antipsychotic Treatment Indications, Effectiveness and Tolerability in Youth (SATIETY) study, in addition to providing a comprehensive analysis of weight and metabolic change in early treatment in youth, shed some light on this issue [65]. In this study, children aged 7 to 19 were followed for 12 weeks as they started antipsychotic treatment. The study was naturalistic in that medication assignment was done by community psychiatrists based on their own clinical practice. Data from the 338 children in this study demonstrated significant weight gain in children on all antipsychotic medication including aripiprazole 4.4 kg, 58.4% gained ≥7% weight; risperidone 5.3 kg, 64.4% gained ≥7% weight; quetiapine 6.1 kg, 55.6% gained ≥ 7% weight and olanzapine 8.5 kg, 84.4% gained ≥ 7% weight during the 12-week period with increases in cholesterol (total and non High density lipoprotein) with olanzapine and quetiapine and increases in triglycerides on these medications as well as on risperidone. What made this uncontrolled sample particularly informative was that children were excluded if they had any more than 1 week of prior exposure to medication. The authors further posited that the sizes of these increases are better accounted for by the lack of prior exposure to antipsychotic medication than the absolute age of the subjects.

The health and metabolic impact of this weight gain has been further delineated by studies relating antipsychotic medication to increased risk of diabetes and cardiovascular disease [66], with some data suggesting that children on antipsychotic medication had a 14% prevalence of developing cardiovascular disease, more than four times the prevalence rate in matched controls (3%). Data obtained from Medicare registries in South Carolina showed that children prescribed antipsychotic medication were much more likely to have cardiovascular conditions (odds ratio 2.70, and type 2 diabetes odds ratio 3.23) than those not prescribed antipsychotic medication [66].

MECHANISM

The specific etiology and mechanism of weight gain associated with SGA use is still being elucidated. Some have linked these medications to decreased activity, and others with increased caloric intake. Experiments reporting on a rat model for iatrogenic weight gain [67] have shown a decrease in motor activity in the first 10 days of antipsychotic treatment. A pilot study of adolescents [68] demonstrated a trend of decreased movement approaching significance using an accelerometer to measure movement changes. Differential trends in substrate utilization, a measure of the manner in which the body utilizes energy stores, with a decrease in fat oxidation, have been shown in adults on olanzapine [69]. This trend toward increased carbohydrate oxidation has been understood to be part of a putative mechanism for weight gain [70]. The most robust finding regarding mechanism of SGA-induced weight gain has been increased intake evinced by adverse event report [71–73]. In the pilot study of adolescents cited earlier [68], this was measured more precisely by weighing food intake for a 2-day period at baseline and again after 4 weeks of olanzapine treatment. This has been shown in a rat model [74] as well.

The correlation between SGA use and the increased hazard of diabetes and metabolic syndrome is only partially understood. The preponderance of data suggests that this risk of diabetes is mediated by weight gain and adiposity; however, there are data suggesting that insulin resistance, a precursor of diabetes mellitus, may occur even in the absence of weight gain in patients taking SGAs [75].

One theory to account for increased intake and the disproportionate increase in adipose tissue involves leptin. Leptin is a hormone secreted by adipose tissue that acts principally on the hypothalamus to inhibit appetite [76]. It has been argued that a deficit in the reactivity to leptin in patients taking SGAs contributes to their excess weight gain. In one of the few studies looking at SGAs utilizing whole-body MRI, leptin appeared to maintain its inhibitory effects on the accumulation of peripheral adipose tissue, but not on that of visceral adipose tissue, suggesting that an iatrogenic effect of the medication may be to block the usual inhibitory action of leptin on visceral adipose accumulation [77]. The authors further suggested that a serotonin receptor, 5HT2c, may be implicated in the iatrogenic effects of leptin insensitivity. This would suggest that polymorphism of the 5HT2c receptor gene may help predict which children are most vulnerable to weight gain on these medications [78]. It follows that the research on the genetics of vulnerability to SGA-induced weight gain has focused on several polymorphisms in the promoter region of the 5HT2c receptor genes that may help predict which individuals are most vulnerable to weight gain on medications. One study found that antipsychotic-related obesity was three times as likely to be correlated with a combined genotype of four genes in the 5HT2c promoter region. Specifically, the variant (less common polymorphism) HTR2C:c.1−142948(GT)n 13 repeat allele, the common allele rs3813929 C, the variant allele rs518147 C, and the variant allele rs1414334 C—was significantly related to an increased risk of obesity (OR 3.71 (95% confidence interval: 1.24−11.12)) in adults on antipsychotic medications. This finding has been shown in adults but not yet examined in adolescents or children. Likewise a finding involving a polymorphism of a −2548a/g leptin receptor promoter showed effect in conferring long-term resistance to weight gain in combination with a 5HT2c polymorphism [79].

Other receptors that have shown promise as an avenue of investigation for the etiology and treatment of antipsychotic-associated weight gain are the hypothalamic histamine receptor, H1, and the function-related H3 autoreceptor [80]. Both are involved in the regulation of appetite and studies examining the correlation between receptor affinity and orexigenicity (likelihood of causing weight gain) found affinity for the H1 receptor the highest in medications with the most potent weight-gain profiles [81]. Kim et al. [82] examined H1 as the central receptor mediating the orexigenic effects of SGAs through a second messenger, adenosine monophosphate activated kinase (AMPk). They demonstrated this in an elegant experiment, utilizing mice bred without the hypothalamic H1 receptor gene (H1 knockout mice) exposed to clozapine, an SGA and a potent orexigen. In H1 knockout mice, there is no change in AMPk levels or in appetite when they are exposed to clozapine; however, in normal mice, AMPk levels drop and eating behavior is increased by clozapine. Kim et al. [82], citing their findings, suggested that the search for therapeutic agents that would reverse the histamine blockade produced by SGAs would be a fruitful avenue of investigation.

TREATMENTS FOR ANTIPSYCHOTIC ASSOCIATED WEIGHT GAIN

Research of treatments for antipsychotic associated weight gain have been conducted almost exclusively in adults [83] with only two randomized trials and a handful of open-label studies published in youth. Baptista and colleagues, authors of several trials of agents to treat antipsychotic-associated weight gain [84], performed a systematic review of 25 pharmacological weight loss intervention studies (N = 1221). They considered results promising for amantadine, metformin, reboxetine, sibutramine, and topiramate noting, however, that the field was hindered by small sample sizes and heterogeneous populations. Indeed, the lack of head-to-head studies comparing different medications for the treatment or prevention of antipsychotic-induced weight gain and the limited number and sample size of randomized, placebo-controlled trials has made it difficult to evaluate the effectiveness of individual pharmacological agents.

Because of its relative success, metformin has had the plurality of research with seven placebo-controlled studies [85–93], four of which showed a significant separation from placebo. In the two prevention trials, where individuals started metformin concomitantly with antipsychotic, subjects gained weight in both treatment and placebo groups. In one study [90], subjects gained significantly less weight in the metformin augmentation group. In the other study [88], there was a trend toward metformin ameliorating weight gain but this did not reach statistical significance.

There are two randomized pediatric trials of pharmacological agents to treat antipsychotic associated weight, again, both testing metformin among youth who have already gained body weight. In 2006 Klein et al. [93] published a double-blind placebo-controlled trial of metformin that showed weight stabilization in adolescents receiving a SGA. In this trial, individuals in the placebo group continued to gain approximately 0.3 kg/week during the study, whereas those in the adjunctive metformin group did not gain further weight. Entry criteria required 10% weight gain in the year since the initiation of SGA treatment. In neither group did weight go back down to the baseline levels that subjects had before they had entered the study. The only other published placebo-controlled trial of any agent in youth also used metformin [95]. In this study, patients receiving risperidone were randomized to receive adjunctive metformin or placebo. There was a trend toward metformin ameliorating weight gain in this small (N = 32) study, but this did not reach statistical significance [92].

To date there are no placebo-controlled trials of medications to prevent antipsychotic associated weight gain in youth. In no studies were subjects able to lose sufficient weight to return to baseline.

Regarding nonpharmacological interventions, a meta-analysis of 10 studies (N = 482) [94] examining behavioral interventions to treat antipsychotic-related weight gain demonstrated a 2.56 kg (CI: 1.92, 3.20) greater reduction in weight in subjects compared to treatment as usual. No significant difference was found between nutritional counseling and CBT. None of these studies, however, included children. Assuming that comparable populations are studied, it would appear that nonpharmacological interventions can be more effective than pharmacological interventions. However, in the only randomized study in which these modalities were compared directly [91], the pharmacological intervention—metformin—performed better than the nonpharmacological treatment—that is, −3.2 kg (CI: −2.5, −3.9) versus −1.4 kg (CI: −0.7, −2.0; p < .05). Of note, however, the most efficacious treatment in that study was the combined metformin and behavioral intervention—that is, −4.7 kg (CI: −3.4, −5.7).

In terms of managing weight gain in children on antipsychotics, one resource is the American Academy of Pediatrics' 5-2-1-0 guideline recommending 5 servings of fruits, 2 hours or less of television, video or computer screen time daily, greater than 1 hour of exercise, and 0 soft drinks. Christoph Correll and Harold Carlson outlined another proposed behavioral regimen in a review of the endocrine effects of antipsychotic medications [95]. They proposed a "12-step" program to assist with controlling weight gain as outlined as follows:

- Involve the family in meal planning.
- Drink water instead of sweetened beverages.
- Have four to six separate meals per day.
- Eat breakfast every day.
- Serve small portions.
- Eat foods with low glycemic index slowly.
- Reduce saturated fat intake.
- Consume at least 25 to 30 g of soluble fiber.
- Avoid snacking while sated.
- Limit fast foods to less than one meal per week.
- Limit sedentary activities to less than 2 hours per day.
- Exercise 30 to 60 minutes daily.

They further suggested monitoring fasting blood work for signs of hyperglycemia, insulin resistance, hypercholesterolemia, and hypertriglyceridemia at baseline, after 3 months, and then at 6-month intervals.

FUTURE DIRECTIONS IN RESEARCH

There are several current initiatives to explore the phenomenology and treatment of antipsychotic associated weight gain. An NIH-funded 5-year study examining the efficacy of antipsychotic medication at controlling aggression as well as the metabolic effects of antipsychotic medications in youth using assessments of resting metabolic rate, total body fat, and insulin action in skeletal muscle, liver, and adipose tissue concluded in 2009 [96]. In terms of clinical interventions, a multisite study was launched to examine the effects of switching to a possibly less orexigenic antipsychotic (aripiprazole) versus adding metformin [97]. There is also a study examining the effect of a centrally acting histamine agonist on weight gain in overweight children on antipsychotic medications [98]. A combined behavioral-pharmacological intervention study is being conducted to look at metformin versus a healthy lifestyle intervention consisting of an additional meeting at each psychiatric visit to review weight changes, level of physical activity, and healthy eating behaviors to treat antipsychotic associated weight gain in youth [99].

Developments in obesity research in adults, both behavioral and pharmacological, will also likely be adapted in the coming years in an attempt to ameliorate the metabolic burden on children and adolescents who require antipsychotic treatment.

CONCLUSION

Obesity rates have tripled among children and youth in the United States since the 1970s. Some of this weight gain may be related to psychiatric illness. Psychotropic medications also often have effects on appetite and satiety. This appears especially pronounced with the newer second-generation antipsychotic medications. These medications are popular because of their perceived efficacy at treating severe conditions, such as irritability associated with autism, psychosis, and bipolar disorder and also their utility as augmentative agents in more common child psychiatric disorders such as ADHD, oppositional defiant disorder, and conduct disorder. Their rate of prescription has increased more than five-fold since 1993.

Although certain agents are more likely to cause weight gain than others, all antipsychotics can cause clinically significant weight gain. Mechanisms of antipsychotic weight gain have not yet been clearly established. However, the most robust findings involve increased caloric intake, possibly mediated by histamine (H1) and serotonin (5HT2c) receptors. Work in pharmacogenetics has shown vulnerability conferred by certain polymorphisms in 5HT2c and leptin receptors.

The research conducted on treatment to date has almost exclusively been on adults. Results in those studies have shown a moderate ameliorative effect for metformin. In children, there have been a handful of studies in metformin showing a modest but consistent effect and little data on other agents. There have been no published behavioral studies in children; however, work in adults shows efficacy for behavioral measures with nutritional counseling and cognitive behavioral therapy being equally effective.

Current studies are under way to further delineate mechanisms of weight gain in children and examine novel treatment strategies. As interventions to treat childhood obesity develop further, these can be applied to the treatment of children with psychotropic-related weight gain.

References

1. Ogden CL, Carroll MD, Curtin LR, McDowell MA, Tabak CJ, Flegal KM. Prevalence of overweight and obesity in the United States, 1999–2004. JAMA 2006;**295**(13):1549–55.
2. Cali AM, Caprio S. Obesity in children and adolescents. J Clin Endocrinol Metab 2008;**93**(11 Suppl. 1):S31–6.
3. Ogden CL, Carroll MD, Flegal KM. High body mass index for age among US children and adolescents, 2003–2006. JAMA 2008;**299**(20):2401–5.
4. Huang ES, Basu A, O'Grady M, Capretta JC. Projecting the Future Diabetes Population Size and Related Costs for the U.S. Diabetes Care 2009;**32**(12):2225–9.
5. Flores G, Olson L, Tomany-Korman SC. Racial and ethnic disparities in early childhood health and health care. Pediatrics 2005;**115**(2):e183–93.
6. Davis PH, Dawson JD, Riley WA, Lauer RM. Carotid intimal-medial thickness is related to cardiovascular risk factors measured from childhood through middle age: The Muscatine Study. Circulation 2001;**104**(23):2815–19.
7. Li S, Chen W, Srinivasan SR, Bond MG, Tang R, Urbina EM, et al. Childhood cardiovascular risk factors and carotid vascular changes in adulthood: the Bogalusa Heart Study. JAMA 2003;**290**(17):2271–6.
8. Weiss R, Dziura J, Burgert TS, Tamborlane WV, Taksali SE, Yeckel CW, et al. Obesity and the metabolic syndrome in children and adolescents. N Engl J Med 2004;**350**(23):2362–74.
9. Urbina EM, Kimball TR, McCoy CE, Khoury PR, Daniels SR, Dolan LM. Youth with obesity and obesity-related type 2 diabetes mellitus demonstrate abnormalities in carotid structure and function. Circulation 2009;**119**(22):2913–19.
10. Molnar D. The prevalence of the metabolic syndrome and type 2 diabetes mellitus in children and adolescents. Int J Obes Relat Metab Disord 2004;**28**(Suppl. 3):S70–4.
11. Pinhas-Hamiel O, Dolan LM, Daniels SR, Standiford D, Khoury PR, Zeitler P. Increased incidence of non-insulin-dependent diabetes mellitus among adolescents. J Pediatr 1996;**128**(5 Pt 1):608–15.
12. Rosenbloom AL. Fetal and childhood nutrition in type 2 diabetes in children and adults. Pediatr Diabetes 2000;**1**(1):34–9. discussion 9–40.
13. Jerrell JM, McIntyre RS. Adverse events in children and adolescents treated with antipsychotic medications. Hum Psychopharmacol 2008;**23**(4):283–90.
14. Zito JM, Safer DJ, DosReis S, Gardner JF, Magder L, Soeken K, et al. Psychotropic practice patterns for youth: a 10-year perspective. Arch Pediatr Adolesc Med 2003;**157**(1):17–25.
15. Costello EJ, Egger H, Angold A. 10-year research update review: the epidemiology of child and adolescent psychiatric disorders: I. Methods and public health burden. J Am Acad Child Adolesc Psychiatry 2005;**44**(10):972–86.
16. Birmaher B, Ryan ND, Williamson DE, Brent DA, Kaufman J, Dahl RE, et al. Childhood and adolescent depression: a review of the past 10 years. Part I. J Am Acad Child Adolesc Psychiatry 1996;**35**(11):1427–39.
17. Grunbaum JA, Kann L, Kinchen S, Ross J, Hawkins J, Lowry R, et al. Youth risk behavior surveillance—United States, 2003. MMWR Surveill Summ 2004;**53**(2):1–96.
18. Haavisto A, Sourander A, Ellila H, Valimaki M, Santalahti P, Helenius H. Suicidal ideation and suicide attempts among child and adolescent psychiatric inpatients in Finland. J Affect Disord 2003;**76**(1-3):211–21.
19. Hallfors DD, Waller MW, Ford CA, Halpern CT, Brodish PH, Iritani B. Adolescent depression and suicide risk: association with sex and drug behavior. Am J Prev Med 2004;**27**(3):224–31.
20. Patton GC, Coffey C, Posterino M, Carlin JB, Wolfe R. Adolescent depressive disorder: a population-based study of ICD-10 symptoms. Aust N Z J Psychiatry 2000;**34**(5):741–7.
21. Roberts RE, Lewinsohn PM, Seeley JR. Symptoms of DSM-III-R major depression in adolescence: evidence from an epidemiological survey. J Am Acad Child Adolesc Psychiatry 1995;**34**(12):1608–17.
22. Ryan ND, Puig-Antich J, Ambrosini P, Rabinovich H, Robinson D, Nelson B, et al. The clinical picture of major depression in children and adolescents. Arch Gen Psychiatry 1987;**44**(10):854–61.

23. Fombonne E, Wostear G, Cooper V, Harrington R, Rutter M. The Maudsley long-term follow-up of child and adolescent depression. 2. Suicidality, criminality and social dysfunction in adulthood. Br J Psychiatry 2001;179:218—23.
24. Kessler RC, Walters EE. Epidemiology of DSM-III-R major depression and minor depression among adolescents and young adults in the National Comorbidity Survey. Depress Anxiety 1998;7(1):3—14.
25. Wichstrom L. Predictors of adolescent suicide attempts: a nationally representative longitudinal study of Norwegian adolescents. J Am Acad Child Adolesc Psychiatry 2000;39(5):603—10.
26. Web-based Injury Statistics Query and Reporting System (WISQARS) Atlanta (GA): Centers for Disease Control and Prevention, National Center for Injury Prevention and Control; [cited Dec 1, 2009]; Available from: www.cdc.gov/injury/wisqars/index.html.
27. March J, Silva S, Petrycki S, Curry J, Wells K, Fairbank J, et al. Fluoxetine, cognitive-behavioral therapy, and their combination for adolescents with depression: Treatment for Adolescents with Depression Study (TADS) randomized controlled trial. JAMA 2004;292(7):807—20.
28. Brent D, Greenhill LL, Compton S, Emslie G, Wells K, Walkup J, et al. The Treatment of Adolescent Suicide Attempters Study (TASA): Predictors of Suicidal Events in an Open Treatment Trial. J Am Acad Child Adolesc Psychiatry 2009;48(10):987—96.
29. Miyazaki M, Yoshino A, Nomura S. Diagnosis of multiple anxiety disorders predicts the concurrent comorbidity of major depressive disorder. Compr Psychiatry. 51(1):15—18.
30. Walkup JT, Albano AM, Piacentini J, Birmaher B, Compton SN, Sherrill JT, et al. Cognitive behavioral therapy, sertraline, or a combination in childhood anxiety. N Engl J Med 2008;359(26):2753—66.
31. Woodruff TJ, Axelrad DA, Kyle AD, Nweke O, Miller GG, Hurley BJ. Trends in environmentally related childhood illnesses. Pediatrics 2004;113(4 Suppl):1133—40.
32. Greenhill LL, Swanson JM, Vitiello B, Davies M, Clevenger W, Wu M, et al. Impairment and deportment responses to different methylphenidate doses in children with ADHD: the MTA titration trial. J Am Acad Child Adolesc Psychiatry 2001;40(2):180—7.
33. Greenhill L, Kollins S, Abikoff H, McCracken J, Riddle M, Swanson J, et al. Efficacy and safety of immediate-release methylphenidate treatment for preschoolers with ADHD. J Am Acad Child Adolesc Psychiatry 2006;45(11):1284—93.
34. Kratochvil CJ, Vaughan BS, Daughton J, Lubberstedt B, Murray DW, Chrisman A, et al. A Double-Blind, Placebo-Controlled Study of Atomoxetine in Young Children with ADHD. Chicago, IL: Annual Meeting of the AACAP; October 2008.
35. Pediatric OCD Treatment Study (POTS) Team. Cognitive-behavior therapy, sertraline, and their combination for children and adolescents with obsessive-compulsive disorder. the Pediatric OCD Treatment Study (POTS) randomized controlled trial. JAMA 2004;292(16):1969—76.
36. Sikich L, Frazier JA, McClellan J, Findling RL, Vitiello B, Ritz L, et al. Double-blind comparison of first- and second-generation antipsychotics in early-onset schizophrenia and schizo-affective disorder: findings from the treatment of early-onset schizophrenia spectrum disorders (TEOSS) study. Am J Psychiatry 2008;165(11):1420—31.
37. Mustillo S, Worthman C, Erkanli A, Keeler G, Angold A, Costello EJ. Obesity and psychiatric disorder: developmental trajectories. Pediatrics 2003;111(4 Pt 1):851—9.
38. Cortese S, Angriman M, Maffeis C, Isnard P, Konofal E, Lecendreux M, et al. Attention-deficit/hyperactivity disorder (ADHD) and obesity: a systematic review of the literature. Crit Rev Food Sci Nutr 2008;48(6):524—37.
39. Waring ME, Lapane KL. Overweight in children and adolescents in relation to attention-deficit/hyperactivity disorder: results from a national sample. Pediatrics 2008;122(1):e1—6.
40. Olfson M, Blanco C, Liu L, Moreno C, Laje G. National trends in the outpatient treatment of children and adolescents with antipsychotic drugs. Arch Gen Psychiatry 2006;63(6):679—85.
41. Citrome L. Iloperidone for schizophrenia: a review of the efficacy and safety profile for this newly commercialised second-generation antipsychotic. Int J Clin Pract 2009;63(8):1237—48.
42. Citrome L. Asenapine for schizophrenia and bipolar disorder: a review of the efficacy and safety profile for this newly approved sublingually absorbed second-generation antipsychotic. Int J Clin Pract 2009;63(12):1762—84.
43. Kogan MD, Blumberg SJ, Schieve LA, Boyle CA, Perrin JM, Ghandour RM, et al. Prevalence of Parent-Reported Diagnosis of Autism Spectrum Disorder Among Children in the US, 2007. Pediatrics 2009;124(4):2—8.
44. Burd L, Fisher W, Kerbeshian J. A prevalence study of pervasive developmental disorders in North Dakota. J Am Acad Child Adolesc Psychiatry 1987;26(5):700—3.
45. Costello EJ, Angold A, Burns BJ, Stangl DK, Tweed DL, Erkanli A, et al. The Great Smoky Mountains Study of Youth. Goals, design, methods, and the prevalence of DSM-III-R disorders. Arch Gen Psychiatry 1996;53(12):1129—36.
46. Youngstrom EA, Birmaher B, Findling RL. Pediatric bipolar disorder: validity, phenomenology, and recommendations for diagnosis. Bipolar Disord 2008;10(1 Pt 2):194—214.
47. McCracken JT, McGough J, Shah B, Cronin P, Hong D, Aman MG, et al. Risperidone in children with autism and serious behavioral problems. N Engl J Med 2002;347(5):314—21.
48. Kowatch RA, Fristad M, Birmaher B, Wagner KD, Findling RL, Hellander M. Treatment guidelines for children and adolescents with bipolar disorder. J Am Acad Child Adolesc Psychiatry 2005;44(3):213—35.
49. Armenteros JL, Lewis JE, Davalos M. Risperidone augmentation for treatment-resistant aggression in attention-deficit/hyperactivity disorder: a placebo-controlled pilot study. J Am Acad Child Adolesc Psychiatry 2007;46(5):558—65.
50. Kutcher S, Aman M, Brooks SJ, Buitelaar J, van Daalen E, Fegert J, et al. International consensus statement on attention-deficit/hyperactivity disorder (ADHD) and disruptive behaviour disorders (DBDs): clinical implications and treatment practice suggestions. Eur Neuropsychopharmacol 2004;14(1):11—28.
51. Cooper WO, Hickson GB, Fuchs C, Arbogast PG, Ray WA. New users of antipsychotic medications among children enrolled in TennCare. Arch Pediatr Adolesc Med 2004;158(8):753—9.
52. Staller JA, Wade MJ, Baker M. Current prescribing patterns in outpatient child and adolescent psychiatric practice in central New York. J Child Adolesc Psychopharmacol 2005;15(1):57—61.
53. Constantine R, Tandon R. Changing trends in pediatric antipsychotic use in Florida's Medicaid program. Psychiatr Serv 2008;59(10):1162—8.
54. Allison DB, Mentore JL, Heo M, Chandler LP, Cappelleri JC, Infante MC, et al. Antipsychotic-induced weight gain: a comprehensive research synthesis. Am J Psychiatry 1999;156(11):1686—96.
55. Kahn RS, Fleischhacker WW, Boter H, Davidson M, Vergouwe Y, Keet IP, et al. Effectiveness of antipsychotic drugs in first-episode schizophrenia and schizophreniform disorder: an open randomised clinical trial. Lancet 2008;371(9618):1085—97.

56. Consensus development conference on antipsychotic drugs and obesity and diabetes. *Diabetes Care* 2004;**27**(2):596–601.
57. Kinon BJ, Kaiser CJ, Ahmed S, Rotelli MD, Kollack-Walker S. Association between early and rapid weight gain and change in weight over one year of olanzapine therapy in patients with schizophrenia and related disorders. *J Clin Psychopharmacol* 2005;**25**(3):255–8.
58. Ratzoni G, Gothelf D, Brand-Gothelf A, Reidman J, Kikinzon L, Gal G, et al. Weight gain associated with olanzapine and risperidone in adolescent patients: a comparative prospective study. *J Am Acad Child Adolesc Psychiatry* 2002;**41**(3):337–43.
59. McClellan J, Sikich L, Findling RL, Frazier JA, Vitiello B, Hlastala SA, et al. Treatment of early-onset schizophrenia spectrum disorders (TEOSS): rationale, design, and methods. *J Am Acad Child Adolesc Psychiatry* 2007;**46**(8):969–78.
60. Fleischhaker C, Heiser P, Hennighausen K, Herpertz-Dahlmann B, Holtkamp K, Mehler-Wex C, et al. Clinical drug monitoring in child and adolescent psychiatry: side effects of atypical neuroleptics. *J Child Adolesc Psychopharmacol* 2006;**16**(3):308–16.
61. Safer DJ. A comparison of risperidone-induced weight gain across the age span. *J Clin Psychopharmacol* 2004;**24**(4):429–36.
62. Weiss M, Panagiotopoulos C, Giles L, Gibbins C, Kuzeljevic B, Davidson J, et al. A naturalistic study of predictors and risks of atypical antipsychotic use in an attention-deficit/hyperactivity disorder clinic. *J Child Adolesc Psychopharmacol* 2009;**19**(5):575–82.
63. Correll CU. Weight gain and metabolic effects of mood stabilizers and antipsychotics in pediatric bipolar disorder: a systematic review and pooled analysis of short-term trials. *J Am Acad Child Adolesc Psychiatry* 2007;**46**(6):687–700.
64. Calarge CA, Acion L, Kuperman S, Tansey M, Schlechte JA. Weight gain and metabolic abnormalities during extended risperidone treatment in children and adolescents. *J Child Adolesc Psychopharmacol* 2009;**19**(2):101–9.
65. Correll CU, Manu P, Olshanskiy V, Napolitano B, Kane JM, Malhotra AK. Cardiometabolic risk of second-generation antipsychotic medications during first-time use in children and adolescents. *JAMA* 2009;**302**(16):1765–73.
66. McIntyre RS, Jerrell JM. Metabolic and cardiovascular adverse events associated with antipsychotic treatment in children and adolescents. *Arch Pediatr Adolesc Med* 2008;**162**(10):929–35.
67. Arjona AA, Zhang SX, Adamson B, Wurtman RJ. An animal model of antipsychotic-induced weight gain. *Behav Brain Res.* 2004;**152**(1):121–7.
68. Gothelf D, Falk B, Singer P, Kairi M, Phillip M, Zigel L, et al. Weight gain associated with increased food intake and low habitual activity levels in male adolescent schizophrenic inpatients treated with olanzapine. *Am J Psychiatry* 2002;**159**(6):1055–7.
69. Graham KA, Gu H, Lieberman JA, Harp JB, Perkins DO. Double-blind, placebo-controlled investigation of amantadine for weight loss in subjects who gained weight with olanzapine. *Am J Psychiatry* 2005;**162**(9):1744–6.
70. Zurlo F, Lillioja S, Esposito-Del Puente A, Nyomba BL, Raz I, Saad MF, et al. Low ratio of fat to carbohydrate oxidation as predictor of weight gain: study of 24-h RQ. *Am J Physiol* 1990;**259**(5 Pt 1):E650–7.
71. Basson BR, Kinon BJ, Taylor CC, Szymanski KA, Gilmore JA, Tollefson GD. Factors influencing acute weight change in patients with schizophrenia treated with olanzapine, haloperidol, or risperidone. *J Clin Psychiatry* 2001;**62**(4):231–8.
72. Sikich L, Hamer RM, Bashford RA, Sheitman BB, Lieberman JA. A pilot study of risperidone, olanzapine, and haloperidol in psychotic youth: a double-blind, randomized, 8-week trial. *Neuropsychopharmacology* 2004;**29**(1):133–45.
73. Woods SW, Martin A, Spector SG, McGlashan TH. Effects of development on olanzapine-associated adverse events. *J Am Acad Child Adolesc Psychiatry* 2002;**41**(12):1439–46.
74. Ota M, Mori K, Nakashima A, Kaneko YS, Fujiwara K, Itoh M, et al. Peripheral injection of risperidone, an atypical antipsychotic, alters the bodyweight gain of rats. *Clin Exp Pharmacol Physiol* 2002;**29**(11):980–9.
75. Newcomer JW, Haupt DW, Fucetola R, Melson AK, Schweiger JA, Cooper BP, et al. Abnormalities in glucose regulation during antipsychotic treatment of schizophrenia. *Arch Gen Psychiatry* 2002;**59**(4):337–45.
76. Muldoon MF, Mackey RH, Korytkowski MT, Flory JD, Pollock BG, Manuck SB. The metabolic syndrome is associated with reduced central serotonergic responsivity in healthy community volunteers. *J Clin Endocrinol Metab* 2006;**91**(2):718–21.
77. Zhang ZJ, Yao ZJ, Liu W, Fang Q, Reynolds GP. Effects of antipsychotics on fat deposition and changes in leptin and insulin levels. Magnetic resonance imaging study of previously untreated people with schizophrenia. *Br J Psychiatry* 2004;**184**:58–62.
78. Hosojima H, Togo T, Odawara T, Hasegawa K, Miura S, Kato Y, et al. Early effects of olanzapine on serum levels of ghrelin, adiponectin and leptin in patients with schizophrenia. *J Psychopharmacol* 2006;**20**(1):75–9.
79. Templeman LA, Reynolds GP, Arranz B, San L. Polymorphisms of the 5-HT2C receptor and leptin genes are associated with antipsychotic drug-induced weight gain in Caucasian subjects with a first-episode psychosis. *Pharmacogenet Genomics* 2005;**15**(4):195–200.
80. Deng C, Weston-Green K, Huang XF. The role of histaminergic H1 and H3 receptors in food intake: A mechanism for atypical antipsychotic-induced weight gain? *Prog Neuropsychopharmacol Biol Psychiatry* 2009;**34**(1):1–4.
81. Kroeze WK, Hufeisen SJ, Popadak BA, Renock SM, Steinberg S, Ernsberger P, et al. H1-histamine receptor affinity predicts short-term weight gain for typical and atypical antipsychotic drugs. *Neuropsychopharmacology* 2003;**28**(3):519–26.
82. Kim SF, Huang AS, Snowman AM, Teuscher C, Snyder SH. From the Cover: Antipsychotic drug-induced weight gain mediated by histamine H1 receptor-linked activation of hypothalamic AMP-kinase. *Proc Natl Acad Sci USA* 2007;**104**(9):3456–9.
83. Citrome L, Vreeland B. Schizophrenia, obesity, and antipsychotic medications: what can we do? *Postgrad Med* 2008;**120**(2):18–33.
84. Baptista T, ElFakih Y, Uzcategui E, Sandia I, Talamo E, Araujo de Baptista E, et al. Pharmacological management of atypical antipsychotic-induced weight gain. *CNS Drugs* 2008;**22**(6):477–95.
85. Maayan L, Vakhrusheva J, Correll CU. *Pharmacologic Interventions to Reduce Antipsychotic-Related Weight Gain and Metabolic Abnormalities: A Systematic Review and Meta-analysis*. Hollywood, FL: American College of Neuropsychopharmacology Meeting; December 6–10, 2009.
86. Citrome L. Compelling or irrelevant? Using number needed to treat can help decide. *Acta Psychiatr Scand* 2008;**117**(6):412–19.
87. Baptista T, Martinez J, Lacruz A, Rangel N, Beaulieu S, Serrano A, et al. Metformin for prevention of weight gain and insulin resistance with olanzapine: a double-blind placebo-controlled trial. *Can J Psychiatry* 2006;**51**(3):192–6.
88. Baptista T, Rangel N, Fernandez V, Carrizo E, El Fakih Y, Uzcategui E, et al. Metformin as an adjunctive treatment to control body weight and metabolic dysfunction during

olanzapine administration: a multicentric, double-blind, placebo-controlled trial. *Schizophr Res.* 2007;**93**(1-3):99−108.
89. Carrizo E, Fernandez V, Connell L, Sandia I, Prieto D, Mogollon J, et al. Extended release metformin for metabolic control assistance during prolonged clozapine administration: a 14 week, double-blind, parallel group, placebo-controlled study. *Schizophr Res.* 2009;**113**(1):19−26.
90. Wu RR, Zhao JP, Guo XF, He YQ, Fang MS, Guo WB, et al. Metformin addition attenuates olanzapine-induced weight gain in drug-naive first-episode schizophrenia patients: a double-blind, placebo-controlled study. *Am J Psychiatry* 2008;**165**(3):352−8.
91. Wu RR, Zhao JP, Jin H, Shao P, Fang MS, Guo XF, et al. Lifestyle intervention and metformin for treatment of antipsychotic-induced weight gain: a randomized controlled trial. *JAMA* 2008;**299**(2):185−93.
92. Arman S, Sadramely MR, Nadi M, Koleini N. A randomized, double-blind, placebo-controlled trial of metformin treatment for weight gain associated with initiation of risperidone in children and adolescents. *Saudi Med J* 2008;**29**(8):1130−4.
93. Klein DJ, Cottingham EM, Sorter M, Barton BA, Morrison JA. A randomized, double-blind, placebo-controlled trial of metformin treatment of weight gain associated with initiation of atypical antipsychotic therapy in children and adolescents. *Am J Psychiatry* 2006;**163**(12):2072−9.
94. Alvarez-Jimenez M, Hetrick SE, Gonzalez-Blanch C, Gleeson JF, McGorry PD. Non-pharmacological management of antipsychotic-induced weight gain: systematic review and meta-analysis of randomised controlled trials. *Br J Psychiatry* 2008;**193**(2):101−7.
95. Correll CU, Carlson HE. Endocrine and metabolic adverse effects of psychotropic medications in children and adolescents. *J Am Acad Child Adolesc Psychiatry* 2006;**45**(7):771−91.
96. Metabolic Effects of Antipsychotics in Children (MEAC) [database on the Internet]. Bethesda (MD): National Library of Medicine (US). 2000-. [cited Dec 1, 2009]. Available from: http://clinicaltrials.gov/show/NCT00205699 NLM Identifier: NCT00205699.
97. Reducing Weight Gain and Improving Metabolic Function in Children Being Treated With Antipsychotics [database on the Internet]. Bethesda (MD): national Library of Medicine (US). 2000-. [cited Dec 1, 2009]. Available from: http://clinicaltrials.gov/show/NCT00806234 NLM Identifier: NCT00806234.
98. To Examine the Effect of Betahistine on Antipsychotic Induced Weight Gain in Adolescents [database on the Internet]. Bethesda (MD): National Library of MedIcine (US). 2000-. [cited Dec 1, 2009]. Available from: http://clinicaltrials.gov/show/NCT00709202 NLM Identifier: NCT00709202.
99. Improving Metabolic Parameters of Antipsychotic Child Treatment With Ziprasidone, Aripiprazole, and Clozapine (ZAC) [database on the Internet]. Bethesda (MD): National Library of Medicine (US). 2000-[cited 2009 Dec 1]. Available from: http://clinicaltrials.gov/show/NCT00617058 NLM Identifier: NCT00617058.
100. Sharpe C, Wolfson T, Trauner DA. Weight gain in children treated with valproate. *J Child Neurol* 2009;**24**(3):338−41.
101. Atmaca M, Kuloglu M, Tezcan E, Ustundag B. Weight gain and serum leptin levels in patients on lithium treatment. *Neuropsychobiology* 2002;**46**(2):67−9.
102. Correll CU. Balancing efficacy and safety in treatment with antipsychotics. *CNS Spectr* 2007;**12**(10 Suppl. 17):12−20, 35.
103. Fava M. Weight gain and antidepressants. *The Journal of Clinical Psychiatry* 2000;**61**(Suppl. 11(11)):37−41.
104. Westenberg HG, Sandner C. Tolerability and safety of fluvoxamine and other antidepressants. *Int J Clin Pract* 2006;**60**(4):482−91.
105. Faraone SV, Biederman J, Morley CP, Spencer TJ. Effect of stimulants on height and weight: a review of the literature. *J Am Acad Child Adolesc Psychiatry* 2008;**47**(9):994−1009.
106. Wigal T, Greenhill L, Chuang S, McGough J, Vitiello B, Skrobala A, et al. Safety and tolerability of methylphenidate in preschool children with ADHD. *J Am Acad Child Adolesc Psychiatry* 2006;**45**(11):1294−303.
107. Drugs@FDA. Abilify Label Information. [Internet]: Silver Spring (MD): Food and Drug Administration (US); [2004]; [cited Dec 1, 2009]; Available from: www.accessdata.fda.gov/drugsatfda_docs/label/2009/021436s027lbl.pdf
108. DailyMed. Chlorpromazine Label Information. [Internet]: Bethesda (MD): National Library of Medicine (US). 2000-[cited 2009 Dec 1]; Available from: http://dailymed.nlm.nih.gov/dailymed/drugInfo.cfm?id=11552
109. Chlorprothixene Advanced Consumer Information. [Internet]: Auckland, New Zealand: Drugs.com. 2000-[cited Dec 1, 2009]; Available from: www.drugs.com/cons/thioxanthene-oral-parenteral.html.
110. DailyMed. *Haloperidol Label Information. [Internet].* Bethesda (MD): National Library of Medicine (US); 2000. -[cited Dec 1, 2009]; Available from: http://dailymed.nlm.nih.gov/dailymed/drugInfo.cfm?id=7211.
111. Drugs@FDA. Moban Label Information. [Internet]: Silver Spring (MD): Food and Drug Administration (US); [2004]; [cited Dec 1, 2009]; Available from: www.accessdata.fda.gov/drugsatfda_docs/label/2009/017111s066lbl.pdf.
112. Drugs@FDA. Risperdal Label Information. [Internet]: Silver Spring (MD): Food and Drug Administration (US); [2004]; [cited Dec 1, 2009]; Available from: www.accessdata.fda.gov/drugsatfda_docs/label/2009/020825s034lbl.pdf.
113. DailyMed. *Perphenazine Label Information. [Internet].* Bethesda (MD): National Library of Medicine (US); 2000 [cited Dec 1, 2009]; Available from: http://dailymed.nlm.nih.gov/dailymed/drugInfo.cfm?id=3703.
114. Drugs@FDA. Orap Label Information. [Internet]: Silver Spring (MD): Food and Drug Administration (US); [2004]; [cited Dec 1, 2009]; Available from: www.accessdata.fda.gov/drugsatfda_docs/label/2009/017473s043lbl.pdf
115. DailyMed. Thioridazine Label Information. [Internet], 2000 [cited Dec 1, 2009]; Available from: http://dailymed.nlm.nih.gov/dailymed/drugInfo.cfm?id=3096.
116. Drugs@FDA. Navane Label Information. [Internet]: Silver Spring (MD): Food and Drug Administration (US); [2004]; [cited Dec 1, 2009]; Available from: www.accessdata.fda.gov/drugsatfda_docs/label/2009/016584s059lbl.pdf
117. DailyMed. *Trifluoperazine Label Information. [Internet].* Bethesda (MD): National Library of Medicine (US); 2000 [cited Dec 1, 2009]; Available from: http://dailymed.nlm.nih.gov/dailymed/drugInfo.cfm?id=4815.
118. Hrdlicka M, Zedkova I, Blatny M, Urbanek T. Weight gain associated with atypical and typical antipsychotics during treatment of adolescent schizophrenic psychoses: A retrospective study. *Neuro Endocrinol Lett* 2009;**30**(2):256−61.
119. Verma S, Liew A, Subramaniam M, Poon LY. Effect of treatment on weight gain and metabolic abnormalities in patients with first-episode psychosis. *Aust N Z J Psychiatry* 2009;**43**(9):812−17.
120. Kumra S, Kranzler H, Gerbino-Rosen G, Kester H, De Thomas C, Kafantaris V, et al. Clozapine and "high-dose" olanzapine in refractory early-onset schizophrenia: a 12-week randomized and double-blind comparison. *Biological psychiatry* 2008;**63**(5):524−9.

121. Tohen M, Kryzhanovskaya L, Carlson G, Delbello M, Wozniak J, Kowatch R, et al. Olanzapine versus placebo in the treatment of adolescents with bipolar mania. *The American Journal of Psychiatry* 2007;**164**(10):1547–56.
122. DelBello M, Kowatch R, Adler C, Stanford K, Welge J, Barzman D, et al. A double-blind randomized pilot study comparing quetiapine and divalproex for adolescent mania. *Journal of the American Academy of Child & Adolescent Psychiatry* 2006;**45**(3):305–13.
123. Shaw P, Sporn A, Gogtay N, Overman G, Greenstein D, Gochman P, et al. Childhood-onset schizophrenia: A double-blind, randomized clozapine-olanzapine comparison. *Archives of general psychiatry* 2006;**63**(7):721–30.
124. Biederman J, Mick E, Hammerness P, Harpold T, Aleardi M, Dougherty M, et al. Open-label, 8-week trial of olanzapine and risperidone for the treatment of bipolar disorder in preschool-age children. *Biological psychiatry* 2005;**58**(7):589–94.
125. Biederman J, Mick E, Wozniak J, Aleardi M, Spencer T, Faraone S. An open-label trial of risperidone in children and adolescents with bipolar disorder. *Journal of Child and Adolescent Psychopharmacology* 2005;**15**(2):311–17.
126. Marchand W, Wirth L, Simon C. Quetiapine adjunctive and monotherapy for pediatric bipolar disorder: a retrospective chart review. *Journal of Child and Adolescent Psychopharmacology* 2004;**14**(3):405–11.
127. Masi G, Mucci M, Millepiedi S. Clozapine in adolescent inpatients with acute mania. *Journal of Child and Adolescent Psychopharmacology* 2002;**12**(2):93–9.
128. Frazier JA, Biederman J, Tohen M, Feldman PD, Jacobs TG, Toma V, et al. A prospective open-label treatment trial of olanzapine monotherapy in children and adolescents with bipolar disorder. *Journal of Child and Adolescent Psychopharmacology* 2001;**11**(3):239–50.

SECTION IV

CONSEQUENCES

CHAPTER 26

Childhood Obesity
Public Health Impact and Policy Responses

Rogan Kersh*, *Brian Elbel**,†

*NYU Wagner School, New York, NY 10003 and †NYU Medical School, New York, NY 10016

What do we know about childhood obesity today, after two decades of increasingly urgent research and analysis? That its incidence has risen sharply across demographic groups and regions of the United States as well as most of the world's countries; that the health effects of early-onset obesity—among preadolescent children, for example—are severely detrimental, both physiologically and psychologically; that medical treatment has thus far been ineffective on the whole; that health policy making may be the best route to reversing the increases in obesity and overweight among children—but that few impactful public policies are being implemented, especially at the U.S. national level.

Evidence is emerging, especially from European countries, that the most effective policies to stem the tide of child obesity involve numerous concentrated interventions, implemented simultaneously. In the United States, policy change has been scattershot and episodic, and therefore minimally effective. The American polity, dominated by interest groups and featuring a system of elaborately separated powers, may not permit the type of focused, multiple-approaches policy change that seems necessary. Possibly exacerbating this problem is the nature of evaluation research—testing a single intervention, often during the formative stage of implementation—which may communicate to policy makers and the public alike the wrong signals about the efficacy of achieving sustainable reform.

INCIDENCE OF CHILD OBESITY: UNITED STATES AND GLOBALLY

The most widely used survey of obesity and overweight in the United States is the National Health and Nutrition Examination Survey (NHANES). Data in this study date back to 1970—providing comparative information about obesity (among all age groups) over four decades. Though most health population indicators change comparatively slowly, obesity's growth rate has been so swift that health officials routinely label it an "epidemic," beginning with the U.S. Surgeon General in 2001 [1]. Looking across a 25-year interval (contrasting NHANES's Cycle II, from 1976 to 1980, with the 2003 to 2006 period), the prevalence of obesity increased among 2- to 5-year-old children from 5% to 12.4%; children aged 6 to 11 years saw an increase from 6.5% to 17%; and obesity among adolescents (12 to 19 years old) rose from 5% to 17.6%.

Comparing among demographic and socioeconomic groups of U.S. children, wide variation is evident. In 2008, obesity prevalence was highest among American Indian or Alaska Native (21.2%) and Hispanic (18.5%) children and lowest among white (12.6%), Asian or Pacific Islander (12.3%), and black (11.8%) children [2]. Among white teen girls, the prevalence of overweight decreases with increasing socioeconomic status. In contrast, among black teen girls, the prevalence of overweight remains the same or rises with increasing socioeconomic status [3].

Recent studies suggest that the rate of childhood obesity may be leveling off among some groups in the United States. Among low-income American children aged 2 to 4, for example, the prevalence of obesity grew from 12.4% in 1998 to 14.5% in 2003 but rose to only 14.6% in 2008. At the same time, obesity prevalence among Native American children grew by nearly 15% over the 2003–2008 period. Additional investigation is required to understand the nuances of developing trends. At best, though, childhood obesity rates have begun to plateau in the United States and perhaps a few other advanced democratic countries at present—at what medical professionals widely regard as unacceptably high levels [4].

Global Trends

The World Health Organization (WHO) maintains two databases on childhood health and weight; originally begun to chart malnutrition among children worldwide, the WHO data turned out to provide valuable information about global obesity rates as well. One database covers children under 5 years of age, and the other covers those from 5 to 19. By 2007, an "alarming rate" of increase in childhood obesity (recorded in both databases) led WHO researchers to label it "one of the most serious public health challenges" facing the globe. Though media and some academic accounts into the early 2000s suggested that child obesity was a "rich-country problem," the WHO data indicate that low- and middle-income nations show the sharpest rises in overweight and obesity among children. As of 2007, the WHO estimated, some 22 million children under the age of 5 years were overweight or obese throughout the world—more than three quarters of them residing in low- and middle-income countries [5].

Local studies of regions including Western Europe [6], East-Central Europe [7], the Persian Gulf [8], North/East Asia, South Asia [9], the eastern Mediterranean [10], North Africa, southern Africa [11], the South Pacific, and South America [12]—in a word, nearly everywhere on the globe with substantial human habitation—indicate that obesity is rising, often sharply, among child populations in each. Some of these studies are in early stages, without reliable longitudinal comparisons, and none is without its methodological flaws. But no serious academic analysis suggests that childhood obesity is not a present public health danger, virtually anywhere in the world.

Though norms in cultures across the globe long embraced greater girth and weight among infants and young children as signals of health, contemporary medical evidence—combined with improving early-mortality statistics in many places—strongly suggests that the benefits of size among small children have their limits. We turn now to a review of the health and medical effects of childhood obesity, as presently understood.

HEALTH EFFECTS AND MEDICAL TREATMENT

Overweight adolescents have a 70% chance of becoming overweight or obese adults. This increases to 80% if one or more parent is overweight or obese [13]. Childhood obesity is associated with a wide range of health problems at every stage of life. For children born in the United States in 2000, to take one well-specified example, the lifetime risk of being diagnosed with type 2 diabetes at some point in their lives is estimated at around 30% for boys and 40% for girls [14].

Other well-documented health effects directly or indirectly caused by child obesity include cardiovascular disease, hypertension, high cholesterol, and even, in a particularly distressing example, heart attacks in children as young as age 5 [15]. Psychological effects have also been found to be significant: one well-specified study found that severely obese children aged 5 to 18 described their quality of life in terms similar to those of cancer patients undergoing chemotherapy [16].

Early-stage research suggests, to cap a long roster of discouraging health effects, that the current under-18 generation of Americans may be the first in the nation's history to live shorter life spans than their parents, on average [17]. Although multiple factors contribute to this actuarial claim, the most significant one is the prevalence of obesity among U.S. youth.

Medical Treatment: Costs and Efficacy

In the United States, obesity-associated annual hospital costs for children and youth more than tripled between 1981 and 2000, growing from $35 million to $127 million [18]. Most of this care was and remains palliative, treating illnesses exacerbated by obesity such as diabetes and asthma that will likely be chronic conditions lasting a lifetime.

Global costs of childhood obesity are difficult to ascertain with any precision but appear to be on the sharp rise as well. The World Health Organization in 2000 estimated the cost of obesity at up to 7% of countries' total healthcare costs around the globe, with costs of child obesity contributing roughly a third of that total [19].

The abovementioned chronic health conditions among obese U.S. children are on average exacerbated among lower-income youth—a group with higher rates of uninsurance. Completing this unvirtuous cycle, adolescents with no insurance or public insurance such as Medicaid are more likely than those covered by other insurance to be overweight [20].

Despite rising attention to—and spending on—childhood obesity, no reliable medical treatment to arrest or reverse this condition has been identified. As one medical journal article's title pithily summarized in 2002, "Childhood obesity: public-health crisis, common sense cure" [21]. Lacking a reliable means of addressing obesity through pharmaceutical or even surgical intervention, medical authorities continue to recommend preventive measures wherever possible. This turns our attention to the *causal* factors affecting overweight and obesity in children.

CAUSAL FACTORS

Since the rise in childhood obesity became a source of widespread public concern early in the present century, a fierce debate has centered around *causes*: What are the principal elements contributing to this "epidemic"? The increasingly inactive lifestyle of American children is the primary culprit, according to one well-publicized view—a position encouraged, as it happens, by the food and beverage industries [22]. Efforts to enhance exercise among youth have thus been the predominant public response to rising childhood obesity rates. But a host of recent research suggests that altering American children's relatively sedentary lives—through school-based physical activity interventions, for example—has at most limited benefits, without simultaneous and dedicated attention to the effects of caloric overconsumption [23]. A prospective study involving middle school students over the course of two academic years showed that the risk of becoming obese increased by 60% for every additional serving of sugar-sweetened beverages per day, an effect that remained significant across different levels of exercise [24].

Thus, attention to the reasons for spreading childhood obesity must also extend to food and dietary practices—both *what* children are consuming and *how much*. Ultimately, an immense ongoing effort to pin down causes and solutions boils down to age-old verities: a combination of improved diet and expanded exercise seems to be the ideal response to rising body mass index (BMI) rates among youth. But achieving this grail has eluded public health experts, school officials, concerned parents, and other advocates striving to make a difference. Enter, if reluctantly, public policy makers.

Political discussions in the United States about child obesity broadly follow the two primary frames shaping obesity politics more generally. The first and, until recently, dominant perspective emphasizes *personal responsibility*. Food consumption is, on this view, a deeply personal matter and up to individuals to decide (or, in the case of children, their parents). More recently, with obesity rates rising despite efforts to appeal to personal choices, a competing frame has gained adherents among policy makers: the *obesogenic environment* in which individuals, perhaps especially children, find their food choices conditioned and even manipulated by availability, price, and advertising.

Personal Responsibility

With respect to child obesity, the personal-responsibility view holds that parents and eventually adolescents themselves are best situated to know and shape consumption decisions [25]. This liberty-maximizing perspective has been advanced, during the era of obesity's presence on the policy agenda, by conservative politicians and food/beverage industry representatives.

As reviewed in the "U.S. Solutions in Practice" section presented later in the chapter, the roster for policy action suggested by personal-responsibility views is rather thin: Emphasize, on a voluntary basis, exercise and healthy diets—but not too strenuously, lest the "nanny-state" label be applied [26]. Government efforts to regulate or restrict dietary practices are off limits, on this account: too much interference with the core value of individual liberty.

Obesogenic Environment

Descriptions of the "obesogenic" environment facing children—with a flood of advertising of high-fat, low-nutrition processed foods targeting youth from an early age, as well as ubiquitous availability of such foods everywhere children congregate including near and even at school—are extensive. A recent *Pediatrics* study shows that children in Philadelphia who attended public schools and shopped at corner stores before or after school purchased almost 360 calories of foods and beverages per visit. This analysis is the first to document in detail what foods and beverages children purchase in local corner stories and consume on their way to and from school, as well as the nutritional content of those items. Chips, candy, and sugar-sweetened beverages were the items most frequently purchased, affirming one researcher's description of the "toxic food environment" inhabited by many children in urban settings [27].

If childhood obesity is seen as having an environmental component, a stronger collection of policy responses appears worth contemplating. In this frame, public officials have a responsibility to actively reduce the high-calorie, low-nutrition foods readily available to children, along with discouraging their consumption in favor of healthier alternatives. Around the globe, such options have included *controlling the conditions of sale*, as in limits on what schools may offer in cafeterias or elsewhere on school grounds; *restricting advertising* of high-fat, low-nutrition foods that targets young children, as numerous countries presently do [28], or through "softer" alternatives like requiring calorie labels on menus; expanding access to healthier foods, through economic incentives and zoning regulations; *subsidizing healthier alternatives*, such as fruits and vegetables, which have much higher per-calorie costs than do most other foods, many of which are (or have ingredients like corn syrup and sugar that are) subsidized under current U.S. farm policies; or *restricting or banning certain ingredients*, such as trans fats.

The effort to frame obesity policy remains a contested struggle in the United States as well as many other nations, with one or the other primary view gaining preeminence in different jurisdictions. Researchers have also identified a variety of alternative frames, each suggesting a distinctive array of policy options and some gaining in currency as obesity remains a widely debated topic [29]. The relative popularity of personal-responsibility views among American public and policy makers likely helps explain the dearth of implemented policies, especially at the U.S. national level.

U.S. SOLUTIONS IN PRACTICE

Focusing specifically on the United States, what policies might be most effective in responding to the spread of childhood obesity? One group of researchers attempted to narrow the sprawling field of proposed responses by undertaking a novel "impact-feasibility" study. The authors compiled a list of 70 programs under consideration at the U.S. national level then asked a varied set of obesity/nutrition researchers to rate each policy based on the impact it would have, in their estimation, if enacted, using a standard 7-point impact scale. Separately and simultaneously, a similarly sized set of policy makers (varying by party, elective branch, and level of government—national and state) were asked to rate each of the 70 policies' feasibility: how likely it was to pass their jurisdiction, again based on a 7-point scale. The results were analyzed via simple cross-tabulation, yielding a list of the most promising (highest impact and feasibility) policies [30].

Next we examine in detail three of the highest-scoring policies designed to alleviate childhood obesity, each implemented in at least one U.S. jurisdiction. We report as well on any scholarly evaluations of such policies. The results in each case are mixed at best, leading some respondents—especially those in the personal-responsibility camp—to conclude that the policy in question has limited or no efficacy in practice. Our conclusion is rather different and draws on other findings in the healthcare arena: multiple solutions, implemented in tandem, are generally preferable to a single intervention carried out in a vacuum.

Calorie Labeling on Menus

At the beginning of 2008, no town, city, or state in the United States required fast-food restaurants to publicly post calorie labels on their menus. Two years later, more than 50 jurisdictions—including the nation's three largest cities, New York, Los Angeles, and Chicago, as well as the largest state, California—had enacted menu-labeling laws, with dozens of other state and local legislatures currently debating doing so. At the national level, the new health-reform law requires menu labeling for all restaurants with more than 20 outlets nationwide.

Few scientific studies have been undertaken to evaluate the influence of menu labeling on fast-food choices or calorie consumption. Those that have been carried out rarely focus primarily (if at all) on childhood obesity. One research project surveyed adolescents aged 11 to 18 who ordered meals from one of three fast-food chains: McDonald's, Denny's, or Panda Express. Utilizing sample variation and with the cooperation of the chains, some respondents were exposed to calorie menu labels. The surveys indicated that calorie information was not a major consideration for the young respondents' meal choices; instead, taste and hunger were each more important [31].

More recently, researchers carried out a randomized, controlled experiment in a Seattle primary-care pediatric clinic, on parents of children 3-6 years old. The experimental study suggested that calorie labeling did make a significant difference in parents' decisions on food choices for their children.

New York City's implementation of calorie labeling opens the way to research evaluations of the policy in practice, including among adolescent consumers of fast food. The present authors conducted one such study, which involved data gathering before and after calorie labeling was introduced in fast-food restaurants in New York and a comparison city—Newark, New Jersey—which has not adopted calorie labeling. The study was carried out in low-income neighborhoods, given that poverty is an established risk factor for obesity and that racially and ethnically diverse populations bear a greater burden of obesity and related health problems in the United States—a status exacerbated among lower-income children and youth [33].

One focus of the project was the influence of citywide calorie labeling on adolescents' food choices. Surveys and receipts were collected from 349 children and adolescents who either visited our sampled set of fast-food restaurants alone or with their parents, before and after labeling was introduced in New York City. Although we did not see statistically significant differences in caloric intake before and after labeling was implemented, many respondents reported noticing the labels, some of whom considered the calorie information in making their meal selection. These results were similar to those for adults in our sample, among whom calorie labeling appears to increase awareness of caloric content but does not appreciably affect the calories consumers purchase [34].

With implementation of calorie labeling beginning to take place in jurisdictions nationwide, other evaluation studies are under way—including across neighborhoods of differing income levels. New York City's Department of Health and Mental Hygiene (DOHMH) also carried out evaluation research before and after the instantiation of menu labeling; though the results have not been formally published, as with the present authors' study, the DOHMH found minimal effect of labels. Both these studies, it should be noted, were carried out during and immediately after New York's introduction of calorie labeling—a policy implemented in something of a vacuum without the accompaniment of either other strong policy measures or targeted efforts such as consumer education about calorie consumption. We return to this important caveat in the conclusion.

Soft Drink Tax

Forty U.S. states and several cities currently levy small taxes on one or more categories of less healthy foods, such as soft drinks, snack foods like potato chips, candy, chewing gum, and the like. In controlled experimental settings, manipulations of price have yielded substantial changes in consumption practices: participants shifted from unhealthy, calorie-dense foods to healthy, low-energy-dense foods. For example, one experiment in a high school cafeteria slashed fruit and salad prices in half; fruit sales quadrupled and carrot sales doubled as a result (though overall salad sales did not change) [35]. Extending research from these laboratory-style settings to the real world—where participants may consume more calories outside the experimental location to compensate—has been difficult; one extensive review of articles investigating food or beverage prices and obesity, in locations around the globe, found only a handful of empirical studies, with inconclusive results to date. None of these focused specifically on child or adolescent consumers [36].

Among U.S. policy makers, the primary efforts in this vein are focused on enacting soft drink taxes—or, in many places, reenacting them: the number of American jurisdictions featuring soda taxes has dropped in recent years, owing primarily to successful lobbying efforts by the food and beverage industries [37]. Given that adolescents and even young children consume sodas and other "junk foods" at high rates on average, many nutrition and health professionals have embraced this approach to addressing high obesity rates.

What are the effects of a penny or half-penny levy per can or bottle of soda? Two nutrition and obesity experts prospectively summarize the case as follows: "A tax on sugar-sweetened beverages would have strong positive effects on reducing consumption. In addition, the tax has the potential to generate substantial revenue to prevent obesity and address other external costs resulting from the consumption of sugar-sweetened beverages, as well as to fund other health related programs" [38]. The frequent comparison is to levies on tobacco, in terms of revenue generation and public health benefits.

In practice, the benefits of a soda tax—again, considered as a stand-alone intervention—are less clear. As Brownell et al. point out, most current state soda taxes are too small—generally a penny per can or bottle—to shift consumption practices very much [38]. One recent study utilized multivariate analysis to assess the effect of grocery store and vending machine soda taxes on adolescents' body mass, drawing BMI data from a set of long-running Monitoring the Future surveys. The results indicated no statistically significant connection between grocery store soda taxes and adolescent BMI, and only a weak causal relationship between vending machine soda tax rates and BMI among teens at risk for overweight. Taxes would have to be raised "substantially," the authors concluded, for a significant effect to be shown on BMI among adolescents [39]. (This evaluation did not measure revenue effects; other studies have affirmed the Brownell et al. observation that even small taxes on soda bring in significant revenue.) A more recent evaluation affirmed that only a fairly substantial tax would meaningfully shift comsumption behaviour, although certain at-risk groups of children may be more sensitive to soda taxes [40].

Competitive Foods/School-Based Policies

Meals and snacks consumed in school are a major source of nutrition for U.S. children and adolescents. The federally subsidized National School Lunch Program (NSLP), since its inception in 1969, has grown from serving fewer than 20 million to more than 30 million schoolchildren each day—or nearly 60% of children in participating schools [41]. Although students in the NSLP consume more milk, fruit, and vegetables and have lower intakes of sweetened beverages and candy than students outside or only occasionally in the program, they also consume more sodium, fat, and saturated fat—and their calorie intake is on average higher [42]. In short, NSLP lunches and breakfasts continue to provide too many calories from fat and fewer fresh fruits and vegetables than nutritional experts recommend.

Of greater concern to advocates of healthier food in schools: many U.S. school districts' practice of contracting with private beverage and food companies to sell "competitive foods" in cafeterias and vending machines. The leading soft drink companies have for years competed with one another to sign school districts to "pouring rights" agreements to sell only their soda in schools. As Brownell and Horgan summarized: "Schools need money and the soft drink companies offer a way to get it" [43]. The conclusion, primarily from anecdotal and qualitative studies, is that competitive foods are a significant source of unhealthy food and drink items consumed at school, contributing directly to the child obesity problem [44].

Given this dim view of competitive foods in schools, a host of policy initiatives to regulate or eliminate the availability of competitive foods have been introduced at all levels of government. As with menu labeling and soda taxes, researchers are just beginning to investigate the practical effects of these policies.

One recent evaluation study assesses the causal effect of competitive food availability on the BMI of a large national sample of U.S. fifth graders. Unsurprisingly, the authors found, the ready availability of competitive foods does boost in-school purchases of junk foods. Yet, contrary to widely held assumptions, no increase in BMI attributable to competitive foods was registered among the fifth graders in the study. The evaluation also assessed information beyond BMI, finding that the presence of competitive foods did not lead to substantial changes in the overall consumption of healthy and unhealthy foods or even in levels of physical activity. The authors concluded that there may *not* be "broader effects of junk foods in school on social/behavioral and academic outcomes," although a wide range of experimental and ethnographical studies have found otherwise [45].

CONCLUSION: MULTIPLE-FRONT APPROACHES NEEDED

Public policies such as menu labels, soft drink taxes, and reducing competitive foods in schools each have been promoted by nutrition and health advocates as a promising means of addressing the obesity crisis among children. Yet initial evaluation studies of each suggest that, at least in isolation, the policy falls short of advocates' hoped-for benefits. Does this imply that public health officials are promoting the wrong policies, or that no currently imagined interventions are likely to be successful in reversing the current dangerous rates of childhood obesity?

Our conclusion is (cautiously) otherwise. Medical experts know well that a single type of treatment often fails to address a health problem and that several strong simultaneous interventions are instead preferable: this practice is presently de rigueur in treating diseases from asthma to zoster (a form of shingles) [46]. The same multiple-solutions approach also may be the most promising means of systematically addressing childhood obesity. In one experimental study, combining calorie labels *and* nutrition education information—to wit, an "anchoring" reminder that 2000 calories is the Food and Drug Administration's average recommended daily allowance—made a significant difference in consumption practices, much more so than the use of labels alone [47]. (This finding was powerful enough to help encourage federal officials to include the "2000 per day" requirements in the 2010 health-reform law, along with mandated calorie labeling.) European health officials have found that a combination of banning junk-food TV advertising to children, taxing unhealthful foods, and substituting healthier foods at school together help to reduce child obesity rates: for example, the EPODE program launched in France in 2003 has yielded promising results [48]. Studies of broad interventions, involving several different alterations in food environments, at U.S. schools have seen at least modest declines in obesity rates [49].

If this insight has merit, an associated concern is that the American polity is traditionally resistant to large-scale, multiple-approach policy interventions. The separated-powers U.S. system—with multiple "veto points" that must be negotiated by any substantial legislative initiative—combined with dedicated interest-group resistance to any attempts to regulate food or beverage policies make it difficult to pass even a single program like menu labeling, much less a roster of concerted national approaches to childhood obesity.

Exacerbating this difficulty may be the very nature of quantitative evaluation research. By focusing on a single intervention in isolation, holding all other factors constant, each individual policy change is likely to appear ineffective. To fully explore this notion would require a battery of separate studies; suffice it to say that concerned inquiries into the nature and impact of evaluation studies themselves have recently been raised in evaluation-research literature [50].

The state of childhood obesity in the United States and worldwide is widely described with terms like "alarming" and "devastating." Unless and until medical responses are devised, the public policy arena appears to hold the most promising response. Yet, especially in the United States, policy tools to address this epidemic situation are underemployed in nearly every jurisdiction. The time-honored American policy-making practices of incrementalism and "muddling through" [51] are proving inadequate in the present crisis.

References

1. Office of the Surgeon General. "A Call to Action: Prevent and Decrease Overweight and Obesity". Washington, D.C.: US Government Printing Office; 2001.
2. Centers for Disease Control. "Obesity Prevalence Among Low-Income, Preschool-Aged Children 1998–2008". *Morbidity & Mortality Weekly Report* 2009;**58**(28):769–96.
3. Gordon-Larsen P, Adair L, Popkin BM. "The Relationship of Ethnicity, Socioeconomic Factors, and Overweight in US Adolescents". *Obesity Research* 2003;**11**:121–9.

REFERENCES

4. Institute of Medicine. *Preventing Childhood Obesity: Health in the Balance*. Washington, DC: National Academies Press; 2005. On physicians' concerns see also de Vries J. "The Obesity Epidemic: Medical and Ethical Considerations," *Science and Engineering Ethics* 13:1, 2007.
5. Direct access to the WHO data is at who.int/nutgrowthdb/en.
6. Jackson-Leach R, Lobstein T. "Estimated Burden of Pediatric Obesity and Co-Morbidities in Europe". *International Journal of Pediatric Obesity* 2006;**1**(1):26–32.
7. Knai Cécile. *"Obesity in Eastern Europe: An Overview of its Health and Economic Implications"*. Geneva: World Health Organization; 2007.
8. Ayatollahi SM, Mostajabi F. "Prevalence of Obesity Among Schoolchildren in Iran". *Obesity Review* 2007;**8**:289–91.
9. Jafar TH, Qadri Z, Islam M, Hatcher J, Bhotta ZA, Chaturvedi N. "Rise in Childhood Obesity With Persistently High Rates of Undernutrition Among Urban School-Aged Indo-Asian Children". *Archives of Disease in Childhood* 2008;**93**:373–8.
10. Musaiger AO. "Overweight and Obesity in the Eastern Mediterranean Region: Can We Control It?" *Eastern Mediterranean Health Journal* 2004;**10**(6):789–93.
11. Du Toit G, van der Merwe MT. "The Epidemic of Childhood Obesity". *South African Medical Journal* 2003;**93**:1.
12. For childhood obesity rates in other regions, see Wang Y and Lobstein T, 2006. "Worldwide Trends in Childhood Overweight and Obesity." *International Journal of Pediatric Obesity* 1:1, 11–25.
13. Office of the Surgeon General, "Call to Action," op. cit.
14. Institute of Medicine. *"Preventing Childhood Obesity: Health in the Balance"*. Washington, DC: Institute of Medicine; 2005.
15. Brownell KD, Horgan KB. *Food Fight*. New York: McGraw-Hill; 2004.
16. Schwimmer JB, Burwinkle TM, Varni JW. "Health-Related Quality of Life of Severely Obese Children and Adolescents". *Journal of the American Medical Association* 2003;**289**:1813–19.
17. Olshansky JS, Passaro DJ, Hershow RC, et al. "A Potential Decline in Life Expectancy in the United States in the 21st Century". *New England Journal of Medicine* 2005;**352**:1138–45.
18. Institute of Medicine, "Preventing Childhood Obesity," op. cit.
19. World Health Organization, 2000. *Obesity: Preventing and Managing the Global Epidemic*. WHO TRS-894.
20. Haas JS, Lee LB, Kaplan CP, Sonneborn D, Phillips KA, Liang SY. "The Association of Race, Socioeconomic Status, and Health Insurance Status with the Prevalence of Overweight Among Children and Adolescents". *American Journal of Public Health* 2003;**93**:2105–10. C.
21. Ebbeling C, Pawlak D, Ludwig D. "Childhood Obesity: Public-Health Crisis, Common Sense Cure". *The Lancet* 2002;**360** (9331):473–82.
22. Brownell and Horgan, *Food Fight*, op. cit.
23. Harris KC, Kuramoto LK, Schulzer M, Retallack JE. "Effect of School-based Physical Activity on Children's BMI". *AAP Grand Rounds* 2009;**22**:17.
24. Ludwig DS, Peterson KE, Gortmaker SL. "Relation between Consumption of Sugar-Sweetened Drinks and Childhood Obesity: A Prospective, Observational Analysis". *Lancet* 2001;**357**:505–8.
25. Kersh R and Morone J. "Obesity, Courts, and the New Politics of Public Health". *Journal of Health Politics, Policy, & Law* 2005;**30**:5.
26. For more on the public policies suggested by personal-responsibility frames see Kersh and Morone, "Obesity, Courts," op. cit.
27. Borradaile KE, Sherman S, Vander Veur SS, McCoy T, Sandoval B, Nachmani J, Karpyn A, Foster GD. 2009, "Snacking in Children: The Role of Urban Corner Stores." Pediatrics 10: 1542/peds. 2009-0964. Brownell coined the "toxic food environment" term; see *Food Fight*, op. cit.
28. A good overview is in Hawkes C. *Marketing Food to Children: Changes in the Global Regulatory Environment, 2004–2006*. Geneva: World Health Organization; 2007.
29. Barry CL, Brescoll VL, Brownell KD, Schlesinger M. "Obesity Metaphors: How Beliefs about the Causes of Obesity Affect Support for Public Policy". *Milbank Quarterly* 2009;**87**:1.
30. Brescoll VL, Kersh R, Brownell KD. "Assessing the Impact and Feasibility of Federal Childhood Obesity Policies". *Annals of the American Academy of Political and Social Science* 2008;**615**:178–94.
31. Yamamoto JA, Yamanoto JB, Yamanoto BE, Yamanoto LG. "Adolescent Fast Food and Restaurant Ordering Behavior With and Without Calorie and Fat Content Menu Information". *Journal of Adolescent Health* 2005;**37**:397–402.
32. Tandon P, Wright J, Zhou C, Rogers CB, Christakis D. "Nutrition Menu Labeling May Lead to Lower-Calorie Restaurant Meal Choices for Children". *Pediatrics* 2010;**125**:244–48.
33. Ogden CL, Flegal KM, Carroll MD, Johnson CL. "Prevalence and Trends in Overweight Among US Children and Adolescents, 1999–2000". *Journal of the American Medical Association* 2002;**288**:1728–32.
34. The full study is described in Elbel B, Kersh R, Brescoll V, and Dixon LB, 2009. "Calorie Labeling and Food Choices: A First Look at the Effects on Low-Income People in New York City." *Health Affairs* 28:6, w1110-21.
35. French SA, Story M, Jeffery RW, Snyder P, Eisenberg M, Sidebottom A. "Pricing Strategy to Promote Fruit and Vegetable Purchase in High School Cafeterias". *Journal of the American Dietetic Association* 1997;**97**(9):1008–10.
36. Powell LM, Chaloupka FJ. "Food Prices and Obesity: Evidence and Policy Implications for Taxes and Subsidies". *Milbank Quarterly* 2009;**87**(1):229–57.
37. For a partial list of taxes "rolled back" in the face of lobbying efforts, see Jacobson MF. and Brownell KD. 2000. "Small Taxes on Soft Drinks and Snack Foods to Promote Health." *American Journal of Public Health* 90:6, 854–857.
38. Brownell KD, Forley T, Willett WC, et al. "The Public Health and Economic Benefits of Taxing Sugar-Sweetened Beverages". *New England Journal of Medicine* 2009;**361**:16.
39. Powell LM, Criqui J, Chaloupka FJ. "Associations Between State-Level Soda Taxes and Adolescent Body Mass Index". *Journal of Adolescent Health* 2009;**45**:S57–63.
40. Sturm R, Powell LM, Chriqui JF, Chaloupka FJ. "Soda Taxes, Soft Drink Consumption, and Children's Body Mass Index". *Health Affairs* 2010;**29**(5):1052–58.
41. Musiker Melissa. "National School Lunch Program Participation Up 57 Percent Since 1969". *Amber Waves* (Washington DC: *U.S. Department of Agriculture*) 2009;**7**:1.
42. Cullen K, Watson K, Zakeri I. *"Middle School Student Lunch Consumption: Impact of National School Lunch Program Meal and Competitive Foods"*. Washington, DC: USDA/ERS Contractor and Cooperator Report No. 30; 2007.
43. Brownell and Horgen, *Food Fight*, op. cit., 161.
44. Story M, Kaphingst KM, French S. "The Role of Child Care Settings in Obesity Prevention". *Childhood Obesity* 2006;**16** (1):109–42.
45. Datar A, and Nicosia N, 2009. "Junk Food in Schools and Childhood Obesity: Much Ado About Nothing?" RAND Working Paper WR-672. Santa Monica, California: RAND Corp.
46. Cabana MD, Ebel BE, Cooper-Patrick L, Powe NR, Rubin HR, Rand CS. "Barriers Pediatricians Face When Using Asthma Practice Guidelines". *Archives of Pediatrics & Adolescent Medicine* 2000;**154**:685–93.

Johnson RW, Dworkin RH. "Treatment of Herpes Zoster and Postherpetic Neuralgia". *British Medical Journal* 2003;**326**: 748–50.

47. Roberto CA, Larsen PD, Agnew H, Baik J, Brownell KD. "Evaluating the Effect of Menu Labeling on Food Choices and Intake". *American Journal of Public Health* 2010;**100**(2):312–18.

48. 1er Symposium EEN, 2009. "EPODE Community-Based Interventions Aimed at Preventing Childhood Obesity." Brussels: EPODE European Network.

49. Gortmaker SL, Peterson K, Wiecha J, Sobol AM, Dixit S, Fox MK, Laird N. "Reducing Obesity via a School-Based Interdisciplinary Intervention Among Youth". *Archives of Pediatric & Adolescent Medicine* 1999;**153**:409–18.

50. See, e.g., Johnson K, Greenseid LO, Toal SA, et al. "Research on Evaluation Use: A Review of the Empirical Literature From 1986 to 2005". *American Journal of Evaluation* 2009;**30**(3):377–410.

51. Lindblom CE. "The Science of 'Muddling Through'". *Public Administration Review* 1959;**19**(2):79–88.

CHAPTER 27

Childhood Obesity and Juvenile Diabetes

Mikael Knip

Hospital for Children and Adolescents and Folkhälsan Research Center, University of Helsinki, Helsinki, and Department of Pediatrics, Tampere University Hospital, Tampere, Finland

INTRODUCTION

Juvenile diabetes (i.e., type 1 diabetes) is considered to be a chronic immune-mediated disease with a subclinical prodrome of variable duration [1]. It is characterized by selective loss of insulin-producing beta cells in the pancreatic islets in genetically susceptible subjects. The most important genes contributing to disease susceptibility are located in the Human Leukocyte Antigen (HLA) class II locus on the short arm of chromosome 6, and the HLA genes have been estimated to explain about half of the familial clustering of type 1 diabetes. In addition, there are more than 40 other non-HLA genes that account for the remaining genetic predisposition [2].

Several lines of evidence support a crucial role of environmental factors in the pathogenesis of type 1 diabetes. Studies in monozygotic twins suggest that only 13% to 33% are pair-wise concordant for the disease [3, 4], implying that there is either acquired postconceptional genetic discordance or differential exposure to the putative environmental factor(s). The geographical variation in the incidence of type 1 diabetes in children is conspicuous even among Caucasians, with the lowest annual rate in Europe reported from Macedonia amounting to 3.2/100,000 children under the age of 15 years [5] and the highest rate observed in Finland reaching 63 in 2006 [6]. This almost 20-fold difference in incidence can hardly be explained by genetic factors. The substantial increase in the incidence of type 1 diabetes among children emerging over the past decades cannot be the consequence only of enhanced genetic disease susceptibility in the population but must mostly be due to changes in lifestyle and environment.

Migrant studies indicate that the incidence of type 1 diabetes has increased in population groups who have moved from a low-incidence region to a high-incidence area emphasizing the influence of environmental conditions. Accumulating evidence suggests that the proportion of subjects with high-risk HLA genotypes has decreased over the past decades among children with newly diagnosed type 1 diabetes, whereas the proportion of those with low-risk or even protective HLA genotypes has increased [7]. These data are compatible with an increased environmental pressure resulting in progression to clinical diabetes with less genetic predisposition.

Overweight and obesity are related to juvenile diabetes in terms of a series of aspects. They may be a risk factor for type 1 diabetes, and obesity can be a therapeutic challenge in the treatment of the disease. Overweight and obesity also increase the risk of macro- and microvascular complications of type 1 diabetes. Such problems may emerge in adolescence and become more common among young adult patients. This article aims at addressing the impact of overweight and obesity in juvenile diabetes from various perspectives.

WEIGHT, WEIGHT GAIN, AND RISK OF TYPE 1 DIABETES

According to a recent meta-analysis based on 12 studies including almost 2.4 million persons, out of whom 7491 were affected by type 1 diabetes, showed that high birth weight (>4000 g) was associated with an increased risk of type 1 diabetes with an odds ratio (OR) of 1.17 (95% confidence interval [CI] 1.09−1.26) [8]. This meta-analysis has, however, been criticized based on poor coverage of published studies, unsatisfactory adjustment for confounders, and inclusion of duplicate cases [9]. Accordingly, the impact of a high birth weight on subsequent risk of juvenile diabetes remains still open, and if there is an effect the increased risk is modest.

A recent Norwegian case-control study reported that maternal obesity before pregnancy and maternal weight gain during pregnancy was associated with higher risk of beta-cell autoimmunity in the offspring [10]. The number of children with positivity for multiple autoantibodies was, however, only 36 in that study. In a Swedish study, maternal weight gain during pregnancy did not differ between cases and controls [11], whereas a survey from the United Kingdom found that excessive maternal weight gain during pregnancy is a risk factor for type 1 diabetes in children [12]. In our own study including 175 cases with advanced beta-cell autoimmunity, we could not find any association between initial maternal weight or weight gain during pregnancy and seroconversion to positivity for multiple diabetes-predictive autoantibodies in the offspring [13]. These controversial data indicate that additional studies are needed to determine whether maternal weight or weight gain during pregnancy is a risk factor for preclinical or clinical type 1 diabetes in the offspring.

Increased weight gain in infancy has repeatedly been reported to be a risk factor for type 1 diabetes later in childhood [8]. A Finnish study showed that those children who presented with type 1 diabetes had been heavier and also taller in infancy [14]. Increased weight and height later in childhood turned out to be definite risk factors for type 1 diabetes as well [15]. Accelerated weight gain and linear growth result in an enhanced beta-cell load and increasing insulin resistance [16]. It has been shown experimentally that active beta cells are more prone to cytokine-induced damage than resting cells [17]. Taken together, these observations imply that rapid growth induces beta-cell stress. According to the accelerator hypothesis presented by Wilkin [18] some years ago, insulin resistance is an important factor affecting the rising incidence of both type 1 and type 2 diabetes. In such a scenario the only differences between these two forms of diabetes would be the pace of progression to overt disease and the fact that those who present with type 1 diabetes carry genetic susceptibility to autoimmunity.

Children in the developed world grow linearly and gain weight faster now than some decades ago. They also reach adult height at a younger age than in earlier decades. The average body mass index (BMI) in 15-year-old Finnish children increased e.g., over a 12-year period from 20 kg/m^2 in 1980 to 21.3 kg/m^2 in 1992 [19]. This is a conspicuous change, and if such a trend would continue over the next decades the mean body mass index would be 25 kg/m^2 in this age group in 2030. There was a significant correlation between the increase in the type 1 diabetes incidence rate among children younger than 15 years of age in Finland and the change in body mass index in adolescents from 1980 to 1992 (Fig. 27.1). As mentioned earlier, rapid growth and weight gain induce beta-cell stress and could thereby lead to an earlier presentation of clinical type 1 diabetes and also an increasing incidence by expanding the proportion of susceptible individuals progressing to overt disease.

WEIGHT GAIN AND OBESITY IN CHILDREN AND ADOLESCENTS WITH TYPE 1 DIABETES

Children with newly diagnosed type 1 diabetes are classically slim, because they have lost weight before the diagnosis, and about half of the patients are to some degree dehydrated as a consequence of increased diuresis and metabolic decompensation at disease manifestation. Overweight and obesity do not, however, protect against beta-cell autoimmunity and progression

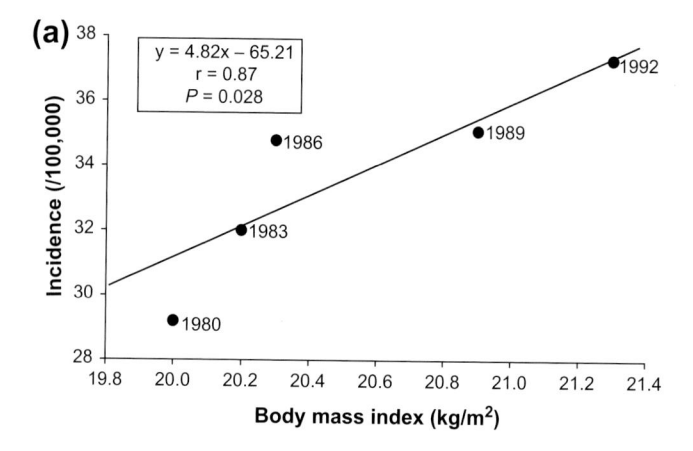

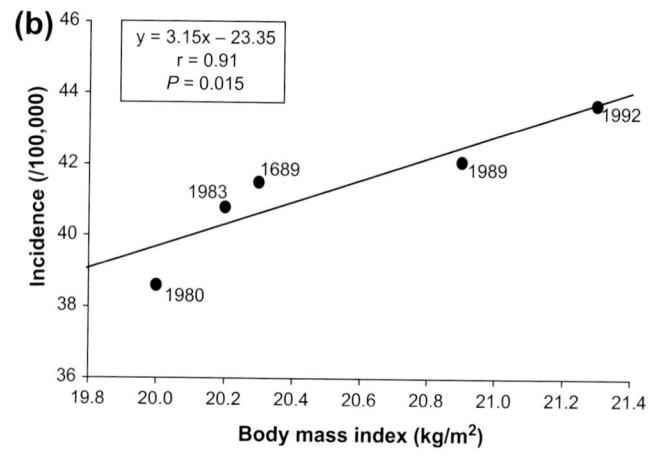

FIGURE 27.1 Correlation between triennially averaged incidence rates for type 1 diabetes in children below the age of 15 years (a) and in children aged 10 to 14.99 years (b) in Finland over a 15-year period (1979–1993) and mean body mass indices in 15-year-old Finnish children in 1980, 1983, 1986, 1989, and 1992.

to type 1 diabetes. As a consequence of the increasing prevalence of overweight and obesity in the childhood population, the number of overweight and obese children with newly diagnosed type 1 diabetes has increased over time. From a physiological point of view, the time of disease presentation is determined by the balance between insulin secretion and peripheral insulin sensitivity. If the child is very insulin sensitive, he or she can manage with a conspicuously reduced insulin secretory capacity, but because overweight and obesity result in insulin resistance, an obese child presents with clinical symptoms earlier at a higher level of residual beta-cell function.

Because the number of obese children with signs of beta-cell autoimmunity at diagnosis has been increasing, especially in the United States, the term "double diabetes" or "hybrid diabetes" has been coined to cover the combination of beta-cell dysfunction and insulin resistance [20, 21]. One may, however, question whether this represents any new disease entity, as insulin resistance has always been a player in type 1 diabetes together with impaired insulin secretion.

Table 27.1 shows the frequency of overweight and obesity among children and adolescents with type 1 diabetes in the United States and in the Netherlands [22, 23]. The combined frequency of overweight and obesity was somewhat higher in the Netherlands than in the United States (38.5% versus 34.7%). The highest frequency of obesity was seen among African American children (20.1%), whereas the highest frequency of overweight was observed among Dutch children (29.3%). These data show that more than one third of children with type 1 diabetes have excess weight. The long-term implications and consequences of overweight and obesity in children and adolescents with type 1 diabetes will be considered in a subsequent chapter.

Studies of body composition in children with type 1 diabetes have demonstrated progressive increases in

TABLE 27.1 The Frequency of Overweight and Obesity in Children and Adolescents with Type 1 Diabetes (T1D) in the Netherlands [22] and in the United States [23]

Country	N (male/female)	Ethnicity	Age	T1D duration	Obesity/ overweight	Definition	Frequency (percentage)
The Netherlands	283 (138/145)	Dutch native 77%	Median 12.8 years	Median 5.3 years	Obesity	BMI ≥ 95th percentile	9.2
		Moroccan 7.1% Turkish 3.5%	Range 3−18 years		Overweight	86th percentile < BMI < 95th percentile	29.3
		Other 12.4%					
United States	3371 (1697/1674)	All	Range 3−19 years	Range < 1−18.4 years	Obesity	BMI ≥ 95th percentile	12.6
					Overweight	85th percentile < BMI < 95th percentile	22.1
	2647 (1354/1293)	NHW			Obesity	BMI ≥ 95th percentile	10.7
					Overweight	85th percentile < BMI < 95th percentile	20.8
	310 (133/177)	AA			Obesity	BMI ≥ 95th percentile	20.1
					Overweight	85th percentile < BMI < 95th percentile	23.4
	414 (210/204)	Hispanic			Obesity	BMI ≥ 95th percentile	18.3
					Overweight	85th percentile < BMI < 95th percentile	28.0

NHW = Non-Hispanic white, AA = African American.

body fat, particularly in girls [24, 25], which appear to be related to the dose of exogenous insulin, the number of insulin injections, and intensified insulin therapy. Longitudinal studies have shown that pubertal children with type 1 diabetes have relative leptin resistance (i.e. higher leptin concentrations for fat mass or BMI than unaffected peers) [25, 26]. The increased leptin levels are, however, associated with excessive weight gain only in girls with type 1 diabetes.

Intensified insulin treatment results often in excess weight gain. In a German study, both girls and boys developed overweight during puberty [27]. In that study the daily dose of exogenous insulin and long-term metabolic control had a minor impact on the development of overweight, whereas multiple injection therapy was strongly associated with weight gain. The use of long-acting insulin analogs has become more and more common among children and adolescents with type 1 diabetes. Detemir insulin has been reported to be related to a smaller weight gain in adults with type 1 diabetes when compared to human intermediate-acting insulin [28]. This has been observed in affected children and adolescents as well [29]. A recent meta-analysis based on more than 6000 pediatric and adult patients with type 1 diabetes showed that detemir insulin was associated with a smaller weight gain than Neutral Protamine Hagedorn (NPH) human insulin, whereas no difference was seen when comparing the latter to glargine insulin [30]. Weight gain has been observed to be of the same magnitude when comparing continuous subcutaneous insulin infusion (CSII) with multiple daily insulin injections [31, 32] in children and adolescents with type 1 diabetes.

Traditionally, oral antidiabetic drugs have not played any role in the treatment of type 1 diabetes. Metformin, which primarily reduces hepatic glucose output, has been tested for a 3-month period as an adjunct therapy in adolescents with type 1 diabetes in two small randomized trials. The Canadian trial showed that metformin lowered the glycated hemoglobin and decreased the dose of exogenous insulin, although no change in insulin sensitivity was demonstrated [33]. Särnblad et al. reported that metformin improved glycemic control and that the effect seen was associated with increased insulin-induced glucose uptake [34]. Thiazolidinediones are insulin sensitizers that are used in the treatment of patients with type 2 diabetes. Zdravkovic and coworkers assessed whether the combination of one of the thiazolidinediones, pioglitazone, with standard therapy improves metabolic control in adolescents with type 1 diabetes. They observed that the addition of pioglitazone was ineffective in improving glycemic control in their patients, and as a matter of fact pioglitazone was associated with an increase in BMI [35]. An Australian study tested another of the thiazolidinediones (rosiglitazone) as adjunct therapy in poorly controlled adolescents with type 1 diabetes and normal weight. The outcome was that the addition of rosiglitazone reduced modestly the insulin dose but had no impact on metabolic control or BMI [36].

OVERWEIGHT AND OBESITY AND COMPLICATIONS OF TYPE 1 DIABETES IN CHILDREN AND ADOLESCENTS

The long-term vascular complications of diabetes consist of retinopathy, nephropathy, neuropathy, and macrovascular disease. Clinically apparent diabetes-related vascular complications are rare in childhood and adolescence [37]. Early functional and structural abnormalities may, however, be observed already a few years after the diagnosis of type 1 diabetes. Zhang et al. reported, based on the patients taking part in the Diabetes Control and Complications Trial (DCCT), a majority of whom were adults, that in addition to metabolic control and duration of follow-up, initial glycated hemoglobin and body mass index (BMI) were significant predictors of diabetic retinopathy [38]. In a Belgian study, an increased BMI was associated with the development of proliferative retinopathy [39].

Stone and coworkers studied the natural history and risk factors for microalbuminuria in adolescents with type 1 diabetes [40]. They found that the incidence of persistent microalbuminuria was 4.6 per 1000 patient-years. Impaired glycated hemoglobin, obesity, and a high insulin dose were predictors of persistent microalbuminuria. Overweight was associated with a higher prevalence of both retinopathy and neuropathy in adult patients with type 1 diabetes, although disease duration and metabolic control were the main determinants of these microvascular complications in a logistic regression analysis [41]. Altogether most studies addressing the prognostic role of overweight and obesity for the development of microvascular complications suggest that increased weight has an adverse impact and increases the cumulative incidence of such complications.

The development of atherosclerosis is initiated in childhood and adolescence. It has been shown that children with type 1 diabetes have endothelial dysfunction and increased arterial intima-media thickness when compared to nondiabetic peers [42]. Silent coronary atherosclerosis has been observed by intravascular ultrasound in young adults with their diabetes diagnosed in childhood [43]. A recent Norwegian study showed a high prevalence of risk factors for cardiovascular disease among children with type 1 diabetes [44]. More than one third had increased low-density lipoprotein-cholesterol concentrations, and about 7% had a low high-density lipoprotein-cholesterol. In an extensive German survey, close to 30% of children and young adults with type 1 diabetes had dyslipidemia, and approximately 8% had hypertension [45]. A Dutch study analyzed the prevalence of the metabolic syndrome among children and adolescents in relation to weight [22]. As mentioned earlier, close to 40% of the patients were overweight or obese. The prevalence of the metabolic syndrome was about four times higher in that group when compared to the normal-weight patients. The overweight/obese patients suffered also from hypertension six times more frequently, and they had an increased alanine aminotransferase concentration four times more often than the normal-weight subjects. In adult patients with their diabetes diagnosed in childhood obesity, abdominal obesity in particular is an important risk factor for cardiovascular disease [46].

A potential therapeutic dilemma is the fact that intensified insulin treatment aimed at improved glycemic control often results in excessive weight gain as an adverse effect [47]. This weight gain can be accompanied by components of the metabolic syndrome, such as increased visceral adiposity, hypertension, dyslipidemia, and increasing insulin resistance [48]. Concerns have been voiced that the development of the metabolic syndrome could lead in some patients to an increased risk for cardiovascular disease despite better metabolic control. One analysis showed, however, that although intensive insulin therapy was associated with an increased frequency of the metabolic syndrome over the course of DCCT, baseline metabolic syndrome did not predict subsequent macrovascular disease [49]. Accordingly it seems that the cardiovascular benefits of improved metabolic control achieved through intensive insulin therapy in patients with type 1 diabetes outweigh the risks associated with increased weight gain and the development of the metabolic syndrome.

CONCLUSION

Accumulated data suggest that excessive weight gain is an undesired companion to type 1 diabetes. Overweight and obesity, during both infancy and childhood, have been shown to be risk factors for progression to type 1 diabetes. Because obesity is associated with increasing insulin resistance, it is logical that increased weight results in an earlier clinical presentation of type 1 diabetes and an increasing penetrance of the disease among children and adolescents. Heavy body mass increases the need of exogenous insulin in patients with established diabetes and may complicate the daily treatment of the disease. Overweight and obesity are associated with various risk factors of micro- and macrovascular complications, such as poor metabolic control, dyslipidemia, and hypertension. In addition, excessive weight gain appears to be an independent predictor of diabetic complications. Taken together, these observations emphasize the need of developing effective measures for the prevention of childhood overweight and obesity. Such measures are needed to combat excessive weight gain both at the population level and among young patients with type 1 diabetes. Successful prevention at the population level can be expected to reduce the increasing incidence rate of type 1 diabetes among children, whereas such an achievement among patients would result in a reduction of the micro- and macrovascular complications of juvenile diabetes.

Acknowledgments

Some of this research was supported by the Juvenile Diabetes Research Foundation International, the Sigrid Jusélius Foundation, the Novo Nordisk Foundation, and the Liv och Hälsa Fund.

References

1. Knip M, Veijola R, Virtanen SM, Hyöty H, Vaarala O, Åkerblom HK. Environmental triggers and determinants of β-cell autoimmunity and type 1 diabetes. *Diabetes* 2005;**54**(Suppl. 2): S125—36.
2. Barrett JC, Clayton DG, Concannon P, Akolkar B, Cooper JD, Erlich HA, Julier C, Morahan G, Nerup J, Nierras C, Plagnol V, Pociot F, Schuilenburg H, Smyth DJ, Stevens H, Todd JA, Walker NM, Rich SS. The Type 1 Diabetes Genetics Consortium. Genome-wide association study and meta-analysis find that over 40 loci affect risk of type 1 diabetes. *Nat Genet* 2009;**41**:703—7.
3. Barnett AH, Eff C, Leslie RDG, Pyke DA. Diabetes in identical twins. A study of 200 pairs. *Diabetologia* 1981;**20**:87—93.
4. Kaprio J, Tuomilehto J, Koskenvuo M, Romanov K, Reunanen A, Eriksson J, Stengård J, Kesäniemi YA. Concordance for Type 1 (insulin-dependent) and Type 2 (non-insulin-dependent) diabetes mellitus in a population-based cohort of twins in Finland. *Diabetologia* 1992;**35**:1060—7.
5. The EURODIAB ACE Study Group. Variation and trends in incidence of childhood diabetes in Europe. *Lancet* 2000;**355**:873—6.
6. Knip M, Siljander H. Autoimmune mechanisms in type 1 diabetes. *Autoimmun Rev* 2008;**7**:550—7.
7. Hermann R, Knip M, Veijola R, Simell O, Laine AP, Åkerblom HK, Groop PH, Forsblom C, Petterson-Fernholm K, Ilonen J, and the FINDIANE Study Group. Temporal changes in the frequencies of HLA genotypes in patients with type 1 diabetes — indication of an increased environmental pressure? *Diabetologia* 2003;**46**:420—5.
8. Harder T, Roepke K, Diller N, Stechling Y, Dudenhausen JW, Plagemann A. Birth weight, early weight gain and subsequent risk of type 1 diabetes: systemic review and meta-analysis. *Am J Epidemiol* 2009;**169**:1428—36.
9. Cardwell CR, Patterson CC. Re: "Birth weight, early weight gain and subsequent risk of type 1 diabetes: systemic review and meta-analysis". *Am J Epidemiol* 2009;**170**:529—30.
10. Rasmussen T, Stene LC, Samuelsen SO, Cinek O, Wetlesen T, Torjesen PA, Rönningen KS. Maternal BMI before pregnancy, maternal weight gain during pregnancy, and risk persistent positivity for multiple diabetes-associated autoantibodies in children with the high-risk HLA genotype: the MIDIA study. *Diabetes Care* 2009;**32**:1904—6.

11. Dahlquist G, Källen B. Maternal-child blood group incompatibility and other perinatal events increase the risk for early-onset type 1 (insulin-dependent) diabetes mellitus. *Diabetologia* 1992;**35**:671–5.
12. McKinney PA, Parslow R, Gurney K, Law G, Bodansky HJ, Williams DR. Antenatal risk factors for childhood diabetes mellitus; a case-control study of medical record data in Yorkshire, UK. *Diabetologia* 1997;**40**:933–9.
13. Arkkola T, Kautiainen S, Takkinen HM, Kenward MG, Nevalainen J, Uusitalo U, Simell O, Ilonen J, Knip M, Veijola R, Virtanen SM (2009) Relationship of maternal weight status in pregnancy to the development of advanced beta-cell autoimmunity in the offspring; A prospective birth cohort study. *Pediatr Diabetes* 2010;**11**:in press.
14. Hyppönen E, Kenward MG, Virtanen SM, Piitulainen A, Virta-Autio P, Knip M, Åkerblom HK, and the Childhood Diabetes in Finland Study Group. Infant feeding, early weight gain and risk of type 1 diabetes. *Diabetes Care* 1999;**22**:1961–5.
15. Hyppönen E, Virtanen SM, Kenward MG, Knip M, Åkerblom HK, and the Childhood Diabetes in Finland Study Group. Obesity, increased linear growth and risk of type 1 diabetes mellitus in children. *Diabetes Care* 2000;**23**:1755–60.
16. Hindmarsh PC, Matthews DR, Di Silvio L, Kurz AB, Brook CG. Relation between height velocity and fasting insulin concentrations. *Arch Dis Child* 1988;**63**:665–6.
17. Palmer JP, Helquist S, Spinas GA, Mølvig J, Mandrup-Poulsen T, Andersen HU, Nerup J. Interaction of beta-cell activity and IL-1 concentration and exposure time in isolated rat islets of Langerhans. *Diabetes* 1989;**38**:1211–16.
18. Wilkin TJ. The accelerator hypothesis: weight gain as the missing link between type 1 and type 2 diabetes. *Diabetologia* 2001;**44**:914–22.
19. Knip M, Reunanen A, Virtanen SM, Nuutinen M, Viikari J, Åkerblom HK. Does the secular increase in body mass in children contribute to the increasing incidence of type 1 diabetes. *Pediatr Diabetes* 2008;**9**:46–9.
20. Libman IM, Becker DJ. Coexistence of type 1 and type 2 diabetes mellitus: "double" diabetes. *Pediatr Diabetes* 2003;**4**:110–13.
21. Wenthworth JM, Fourlanos S, Harrison LC. Reappraising the stereotypes of diabetes in the modern diabetogenic environment. *Nat Rev Endocrinol* 2009;**5**:483–9.
22. van Vliet M, van der Heyden JC, Diamant M, von Rosenstiel IA, Schindhelm RK, Aanstoot HJ, Veeze HJ. Overweight is highly prevalent in children with type 1 diabetes and associates with cardiometabolic risk. *J Pediatr* 2010;**156**:923–9.
23. Liu LL, Lawrence JM, Davis C, Liese AD, Pettitt DJ, Pihoker C, Dabelea D, Hamman R, Waitzfelder B, Kahn S. Prevalence of overweight and obesity in youth with diabetes in USA: the SEARCH for Diabetes in the Youth Study. *Pediatr Diabetes* 2010;**11**:4–11.
24. Gregory JW, Wilson AC, Greene SA. Body fat and overweight among children and adolescents with diabetes mellitus. *Diabet Med* 1992;**9**:344–8.
25. Ahmed ML, Ong KK, Watts AP, Morrell DJ, Preece MA, Dunger DB. Elevated leptin levels are associated with excess gains in fat mass in girls, but not boys, with type 1 diabetes: Longitudinal study during adolescence. *J Clin Endocrinol Metab* 2001;**86**:1188–93.
26. Kiess W, Anil M, Blum WF, Englaro P, Juul A, Attanasio A, Dotsch J, Rascher W. Serum leptin levels in children and adolescents with insulin-dependent diabetes mellitus in relation to metabolic control and body mass index. *Eur J Endocrinol* 1998;**138**:501–9.
27. Holl RW, Grabert M, Sorgo W, Heinze E, Debatin KM. Contributions of age, gender and insulin administration to weight gain in subjects with IDDM. *Diabetologia* 1998;**41**:542–7.
28. Pieber TR, Treichel HC, Hompesch B, Philotheou A, Mordhorst L, Gall MA, Robertson LI. Comparison of insulin detemir and insulin glargine in subjects with type 1 diabetes using intensive insulin therapy. *Diabet Med* 2007;**24**:635–42.
29. Robertson KJ, Schoenle E, Gucev Z, Mordhorst L, Gall MA, Ludvigsson J. Insulin detemir compared with NPH insulin in children and adolescents with type 1 diabetes. *Diabet Med* 2007;**24**:27–34.
30. Monami M, Marchionni N, Mannucci E. Long-acting insulin analogues vs. NPH human insulin in type 1 diabetes. A meta-analysis. *Diabetes Obes Metab* 2009;**11**:372–8.
31. Nahata L. Insulin therapy in pediatric patients with type 1 diabetes: continuous subcutaneous insulin infusion versus multiple daily injections. *Clin Pediatr* 2006;**45**:503–8.
32. Doyle EA, Weinzimer SA, Steffen AT, Ahern JA, Vincent M, Tamborlane WV. A randomized prospective trial comparing the efficacy of continuous subcutaneous insulin infusion with multiple daily injections using insulin glargine. *Diabetes Care* 2004;**27**:1554–8.
33. Hamilton J, Cummings E, Zdravkovic V, Finegood D, Daneman D. Metformin as an adjunct therapy in adolescents with type 1 diabetes and insulin resistance: a randomized controlled trial. *Diabetes Care* 2003;**26**:138–43.
34. Särnblad S, Kroon M, Åman J. Metformin as additional therapy in adolescents with poorly controlled type 1 diabetes: randomised placebo-controlled trial with aspects on insulin sensitivity. *Eur J Endocrinol* 2003;**149**:323–9.
35. Zdravkovic V, Hamilton JK, Daneman D, Cummings EA. Pioglitazone as adjunctive therapy in adolescents with type 1 diabetes. *J Pediatr* 2006;**149**:845–9.
36. Stone ML, Walker JL, Chisholm D, Craig ME, Donaghue KC, Crock P, Anderson D, Verge CF. The addition of rosiglitazone to insulin in adolescents with type 1 diabetes and poor glycaemic control: a randomized-controlled trial. *Pediatr Diabetes* 2008;**9**:326–34.
37. Donaghue KC, Chiarelli F, Trotta D, Allgrove J, Dahl-Jorgensen K. Microvascular and macrovascular complications associated with diabetes in children and adolescents. *Pediatr Diabetes* 2009;**10**(Suppl. 12):195–203.
38. Zhang L, Krzenotowski G, Albert A, Lefebvre P. Risk of developing retinopathy in Diabetes Control and Complications Trial type 1 diabetic patients with good or poor metabolic control. *Diabetes Care* 2001;**24**:1275–9.
39. Dorchy H, Claes C, Verougstraete C. Risk factors of developing proliferative retinopathy in type 1 diabetic patients. *Diabetes Care* 2002;**25**:798–9.
40. Stone ML, Craig ME, Chan AK, Lee JW, Verge CF, Donaghue KC. Natural history and risk factors for microalbuminuria in adolescents with type 1 diabetes: a longitudinal study. *Diabetes Care* 2006;**29**:2072–7.
41. deBlock CE, de Leeuw IH, van Gaal LF. Impact of overweight on chronic microvascular complications in type 1 diabetic patients. *Diabetes Care* 2005;**38**:1649–55.
42. Järvisalo MJ, Raitakari M, Toikka JO, Putto-Laurila A, Rontu R, Laine S, Lehtimäki T, Rönnemaa T, Viikari J, Raitakari OT. Endothelial dysfunction and increased arterial intima-media thickness in children with type 1 diabetes. *Circulation* 2004;**109**:1750–5.
43. Larsen J, Brekke M, Sandvik I, Arnesen H, Hanssen K, Dahl-Jorgensen K. Silent coronary atheromatosis in type 1 diabetic patients and its relation to long-term glycemic control. *Diabetes* 2002;**51**:2637–41.
44. Margeirsdottir HD, Larsen JR, Brunborg C, Overby NC, Dahl-Jørgensen K, and Norwegian Study Group for Childhood Diabetes. High prevalence of cardiovascular risk factors in children

and adolescents with type 1 diabetes: a population-based study. *Diabetologia* 2008;**51**:554–61.

45. Schwab KO, Doerfer J, Hecker W, Grulich-Henn J, Wiemann D, Kordonouri O, Beyer P, Holl RW, and DPV Initiative of the German Working Group for Pediatric Diabetology. (2006). Spectrum and prevalence of atherogenic risk factors in 27,358 children, adolescents, and young adults with type 1 diabetes: cross-sectional data from the German diabetes documentation and quality management system (DPV). *Diabetes Care* 29, 218–225.

46. Mäkinen VP, Forsblom C, Thorn LM, Wadén J, Gordin D, Heikkilä O, Hietala K, Kyllönen L, Kytö J, Rosengård-Bärlund M, Saraheimo M, Tolonen N, Parkkonen M, Kaski K, Ala-Korpela M, Groop PH, 2nd FinnDiane Study Group. Metabolic phenotypes, vascular complications, and premature deaths in a population of 4,197 patients with type 1 diabetes. *Diabetes* 2008;**57**:2480–7.

47. Purnell JQ, Hokanson JE, Marcovina SM, Steffes MW, Cleary PA, Brunzell JD. Effect of excessive weight gain with intensive therapy of type 1 diabetes on lipid levels and blood pressure: results from the DCCT. Diabetes Control and Complications Trial. *JAMA* 1998;**280**:140–6.

48. Retnakaran R, Zinman B. Type 1 diabetes, hyperglycemia, and the heart. *Lancet* 2008;**371**:1790–9.

49. Kilpatrick ES, Rigby AS, Atkin SL. Insulin resistance, the metabolic syndrome, and complication risk in type 1 diabetes: "double diabetes" in the Diabetes Control and Complications Trial. *Diabetes Care* 2007;**30**:707–12.

CHAPTER 28

Bone Health in Obesity and the Cross Talk between Fat and Bone

Sowmya Krishnan[*], Venkataraman Kalyanaraman[†]

[*]Department of Pediatrics, University of Oklahoma Health Sciences Center, Children's Medical Research Institute Diabetes and Metabolic Research Program, Harold Hamm Oklahoma Diabetes Center, Oklahoma City, OK, USA and
[†]Department of Medicine, University of Oklahoma Health Sciences Center, Harold Hamm Oklahoma Diabetes Center, Oklahoma City, Oklahoma; VA Medical Center, Oklahoma City, Oklahoma

INTRODUCTION

The problem of obesity is burgeoning all over the world and is increasingly affecting children in both developed and developing countries [1]. Childhood obesity carries with it a huge morbidity including early atherosclerotic changes in major vessels [2]. Paralleling the obesity epidemic is the prevalence of type 2 diabetes, which is being increasingly diagnosed in children [3]. This has brought a lot of attention to the cardiovascular burden imposed by early childhood obesity. That there could be other ramifications of childhood obesity, apart from cardiovascular health, is also now being recognized. Both type 1 and type 2 diabetes are associated with an increase risk for fractures [4–6]. There were an estimated 1.31 million new hip fractures in 1990, and the prevalence of disability resulting from hip fractures was estimated to be 4.48 million [7]. Worldwide osteoporotic fractures accounted for 0.83% of the global burden of noncommunicable disease. In Europe, osteoporotic fractures accounted for more disability-adjusted life years than many other chronic noncommunicable diseases [8]. All these data underscore the importance of paying attention to bone health in this population. In this chapter we will briefly address the issue of bone health in obesity and diabetes, especially in relation to children, and discuss the recently described link between bone and energy metabolism.

BONE MINERAL DENSITY AS A SURROGATE MARKER FOR BONE STRENGTH

Osteoporosis is defined as a "skeletal disorder characterized by compromised bone strength, predisposing to an increased risk of fracture" [9]. In adults, the use of densitometry has been shown to predict probability of fractures [10]. Dual-energy x-ray absorptiometry (DXA) is the most commonly used tool to measure bone density, as it is safe, noninvasive, and has low radiation exposure. Most of the data on the use of densitometry come from studies on postmenopausal women where densitometry has been shown to be especially useful to detect threshold levels for at risk individuals. The World Health Organization has developed criteria for the diagnosis of osteoporosis in postmenopausal women based on bone mineral density measurements (BMD) that is 2.5 standard deviations or more below the average value for a young adult (T-score ≤ 2.5).

Increasingly, DXA as a tool to measure bone density is being used in other populations like elderly men and at-risk children. A word of caution is in order before we delve into the data on bone density measurements in the obese population. The utility of DXA to detect subjects at risk for clinically significant fracture in this population is still to be proven. One should also keep in mind that DXA is just a measurement of bone mineral density and various other markers of bone strength like bone size, shape, geometry, and microarchitecture are not being measured. But DXA measurements of bone density is the best available tool for us so far, and it can be used as a surrogate marker of bone strength and most of the clinical data available to date uses this instrument.

RELATION OF BONE MASS TO BODY WEIGHT

That there is a relationship between body mass index (BMI) and bone density is clearly evident in conditions like anorexia nervosa in which this has been extensively studied. This condition, which is characterized by distorted body image and extreme thinness, also is associated with low BMD [11]. BMD improvement can lag behind weight gain in this condition [12]. Various other studies have documented a direct relationship between body mass index and BMD [13], though this effect tends to plateau after a certain BMI. Studies on the association between body mass index and BMD are listed in Table 28.1. In general, body fat tends to be protective against postmenopausal osteoporosis. This could be due to the possible aromatization of circulating androgens by the adipose tissue to estrogens.

FAT MASS OR LEAN MASS: WHAT INFLUENCES BONE MASS?

Recent years have shown an explosion of studies trying to delineate the exact relationship between each body composition variable with bone mineral density. Most studies support the conclusion that lean body mass (LBM) influences bone density positively [14, 15], though the effect may depend on the bone mass parameter being used and the bone site being measured. The influence of fat mass on bone density is still unclear with some studies showing a positive association [15, 16] and some a negative association [14, 17] (Table 28.2). Khosla et al. reported that the relationship between bone mass and body composition variable is dependent on the area of bone mass being measured with varying relationship of bone mass at different sites in relation to these body composition variables. They also showed that the relationship was affected by the menopausal status of these women [16]. Similarly Chen et al. showed that bone mineral mass status is more closely related to LBM than fat mass, though changes in regional BMD

TABLE 28.1 Relationship between Body Mass Index with Bone Mineral Density

Study	Results	Age of subjects
Felson et al. (1993) [51]	Body mass index explained variation in BMD for all sites in women and BMD in weight bearing sites in men	Mean age 76 years
Chen et al. (1997) [18]	Increased body weight associated with increased bone density	Postmenopausal Chinese women
Ravn et al. (1999) [13]	Women in the lowest tertiles of body fat or BMI had 12% lower BMD at baseline	Postmenopausal women
Goulding et al. (2001) [22]	Children with history of fractures were more obese and had lower areal and volumetric BMD	3 to 19 years of age
Rocher et al. (2008) [52]	Whole body bone mineral areal density (BMAD) lower but lumbar spine BMAD higher in obese children	9- to 12-year-old children

TABLE 28.2 Relationship between Various Body Composition Variables to Body Mineral Density

Study	Results	Comments
Khosla et al. [16] (1996)	Both fat mass and lean body mass affect bone mass and the effect depends on the bone mass parameter used, skeletal site measured, and menopausal status of women	Premenopausal and postmenopausal women (21 to 94 years)
Zhao et al. [53] (2007)	Negative correlation between fat mass and bone mass	Young adults of Chinese and Caucasian descent
Janicka et al. [14] (2007)	Lean mass has a significant correlation with bone mass but negative to no effect of fat mass on bone mass	Sexually mature adolescents and young adults (13 to 21 years)
Sayers et al. [15] (2009)	Lean mass has a positive relation with cortical bone mineral content	Mean age of 15.5 years

annually correlated with fat mas [18]. This differential effect of fat mass and LBM on different parts of the skeleton could be due to varying mechanism of actions of these body composition variables. Although LBM may contribute to the muscle mass and the skeletal loading and thus provide a direct mechanical affect on the bone, the fat mass may exert its effect by various adipokines secreted and by production of estrogen through aromatization [16].

BONE MASS IN OBESE CHILDREN

Data on BMD in obese children are conflicting with some reports of increased BMD [19—20] and some of decreased BMD [21, 22] when adjusted for fat mass. This could be due to different sites of measurement as obesity could exhibit differential effects on the skeleton depending on the site of measurement. Childhood is characterized by intense acquisition of bone mineral. Furthermore, studying bone mineral density during this period has inherent biases because of the influence of sexual maturity and height on bone mineral density interpretations. Most studies are cross-sectional in nature and the effect of fat mass on BMD may very well depend on the duration of obesity and possibly various other factors including genetically determined bone mass and associated inflammation.

There have also been reports of increased fracture incidence in obese children [22, 23]. It is unclear at this time if this is due to defective bone density or a higher load sustained on fall by obese children. These results need to be replicated in further longitudinal studies.

BMD AND FRACTURE RISK IN DIABETES

Both type 1 diabetes and type 2 diabetes are characterized by a higher incidence of fractures [4]. Bone mineral density data, though, are conflicting in these two types of diabetes. Type 1 diabetes has always been associated with decreased BMD [24], whereas the data in type 2 diabetes are unclear with some studies showing it to be increased [25] and some showing it to be decreased [26]. The picture is further complicated by the presence of obesity in most patients with type 2 diabetes and the varying duration of type 2 diabetes before diagnosis that is characteristic in this condition. Kinjo et al. looked at BMD in subjects with and without the metabolic syndrome in a large cohort from the third National Health and Nutrition Examination Survey (NHANES III) [27]. They found that the femoral neck BMD was higher in patients with metabolic syndrome than in those without ($p < 0.0001$). Additionally they found that the subgroup of patients with diabetes had higher femoral neck BMD compared to those without, independent of abdominal obesity. Animal studies have shown altered bone mass, geometry, and mechanical properties with type 2 diabetes [28]. This warrants concern, and the increased fracture incidence seen with type 2 diabetes may be secondary to other defects in bone health apart from bone mineralization.

VITAMIN D

Any discussion about bone health is not complete without highlighting the role of vitamin D. Vitamin D plays a critical role in bone mineralization and its deficiency is known to cause rickets. Recently though, the role of Vitamin D in insulin sensitivity and secretion has garnered a lot of interest. Low vitamin D levels have been described in relation to increased adiposity [29]. It has been postulated that increased body fat sequesters the vitamin D, leading to decreased bioavailability as it is a fat-soluble vitamin. Additionally, vitamin D status has been linked to insulin sensitivity [30] with short-term trials of vitamin D shown to improve insulin sensitivity in obese men [31]. Vitamin D deficiency could be the possible link behind the increased fracture frequency seen in obese children, though this hypothesis needs to be tested. Vitamin D is the "hot" vitamin of this period, and we are sure to see more research elucidating the link between vitamin D status and various metabolic parameters related to obesity.

BONE AND ENERGY METABOLISM

Osteoblasts and adipocytes originate from common precursor bone marrow mesenchymal cells. Complex signaling cascades direct their development into either osteoblasts or adipocyte cell lineage. Conditions associated with enhanced bone marrow adiposity are associated with low bone mineral content [32, 33]. Medications like thiazolidinediones that enhance the differentiation of bone marrow mesenchymal cells into adipocyte lineage are associated with increased marrow adiposity and heightened risk of fractures [34]. Though the close relation between fat and bone cells has been recognized for a long time, recent discoveries suggest that the skeleton plays an important role in energy metabolism. Hormones secreted from the adipocyte (adipokines) influence bone mass and similarly hormones secreted from osteoblasts have been shown to influence insulin secretion, sensitivity, and the action of adipokines in mice studies. We will briefly review these agents here.

Adipocyte-Derived Hormones (Adipokines)

Leptin

Leptin is one of the well-known adipokine (hormones secreted from adipose tissue), and its role in energy metabolism has been well described. Specifically it is secreted after eating and acts on the ventromedial hypothalamus to cause satiety. Various investigators have studied Leptin's action on bone. Specifically Gordeladze et al. showed the effect of leptin on bone mineralization and osteoclastic signaling [35]. Cultured iliac cell osteoblasts were incubated with leptin and studied for markers of various cell proliferation markers, cell apoptosis, and collagen synthesis. Leptin exposure was shown to increase the expression of transforming growth factor, insulin-like growth factor-1, collagen-1α, and osteocalcin mRNA. The CD44 osteocyte marker gene expression was increased, and they postulated that leptin exposure enhances transition of osteoblasts to preosteocytes.

Leptin also inhibits osteoclast generation and increases osteoprotegerin messenger RNA and protein expression in peripheral blood mononuclear cells [36]. Leptin treatment in leptin deficient *ob/ob* mice increases whole body bone mineral content (BMC) [37]. That leptin can have the opposite effect of enhancing bone resorption when administered centrally was shown by elegant experiments done by Ducy et al. [38]. This was postulated to be due to its action via the sympathetic nervous system. In vivo, the peripheral action of leptin seems to dominate, as evidenced by increased bone mass seen with leptin treatment in leptin-deficient *ob/ob* mice [39].

Adiponectin

Adiponectin is another adipokine secreted by adipocytes. Its levels decrease in obesity and diabetes and may increase with weight loss. Higher adiponectin levels are seen with decreased BMD in cross-sectional studies [40] and need to be clarified by further longitudinal studies.

Resistin

Resistin levels are increased proportional to obesity status. An inverse relationship has been described between resistin levels and BMD [41].

Pancreatic Hormones

Insulin

BMD is directly related to fasting insulin concentration [42]. Osteoblasts have been shown to have insulin receptors that may mediate the anabolic action of insulin on bone. Additionally the influence of insulin on bone may be mediated by indirect effects via its action on sex hormone production in ovary and sex hormone binding globulin production from liver.

Amylin

Amylin is cosecreted with insulin. It causes proliferation of osteoblasts and increases indices of bone formation [43]. Increased amylin levels seen in adiposity may be associated with the increase in bone mass.

Preptin

Preptin is a hormone secreted by beta cells of the pancreas and has been shown to be anabolic to bone [44].

Others

IL-6 levels are increased in overweight and obese children and adults. It has been shown to be an osteoresorptive factor and could cause decreased BMD associated with inflammation [45]. IL-6 knockout mice, though, have normal bone pathology.

Various other peptides have been shown to have an effect on bone, especially glucagon-like peptides 1 and 2 (GLP-1, GLP-2) [46, 47] and glucose dependent insulinotropic polypeptide (GIP). These peptides are secreted with feeding and may mediate the decreased bone resorption seen after feeding. In addition, ghrelin has an important anabolic action on bone [48].

Osteocalcin

Osteocalcin is a protein secreted by osteoblasts that has been known to play a major part in bone mineralization. Animal experiments have shown that the uncarboxylated form to increase beta cell proliferation, insulin secretion, insulin sensitivity, and adiponectin expression [49]. Human studies have shown that osteocalcin level is inversely related to insulin resistance as measured by homeostasis model assessment of insulin resistance [50]. Osteocalcin receptors have not yet been described in humans, and elucidation of its role in energy metabolism in humans needs further research.

CONCLUSION

The association between adiposity status and BMD is still not very clear. Although body fat seems to be protective against postmenopausal osteoporosis, childhood obesity seems to have an adverse affect on bone health. This difference could be because of the different sites being measured and different hormonal milieu (premenopausal/postmenopausal status, Tanner stages). Similarly, the bone mineral density data in type 2 diabetes is unclear, but this population seems to be definitely at risk for fractures at all locations including hip fractures. There have been few reports already of increased fractures in obese children, but there are no data on children or young adults with type 2 diabetes. This is concerning, and childhood obesity may be one of the most important modifiable factors to prevent later osteoporotic fractures.

The recently described link between bone and energy metabolism is intriguing and holds tremendous therapeutic potential. There yet may be other hormones that have not been described so far that link bone and energy metabolism.

References

1. Kopelman PG. Obesity as a medical problem. Nature 2000;404:635.
2. McGill Jr HC, McMahan CA, Herderick EE, Zieske AW, Malcom GT, Tracy RE, Strong JP, for the Pathobiological Determinants of Atherosclerosis in Youth Research, G. Obesity Accelerates the Progression of Coronary Atherosclerosis in Young Men. Circulation 2002;105:2712−18.
3. Liese AD, D'Agostino RB, Jr., Hamman RF, Kilgo PD, Lawrence JM, Liu LL, Loots B, Linder B, Marcovina S, Rodriguez B, Standiford D & Williams DE (2006). The burden of diabetes mellitus among US youth: prevalence estimates from the SEARCH for Diabetes in Youth Study. Pediatrics 118, 1510−18.
4. Janghorbani M, Van Dam RM, Willett WC, Hu FB. Systematic Review of Type 1 and Type 2 Diabetes Mellitus and Risk of Fracture. Am J Epidemiol 2007;166:495−505.
5. Schwartz AV, Sellmeyer DE, Ensrud KE, Cauley JA, Tabor HK, Schreiner PJ, Jamal SA, Black DM, Cummings SR, for the Study of Osteoporotic Fractures Research, G. Older Women with Diabetes Have an Increased Risk of Fracture: A Prospective Study. Journal of Clinical Endocrinology & Metabolism 2001;86:32−8.
6. Khazai NB, Beck Jr GR, Umpierrez GE. Diabetes and fractures: an overshadowed association. Current Opinion in Endocrinology, Diabetes & Obesity 2009;16:435−45.
7. Johnell O, Kanis J. An estimate of the worldwide prevalence and disability associated with osteoporotic fractures. Osteoporosis International 2006;17:1726−33.
8. Cole Z, Dennison E, Cooper C. Osteoporosis epidemiology update. Current Rheumatology Reports 2008;10:92−6.
9. Osteoporosis prevention, diagnosis, and therapy. NIH Consensus Statement 2000;17(1):1−45.
10. Kanis JA, Johnell O, Oden A, Dawson A, De Laet C, Jonsson B. Ten year probabilities of osteoporotic fractures according to BMD and diagnostic thresholds. Osteoporosis International 2001;12: 989−95.
11. Grinspoon S, Thomas E, Pitts S, Gross E, Mickley D, Miller K, Herzog D, Klibanski A. Prevalence and Predictive Factors for Regional Osteopenia in Women with Anorexia Nervosa. Annals of Internal Medicine 2000;133:790.
12. Heer M, Mika C, Grzella I, Heussen N, Herpertz-Dahlmann B. Bone turnover during inpatient nutritional therapy and outpatient follow-up in patients with anorexia nervosa compared with that in healthy control subjects. Am J Clin Nutr 2004;80:774−81.
13. Ravn P, Cizza G, Bjarnason NH, Thompson D, Daley M, Wasnich RD, Mcclung M, Hosking D, Yates AJ, Christiansen C, For The Early Postmenopausal Intervention Cohort Study, G. Low Body Mass Index Is an Important Risk Factor for Low Bone Mass and Increased Bone Loss in Early Postmenopausal Women. Journal of Bone and Mineral Research 1999;14:1622−7.
14. Janicka A, Wren TAL, Sanchez MM, Dorey F, Kim PS, Mittelman SD, Gilsanz V. Fat Mass Is Not Beneficial to Bone in Adolescents and Young Adults. Journal of Clinical Endocrinology & Metabolism 2007;92:143−7.
15. Sayers A, Tobias JH. Fat Mass Exerts a Greater Effect on Cortical Bone Mass in Girls than Boys. Journal of Clinical Endocrinology & Metabolism 2010;95:699−706.
16. Khosla S, Atkinson EJ, Riggs BL, Melton 3rd LJ. Relationship between body composition and bone mass in women. Journal of Bone & Mineral Research 1996;11:857−63.
17. Zhao L-J, Liu Y-J, Liu P-Y, Hamilton J, Recker RR, Deng H-W. Relationship of Obesity with Osteoporosis. Journal of Clinical Endocrinology & Metabolism 2007;92(5):1640−6.
18. Chen Z, Timothy GL, William AS, Ritenbaugh C, Aickin M. Fat or lean tissue mass: Which one is the major predictor of bone mineral mass in healthy postmenopausal women? Journal of Bone & Mineral Research 1997;12:144−51.
19. Ellis KJ, Shypailo RJ, Wong WW, Abrams SA. Bone mineral mass in overweight and obese children: diminished or enhanced? Acta Diabetologica 2003;40(Suppl. 1):S274−7.
20. Leonard MB, Shults J, Wilson BA, Tershakovec AM, Zemel BS. Obesity during childhood and adolescence augments bone mass and bone dimensions. American Journal of Clinical Nutrition 2004;80:514−23.
21. Goulding A, Taylor RW, Jones IE, McAuley KA, Manning PJ, Williams SM. Overweight and obese children have low bone mass and area for their weight. International Journal of Obesity & Related Metabolic Disorders: Journal of the International Association for the Study of Obesity 2000;24:627−32.
22. Goulding A, Jones IE, Taylor RW, Williams SM, Manning PJ. Bone mineral density and body composition in boys with distal forearm fractures: A dual-energy x-ray absorptiometry study. The Journal of Pediatrics 2001;139:509−15.
23. Goulding A, Jones IE, Taylor RW, Manning PJ, Williams SM. More Broken Bones: A 4-Year Double Cohort Study of Young Girls With and Without Distal Forearm Fractures. Journal of Bone and Mineral Research 2000;15:2011−18.
24. Vestergaard P. Discrepancies in bone mineral density and fracture risk in patients with type 1 and type 2 diabetes—a meta-analysis. Osteoporosis International 2007;18:427−44.
25. van Daele PLA, Stolk RP. Bone density in non-insulin-dependent diabetes. Annals of Internal Medicine 1995;122:409.
26. Yaturu S, Humphrey S, Landry C, Jain SK. Decreased bone mineral density in men with metabolic syndrome alone and with type 2 diabetes. Medical Science Monitor 2009;15:CR5−9.
27. Kinjo M, Setoguchi S, Solomon DH. Bone mineral density in adults with the metabolic syndrome: analysis in a population-based U.S. sample. Journal of Clinical Endocrinology & Metabolism 2007;92:4161−4.
28. Prisby RD, Swift JM, Bloomfield SA, Hogan HA, Delp MD. Altered bone mass, geometry and mechanical properties during the development and progression of type 2 diabetes in the Zucker diabetic fatty rat. Journal of Endocrinology 2008;199:379−88.
29. Wortsman J, Matsuoka LY, Chen TC, Lu Z, Holick MF. Decreased bioavailability of vitamin D in obesity. Am J Clin Nutr 2000;72: 690−3.
30. Ashraf A, Alvarez J, Saenz K, Gower B, McCormick K, Franklin F. Threshold for effects of vitamin D deficiency on glucose metabolism in obese female African-American adolescents. Journal of Clinical Endocrinology & Metabolism 2009;94:3200−6.
31. Nagpal J, Pande JN, Bhartia A. A double-blind, randomized, placebo-controlled trial of the short-term effect of vitamin D_3 supplementation on insulin sensitivity in apparently healthy, middle-aged, centrally obese men. Diabetic Medicine 2009;26:19−27.

32. Verma S, Rajaratnam JH, Denton J, Hoyland JA, Byers RJ. Adipocytic proportion of bone marrow is inversely related to bone formation in osteoporosis. *Journal of Clinical Pathology* 2002;**55**:693–8.
33. Moerman EJ, Teng K, Lipschitz DA, Lecka-Czernik B. Aging activates adipogenic and suppresses osteogenic programs in mesenchymal marrow stroma/stem cells: the role of PPAR-gamma2 transcription factor and TGF-beta/BMP signaling pathways. *Aging Cell* 2004;**3**:379–89.
34. Benvenuti S, Cellai I, Luciani P, Deledda C, Baglioni S, Giuliani C, Saccardi R, Mazzanti B, Dal Pozzo S, Mannucci E, Peri A, Serio M. Rosiglitazone stimulates adipogenesis and decreases osteoblastogenesis in human mesenchymal stem cells. *Journal of Endocrinological Investigation* 2007;**30**:RC26–30.
35. Gordeladze JO, Drevon CA, Syversen U, Reseland JE. Leptin stimulates human osteoblastic cell proliferation, de novo collagen synthesis, and mineralization: Impact on differentiation markers, apoptosis, and osteoclastic signaling. *Journal of Cellular Biochemistry* 2002;**85**:825–36.
36. Holloway WR, Collier FM, Aitken CJ, Myers DE, Hodge JM, Malakellis M, Gough TJ, Collier GR, Nicholson GC. Leptin inhibits osteoclast generation. *Journal of Bone & Mineral Research* 2002;**17**:200–9.
37. Hamrick MW, Della-Fera MA, Choi Y-H, Pennington C, Hartzell D, Baile CA. Leptin treatment induces loss of bone marrow adipocytes and increases bone formation in leptin-deficient ob/ob mice. *Journal of Bone & Mineral Research* 2005;**20**:994–1001.
38. Ducy P, Amling M, Takeda S, Priemel M, Schilling AF, Beil FT, Shen J, Vinson C, Rueger JM, Karsenty G. Leptin Inhibits Bone Formation through a Hypothalamic Relay: A Central Control of Bone Mass. *Cell* 2000;**100**:197–207.
39. Cornish J, Callon KE, Bava U, Lin C, Naot D, Hill BL, Grey AB, Broom N, Myers DE, Nicholson GC, Reid IR. Leptin directly regulates bone cell function in vitro and reduces bone fragility in vivo. *Journal of Endocrinology* 2002;**175**:405–15.
40. Lenchik L, Register TC, Hsu FC, Lohman K, Nicklas BJ, Freedman BI, Langefeld CD, Carr JJ, Bowden DW. Adiponectin as a novel determinant of bone mineral density and visceral fat. *Bone* 2003;**33**:646–51.
41. Ki Won O, Won Young L, Eun Jung R, Ki Hyun B, Kun Ho Y, Moo Il K, Eun Joo Y, Cheol Young P, Sung Hee I, Moon Gi C, Hyung Joon Y, Sung Woo P. The relationship between serum resistin, leptin, adiponectin, ghrelin levels and bone mineral density in middle-aged men. *Clinical Endocrinology* 2005;**63**:131–8.
42. Barrett-Connor EMD, Kritz-Silverstein DP. Does Hyperinsulinemia Preserve Bone? *Diabetes Care* 1996;**19**:1388–92.
43. Cornish J, Naot D. Amylin and Adrenomedullin: Novel Regulators of Bone Growth. *Current Pharmaceutical Design* 2002;**8**:2009.
44. Cornish J, Callon KE, Bava U, Watson M, Xu X, Lin JM, Chan VA, Grey AB, Naot D, Buchanan CM, Cooper GJS, Reid IR. Preptin, another peptide product of the pancreatic beta-cell, is osteogenic in vitro and in vivo. *Am J Physiol Endocrinol Metab* 2007;**292**:E117–22.
45. Rodan GA. Introduction to bone biology. *Bone* 1992;**13**:S3–6.
46. Bollag RJ, Zhong Q, Phillips P, Min L, Zhong L, Cameron R, Mulloy AL, Rasmussen H, Qin F, Ding KH, Isales CM. Osteoblast-Derived Cells Express Functional Glucose-Dependent Insulinotropic Peptide Receptors∗. *Endocrinology* 2000;**141**:1228–35.
47. Bollag RJ, Zhong Q, Ding KH, Phillips P, Zhong L, Qin F, Cranford J, Mulloy AL, Cameron R, Isales CM. Glucose-dependent insulinotropic peptide is an integrative hormone with osteotropic effects. *Molecular and Cellular Endocrinology* 2001;**177**:35–41.
48. Nobuhiro F, Reiko H, Hitoshi T, Yoshihiko F, Toshiaki T, Hiroshi I, Shu T, Yasuhiro T, Seiji F, Kenji K, Kensei N, Masayasu K. Ghrelin Directly Regulates Bone Formation. *Journal of Bone and Mineral Research* 2005;**20**:790–8.
49. Lee NK, Sowa H, Hinoi E, Ferron M, Ahn JD, Confavreux C, Dacquin R, Mee PJ, McKee MD, Jung DY, Zhang Z, Kim JK, Mauvais-Jarvis F, Ducy P, Karsenty G. Endocrine regulation of energy metabolism by the skeleton. *Cell* 2007;**130**:456–69.
50. Hwang Y-C, Jeong I-K, Ahn KJ, Chung HY. The uncarboxylated form of osteocalcin is associated with improved glucose tolerance and enhanced beta-cell function in middle-aged male subjects. *Diabetes/Metabolism Research Reviews* 2009;**25**:768–72.
51. Felson DT, Zhang Y, Hannan MT, Anderson JJ. Effects of weight and body mass index on bone mineral density in men and women: the Framingham study. *Journal of Bone & Mineral Research* 1993;**8**:567–73.
52. Rocher E, Chappard C, Jaffre C, Benhamou C-L, Courteix D. Bone mineral density in prepubertal obese and control children: relation to body weight, lean mass, and fat mass. *Journal of Bone & Mineral Metabolism* 2008;**26**:73–8.
53. Zhao C, Timothy GL, William AS, Cheryl R, Mikel A. Fat or Lean Tissue Mass: Which One Is the Major Determinant of Bone Mineral Mass in Healthy Postmenopausal Women? *Journal of Bone and Mineral Research* 1997;**12**:144–51.

SECTION V

PREVENTION AND TREATMENT

CHAPTER 29

A Community-Level Perspective for Childhood Obesity Prevention

Christina Economos, Erin Hennessy

John Hancock Research Center for Physical Activity, Nutrition, and Obesity Prevention,
Gerald J. and Dorothy R. Friedman School of Nutrition Science and Policy,
Tufts University, Boston, MA, USA

It is unreasonable to expect people to change their behavior when the social, cultural and physical environments around them fully conspire against them. —*Sir Michael Marmot*
Marriott MA, Wilkinson R, Social Determinants of Health. The Solid Facts, 2nd edition. World Health Organization for Europe. Denmark 2003.

INTRODUCTION

Current trends in the field of health promotion emphasize community-based programs employing multiple interventions as the main strategy for achieving population-level change in risk behaviors and health [1]. There is broad agreement that to reduce obesity, priority needs to be given to multistrategy, multisetting prevention efforts, particularly in children [2–4]. Controlled obesity prevention trials in childhood are few in number, mostly short term (1 year or less), implement a limited number of strategies (education or social marketing), focus in single settings (school-based or childcare), and, in large part, show little or no impact [5–7]. Until recently, the studies that did show an impact tended to be high-intensity, less sustainable approaches (e.g., extensive classroom time promoting individual behavior change) [5–7]. It is clear that if "we keep doing what we have been doing we are going to keep on getting what we have been getting" [8, p.171]. Innovative approaches that work at multiple levels and are flexible, effective, cost-effective, equitable, and sustainable are urgently needed. As will be discussed in this chapter, multisetting community-based interventions hold promise as one such option [2, 3, 7, 9, 10].

Defining "Community" and "Community-Based" Interventions

The concept of community is integral to the discussion of community-based interventions for obesity prevention. Within the community health arena, debates often center on whether it is best to define communities as "communities of place" (defined as those who live or work in geographically bounded spaces) or "communities of identity" (defined in terms of people who share a common social identity such as religious communities) [11]. Communities have been defined as (1) functional spatial units meeting basic needs for sustenance, (2) units of patterned social interaction, (3) symbolic units of collective identity, and (4) a social unit where people come together politically to make changes [12]. For instance, a "community" may be defined as any social entity that can be classified spatially on the basis of where persons live, work, learn, worship, and play (e.g., homes, schools, parks, roads, and neighborhoods) [13].

Naturally, all individuals are embedded within multiple communities so a distinction must be made between community interventions and interventions *in* a community. One could conceptualize the different types of community research as a continuum. At one end of this continuum is "community-placed" research (CPR). This refers to targeted research that takes place *in* a community (such as in an after-school program or church), but does not integrate any level of change (via changes to policy or environment) that expands across the community. Community-based research (CBR) lies in the middle of the continuum and interventions occur either *with* community members or occur *on* the community. For instance, interventions that are implemented on a community-wide basis, such as mass media or social marketing campaigns (e.g., the VERB™ campaign [14]), would be classified as occurring *on* a community because they do not incorporate input or participation *with* the community itself. To conduct research *with* communities, one must take into account the varied nature of relationships, networks, and how they may all work together synergistically [15].

However, simply because one is working *in* a community and interacting *with* community members in various ways does not mean that one is engaged in participatory or collaborative research [16]; thus, community-based participatory research (CBPR) lies at the other end of the continuum from CPR. This type of research is an approach, not a method, and allows for shared power and decision making between researchers and community members [17]. Regardless of whether one conceptualizes communities as social entities or as groups of people who live within certain geographical boundaries, all communities have a shared sense of place, belonging, and identity. This collective sense of identity represents an important resource for fostering change among members of a community and for designing or adapting interventions to improve a community. Thus, CBPR is designed to ensure and establish structures for participation by communities affected by the issue being studied. Community members as well as representative organizations and researchers become involved in all aspects of the research process. One caveat is that there is a confusing mix of nomenclature used to describe this kind of research: participatory research, action research, participatory action research, collaborative action research, community based inquiry, and so on [18]. A common theme to these various forms of research is that they evolved with the intention to address a need not typically acknowledged by conventional research, and most of them include a collaborative component between the researcher and the community or organization participating in the research [19].

For the purposes of this chapter, a community-based child obesity intervention is defined as an intervention to prevent overweight or obesity that (1) was implemented within one or more community groups (ad hoc or formal); (2) promoted change through policy, social marketing, or environmental change, and (3) targeted members of certain groups or community members at large (excluding schools, which are covered in a previous chapter). This includes, but is not limited to, studies that also utilize a participatory research approach. The definition that guides this chapter is similar to other reviews on this topic [4].

THEORY AND RATIONALE

A number of systematic reviews have shown that using theory in crafting interventions can lead to more powerful effects than interventions developed without theory [20, 21]. However, though it is generally accepted that modest changes in health behavior can be achieved with carefully designed and theoretically informed interventions, the extent to which behavior change is lasting or translates into health improvements at a population level is considerably less clear [22, 23]. One reason for this may be that previous intervention studies have largely ignored the social context that shapes behaviors.

An understanding of the functioning of communities (and the groups, organizations, and institutions within communities) is vital to health enhancement [24]. The collective well-being of communities can be fostered by creating structures and policies that support healthy lifestyles and by reducing or eliminating health hazards and constraints in the social and physical environments. These approaches require an understanding of how social systems operate, how change occurs within and among systems, and how community changes influence individual behavior and health [24]. Community-level models (community organization and community building, diffusion of innovations, theories of organizational change, communication theory, and others) offer a framework for understanding how social institutions (such as communities) function and change, and how they can be activated. These models complement individually oriented behavior change theories. For a detailed review, readers are referred to the *Health Behavior and Health Education: Theory, Research, and Practice* manual [25].

Ecological Models of Health Behavior

We all live in environments that influence and affect our health [26, 27]. Delineation of how this occurs has been challenging because of the multilevel, multistructural, multifactorial, and multi-institutional nature of the influences and interrelationships among these influences. The socioecological model recognizes that a complex, reciprocal, and interactive relationship exists between individuals and their environment. It assumes that behavior is affected by, and affects, multiple levels of influence including (1) intrapersonal factors, (2) interpersonal factors, (3) organizational/institutional factors, (4) community factors, and (5) public policy factors [27]. These models recognize that children's obesity-promoting behaviors cannot be understood nor can interventions to change them succeed without taking into consideration the complex and multidimensional micro- and macrolevel contexts in which their obesity-related behaviors are shaped, mediated, moderated, and maintained [28, 29]. A multilevel research approach for obesity prevention frames obesity as a complex systems problem, for which obesity-related behaviors (diet, physical activity) are not only a matter of individual choice but are also strongly influenced by multiple levels of socioenvironmental risk as defined by the socioecological model [23, 30].

Social Change Models

Population behavior is influenced by several societal subsystems, including the economy, the political system, social institutions, and culture. To influence behavior on a broad societal level, multiple subsystems must be targeted and communities can be seen as important social forces in the process of change. As societies develop their strategies to tackle the epidemic of obesity in children, they will be able to draw on the types of strategies, polices, and programs that have worked to control other epidemics [31]. Understanding how to prevent a further rise in obesity can be informed by lessons learned from a range of successful models of social change, including increasing breast-feeding rates, seat belt use, smoking cessation, and recycling [32]. Key elements identified as essential from these past successes include the following:

- Recognition that there was a crisis
- Major economic implications associated with the crisis
- A science base including research, data, and evidence
- Sparkplugs, or leaders who can work for their cause through their knowledge, competence, talents, skills, and even charisma
- Coalitions to move the agenda forward and a strategic, integrated media advocacy campaign
- Involvement of the government at the state level to apply regulatory and fiscal authority and at the local level to implement change
- Mass communication that includes consistent positive messages supported by scientific consensus and repeated in a variety of venues
- Policy and environmental changes that promote healthy lifestyle behaviors
- A plan that includes many components that work synergistically

Applying these social change strategies to the community environment to encourage healthful eating, increased levels of physical activity, and decreased sedentary behaviors is emerging as a practical way to address obesity on a large scale [10, 33].

COMMUNITY-BASED RESEARCH: DESIGN, METHODS, AND ANALYSIS

Advances in community-based obesity prevention research are highly dependent on the quality and applicability of study designs, measures, and data analysis methodology. To extract the most useful information from these studies, the field requires development or adaptation of these research components. Given the challenges inherent in community-based research—such as cultural differences among participants, widely variant preferences for treatment, lost to follow-up, and the need for succinct assessments—it is imperative that investigators conducting community-based research consider and test advances that emanate from any scientific discipline.

Research Design

Although there is a national call for community-based interventions that integrate a participatory approach [34], some stakeholders have viewed the involvement of community members in research as a threat to the objectivity of the research endeavor. Concerns have also been raised that this type of research process—in an effort to become more accessible—is not as rigorous or sophisticated as it could be [16]. Additional concerns include whether one could test intervention effectiveness and the generalizability of the results beyond the community in which the study was involved. However, CBPR is an approach, not a method. It has the potential to be as good or as bad as the research design, data collection methods, analysis, and interpretation of results allow [16].

Traditional research methods suggest that randomized controlled trials (RCTs), when well designed and executed, offer the strongest level of scientific evidence; yet, in practice, an ideal obesity prevention trial is virtually impossible in the community [35]. Determinants of obesity are embedded in, and interventions are fielded in, complex and multilevel systems [36]. Thus, it is not surprising that there is debate on how best to design, implement, and evaluate complex, multilevel, multicomponent, community-based interventions. The overarching question is clear: when complex, field-based interventions are the object of inquiry, what research designs are most likely to yield the best evidence on the extent to which interventions are effective? [37]

Quasi-experimental designs (e.g., matched group) offer a viable alternative to traditional RCTs. The goal for multilevel research is to use designs with hierarchical analytical models (with attention to nesting and cluster sampling) and long-term designs to test for change and sustainability of effects. When controlled experiments cannot be mounted, other quantitative designs can and should be considered, such as approximating randomized experiments with propensity score matching, instrumental variables, regression discontinuity designs, and so on [37]. Community-based interventions are also uniquely positioned to take advantage of "natural experiments" (e.g., policy or environmental changes initiatives in a community).

Challenges to multilevel community-based research [35, 38, 39] include the following:

- Design and measurement (e.g., feasibility of RCTs, acceptability and social or cultural validity of evaluation procedures)
- Isolating context from composition (e.g., evaluating implementer, recipient, and contextual variations, specifying and operationalizing the relevant "contexts," measuring group-level attributes)
- Time (e.g., time lags, changing contexts)
- Dynamic relationships (e.g., unanticipated changes or conditions, assessing interactions among levels, engaging multiple stakeholders in a participatory process)

Many questions need to be addressed in the area of community-based obesity prevention trials. For instance, what is a realistic time frame for how long a community-level intervention should take to produce changes in children's body mass index (BMI) levels? How do we adapt interventions to fit the local context and be culturally relevant? Research designs must account for this and perhaps focus energy on other influential factors that impact short-term outcomes (e.g., changing policies to support obesity prevention) and intermediate outcomes (e.g., increasing the proportion of children involved in physical activity on a daily basis) [34]. Additionally, individual communities across the nation are at different stages of engagement and action in addressing childhood obesity, and this remains a challenge to comparing interventions across communities. Tools such as the Community Readiness Model may offer some guidance on how to account for these differences [40].

Measures

As much as researchers need data, so do communities to be able to make the case for action to local decision makers. This calls in to light challenges with creating reliable and valid community-level measures. An absence of measurement tools to assess policy and environmental changes at the community level has impeded efforts to assess the implementation of these initiatives for preventing obesity [13]. In general, the measurement field to evaluate community level change is challenged by a lack of validated measures, measures that are unidimensional despite the complexity of the environment and policies, no established standards by which to assess and compare different communities on a particular measure, and a lack of sensitivity to measures to assess change. For example, after a community has a desired policy in place, if the appropriate measurement tools are available, several years might elapse before any verifiable change can be detected, quantified, and reported. The Centers for Disease Control and Prevention recently released a report highlighting recommended community strategies and measurements to prevent obesity (Table 29.1) [13]; however, more work is needed in the measurement area to provide researchers with reliable and valid tools that are sensitive enough to detect change at the community level.

Analysis

Data generated from community-based interventions are often nested or complex, and may require multilevel or spatial statistics. Group randomized trials offer investigators an alternative to individually randomized trials and offer the feasibility to make large-scale environmental change without risking contamination [35]. However, analyses must account for the within-group correlation that occurs because of this research design. In other words, analyses need to adjust for the fact that people within groups are similar to each other.

What becomes critical in multilevel intervention work is consideration of the levels that are targeted via intervention and evaluation [38]. In multilevel interventions, one can construct an intervention to be delivered at one level, while measuring impact at multiple levels. Alternatively, one could intervene at multiple levels and evaluate at individual or multiple levels. Nastasi and Hitchcock identified [38] four possibilities for framing intervention-outcome: Individual—Individual (I—I), Individual—Multilevel (I—M), Multilevel—Individual (M—I), and Multilevel—Multilevel (M—M). The first of these, I—I, is the traditional model in social sciences, exemplified by a single-level RCT: an intervention is directed at changing the behavior of the individual, and outcome is measured via documenting changes in the individuals' behaviors. By contrast, cluster trials are becoming increasingly prevalent, where groups (e.g., communities) are randomized but outcomes at the individual level are of interest and can be studied via M—I and M—M approaches. If a given comprehensive intervention is meant to change, for example, child nutritional knowledge only, it may be classified as M—I. If, however, the intervention might impact child nutritional knowledge and teacher practice (with the hopes of enacting long-term instructional change), this might be thought of as an M—M scenario [38].

In general, there is a need to develop innovative statistical models tailored to the demands of community-based research studies [41]. A growing commitment in community-based obesity intervention research is to investigate how analysis at the community level can contribute to our understandings of the social context of health and how action at the community level can contribute to the development of community contexts that are enabling and supportive of health

TABLE 29.1 Recommended Community Strategies and Measurements to Prevent Obesity [13]

Strategy	Measurement
1. Strategies to promote the availability of affordable healthy food and beverages	A policy exists to do the following: — Apply nutrition standards that are consistent with the Dietary Guidelines for Americans [66] to all food sold (e.g., meal menus and vending machines) within local government facilities in a local jurisdiction or on public school campuses during the school day within the largest school district in a local jurisdiction. — Affect the cost of healthier foods and beverages (as defined by IOM [67]) relative to the cost of less healthy foods and beverages sold within local government facilities in a local jurisdiction or on public school campuses during the school day within the largest school district in a local jurisdiction. — Encourage the production, distribution, or procurement of food from local farms in the local jurisdiction. The number of full-service grocery stores and supermarkets per 10,000 residents located within the three largest underserved census tracts within a local jurisdiction. Local government offers at least one incentive to new or existing food retailers to offer healthier food and beverage choices [67] in underserved areas. The total annual number of farmer-days at farmers' markets per 10,000 residents within a local jurisdiction.
2. Strategies to support healthy food and beverage choices	A policy exists to do the following: — Prohibit the sale of less healthy foods and beverages [67] within local government facilities in a local jurisdiction or on public school campuses during the school day within the largest school district in a local jurisdiction. — Limit the portion size of any entree (including sandwiches and entrée salads) by either reducing the standard portion size of entrees or offering smaller portion sizes in addition to standard portion sizes within local government facilities within a local jurisdiction. — Limit advertising and promotion of less healthy foods and beverages [67] within local government facilities in a local jurisdiction or on public school campuses during the school day within the largest school district in a local jurisdiction. Licensed childcare facilities within the local jurisdiction are required to ban sugar-sweetened beverages (including flavored/sweetened milk) and limit the portion size of 100% juice.
3. A strategy to encourage breast-feeding	A policy exists to do the following: — Require local government facilities to provide breast-feeding accommodations for employees that include both time and private space for breast-feeding during working hours.
4. Strategies to encourage physical activity or limit sedentary activity among children and youth	The largest school district located within the local jurisdiction has a policy that requires the following: — A minimum of 150 minutes per week of physical education (PE) in public elementary schools and a minimum of 225 minutes per week of PE in public middle schools and high schools throughout the school year. — K-12 students to be physically active for at least 50% of time spent in PE classes in public schools. — A percentage of public schools within the largest school district in a local jurisdiction to allow the use of their athletic facilities by the public during nonschool hours on a regular basis. — Licensed childcare facilities within the local jurisdiction to limit screen time to no more than 2 hours per day for children aged ≥2 years.
5. Strategies to create safe communities that support physical activity	A percentage of residential parcels within a local jurisdiction located within a half-mile network distance of at least one outdoor public recreational facility. Total miles of designated shared-use paths and bike lanes relative to the total street miles (excluding limited access highways) that are maintained by a local jurisdiction. Total miles of paved sidewalks relative to the total street miles (excluding limited access highways) that are maintained by a local jurisdiction. The largest school district in the local jurisdiction has a policy that supports locating new schools, and/or repairing or expanding existing schools, within easy walking or biking distance of residential areas. A percentage of residential and commercial parcels in a local jurisdiction that are located either within a quarter-mile network distance of at least one bus stop or within a half-mile network distance of at least one train stop (including commuter and passenger trains, light rail, subways, and street cars). Percentage of zoned land area (in acres) within a local jurisdiction that is zoned for mixed use that specifically combines residential land use with one or more commercial, institutional, or other public land uses. The number of vacant or abandoned buildings (residential and commercial) relative to the total number of buildings located within a local jurisdiction. Local government has a policy for designing and operating streets with safe access for all users, which includes at least one element suggested by the National Complete Streets Coalition.
6. A strategy to encourage communities to organize for change	Local government is an active member of at least one coalition or partnership that aims for environmental and policy change to promote active living and/or healthy eating (excluding personal health programs such as health fairs).

enhancing behaviors [11]. This requires analyses with community as the level of analysis or other types of analyses such as propensity score matching, time series, case-comparison, mixed methods, and others [42]. Additionally, community-based obesity intervention research could also include analyses to identify associations between characteristics of programs and policies and impacts/outcomes desired for reducing childhood obesity rates and for determining how effective and cost-effective such interventions are likely to be. Evidence needs to be collected to inform estimates of the relative population impact (with levels of uncertainty) and costs for the intervention so that the most promising ones can be considered for wide-scale implementation [43].

COMMUNITY INTERVENTIONS: PROGRESS AND PROMISE

The premise of this chapter is that improvements in health require understanding both the multilevel determinants of health behavior and a range of change strategies at the individual, interpersonal, and macro levels [44]. Macrolevel models and the different types of models available emphasize community assets and strengths rather than being driven solely by problems. They are not simply community based but community driven. The view that societal-level changes and supportive environments are necessary serves as the foundation for the few interventions that have been conducted to date.

Previous community-based approaches to change behavior and prevent disease give promise for the future of community intervention work [45–52]. Evidence in support of health improvement and disease reduction by way of community involvement began gaining ground by the 1970s. The North Karelia Project [53] and the Stanford Three Community Study [50–54] were among the first to break ground in this area. Each proved effective in translating educational messages into significant positive changes and cardiovascular disease risk reduction in the populations that received the interventions, as compared to control populations. The intervention strategies of these projects used mass media, low-cost lifestyle modifications, and the involvement of community members. Subsequently, the National Institutes of Health (NIH) financed three major community-based intervention projects: the Stanford Five-City Project [49], the Minnesota Heart Health Program [55], and the Pawtucket Heart Health Program [46]. These trials essentially provided community-wide health education over several years. The Stanford Project integrated social learning theory, a communication-behavior change model, community organization principles, and social marketing methods to create its comprehensive program [49]. Minnesota's multiple strategy approach provided systematic population screening for hypertension, mass media campaigns, adult and youth education programs, physician and health professional programs, and community organization efforts [11]. Pawtucket provided multilevel education, screening, and counseling programs throughout the community [46]. This literature demonstrates that community-wide strategies offer a comprehensive, equitable, and intergenerational response to the problem and potentially a means of treatment and prevention. Based on this work and the ongoing work of communities in the United States, the Institute of Medicine recently released a report highlighting the key elements of community-based strategies (Table 29.2) [34], which echo those described by other social change models [32].

In general, community-based programs focused on youth have been carried out to increase contraception use [36] and physical activity [56]. There are very few examples of community-based interventions focused on obesity because of the complex nature of both the etiology and the solution. The discussion that follows reviews the approaches utilized by the few community-based obesity prevention interventions that have been published to date.

Pathways

The modest numbers of community-based childhood obesity interventions are paving the way for future approaches to managing the childhood obesity epidemic. The Pathways intervention was a randomized controlled trial conducted within Native American communities, the first of its kind to take into account cultural, theoretical, and operational viability in the study population and to operate on a large scale (1704 participants) in 41 schools over the span of 6 years, including 3 years of feasibility testing and 3 years of intervention. The aim of the project was to reduce body fat by promoting behavioral change and a holistic view of health among Native American children in third, fourth, and fifth grades. Although the intervention was largely carried out within the schools, care was taken to enlist the support of community and tribal leaders, as well as parents. The intervention was developed through a collaboration of universities and American-Indian nations, schools, and families. The focus was on individual, behavioral, and environmental factors and merged constructs from the social learning theory with American-Indian customs and practices. Pathways was successful in reducing the energy density of foods consumed by changing the school food environment. Although the main outcome of the study, change in percentage body fat, produced no significant difference between intervention and

TABLE 29.2 Key Elements of Community-Based Strategies [34]

Leadership	Community-wide obesity prevention efforts require the investment of adequate resources and the commitment of the institutions and organizations that operate within a community; sparkplugs are needed to serve as a driving force behind sustaining collaborative efforts, dedicating resources, and working to change social norms that support healthier lifestyles
Building Community Coalitions	The efforts needed to prevent childhood obesity require a diverse set of skills and expertise—from renovating community recreational facilities to developing multimedia campaigns to promote healthy lifestyles. Because childhood obesity prevention is central to the health of the community's children and youth, the development of community coalitions is a particularly relevant means of addressing this issue.
Cultural Relevance	Culturally appropriate intervention strategies and elements are necessary and fundamental to the promotion of grassroots involvement. They can be peripheral, evidential, linguistic, constituency based, and sociocultural and can greatly affect intervention and policy outcomes.
Sufficient Resources and Sustained Commitment	Community-based childhood obesity prevention efforts require careful planning and coordination, well-trained staff, and sufficient resources. Insufficient resources may result in an intervention that is inadequate, whereas certain policy and environmental change initiatives are often time and resource intensive requiring sustained commitment from local leaders.
Focus on Safety	Addressing safety concerns—both real and perceived—is a necessary component of many childhood obesity prevention efforts, especially those at the community level. Combining community safety and childhood obesity prevention efforts is synergistic and mutually beneficial for a community.
Community-Based Participatory Research (CBPR)	Although not a required component of community-based childhood obesity prevention research, CBPR is an excellent approach to this public health issue because it is, by nature, culturally competent and congruent with the needs and values of a target group.
Building on Multiple Social and Health Priorities	Community-based efforts to address childhood obesity can find common ground with other factors that may require for a community's attention (poverty, crime, violence, limited access to healthcare, underperforming schools, etc.). Many of the efforts and strategies to tackle these common problems have mutual benefits (e.g., improving playgrounds and recreational facilities may enhance safety, reduce crime, and increase physical activity of children). Finding common ground is a key element in garnering sufficient investment for sustained efforts.

control schools, other measurable benefits were demonstrated. Twenty-four-hour dietary intake measures showed a significantly lower total daily energy intake (1892 compared with 2157 kcal/d) and percentage of energy from total fat (31.1% compared with 33.6%) in the intervention group than in the control group. Further, the percentage of energy as fat shown in school lunches was 28.2% in the intervention schools compared to 32% in controls, and self-reported physical activity (as assessed via Physical Activity Questionnaire), and healthy food choice intentions were conversely higher for intervention verses control schools. Finally, Pathways curricula knowledge increased significantly in children involved in the intervention. The Pathways study demonstrated a successful marriage of theoretical underpinnings, community and family involvement, and cultural and situational appropriateness. In this manner, Pathways provided an excellent community research framework upon which to build.

Shape up Somerville

Informed by previous social change models and the Pathways study, *Shape up Somerville (SUS): Eat Smart, Play Hard*, conducted in Somerville, Massachusetts, was one of the first CBPR initiatives designed to change the environment to prevent obesity in early elementary school-aged children [48]. Academics partnered with community members of three culturally diverse urban communities to conduct a controlled trial evaluating whether an environmental change intervention could prevent a rise in body mass index (BMI) z-scores in young children through enhanced access and availability of physical activity options and healthy food throughout their entire day. The SUS intervention focused on creating multilevel environmental change to support behavioral action and maintenance and to prevent weight gain among early elementary school children through community participation. Specific changes within the before-, during-, and after-school environments provided a variety of increased opportunities for physical activity. The availability of lower energy dense foods, with an emphasis on fruits, vegetables, whole grains, and low-fat dairy, was increased; foods high in fat and sugar were discouraged. Additional changes within the home and the community, promoted by the intervention team, provided reinforced opportunities for increased physical activity and improved access to healthier food. To achieve this level of change, many groups and individuals within the community (including children, parents, teachers, school food service providers, city departments, policy makers, healthcare providers, before- and after-school programs, restaurants, and the media) were engaged in the intervention (see http://nutrition.tufts.edu/research/shapeup for details). These changes were intended to bring the overall energy equation into balance. Specifically, this intervention aimed to increase energy expenditure of up to 125 kcals per day beyond the increases in energy expenditure and energy intake accompanying growth. A central aim of the intervention was to create a community model that could be replicated nationwide as a cost-effective, community-based action plan to prevent obesity at local levels. After the first school year of intervention (8 months) in the intervention community, BMI z-scores decreased by -0.1005 (P = 0.001, 95% confidence interval -0.1151 to -0.0859) compared to children in the control communities after controlling for baseline covariates [48]. Analyses are currently being conducted to evaluate the effect of the intervention after the second school year.

Be Active, Eat Well

Community-based interventions are also being effectively implemented in other parts of the world. Recently, an Australian intervention program utilizing the socio-ecological model, *Be Active, Eat Well*, was evaluated and found to be successful in a number of areas [57]. This was a multifaceted community capacity-building program promoting physical activity and healthy eating for children aged 4 to 12 years in one Australian town. Using a quasi-experimental, longitudinal design, anthropometric data were collected from four intervention preschools and six primary schools at baseline (2003) and follow-up (2006). A comparison sample included a stratified random sample of preschoolers and primary school children from a neighboring community. The intervention was designed to build the community's capacity to create its own solutions to obesity-related behaviors (diet, physical activity) among children. The program was designed, planned, and implemented by key community organizations with technical support, training, and evaluation provided by academic researchers. The objective was to include broad actions around governance, partnerships, coordinating, training, and resource allocation. Five objectives targeted evidence-based behavior changes and each objective had a variety of strategies (increase fruit and vegetable consumption [objective] was met by the creation of a community garden, changes in school nutrition policies, menu changes, etc.). In the end, children in the intervention community had significantly lower increases in body weight, waist, waist/height, and BMI z-score than comparison children [57]. Further, the intervention was shown not to increase health inequalities related to obesity and was also deemed to be safe as changes in underweight and attempted weight loss were not different between the two groups of children [57].

Fleurbaix Laventie Ville Santé (FLVS) Study (2002–2007)

Three consecutive studies took place in two small towns located in northern France: Fleurbaix and Laventie (FL) against two matched control communities. The first period (1992–1997) focused on nutrition education; the second period (1997–2002) was a longitudinal observational study on the determinants of weight changes; and the third period (2002–2007) targeted physical activity and nutrition in the FL population as a whole via a series of community-based actions [58]. Because of the consecutive nature of these studies, momentum and support of community residents for the intervention grew and the community became increasingly committed. The "intervention" included the employment of two dietitians in the schools to perform various interventions as well as attend various meetings in the town targeting both children and adults. Town councils supported actions in favor of physical activity, such as building new sports facilities, supporting new sports educators to develop programming in the schools, and organizing walk-to-school campaigns and family activities. Various stakeholders in the community (physicians, shopkeepers, and organizations) also created family activities focused on a "healthy lifestyle." Media interest of this "social change movement" grew and included articles in the local newspaper, medical press, and national press as well as television and radio reports. Height, weight, and sociodemographic data were collected from the intervention and comparison communities over multiple years. After an initial rise in the previous year, the overweight prevalence was significantly lower in FL (8.8%) during the 2004 school year than in the comparison towns (17.8%, p < 0.0001). The authors noted that the first wave of studies, which focused on school-based obesity prevention, served as a catalyst for raising awareness of the issue. Moreover, this awareness-raising process gradually intensified over time and prompted the initiation of a whole-community intervention program. Although there are limitations to this study, it provides evidence that community-based interventions take time but may also be successful in reducing the prevalence of childhood obesity at a population level.

Ongoing Studies

Few community-based obesity prevention studies have been conducted, but several are currently under way. For example, the SWITCH™ study is a community-, school-, and family-based intervention aimed at modifying key behaviors (physical activity, television viewing/screen time, and nutrition) related to childhood obesity in third through fifth graders residing in two Midwestern cities [59]. This program used the socioecological model to guide its multilevel intervention components. At the community level, one intervention strategy was to increase community awareness and knowledge about preventing childhood obesity through public education including public service announcements, news columns, public information sessions, and so on. The full randomized intervention was conducted from January 2005 through May 2006 and included 10 schools (5 assigned to intervention group, and 5 assigned to control group). Main outcome measures include physical activity, screen time, fruit and vegetable consumption, body mass, and waist circumference of the target age group (third through fifth graders), and results have not yet been released. Additionally, the Shape up Somerville (SUS) intervention model [48] is currently being replicated in two separate studies. The Balance Project replicates SUS in three underserved, urban U.S. communities in a 2-year, controlled trial targeting first through third graders and their families. Six communities were selected from a rigorous Request for Application process with similar populations and levels of readiness to participate in the research trial. Three were randomized to receive the intervention and three to be monitored (control communities). The three intervention cities are receiving training, tools, and funding that will enable them to create an environment that surrounds children with healthier food options and opportunities for active living. By choosing intervention and control communities at the same level of readiness, researchers can determine what happens over a 2-year period with and without an investment of resources and inputs. Data are being collected at the policy and environmental level; no individual measures will be evaluated. The CHANGE Study is a collaborative effort among Tufts University; Save the Children, U.S. Programs; and four low-income rural communities located in the regions of Central Valley, California, Mississippi River Delta, Appalachia, and South Carolina. Individual level measures include BMI as well as dietary intake and physical activity behavior of elementary school-aged children. The goal is to adapt the SUS model for rural communities to understand the modifications necessary to make the intervention culturally relevant for rural areas, which face additional challenges with respect to healthcare professional shortages and the built environment [60].

Discussion

Community-based interventions allow for the wealth of assets present in any community to be tapped and used with efficiency and direction. One of the most important assets found in communities is, naturally, the vast array of human resources. From vested community leaders, to service and information providers, to organizations and faith-based groups, to community members seeking employment, the opportunities to partner, collaborate, expand, and enrich initiatives are numerous. Additionally, the depth of community understanding possessed by its members cannot be matched by efforts made by individuals from the outside. Soliciting community input can be invaluable in shaping and implementing research and programmatic activity. Indeed, allowing community members to participate in the work offers several advantages to investigator driven research and programming. Knowledge of the resources and dynamics existing within communities is best acquired directly from community members. One potential reason why previous interventions have not been successful at preventing childhood obesity may be due to the fact that many studies have not adequately integrated community assets and members into the study design and implementation process.

In their comprehensive synthesis of evidence of reducing obesity and related chronic disease risk in children and youth, Flynn et al. [7] presented recommendations for a broad range of sectors, organizations, and health professionals, which are based on the available evidence and gaps in knowledge identified during the synthesis. With regard to intervention activities, the recommendations can be summarized into the following points:

- Population-based interventions should be developed to balance, support, and extend the current emphasis on individual-based programs.
- Obesity prevention programs need to be developed with rigorous evaluation components in community and home settings where limited program activity is evident and effectiveness is unknown.
- Interventions need long-term implementation and follow-up to determine the sustainability of program impacts as on body weight.
- To maximize funding and health impact, interventions should be developed within an integrated chronic disease prevention model and with a CBPR framework.
- Program design process should be developed to allow continual incorporation of new elements associated with greater program effectiveness, using an action research model.

The success of a multisetting intervention approach may be the result of a number of factors. An approach such as this works within a framework, recognizing that multiple factors affect a community's function and, in turn, the health of the individuals within. Reviews of the intervention literature, particularly in obesity prevention, have shown that interventions that use these frameworks to guide their design are more likely to be successful [48, 57]. Interventions that are community based and community wide can also address risk factors that are common to a number of chronic diseases. The integrated chronic disease prevention (CDP) model has developed from recognition of the preventable risk factors shared by leading chronic diseases [61]. Key concepts in the integrated CDP model include an ecological perspective, intersectoral action, multilevel intervention, and collaborative processes. The multiplicity and complexity of this approach is captured in a definition put forward by Shiell: "[Integrated chronic disease prevention is an approach] that targets more than one risk factor or disease outcome, more than one level of influence, more than one disciplinary perspective, more than one type of research method, or more than one societal sector, and which targets populations—rather than individuals—as a unit." [61, p. 2]. The influence of the ecological perspective is evident in that integrated CDP frameworks consider the interdependence between individuals and the broader socioenvironmental context. For example, a community-wide intervention to improve the delivery of preventative services to children in the United States achieved far reaching changes [62]. The intervention approach was based on systems theory, which suggests that many opportunities for improvement exist in the interactions between elements of a system. For this intervention, the application of this theory resulted in viewing care delivery as a series of processes extending from the home to the primary care practice and other community health and social services. The intervention activities were directed at the community, practice, and family level. At the community level, positive effects were seen in state and community policies that led to sustainable changes in organization practices and funding approaches. At the practice level, alignment and integration of services delivered by multiple practices resulted in reduced duplication, improved coordination, and changes in service delivery. At the family level, the intervention resulted in improved child and maternal health outcomes [62].

An additional benefit of a multisetting community-wide approach is its potential to improve the health and development of all children in the community. Interventions that attempt to address at least some of the social determinants of health have the potential to address population-level determinants of ill health, rather than individual characteristics. They can be equity focused and reduce the socioeconomic gradient that currently exists for almost all health outcomes. This approach can also positively influence individual behaviors through addressing the societal and environmental influences at the community level. Interventions that target multiple aspects of individual environments have the ability to make health-promoting options easier and, over time, can also shift behavioral and cultural norms in a sustainable manner. Targeting environments also represents an upstream approach, as children in low-income families live in environments that limit social and economic opportunities, access to healthful foods, and opportunities for physical activity. In the Shape up Somerville intervention program, a significant reduction in z-BMI was seen after 1 year in the intervention children [48]. This intervention engaged the community widely and was specifically focused on changing children's environments at school and also enhancing access and availability of healthy eating and physical activity options throughout the entire day for children, including before- and after-school programs [48]. Also as a result of the intervention, there were changes in the home and community, which provided reinforced opportunities for increased physical activity and improved access to more nutritious food.

FUTURE DIRECTIONS

Community-based obesity prevention research designs and analyses should incorporate multilevel intervention and multilevel evaluations. For instance, in a hypothetical community-based obesity intervention study,[1] three levels could be targeted: (1) community as a whole changing norms within community context at an aggregate level as well as cognitions and behaviors of individuals; (2) schoolteachers changing their knowledge and practices, and (3) children changing their cognitions and behaviors. Components of the intervention are directed at all three levels. Although evaluation could focus on just the individual (child), it could also entail (1) measuring changes at multiple levels, (2) testing the paths of change (direct and indirect), and (3) documenting the cultural and contextual factors that either defined the intervention or may have influenced either the intervention or outcomes.

In general, the future of community-based obesity intervention research may include the following [23, 41]:

- A global perspective on obesity research
- Cross-disciplinary efforts to connect multiple levels of risk factors across the socioecological continuum

---

[1]This hypothetical example was adapted from Nastasi and Hitchock (2009).

- Testing of multiple levels of socioecological model and evaluating interactions of variables across levels
- Understanding how local communities can be mobilized to initiate policy change
- Capacity building and rigorous training of a new generation of multilevel scientists to design and analyze complex, multilevel community interventions
- Integration of community-based participatory research approaches, which the Institute of Medicine named as one of eight new competency areas essential for breadth in public health training

Systems Perspective

As previously mentioned, systems science is increasingly being utilized in chronic disease research. We know that the obesity epidemic cannot be prevented by individual action alone; rather, it demands a societal approach. Developing an understanding of the whole system is a critical first step in tackling the problem more effectively [64]. Because of the complex system that affects obesity, researchers also need to use a systems-oriented approach to address the multiple factors and levels [3]. Systems science may also help to identify what structure or set of relationships might be driving the behavior and what changes would lead to more desirable behavior. It helps to map out the processes and mechanisms that are needed to change and alter the social relations that are damaging to health.

Glass and McAtee have also developed a multilevel, three-dimensional framework to examine health behaviors and disease in social and biological context. They challenge us to develop better theory and data to understand how social factors regulate behaviors or distribute individuals into risk groups and how these social factors come to be embodied [23]. This is necessary because although we are knowledgeable about the behaviors that lead to ill health and disease, relatively little is known about how these behaviors arise, are maintained, and can be changed. By advancing the study of the social determinants, Glass and McAtee suggested that more effective population interventions can be developed. Accordingly, continuing to conduct interventions that attempt to alter health behaviors in isolation from the broader social and environmental context will continue to provide disappointing results. The authors emphasized the need to focus on the health behaviors and the mediating structures that lie between the behavioral sphere and the macrosocial context.

In fact, a major limitation of most current community interventions is the failure to address potential mediators and outcomes adequately [25]. These mediating structures are termed "risk regulators" and in the obesity context are, for example, cultural norms, area deprivation, food availability, laws and policies, and workplace conditions [23]. These risk regulators influence the two key behaviors related to obesity, nutrition and physical activity, in a way that is dynamic and extends over the life course. Accordingly, population interventions to prevent obesity cannot attempt to influence health behaviors without attempting to address at least some of these risk regulators; a more contextual understanding of health behaviors and health service usage, for example, would increase the effectiveness of obesity prevention interventions and public health policies [23]. Again, systems science may provide us with a better understanding of the necessary levers to target in obesity prevention efforts. The Institute of Medicine recently convened a panel to develop a framework for evidence-informed decision-making in obesity prevention efforts [36], which will be guided, in part, by the need for a systems approach that explicitly takes into account the social contexts in which decisions are made and the multiple interacting determinants of policy and community action.

Agent-Based Modeling

This chapter has touched on the fact that traditional epidemiological study designs and analytical approaches are unable to adequately examine the dynamic processes that occur between individuals and their communities, which both adapt and change over time. Agent-based models (ABMs) and other systems-dynamics models may help to address some of these challenges [65] and lead to an understanding of the processes that may help to identify more effective interventions. Agent-based models offer computer representations of complex systems and provide a venue to test interventions, which are not yet feasible in the real world, and allow one to evaluate intervention effects under conditions different than those observed [39]. Their strengths are that they can account for the interrelatedness of individuals and their environment—both the reciprocal and dynamic nature of these relationships—and force investigators to think about processes. However, a number of challenges and limitations exist for ABMs: making them simple enough to yield useful insights and complex enough to not misrepresent what is occurring in the real world; no agreed-upon formula for what to include in an ABM; and the validity of the data, because locating the relevant data with which to parameterize the model is difficult [65]. At this time, though, ABMs offer promise, provide a complement to traditional epidemiological techniques, and yield additional insight into the processes involved and the interventions that may be most useful in addressing the current obesity epidemic.

SUMMARY

Childhood obesity prevention interventions are few in number, but those that do exist offer promise and direction for future research efforts.

CONCLUSION

Community research increases the breadth of the target audience in a cost-effective manner. Communities share proximity and problems; they also share resources and unique attributes that can be harnessed and used in positive ways. The Social Ecological model provides an excellent structure for framing change efforts on multiple levels and is the most effective manner in which to support and maintain positive behavior change in individuals. Involving the community in any initiative helps researchers pinpoint the specific needs of the community as well as identify assets and untapped resources and solutions. Additionally, involving communities in the intervention or project development process can be, in and of itself, a motivating factor.

To date, few research-based community interventions have addressed obesity, despite the need for this work emphasized in the literature and calls for such efforts from government agencies and private foundations. More interventions that focus on multifaceted community-based environmental change approaches using key elements of other successful social change models (a recognized crisis, economic impact, evidence based, government involvement) are needed [32]. Advanced community-based research approaches to turn the tide on childhood obesity will require training future leaders in community research methodology, increased funding to conduct rigorous trials, and acceptance of the study model as viable from the broad scientific community [63].

Preventing obesity is a societal challenge, similar to climate change. It requires partnership between government, science, business, and civil society. From a proximal standpoint, community-based interventions are a unique opportunity to create this type of social change because we know that tackling obesity requires far greater change than the majority of trials that have been conducted thus far have attempted to implement. Community-based, multilevel interventions are needed to create change at the personal, family, community, and, eventually, national level. There is a need for long-term, sustained interventions and efforts to focus on ongoing evaluation and continuous improvement [64].

References

1. Merzel C, D'Afflitti J. Reconsidering community-based health promotion: promise, performance, and potential. *Am J Public Health* 2003;**93**:557–74.
2. Position of the American Dietetic Association: individual-, family-, school-, and community-based interventions for pediatric overweight. *J Am Diet Assoc* 2006;**106**:925–45.
3. Huang TT, Drewnowski A, Kumanyika SK, Glass TA. A systems-oriented multilevel framework for addressing obesity in the 21st century. *Prev Chronic Dis* 2009;**6**:A97.
4. Ritchie LD, Crawford PB, Hoelscher DM, Sothern MS. Position of the American Dietetic Association: individual-, family-, school-, and community-based interventions for pediatric overweight. *J Am Diet Assoc* 2006;**106**:925–45.
5. Summerbell CD, Waters E, Edmunds LD, Kelly S, Brown T, Campbell KJ. Interventions for preventing obesity in children. *Cochrane Database Syst Rev*; 2005. CD001871.
6. Doak CM, Visscher TL, Renders CM, Seidell JC. The prevention of overweight and obesity in children and adolescents: a review of interventions and programmes. *Obes Rev* 2006;**7**:111–36.
7. Flynn MA, McNeil DA, Maloff B, Mutasingwa D, Wu M, Ford C, Tough SC. Reducing obesity and related chronic disease risk in children and youth: a synthesis of evidence with "best practice" recommendations. *Obes Rev* 2006;**7**(Suppl. 1):7–66.
8. Wandersman A, Duffy J, Flaspohler P, Noonan R, Lubell K, Stillman L, Blachman M, Dunville R, Saul J. Bridging the gap between prevention research and practice: the interactive systems framework for dissemination and implementation. *Am J Community Psychol* 2008;**41**:171–81.
9. Sorensen G, Emmons K, Hunt MK, Johnston D. Implications of the results of community intervention trials. *Annu Rev Public Health* 1998;**19**:379–416.
10. French SA, Story M, Jeffery RW. Environmental influences on eating and physical activity. *Annu Rev Public Health* 2001;**22**:309–35.
11. Campbell C, Murray M. Community health psychology: promoting analysis and action for social change. *J Health Psychol* 2004;**9**:187–95.
12. Minkler M, Wallerstein N. *Community-based participatory research for health*. San Francisco, CA: Jossey-Bass; 2008.
13. Kettel Khan L, Sobush K, Keener D, Goodman K, Lowry A, Kakietek J, Zaro S. Recommended community strategies and measurements to prevent obesity in the United States. *Morbidity and Mortality Weekly Report* 2009;**58**:1–26.
14. Wong F, Huhman M, Heitzler C, Asbury L, Bretthauer-Mueller R, McCarthy S, Londe P. VERB - a social marketing campaign to increase physical activity among youth. *Prev Chronic Dis* 2004;**1**:A10.
15. Wellman Ba W, S. Different Strokes from Different Folks: Community Ties and Social Support. *American Journal of Sociology* 1990;**96**:558.
16. Lantz PM, Israel BA, Schulz AJ, Reyes A. Community-based participatory research: rationale and relevance for social epidemiology. In: Oakes JM, Kaufman JS, editors. *Methods in Social Epidemiology*. San Francisco: John Wiley & Sons, Inc.; 2006.
17. Israel B, Eng E, Schulz A, Parker E. *Methods in community-based participatory research for health*. San Francisco: Jossey-Bass; 2005.
18. Ansley F, Gaventa J. Researching for democracy and democratizing research. *Change* 1997;**29**:46–53.
19. Kemmis S, McTaggert R. Participatory action research. In: Denzin NK, Lincoln YS, editors. *Handbook of qualitative research*. Thousand Oaks, CA: Sage Publications; 2000.

20. Ammerman AS, Lindquist CH, Lohr KN, Hersey J. The efficacy of behavioral interventions to modify dietary fat and fruit and vegetable intake: a review of the evidence. *Prev Med* 2002;**35**(1):25—41.

21. Legler J, Meissner HI, Coyne C, Breen N, Chollette V, Rimer BK. The effectiveness of interventions to promote mammography among women with historically lower rates of screening. *Cancer Epidemiol Biomarkers Prev* 2002;**11**(1):59—71.

22. Glasgow RE, Klesges LM, Dzewaltowski DA, Bull SS, Estabrooks P. The future of health behavior change research: what is needed to improve translation of research into health promotion practice? *Ann Behav Med* 2004;**27**:3—12.

23. Glass TA, McAtee MJ. Behavioral science at the crossroads in public health: extending horizons, envisioning the future. *Soc Sci Med* 2006;**62**:1650—71.

24. Glanz K. Community and group models of health behavior change. In: theory, research, practice Glanz K, Rimer BK, Viswanath K, editors. *Health behavior and health education*. San Francisco: Jossey-Bass; 2008. pp. 283—5.

25. Glanz K, Rimer BK, Viswanath K. *Health behavior and health education: theory, research, and practice*. San Francisco: Jossey-Bass; 2008.

26. Baranowski T, Cullen KW, Nicklas T, Thompson D, Baranowski J. Are current health behavioral change models helpful in guiding prevention of weight gain efforts? *Obes Res* 2003;**11**(Suppl):23S—43S.

27. Sallis JF, Owen N, Fisher EB. Ecological models of health behavior. In: theory, research, practice Glanz K, Rimer BK, Viswanath K, editors. *Health behavior and health education*. San Francisco: Jossey-Bass; 2008. pp. 465—82.

28. Davison KK, Birch LL. Childhood overweight: a contextual model and recommendations for future research. *Obes Rev* 2001;**2**:159—71.

29. Livingstone MB, McCaffrey TA, Rennie KL. Childhood obesity prevention studies: lessons learned and to be learned. *Public Health Nutr* 2006;**9**:1121—9.

30. Huang TT, Glass TA. Transforming research strategies for understanding and preventing obesity. *JAMA* 2008;**300**:1811—13.

31. Swinburn B. Obesity prevention in children and adolescents. *Child Adolesc Psychiatric Clin N Am* 2008;**18**:209—23.

32. Economos CD, Brownson RC, DeAngelis MA, Novelli P, Foerster SB, Foreman CT, Gregson J, Kumanyika SK, Pate RR. What lessons have been learned from other attempts to guide social change? *Nutr Rev* 2001;**59**:S57—65. S40—56; discussion.

33. Hill JO, Peters JC. Environmental contributions to the obesity epidemic. *Science* 1998;**280**:1371—4.

34. Medicine IO. Communities. In: Koplan JP, Liverman CT, Kraak VI, Wisham SL, editors. *Progress in Preventing Childhood Obesity*. Washington, DC: The National Academies Press; 2007.

35. Stevens J, Taber DR, Murray DM, Ward DS. Advances and controversies in the design of obesity prevention trials. *Obesity (Silver Spring)* 2007;**15**:2163—70.

36. Medicine IO. *A framework for decision-making for obesity prevention: integrating action with evidence*; 2009.

37. Chatterji M. Alternative and trade-offs in generating and evaluating evidence: perspectives from education. In Workshop on Meeting the Challenges of Generating Useful Evidence and Using it Effectively in Obesity Prevention Decision-making, Washington, DC; January 8, 2009.

38. Nastasi BK, Hitchcock J. Challenges of evaluating multilevel interventions. *Am J Community Psychol* 2009;**43**:360—76.

39. Diez Roux AV. Multi-level approaches to understanding and preventing obesity: analytical challenges and new directions. In Workshop on the Application of Systems Thinking to the Development and Use of Evidence in Obesity Prevention Decision-Making Irving, CA; March 16, 2009.

40. Findholt N. Application of the Community Readiness Model for childhood obesity prevention. *Public Health Nurs* 2007;**24**:565—70.

41. Sallis JF, Story M, Lou D. Study designs and analytic strategies for environmental and policy research on obesity, physical activity, and diet: recommendations from a meeting of experts. *Am J Prev Med* 2009;**36**:S72—7.

42. Oakes JM, Kaufman JS. *Methods in Social Epidemiology*. San Francisco, CA: Jossey-Bass; 2006.

43. Swinburn B, Gill T, Kumanyika S. Obesity prevention: a proposed framework for translating evidence into action. *Obes Rev* 2005;**6**:23—33.

44. Marmot M. Social determinants of health: from observation to policy. *Med J Aust* 2000;**172**:379—82.

45. Community Intervention Trial for Smoking Cessation (COMMIT): summary of design and intervention. COMMIT Research Group. *J Natl Cancer Inst* 1991;**83**:1620—8.

46. Carleton RA, Lasater TM, Assaf AR, Feldman HA, McKinlay S. The Pawtucket Heart Health Program: community changes in cardiovascular risk factors and projected disease risk. *Am J Public Health* 1995;**85**:777—85.

47. DeMattia L, Denney S. Childhood Obesity Prevention: Successful Community-Based Efforts. Annals. *AAPSS* 2008;**615**:83.

48. Economos CD, Hyatt RR, Goldberg JP, Must A, Naumova EN, Collins JJ, Nelson ME. A community intervention reduces BMI z-score in children: Shape Up Somerville first year results. *Obesity (Silver Spring)* 2007;**15**:1325—36.

49. Farquhar JW, Fortmann SP, Flora JA, Taylor CB, Haskell WL, Williams PT, Maccoby N, Wood PD. Effects of communitywide education on cardiovascular disease risk factors. The Stanford Five-City Project. *JAMA* 1990;**264**:359—65.

50. Fortmann SP, Williams PT, Hulley SB, Haskell WL, Farquhar JW. Effect of health education on dietary behavior: the Stanford Three Community Study. *Am J Clin Nutr* 1981;**34**:2030—8.

51. Killen JD, Robinson TN, Telch MJ, Saylor KE, Maron DJ, Rich T, Bryson S. The Stanford Adolescent Heart Health Program. *Health Educ Q* 1989;**16**:263—83.

52. Zahuranec DB, Morgenstern LB, Garcia NM, Conley KM, Lisabeth LD, Rank GS, Smith MA, Meurer WJ, Resnicow K, Brown DL. Stroke Health and Risk Education (SHARE) Pilot Project. Feasibility and Need for Church-Based Stroke Health Promotion in a Bi-Ethnic Community. *Stroke; a journal of cerebral circulation* 2008;**39**(5):1583—5.

53. Puska P, Tuomilehto J, Nissinen A, Salonen JT, Vartiainen E, Pietinen P, Koskela K, Korhonen HJ. The North Karelia project: 15 years of community-based prevention of coronary heart disease. *Ann Med* 1989;**21**:169—73.

54. Stern MP, Farquhar JW, McCoby N, Russell SH. Results of a two-year health education campaign on dietary behavior. The Stanford Three Community Study. *Circulation* 1976;**54**:826—33.

55. Mittelmark MB, Luepker RV, Jacobs DR, Bracht NF, Carlaw RW, Crow RS, Finnegan J, Grimm RH, Jeffery RW, Kline FG, et al. Community-wide prevention of cardiovascular disease: education strategies of the Minnesota Heart Health Program. *Prev Med* 1986;**15**:1—17.

56. Hoehner CM, Soares J, Perez DP, Ribeiro IC, Joshu CE, Pratt M, Legetic BD, Malta DC, Matsudo VR, Ramos LR, Simoes EJ, Brownson RC. Physical activity interventions in Latin America: a systematic review. *Am J Prev Med* 2008;**34**:224—33.

57. Sanigorski AM, Bell AC, Kremer PJ, Cuttler R, Swinburn BA. Reducing unhealthy weight gain in children through community capacity-building: results of a quasi-experimental intervention program, Be Active Eat Well. *Int J Obes (Lond)* 2008;**32**:1060—7.

58. Romon M, Lommez A, Tafflet M, Basdevant A, Oppert JM, Bresson JL, Ducimetiere P, Charles MA, Borys JM. Downward trends in the prevalence of childhood overweight in the setting of 12-year school- and community-based programmes. *Public Health Nutr* 2009;**12**:1735−42.
59. Eisenmann JC, Gentile DA, Welk GJ, Callahan R, Strickland S, Walsh M, Walsh DA. SWITCH: rationale, design, and implementation of a community, school, and family-based intervention to modify behaviors related to childhood obesity. *BMC Public Health* 2008;**8**:223.
60. Filbert E, Chesser A, Hawley SR, St Romain T. Community-based participatory research in developing an obesity intervention in a rural county. *J Community Health Nurs* 2009;**26**: 35−43.
61. Minke SW, Smith C, Plotnikoff RC, Khalema E, Raine K. The evolution of integrated chronic disease prevention in Alberta, Canada. *Preventing Chronic Disease* 2006;**3**:1−12.
62. Margolis PA, Stevens R, Bordley WC, Stuart J, Harlan C, Keyes-Elstein L, Wisseh S. From concept to application: the impact of a community-wide intervention to improve the delivery of preventive services to children. *Pediatrics* 2001;**108**:E42.
63. Economos CD, Irish-Hauser S. Community interventions: a brief overview and their application to the obesity epidemic. *J Law Med Ethics* 2007;**35**:131−7.
64. Foresight. *Tackling Obesities: Future Choices—Project Report*. London: UK Government Office for Science; 2007.
65. Auchincloss AH, Diez Roux AV. A new tool for epidemiology: the usefulness of dynamic-agent models in understanding place effects on health. *Am J Epidemiol* 2008;**168**:1−8.
66. US Department of Health and Human Services, U.D. o. A. *Dietary Guidelines for Americans*. Washington, DC: U.S. Government Printing Office; 2005.
67. Medicine IO. *Preventing childhood obesity: health in the balance*. Washington, DC: The National Academies Press; 2005.

CHAPTER 30

School-Based Obesity-Prevention Programs

Genevieve Fridlund Dunton, Casey P. Durand, Nathaniel R. Riggs, Mary Ann Pentz

Department of Preventive Medicine, University of Southern California, Alhambra, CA, USA

INTRODUCTION

Overweight and obesity during childhood and adolescence increase the risk for a number of serious health conditions including cancer, type 2 diabetes, cholesterol levels, and cardiovascular complications [1, 2]. Despite global attention directed toward the problem, rates of overweight and risk of overweight among youth have risen to over 30% in many developed and developing countries [3–5]. Researchers, educators, and policy makers have taken steps to address concerns over these disturbing trends through the development and implementation of obesity-prevention programs and policies across a variety of settings. Schools have been identified as a particularly relevant context for obesity prevention because of the substantial amount of time that children spend in this setting and the opportunity to integrate physical activity and nutrition education into existing curricula.

Despite the potential schools have to substantially impact the development of healthy energy balance habits and to stem the progression of overweight and obesity in children, there is some question as to whether school-based obesity-prevention programs can effectively achieve these outcomes. This chapter provides a backdrop for the focus on school settings as a critical setting for obesity prevention; describes the types of strategies and approaches often used in school-based obesity-prevention programs; and summarizes the results of studies evaluating the effectiveness of school-based interventions to increase physical activity, decrease sedentary behavior, improve dietary habits, and reduce obesity risk. It also seeks to guide further research and discussion in this area by highlighting the conceptual gaps and methodological limitations of studies conducted to date and making recommendations for future evaluation and program/policy development.

THE SCHOOL AS A CRITICAL SETTING FOR OBESITY PREVENTION

Public health researchers have mobilized efforts to stem the tide of increasing rates of overweight and obesity in youth. To date, a number of contexts and settings have been targeted for the implementation of intervention strategies. For example, hospitals and clinics have been identified as playing an important role in the treatment of obesity in youth currently overweight [6]. Because many aspects of food intake, physical activity, and sedentary behavior involve behaviors learned from parents and reinforced by siblings, families have also been targeted to break the familial cycle of overweight and obesity [7]. Also targeted is the modification of unhealthy media portrayals of physical activity, sedentary behavior, and food intake, as well as social marketing campaigns aimed at increasing the perceived benefits of eating healthy and being physically active [8].

Schools have also been identified as a context critical in the development and prevention of youth obesity because of a number of structural and logistical advantages inherent to this environment [9]. First, schools contain large concentrations of students for extended periods of time, sometimes up to 6 hours per day for 180 days per year. With the exception of the family context, there is perhaps no other context or setting in which youth spend more time. Furthermore, the broad ethnic and socioeconomic representation in many schools allows school-based public health interventions to reach at-risk youth.

Second, children attend school during important periods in the development of overweight and obesity. Two childhood developmental periods have been identified as high-risk periods for both development of and potential intervention with obesity. The first is adiposity rebound in early childhood, approximately age 6 [10]. The second is late childhood/early adolescence, about age 10, when obesogenic trajectories defined as the temporal progression toward overweight and obesity rise sharply across both males and females and different ethnic groups [11]. These periods of risk for obesity strongly argue for the potential of elementary school-based obesity-prevention programs.

Third, schools typically have preexisting settings and procedures that can serve as logical mechanisms for the implementation of obesity prevention. Here, schools play an active role in the delivery of formal health and physical education (PE) curricula, which can serve as vehicles for intervention delivery. In addition, school-based obesity-prevention appears to have public support, with one national survey showing that 65% of parents support the sentiment that schools should play a major role in obesity-prevention efforts [12].

OVERVIEW OF SCHOOL-BASED INTERVENTION STRATEGIES

A recent increase in the number of school-based obesity-prevention programs has occurred in large part as a result of these potential advantages for intervention implementation. However, there is a great deal of heterogeneity among the types of school-based obesity-prevention interventions in terms of approach. Fortunately, a growing number of review articles and meta-analyses have assisted in the organization of trends and patterns in obesity-prevention program structure and function. Yet even among these reviews, there is considerable variability in study focus.

Despite differences among school-based obesity programs, some common dimensions of program variation can be identified. One dimension is the behavior that is being targeted as a potential mediating mechanism for ultimate reduction in youth overweight and obesity. Typically, obesity-prevention programs aim to address some combination of enhanced physical activity, decreased sedentary behavior, or improved dietary intake. An appraisal of current review and meta-analytic articles suggests that school-based obesity interventions often target more than one of these behaviors thought to influence overweight and obesity. For example, Zenzen and Kridli's [13] review demonstrated that 14 of 16 interventions included both a healthy lifestyle education content and physical activity component, with only two implementing healthy lifestyle education only. Similarly, Kropski and colleagues' [14] review of universal, experimental, or quasi-experimental school-based obesity-prevention programs found that of 14 programs that met their inclusion criteria, 11 contained both nutritional and physical activity components. Finally, Peterson and Fox [15] found that 70% of studies that fit their review criteria contained a dual focus on physical activity and nutrition.

A second dimension upon which programs can vary is the type of program (e.g., curriculum/educational, environmental, policy, family, or multicomponent). Naylor and McKay's [16] review of school-based physical activity promotion programs found that these interventions typically fell into four main categories: educational, environmental, policy changes, and multicomponent or what they termed "whole school" approaches. Table 30.1 shows a variety of intervention approaches, and components that fall within each category. Among these approaches, curriculum-based educational interventions, with classroom or PE instructors teaching the lessons, are commonly used [15]. Curriculum-based programs tend to focus on the intra-individual cognitive contributors to these behaviors including children's knowledge and attitudes toward behavioral mediators of obesity [17–21]. For example, Argon and colleagues [17] trained 10th graders in basic nutrition and physical activity knowledge and attitudes over a 9-week period, and Muller and colleagues' [19] intervention employed nutritionists and teachers to promote knowledge of benefits of being physically active, eating more fruit and vegetables, and decreasing intake of high-fat foods. Less often addressed are curriculum-based skill development programs that promote health behaviors such as affect regulation and self-control [22]. Notable exceptions include Project SPARK [23], which includes both self-regulation and direct physical activity curricula, and the Pathways to Health program that focuses in large part on the promotion of affective self-regulation skills related to food intake and physical activity [24].

Recently, environmental and policy changes at the school level have been suggested as a critical measure to address childhood obesity [25]. Common environmental approaches to obesity-prevention are playground and neighborhood improvements. For example, Safe Routes to School (SR2S) programs mobilize community leaders, schools, and parents to improve neighborhood safety and encourage children to safely walk and bicycle to school [26]. Such strategies are predicated on the argument that even small pedestrian or bicycle facility improvements, if strategic, may increase the propensity of children to walk or bicycle to school. School-based obesity-prevention policies, on the other hand, can be

TABLE 30.1 Types of School-Based Obesity-Prevention Strategies

CURRICULUM

1. Stand-alone nutrition and physical activity classroom-based curriculum
2. Integration of nutrition and physical activity concepts into existing curricula (e.g., home economics, biology, mathematics)
3. Required or modified physical education
4. Peer-led education, peer mentoring, student-led seminars on nutrition and physical activity
5. Cooking classes
6. Inclusion of nutrition education and physical activity into after-school programs
7. Offer intramural and intrascholastic sports programs
8. Offering noncompetitive activities during physical education or after school (e.g., dance, yoga)
9. Computer and video game-based programs to promote physical activity and healthy eating

PARENT/FAMILY

1. Postcards/newsletters with nutrition and physical activity information sent to parents
2. Parent night with family-based nutrition and physical activity educational sessions

SCHOOL ENVIRONMENT/POLICY

1. Safe routes for walking and biking to school
2. School facilities made available for physical activity outside of school hours
3. Modification to playgrounds, playing fields, equipment on school grounds
4. Fruit carts or farmers' markets
5. Short (5- to 10-minute) activity breaks integrated throughout the school day
6. Structured, longer, more frequent recess
7. School garden
8. Health fairs
9. Taste-testing of novel fruits and vegetables
10. Healthy snack breaks
11. Healthy eating zones (free of fast food) in neighborhood surrounding schools
12. Improved nutritional content of school lunch and breakfast
13. Reduced access to vending machines with sugar-sweetened beverages and high fat/sugar snacks
14. Prohibition of in-school advertising of restaurants or brands that sell high-fat/sugar foods
15. Annual assessments of student height and weight by school health personnel
16. School site health promotion for faculty and staff
17. Restrictions on high-sugar/fat food served at school parties
18. Pedometer distribution with related games and activities
19. School fundraising to consist of group walks/runs and sale of healthy foods

categorized into one of three domains [27]. The first area involves nutrition guidelines, which are those policies that guide standards for menu planning applied to school meal programs or other meals sold at schools. The second domain includes regulations of food or beverage availability, which limit access to unhealthy foods by controlling the type of food and beverages sold or otherwise provided at schools. The third area consists of price intervention policies, which target free or subsidized foods or control the price of foods and beverages sold to students. The challenge with assessing the role of policy change in school-based obesity prevention is that changes in policy can be targeted directly at schools or at any number of state or federal levels, which may indirectly influence schools.

School-based obesity-prevention programs can also exercise a multicomponent approach. For example, because parental involvement in intervention is critical to achieving long-term healthy developmental benefits [28], the Pathways to Health Program combines a school-based curriculum with a Parent Skills Night that focuses on activities targeting healthy parent-child communication, rules, and expectations related to food intake and physical activity. Similarly, the Coordinated Approach to Child Health (CATCH) program used a three-pronged approach—physical activity intervention, family involvement, and school food service intervention [29].

THEORETICAL FOUNDATIONS TO SCHOOL-BASED OBESITY-PREVENTION PROGRAMS

Because it appears that schools are a logical context for obesity-prevention programs, it is important that these programs be grounded in established health, developmental, educational, and intervention theory. Having a strong theoretical foundation is important for two reasons. The first is that theory helps to guide the content and strategies to be used in interventions. The second is that theory, along with theoretically informed evaluation, assists in the understanding of the mediating mechanisms through which interventions work to prevent obesity. The application of theory to obesity intervention, however, is not universally applied [13]. Thus, it is often difficult to determine how theory informs many interventions [30]. A review of obesity preventive interventions indicated that the most prevalent theories on which programs are based are social learning theories [31, 32] (including social cognitive theory), which attempt to modify the reciprocal relationship between youth behavior and the environment. In Zenzen and Kridli's [13] review of school-based obesity-prevention programs, half of the 8 studies out of a total of 16, utilized social cognitive theory. Other less frequently used theories include theories of reasoned action or planned behavior that address attitudes, subjective norms, and perceived power in affecting health outcomes [33]; the transtheoretical model, which attempts to move participants through the stages of health behavior change [34]; and theories

TABLE 30.2 Summary of Review Articles on Effectiveness of School-Based Interventions on Physical Activity Outcomes

	Curriculum	Parent/family	School environment/policy	Combined
Kropski et al. [14]	1/1 (100%)	—	—	6/6 (100%)
Peterson et al. [15]	1/1 (100%)	—	—	2/3 (67%)
Sharma et al. [55]	4/5 (80%)	—	—	1/2 (50%)
Sharma et al. [80]	3/4 (75%)	—	1/1 (100%)	3/5 (60%)
Summerbell et al. [61]	3/3 (100%)	—	—	1/5 (20%)
Van Sluijs et al. [39]	5/36 (14%)	—	2/5 (40%)	6/16 (38%)
Average percentage	**34%**	—	**50%**	**51%**

Ratios (and percentages) indicate the number of studies with a statistically significant finding in the expected direction divided by the total number of studies in that category included in the review paper. The average percentage represents the mean of the weighted individual percentages across all of the review papers. Weights were assigned according to the total number of studies within each review paper for that category.

TABLE 30.3 Summary of Review Articles on Effectiveness of School-Based Intervention on Dietary Intake

	Curriculum	Parent/family	School environment/policy	Combined
de Sa et al. [49]	7/8 (88%)	—	3/3 (100%)	10/12 (83%)
Jaime et al. [27]	—	—	11/13 (85%)	8/10 (80%)
Kropski et al. [14]	4/4 (100%)	—	—	3/3 (100%)
Peterson et al. [15]	2/2 (100%)	—	—	1/4 (25%)
Sharma et al. [55]	4/5 (80%)	—	—	1/1 (100%)
Sharma et al. [80]	3/3 (100%)	—	3/3 (100%)	1/1 (100%)
Summerbell et al. [61]	2/3 (67%)	—	—	2/4 (50%)
Average percentage	**88%**	—	**89%**	**74%**

Ratios (and percentages) indicate the number of studies with a statistically significant finding in the expected direction divided by the total number of studies in that category included in the review paper. The average percentage represents the mean of the weighted individual percentages across all of the review papers. Weights were assigned according to the total number of studies within each review paper for that category.

that address the role of emotion as it relates to impulse control, affect regulation, or healthy planning and goal setting [24, 30, 35].

EFFECTIVENESS OF SCHOOL-BASED OBESITY-PREVENTION PROGRAMS

At this time, there is not a coherent understanding of precisely what works in school-based childhood obesity-prevention efforts. Though the number of studies published on this topic seems to increase exponentially every year, public health research has not been able to pinpoint particular strategies and intervention components that are truly effective across a variety of populations. To better understand what the current evidence shows on this topic, we have synthesized a number of current review papers on school-based interventions to modify physical activity, diet, and body composition. For each review article, we examined the total number of individual studies targeting each outcome and the percentage of those studies that were effective (i.e., found significant results in the expected direction). We then calculated an average percentage that represents the mean of the weighted individual percentages across all of the review papers. Weights were assigned according to the total number of studies within each review paper for that category. To aid in understanding, we stratified these results by the type of intervention strategy used (i.e., curriculum, parent or family, school environment and policy, and combined) (Tables 30.2 through 30.4).

Physical Activity

Table 30.2 shows that the majority of studies targeting physical activity used a curriculum (50 studies) or combined intervention (37 studies) approach. In contrast, relatively few studies used an environment or policy approach alone to change physical activity, and none used parent or family-only methods.

TABLE 30.4 Summary of Review Articles on the Effectiveness of School-Based Intervention on Body Composition Outcomes

	Curriculum	Parent/family	School environment/policy	Combined
Baranowski et al. [30]	7/20 (35%)	—	—	—
Brown et al. [49]	7/20 (35%)	—	1/1 (100%)	9/17 (53%)
Budd et al. [50]	3/6 (50%)	—	—	1/6 (17%)
Harris et al. [81]	4/9 (44%)	—	—	2/6 (33%)
Kropski et al. [14]	2/6 (33%)	—	0/1 (0%)	3/6 (50%)
Li et al. [82]	8/11 (73%)	—	—	8/11 (73%)
Peterson et al. [15]	1/4 (25%)	—	—	3/6 (50%)
Sharma et al. [55]	4/6 (67%)	—	—	1/2 (50%)
Sharma et al. [80]	2/6 (33%)	—	—	4/5 (80%)
Story et al. [83]	7/7 (100%)	0/1 (0%)	—	4/4 (100%)
Summerbell et al. [61]	3/9 (33%)	—	—	1/6 (17%)
Average percentage	**41%**	**0%**	**50%**	**53%**

Ratios (and percentages) indicate the number of studies with a statistically significant finding in the expected direction divided by the total number of studies in that category included in the review paper. The average percentage represents the mean of the weighted individual percentages across all of the review papers. Weights were assigned according to the total number of studies within each review paper for that category.

Approximately 34% of curriculum-only interventions resulted in either an increase in physical activity or a decrease in sedentary time among children. Effective curricula included those that focused on reducing screen time (television, video games, and computers) through classroom lessons, and others that aimed to increase physical activity through lessons on self-management behavior and skill building [23, 36]. Combined interventions show somewhat stronger effects than curriculum-only approaches, with 51% of studies finding results in the expected direction. Most of these combined programs included curriculum and either a parent component or school policy change. The parent-focused elements included such strategies as take-home activity packets and parent information sessions [29, 37]. The school environment and policy component usually involved an increase in the number of required PE classes or the incorporation of more vigorous levels of activity into existing PE classes [38, 39]. Despite the fact that three of six studies found school environment and policy change alone to be effective, it may be best to withhold judgment on this approach until a stronger evidence base is built.

Dietary Intake

A total of 79 school-based obesity-prevention studies measured dietary intake, making it the least measured of the three outcomes (see Table 30.3). Although numerous programs have elements that target diet and eating behavior, not all measure dietary change as an intervention outcome. Nonetheless, we can begin to make some initial inferences about what program strategies are particularly effective. Unlike with physical activity, there is a more even split of studies using curriculum (25 studies), school environment and policy (19 studies), and combined (35 studies) interventions. There are no studies that are parent focused only. Of the curriculum-focused studies, 88% showed significant results in the expected direction. These programs used educational components such as games, tasting opportunities to increase preference for fruit, integration of nutrition education with the standard science curriculum, and positive messages about the benefits of a healthy diet [36, 40, 41]. With an equivalent level of effectiveness, 89% of school environment and policy-only programs successfully improved dietary intake. These programs generally took the form of school food service interventions, including price reductions for healthier foods, decreased sugar-sweetened beverage availability, or wholesale changes to cafeteria offerings (e.g., lower fat and sodium and higher fiber content offerings) [42–44]. A somewhat lower percentage of combined interventions (74%) had a positive effect on diet as compared to the curriculum- and environment-only programs. Similar to the combined physical activity interventions, most of these programs included a classroom education component, along with a parent component or an environment or policy change. Parent components consisted of activities such as involvement with the child's food-related homework and family fun nights [45, 46]. Environment and policy changes consisted of the previously listed food service interventions as well as other methods, such as point-of-purchase education and increased availability of fruits and vegetables [47, 48].

Body Composition

The majority of studies targeted body composition (e.g., body mass index [BMI], body weight, skinfolds), and thus the largest amount of evidence is available for this outcome (see Table 30.4). Curriculum-based programs were the most frequent (104 studies), followed by combined interventions (69 studies), school environment and policy only (2 studies), and parent or family only (1 study). For curriculum-based studies, approximately 41% of the programs were found to be effective. A larger percentage of combined interventions (53%) found significant results in the expected direction with respect to BMI. Both of these percentages are similar to what was found for physical activity, but they were substantially lower than results for diet-focused interventions. Only one study took a parent-only approach to modifying body composition, and two studies used school environment or policy-only strategies. As a result of the low numbers, it is not possible to draw conclusions about the effectiveness of these strategies. Studies focusing on body composition outcomes used intervention strategies similar to those previously described. Curriculum components included skill building and educational handouts or worksheets; parent involvement used newsletters, homework, and education nights; school environment and policy involved changes to food service and physical activity requirements; and combined interventions utilized multiple elements.

Summary of Effectiveness Studies

Results indicate that among school-based obesity-prevention programs, multicomponent interventions appear to be the most effective, especially in terms of their impact on physical activity and body composition. These programs work by combining at least two of the following approaches: curriculum, family or parent involvement, or modification to the school environment or policy. Curriculum-only programs have also proven to be effective, particularly for diet-focused interventions. Currently, there is insufficient evidence to make conclusions about the effectiveness of family or environment-only interventions to prevent obesity in the school setting. We note that this synthesis is not intended to be a comprehensive review of reviews. Rather, it is intended to assist the reader in understanding which school-based intervention strategies show the most potential for successfully modifying physical activity, dietary intake, and body composition.

FACTORS THAT MAY INFLUENCE THE EFFECTIVENESS OF SCHOOL-BASED PROGRAMS

Evidence suggests that interventions to halt the progression of overweight and obesity in the school setting may not be universally effective. Instead, the success of the program may depend on a variety of student, programmatic, and institutional characteristics. An area that has received attention is whether certain types of programs or intervention strategies may be more effective for younger as compared to older children. Two recently published reviews suggest that interventions aiming to increase physical activity or reduce sedentary behavior may be particularly successful in younger children [49, 50], although one review concluded the opposite—that there was more evidence for an effect of physical activity interventions among adolescents than among children [39]. Older children are also thought to be more responsive to curriculum interventions delivered through classroom instruction because they have the necessary cognitive competencies to develop the planning and problem-solving skills used in intentional health-behavior change [14, 50]. Research further indicates that multicomponent programs involving a combination of classroom-based, environmental/policy, and family may be more effective for the children in higher grades who may have more choice over their own behavior in and outside of the school setting [50]. There is some evidence to suggest that school-programs targeting younger children are generally not effective in terms of reducing BMI or obesity prevalence [14]. It is possible that the effects of obesity-prevention interventions on body composition are attenuated during the developmental period before adiposity rebound in childhood [51]. Taken together, these studies suggest that school-based obesity-prevention programs should take different strategies depending on the age of the students being targeted. However, further research is necessary before we understand which approaches are the most effective with each age group.

Another factor that has been considered as a potential point of divergence for the effectiveness of school-based obesity-prevention studies is gender. A small body of research has observed differential results for boys as compared to girls. These studies suggest that girls versus boys or vice versa are more responsive to certain types of intervention strategies or that the size of intervention effects on particular outcomes differs by gender. For example, in a review, Kropski and colleagues [14] concluded that school-based obesity-prevention interventions grounded in social learning theory such as Planet Health [36] appear to be more successful among girls than boys. Also, short-term changes in dietary intake as a result of school-based obesity-prevention programs were more prominent in girls as opposed to boys [52]. In contrast, the review conducted by Kropski and colleagues [14] found that boys may be more responsive to structural and environmental interventions in the school setting to promote physical activity. Overall, a general pattern suggesting that curriculum- and instruction-based interventions are more effective for changing behavior among girls whereas programs aiming to modify features of the school grounds and policies are more successful in boys has been identified. Additional research studies are needed to replicate these findings across a wider range of population subgroups and settings. Taken together, these initial findings indicate that researchers and educators should consider utilizing different intervention strategies for boys as compared to girls in order to successfully impact obesity.

Emerging evidence suggests that the effectiveness of school-based obesity-prevention interventions may also partially depend on the socioeconomic resources of the target population. Several review studies have found that children from moderate to high socioeconomic backgrounds benefit more from obesity-prevention programs delivered in the school setting than children from less well-off families [39, 52, 53]. For example, a school-based program targeting body weight found a reduced cumulative 4-year incidence of overweight only in children from families with high socioeconomic status [54]. Also, children from intact families appear to respond more favorably to school-based obesity-prevention strategies than those with divorced or single parents [52]. Although explanations for these findings have not necessarily been tested empirically, it is likely that children from families with greater socioeconomic resources have more opportunities for reinforcement and follow-through of intervention concepts at home. For instance, higher-income families may have greater access to or are better able to purchase fresh fruits and vegetables, whole grains, and low-fat foods that are promoted in the nutritional curriculum completed by their children. Furthermore, families with greater economic resources or two-parent households may have more discretionary time for the extension of physical activity outside of the school day.

INTERNATIONAL PERSPECTIVES ON SCHOOL-BASED OBESITY PREVENTION

School-based obesity-prevention programs conducted internationally share many of the same characteristics as programs offered in the United States. A review paper summarizes findings from published evaluations of interventions taking place in Europe, Canada, Singapore, Australia, and New Zealand [55]. According to this review, a large number of international programs aim to change both physical activity and dietary intake. Also, similar to U.S. studies, most programs utilize existing teachers to deliver the intervention. Programs that incorporate parental involvement appear to be particularly successful in international settings. Greater parental influence on children's nutritional and physical activity habits in other countries underscores the importance of family participation in school-based programs conducted internationally. A notable difference between programs conducted outside as compared to within the United States is the lack of international interventions with an environmental or policy focus [55]. Few international school-based interventions have a clear theoretical basis, which is also dissimilar from U.S. programs. Overall, there is a lack of evidence on the success of school-based obesity-prevention programs in developing and underdeveloped countries [46]. The research available is largely limited to developed countries in North America, Europe, and Australia. Whether and which types of school-based strategies to increase physical activity, improve diet, or decrease or maintain BMI conducted in underdeveloped and developing countries are effective is an important and unanswered question.

GAPS IN RESEARCH ON SCHOOL-BASED OBESITY-PREVENTION INTERVENTIONS

Despite the sizable body of research studies evaluating the effectiveness of obesity-prevention programs delivered in the school setting, a number of areas remain understudied. Empirical evidence evaluating policy approaches to prevent obesity in the school environment is severely lacking. A number of policies have been proposed in recent years such as the regulation of the sale of sugar-sweetened beverages in schools [56], oversight of school breakfast and lunch menu content [57], and physical education requirements [58]. For example, sugar-sweetened beverage regulations in schools may include content restrictions (e.g., added sweeteners, percentage juice), portion restrictions (e.g., size of container [8–12 oz]), ratio rules (e.g., < 66 calories per ounce for sports drinks and light juices), time and event requirements (e.g., meal times, entire school day, parties), age or grade requirements (e.g., elementary allowed water, milk, 100% juice only), marketing provisions (e.g., honoring existing beverage contracts, marketing), and access to water provisions [56]. However, few of these policies have been systematically evaluated to determine the extent to which they have been successfully implemented and are effective at reducing obesity risk.

Another area that has received less research attention is the evaluation of school space and microenvironmental interventions. Programs that redesign the architecture of indoor and outdoor spaces within school grounds to promote physical activity and healthy eating have not been extensively studied. These interventions include the provision of weather-protected spaces (porches, overhangs, covered courts) to encourage activity during unfavorable weather, walking or nature trails, outdoor auditoriums, signage and instructions to educate children on how to use activity equipment, school gardening programs, standing desks and activity ball chairs, improvements to stairwells to promote use, and commercial teaching kitchens [59]. Studies are needed to understand whether these and other modifications to school microenvironments can have a substantial impact on obesity.

RESEARCH LIMITATIONS OF SCHOOL-BASED OBESITY-PREVENTION STUDIES

Many of the inconsistencies in the results of effectiveness studies could be resolved through improvements in the design and methodology of school-based obesity-prevention evaluation studies. In particular, concern has been raised about the lack of information provided about how programs were developed and initially tested [60]. Findings from formative research and pilot studies should be reported as stand-alone papers or incorporated into outcome evaluation articles. Published studies also often inadequately describe or fail to report altogether the theoretical underpinnings of obesity-prevention programs. Greater effort should be made to explain how intervention components map into theoretical constructs. Furthermore, the design of evaluation studies could be improved to reduce threats to internal validity. Common design weaknesses include a lack of randomization, the failure to include an attention-equivalent control group, and post-only assessments.

Other methodological limitations include inadequate power analyses that leave studies without the statistical power to detect significant group differences [49, 50] and unit of analysis problems (i.e., randomization in conducted at the classroom level and analyses are done at the individual level) [50, 61]. Evaluation studies of school-based obesity-prevention programs also lack sufficient process data, staff/teacher training, program delivery and implementation, and fidelity to the intervention design [27, 49]. For example, studies rarely assess student, teacher, or parent level of engagement or satisfaction with the program [49]. The quality of and lack of comparability among outcome measures has also been criticized [46, 49, 61, 62]. Studies often rely on self-report of height, weight, and physical activity instead of using more reliable and valid measures such as skinfold assessments, scales, stadiometers, and accelerometers. Another concern is that measuring behaviors and body composition informs control group participants of the study objectives, resulting in possible demand characteristics and unintended behavior change [50, 61]. Similar to other areas of research, the evaluation of school-based obesity-prevention programs most likely suffers from a file drawer problem. Statistically insignificant results are either not reported within published studies or rejected from publication altogether, which would lead to an overestimation of the overall effectiveness.

Several other methodological limitations should be addressed in future studies to improve the quality of research findings. There is widespread concern that obesity-prevention programs implemented in schools are not of a sufficient length or intensity to produce a change in body weight or BMI [27, 49, 50, 61]. Although behavioral changes may be evident after a few months, interventions should last over a year or more in order to significantly impact body composition in children. Along a similar line, few studies have a sufficient follow-up time period to determine whether initial changes can be maintained after the program has ended [27, 60]. Research examining factors that predict successful dissemination and diffusion of school-based obesity-prevention studies at the population level are also lacking. Another problem is that intervention studies often target homogeneous groups who are fairly healthy and well educated [61]. The effect of culture and risk level on the effectiveness of programs is rarely considered [60]. Lastly, the overall effectiveness of school-based obesity-prevention programs could be better assessed through the generation of cost-efficacy data. A cost-benefit analysis of Planet Health demonstrated modest results. At an intervention cost of $33,677 or $14 per student per year, the program would prevent an estimated 1.9% of the female students from becoming overweight adults. As a result, this translated to an estimated cost saving of $534 per case of adulthood overweight prevented [63]. Further research evaluating the costs of school-based interventions in comparison to their direct health benefits would help to inform school administrators and policy makers about which programs should be selected for implementation.

SUMMARY AND FUTURE DIRECTIONS

This chapter has thus far focused on reviewing the types and effectiveness of school-based programs for childhood obesity prevention and the limitations of studies that evaluate these programs. Reviews of studies indicate that school programs vary widely in terms of focus on eating or physical activity (or both), theoretical base, and inclusion of policy or environmental change as part of intervention [13, 61, 64]. On balance, school-based programs appear to have some mixed effects on obesity risk factors related to eating or physical activity [13, 61]. However, the reported effectiveness of programs varies widely across individual reviews, with some reviews concluding that school-based programs yield no effects on "hard" indicators of obesity risk such as BMI, and others concluding that school-based programs produce changes in obesity prevalence or weight [66, 67]. The variable conclusions about effectiveness may be related to differences and limitations across studies in terms of measures or outcomes used, unit of assignment and analysis, theory, and program length, among other factors [67]. The last part of this chapter frames these variations in terms of barriers to effective school-based obesity prevention, assuming that school-based obesity-prevention programs are or could be more effective if certain conditions for program delivery are met. Finally, recommendations for future obesity-prevention programs and studies of effectiveness are discussed.

Barriers to Effective Program Delivery

At least four classes of factors pose barriers to achieving more effective school-based prevention programs. These consist of individual, programmatic, policy, and environmental factors. *Individual*-level barriers include sensitivity about weight for those youth who are overweight or obese compared to their peers, and a lack of attention to individual differences in patterns of eating and activity [67]. This issue constitutes a barrier to youth (and their parents) who might not want to be measured or drawn attention to relative to peers. Unlike the field of drug abuse prevention, for example, in which drug use is illegal and thus to be prohibited by all youth, eating and physical activity are normal functions in which all youth engage. A child who is obese relative to peers might perceive herself as abnormal. The second individual-level barrier is a lack of tailoring of programs to idiographic patterns of eating and activity. For example, recent work using population-based samples of fourth-grade children shows four patterns of energy intake and expenditure: (1) moderate eating and physical activity, with some sedentary behavior; (2) low food intake and low physical activity; (3) high junk food and sugar intake and high sedentary behavior; and (4) high fruit and vegetable intake and high physical activity [68]. Furthermore, others have shown that obesogenic trajectories differ among children [69]. Yet most school-based programs necessarily take a universal prevention approach (i.e., "one size fits all") because of time constraints for program delivery, the added complexity of delivering four or more program variations, and a concern about negative labeling of some subgroups that are defined by their pattern of eating and activity.

Programmatic barriers largely revolve around the keen competition for time, resources, and educational requirements that teachers and administrators face each day in school. First, there are no educational requirements that specifically target obesity prevention [70]. The closest requirement would be health education under which nutrition and physical health might fall. Although there are both federal and state health education standards that encompass kindergarten through 12th grade, there are no clear guidelines as to where obesity prevention fits or in which grade(s). Faced with a clear math requirement to meet within the limited hours of a school day, for example, teachers might opt out of delivery of an obesity-prevention program. Second, there are no funds available to schools for teaching obesity prevention. Previous research on evidence-based drug and tobacco use prevention programs suggests that it was only after schools received specific funding for these programs from the Drug Free Schools and Communities Act did they use them [71]. This example argues strongly for the development of policies that set aside specific funds for obesity prevention. Finally, there are not yet evidence-based programs for obesity prevention or national registries of programs that consistently show effects on reducing obesity risk [3, 69–72]. The lack of evidence-based programs makes it difficult for a curriculum coordinator—whose job it is to select a program for a school district—to make informed decisions about obesity prevention.

There are also *policy* barriers. One is that the selection of foods available in school cafeterias and vending machines are often dependent on economic considerations, convenience, and commercial marketing rather than student health considerations [65, 71]. Most of these selections are not healthy foods, and the movement toward school policies to restrict high sugar/high fat foods has been slow. Furthermore, the ready availability of these foods counteracts the beneficial effects that could be derived from an obesity-prevention program focusing on healthy food choices. A similar barrier occurs for physical activity. Current federal guidelines recommend that children participate in 60 minutes of physical activity per day. Yet increasingly, schools have cut back on recess and physical education time because of pressures to improve student academic performance, and with rare exception, no formal policies exist for set aside physical activity in a school regardless of number of minutes. Other policy-related barriers include a lack of awareness by teachers, students, and parents of school guidelines for eating and physical activity, a lack of consequences to the school for violating guidelines or policies, and a lack of coordination of eating and physical activity efforts within the school.

Finally, there are barriers that could be considered *environmental*. One is the immediate environment surrounding the school, such as parks, convenience stores, fast-food outlets, and vendor carts, all of which represent the impact of community on child obesity risk [13, 65]. Tobacco-prevention studies have shown that activism oriented toward prohibiting local store sales to minors has had some prevention effect on students. No such activism exists yet for providing more healthy food and physical activity choices for students, nor for community policies that could align with and support school obesity-prevention programs [73]. A second is the home environment. Students learning skills and benchmarks for healthy food choices and exercise will not get the opportunity to practice these skills if healthy choices are not offered at home or if parents are not also engaged in the school program, for example, through homework activities. Finally, media constitutes an environmental barrier. The ready availability of television and video games at home invite sedentary behavior, which could directly counteract the effects of a physical activity program offered in school. Local and national media promoting inexpensive high-fat foods at fast-food outlets would compete with nutrition programs at school.

Programmatic, Policy, and Research Recommendations

The barriers just summarized are likely to continue until such time that sound policies are in place to recognize and institutionalize evidence-based school programs for obesity prevention [73]. Nevertheless, several recommendations can be followed now. These recommendations can be grouped into sets representing educational, community, and marketing domains. The first set of recommendations involves the *educational* enterprise. One is that national and state departments of education start the process of infusing obesity prevention into health education objectives and curricula at each grade level from K through 12 so that they become part of normative education. This process involves both intervention mapping and curriculum integration, strategies that are already used widely in education [69, 71]. A second is to begin implementing school-based programs that are most efficient and most likely to yield positive outcomes based on social behavioral considerations. For example, schools may have to directly address changing social norms for weight acceptability before obesity-prevention programs will be widely supported by parents, teachers, and administration [74]. One possible benchmark to consider is based on diffusion of innovation theory as well as social normative theory: once obesity rates rise above a certain threshold, they may produce their own forward motion unless intervened upon [72].

The second set of recommendations involves the broadening of school-based interventions to include *community* and other intervention components that represent additional influences on child obesity. One is to treat school-based programs as one of several program components, along with community organization, media programming, parent programs, and local policy changes that support obesity prevention [66, 75]. Another is to coordinate school programs with other health-related school enterprises—for example, integrating a school program with BMI measurement and clinical counseling in school-based health centers—and with physical fitness tests in physical education classes [73, 76]. A third is to reexamine the concept of how schools might function more as health-promoting centers in the community rather than providing limited teaching of health education [77].

The third set of recommendations addresses *marketing and policy* change. On a macrolevel, the more the public pays attention to mass media messages about rising and nondiscriminating rates of child obesity, the greater the likelihood that federal and state departments of education will allocate per capita funds for obesity prevention as part of obesity policy [71]. On a more microlevel, teachers, administrators, and parents could be familiarized with research showing how student wakefulness, attention, and academic achievement in school could improve with better nutrition and exercise [78, 79].

Several of these recommendations naturally generate opportunities for future research. One opportunity is to evaluate whether current school policies—as they are in short supply—are effective relative to curriculum-based programs. For example, although 13 states require measurement of BMI in schools, little is known about whether this legislation is effective relative to a curriculum-based program or whether it is implemented with fidelity [67]. Similarly, little is known about whether school policy is more or less effective than environmental change or which types of school policies are most effective [65]. There is little research on how school-based programs should be sequenced to take advantage of child development of obesity risk factors, for example, which combination of physical activity and eating behaviors and in which order should be addressed. Finally, little is known about different patterns of eating and physical activity and different trajectories of obesity among children that could inform the development of more tailored prevention programs than are currently available in schools.

CONCLUSION

The aims of this chapter were to provide an overview of school-based obesity-prevention strategies in the United States and other countries, summarize the results of program effectiveness research, and offer recommendations for future work in this domain. Overall, school-based programs most frequently used curriculum-only strategies. However, combination intervention approaches—which incorporated multiple aspects of curriculum, family-parent involvement, and policy and environmental components—were the most effective at changing physical activity and body composition. Program success varied according to the gender, age, and socioeconomic resources of students. Generally speaking, limitations in the research design and methodology of evaluation studies hampered the ability to make broad conclusions about program effectiveness. Information is also lacking about the implementation and outcomes of school-based obesity-prevention programs in developing countries, policy interventions, and school microenvironmental modifications. The effective delivery of school-based obesity-prevention interventions faces various programmatic and institutional barriers that are inherent to educational systems. However, success may be achievable through strategies that integrate obesity prevention into existing curriculum, change school social norms, build educator and community support, and raise overall awareness of the benefits improved nutrition and physical activity can provide.

References

1. Strong WB, Malina RM, Blimkie CJ, Daniels SR, Dishman RK, Gutin B, Hergenroeder AC, Must A, Nixon PA, Pivarnik JM, Rowland T, Trost S, Trudeau F. Evidence based physical activity for school-age youth. *J Pediatr* 2005;**146**:732–7.
2. Dietz WH. Health consequences of obesity in youth: childhood predictors of adult disease. *Pediatrics* 1998;**101**:518–25.
3. Ogden CL, Carroll MD, Flegal KM. High body mass index for age among US children and adolescents, 2003–2006. *JAMA* 2008;**299**:2401–5.
4. Troiano RP, Flegal KM, Kuczmarski RJ, Campbell SM, Johnson CL. Overweight prevalence and trends for children and adolescents. The National Health and Nutrition Examination Surveys, 1963 to 1991. *Arch Pediatr Adolesc Med* 1995;**149**:1085–91.
5. WHO Consultation on Obesity. "Obesity: preventing and managing the global epidemic." WHO technical report series 894. Geneva, Switzerland; 1999.
6. National Institutes of Health, National Heart, Lung, and Blood Institute. Clinical guidelines on the identification, evaluation, and treatment of overweight and obesity in adults: the Evidence Report. *Obes Res* 1998;**6**:64–82.
7. White MA, Martin PD, Newton RL, Walden HM, York-Crowe EE, Gordon ST, Ryan DH, Williamson DA. Mediators of weight loss in a family based intervention presented over the internet. *Obes Res* 2004;**12**:1050–9.
8. Wardle J, Rapoport L, Miles A, Afaupe T, Duman M. Mass education for obesity prevention: the penetration of the BBC's Fighting Fat, Fighting fit campaign. *Health Educ Res* 2001;**16**:343–55.
9. St. Leger LH, Kolbe L, Lee A. School health promotion: achievements, challenge and priorities. In: McQueen DV, Jones CM, editors. *"Global perspectives on health promotion effectiveness"*. New York: Springer Science; 2007.
10. Dietz WH, Gortmaker SL. Preventing obesity in children and adolescents. *Annu Rev Public Health* 2001;**22**:337–53.
11. Berhane K, Gauderman WJ, Stram DO, Thomas DC. Statistical issues in studies of the long term effects of air pollution: The Southern California Children Health Study. *Statistical Science* 2004;**19**:414–49.
12. Lake Snell Perry & Associates, http://www.healthinschools.org/Publications-and-Resources/Polls-and-Surveys/Public-Opinion-Polls/Parents-Speak-Out-on-Health-and-Health-Care-in-Schools.aspx; 2003. Accessed at On Nov. 13 2009.
13. Zenzen W, Kridli S. Integrative review of school-based childhood obesity prevention programs. *J Pediatr Health Care* 2008;**23**:242–58.
14. Kropski JA, Heckley PH, Jensen G. School-based obesity prevention programs: an evidence based review. *Obes Rev.* 2008;**16**:1009–18.
15. Peterson KE, Fox MK. Addressing the epidemic of childhood obesity through school-based interventions: what has been done and where do we go from here. *J Law Med Ethics* 2007;**35**:114–30.
16. Naylor PJ, McKay HA. Prevention in the first place: schools a setting for action on physical inactivity. *Br J Sports Med* 2009;**43**:10–13.
17. Argon P, Takada E, Purcell A. California Project LEAN's food on the run program: an evaluation of high school-based student advocacy nutrition and physical activity program. *J Am Diet Assoc.* 2002;**102**:103–5.
18. Cason K, Logan BN. Educational intervention improves 4th grade school children's nutrition and physical activity knowledge and behaviors. *Top Clin Nutr* 2006;**21**:234–40.
19. Muller MJ, Asbeck I, Mast M, Lagnase K, Grund A. Prevention of obesity—more than an intention. *Int J Obes* 2001;**25**:66–74.
20. Warren JM, Henry CJ, Lightowler HJ, Bradshaw SM, Perwaiz S. Evaualtion of a pilot school program aimed at the prevention of obesity in children. *Health Promot Int* 2003;**18**:287–96.
21. Whelling-Weepie AK, McCarthy AM. A healthy lifestyle program: promoting child heath in schools. *J Sch Nurs* 2002;**18**:322–8.
22. Riggs NR, Spruijt-Metz D, Sakuma KL, Chou CP, and Pentz MA. Executive cognitive function and food intake in children. *Journal of Nutrition Education and Behavior*. In press.
23. Sallis JF, McKenzie TL, Alcaraz JE, Kolody B, Faucette N, Hovell MF. The effects of a 2-year physical education program (SPARK) on physical activity and fitness in elementary school students. Sports, play and active recreation for kids. *Am J Public Health* 1997;**87**:1328–34.
24. Riggs NR, Kobayakawa-Sakuma KL, Pentz MA. Preventing risk for obesity by promoting self regulation and decision making skills: Pilot results from the Pathways to Health Program. *Evaluation Review* 2007;**31**:287–301.
25. Gostin LO. Law as a tool to facilitate healthier lifestyles and prevent obesity. *JAMA* 2007;**297**:87–90.
26. Boarnet MG, Anderson CL, Day K, McMillan T, Alfonzo M. Evaluation of the California Safe Routes to School legislation: urban form changes and children's active transportation to school. *Am J Prev Med* 2005;**28**:134–40.
27. Jaime PC, Lock K. Do school based food and nutrition policies improve diet and reduce obesity? *Prev Med* 2009;**48**:45–53.

28. Pyle SA, Sharkey J, Yetter G, Felix E, Furlong MJ, Carlos Poston WS. Fighting an epidemic: the role of schools in reducing childhood obesity. *Psychology In Schools* 2006;**43**:361–76.
29. Coleman KJ, Tiller CL, Sanchez J, Heath EM, Sy O, Miliken G, Dzewaltowski DA. Prevention of the epidemic increase in child risk of overweight in low-income school: The El Paso coordinated approach to child health. *Arch Pediatr Adolesc Med* 2005;**159**:21–224.
30. Baranowski T, Cullen KW, Nicklas T, Thompson D, Baranowski J. School-based obesity prevention: A blueprint for taming the epidemic. *Am J Health Behav* 2002;**26**:486.
31. Bandura A. *Social Learning Theory*. Englewood Cliffs, New Jersey: Prentice Hall; 1977.
32. Caballero B. Obesity prevention in children: opportunities and challenge. *Int J Obes* 2004;**28**:90–5.
33. Ajzen I. The Theory of planned behavior. *Organ Behav Hum Decis Process* 1991;**50**:179–211.
34. Prochaska JO, Velicer WF. Behavior Change: The Transtheoretical Model of Health Behavior Change. *Am J Health Behav* 1997;**12**:38–48.
35. Irwin Jr CE, Eyre S, Millstein S. Risk-taking behavior in adolescent: The paradigms. *Annals of the New York Academy of Science* 1997;**817**:1–35.
36. Gortmaker SL, Peterson K, Wiecha J, Sobol AM, Dixit S, Fox MK, Laird N. Reducing obesity via school based interdisciplinary intervention among youth. Planet Health. *Arch Pediatr Adolesc Med* 1999;**153**:409–18.
37. Muller MJ, Asbeck I, Mast M, Langnase K, Grund A. Prevention of obesity—more than an intention. Concept and first results of the Kiel obesity prevention study (KOPS). *Int J Obes Relat Metab Disord.* 2001;**25**:S66–74.
38. Nader PR, Stone EJ, Lytle LA, Perry CL, Osganian SK, Kelder S, Webber LS, Elder JP, Montgomery D, Feldman HA, Wu M, Johnson C, Parcel GS, Luepker RV. Three-year maintenance of improved diet and physical activity: The CATCH cohort. *Arch Pediatr Adolesc Med* 1999;**153**:695–704.
39. van Sluijs EMF, McMinn AM, Griffin SJ. Effectiveness of interventions to promote physical activity in children and adolescents: Systematic review of controlled trials. *Br J Sports Med* 2008;**42**:653–7.
40. James J, Thomas P, Cavan D, Kerr D. Preventing childhood obesity by reducing consumption of carbonated drinks: cluster randomized controlled trial. *BMJ* 2004;**328**:1237.
41. Taylor RW, McAuley KA, Barbezat W, Strong A, Williams SM, Mann JI. APPLE project: 2-y findings of a community-based obesity prevention program in primary school age children. *Am J Clin Nutr* 2007;**86**:735–42.
42. Osganian SK, Ebzery MK, Montgomery DH, Nicklas TA, Evans MA, Mitchell PD, Lytle LA, Snyder MP, Stone EJ, Zive MM, Bachman KJ, Rice R, Parcel GS. Changes in the nutrient content of school lunches: Results from the CATCH eat smart food service intervention. *Prev Med* 1996;**25**:400–12.
43. French S, Jeffery R, Story M, Breitlow K, Baxter J, Hannan P, Snyder M. Pricing and promotion effects on low-fat vending snack purchases: The CHIPS study. *Am J Public Health* 2001;**91**:112–17.
44. Cullen KW, Hartstein J, Reynolds KD, Vu M, Resnicow K, Greene N, White MA. Improving the school food environment: Results from a pilot study in middle schools. *J Am Diet Assoc* 2007;**107**:484–9.
45. Stone EJ, Osganian SK, McKinlay SM, Wu MC, Webber LS, Luepker RV, Perry CL, Parcel GS, Elder JP. Operational design and quality control in the CATCH multicenter trial. *Prev Med* 1996;**25**:384–99.
46. de Sa J, Lock K. Will European agricultural policy for school fruit and vegetables improve public health? A review of school fruit and vegetable programs. *Eur J Public Health* 2008;**18**:558–68.
47. Baranowski T, Davis M, Resnicow K, Baranowski J, Doyle C, Lin LS, Smith M, Wang DT. Gimme 5 fruit, juice, and vegetables for fun and health: Outcome evaluation. *Health Educ Behav* 2000;**27**:96–111.
48. te Velde SJ, Brug J, Wind M, Hildonen C, Bjelland M, Pérez-Rodrigo C, Klepp K. Effects of a comprehensive fruit- and vegetable-promoting school-based intervention in three European countries: The pro children study. *Br J Nutr* 2008;**99**:893–903.
49. Brown T, Summerbell C. Systematic review of school-based interventions that focus on changing dietary intake and physical activity levels to prevent childhood obesity: An update to the obesity guidance produced by the national institute for health and clinical excellence. *Obes Rev* 2009;**10**:110–41.
50. Budd GM, Volpe SL. School-based obesity prevention: Research, challenges, and recommendations. *J Sch Health* 2006;**76**:485–95.
51. Adair LS. Child and adolescent obesity: epidemiology and developmental perspectives. *Physiol Behav* 2008;**94**:8–16.
52. Muller MJ, Asbeck I, Mast M, Lagnase K, Grund A. Prevention of obesity — more than an intention. *Int J Obes* 2001;**25**(Suppl. 1): S66–74.
53. Thomas H, Ciliska D, Micucci S, Wilson-Abra J, Dobbins M. *Effectiveness of Physical Activity Enhancement and Obesity Prevention Programs in Children and Youth*. Hamilton, ON: Effective Public Health Practice Project (EPHPP); 2004.
54. Plachta-Danielzik S, Pust S, Asbeck I, Czerwinski-Mast M, Langnase K, Fischer C, Bosy-Westphal A, Kriwy P, Muller MJ. Four year follow up of school- based intervention on overweight children: the KOPS study. *Obes Rev* 2007;**15**:3159–69.
55. Sharma M. International school-based interventions for preventing obesity in children. *Obes Rev* 2006;**8**(2):155–67.
56. Michelle MM, Jennifer Pomeranz JD, Patricia M. The Interplay of Public Health Law and Industry Self Regulation: The Case of Sugar Sweetened Beverage Sales in School. *Am J Public Health* 2008;**98**:595–604.
57. Goldberg JP, Collins JJ, Folta SC, McLarney MJ, Kozower C, Kuder J, Clark V, Economos CD. Retooling food service for early elementary school students in Somerville, Massachusetts: the Shape Up Somerville experience. *Prev Chronic Dis* 2009;**6**:103.
58. Masse LC, Chriqui JF, Igoe JF, Atienza AA, Kruger J, Kohl HWIII, Frosh MM, Yaroch AL. Development of a Physical Education Related State Policy Classification System (PERSPCS). *Am J Prev Med* 2007;**33**:264–76.
59. Gorman N, Lackney JA, Rollings K, Huang TT. Designer schools: the role of school space and architecture in obesity prevention. *Obes Rev* 2007;**15**:2521–30.
60. Gittelsohn J, Kumar MB. Preventing childhood obesity and diabetes: is it time to move out of the school? *Pediatr Diabetes* 2007;**9**:55–69.
61. Summerbell CD, Waters E, Edmunds LD, Kelly S, Brown T, Campbell KJ. Interventions for preventing obesity in children. *Cochrane Database Syst Rev* 2005;**20**.
62. Katz DL, O'Connell M, Yeh M, Nawaz H, Njike V, Anderson LM, Cory S, Dietz W. Task Force on Community Preventive Services. Public health strategies for preventing and controlling overweight and obesity in school and worksite settings: a report on recommendations of the task force on community preventive services. *MMWR Recomm Rep* 2005;**54** (RR-10):1–12.

63. Wang LY, Yang Q, Lowry R, Wechsler H. Economic analysis of a school-based obesity prevention program. *Obes Res* 2003;**11**:1313−24.
64. Gonzalez SC, Worley A, Grimmer SK, Dones V. School based interventions on childhood obesity a meta-analysis. *Am J Prev Med* 2009;**37**:418−27.
65. Story M, Nanney MS, Schwartz MB. Schools and obesity prevention: creating school environments and policies to promote healthy eating and physical activity. *Milbank Q* 2009;**87**:71−100.
66. Lytel LA. School based interventions: where do we go next? *Arch Pediatr Adolesc Med* 2009;**163**:388−90.
67. Nihiser AJ, Lee SM, Wechsler H, McKenna M, Odom E, Reinold C, Thompson D, Grummer SL. BMI measurement in schools. *Pediatrics* 2009;**124**:89−97.
68. Huh J, Riggs NR, Spruijt-Metz D, Chou C, Huang Z, Pentz M. Identifying patterns of eating and physical activity in children: A latent class analysis of pediatric obesity risk. Presented at: *Society of Behavioral Medicine Annual Meeting*. Seattle WA; 2010
69. Pentz MA. Understanding and preventing risks for adolescent obesity. In: Crosby R, Santelli J, editors. *Adolescent Health: Understanding and Preventing Risks*. Hoboken, NJ: John Wiley & Sons; 2008.
70. Katz DL. School based interventions for health promotion and weight control: not just waiting on the world to change. *Annu Rev Public Health* 2009;**29**:253−72.
71. Pentz MA, Mares D, Schinke S, Rohrbach LA. Political Science, Public Policy, and Drug Prevention. *Subst Use Misuse* 2004;**39**:1821−65.
72. Pentz MA. Evidence Based Prevention: Characteristics, Impact, and Future Direction. *J Psychoactive Drugs* 2003;**35**:143−52.
73. Pentz MA. The school community interface in comprehensive schools health education. In: Stanfield S, editor. *Institute of Medicine Annual Report, Committee on Comprehensive School Health Programs, Institute of Medicine, Bethesda Maryland*. Washington DC: National Academy Press; 1995.
74. Pentz MA. Institutionalizing community-based prevention through policy change. *J Community Psychol* 2000;**28**:257−70.
75. Pentz MA. Preventing drug abuse through the community: Multi component programs make the difference. In Sloboda A, and Hansen WB (Eds.), *Putting research to work for the community* (NIDA Publication No. 98-4293;73-86). Rockville, MD: National Institute on Drug Abuse, 1998.
76. Oetzel KB, Scott AA, McGrath J. School based health centers and obesity prevention: changing practice through quality improvement. *Pediatrics* 2009;**123**:267−71.
77. Lee A. Health promoting schools: evidence for a holistic approach to promoting health and improving health literacy. *Appl Health Econ Health Policy* 2009;**7**:11−17.
78. Azrin NH, Ehle CT, Beaumont AL. Physical exercise as a reinforcer to promote calmness of an ADHD child. *Behav Modif* 2006;**30**:564−70.
79. Kwak L, Kremers S, Bergman P, Ruiz JR, Rizzo NS, Sjöström M. Associations between physical activity, fitness, and academic achievement. *J Pediatr* 2009;**155**:914−18.
80. Sharma M. School-based interventions for childhood and adolescent obesity. *Obesity Reviews* 2006;**7**:261−9.
81. Harris KC, Kuramoto LK, Schulzer M, Retallack JE. Effect of school-based physical activity interventions on body mass index in children: a meta-analysis. *CMAJ* 2009;**180**:719−26.
82. Li M, Li S, Baur LA, Huxley RR. A systematic review of school-based intervention studies for the prevention or reduction of excess weight among Chinese children and adolescents. *Obes Rev* 2008;**9**:548−59.
83. Story M. School-based approaches for preventing and treating obesity. *Int J Obes Relat Metab Disord* 1999;**23**:S43−51.

CHAPTER 31

School-Based Obesity Prevention Interventions Show Promising Improvements in the Health and Academic Achievements among Ethnically Diverse Young Children

Danielle Hollar*, Sarah E. Messiah†, Gabriela Lopez-Mitnik†, T. Lucas Hollar‡, Michelle Lombardo§

*Department of Pediatrics, University of Miami Miller School of Medicine, Mississippi Food Network, Miami, FL, USA,
†University of Miami, Miller School of Medicine, Batchelor Children's Research Institute, Miami, FL, USA,
‡Department of Government, Stephen F. Austin State University, Nacogdoches, TX, USA and
§The OrganWise Guys, Inc., Duluth, GA, USA

INTRODUCTION

In the United States, the prevalence of obesity remains high among all age and racial groups in the United States, with a disproportionately high prevalence among African Americans and Hispanic/Mexican Americans [1–3]. Because obesity and associated chronic disease risk factors are relatively stable characteristics that tend to track from childhood into adulthood [4–10], the identification of children and adolescents with elevated risk factors is of great interest from both clinical and public health standpoints. Even among children considered in the normal weight category, childhood weight gain is associated strongly with risk of future cardiovascular disease, including elevated blood pressure and lipids [11, 12]. In addition to cardiovascular disease, childhood obesity can lead to neurological, endocrine, pulmonary, gastrointestinal, renal, and musculoskeletal complications [13], as well as lower self-esteem, higher rates of anxiety disorders, depression, and other psychopathology, which in turn may affect academic performance [14–17].

The etiology of the childhood obesity epidemic is evolving and multifaceted and has been evolving for a while now. The increase in sedentary lifestyles, including television viewing and computer use, as well as advertisements aimed at children promoting calorie-dense, lower-nutrient foods, socialize children into unhealthy lifestyle habits that follow into adulthood [18, 19]. Because of the focus on standardized testing, recommendations for daily physical activity at school and instruction regarding nutrition and healthy living often are not offered [20, 21].

In the United States, schools can play a crucial role in improving the health of children. Because children generally attend school 5 days per week during nine months of the school year, and schools are located in communities of every socioeconomic and racial/ethnic group, they provide ideal locales for interventions. Also, school-age children, particularly those from low-income backgrounds who participate in the United States Department of Agriculture (USDA) National School Lunch Program (NSLP) and the School Breakfast Program, receive a substantial proportion of their daily nutrient requirements at school, often resulting in as much as 51% of daily energy intake [22].

Healthier Options for Public Schoolchildren (HOPS) was designed to pilot-test a school-based obesity prevention intervention with nutrition and physical activity components, targeting a large, multiethnic population of 6- to 13-year-olds. The overall goal was to improve overall health status (body mass index [BMI] percentile, weight, and blood pressure) and academic achievement using strategies that can be replicated in other school settings. The hypothesis was that the intervention would maintain healthy weight/BMI percentiles, improve diastolic and systolic blood pressure and result in higher standardized test scores in intervention children as compared to control children.

METHODS

Design

The study was implemented in August 2004 and included approximately 3769 (50.2% Hispanic) attending five elementary schools (four intervention, one control) in central Florida. Demographic, anthropometric (height, weight, BMI), clinical (systolic and diastolic blood pressure), and academic (Florida Comprehensive Assessment Test) data were collected during the 2-year study period (2004–2006). All schools were chosen from a sample of convenience and had similar demographic and socioeconomic characteristics of the student body. In a quasi-experimental design, schools were assigned nonrandomly to one of four intervention schools or one of two control schools by school district administration. One control school was removed from the sample (after the study began) because it was found to have an exceptional physical education program, including state and federal grants, such as the Carol M. White Physical Education Program (PEP) grant, that could potentially confound results, ultimately supported by post hoc analyses. To ensure exposure to the interventions was consistent over time, students who moved among schools of different treatment status were dropped from the sample. The interventions included modified dietary offerings, nutrition and healthy lifestyle educational curricula, a physical activity component, and other school-based wellness projects. One portion of the analyses presented here focuses only on children from low-income families, which was measured by a child's qualification for free or reduced price meals in the USDA NSLP proxy. This program provides free meals to children from families with incomes at or below 130% of the federal poverty level and reduced-price meals to children from families with incomes between 130% and 185% of the poverty level. For the period July 1, 2008, through June 30, 2009, 130% of the poverty level was $27,560 for a family of four; 185% was $39,220 [23]. By including children who most likely received school-provided lunch every day, we improved the intervention's internal validity and thus decreased potential confounders (e.g., higher socioeconomic status children likely eat better in general [24], regardless of eating the school lunch or not, and are more likely to bring lunch from home).

The Sterling Institutional Review Board (Atlanta, Georgia), which reviewed the study protocol and procedures to ensure the protection of study participants, approved the study. Letters were sent home to parents of students attending the six study schools. Parents signed consents for their minor children if they did not want their child to participate.

Intervention Components

The study included a replicable set of multifaceted intervention components including (1) the provision of nutrient-dense ingredients and whole foods (acquired via existing public school food distribution networks implementing USDA NSLP) in breakfasts, lunches, and extended day snacks, which modeled nutrition education in the classrooms; (2) the implementation of a holistic curricula that taught children, parents, and school staff about good nutrition, healthy lifestyle management, and the importance of increased levels of physical activity; and (3) the commencement of other school-based wellness activities such as fruit and vegetable gardens and walking clubs. The primary objective of the interventions was to improve the health and academic achievement of children in a replicable and sustainable manner. Replication and sustainability were assisted by incorporating USDA nutrition education materials (Team Nutrition, etc.) that are available to schools throughout the United States, USDA feeding programs, and the OrganWise Guys (OWG) curricula [25] that are used by many USDA county extension agents who conduct nutrition education in schools and their surrounding communities.

Dietary Intervention: Provision of Nutrient-Dense Foods That Model Nutrition Lessons

The dietary intervention included rigorous modifications to school-provided breakfasts, lunches, and extended-day snacks in all intervention schools. Menus were modified to include more nutrient-dense foods, fewer calorie-dense foods, and healthy amounts and types of fats. This was operationalized by including more high-fiber items, such as whole grains, fresh fruits and vegetables; fewer items with high-glycemic effects, such as high-sugar cereals, processed flour bakery goods; and lower amounts of total, saturated, and trans fats, thus modeling the nutrition messages being shared in classrooms and in parent outreach information that reflect the core tenets of the Dietary

Guidelines for Americans [26], and thus in compliance with USDA NSLP guidelines [27]. Accordingly, the majority of dietary changes were due to the substitution of healthier ingredients for less healthy ingredients, rather than an outright ban on "child-friendly" food items. For example, processed white flour coated chicken patties were replaced by whole grain flour coated patties; whole milk (higher fat) products were replaced by reduced fat dairy products, including USDA Foods (also known as "USDA Commodities"). Menu offerings, created under the direction of a registered dietitian (RD), provided an especially important component of the interventions whereby good eating practices, being taught in the classrooms, were modeled every day in school-provided meals. Study staff worked closely with the USDA Food and Nutrition Service (FNS), and school administration and cafeteria staff to ensure fidelity of the intervention. Nutrition analyses of breakfast and lunch menus showed intervention menus, on average, contained approximately two times more fiber and 23% less fat than those served in control schools [28–30].

Nutrition and Healthy Living Curricula

The nutrition and healthy living curricula intervention consisted of a school-based holistic nutrition and healthy lifestyle management program for schoolchildren, their parents, teachers, and staff. The curricula included a thematic set of nutrition educational activities developed by study staff, including an RD, in collaboration with elementary school education experts and USDA FNS staff. A multimedia set of materials, highlighting especially nutrient-dense foods and healthy lifestyle habits, was sent to intervention schools, including Foods of the Month (FoM) posters, tips for FoM tastings, FoM parent newsletter inserts, FoM activity packets, healthy lifestyle handouts, school gardening instructions, and other materials aligned with special programming, such as National Heart Health Month, National Nutrition Month, and National School Breakfast and Lunch Weeks were provided to intervention schools. These curricula now are disseminated by the OrganWise Guys Inc. [25] (see Chapter 33 for more information about these curricula and how they are used in schools and community-based settings). Classroom teachers, after-school staff, food service personnel, and others who taught and cared for children were trained to use these materials to teach children about the nutrient-dense foods served in their cafeterias, as well as outside of the school setting. Food service staff, who also received training, included the foods of the month on the school menus as much as possible and periodically hosted food tastings to provide children with experiential opportunities that allowed children to taste foods they were learning about via the curricula.

In addition to the monthly educational programming just described, each intervention school received an OWG Core Kit. The OWG Core Kit brings together nutrition, physical activity, and other lifestyle behavior messages to help children understand the importance of making healthy lifestyle choices and to motivate them to make these choices daily. In previous studies, OWG Core Kit implementation resulted in improvements in body mass index percentiles of OWG children, as well as evidence that parents increasingly are engaged in their children's nutrition and healthy food choices ([31]; see Chapter 33 by Dr. Michelle Lombardo et al. for more information about these study results). The OWG Core Kit includes print (books, posters, etc.) and electronic media materials (videos, Internet activities), a physical activity program (WISERCISE [25]), and school assembly materials.

Nutrition and healthy living activities also included the cultivation of fruit and vegetable gardens at intervention schools. The goal of the garden intervention was to teach children how the nutritious fruits and vegetables served in their school cafeterias, their homes, and in restaurants are grown, cultivated, and harvested. USDA master gardeners, who are part of the cooperative extension in each county, assisted with this intervention. USDA master gardeners assist communities with gardening activities, including education about planting gardens, pest management, and general garden maintenance. Each USDA master gardener must perform volunteer service hours to maintain USDA master gardener status, which provides an ongoing, sustainable technical assistance resource for schools growing fruit and vegetable gardens.

Physical Activity Component

The physical activity intervention included increased opportunities for physical activity during the school day, as feasible within the constraints of testing mandates. Thus, the amount and types of physical activity varied among intervention schools throughout the study. Buy-in for allocating more time to physical activity in study schools was difficult until the governor of Florida mandated 150 minutes of physical activity, per week, for elementary schoolchildren, which was not passed until Fall 2007. To encourage increased amounts of physical activity during year 2 of the study, students were provided pedometers and OWG tracking books to track the number of steps they took each day. However, students often lost the pedometers or broke them. Therefore, although a previous study showed the OWG pedometer program was useful in increasing daily physical activity of children participating in the program by approximately

1000 more steps per day as compared to nonparticipants [32], the use of pedometers in this study was discontinued. Instead, schools were encouraged to implement daily physical activity in the classroom using a 10- to 15-minute desk-side physical activity program (WISERCISE [25] or TAKE10! [33]) during regular teaching time. To encourage adoption of daily physical activity in addition to recess and physical education time, these desk-side physical activities are matched with core academic areas, such as spelling and math. As much as possible, schools were asked to implement structured physical activity during recess time, as well as other physical activities such as walking clubs, to encourage children and adults to walk before or after each school day.

DATA ANALYSES

Measures

Demographic, Anthropometric, and Physiological

Demographic information, including date of birth, gender, grade, and race/ethnicity, were collected by study coordinators at baseline (Fall 2004) and each fall and spring (2004–2006). Anthropometric data included an age and gender-specific BMI, weight in kg/height in meters squared) calculated using height (Seca 214 Road Rod Portable Stadiometer) and weight (LifeSource 321 Scale). Children were asked to remove their shoes and heavy outer clothing and to empty their pockets prior to being measured and weighed. BMI percentiles for age and sex were determined in accordance with Centers for Disease Control and Prevention standardized groups as follows: (1) normal weight (BMI < 85th percentile); (2) at risk for overweight (BMI $\geq$ 85th percentile but < 95th percentile); and (3) obese (BMI $\geq$ 95th percentile) (National Center for Health Statistics, National Health and Nutrition Examination Survey, Z score data files. Available at www.cdc.gov/nchs/about/major/nhanes/growthcharts/zscore/zscore.htm; accessed November 7, 2008). Systolic and diastolic blood pressure, as well as pulse, were measured three times during each data-collection session using WelchAllyn Spot Vital Signs automated measurement machines, which included cuff sizes from very small child through large adult. The three measures were averaged to create one measurement of each type (systolic, diastolic, and pulse), which were used in analyses.

Academic

The Florida Comprehensive Achievement Test (FCAT) is a standardized measurement of student achievement administered to all Florida public schoolchildren beginning in the third grade. School administration provided the FCAT reading and math scores for each child.

Procedures

Presented below are two sets of analyses: (1) all children in the four intervention schools and one control school (N = 3769); and (2) a subset of children of low-income background in the four intervention schools and one control school (N = 1172), which was determined by a child's qualification for Free or Reduced Price Meals in the USDA NSLP proxy.

Because the unit of analysis for this pilot study was a school, rather than individual-level data, cluster randomization was taken into account. With cluster randomization, the mean response under each experimental condition is subject to two sources of variation: cluster to cluster and across individuals within a cluster. Approaching the analytical plan from an individual-level only, rather than a cluster-level, would not take into account the between-cluster variation and can cause an inflation of type 1 errors where any intervention effect may become confounded with the natural cluster-to-cluster variability. Although we realize that this trial did not include a large number of schools to conduct a robust cluster analysis, we applied a two-stage approach to the data analysis:

First stage: Individual level. In the first stage, we analyzed all individual-level covariates to derive school-specific means that are adjusted for individual-level covariates.

Second stage: School level. In the second stage, we analyzed school-specific means and appropriately adjusted for school-specific covariates to evaluate any intervention effects. Univariate analysis consisted of simple frequency statistics for all demographic variables. Chi squared analyses were performed to test for associations between intervention condition and demographic characteristics. Tests for independent samples were applied to capture differences in the percentages of change in BMI percentile group from baseline to the end of the intervention.

Repeated measures analysis tested for changes in trends over time (the 2-year study period or 4 points in time) in BMI percentile group and FCAT scores. For the repeated measures analysis, only those children with data in all years were retained. P-value was significant if less than .05. All tests were two-tailed. The SAS statistical software package version 9.1 (Cary, North Carolina) and SPSS version 15 SAS 9.1 was used for all statistical analyses.

RESULTS

All Children

The majority of the sample was Hispanic (50.2%), and the rest were 33.4% white, 8% black, and 8.4% other (multi-ethnic, Asian, American Indian). The average age was 8 years (range 4 to 13) and 51% were females. Ethnicity by specific school site is described in Table 31.1. There were no significant differences by ethnicity, baseline BMI percentile, or baseline average FCAT scores between treatment arms.

Anthropomorphic and Physiological Results

A greater decrease in BMI percentiles occurred in intervention children as compared to control children during year 1 (2004—2005) of the study, but it was not until year 2 (2005—2006) that the difference between improvements in BMI percentiles reached statistical significance, with intervention children improving more than control children (P = .007) [34].

With respect to girls, BMI z-score and weight z-score significantly decreased in the intervention schools as compared to controls (P < 0.01; P < 0.005, respectively) over the 2-year study period. The mean BMI z-score for boys in intervention schools decreased slightly over the 2-year study period from 0.73 to 0.72, whereas mean BMI z-scores increased from 0.77 to 0.87 for boys in the control schools over the 2-year period, but the change was not significant. Weight z-scores among boys trended in the same direction [35] (Table 31.2).

With regard to blood pressure, girls in the intervention schools experienced a decrease in systolic blood pressure (SBP) from 100.07 mm Hg at baseline (Fall 2004) to 98.3 mm Hg by Fall 2005 and ended at 98.5 mm Hg in Spring 2006 (P = 0.03 for Fall 2004 to Fall 2005, not significant difference for overall difference). A very slight rise in SBP was experienced by girls in control schools over the 2-year study period. Over the 2-year study period, there were no significant changes in SBP noted for boys in the intervention versus control schools. With regard to diastolic blood pressure (DBP), over the 2-year study period, repeated measures analysis showed girls at intervention schools experienced a significant decrease in DBP as compared to girls in the control school (P < 0.05). Among boys, there were no significant changes in DBP by treatment group [35] (Table 31.2). An interesting point to note regarding DBP is related to the significant decreases in both weight and DBP in girls in the intervention group versus controls. This may be an indication that DBP is more correlated with weight than SBP because, although

TABLE 31.1 Healthier Options for Public School Children (HOPS)/The OrganWise Guys Ethnic Distribution by School and Intervention Arm

	School	Black n %	Hispanic n %	White n %	Other n %	Total number of children	Black n %	Hispanic n %	White n %	Other n %	Total number of children
		Total number of children enrolled					**Total number of children enrolled in free/reduced lunch**				
Intervention Schools	#1	29 / 6.07	301 / 62.97	101 / 21.13	47 / 9.83	478	9 / 6.04	119 / 79.87	8 / 5.37	13 / 8.72	149
	#2	64 / 8.89	355 / 49.31	230 / 31.94	71 / 9.86	720	18 / 8.78	138 / 67.32	32 / 15.61	17 / 8.29	205
	#3	53 / 5.61	484 / 51.22	352 / 37.25	56 / 5.93	945	12 / 4.58	212 / 80.92	25 / 9.54	13 / 4.96	262
	#4	102 / 11.47	442 / 49.72	268 / 30.15	77 / 8.66	889	47 / 13.06	210 / 58.33	69 / 19.17	34 / 9.44	360
	Intervention Totals	248 / 8.2	1582 / 52.17	951 / 31.36	251 / 8.27	3032	86 / 8.8	679 / 69.9	134 / 13.7	77	976
Control School	#1	53 / 7.19	310 / 42.06	309 / 41.93	65 / 8.82	737	16 / 8.16	122 / 62.24	45 / 22.96	13 / 6.63	196
	Control Totals	53 / 7.19	310 / 42.06	309 / 41.93	65 / 8.82	737	16 / 8.16	122 / 62.24	45 / 22.96	13 / 6.63	196
Grande Total		301 / 8.0	1892 / 50.20	1260 / 33.43	316 / 8.37	3769	102 / 8.7	801 / 68.3	179 / 15.3	90 / 7.7	1172

Source: Hollar D, Lombardo M, Lopez-Mitnik G, Almon M, Hollar TL, Agatston AS, Messiah SE. *Effective multilevel, multi-sector, school-based obesity prevention programming improves weight, blood pressure, and academic performance, especially among low income, minority children.* Journal of Health Care for the Poor and Underserved 2010;21(2) 93—108.

TABLE 31.2 Change in Blood Pressure and Weight by Gender and Intervention Condition, HOPS[a] Fall 2004 through Spring 2006

	Gender	Intervention	Fall 2004	Spring 2005	Fall 2005	Spring 2006	P-value Fall 2004 vs. Spring 2005	P-value Fall 2004 vs. Fall 2005	P-value Fall 2004 vs. Spring 2006	P-value Fall 2004 to Spring 2006
BMI[b] (z-score)	Male	Intervention (4 schools)	0.73(1.20)	0.65(1.22)	0.78(1.09)	0.72(1.13)	0.09	0.87	0.88	0.86
		Control (1 school)	0.77(1.19)	0.89(0.99)	0.85(1.09)	0.87(1.06)				
	Female	Intervention (4 schools)	0.57(1.19)	0.51(1.17)	0.63(1.10)	0.54(1.12)	*0.0123*	*0.0054*	*0.0008*	*0.0031*
		Control (1 school)	0.78(0.98)	0.70(1.02)	0.74(1.08)	0.78(1.04)	0.55	0.67	0.38	0.3
Systolic Blood Pressure	Male	Intervention (4 schools)	101.20(9.76)	100.85(10.00)	100.51(10.50)	100.27(10.89)				
		Control (1 school)	101.52(9.82)	99.81(9.11)	101.98(10.26)	101.31(10.13)	0.46	*0.0343*	0.14	0.15
	Female	Intervention (4 schools)	100.07(10.42)	99.22(10.57)	98.26(10.06)	98.47(10.49)				
		Control (1 school)	99.77(11.04)	98.54(9.12)	100.33(10.56)	99.97(9.40)	0.32	0.76	0.31	0.79
Diastolic Blood Pressure	Male	Intervention (4 schools)	60.99(6.55)	59.78(6.24)	60.33(6.53)	60.00(6.95)				
		Control (1 school)	60.64(6.46)	59.34(6.40)	61.98(6.83)	60.25(6.61)	0.21	*0.0077*	0.25	*0.0368*
	Female	Intervention (4 schools)	61.30(6.58)	59.76(6.40)	59.96(6.54)	59.55(6.51)				
		Control (1 school)	60.59(6.75)	59.49(5.70)	62.67(6.73)	60.63(5.93)	0.88	0.52	0.57	0.59
Weight (z-scores)	Male	Intervention (4 schools)	0.74(1.14)	0.72(1.13)	0.68(1.14)	0.68(1.13)				
		Control (1 school)	0.68(1.19)	0.76(1.14)	0.72(1.16)	0.72(1.16)	0.07	*0.0098*	*0.0058*	*0.011*
	Female	Intervention (4 schools)	0.56(1.13)	0.55(1.11)	0.53(1.11)	0.51(1.10)				
		Control (1 school)	0.71(1.03)	0.68(1.11)	0.65(1.13)	0.68(1.12)				

[a]*Healthier Options for Public School Children (HOPS).*
[b]*Body mass index (BMI).*
This table was published in the Journal of the American Dietetic Association, Hollar D, Messiah SE, Lopez-Mitnik G, Almon M, Hollar TL, Agatston AS, Effect of a school-based obesity prevention intervention on weight and blood pressure in 6–13 year olds, 2010;**110**(2),261–67. Copyright Elsevier 2010.

similar trends in SBP were noted, they were only significant for the first year among girls, and only modestly so [35]. This is contrary to previous research that has shown a high correlation between SBP and weight by measures of BMI and waist circumference [36–39].

Academic Results

At baseline, no significant differences were found for either math or reading FCAT scores between intervention and control schools (P = 0.46, P = 0.68, respectively). Overall, significantly higher FCAT math scores were found among intervention children, in both years of the study, versus control children (P < 0.001), and a nonsignificant trend was found for FCAT reading scores in the overall sample (P = 0.08). Repeated measures ANOVA, controlling for race/ethnicity, found that all three ethnic intervention groups showed a statistically significant improvement in FCAT math scores versus controls in both study years. Specifically, whereas controls experienced decreases over the same period, Hispanic children in intervention schools showed a more than 20-point gain in FCAT math scores (P = 0.006). Similarly, both black and white students in intervention schools experienced statistically significant gains of more than 40 points (P < 0.05) and more than 20 points (P < 0.02), respectively, as compared to the same ethnic groups in the control school [40] (Table 31.3).

With respect to FCAT reading scores, though not statistically significant (P = 0.08), the same overall trends were seen whereby intervention children showed gains in both years of the intervention, whereas control schoolchildren experienced a decrease in mean FCAT reading scores during the same time period. With respect to race/ethnicity, Hispanic children in intervention schools increased their FCAT reading scores over the 2-year intervention, whereas white and black control schoolchildren showed decreases in scores. The same trends were found in the control school FCAT reading results, with scores for the control school being lower than scores of children in intervention schools [40] (Table 31.3).

Subsample (USDA Free and Reduced-Price Meals, Children Only)

Anthropomorphic and Academic Results

Subsample analyses included 1197 children who qualified for the USDA Free and Reduced Meals Program (68% Hispanic, 9% black, 15% white, 8% other; mean age 7.84 + 1.67). Raw FCAT math and reading

TABLE 31.3 Change in Raw Math and Reading by HOPS Intervention Condition from 2003–2004 to 2005–2006 School Year for Overall Sample and by Ethnicity

Ethnicity	FCAT subject	Intervention condition	FCAT raw score 2003–2004	FCAT raw score 2004–2005	FCAT raw score 2005–2006	P-value from Fall 2004 to Spring 2006
All	Math	Intervention	285.6(58.7)	296.4(59.3)	307.9(51.3)	**0.0005**
		Control	279.2(45.0)	285.5(53.8)	276.2(60.9)	
	Reading	Intervention	286.7(64.2)	291.3(59.8)	292.4(57.7)	0.08
		Control	282.9(55.4)	279.9(65.7)	281.7(55.8)	
Hispanic	Math	Intervention	281.7(61.0)	290.8(62.4)	303.4(52.7)	**0.006**
		Control	277.9(46.8)	281.2(59.8)	270.1(67.6)	
	Reading	Intervention	282.4(65.5)	284.7(61.6)	288.2(57.7)	0.09
		Control	275.7(62.2)	269.9(72.1)	276.8(58.1)	
White	Math	Intervention	309.3(54.8)	319.8(43.5)	330.8(39.7)	**0.016**
		Control	292.9(37.4)	304.7(29.1)	299.7(36.6)	
	Reading	Intervention	308.5(60.8)	320.0(43.4)	315.5(54.6)	0.16
		Control	297.6(23.2)	306.4(45.1)	294.7(53.9)	
Black	Math	Intervention	270.9(34.0)	306.8(46.4)	311.5(41.5)	**0.04**
		Control	243.8(22.3)	264.8(52.2)	267.6(44.1)	
	Reading	Intervention	265.5(51.8)	302.1(51.2)	294.9(53.3)	0.53
		Control	284.8(59.2)	287.8(54.6)	279.6(33.2)	

*This table was published by the American Journal of Public Health: Hollar D, Messiah SE, Lopez-Mitnik G, Almon M, Hollar TL, Agatston AS. Effect of an elementary school-based obesity prevention intervention on weight and academic performance among low income children. Am J Public Health. 2010;**100**:646–53.*

scores were not significantly different between groups before commencement of interventions. With respect to weight measures, repeated measures ANOVA for the 2-year period found children in the intervention schools were significantly more likely to reduce their body mass index Z score ($p < .01$) and their weight Z score ($p < .05$) in comparison to children in the control schools [41] (Table 31.4). With respect to academic achievement, repeated measures ANOVA, after controlling for race, showed that in both study years, Hispanic and white children in intervention schools were significantly more likely to have higher FCAT math scores ($P < .001$) than their counterparts in the control school. Although not statistically significant, intervention children had higher FCAT reading scores in both years of the intervention as compared to control children [40] (Table 31.3).

DISCUSSION

The longitudinal analyses of a school-based obesity prevention intervention among elementary school-aged children described in this chapter show healthy, smart results. Overall, weight measures (BMI percentiles, BMI z-scores, weight z-scores) and blood pressure measures improved during the school year for all children, with significant improvements experienced by intervention children. With respect to sex, significant decreases in weight and blood pressure among girls, over a 2-year study period, were experienced by those in intervention versus control schools. Although no significant differences were noted among boys, intervention boys experienced improvements in weight and blood pressure, whereas boys in controls schools did not. Overall, these weight and blood pressure improvements were strongest among Hispanic and white children in intervention schools.

With respect to low-income children who qualified for free and reduced-price meals through the USDA NSLP, significant improvements in weight measures and significantly higher standardized test scores were associated with the nutrition and physical activity interventions. Specifically, improvements in BMI z-scores and weight z-scores were found in low-income intervention schools as compared to the control. Two-year longitudinal analyses showed low-income children attending intervention schools, regardless of ethnic background, were significantly more likely to have higher FCAT math scores as compared to children in the control school. A similar trend was found for FCAT reading scores, although not statistically significant. These findings indicate that school-based interventions targeting obesity prevention can have direct health benefits and indirect positive effects on academic performance, particularly among low-income children who are at high risk for both obesity and poor academic achievement. This is particularly encouraging given that the majority of children in the United States attend school and thus intervention exposure can be maximized.

Currently, evidence regarding efficacy of school-based obesity interventions for health promotion and weight control is limited [42]. Probably the most widely known school-based intervention program was the Child and Adolescent Trial for Cardiovascular Health (CATCH), a National Heart, Lung, and Blood Institute-sponsored multicenter, school-based intervention study promoting healthy eating, physical activity, and tobacco nonuse by elementary school students (1991–1994, with 3-year follow-up) [43]. The reduction of serum total cholesterol levels was the primary physiological goal. Behavioral goals included reduction of dietary fat (total, saturated) and sodium intake, increased physical activity, and smoking prevention. Overall, no statistically significant changes in body size/weight measures, blood pressure, or serum lipids in the intervention group compared with the control group were found [44, 45], unlike the study presented in this chapter that did find significant differences in blood pressure and weight. However, different risk factor patterns for sex

TABLE 31.4 Change in BMI Z-Scores by Intervention Condition from 2004 to 2006 School Years for Children Qualified for Free or Reduced-Priced Meals/Low-Income Children

Measure	Treatment (number of schools)	Fall 2004	Spring 2005	Fall 2005	Spring 2006	P-value (Fall 2004 to Spring 2006)
BMI (z-score)	Intervention (4 schools)	0.61(1.19)	0.56(1.18)	0.76(1.07)	0.71(1.09)	0.0013
	Control (1 school)	0.98(0.88)	0.97(0.87)	1.02(0.87)	1.05(0.85)	
Weight (z-scores)	Intervention (4 schools)	0.61(1.14)	0.61(1.13)	0.64(1.14)	0.65(1.12)	0.011
	Control (1 school)	0.90(0.98)	0.89(1.01)	0.90(1.01)	0.95(1.00)	

Source: Hollar D, Lombardo M, Lopez-Mitnik G, Almon M, Hollar TL, Agatston AS, Messiah SE. Effective multilevel, multi-sector, school-based obesity prevention programming improves weight, blood pressure, and academic performance, especially among low income, minority children. Journal of Health Care for the Poor and Underserved 2010 (August); 21.3 Suppl.

were noted [44, 45], as were ethnic group differences. Specifically with regard to ethnic differences, the El Paso CATCH study (four intervention and four control Title 1 [low-income] primarily Hispanic schools) reported slowing the increase in risk of overweight or overweight in intervention children as compared to controls [46]. However, unlike the study presented here, which also included schools with predominantly Hispanic student populations, El Paso CATCH did not result in decreases in weight measures during the study period.

Strengths

The strengths of the study presented here are the large sample size overall (~3700 children), and with respect to the low-income subgroup (~1200), the diversity of the sample, and the use of objective measures of health improvement (BMI z-scores and percentiles that appear to correlate well with blood pressure measurements) and academic achievement (FCAT, a standardized test), and multiple measures of the same group of children over an extended time period (2 years). Certainly, these results argue for a large-scale randomized, multicenter study similar to that presented here.

Limitations

Some limitations of this research are worth noting. First, the study was a school-based prevention intervention. As such, out-of-school eating or exercise could not be controlled, neither during the school year nor during holiday breaks. Similarly, there are concerns about lack of study control over eating and physical activity during extended periods of out-of-school time (holidays and summer vacation). Because children appeared to increase their weight and blood pressure during summer break [47, 48], it appears consistent implementation of interventions was not possible. However, it is worth pointing out that despite these limitations regarding control of out-of-school eating and exercise, children improved their overall weight and blood pressure measures during the 2-year intervention, particularly girls. Second, despite trainings on blood pressure measurement methodology before each data-collection period, and the use of simple-to-use blood pressure measurement equipment, the measurements were taken by study coordinators in nonclinical settings; thus measurement may be susceptible to some errors. Additionally, despite a standardized methodology for measuring blood pressure four times over 2 years, study findings are susceptible to error from measurement and from variation in blood pressure between measurement periods. However, the longitudinal data-collection period and the large sample size have assisted in overcoming this limitation. Third, the study population was not selected at random, was of limited geographical variability (one school district), and only one school served as control. Fourth, the design did not include assessment of intervention exposures (minutes curricula used, minutes of physical activity, etc.). Lastly, considerable debate exists regarding the validity of standardized tests, such as the FCAT, in adequately measuring academic achievement, particularly among minority children [49–51].

CONCLUSION

School-based obesity prevention programs—which include a combination of changes to school-provided meals, nutrition and healthy lifestyle education, and physical activity—show promise in improving health and academic achievement of young children. This is particularly true among school-aged children from low-income backgrounds. In light of recent dramatic increases in the prevalence of obesity in the United States, the results presented in this chapter are quite encouraging, given that many children from low-income backgrounds receive a significant proportion of their daily nutrition requirements at school.

Obesity prevention programming based on the research presented here is resulting in the creation of "obesity prevention laboratories," whereby schools are hubs of prevention activity. As described with more specificity in Chapter 33 by Dr. Michelle Lombardo et al., such laboratories are especially important in our current agriculture, school policy, and public health-based obesity prevention context.

Poststudy programmatic expansion efforts, such as the HOPE2 Project, a $2 million obesity prevention project recently funded by the W.K. Kellogg Foundation, are attempting to address this concern through the development of community-based partnerships to expand on and extend outward (from schools) the nutrition and healthy living interventions. This type of collaborative takes a multilevel, multiagency approach to obesity prevention and treatment by creating "obesity prevention laboratories," whereby synergies of combining proven-effective programs operated by multidisciplinary collaborators are achieved. In so doing, *laboratories* are created that include elementary schools, university extension, nonprofit foundations and organizations, memberships of professional associations (American Dietetic Association Foundation, School Nutrition Association), state departmental agencies (Agriculture, Education, and Health), federal agencies (USDA), national foundations (W.K. Kellogg Foundation), state and regional foundations/

corporations (Health Care Service Corporation, Blue Foundation for a Healthier Florida), community-based service organizations, and for-profit companies, among others. These multilevel, multiagency "laboratory" partners bring strong sets of skills (including nutrition education and outreach, program evaluation, and dissemination of best practices/results) and the potential for leveraging of skills and resources, to shape policies and programs affecting the health of the diverse populations of children and families in sustainable ways all year long.

Indeed, school-based nutrition education and feeding programs, such as the model tested during our study, offer opportunities to improve the health and academic achievement of young children while at the same time assisting in the alleviation of poor nutrition and food insufficiency. The Nutrition and WIC Reauthorization Act of 2004 (enacted in 2004) mandated the development of wellness policies at every elementary school that participates in the USDA NSLP. Other federal nutrition-based initiatives—such as USDA technical assistance to school food-service departments, USDA Team Nutrition curricula, the Supplemental Nutrition Assistance Program Education Program (SNAP-Ed), the Institute of Medicine's Committee to Review the National School Lunch and School Breakfast Programs Meal Patterns and Nutrient Standards, and increases in fresh fruit, vegetable, and whole-grain offerings and education opportunities as part of the 2008 Farm Bill (H.R. 2419 [110th]: Food, Conservation, and Energy Act of 2008; www.govtrack.us/congress/billtext.xpd?bill=h110-2419, accessed July 20, 2009)—support improvements in the nutrition well-being and knowledge of schoolchildren. Together, these initiatives enhance the meals and snacks provided to schoolchildren through the USDA NSLP programs (and associated breakfast, snack, and supper feeding programs) and offer opportunities for children to become familiar with healthy eating habits. Indeed, school-based programming can play a strong role in addressing the childhood obesity crisis, child nutrition status, food insecurity, and the attendant health and academic achievement implications. Focusing on the development of "obesity prevention laboratories" to engage communities surrounding schools can help fill the need for focusing prevention efforts both in and out of school time and thus help prevent the development cardiovascular disease in early adulthood.

References

1. *"Preventing Childhood Obesity. Health in the Balance"*. Washington, DC: National Academy Press; 2004.
2. Ogden CL, Carroll MD, Curtin LR, McDowell MA, Tabak CJ, Flegal KM. Prevalence of overweight and obesity in the United States, 1999–2004. *JAMA* 2006;**295**(13):1549–55.
3. New CDC Study Finds No Increase in Obesity Among Adults; But Levels Still High. Centers for Disease Control and Prevention. www.cdc.gov/nchs/pressroom/07newsreleases/obesity.htm. November 28, 2007. Accessed November 9, 2008.
4. Ford ES, Chaoyang L. Defining the metabolic syndrome in children and adolescents: will the real definition please stand up? *J Pediatr* 2008;**152**(2):160–4.
5. Cook S, Auinger P, Li C, Ford ES. Metabolic syndrome rates in United States adolescents, from the National Health and Nutrition Examination Survey, 1999–2002. *J Pediatr* 2007;**152**(2):165–70. Epub 2007 Oct 22.
6. *"The Third Report of the National Cholesterol Education Program Expert Panel on Detection, Evaluation, and Treatment of High Blood Cholesterol in Adults (Adult Treatment Panel III)"*. Bethesda, MD: National Institutes of Health; NIH Publication 01-3670; 2001.
7. Vanhala M, Vanhala P, Kumpusalo E, Halonen P, Takala J. Relation between obesity from childhood to adulthood and the metabolic syndrome: population-based study. *BMJ* 1998;**317**(7154):319.
8. Guo SS, Roche AF, Chumlea WC, Gardner JD, Siervogel RM. The predictive value of childhood body mass index values for overweight at 35y. *Am J Clin Nutr* 1994;**59**(4):810–19.
9. Whitaker RC, Wright JA, Pepe MS, Seidel KD, Dietz WH. Predicting obesity in young adulthood from childhood and parental obesity. *N Engl J Med* **337**(13):859–73.
10. Ford ES, Giles WH, Dietz WH. Prevalence of the metabolic syndrome among US adults: findings from the third National Health and Nutrition Examination Survey. *JAMA* 2002;**287**(3):356–9.
11. de Ferranti S, Ludwig DS. Storm over statins – the controversy surrounding pharmacologic treatment of children. *N Engl J Med* 2008;**359**(13):1309–12.
12. Baker JL, Olsen LW, Sørensen TIA. Childhood body-mass index and the risk of coronary disease in adulthood. *N Engl J Med* 2007;**357**(23):2329–37.
13. Ludwig DS. Childhood obesity: the shape of things to come. *N Engl J Med* 2007;**357**(23):2325–7.
14. Zametkin AJ, Zoon CK, Klein HW, Munson S. Psychiatric aspects of child and adolescent obesity: a review of the past 10 years. *J Am Acad Child Adolesc Psychiatry* 2004;**43**(2):134–50.
15. Vila G, Zipper E, Dabbas M, Bertrand C, Robert JJ, Ricour C, Mouren-Siméoni MC. Mental disorders in obese children and adolescents. *Psychosom Med* 2004;**66**(3):387–94.
16. Taras H, Potts-Datema W. Obesity and student performance at school. *J Sch Health* 2005;**75**(8):291–5.
17. Mustillo S, Worthman C, Erkanli A, Keeler G, Angold A, Costello EJ. Obesity and psychiatric disorder: developmental trajectories. *Pediatrics* 2003;**111**(4 pt 1):851–9.
18. Ludwig DS, Gortmaker S. Programming obesity. *Lancet* 2004;**364**(9430):226–7.
19. Kelder SH, Perry CL, Klepp KI, Lytle LL. Longitudinal tracking of adolescent smoking, physical activity, and food choice behaviors. *Am J Public Health* 1994;**84**(7):1121–6.
20. Taras H, Duncan P, Luckenbill D, Robinson J, Wheeler L, Wooley S. *Health, Mental Health and Safety Guidelines for Schools [Guideline 3-01]*. Available at www.nationalguidelines.org; 2004. Accessed August 5, 2008.
21. *"Moving Into the Future: National Standards of Physical Education"*. 2nd ed. Reston, Va: National Association for Sport and Physical Education; 2004.
22. Briefel RR, Wilson A, Gleason PM. Consumption of low-nutrient, energy-dense foods and beverages at school, home, and other locations among school lunch participants and nonparticipants. *J Am Diet Assoc* 2009;**109**:S79–90.

23. United States Department of Agriculture Food & Nutrition Service National School Lunch Program Fact Sheet. www.fns.usda.gov/cnd/Lunch/AboutLunch/NSLPFactSheet.pdf Accessed February 6, 2009.
24. Patrick H, Nicklas TA. A review of family and social determinants of children's eating patterns and diet quality. *J Amer Col Nut* 2005;**24**(2):83–92.
25. The OrganWise Guys Inc., Duluth, GA; www.organwiseguys.com.
26. U.S. Department of Health and Human Services, U.S. Department of Agriculture. Dietary guidelines for Americans 2005. www.health.gov/DietaryGuidelines/dga2005/document/default.htm. Accessed on July 14, 2009.
27. Code of Federal Regulations 7CFR210, Subchapter A-Child Nutrition Programs, Part 210-National School Lunch Program. www.fns.usda.gov/cnd/governance/regulations/7cfr210.pdf. Accessed on July 14, 2009.
28. Almon M, Gonzalez J, Agatston AS, Hollar TL, Hollar D. *The HOPS Study: dietary component and nutritional analyses*. Los Angeles: Annual Nutrition Conference of the School Nutrition Association; July 17, 2006. CA (poster, copy available from corresponding author upon request).
29. Almon M, Gonzalez J, Agatston AS, Hollar TL, Hollar D. The dietary intervention of the Healthier Options for Public Schoolchildren Study: A school-based holistic nutrition and healthy lifestyle management program for elementary-aged children. *J Am Diet Assoc* 2006;**106**(8):A53.
30. Gonzalez J, Almon M, Agatston A, Hollar D. The continuation and expansion of dietary interventions of the Healthier Options for Public Schoolchildren Study: a school-based holistic nutrition and healthy lifestyle management program for elementary-aged children. *J Am Diet Assoc* 2007;**107**(8) (Suppl. 3):A76.
31. Lombardo M. *The Delta H.O.P.E. Tri-State Initiative*. San Diego: Annual Meeting of the American Public Health Association; 2008. CA (presentation, copy available from corresponding author upon request).
32. "Delta H.O.P.E. Tri-State Initiative. Final Report to the Mississippi Alliance for Self-Sufficiency for the period: August 2003 to June 2007". Washington, DC: ILSI Research Foundation; 2007.
33. ILSI Research Foundation (2007). Delta H.O.P.E. Tri-State Initiative Final Report to the Mississippi Alliance for Self-Sufficiency for the period: August 2003 to June 2007. Washington, DC.
34. Hollar D, Hollar TL, Agatston AS. School-based early prevention interventions decrease body mass index percentiles during school year, but children experience increase in percentiles during summer. *Circulation* 2007;**116**. II_843-II_844.
35. Hollar D, Messiah SE, Lopez-Mitnik G, Almon M, Hollar TL, Agatston AS. Effect of a school-based obesity prevention intervention on weight and blood pressure in 6–13 year olds. *Journal of the American Dietetic Association* 2010;**110**(2):261–7.
36. Sorof JM, Lai D, Turner J, Poffenbarger T, Portman RJ. Overweight, ethnicity, and the prevalence of hypertension in school-aged children. *Pediatr* 2004;**113**(3):475–82.
37. Weiss R, Dziura J, Burgert TS, Tamborlane WV, Taksali SE, Yeckel CW, Allen K, Lopes M, Savoye M, Morrison J, Sherwin RS, Caprio S. Obesity and the metabolic syndrome in children and adolescents. *N Engl J Med* 2004;**350**(23):2362–74.
38. Paradis G, Lambert M, O'Loughlin J, Lavallee C, Aubin J, Delvin E, Levy E, Hanley JA. Blood pressure and adiposity in children and adolescents. *Circulation* 2004;**110**(13):1832–8.
39. Messiah SE, Arheart KL, Luke B, Lipshultz SE, Miller TL. Relationship between body mass index and metabolic syndrome risk factors among US 8- to 14-year-olds, 1999 to 2002. *J Pediatr* 2008;**153**(2):215–21.
40. Hollar D, Messiah SE, Lopez-Mitnik G, Almon M, Hollar TL, Agatston AS. Effect of an elementary school-based obesity prevention intervention on weight and academic performance among low income children. *Am J Public Health* 2010;**100**:646–53.
41. Hollar D, Lombardo M, Lopez-Mitnik G, Almon M, Hollar TL, Agatston AS, Messiah SE. Effective multilevel, multi-sector, school-based obesity prevention programming improves weight, blood pressure, and academic performance, especially among low income, minority children. *Journal of Health Care for the Poor and Underserved* 2010;**21**(2)93–108.
42. Katz DL. School-based interventions for health promotion and weight control: not just waiting on the world to change. *Annu Rev Pub Health* 2009;**30**:253–72.
43. Webber LS, Osganian SK, Feldman HA, Wu M, McKenzie TL, Nichaman M, Lytle LA, Edmundson E, Cutler J, Nader PR, Luepker RV. Cardiovascular risk factors among children after a 2 1/2-year intervention—The CATCH Study. *Prev Med* 1996;**25**(4):432–41.
44. Luepker RV, Perry CL, McKinlay SM, Nader PR, Parcel GS, Stone EJ, Webber LS, Elder JP, Feldman HA, Johnson CC. Outcomes of a field trial to improve children's dietary patterns and physical activity. The Child and Adolescent Trial for Cardiovascular Health (CATCH). *JAMA* 1996;**275**(10):768–76.
45. Webber LS, Osganian SK, Feldman HA, Wu M, McKenzie TL, Nichaman M, Lytle LA, Edmundson E, Cutler J, Nader PR, Luepker RV. Cardiovascular risk factors among children after a 2 1/2-year intervention—The CATCH Study. *Prev Med* 1996;**25**(4):432–41.
46. Coleman KJ, Tiller CL, Sanchez J, Heath EM, Sy O, Milliken G, Dzewaltowski DA. Prevention of the epidemic increase in child risk of overweight in low-income schools: the El Paso coordinated approach to child health. *Arch Peds & Adol Med* 2005;**159**(3):217–24.
47. Hollar D, Hollar TL, Agatston AS. School-based early prevention interventions decrease body mass index percentiles during school year, but children experience increase in percentiles during summer. *Circulation* 2007;**116:II**:843–4.
48. Hollar D, Messiah SE, Lopez-Mitnik GL, Hollar TL, Almon M, Agatston AS. The Effect of Summer Vacation on Weight and Blood Pressure in Multiethnic Elementary Aged Children Participating in a School-based Wellness and Nutrition Program. *JADA* 2008;**108**(9) (Suppl. 3):A12.
49. Linn RL. A century of standardized testing: controversies and pendulum swings. *Educational Assessment* 2001;**7**(1):29–38.
50. Kubiszyn T, Borich G. *"Educational Testing and Measurement: Classroom Application and Practice"*. New York: John Wiley & Sons, Inc; 2007.
51. Perrone V. *Association for Childhood Education International Position Paper on Standardized Testing*. Accessed on July 20, 2009, www.acei.org/onstandard.htm#question; 1991.

CHAPTER 32

School and Community-Based Physical Education and Healthy Active Living Programs
Holistic Practices in Hong Kong, Singapore, and the United States

Ming-Kai Chin*, Christopher R. Edginton*, Mei-Sin Tang[†],
Kia-Wang Phua[‡], Jing-Zhen Yang[§]

*School of Health, Physical Education and Leisure Services, University of Northern Iowa, Cedar Falls, IA, USA,
[†]Baptist (Sha Tin Wai) Lui Ming Choi Primary School, Hong Kong, China, [‡]North Vista Primary School, Singapore and
[§]Department of Community and Behavioral Health, College of Public Health, University of Iowa, Iowa City, IA, USA

INTRODUCTION

Significant changes in physical education have taken place since the early 1970s with a transition from a traditional sports skill-orientation to a broader emphasis on health-related fitness and lifelong physical activity [1, 2]. In the 1970s, as interest in aerobic fitness, strength, leanness, and flexibility began to grow, the focus in physical education shifted toward achieving good general health. It is believed that the processes that lead to chronic degenerative diseases of adulthood are often set in motion during childhood and adolescence [3]. Therefore, it is reasonable to pursue health-related fitness at an early age.

The global epidemic of overweight and obesity is evident in many parts of the world [4, 5], and the worldwide prevalence of obesity in childhood is also increasing [6]. This chapter presents an integrative approach to addressing current trends and directions of the physical education profession, related to the growing burden of childhood overweight and obesity with physical activity, diet, and physical education in schools from the Asia-Pacific perspective. Three model physical education programs, two in Asia and one in North America, are highlighted to illustrate innovative, integrative, and holistic approaches in promoting lifelong healthy active living and wellness through physical education.

GLOBAL EPIDEMIC OF OBESITY

The British anthropologist Ashley Montagu once wrote, "The goal in life is to die young as late as possible" [7]. This notion, although glamorized in the media worldwide, has implications for how we live and maintain our lives in a healthy fashion. To live a healthy, vigorous life requires one to sustain a program of physical activity, to regulate one's dietary habits, and to reduce stress factors and other threats to daily living that impede individual well-being. In the past several decades, rapid modernization, dramatic changes in lifestyle, diets high in fat and sugar, and reduced physical activity have resulted in obesity as the single most contributing factor to the most frequent global metabolic disease [8]. If, in fact, obesity continues as the most dominant factor contributing to metabolic disease throughout the world, Montagu's prophecy for us will be a hollow one.

According to recent estimates from the International Obesity Task Force (IOTF), one in every four individuals, worldwide, is either overweight or obese [9]. The World Health Organization (WHO) predicts that by 2015 approximately 2.3 billion adults will be overweight and more than 700 million will be obese [10]. We live in what has been called an "obesogenic environment" (obesity promoting) [11–13], and the globalization of Western culture encourages an unhealthy lifestyle by increasing energy consumption and discouraging energy expenditure with a reliance on convenience [14].

The direct and indirect cost of obesity to health systems and the social costs to communities and individuals are escalating. In the United States, estimates show that the annual medical burden of obesity rose to $147 billion in 2008 (10% of the national healthcare budget) [15]. The costs arising from obesity-associated illness in children in the United States have also risen, from $125.9 million to $237.6 million between 2001 and 2005 [16]. The medical costs in 1 year of diagnosis follow-up and management of 8.5 million overweight or obese youth in the United States is estimated at nearly $820 million [17].

EPIDEMIC OF CHILDHOOD OBESITY

On a global basis, the childhood and adolescent overweight epidemic is a startling phenomenon and continues to be a major and increasing public health concern [18]. It is estimated that 1 in 10 children worldwide, show symptoms of being overweight or obese [9]. In 2010, the number of overweight children under the age of five is estimated to be more than 43 million according to the World Health Organization [19]. Ogden et al. [20] reported that 25 million U.S. children are overweight or obese. The prevalence of overweight adolescents in the United States is increasing at such an extent that a high proportion of such individuals would qualify for weight-loss surgery [21]. It has also been postulated that the figure of actual prevalence of childhood obesity is higher than reported [22]. In the United States and the United Kingdom, for the first time, the current generation is projected to have a shorter life span than the previous one—the first such possibility in history [23, 24].

The prevalence of overweight and obesity amongst children appears to be rising rapidly in many countries around the world, including countries in Asia [6]. The prevalence of childhood and youth obesity varies from 6.7% in Thailand [25], to 7.3% in a local Malaysian study of schoolchildren in an urban area [26], 10% to 15% in Singapore [27], 10.6% in Japan [28], 11.3% in Korea [29], 12.8% in Hong Kong [30], 14.9% in Taiwan [31], 16.6% in China [32], and 24.0% in a study of urban Indian children in New Delhi [33].

Major consequences of obesity in youth, such as clustering of cardiovascular risk factors, dyslipidemia, hypertension, type 2 diabetes mellitus, polycystic ovarian syndrome, joint stress, obstructive sleep apnea, and other social, emotional, and psychological difficulties are many and far reaching [3, 34, 35]. A study conducted by Yach, Stuckler, and Browell [36] estimated that by the early 2030s, the prevalence of type 2 diabetes (caused mostly by diet, inactivity, and obesity) is expected to increase by 36.5% in the United States, 75.5% in China, and 134% in India. Because the problem of childhood obesity is so severe, the Institute of Medicine's (IOM) Committee of Obesity in Children and Youth suggested that immediate actions are warranted, "based on the best *available* evidence—as opposed to waiting for the best *possible* evidence," and stressed that it is the responsibility of national governments to take steps to reverse the obesity trend [37].

CHANGES AND SHIFTS IN DIET AND PHYSICAL ACTIVITY PATTERNS

The shifts in dietary and activity patterns and body composition seem to be occurring at a rapid pace because of globalization. The linkage between obesity, physical activity, and unhealthy eating is well documented [38]. Physical inactivity and excessive consumption of high-calorie, nutrient-poor foods result in the storage of body fat, leading to obesity in adults and in children [39]. It is likely that both physical inactivity and Western eating patterns act synergistically [40].

Dietary Trends

Rapid economic development in Asia, together with raised standards of living since the 1980s, have resulted in increased nutrient availability to many countries in the region and also improved health facilities. In China and elsewhere in developed and developing countries in East Asia, rapid changes in dietary habits such as the convenient availability of high-energy foods and fast foods and reduced complex carbohydrates are a cause for concern as these changes contribute definitively to obesity among youth and adults [41, 42]. Sweetened or carbonated drink consumption has also increased significantly in China and other Asian countries. Such dietary trends are considered one of the risk factors linked to the prevalence of increased obesity [43, 44, 45–48]. Familial factors, the nature of food available at home and school, and frequent patronage of fast-food establishments are found to be the most significant influences on the eating habits of children and youth [49]. In the United States, almost 50% of total family food dollars were spent at restaurants and on fast food [37]. Bowman and colleagues [43] reported that 30.3% of children aged 4 to 19 consumed at least one meal per day that was purchased at a fast-food establishment. The growth of the fast-food market in the Asia Pacific region is alarming. According to an ACNielsen Online Survey [50], 30% of Asia Pacific consumers claimed to eat takeaway at least once a week, closely behind the United States (33%). There are more than 2870 Kentucky

Fried Chicken (KFC) fast-food establishments [51] and 960 McDonald's restaurants in China [52]. A survey conducted under the auspices of the National Institute of Education [53] found that the total number of fast-food chains in Singapore (79 McDonalds, 70 KFCs, and 46 Burger Kings) is higher than the number of primary schools. Austin et al. [54] reported that there is a high concentration of fast-food restaurants within a short walking distance from schools, and, as a result, children are exposed to poor-quality food environments in their school neighborhoods. Horgen, Choate, and Brownell [55] stated that all of these changes in the availability, composition, and marketing of food in developed countries have led some to describe today's situation as a "toxic food environment."

Physical Inactivity

When examining the etiology of pediatric overweight, some evidence suggests that physical inactivity rather than high-fat diets are a major determinant of obesity [56–58]. The findings on the gradual decline in physical activity between childhood and adolescence are disturbing. An age-related decline of 26% to 37% in total physical activity during adolescence has been documented in longitudinal studies, and this decline is of particular concern among girls [59, 60].

Screen Time

Indicators of physical inactivity include the hours spent in screen-based activities such as viewing television, playing video games, and using computers. Such sedentary leisure pursuits have multiplied throughout the world [59, 61]. Surveys have reported that the time children spend on television, videos, video games, and computers exceeds 5 hours per day [62, 63]. Studies linking "screen time" with obesity, cardiovascular risk factors, negative health indicators, and physical inactivity have been well documented [64–66]. Studies also showed that television viewing increases the motivation to increase food and energy intake in children [66, 67].

AN INTEGRATED APPROACH OF PHYSICAL EDUCATION, PHYSICAL ACTIVITY, AND WELLNESS IN SCHOOL

As children spend approximately 6 to 8 hours a day for 9 to 10 months a year in a school setting [68, 69], schools are often suggested as the ideal and key settings for promotion of physical activity, healthy eating, and active lifestyles to prevent overweight and obesity [22, 70, 71]. The U.S. Dietary Guidelines for Americans recommend that young people (aged 6 to 19) participate in at least 60 minutes of moderate-to-vigorous physical activity (MVPA) on most, if not all, days of the week [72]. A recent European study suggested an accumulation of 90 minutes of MVPA and 11 to 14 thousand steps daily in order to gain the health benefits for young people [56].

Increasing physical activity through physical education is also a proposed public health strategy to reduce obesity in childhood and adolescence [73]. A survey of state chronic disease directors in the United States reported that school-based approaches such as "increasing physical education classes, allocating more recess/playtime, or improving the nutritional content of foods sold in schools" were ranked as top priorities in the prevention of obesity policies [69]. In many developed countries, school physical education programs have become the major source of MVPA for a majority of children and adolescents, though the time allocated to this subject is far from adequate according to the most recent international surveys [74, 75].

In other words, schools may be best positioned to creatively address physical inactivity by going beyond the provision of quality physical education and maximizing other opportunities by building up a Comprehensive School Physical Activity Program (CSPAP) as suggested by the National Association for Sport and Physical Education (NASPE), and other researchers and professional health organizations [76, 77]. NASPE recommends that a CSPAP include four key components: quality physical education, school-based physical activity opportunities (recess, extracurricular activity, and interscholastic sports programs), school employee wellness and involvement, and family and community involvement.

To illustrate the actual implementation of the aforementioned concepts, physical education programs at three schools—one in Hong Kong, one in Singapore, and one in the United States—will be presented as case studies. Each of these schools represents what we would refer to as "best practices." They have distinguished themselves through their innovation in the provision of physical education programs that have extended themselves beyond traditional offerings into the community. They all reflect the aforementioned four key components that the authors believe are essential in providing physical education programs to meet 21st-century needs.

BAPTIST (SHA TIN WAI) LUI MING CHOI PRIMARY SCHOOL (HONG KONG-CHINA): A HOLISTIC APPROACH

In Hong Kong-China, in order to formulate a curriculum paradigm that fosters lifelong learning and focuses on whole-person development, physical education is included as one of the Key Learning Areas (KLAs) [78, 79]. Physical education curricula in Hong Kong-China have recently been the focus of major transformation. According to the Curriculum Development Council [80], the overall aims of physical education are "to help students to develop an active lifestyle and acquire good health, physical fitness, and body coordination through learning various physical and sport skills and knowledge."

Promoting Quality Physical Education

Baptist (Sha Tin Wai) Lui Ming Choi Primary School (LMC) of Hong Kong-China is one of the few primary schools with more than 1000 students aged 6 to 12 years offering three physical education classes per week. The mission statement of LMC's physical education and health programs affirms that the goals for the students are (1) to have fun with a variety of physical activities; (2) to develop the knowledge, skills, attitudes, and responsibility for their own health and well-being; (3) to maximize physical activities in physical education lessons to enhance health and fitness; and (4) to be challenged to develop generic skills such as creativity, problem solving, cooperation, and critical thinking.

The mission statement is, in fact, directly linked to current research findings and the emerging educational reform in Hong Kong-China and worldwide. For example, the research findings of Sallis et al. [81] suggested that to have fun in physical education was one of the strongest and most consistent correlates supporting the first mission statement. These researchers concluded that "enjoyment of physical education should be a health-related goal because it is related to physical activity out of school" (p. 415). Research findings also support the notion that physical education may, in fact, empower children and youth to take responsibility to develop skills and gain knowledge to develop an appreciation of the importance of physical activity [82, 83]. Further, other research findings suggest that the responsibility of physical education is to "educate" the body, giving knowledge about the potential of movement for developing the skills to participate with enjoyment in many kinds of physical activity [84].

Studies by Fairclough and Stratton [85], Van Beurden et al. [86], and McKenzie et al. [87] reported that, on average, children and youth spend only 34%, 35%, and 37.9% of their physical education lessons, respectively, engaged in moderate to vigorous intensity physical activity (MVPA). These studies support the mission statement focused on maximizing physical activities in physical education lessons to enhance health and fitness. Last, one of the main objectives in the physical education curriculum reform is to strengthen generic skills in the physical education context with a carryover value to lifelong learning and pursuit of a quality adult life [79, 80]. The program directly addresses this desire for educational reform in Hong Kong-China in its mission statement.

There are eight certified physical education teachers with bachelor's degrees in physical education and a swimming teacher on the faculty of the school. The importance of lifelong skill enhancement and health-related fitness is emphasized in the program by providing two physical education lessons per week devoted to swimming and utilizing the "Physical Best" program in alternative weeks. All students have swimming lessons throughout the year during their first 6 years of education. The content of the program includes a focus on various swimming techniques, aquatic games/activities, and water fitness training. Physical Best, a program design drawn from the National Association of Sport and Physical Education (NASPE) and the American Alliance of Physical Education, Recreation and Dance (AAHPERD) is a comprehensive health-related fitness education program operated as a part of the physical education curriculum. The Physical Best program is a standardized curriculum directed toward moving students from a dependent state to an independent one and encouraging individuals to assume the responsibility for their own fitness and health by promoting regular, enjoyable physical activity [88, 89]. Physical education teachers throughout the United States have been trained in this program. For example, from 2005 to 2006, more than 400 elementary school teachers with a standardized curriculum in the New York City school district were trained in the Physical Best program [90].

Under a school and university partnership, a number of local and overseas university professors are invited to come to the school to support the development of existing staff and the physical education teachers. As a result, physical education teachers can greatly enhance their teaching skills. Over the past three summers, physical education teachers at LMC have participated in a professional development program emphasizing the Physical Best curriculum design. They are trained by an expert from Montclair State University (United States). LMC has two complete sets of Physical Best equipment to implement the curriculum. In addition, sufficient modified ballgame equipment is available so that two physical education classes would have adequate equipment to be used at the same time. The other physical education lesson emphasizes fundamental movement directed toward lower primary students and athletics, ballgames, gymnastics, and dances to upper primary students. Modified ballgames are taught through different teaching strategies such as Teaching Games for Understanding (TGfU) [91] and sport education [92]. These teaching strategies enable all students, irrespective of their physical and motor abilities, to enjoy the physical education experience with active participation in health enhancing physical activities.

School-Based Physical Activity Opportunities

The LMC physical education program provides many opportunities for school-based physical activities beyond the classroom setting including activities during recess and in extracurricular settings and interscholastic programs. For elementary school students, recess can be utilized to provide opportunities for students to accumulate meaningful amounts of physical activity, preferably engaging in MVPA for 40% of playtime [93, 94]. Beighle et al. [95] used pedometers to asses physical activity and reported that children spend the majority (>60%) of their recess time in physical activity and a smaller proportion of their outside of school time in activity (about ≈20%). Results suggest that recess is an important source of physical activity for youth and should be a part of each school day. Children are more active and tend to increase their MVPA during their lunch break when game equipment is available (basketballs, hoops, etc.), improvements are made in playgrounds, and a teacher is present to provide supervision and encourage involvement in organizing active game activities [96, 97]. During recess at LMC, some of the physical activities provided include rock climbing, 3-on-3 basketball (primary school students in grades 4 through 6), hula hoops, minigames (primary school students in grades 1 through 3) and a Quick Walk around a "Great Wall." Immediately following the dynamic recess period for 5 minutes every day, all students and teachers in the school engage in a program featuring various dances such as Chu Shang de Taiyang, Qingchun de Huoli, poem chanting, worship dance, modern dance, and jazz. This program is the only one of its kind at any school in all of Hong Kong and has been continuously implemented since 2003 with great success.

Extracurricular and after-school physical activity programs have been used extensively in schools in an attempt to promote ongoing active lifestyles and lifelong participation in sport and physical activity [98–100]. Extracurricular settings at LMC feature physical activities organized in a club format such as badminton, table tennis, Mandarin basketball, Wu Shu, skipping, Chinese dance, ballet, modern dance, gymnastics, rock climbing, and fencing. Interscholastic sports programs include athletics (track and field), volleyball, football, table tennis, badminton, skipping (jumping rope), handball, swimming, and basketball. Programs in swimming have been particularly successful at LMC where the school has excelled by winning many individual medals and the overall district championship. These physical activities have provided a well-rounded program that is comprehensive in nature and interconnected for students. The emphasis is to integrate physical activity in as many settings linked to the school as possible, especially ones that promote lifelong leisure skill acquisition.

School Employee Wellness and Family and Community Involvement

LMC's School Employee Wellness program and the involvement of family and community members represent another dimension of the effort, attesting to its comprehensive integrative nature. Further, the school administration and members of the community have provided great leadership. For example, the principal solicited support and collaboration with a swimming school, and community members and other sponsors raised funds to build a heated indoor swimming pool (U.S. $1.3 million) and build an employee fitness center (U.S. $32,050) through the Quality Education Fund. In addition, parents of LMC are extremely supportive, especially to ensure that healthy, nutritious meals are provided. Every day parents come to school to check the content of the lunch boxes provided to the pupils. Parental involvement is essential for the success of the implementation of strategies for child obesity prevention [22, 101]. Dieticians plan the nutrition facts of the daily lunch to conform to the food pyramid. Calories, fat, and fiber proportions are carefully calculated to ensure that the children have a balanced diet. Each lunch box is treated in the ratio 3:2:1 (i.e., half of the food is cereal, one third of the food is vegetable, and one sixth of the food is meat). The preparation of the meal (cooking) follows the "3 low 1 high" formula (i.e., low sugar, low salt, low oil, but high fiber). The food provided to children is fresh, nutritious, and delicious. The tuck shop (a small separate food service area) of the school is known as the Chung Ming Hut. It is a social enterprise operated by individuals with impaired hearing to provide only healthy food to the pupils. A research study conducted by Foster et al. [102] reported that a multicomponent school-based nutrition intervention can be effective in preventing overweight among children. The overall program design has also featured the creation of a school health team. This team consists of panels of individuals focused on student health services, religious education, health curriculum, school ethos and interpersonal relationships, healthy school environments, and community relationships, as well as individuals with medical backgrounds, physical education teachers, a school counselor, psychologist, and speech therapist. This group provides advice and counsel to the effort in a holistic fashion.

NORTH VISTA PRIMARY SCHOOL (SINGAPORE): THE COMMUNITY OF LEARNERS AT THE SCHOOL OF THE FUTURE

Preparing children for the future is a vital investment in the city-state of Singapore where natural resources are scarce. In Singapore, human resources are its most vital asset. Becoming a first world nation from a third world country in less than 40 years after its independence has called for ingenuity and innovation on the part of Singaporeans. North Vista Primary School (NVPS) is located in the northeast region of this land-scarce country of only 710 square kilometers. Approximately 5 million people live in high-rise apartments. NVPS is actively harnessing the human and other resources of the community to help assist it in building a model program of the future. By drawing from best practices from throughout its global network, the school has provided a recognized world-class program in physical health featuring strong community support. Employing findings found in the research literature, the school curriculum is designed to produce students who are confident, self-directed learners, good citizens, and active contributors to the nation. The emphasis is on providing them with the knowledge, skills, and values needed for a productive life in the 21st century. The wealth of this nation hinges highly on the health of her people to protect and defend this small nation-state and at the same time be at its peak in productivity to engage in various enterprises throughout the world. It is in this context that the school aims to seamlessly integrate its physical health program deeply into its curriculum.

Physical education is conducted three times a week for 50 minutes in each period. As in LMC, the utilization of the Physical Best program promotes fun in physical activities, self-directed learning, confidence building, collaboration, and social responsibilities in an environment of continual active learning. Students are encouraged to make decisions, display good sportsmanship, think critically, and track their own progress through the use of heart-rate monitors (HRMs). Through 1:1 computing, where every child owns a personal notebook, the HRM data can be easily downloaded and students are encouraged to take ownership of their own fitness regime. This has transformed learning from that of forced physical activities to self-directed learning that is personalized for every child. As one child at the school stated, "There is never a dull moment in physical education." "Physical Education is Fun!" workshops are conducted for parents so that they will gain an understanding and appreciation for the program's goals and objectives. In this way, parents become partners in the educational process. They participate in the same activities as their children, gaining and understanding the concepts of Physical Best. This collaborative effort enables parents to work with the school to keep their children fit and healthy. Parents and children track their progress through the HRM data and develop strategies for an optimal healthy lifestyle.

To encourage parents and children to get out and play, the school opens its doors on Wednesday evenings and Saturday mornings, giving parents and children the opportunity to line-blade or play games such as badminton. Whereas most schools in Singapore have only a short break of 20 minutes for snack, NVPS increases playtime by providing two breaks: one at morning tea of 20 minutes and another, longer 40-minute lunch break. This has increased playtime for students. Students are encouraged to become engaged in self-organized forms of play, such as inline skating, skate boarding, basketball, and badminton in the school fields, courtyards, and indoor sports hall. For those who prefer to stay in shaded areas, NVPS has invested in eight Wii stations placed at the Galaxy, a strategic location for students to gather during breaks. Students may borrow, from the school library, game simulations played on the Nintendo Wii, allowing them to engage in technology-aided fitness activities with their friends during breaks. This enables students to discover for themselves how they can use television and the electronic simulations presented as a tool for a quick workout. This encourages physical activity rather than the inactivity that often comes when playing computer games. Students learn game concepts and, because of the high interest of such individuals and the effectiveness of the use of the technology in imparting games concepts, Wii has been incorporated into NVPS physical education curriculum.

Community as Partners, Teachers, as Researchers

There is an old African proverb that states, "It takes a village to raise a child." NVPS engages extensively with its community partners. The National Health Promotion Board (HPB) assists NVPS in training bistro vendors to prepare nutritious and healthy food. HPB monitors and tracks food sold in the bistro, ensures that food products meet required standards (e.g., low sugar, salt, and oil content in the preparation of food and drinks), and encourages a healthy balanced diet for students. Teachers from NVPS work collaboratively with governmental agencies and the Ministry of Education on new pedagogical approaches and initiatives to promote holistic health. Collaborative initiatives, such as the Fruttie-Veggie Bites, are aimed at increasing student intake of fruits and vegetables. Further, the Model School Tuck Shop Program (MSTP) is aimed at monitoring and meeting the nutritional needs of students. NVPS started with only one teacher trained in physical education. To build the capacity of NVPS teachers, the school has opted for co-teaching in the development of teachers who are not specialized in the training of physical education. This 1-year mentoring and coaching program allows teachers who are untrained in physical education to become involved in co-teaching with the head of physical education and to gain knowledge, skills, and experience in this area. Teachers only "graduate" when they have been observed and appraised by consultants from Montclair State University (United States) and the University of Northern Iowa (United States). The school has now structured tabled time for teachers to meet as professionals to discuss research on the progress of teaching and learning physical education. Results have shown that obesity rates have fallen from 12% to 8%. In addition, 97% of students pass the annual National Physical Fitness Test.

GRUNDY CENTER (IOWA, UNITED STATES) COMMUNITY SCHOOLS/POLAR ELECTRO, INC./UNIVERSITY OF NORTHERN IOWA: A PARTNERSHIP OF EXCELLENCE

Collaboration, cooperation, and the building of partnerships are hallmarks for success for organizations as we move into the 21st century. Schools, universities, nonprofit organizations, and commercial enterprises are all being challenged to find ways to work with one another to advance the well-being of society. In recent years, individual and community health and well-being has declined as a result of a variety of factors including diet, lack of exercise, use of tobacco or alcohol, and other behaviors. Consequently, there has been a reduction in longevity as well as the satisfaction that one draws from maintaining a robust lifestyle. Individual health contributes to or draws down on community resources, affecting the way in which we live collectively. Further, without a healthy, productive workforce, businesses and commercial enterprises cannot prosper. These and other challenges have become the focal point for the development of a unique school and community-based learning opportunity involving multiple entities including the Grundy Center (Iowa) Community Schools, POLAR Electro, Inc., HOPSports Training Systems, and the University of Northern Iowa's School of Health, Physical Education and Leisure Services.

The Grundy Center physical education program has gained national attention in the United States. The U.S. Secretary of Education Arne Duncan witnessed the program in 2009 in an effort to gain an awareness and understanding of the uniqueness and importance of this program. As Duncan noted in an interview for a local community newspaper:

> I love the innovation, I loved the engagement, and these students are getting a great background, and a great education. It was just really inspiring to see. These students [in Grundy Center]—because of these types of activities—they're going to take ownership for their own health for the rest of their lives. [103]

Building a Partnership

The Grundy Center is a small rural community located in the state of Iowa in the United States that prides itself in promoting the "good life" for its residents through the quality of its school system, the safety of the community, the outpouring of neighborly support, and the activities available for families [104]. The Grundy Center Community School system focuses its efforts on empowering "individuals with the attitudes, skills, and knowledge to become responsible, productive and fulfilled citizens" [105]. Its vision and belief statements are punctuated with terms like "collaboration," "cooperation," "communication," "problem solving," "quality connectedness across disciplines," "use of technology," "meaningful experiences," "mutual respect," "high expectations," "climate of success," and "opportunities for all children to learn." The University of Northern Iowa is one of three state-assisted universities in the state of Iowa. With historical roots in teacher education, today it is a comprehensive university emphasizing the tripartite mission of teaching, research, and service. The School of Health, Physical Education and Leisure Services traces its founding to 1896 and offers one of the more highly regarded physical education teacher preparation programs in the United States. POLAR Electro, Inc. [106], is the leading brand in sports instruments and heart rate monitoring. HOPSports Training Systems utilize 21st-century technology in educating for physical activity, promoting proper nutritional habits, and encouraging other social messaging by employing a dynamic multimedia format used in the classroom.

Initially conceived in a holistic fashion, these entities have collaborated to build a partnership to prepare physical educators for the 21st century with a focus on the use of technology. Emphasis was placed on developing an integrated effort to involve all entities in the preparation of physical education teachers that was not just school bound but was a program that would be supported by and permeated throughout the entire community. As such, the collaborative effort was designed with a deep commitment for promoting a healthy, active lifestyle and improving the quality of individual and community life as contrasted with programs that focus exclusively on the preparation of physical education teachers without a mandate to influence the community beyond the classroom. Thus, the program involved the development of relationships with the local hospital, the YMCA and other entities to promote healthy active lifestyles as a community focus. In fact, the YMCA is embedded in the school system, utilizing its resources and sharing professional staffing to provide a community-wide perspective and program focus.

THE INNOVATIVE POLAR SCHOLARS PROGRAM

On an annual basis, the University of Northern Iowa's School of Health, Physical Education and Leisure Services and the Grundy Center Community Schools recruit worldwide and select a small, highly qualified group of individuals to participate in the program. The design of the teacher preparation program is significantly different than others found throughout the world. The program is organized to engage students as full time-teachers in a contextually based, full-immersion graduate program. Key elements in the program are that of linking practice to theory [107] involvement with a master teacher, the organization of students as a cohort group, emphasis on reflective thinking, and a deep embedding in community activities outside of the school. The individuals participating in this program are designated as POLAR Scholars.

POLAR Scholars teach elementary and secondary physical education with a heavy emphasis on the use of technology as well as educating the whole community about health-related concerns. For example, POLAR Scholars lead adult and senior life fitness classes in school facilities to help to promote healthier living for all community members. The community shares the facilities and the teaching staff with what might be the smallest YMCA in the nation. The POLAR Scholars also serve as sport coaches and fitness leaders for students after school hours to ensure opportunities for maximum physical activity, which encourages the acquisition of lifelong learning of fitness and leisure skills.

Promoting Leadership in Sports Technology

The great success of the program can be attributed to the quality of instruction and leadership provided by the extraordinary Grundy Center physical education professional staff and partnering individuals. These individuals have been recognized by American Alliance of Health, Physical Education, Recreation and Dance (AAHPERD), the National Association of Sport and Physical Education (NASPE), the U.S. Department of Education, and many other professional associations and societies. Like the LMC program mentioned previously, great administrative support has impacted the success of this program in many positive ways. In particular, the superintendent of schools, as well as principals and teachers in other content and professional areas, has provided direct and indirect support for the effort.

The quality of the program is also enhanced through the use of technology, in particular the use of heart rate monitors, personal digital assistants (PDAs) and TriFit Assessment Systems in the physical education curriculum. This technology enables the program to objectively assess each student and to develop personalized health and fitness portfolios for each individual [108, 109]. As a result, students in physical education classes are highly motivated, self-directed, and engaged in a very individualized program of activity. With the use of heart rate monitors, each student knows what he or she is seeking in terms of target heart rate intensity during each physical education session. For example, students in elementary school wear heart rate monitors during physical education classes to ensure that they are exercising within their target heart rate zone. This method provides instant feedback to students regarding their cardiovascular activity and encourages students to strive for their personal best. All of the data are downloaded and stored for the purposes of enabling students to monitor their performance over time and as a measure of accountability for reporting accurately their progress to parents. Data can be retrieved on individual student achievement and used for grading the results of their effort objectively.

The Grundy Center POLAR Scholar program has drawn great interest in the United States and internationally [110, 111]. Not only are educators and researchers interested in the use of technology in the design of physical education curriculums, but the program has also created a new dynamic pedagogy in the preparation of physical education teachers. The linkage of the program in a holistic sense to the community has created great benefits in advancing fitness and other quality-of-life concerns. As the community as a whole has embraced the effort, recognition has spread and efforts have increased in regard to combating child and youth overweight and obesity. The entire community and its other health-related resources, including the hospital and YMCA, are working and in a cooperative fashion to create a partnership that advances strategies aimed at ensuring that Grundy Center's current and future citizens achieve the "good life."

GLOBAL FORUM FOR PHYSICAL EDUCATION PEDAGOGY (2010) (GOFPEP 2010)

In May 2010, the University of Northern Iowa's School of Health, Physical Education and Leisure Services (Iowa, United States) and the Grundy Center (Iowa, United States) Community Schools hosted the Global Forum for Physical Education Pedagogy 2010 (GoFPEP 2010). The event focused on the theme of "Revitalizing Health and Physical Education through Technology." Organized to examine new forms of pedagogy, GoFPEP 2010 sought to review the use of technology, ways of linking practice to theory, and the importance of contextually based education embedded in community life as a way to reshape and redesign the future of health and physical education. GoFPEP 2010 drew 70 invited delegates from 30 countries representing 64 universities, institutions, organizations, and schools globally to examine (1) a new pedagogy for preparing physical education teachers (one that uses full immersion, is contextually based, and enhances the use of technology), (2) the utilization of technology to teach physical education, and (3) the building of school, university, community, and corporate partnerships.

The GoFPEP 2010 program featured presentations regarding the three aforementioned model school's physical education programs: Baptist (Sha Tin Wai) Lui Ming Choi Primary School (Hong Kong-China), North Vista Primary School (Singapore), and Grundy Center (Iowa, United States) Community Schools/Polar Electro, Inc./University of Northern Iowa. Not only were the physical education programs highlighted by teachers and principals, but strategies used in building partnerships were also offered by key individuals such as the superintendent of schools and corporate partners. In addition, a commentary was introduced regarding a model program for preparing physical education teachers.

During GoFPEP 2010, a consensus statement will be issued from the discussion of the participants and a proceeding will be published and distributed globally. It is the objective of GoFPEP 2010 to stimulate the interest of colleagues globally on this unique model of health and physical education for future diffusion to various communities and school systems internationally. GoFPEP 2010 has been endorsed by 14 local and world-renowned international professional organizations in physical education, physical activity, exercise science, and health.

CONCLUSION

The increasing incidence of overweight and obesity calls for an integrative and interconnected solution to this 21st-century challenge. There is a need to connect across disciplines and professional areas to seek solutions to the growing epidemic leading to a rapid rise in the metabolic disease of obesity [112, 113]. Throughout the world, there is growing evidence that lack of physical activity and poor nutritional habits are contributing to this major problem. Rapid modernization and changes in lifestyle reflected on a global scale are now significantly impacting the health of individuals, communities, and nations in the Asian Pacific Region. Developed and developing countries are likewise being affected by these changes. As living standards throughout the world provide greater opportunities to achieve the good life, poorly developed values, attitudes, and behaviors regarding lifestyle issues are, at the same time, reducing the life span and quality of living for many individuals.

Recently, the First Lady of the United States of America, Michelle Obama, declared that her major focus will be addressing the area of childhood obesity and overweight. In February 2010, she unveiled a nationwide campaign known as "Let's Move." This program will develop a national action plan to address this rising concern. Her comprehensive campaign is supported by President Obama, who established an interagency task force to "solve the problem of childhood obesity within a generation of a comprehensive approach that builds effective strategies, engages families and communities, and mobilizes both public and private sector resources" [114].

The challenge to physical education is one for immediate, dynamic, and powerful change. Charles Darwin [115] reminds us that, "It is not the strongest of the species that survives, nor the most intelligent that survives. It is the one that is the most adaptable to change." The pathways of the past must give way to a new set of innovative and creative solutions, methods, and strategies to address this emerging and now significant problem of overweight and obesity especially among children and youth. We are robbing today's children and youth of their future by continuing traditional approaches to teaching physical activities. A new set of best practices must be found and implemented that emphasizes a multidisciplinary approach to promoting healthy, active living. Research and scholarship in physical education must be connected more effectively to the application and implementation of programs. Holistic, integrative solutions must be explored and new collaborative, cooperative partnerships are required to advance physical education in the context of not only the school, but one's entire community life.

Edginton [116] has asked the question, "Has physical education failed?" This question must be addressed in a forthright manner. The evidence is now clear that physical education programs are not only failing to address current challenges, but are rapidly being dismissed throughout the world as a priority for individuals within the schools and in community life in general. Can the profession as a whole respond? Is there a need for an entire new paradigm for teaching physical education, especially one that is designed in a holistic fashion; one that embraces technology as a means for effectively reaching, relating to, and communicating with children and youth; and one that promotes accountability? What is needed is a curriculum design that enables teachers to explain with precision the performance needs of children and youth and their results to parents. Is there a need to rethink the way in which we prepare future physical education teachers so that they have a broader perspective embracing 21st-century themes? If we are to combat the epidemic of overweight and obesity, these challenges must be addressed in a direct and immediate fashion.

AUTHORS' NOTE

Part of this chapter was drawn and modified with permission from the original version of the publication: Chin, M.K., Edginton, C.R., Mok, M.C., Tang, M.S., and Masterson, C. (2009). Obesity Prevention, Physical Activity, Diet and Physical Education in Schools—Current Research, Challenges and Best Practice in the Asia-Pacific Context. Proceeding of 12th World Sport for All Congress on "Sport for All − for Life" organized by the Olympic Council of Malaysia, International Olympic Committee (IOC), World Health Organization (WHO) and General Association of International Sports Federations (GAISF), Genting Highlands, Malaysia, November 3−6, 2008, 25−39.

References

1. Bocarro J, Kanters MA, Casper J, Forrester S. School physical education, extracurricular sports and lifelong active living. *JTPE* 2008;**27**:155−66.
2. McKenzie T, Kahan D. Physical activity, public health, and elementary schools. *ESJ* 2008;**3**:171−9.
3. Freedman DS, Mei Z, Srinivasan SR, Berenson GS, Dieta WH. Cardiovascular risk factors and excess adiposity among overweight children and adolescents: The Bogalusa heart study. *J Pediatr* 2007;**150**:12−17.
4. Hossain P, Kawar B, Nahas EL. Obesity and diabetes in the developing world: a growing challenge. *N Eng J Med* 2007;**356**(3):213−15.
5. World Health Organization. Nutrition Data Banks. *Global data base on obesity and body mass index (BMI) in adults*; 2002. Retrieved April 12, 2002, from http://who.int/nut/obs/htm.
6. Wang Y, Lobstein T. Worldwide trends in childhood overweight and obesity. *Int J Ped Pbesity* 2006;**1**:11−25.
7. Montagu A. *Growing Young*. 2nd eds. CA: Greenwood Publishing Group; 1989.
8. Bauman A, Allman-Farinelli M, Huxley R, James WPT. Leisure-time physical activity alone may not be a sufficient public health approach to prevent obesity: a focus on China. *Obes Rev* 2008;**9**(Suppl.):119−26.
9. International Obesity Task Force. *About obesity*; 2008. Retrieved September 15, 2008, from www.iotf.org.
10. World Health Organization. *Obesity*; 2006. Retrieved March 9, 2010, from http://who.int/mediacentre/factsheets/fs311/en/index.html.
11. Harrington DW, Elliott SJ. Weighing the importance of neighborhood: a multilevel exploration of the determinants of overweight and obesity. *Soc Sci Med* 2009;**68**:593−600.
12. Heber D. An integrative view of obesity. *Am J Clin Nutr* 2010;**91**(Suppl.):280S−3S.
13. Ludwig DS, Pollack HA. Obesity and the economy: from crisis to opportunity. *JAMA* 2009;**301**(5):533−5.
14. Hills AP, King NA, Armstrong TP. The contribution of physical activity and sedentary behaviours to the growth and development of children and adolescents. Implications for overweight and obesity. *Sports Med* 2007;**37**:533−45.
15. Finkelstein EA, Trogdon JG, Cohen JW, Dietz W. Annual medical spending attributable to obesity: payer- and service-specific estimates. *Health Aff* 2009;**28**:W822−31.
16. Trasande L, Liu Y, Fryer G, Weitzman M. Effects of childhood obesity on hospital care and costs, 1999−2005. *Health Affairs* 2009;**28**(4):w751−60.
17. Cook S, Blumkin A, Szilagyi SB. Medical costs of implementing childhood obesity expert recommendations. *Circulation* 2009;**120**:S405.
18. Popkin BM. Recent dynamics suggest selected countries catching up to US obesity. *Am J Clin Nutr* 2010;**91**(Suppl.):284S−8S.
19. World Health Organization. *Global strategy on diet, physical activity and health: childhood overweight and obesity*; 2010. Retrieved March 25, 2010, from www.who.int/dietphysicalactivity/childhood/en.
20. Ogden CL, Carroll MD, Curtin LR, McDowell MA, Tabak CJ, Flegal KM. Prevalence of overweight and obesity in the United States, 1999−2004. *JAMA* 2006;**295**(13):1549−55.
21. Lenders CM, Wright JA, Ludwig DS, Hess DT, Shukla RR, Adams WG, Lee K. Weight loss surgery eligibility criteria according to various BMI criteria in adolescents. *Obesity (Silver Spring)* 2009;**17**:150−5.
22. Katz DL. School-based intervention for health promotion and weight control: not just waiting on the world to change. *Annu Rev Public Health* 2009;**30**:253−72.
23. House of Commons Health Committee. *Obesity: third report of session 2003−04 [online]*; 2003. Retrieved April 30, 2007, from www.publications.parliament.uk/pa/cm200304/cmselect/cmhealth/23/23.pdf.
24. Olshansky SJ, Passaro DJ, Hershow RC, Layden J, Carnes BA, Brody J, Hayflick L, Butler RN, Allison DB, Ludwig DS. A potential decline in life expectancy in the United States in the 21st century. *N Eng J Med* 2005;**352**(11):1138−45.
25. Aekplakorn W, Mo-Suwan L. Prevalence of obesity in Thailand. *Obes Rev* 2009;**10**(6):589−92.
26. Foong MM, Chong YG, Mohd KSZ. Body mass status of school children and adolescents in Kuala Lumpur, Malaysia. *Asia Pac J Clin Nutr* 2004;**13**(4):324−9.
27. Tang JP. Obesity and obstructive sleep apnea hypoponea syndrome in Singapore children. *Ann Acad Med Singapore* 2008;**37**(8):710−14.
28. Matsushita Y, Yoshiike N, Kaneda F, Yoshita K, Takimoto H. Trends in childhood obesity in Japan over the last 25 years from the National Nutrition Survey. *Obes Res* 2004;**12**:205−14.
29. Kim HM, Park J, Kim HS, Kim DH, Park SH. Obesity and cardiovascular risk factors in Korean children and adolescents aged 10−18 years from the Korean National Health and Nutrition Examination Survey, 1998 and 2001. *Am J Epidemiol* 2006;**164**(8):787−93.

30. Chin MK, Yang JZ, Girandola RN, Ding K, Peek-Asa C. Prevalence of obesity and body composition in Hong Kong school children. *JESF* 2006;**4**(2):85—95.
31. Chu NF, Pan WH. Prevalence of obesity and its comorbidities among schoolchildren in Taiwan. *Asia Pac J Clin Nutr* 2007;**16** (S2):601—7.
32. Zhou H, Yamauchi T, Natsuhara K, Yan Z, Lin H, Ichimaru N, Kim SW, Ishii M, Ohtsuka R. Overweight in urban schoolchildren assessed by body mass index and body fat mass in Dalian, China. *J Physiol Anthropol* 2006;**25**(1):41—8.
33. Bhardwaj S, Misra A, Khurana L, Gulati S, Shah P, Vikram NK. Childhood obesity in Asian Indians: a burgeoning cause of insulin resistance, diabetes and sub-clinical inflammation. *Asia Pac J Clin Nutr* 2008;**17**(S1):172—5.
34. Anderson SE, Cohen P, Naumova EN, Jacques PF, Must A. Adolescent obesity and risk for subsequent major depressive disorder and anxiety disorder: prospective evidence. *Pschosom Med* 2007;**69**:740—7.
35. DeMattia L, Denney SL. Childhood obesity prevention: successful community based efforts. *Ann Amer Acad Polit Soc Sci* 2008;**615**(1):83—9.
36. Yach D, Strucker D, Brownell KD. Epidemiologic and economic consequences of the global epidemics of obesity and diabetes. *Nat Med* 2006;**12**:62—6.
37. Committee on Prevention of Obesity in Children and Youth, Food and Nutrition Board, Institute of Medicine (IOM). *Preventing Childhood Obesity: health in the balance*. Washington, D.C: The National Academic Press; 2004.
38. Morrill AC, Chinn CD. The obesity epidemic in the United States. *J Pub Health Policy* 2004;**25**(3-4):353—66.
39. Blackburn GL, Wollner S, Heymsfield SB. Lifestyle interventions for the treatment fo class III obesity: a primary target for nutrition medicine in the obesity epidemic. *Am J Clin Nutr* 2010;**91**(Suppl.):289S—92S.
40. Prentice AM, Jebb S. Energy intake/physical activity interactions in the homeostasis of body weight regulation. *Nutr Rev* 2004;**62**(2):S 98—104.
41. Ismail MN, Chee SS, Nawawi H, Yusoff K, Lim TO, James WPT. Obesity in Malaysia. *Obes Rev* 2002;**3**(3):203—8.
42. Stookey JD. Energy density, energy intake and weight status in a large free-living sample of Chinese adults: Exploring underlying roles of fat, protein, carbohydrate, fiber and water intakes. *Eur J Clin Nutr* 2001;**55**:192—9.
43. Bowman SA, Gortmaker SL, Ebbeling CB, Pereira MA, Ludwig DS. Effects of a fast food consumption on energy intake and diet quality among children in a national household survey. *Pediatrics* 2004;**113**(1):112—18.
44. Malik VS, Schulze MB, Hu FB. Intake of sugar-sweet-ended beverages and weight gain: a systemic review. *Am J Clin Nutr* 2006;**84**(2):274—88.
45. Briefel RR, Crepinsek MK, Cabili C, Wilson A, Gleason PM. School food environment and practices affect dietary behaviors of US public school children. *J Am Diet Assoc* 2009;**109(2)** (Suppl. 1):S91—107.
46. Ebbeling CB, Feldman HA, Osganian SK, Chomitz VR, Ellenbogen SJ, Ludwig DS. Effects of decreasing sugar-sweetened beverage consumption on body weight in adolescents: a randomized, controlled pilot study. *Pediatrics* 2006;**117**(3):673—80.
47. Vartanian LR, Schwartz MB, Brownell KD. Effects of soft Drink consumption on nutrition and health: a systemic review and meta-analysis. *Am J Public Health* 2007;**97**:667—75.
48. Wang YC, Ludwig DS, Sonneville K, Gortmaker SL. Impact of change in sweetened caloric beverage consumption on energy intake among children and adolescents. *Arch Pediatr Adolesc Med* 2009;**163**(4):336—43.
49. Taylor JP, Evers S, McKenna M. Determinants of healthy eating in children and youth. *Can J Public Health* 2005;**96**(Suppl. 3): S20—6, S22—9.
50. ACNielsen Online Survey. *A 360° view of fast food and impulse habits*; 2004. Retrieved March 29, 2009, from http://asiapacific.acnielsen.com/pubs/2005_q2_ap_fastfood.shtml.
51. Yum Brands. *Yum! China*; 2010. Retrieved March 10, 2010, from www.yum.com/company/china.asp.
52. CHINAdaily. *McDonald's growing in China*; 2008. Retrieved March 10, 2010, from www.yum.com/company/china.asp.
53. Ho A, Gupta N, Musa H, Giet KM, Huang LL, Sin WL, Thor. D. *Survey on the fast food habits of Singaporean children. Paper presented at the Graduate Seminar of Physical Education and Sports Science*. Nanyang Technological University, Singapore: National Institute of Education; 2007, November.
54. Austin SB, Melly SJ, Sanchez BN, Patel A, Buka S, Gortmaker SL. Clustering of fast-food restaurants around schools: a novel application of spatial statistics to the study of food environments. *Am J Public Health* 2005;**95**(9):1576—81.
55. Horgen KB, Choate M, Brownell KD. Food advertising: targeting children in a toxic environment. In: Singer DG, Singer JL, editors. *Handbook of Children and the Media*. Thousand Oaks, CA: Sage; 2001. pp. 447—62.
56. Andersen LB, Harro M, Sardinha LB, Froberg K, Ekelund U, Brage S, Anderssen SA. Physical activity and clustered cardiovascular risk in children: a cross-sectional study (the European Youth Heart Study). *Lancet* 2006;**368**:299—304.
57. Blair S, Nichaman M. The public health problem of increasing prevalence rates of obesity and what should be done about it. *Mayo Clin Proc* 2002;**77**:109—13.
58. Patrick K, Norman GJ, Calfas KJ, Sallis JF, Zabinski MF, Rupp J, Cella J. Diet, physical activity, and sedentary behaviors as risk factors for overweight in adolescence. *Arch Pediat Adolesc Med* 2004;**158**:385—90.
59. Nelson MC, Neumark-Stzainer D, Hannan PJ, Sirard JR, Story M. Longitudinal and secular trends in physical activity and sedentary behavior during adolescence. *Pediatrics* 2006;**118** (6):e1627—34.
60. Sallis JF, Prochaska JJ, Taylor WC. A review of correlates of physical activity of children and adolescents. *Med Sci Sports Exerc* 2000;**32**(5):309—13.
61. Hardy LL, Bass SL, Booth ML. Changes in sedentary behavior among adolescent girls: a 2.5-year prospective cohort study. *J Adolesc Health* 2007;**40**:158—65.
62. Jordan AB, Hersey JC, McDivtt JA, Heitzler CD. Reducing children's television-viewing time: a qualitative study of parents and their children. *Pediatrics* 2006;**118**(5):1303—10.
63. Rideout VJ, Roberts DF, Foehr UG. *Generation M: media in the lives of 8-18 year-old. Executive summary*. Menlo Park, CA: Henry J. Kaiser Family Foundation; 2005.
64. Boone JE, Gordon-Larsen P, Adair LS, Popkin BM. Screen time and physical activity during adolescence: longitudinal effects on obesity in young adults. *Int J Behav Nutr Phys Act* 2007;**4**:26.
65. Iannotti RJ, Kogan MD, Janssen I, Boyce WF. Patterns of adolescent physical activity, screen-based media use, and positive and negative health indicators in the U.S. and Canada. *J Adolesc Health* 2009;**44**:493—5.
66. Jackson DM, Djafarian K, Stewart J, Speakman JR. Increased television viewing is associated with elevated body fatness but not with lower total energy expenditure in children. *Am J Clin Nutr* 2009;**89**:1—6.
67. Temple JL, Giacomelli AM, Kent KM, Roemmich JN, Epstein LH. Television watching increases motivated responding for food and energy intake in children. *Am J Clin Nutr* 2007;**85**:355—61.

68. Institute of Medicine. *Progress in preventing childhood obesity: how do we measure up?* Washington, DC: National Academy Press; 2006.
69. Trust for America's Health. *F as in fat: how obesity policies are failing in America.* Washington, DC: Trust for America's Health; 2006. Retrieved June 29, 2007, from http://healthyamericans.org/reports/obesity2006.
70. Committee on Progress in Preventing Childhood Obesity. Schools. In: Koplan JP, Liverman CT, Kraak VL, Wosja SL, editors. *Progress in preventing childhood obesity: how do we measure up?* Washington, DC: National Academies Press; 2007. pp. 280–325.
71. Pate RR, Davis MG, Robinson TN, Stone EJ, McKenzie TL, Young JC. Promoting PA in children and youth: a leadership role for schools: a scientific statement from the American Heart Association Council on Nutrition, Physical Activity, and Metabolism (Physical Activity Committee) in collaboration with the Councils on Cardiovascular Disease in the Young and Cardiovascular Nursing. *Circulation* 2006;**114**(11):1214–24.
72. Strong WB, Malina RM, Blimkie CJR, Daniels SR, Dishman RK, Gutin B, Hergenroeder AC, Must A, Nixon PA, Pivarnik JM, Rowland T, Trost S, Trudeau F. Evidence based physical activity for school-age youth. *J Pediatr* 2005;**146**:732–7.
73. Jago R, McMurray RG, Bassin S, Pyle L, Bruceker S, Jakicic JM, Moe E, Murray T, Volpe SL. Modifying middle school physical education: piloting strategies to increase physical activity. *Pediatr Exerc Sci* 2009;**21**(2):171–85.
74. Marshall J, Hartman K. The state and status of physical education in schools international context. *Eur Phys Educ Rev* 2006;**6**:203–29.
75. Puhse U, Gerber W. *International comparison of physical education.* Oxford: Meyer & Meyer; 2005. p. 779.
76. National Association for Sport and Physical Education. *Comprehensive School Physical Activity Program [Position statement].* Reston, VA: National Association for Sport and Physical Education; 2003.
77. Burgeson CR. Physical education's critical role in educating the whole child and reducing childhood obesity. *The State Educ Standard* 2004;**5**(2):27–32.
78. Education Bureau. *Key learning areas*; 2007. Retrieved April 1, 2009, from www.edb.gov.hk/index.aspx?langno=1&;nodeID=2879.
79. Education Bureau. *Physical education*; 2007. Retrieved April 1, 2009, from www.edb.gov.hk/index.aspx?nodeID=2408&;langno=1.
80. Curriculum Development Council. *Learning to learn (consultation document), key learning area-physical education [Electronic version]*; 2000. Retrieved February 18, 2007, from www.emb.gov.hk/FileManager/EN/Content_4079/pe-e.pdf.
81. Sallis JF, Prochaska JJ, Taylor WC, Hill JO. Correlates of physical activity in a notional sample of girls and boys in grade 4 through 12. *Health Psychol* 1999;**18**:410–15.
82. Nilges L. Sport philosophy: implications for increasing the activity level of postsecondary adults. *JOPERD* 2005;**76**(8):22–3.
83. Pangrazi R. *Dynamic physical education for elementary school children.* 15th ed. San Francisco: Pearson Benjamin Cummings; 2007.
84. Stodden DF, Goodway JD. The dynamic association between motor skill development and physical activity. *JOPERD* 2007;**78**(8):33–4.
85. Fairclough SJ, Stratton G. Physical education makes you fit and healthy: physical education's contribution to young people's physical activity levels. *Health Educ Res* 2005;**20**(1):14–23.
86. Van Beurden E, Barnett LM, Zask A, Dietrich UC, Brooks LO, Beard J. Can we skill and activate children through primary school physical education lessons? "Move it Groove it": a collaborative health promotion intervention. *Prev Med* 2003;**36**:493–501.
87. McKenzie TL, Catellier DJ, Conway T, Lytle LA, Grieser M, Webber AA, Pratt CA, Elder JP. Girls' activity levels and lesson contexts in middle school PE: TAAG baseline. *Med Sci Sports Science* 2006;**38**:1229–35.
88. American Alliance for Health, Physical Education, Recreation and Dance. *Physical Best activity guide: elementary level.* 2nd ed. Champaign, IL: Human Kinetics; 2005.
89. Chin MK, Yang JZ, Masterson C. Connection between physical education and Physical Best in Hong Kong: an alternative new model of innovative teaching health-related fitness in Asia? *J of ICHPER.SD* 2003;**39**(3):60–4.
90. Cook G. *Killing PE is killing our kids the slow way.* Ed Digest 2005;**71**(2):25–32.
91. Chow JY, Davids K, Button C, Shuttleworth R, Renshaw I, Araujo D. The role of nonlinear pedagogy in physical education. *Rev Educ Res* 2007;**77**:251–78.
92. Dyson B, Griffin LL, Hastie P. Sport education, tactical games and co-operative learning: theoretical and pedagogical considerations. *Quest* 2004;**56**:226–40.
93. Mota J, Silva P, Santos MP, Ribeiro JC, Duarette JA. Physical activity and school recess time: differences between sexes and the relationship between children's playground physical activity and habitual physical activity. *J Sport Sci* 2005;**23**:269–75.
94. Ridgers ND, Stratton G, Fairclough SJ. Assessing physical activity levels during recess using accelerometry. *Prev Med* 2005;**41**(1):102–7.
95. Beighle A, Morgan CF, Masurier GL, Pangrazi RP. Children's physical activity during recess and outside of school. *J Sch Health* 2006;**76**(10):516–20.
96. Sallis JF, Conway TL, Prochaska JJ, McKenzie TL, Marshall SJ, Brown M. The association of school environment with youth physical activity. *AJPH* 2001;**91**(4):618–20.
97. Verstraete SIM, Cardon GM, De Clercq DLR, De Bourdeauhidl IMM. Increasing children's physical activity levels during recess periods in elementary schools: the effects of providing game equipment. *EJPH* 2006;**16**:415–19.
98. Pate RR, O'Neil RR. After-school interventions to increase physical activity among youth. *Br J Sports Med* 2009;**43**:14–18.
99. Salmon J, Booth ML, Phongsavan P, Murphy N, Timperio A. Promoting physical activity participation among children and adolescents. *Epidemiol Rev* 2007;**29**:144–59.
100. Trost SG, Rosenkranz R, Dzewaltowski D. Physical activity levels among children attending after-school programs. *Med Sci Sports Exerc* 2008;**10**(4):622–9.
101. Wofford LG. Systematic review of childhood obesity prevention. *J Ped Nursing* 2008;**23**:5–19.
102. Foster GD, Sherman S, Borradale KE, Grundy KM, Vander SS, Nachmani J, Karpyn A, Kumanyika S, Shults J. A policy-based school intervention to prevent overweight and obesity. *Pediatrics* 2008;**121**:2794–e802.
103. Harringa A. U.S. Secretary of Education inspired by Grundy Center Schools. *The Grundy Register (April, 2009)*; 2009:p.1.
104. Grundy Center City Government. *The Good Life*; 2009. Retrieved March 28, 2009, from www.grundycenter.com/govt/default.asp.
105. Grundy Center Community Schools. *Mission and Vision*; 2009. Retrieved March 13, 2009, from www.grundy-center.k12.ia.us/index.php?option=com_content&;view=frontpage&Itemid=1.
106. POLAR Electro, Inc. *About Polar*; 2009. Retrieved March 13, 2009, from www.polarusa.com/us-en.
107. Korthagen FAJ. *Linking practice and theory: the pedagogy of realistic teacher education.* New York: Routledge; 2001.
108. Juniu S. Implementing handheld computing technology in physical education. *JOPERD* 2002;**73**(3):43–8.

REFERENCES

109. Morgan CF, Pangrazi RP, Beighie A. Using pedometers to promote physical activity in physical education. *JOPERD* 2005;**74**(7):33—8.
110. Edginton CR. (2008, August) Teaching with technology: leading physical education into the 21st century. A paper presented at the 2008 International Convention on Science, Education and Medicine in Sport. Guangzhou, The People's Republic of China.
111. Weir T. *New PE objective: get kids in shape. USA Today*; 2004. Retrieved March 17, 2009, from www.acfn.org/news/121504.
112. Fox KR, Hillsdon M. Physical activity and obesity. *Obes Rev* 2007;**8**(Suppl. 1):115—21.
113. Huang TT, Drewnowski A, Kumanyika SK, Glass TA. A system-oriented multilevel framework for addressing obesity in the 21st century. *Prev Chronic Dis* 2009;**6**(3). Retrieved March 6, 2010, from www.cdc.gov/pcd/issues/2009/jul/09_0013.htm.
114. Teehee K. *Combating childhood obesity in Indian country*; 2010. Retrieved on March 13, 2010, from http://letsmove.gov/blog/obesity_in_indian_country_1.html.
115. Darwin C. Origin of species. *Charles Darwin quotes*; 1859. Retrieved March 28, 2009, from www.brainyquote.com/quotes/authors/c/charles_darwin.html.
116. Edginton CR. Has physical education failed? *AJESS* 2007;**3**(1):1—7.

CHAPTER 33

Schools as "Laboratories" for Obesity Prevention
Proven Effective Models

Michelle Lombardo [*], *Danielle Hollar* [†], *T. Lucas Hollar* [‡], *Karen McNamara* [*]

[*] The OrganWise Guys, Inc., Duluth, GA, USA, [†] Department of Pediatrics, University of Miami Miller School of Medicine, Miami, FL, USA and [‡] Department of Government, Stephen F. Austin State University, Nacogdoches, TX, USA

INTRODUCTION

The National Problem: Obesity

Childhood obesity poses a serious long-term threat to the United States and its healthcare system. In the United States, one third of children and two thirds of adults are classified as overweight or obese, and the prevalence of obesity seems likely to continue to increase in the near future [1, 2]. On the current trajectory, by 2030 obesity trends may result in 86.3% of adults being overweight or obese, and 51.1% of children being overweight or obese. The increasing prevalence of childhood and adult obesity has many implications for the development of cardiovascular and other chronic diseases that affect not only our health but also our economy. In fact, if current trends continue, obesity will account for more than $860 billion of healthcare expenditures in the United States by 2030 [3].

In the United States, schools play a vital role in socializing children in many areas, including eating and health behaviors. In so doing, schools provide a unique context for addressing childhood obesity prevention, and thus improving the health of children. Because children generally attend school 5 days per week during 9 months of the school year, and schools are located in communities of every socioeconomic and racial/ethnic group, they provide ideal locales for obesity prevention initiatives. During school time, there are many opportunities for children to be taught about good nutrition and healthy living practices. Practicing good nutrition and thus cultivating healthy eating behaviors also is possible when children consume school meals as part of the United States Department of Agriculture (USDA) National School Lunch Program (NSLP) and the School Breakfast Program. This is especially true for children from low-income backgrounds who participate in the USDA Free and Reduced Priced Meals Program, many of whom receive a substantial proportion of their daily nutrient requirements at school, often resulting in as much as 51% of daily energy intake [4].

SCHOOLS AS "HUBS" OF OBESITY PREVENTION: A MULTILEVEL, MULTIAGENCY APPROACH

Despite the continual increase in the prevalence of obesity, there is hope for reversing these trends. One such approach requires multilevel, multiagency collaboration to address the multiplicity of factors affecting weight management and its attendant good nutrition and healthy living behaviors. Focusing on individual behavior change alone, in isolation from broader social, cultural, physical, economic, and political contexts, will not work. Multilevel approaches thus are required that address the interpersonal level (feeding styles, family demands, etc.), the community level (foods available in schools and other institutional cafeterias, presence of vending machines and fast food, lack of access to physical activity forums, etc.), and the governmental level (policies regarding food, education, urban design, marketing, etc.) [5].

In our experience, a multilevel, multiagency approach to obesity prevention and treatment takes the form of an "obesity prevention laboratory," whereby synergies of combining proven-effective programs, operated by multidisciplinary collaborators, are achieved using the school as the "hub" for community-based obesity prevention initiatives. In so doing, invited into the laboratory are elementary schools, university (county) extension, nonprofit foundations and organizations (Early Childhood Centers, etc.), professional associations (American Dietetic Association Foundation, School Nutrition Association, etc.), state agencies (agriculture, education, and health), federal agencies (United States Department of Agriculture [USDA], the Centers for Disease Control and Prevention [CDC], etc.), national foundations (W.K. Kellogg Foundation), community-based service organizations (community health centers, etc.), and for-profit companies (Blue Cross/Blue Shield, grocery stores, etc.). These multilevel, multiagency laboratory partners bring a strong set of skills (including nutrition education and outreach, program evaluation, dissemination of best practices/results, and resources for ongoing programming) and the potential for leveraging skills and resources in a way that impacts policies and programs affecting the health of the diverse populations of children and families. Here we describe how The Organ-Wise Guys Comprehensive School Program facilitates the important prevention work of "obesity prevention laboratories," the significant health and academic benefits that can result from laboratory activities, and how such initiatives can be sustained.

Obesity Prevention Tools for Young Children: The OrganWise Guys Comprehensive School Program

Evidence-based programming is key to successful obesity prevention laboratory work. One such program illustrated in this chapter is The OrganWise Guys (OWG) Comprehensive School Program (CSP), which synergizes the nutrition education intervention models used in the Healthier Options for Public Schoolchildren (HOPS) Study (see Box 33.1 and Chapter 31 by Dr. Danielle Hollar and colleagues for more information about this study), and the W.K. Kellogg Foundation (WKKF)-funded Delta HOPE Tri-State (Louisiana, Arkansas, and Mississippi) Healthy Options for People through Extension (HOPE) Initiative (see Box 33.2 for descriptions of HOPE interventions). The OWG CSP thematically integrates an evidence-based set of interventions including nutrition and healthy lifestyle educational curricula focusing on core principles of healthy living (high fiber, low fat, lots of water, exercise) and eating (nutrient-dense foods), nutritious dietary offerings in school cafeterias (and other feeding institutions, particularly those that participate in the USDA feeding and nutrition education programs) that model classroom-based and parent nutrition education programming, increased physical activity, and other school-based projects in a proven-effective manner.

The OWG CSP nutrition and healthy lifestyle program includes curricula that are linked to the state standards for all core subject areas in states that implement the full program, and it is designed to teach children and adults about good nutrition and healthy living. The OWG CSP includes [1] the OWG Core Kit, [2] the Foods of the Month (FoM) Club programming, [3] a physical activity program called WISERCISE!, and [4] Take Charge of Your Health (older child/adult program). The OWG Core Kit is a set of evaluated teaching tools that bring the body to life and facilitate the communication of important health issues in a manner understood by children. This innovative, stand-alone curriculum is sustainable long term because it requires little implementation assistance and is linked to core curricula standards, thus allowing health and nutrition concepts to be incorporated very easily into academic core subjects. OWG HOPE, which included obesity prevention via the OWG Core Kit, received a gold rating by the Cooper Institute, an award based on the evaluation of more than 300 childhood obesity projects nationwide. It also was the recipient of an Innovation in Prevention award from the Department of the Health and Human Services (DHHS). The second component of the OWG CSP, the FoM Club, highlights nutrient-dense, healthy foods and food groups (such as whole grains, good fats, cruciferous vegetables) and includes monthly dissemination of FoM parent newsletters (in English and Spanish), student activity packets, cafeteria cards and posters, and other healthy handouts for parents, teachers, and staff. School cafeterias menu FoM Club items as part of their regularly served meals, thus modeling nutrition education taking place in the classrooms. WISERCISE! is a daily physical activity program for use in the classroom during regular teaching time. This 10-minute desk-side physical activity program for grades K through 5 capitalizes on a child's natural desire to be physically active. WISERCISE! is designed to reduce sedentary time during the school day while promoting positive health messages about physical activity and nutrition. WISERCISE!

BOX 33.1

PILOTING THE "LABORATORIES" FOR OBESITY PREVENTION CONCEPT: HOPS

The Healthier Options for Public School Children (HOPS) Study and Program took place in 80 public elementary schools and 28 after-school sites in seven states (Florida, Illinois, Indiana, Mississippi, New York, North Carolina, and West Virginia), including approximately 39,000 elementary school-age children (two thirds of schools participated in research activities including implementation of nutrition and physical activity interventions as well as data collection twice each year on all children; one third participated by implementing interventions, without data collection activities). HOPS schools included large numbers of minority children and many who qualified for free or reduced-priced meals in the USDA National School Lunch Program.

HOPS began as a research study in six elementary schools (four intervention and two controls) in central Florida in the fall of 2004. The aim of HOPS was to pilot test obesity prevention programming, including the OrganWise Guys Core Kit educational curriculum, foods of the month programming, increased physical activity, and school gardens in an elementary school setting. Educational curricula were *modeled every day in each school cafeteria* through meals served to children. Various groups assisted with implementation of interventions, including teachers, staff, parents/PTAs, food service staff, county extension nutrition educators, USDA master gardeners, and many other members of communities surrounding participating schools—thus creating "obesity prevention laboratories." Efficacy of interventions was evaluated using a quasi-experimental, intervention-control group design. Anthropomorphic (height, weight, waist and hip circumferences) and clinical (blood pressure/pulse) measurements and information about physical activity level, location of meal consumption, and standardized test data were collected for all children in research schools each fall and spring. Dietary interventions were evaluated yearly via nutritional analyses of breakfast and lunch menus of intervention and control schools.

Results of the pilot study described here showed significant improvements in weight, blood pressure, and academic test scores of elementary-aged children, especially among ethnically and racially diverse elementary-aged children who are qualified for free or reduced-priced meals in the United States Department of Agriculture (USDA) National School Lunch Program. Specifically, children in the program implementation schools experienced statistically significantly greater improvements in age- and gender-specific body mass index (BMI) percentiles and weight z-scores [11–13], as well as greater improvements in blood pressure measures, as compared to children in schools that did not participate in the interventions [11]. Additionally, children participating in the program achieved statistically significantly higher Florida Comprehensive Assessment Test (FCAT) math scores as compared to children in control schools. Program children achieved higher FCAT reading scores as well, and although the difference did not reach statistical significance, the data are trending in this direction [12]. Nutritional analyses of 6 weeks of 2005–2006 program and nonprogram breakfast and lunch menus showed nutritional benefits of program lunch and breakfast menus as compared to control menus. In 2005–2006, dietary programming, which models nutrition education activities taking place in classrooms, resulted in approximately 28% less total fat, 21% less saturated fat, and about two times more dietary fiber in intervention versus control school menus [14, 15]. Nutrition analyses of 2006–2007 menus yielded similar results: the program menu resulted in approximately 29% less total fat, 21% less saturated fat, and about one and a half times more dietary fiber than control school menus [16]. The model developed during this pilot study now is rolling out throughout the United States, and there is international interest as well.

---

activities are linked to academic curriculum requirements in math, language arts, and health/nutrition. Finally, the Take Charge of Your Health curriculum teaches older children (middle and high school), staff, and parents about preventive lifestyle behaviors and good nutrition utilizing the same OWG characters and messaging that are used in elementary schools to ensure consistency of preventive messaging across target groups. Implementation of OWG Core Kit, FoM Club programming, WISERCISE!, and Take Charge of Your Health through partnerships with child health and nutrition experts such as university extension nutrition educators, school nurses, and other health and school-based agencies has been proven very replicable [6–10] and effective in significant health [11–13] and academic [12, 13] achievements.

> **BOX 33.2**
>
> ## DELTA HOPE* TRI-STATE (LOUISIANA, ARKANSAS, AND MISSISSIPPI) INITIATIVE
> **Healthy Options for People through Extension (HOPE)*
>
> The Mississippi Alliance for Self-Sufficiency (MASS), a cooperative outreach including the Mississippi Food Network, Inc., of Jackson, Mississippi, implemented a project named the Delta "Healthy Options for People through Extension (HOPE) Tri-State Initiative" (HOPE) in 2004 with the goal of addressing the epidemic of childhood obesity in the Delta region of Mississippi, Louisiana, and Arkansas. This tri-state initiative was a unique collaboration among many organizations in the three states that replicated a successful intervention model piloted in Mississippi in 2003. HOPE was funded by a 4-year, $1.57 million grant from the W.K. Kellogg Foundation of Battle Creek, Michigan.
>
> The HOPE activities focused on the implementation of a comprehensive, school-based nutrition and physical activity program to address childhood overweight and obesity. The target audience included children in grades K through 5, primarily Mississippi schoolchildren in Delta counties (63 schools), with smaller-scale implementation in Delta counties in Louisiana (14 schools) and Arkansas (12 schools). The HOPE program implementation utilized The OrganWise Guys curricula, comprised of innovative educational materials such as books, student activity books, videos, CD-ROMs, as well as an in-classroom physical activity component—all of which are matched with core curricula subject areas. All materials include evaluated teaching tools called The OrganWise Guys, a cast of characters that brings the body to life and facilitates the communication of important health issues in a manner understood by children (and adults). Implementation and evaluation of the HOPE project was led by the Mississippi State University Extension Service Family Nutrition Program (FNP) and statewide members of MASS (including the Mississippi Department of Education Child Nutrition Program, and the Mississippi Department of Agriculture), University of Arkansas Cooperative Extension Service, and Louisiana State University (LSU) AgCenter.
>
> BMI analysis on approximately 1400 HOPE participants suggests that the percentage of students in the overweight and obesity categories declined over time. Further, the percentage of students in the healthy weight category increased over the 3-year period (2004–2007). Specifically, between 2005 and 2007, the percentage of students in the obese category declined from 24.43% to 20.24%. In the baseline year of 2005, 53.13% of students fell within the healthy weight category. In the final intervention year of 2007, 59.12% of students were within a healthy BMI for age percentile suggesting students are shifting from the higher categories to the healthy weight category [17].
>
> This innovative nutrition program received a number of awards, including a gold rating by the Cooper Institute, an award based on an evaluation of more than 300 childhood obesity projects around the country, sponsored by the Dell Foundation, as well as the United States Department of Health and Human Services 2005 Innovation in Prevention Award for a school-based prevention program.

Maintenance and Sustainability of Obesity Prevention Laboratories through Strategic Partnerships

The ultimate outcome of a successful obesity prevention intervention is the ability to improve health outcomes in a manner that is cost effective and sustainable. During the past several years, OWG programming has been a successful tool for creating sustainable partnerships for nutrition education and health improvement, especially among land-grant university cooperative extension agencies, as well as other health-oriented entities and the communities they serve. In so doing, obesity prevention laboratories evolve naturally as collaboratives develop. Partners may provide expertise during education activities, host food tastings, conduct school assemblies, and provide other valuable resources to support sustainability. Likely the most widely used model involves the collaboration of cooperative extension universities, which administer the USDA Supplemental Nutrition Assistance Education Program (SNAP-Ed), with schools and other community-based groups. SNAP-Ed programming allows university partners to use nonfederal resources to leverage federal matching dollars when using science-based nutrition education programming as part of their statewide nutrition education plan. Through SNAP-Ed collaboration, extension nutrition educators train

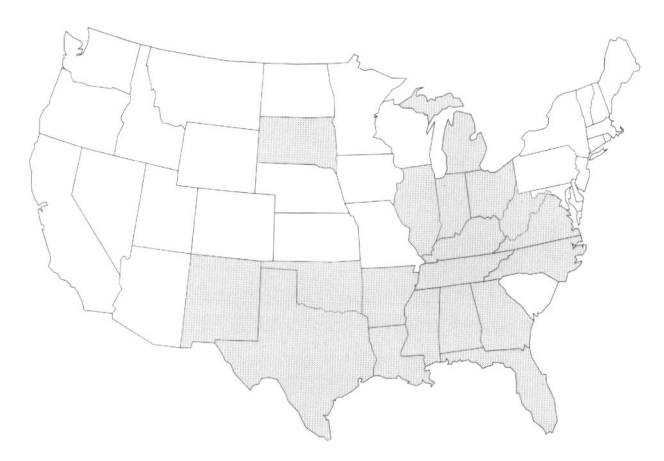

FIGURE 33.1 USDA SNAP-Ed state plans that include OWG programming.

teachers on grade-specific materials, with the aim that teachers conduct nutrition lessons daily as part of their regular lessons. Nutrition instruction by teachers results in federal match funding to further nutrition education efforts and thus provides strong mechanisms for sustained nutrition and health education programming. The OWG CSP is an example of such a program being used in many states as part of their SNAP-Ed state plans, as shown in Figure 33.1. We will describe a few models for SNAP-Ed program implementation that address childhood obesity prevention.

Although the OWG CSP grade-specific curricula remain constant, the method of program implementation can vary from state to state and even county to county within a state. One method is a direct delivery model in which extension nutrition educators deliver the lessons themselves, classroom-by-classroom, leaving behind OWG nutrition-related activities for the classroom teachers to incorporate into their lessons as feasible. This model is an effective tool for nutrition education and is used in a number of locations. However, the human resources required for implementation using this model can limit this method's capacity to reach a large population. Collaboration between the nutrition educator and food service personnel, which takes place in some locations, helps broaden the reach of nutrition programming. This collaboration also provides experiential nutrition education opportunities when children have the opportunity to eat the nutrient-dense foods they learn about during OWG CSP lessons (see Box 33.3 for an example of this collaborative model).

The second method of program dissemination, originally piloted during the WKKF-funded Healthy Options for People through Extension (HOPE) Tri-State Initiative (see Box 33.2), uses a train-the-trainer model whereby classroom teachers deliver the nutrition and healthy lifestyle programming during their daily instruction of language arts, math, science, and the like. In this method, the extension nutrition educator delivers the school assembly, trains teachers on how to use the grade-specific and school-wide OWG materials, supports ongoing nutrition activity, and oversees the program. Being able to energize and inspire classroom teachers to add the OWG CSP to their heavy teaching load has been surprisingly successful. The extension nutrition educator's ability to develop relationships with school administrators and classroom teachers in creating the voluntary commitment to this project is crucial for success. The goal is for teachers to lead some sort of nutrition lesson daily that reinforces healthy lifestyle behaviors, which results in federal match funding being provided to further support extension's efforts in low-income qualified schools. In this model, extension also supports schools through additional individualized classroom education sessions, assistance with school gardening projects, food tastings in classrooms and cafeterias, as well as through a wide variety of other activities addressing the important area of nutrition to the families they serve. In many instances, public-private funding opportunities galvanize this model's implementation.

Public-Private Partnerships

A number of public-private partnerships have developed that create contexts for successful obesity prevention laboratories. Success in implementing these two models, and the attendant healthy, smart results such as those found in the HOPS and HOPE pilot testing projects, namely, significant improvements in health (11–13) and academic achievement [12, 13], increases markedly when these partnerships are in place. Three of the most notable examples are (1) WKKF grant(s), (2) Blue Cross Blue Shield (BCBS) program funding, and (3) the Florida Department of Education and the Blue Foundation for a Healthier Florida statewide project.

In January 2009, the Mississippi Food Network, a food bank system headquartered in Jackson, Mississippi, received a $2 million grant from WKKF to address childhood obesity prevention in six states with large numbers of overweight children: Mississippi, Arkansas, Florida, Louisiana, Michigan, and New Mexico (Fig. 33.2). The project, called Healthy Options for People through Extension Expansion Program 2 (HOPE2), is being implemented in 72 elementary schools where more than 50% of the children qualify for free and reduced-price meals under the United States Department of Agriculture (USDA) National School Lunch Program (NSLP). Led by land-grant extension universities and their local county agents working in

> **BOX 33.3**
>
> ## ST. JOHN'S COUNTY FLORIDA: DIRECT DELIVERY MODEL WITH FOOD SERVICE COLLABORATION
>
> Nutrition education activities in St. Johns County, Florida, schools take place through collaborative efforts of participating schools (including their nurses and cafeterias), USDA master gardeners, other community-based organizations, and the University of Florida Family Nutrition Program, which is the program that implements the Supplemental Nutrition Assistance Program (SNAP) education programming in St. Johns County. This "obesity prevention laboratory," which began as a research site in the Healthier Options for Public Schoolchildren Study, has been very successful, and sustainable, because of the diverse partners.
>
> The OrganWise Guys Comprehensive School Program (OWG CSP) was the primary nutrition intervention tool for the study and has been continued in the poststudy period through efforts of Bonnie Rowe, a St. Johns County extension agent, school nurses, cafeteria managers, and USDA master gardeners. Rowe assists classroom teachers and cafeteria staff in the provision of nutrition education, including hands-on guidance with nutritious food tastings, gardens, and classroom-based nutrition lessons. Food service staff members assist with the food tastings and promote nutrient-dense foods to children. The school nurse and teachers integrate the OWG CSP messages into health and core curricula lessons.
>
> The nutrition education activities of St. Johns County have great impact on the community served through various outreach mechanisms. In addition to the regular nutrition education classes led by Rowe, dissemination of nutrition messages and stories about the program's impact have been the subject of articles in local newspapers and have been presented at a number of national conferences. The Family Nutrition Program itself concluded the school year nutrition lessons at five elementary schools, having presented nutrition education lessons to more than 8000 children. The impact on behavior change is significant—sometimes one may wonder if the program really has an impact on children, and whether food behaviors change. I witness such change quite often. Just a couple of weeks ago, while out shopping, two former students approached me and said, "Aren't you the lady who taught nutrition at my school?" When I answered yes, they both went on to tell me how much it helped them and how they made just one "healthy" change (for both it was to stop drinking soda) and how they had lost weight. One student even said, "You may not recognize me. I used to be kind of fat." That's when I knew our program had made an impact.
>
> *Bonnie Rowe*
> *University of Florida*
> *Family Nutrition Program*

elementary schools, HOPE2 provides the opportunity for these schools and surrounding communities to participate in the OWG CSP evidence-based wellness initiative and is intended to create healthy school environments that reach into the community to address obesity prevention. The creation of obesity prevention laboratories through HOPE2 includes partners such as local grocery stores and produce providers; community health centers; physicians' offices; Women, Infants, and Children (WIC) clinics; Head Start programs; faith-based institutions; food banks; and other institutions that educate and serve children and families. HOPE2 results will be disseminated periodically during the grant period and in final report form in 2012.

The second example of a public-private model developed as a result of the success of the original WKKF HOPE project. Because of the improvements in body mass index (BMI) and nutrition behavior change after HOPE implementation (see Box 33.2 for more information about HOPE results), Louisiana State University (LSU) AgCenter received a 5-year, $1.8 million grant from the Blue Cross and Blue Shield (BCBS) of Louisiana

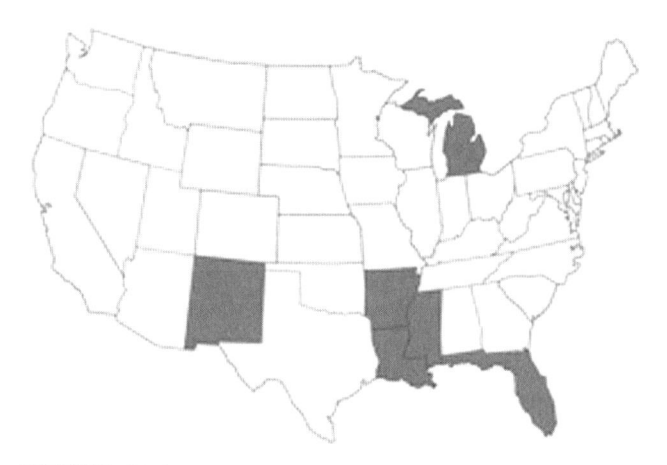

FIGURE 33.2 W.K. Kellogg Foundation-funded HOPE2 state project sites.

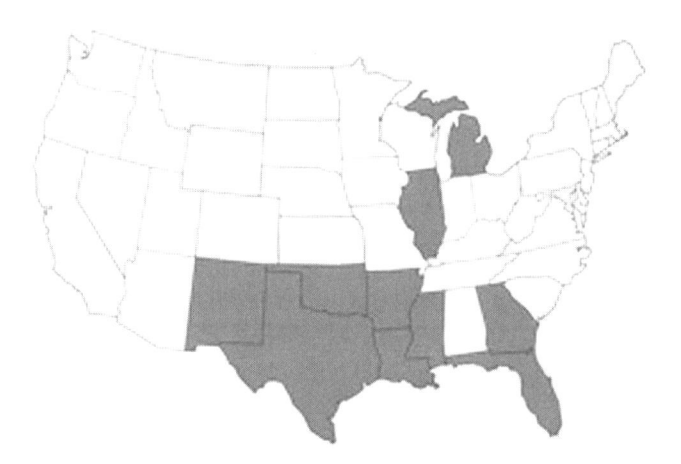

FIGURE 33.3 Public-private partnerships between Blue Cross Blue Shield organizations, university extension (SNAP-Ed), and OWG CSP.

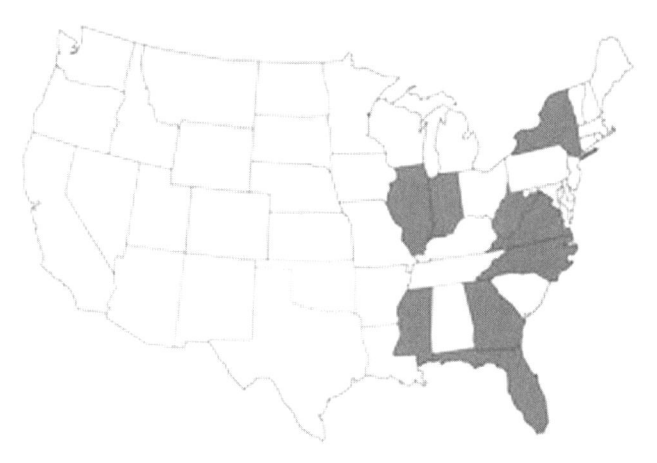

FIGURE 33.4 Locally led OWG CSP obesity prevention initiatives.

Foundation to continue OWG programming (in their signature program entitled Smart Bodies). This led other "Blues" (Fig. 33.3) to fund OWG projects in a variety of models because of the keen interest the health insurance industry has in keeping the insured at a healthy weight. For example, Mississippi State University received multiyear funding support from the BCBS Foundation of Mississippi to increase the reach of OWG programming in its state. In Georgia, the Wellpoint Foundation (BCBS of GA) funded a 3-year OWG project that helped reestablish USDA SNAP-Ed programming in Georgia, which supports sustainability of that project. And in Michigan, BCBS of Michigan uses a grant application process whereby schools apply for the OWG CSP. Implementation includes cultivating relationships between grant recipients and their local extension agents to begin the SNAP-Ed program in their communities, and linkages to other nutrition- and health-supporting local institutions.

In another model, Health Care Service Corporation (HCSC), the parent company of four states' BCBS organizations (Texas, New Mexico, Oklahoma, and Illinois), is funding a 500-school, 5-year rollout of the OWG CSP model as part of its strategic mission to improve the health of its communities as well as its members. Collaboration among schools, university extension (SNAP-Ed), and community-based partners is central to this model. HCSC recently was honored as a finalist of the U.S. Chamber of Commerce's 2009 Corporate Citizenship Award for its work addressing childhood obesity through its OrganWise Guys Community Outreach Program.

In addition to the large-scale projects just described, the final example of a public-private partnership model is evident in locally led initiatives. OWG CSP is being implemented in many locations throughout the United States led by local agencies (Fig. 33.4). Some of these initiatives are small, whereas others have grown organically into large statewide projects. In all of these states, local implementation leaders are cultivating relationships with land-grant universities to leverage their obesity prevention and nutrition education work with USDA SNAP-Ed programming.

One locally led initiative began with the purchase of the OWG Core Kit for 187 elementary schools by the Florida Department of Education/Office of Food and Nutrition Management and Healthy Schools. To enhance nutrition education in these 187 schools, they partnered with University of Florida (UF) Extension, which added these 187 schools into its annual 2009–2010 SNAP-Ed plan. The addition of these schools to the state plan submitted to USDA allows UF to acquire federal match funding to support ongoing nutrition education and outreach. In addition, a grant from the Blue Foundation for a Healthier Florida (the philanthropic affiliate of Blue Cross and Blue Shield of Florida) supports the OWG Foods of the Month nutrient-dense curriculum to all schools with at least 50% of children qualifying for free and reduced-priced meals under the USDA National School Lunch Program. Commencement of this project began in the fall of 2009 when UF extension agents in five counties were trained to implement the program. The agents then trained teachers in their counties on how to use the OWG materials. The amount of time each teacher uses the materials with his or her children will be tracked and reported back to UF extension. UF extension will use its match funds to provide OWG activity books to participating schools as well as to expand and support nutrition education for its intended audience. These activities result in the sustainability of programming as classroom teachers generate additional, substantial match funding for future work. Extension agents also meet with food service personnel to integrate SNAP-Ed nutrition education activities with nutrition and feeding efforts of food service staff with the aim to have seamless, fun programming throughout participating schools. Partnerships with local community-based nonprofit and for-profit organizations, such as Publix Supermarket in Brevard County, Florida, are helping create sustainable obesity prevention laboratories throughout Florida as this program rolls out statewide.

Another example of locally led programming includes collaborative funding from a large national foundation and a regional foundation. In 2007, WKKF and the Oliver Foundation (Houston, Texas) funded a collaborative grant to expand OWG programming nationally. This expansion grant provided for the distribution of 125 OWG Core Kits to elementary schools via a call for proposals (CFP) process whereby a school team, including principals, teachers, and students, completed an application for the kit. The proposals included a plan for how the kit would assist them in strengthening their school's wellness initiatives and policies. As part of the proposal review process, a group of young students, called the Oliver Foundation's Teen Advisory Board (TAB): Youth Excited About Health (YEAH!), was invited to take active roles as "reviewers." All 15 youth took their jobs of "reviewer" seriously and provided specific information that assisted the grant selection team in choosing the grant recipients; at the same time, the students gained experiences and skills needed for success in college, such as managing their time, analyzing information, and providing concise feedback. Active youth involvement was a huge asset to this project, which led to funding nutrition and healthy living programming in 125 schools throughout the United States.

As has been the case with large-scale OWG CSP projects led by university extension, USDA SNAP-Ed programming became a vital component of some of the locally implemented projects, particularly in two states, Indiana and West Virginia. Local organizations in Indiana and West Virginia used their WKKF-Oliver Foundation awards to commence programming in local schools utilizing the OWG CSP as part of USDA SNAP-Ed activities in qualified schools. Because the OWG Core kits are approved by state agencies that administer SNAP-Ed, WKKF-Oliver Foundation awardee schools were able to partner with their states' land-grant university (Purdue University and Marshall University, respectively) to begin the process of including this project into their SNAP-Ed statewide plan, thus allowing for federal dollars to be drawn down for expansion and sustainability of this evidence-based programming throughout their states.

Another aspect of this grant involved the development of 30- and 60-second vignettes (The OrganWise Guys *Shorts!*), essentially public service announcement (PSA)-types of videos, on topics such as eating well, exercise, bone health, drinking water, gardening, smoking cessation, limiting TV, eating breakfast, food safety, healthy snacking/portions, hand washing, and the like. These vignettes have been shown to be useful in providing important health and wellness messages in multiple venues, such as classrooms, school television, after-school sites, community health clinics, and doctors' offices, and they are to be tested soon in grocery stores. Recently, American Public Television began free distribution of the *Shorts!* to public television stations nationwide. Thus, the videos assist in creating obesity prevention laboratories, as messages are available in many locations where people seek services or products. Currently, discussions are in the works for another round of national dissemination of OWG CSP nutrition and healthy living materials using this locally driven model to replicate the successful partnerships, and linkages to SNAP-Ed programming, developed during the WKKF-Oliver Foundation grant period.

Indeed, this public/private partnership model, with its capacity to draw down matching SNAP-Ed funds to leverage and sustain these substantial investments and draw in local partners such as grocery stores and public television stations, has great potential for creating, sustaining, and expanding obesity prevention laboratories.

CONCLUSION

Obesity prevention laboratories are created and sustained through community partners. With the school as a hub of good nutrition and healthy living in action, the messages filter out into the community organically. Using an evidence-based "umbrella" tool such as the OWG CSP and linkages to sustainable funding mechanisms such as the USDA SNAP-Ed nutrition program allows a wide variety of partnerships to develop to share consistent healthy messaging specific to each laboratory partner organizations' causes. Integration of an obesity prevention program that fits well within established programs and agendas, including coordinated school health (Box 33.4), poses the greatest opportunity for community-wide health improvement. The true power of these laboratories lies in community collaborations of diverse organizations (Box 33.5). We, along with our study and program collaborators, continue to test new components in our laboratory with the aim of informing regulatory and programmatic change in nutrition education and feeding policies and programs that serve children in and out of school time, as well as their families. It will take all of us working together to combat the increasing prevalence of obesity in our country and indeed the world at large.

BOX 33.4

EVIDENCE-BASED TOOLS HELP SCHOOLS IMPROVE HEALTH AND ACADEMICS
A Coordinated School Health Approach

Research confirms that good health is important to learning. Although schools don't create the problems students bring with them to school, they need to be part of the solution to improve academic outcomes. In 2004, the Evansville-Vanderburgh School Corporation (EVSC), the third largest urban school district in Indiana with a greater than 53% poverty rate, 38 school buildings, and more than 22,000 students, embarked on a journey utilizing a coordinated school health (CSH) model. This model helps schools assess their level of activity in the areas of health education, nutrition services, physical education, health services, counseling, psychological and social services, a healthy school environment, family/community involvement, and health promotion for staff. All of these areas have an impact on the health and academic achievement of our students. We know there is not often one solution to a problem but many tools that can be utilized to help us help our children to be healthier and achieve the most they can each day. Because of our work implementing a CSH model, in 2009, the Centers for Disease Control and Prevention (CDC) nominated the EVSC as one of six exemplary models in the nation for coordinated school health.

The EVSC began its CSH journey in one school, and based on that school's success, 21 schools now use this evidence-based model. Each school utilized a proven effective school assessment tool, such as the "Healthy School Report Card" or the CDC's "School Health Index," to help identify strengths and weaknesses in the core CSH areas to be addressed. Each school created wellness teams, consisting of staff and community partners who developed 3-year, individualized school action plans. Activities such as these take money and many resources, so grants were applied for (and awarded!) whereby each school committed to complete a set of minimum yet specific activities. These efforts included hiring a wellness coordinator, training PE staff in SPARK (Sports, Play, and Active Recreation for Kids) to improve physical activity during PE class, implementing walking clubs, improving cafeteria food with more fresh fruit, vegetables, and healthier items to choose from, increasing health education for students using community health organizations, exceeding the existing "Wellness Policy of the District," and creating a "climate of wellness within their building." In 2008, the district stopped allowing soft drinks to be sold in schools during the day and went to water, milk products, and 100% juices only. Each school does an extensive evaluation with an outside evaluator; the staff completes health surveys, and for all children in the CSH schools, a number of assessments are conducted twice each school year, including blood pressure, age- and gender-adjusted body mass index percentile, health surveys, and the number of minutes spent in moderate to vigorous physical activity each day. Wide varieties of after-school and summer programs promote healthy physical activities and health education as well as academic programs. Strong collaboration with community health partners have increased health education programs in the schools that are often aligned with state curriculum standards or are research-proven programs. EVSC plans to expand CSH into early childhood development programs beginning in the next few years as well. Outside evaluation of the overall effort leads us to believe these activities are making a profound difference in health and in academics.

With Indiana being one of the most obese states in the nation, nutrition education plays an important role in CSH activities. CSH nutrition education is brought into the classroom, cafeterias, and after-school settings in a variety of forms. One of the newest nutrition education programs, with strong community-based support through our local county extension office that works in low-income elementary schools, is The OrganWise Guys Comprehensive School Program (OWG CSP). The OWG CSP is being implemented in K-5 elementary grades. Utilizing researched-based curricula including a clever doll with the body organs ("OrganWise Guy") that detach, children are learning about the relationship of food and nutrition to the body in a unique and entertaining way. The organs have names like the "Kidney Brothers," "Peter Pancreas," and "Madame Muscle" which endear them to the children. The curriculum is reinforced with visuals that are enchanting to small children. Changing monthly messages go out to staff and parents with information adaptable to school newsletters about nutrient-dense foods we all should consume. Cafeteria posters and placards on tables continue to reinforce the messages in areas where children eat each day. Cafeteria staff members are taught songs to keep the children thinking about the foods they choose. The whole OWG CSP concept is a great, fun way to educate children about the important topic of nutrition without being turned off to the message. Individual schools have a variety of ways of getting the children to try new fruits or vegetables. WISERCISE!, which accompanies the program, encourages teachers to

(Continued)

BOX 33.4 Cont'd

incorporate desk-side exercises into academic subject teaching. As children get restless and tired of sitting, it is often beneficial to have them stand and do a short exercise to get the blood moving again and increase the oxygen flowing to their brains to improve learning. Some schools have staff and students exercise a few minutes during morning announcements. Students on "poster patrol" rotate health and nutrition posters throughout the school to keep messages fresh and for constant reinforcement.

This CSH project has not been an easy journey. It all comes down to building trusting relationships in schools with staff and students and with community organizations. And nothing happens without the buy-in of the superintendent and principals in each school. They are the decision makers. As all districts struggle to improve academics, I would recommend they look at the CSH model. The data collected and the evaluation results are invaluable for several reasons. Kids who are hungry, unhealthy, and sad often come from abusive homes, may be in pain from dental problems, or have not been prepared to begin school, and thus cannot learn to the best of their ability, if at all. A CSH model helps to focus our efforts in a research-proven way and thus make a difference in children's lives every day.

Ginny O'Connor, RN
Former Project Director
EVSC School-Community Council

BOX 33.5

GROWING AN OBESITY PREVENTION LABORATORY THROUGH PUBLIC AND PRIVATE PARTNERSHIPS: NEW MEXICO

New Mexico State University (NMSU) Cooperative Extension Service has conducted nutrition education with limited-resource audiences for 40 years. We use a number of models, including classroom-based instruction by paraprofessional educators (such as our Ideas for Cooking and Nutrition [ICAN]), as well as a "train-the-trainer" model that has enabled NMSU extension to reach more schools without hiring additional staff. Central to our success in the second model, described in more detail below, has been the incorporation of The OrganWise Guys Comprehensive School Program (OWG CSP) into our SNAP-Ed plan.

In this model, our state OWG CSP coordinator and county home economists train school personnel to teach the OWG program to students themselves — thus, thousands of children can be taught about good nutrition and healthy living within the current human resource structure of NMSU extension. Adding OWG CSP to our existing menu of options has enabled us to extend the reach of our program, as well as leverage additional funding. We have been fortunate to receive private funding from Blue Cross Blue Shield of New Mexico (Health Care Service Corporation) and the W.K. Kellogg Foundation to support commencement and expansion of this model. We use these funds to purchase the OWG CSP school kits and the first year of activity books for each new school and to attract federal SNAP-Ed funding match. Also, as teachers use the OWG CSP to teach nutrition education in their classrooms, we are able to track their time and leverage additional federal funds to support sustainability of activities. These additional funds enable us to pay the costs for each school beyond year 1, as well as offer OWG CSP to even more schools in New Mexico each year.

Partnerships with these private entities, as well as the public schools, are strengthened by new alliances with community-based organizations interested in similar nutrition and wellness activities. For example, we have formed an exciting partnership with KRWG-TV, our local public television station. Not only has the station promised to run the OWG interstitials (*Shorts!*), but it plans to feature OWG on a local news show and to film a half-hour special showcasing OWG and other extension health programming. Our "obesity prevention laboratory" is young, but it is growing by leaps and bounds!

Katherine Bachman, MA
New Mexico State University
Cooperative Extension Service

References

1. Ogden CL, Carroll MD, Curtin LR, McDowell MA, Tabak CJ, Flegal KM. Prevalence of overweight and obesity in the United States, 1999−2004. *JAMA* 2006;**295**(13):1549−55.
2. Ogden CL, Carroll MD, Flegal KM. High body mass index for age among US children and adolescents, 2003−2006. *JAMA* 2008;**28**(20):2401−5. 299.
3. Wang Y, Beydoun MA, Liang L, Caballero B, Kumanyika SK. Will all Americans become overweight or obese? Estimating the progression and cost of the US obesity epidemic. *Obesity* 2008;**16**(10):2323−30.
4. Briefel RR, Wilson A, Gleason PM. Consumption of low-nutrient, energy-dense foods and beverages at school, home, and other locations among school lunch participants and nonparticipants. *J Am Diet Assoc* 2009;**109**:S79−90.
5. Huang TTK, Glass TA. Transforming research strategies for understanding and preventing obesity. *JAMA* 2008;**300**(15):1811−13.
6. Hollar D, Agatston AS, McNamara K. *Collaborating on Nutrition Education can be Fun, Simple, and Effective!*. Philadelphia, PA: 2008 Annual Nutrition Conference of the School Nutrition Association; 2008, July.
7. Hollar D, Hollar TL, Agatston AS. *Creating a culture of wellness in elementary schools: An evidence-based prevention study*. Washington, DC: 2007 National Prevention and Health Promotion Summit; 2007, November.
8. Hollar D, McKay J, Campbell J. *Implementing Feasible Wellness Programming…with Outcomes-based Healthy Results*. Orlando, FL: 68th Annual Conference of the National School Board Association; 2008, April.
9. Hollar D, Lombardo M, DiBono M. *Nutrition Education Works! (Especially When Modeled in School Cafeteria Offerings!)*. Atlanta, GA: 2008 Annual Conference of the Society for Nutrition Education; 2008, July.
10. Little D, Lombardo M, Hollar D. *Bringing it All Together Through Extension: The Implementation and Successes of HOPS and HOPE childhood wellness initiatives*. Indianapolis, IN: Galaxy III Educational Programs; 2008, September.
11. Hollar D, Messiah SE, Lopez-Mitnik G, Almon M, Hollar TL, Agatston AS. Effect of a school-based obesity prevention intervention on weight and blood pressure in 6-13 year olds. *Journal of the American Dietetic Association* 2010;**110**(2):261−7.
12. Hollar D, Messiah SE, Lopez-Mitnik G, Almon M, Hollar TL, Agatston AS. Effect of an elementary school-based obesity prevention intervention on weight and academic performance among low income children. *Am J Public Health*. 2010;**100**:646−53.
13. Hollar D, Lombardo M, Lopez-Mitnik G, Almon M, Hollar TL, Agatston AS, Messiah SE. Effective multilevel, multi-sector, school-based obesity prevention programming improves weight, blood pressure, and academic performance, especially among low income, minority children. *Journal of Health Care for the Poor and Underserved* 2010;**21**(2):93−108.
14. Almon M, Gonzalez J, Agatston AS, Hollar TL, Hollar D. *The HOPS Study: dietary component and nutritional analyses*. Los Angeles, CA: Annual Nutrition Conference of the School Nutrition Association; July 17, 2006 (poster, copy available from corresponding author upon request).
15. Almon M, Gonzalez J, Agatston AS, Hollar TL, Hollar D. The dietary intervention of the Healthier Options for Public Schoolchildren Study: A school-based holistic nutrition and healthy lifestyle management program for elementary-aged children. *J Am Diet Assoc* 2006;**106**(8):A53.
16. Gonzalez J, Almon M, Agatston A, Hollar D. The continuation and expansion of dietary interventions of the Healthier Options for Public Schoolchildren Study—a school-based holistic nutrition and healthy lifestyle management program for elementary-aged children. *J Am Diet Assoc Suppl 3* 2007;**107**(8):A76.
17. "Delta H.O.P.E. Tri-State Initiative. Final Report to the Mississippi Alliance for Self-Sufficiency for the period: August 2003 to June 2007". Washington, DC: ILSI Research Foundation; 2007.

CHAPTER 34

Fitness and Fatness in Childhood Obesity
Implications for Physical Activity

Sarah P. Shultz *, *Benedicte Deforche* [†], *Nuala M. Byrne* *, *Andrew P. Hills* *

*Institute of Health and Biomedical Innovation, Queensland University of Technology, Australia and
[†] Department of Human Biometry and Biomechanics, Faculty of Physical Education and Physiotherapy,
Vrije Universiteit Brussel, Belgium; Fund for Scientific Research Flanders (FWO), Belgium;
Department of Movement and Sports Sciences, Ghent University, Belgium

INTRODUCTION

The global epidemic of obesity is widespread and insidious, impacting societies in both developed and developing nations [1]. Overweight and obesity are associated with an increased risk of various health problems including hypertension, hyperlipidemia, diabetes, osteoarthritis, sleep apnea, cardiovascular disease, and some cancers [2]. Physical activity (PA) is health protective and essential for the physical growth and development of children; however, because of increasingly "toxic" and obesogenic environments [3], many young people are not sufficiently active. For many children, sedentary behaviors including television and screen-based games have replaced more active PA behaviors. The decreased level of habitual PA, in combination with poor eating behaviors, has a major impact on positive energy balance and undesirable weight gain in children and adolescents.

Defining Physical Activity, Exercise, and Physical Fitness

The terms "physical activity" and "exercise" are often used interchangeably; however, PA is a broader concept and encompasses "bodily movement that is produced by the contraction of skeletal muscles and that substantially increases energy expenditure" [2 p. 42]. In contrast, exercise is a subset of PA and is defined as "planned, structured, and repetitive bodily movement undertaken to improve or maintain one or more components of physical fitness" [2]. From a broad public health perspective, PA encompasses five main domains, which include leisure time and recreational PA and sport (including exercise), household activity (and yard work), occupational activity, self-powered transportation, and discretionary sedentary activity (including television viewing and playing computer games) [4]. Typically, physical fitness can be considered on the basis of health- and motor- or skill-related components. Health-related components of fitness include body composition, muscular strength and endurance, cardiovascular endurance (aerobic fitness), and flexibility. Motor-related components include balance, power, speed, reaction time, and agility [2]. Numerous health benefits are associated with regular participation in PA including improvements in body composition, cardiometabolic health, and other components of physical fitness [2]. However, significant proportions of many populations are not sufficiently active to gain health benefits and instead suffer from ill-health as a result of physical inactivity [5].

PHYSICAL ACTIVITY, PHYSICAL FITNESS, AND MOTOR COMPETENCE IN OBESE CHILDREN

Physical Activity and Obesity in Children

The consistent trend across a wide range of countries is that obesity is linked to reduced levels of PA. A compilation of data from numerous European countries reported that higher levels of PA participation significantly reduced the likelihood of being overweight in most settings [6]. More recent studies have reported similar findings in non-Western countries such as China [7], Japan [8], South Africa [9], and the Kingdom of Tonga [10]. Because a major limitation of most of these studies is their reliance on self-reported data, objective measurement approaches such as accelerometry have been used to reduce error. Comparisons of PA levels between overweight and normal-weight children using accelerometry have consistently concluded that the overweight are less physically active [11–19]. Further, Wittmeier et al. [20] showed that decreased time spent participating in PA (at both moderate and vigorous intensities) was associated with increased odds of overweight and adiposity. Beyond the results of these cross-sectional studies, available evidence from two recent reviews of longitudinal observational studies suggests that increased PA is protective against relative weight and fatness gains across childhood and adolescence [21, 22]. McMurray et al. [23] found that although PA declined from childhood to adolescence, overweight girls who became normal weight had less of a decline in moderate or vigorous PA than normal-weight girls who became overweight.

The energy expended when performing weight-bearing PA is directly related to body weight [24–26] such that as body weight increases, the energy cost of an activity also increases. Therefore, when the same movement is completed by obese and normal-weight children, the obese will incur a greater absolute energy cost. However, there is considerable confusion in the literature regarding the relationship between PA and obesity in children. In large part, the conflict is due to the lack of comparability between assessment techniques used by studies investigating this relationship. Cross-sectional studies that focused on activity energy expenditure have shown that the proportion of total energy expenditure devoted to PA is comparable in obese and nonobese children [27–30]. Further, longitudinal studies have failed to find any link between reduced energy expenditure and subsequent body weight gain [31–35]. Goran et al. [36] found no relationship between body fat mass and energy cost of PA (using doubly labeled water), whereas time spent performing physical activities (assessed from questionnaire) was inversely related to fat mass. These findings were confirmed by Ekelund et al. [37] who found that accelerometer-derived PA was lower in obese adolescents than controls, whereas energy expenditure did not differ significantly between groups. The increased energy cost of moving a larger body mass explained the lack of between-group differences in activity energy expenditure, despite the fact that the obese group was less physically active. Based on these findings, it has been suggested that activity time rather than activity energy expenditure may be a more important factor in the maintenance of whole body energy stores.

In addition to the inverse relationship between PA levels and obesity, many cross-sectional studies have identified a positive association between overweight status in children and time spent in inactive leisure-time pursuits. A meta-analysis of 39 studies concluded that there was a statistically significant relationship between TV viewing and adiposity among children and adolescents [38]. In comparison to TV viewing, activities such as playing video games and using computers do not appear to be associated with obesity [39, 40]. Several mechanisms have been suggested for the link between TV viewing and overweight and obesity in youth. Because TV viewing can increase dietary intake [41] and expose viewers to food advertisements [42], it is possible to see more of an association with obesity than the "calorie-free" environment found when playing video games [43].

Few studies have investigated the combined influence of PA and TV viewing on the risk of obesity in youth. Sedentary and PA behaviors can coexist so that children who are sufficiently active may also have high screen time. A nationally representative U.S. cross-sectional study found that overweight 4- to 12-year-old children were more likely to have both low levels of self-reported PA and high screen time [44]. A separate representative sample of U.S. youth (14 to 18 years) showed that boys and girls with low levels of TV viewing typically did not have increased risk of overweight regardless of the self-reported PA level; the exception was girls who also had low vigorous-intensity PA levels. Girls who watched moderate and high levels of TV had an increased risk of overweight, regardless of the amount of moderate- or vigorous-intensity PA completed [45]. A third U.S. study [46] found that 7- to 12-year-old children not meeting the PA (13,000 steps/day for boys and 11,000 steps/day for girls) or screen time (no more than 2 hours/day) recommendations were three to four times more likely to be overweight than those complying with both recommendations. Furthermore, those meeting the PA and screen time recommendations were the least likely to be overweight. One longitudinal study investigated the combined effect of PA and sedentary behavior on overweight in youth and found activity level to be protective against overweight regardless of level of inactivity [47].

Physical Fitness in Obese Children

Physical fitness is defined by multiple components that address an individual's ability to perform a task or activity [2]. Body composition is the only health-related fitness component that does not involve a performance-based task; however body composition status indirectly affects other fitness components. For example, fat mass (FM) and fat-free mass (FFM) are positively associated with cardiopulmonary work and should be considered when testing for cardiovascular fitness. Maximum oxygen update (VO_{2max}) is the most common marker of cardiovascular fitness; however, there has commonly been confusion regarding the most appropriate way of expressing VO_{2max} in the obese. Absolute VO_{2max} is increased in obese children [48–50] as a result of both increased FM (associated with increased cardiopulmonary work) [51] and increased FFM (metabolically active tissue, affecting VO_{2max} levels) [52]. Because of the influence of body composition on cardiovascular performance, VO_{2max} should be expressed relative to body mass and FFM. When VO_{2max} is expressed relative to body mass, levels are significantly different between obese and normal-weight children. VO_{2max} relative to body mass explained 37% to 43% and 48% to 49% of variance for body mass index (BMI) and skin fold assessments, respectively, in obese Spanish children [53]. Similarly, a study involving obese Swedish children and adolescents presented a multiple regression analysis in which BMI explained 45% of VO_{2max} relative to body mass [48]. VO_{2max} relative to FFM has been suggested as the optimal method for understanding the capacity of the tissue to maximally consume oxygen and can explain much of the influence of body weight on cardiovascular fitness [54]. In summary, obese children have a higher absolute VO_{2max} and lower relative VO_{2max}, resulting in a poorer performance in weight-bearing activities but a similar performance in non-weight-bearing activities. Because most activities of daily living are weight bearing, the cardiovascular challenge for many obese children could increase the level of difficulty in performing daily tasks and activities.

Health-related fitness also includes flexibility, muscular endurance, and strength. Obese children have shown similar results to normal-weight children when performing flexibility tests, such as the sit-and-reach [55, 56]. Additionally, absolute muscular strength is significantly greater in obese children [55], although no differences exist when strength is normalized to body weight [57]. Muscular endurance tests often include repetitions of gross body movements (e.g., push-ups, curl-ups). Because these tasks involve moving the bulk of body mass quickly and repeatedly, obese children often perform worse [55, 56, 58]. Skill-related physical fitness includes agility, coordination, power, and speed. Agility, power, and speed involve tasks associated with moving body weight, such as shuttle runs, standing broad jumps, and sprints, which are significantly more difficult for obese children and result in lower performance levels [55, 58, 59]. The challenges associated with performing these activities contribute to the promotion of a more sedentary lifestyle and subsequent increase in pediatric obesity.

Fitness tests correlate with habitual PA and are strongly associated with moderate to vigorous PA [16, 60, 61]. Byrd-Williams et al. [62] found that Hispanic boys participate in significantly less moderate to vigorous PA and are at risk of subsequent weight gain related to absolute VO_{2max}. Sports participation and PA outside of school has also been shown to have a protective effect against the accumulation of subcutaneous fat [53], as well as a predictor of 7% of the variance in VO_{2max} [48]. The strong associations found between fitness, PA, and fatness underline the importance of increased levels of PA in obese children. However, the physiological barriers that result in the significant differences in the performance of cardiovascular activities and the inability of the obese to move the excess mass create an environment that promotes physical inactivity.

The associations between physical fitness, PA, and fatness have implications for future health risks in obese children and adolescents. A study investigating children in Denmark, Estonia, and Portugal found that PA levels, fitness (as defined by VO_{2max}), and fatness were independently associated with cardiovascular disease risk [63]. PA levels had the strongest associated risk, which was still significant after adjusting for both fitness and fatness. This was similar to the results of a study investigating associations of fitness, fatness, and PA with cardiovascular disease in Greek children [64]. Additionally, PA levels in Greek children were specifically associated with high-density lipoprotein, the ratio of high-density lipoprotein to total cholesterol, and systolic blood pressure. In a study comparing both fatness and fitness in Taiwanese children, blood pressure was significantly higher in the obese children and obesity had the highest odds risks for hypertension. Taiwanese children with low levels of cardiovascular fitness were also 30% more likely to develop hypertension than their fitter counterparts [56]. Cardiovascular fitness was also inversely correlated to insulin resistance and metabolic syndrome in Italian obese children [65]. Although typically associated with adult obesity, these related health risks have potentially serious consequences for obese children and adolescents.

Balance and Gait in Obese Children

Balance is a skill-related component of physical fitness and is composed of static and dynamic subcategories. Studies based on the adult obese population have shown that excess mass can explain over 50% of the variance for postural control variables [66] and reduce stability in the sagittal plane of leg kinematics during walking [67]. Similar results in the static and dynamic balance systems have been found in obese children. BMI has been negatively correlated to both static and dynamic balance and accounts for 20% of variance for balance-related tasks [68]. Obese children have significantly poorer performance in static balance, specifically when asked to perform a one-legged "stork" stance on a balance beam [69]. Research on adults hypothesized that the heavier weight decreases the sensitivity of the balance control system by providing a constant stimulus to the mechanoreceptors within the plantar aspect of the foot [66]. This is supported by previous research, which has shown mean peak plantar pressures ($N \cdot cm^{-2}$) under the midfoot and metatarsal heads II to V of overweight children [70, 71]. The increased pressures can reduce the sensory feedback associated with the receptors of the foot, thereby decreasing static balance in obese children. Additionally, a greater static balance deficit has been shown in the medial-lateral direction than in the anterior-posterior direction of obese children [72]. The medial-lateral direction is also more heavily influenced by excess mass during dynamic balance, and medial-lateral center of mass displacement is greater in obese children [73]. Directional stability during dynamic balance is controlled by different mechanisms; anterior-posterior stability is maintained through ankle rotation [74], whereas a lateral weight shift from the foot forces is used to stabilize the medial-lateral direction [72]. Additional mass, as well as a greater step width, could affect the ability of an obese child to shift weight laterally and therefore maintain medial-lateral stability. Because activities of daily living and PA create large demands on the balance control system to maintain medial-lateral stability, obese children could find it more difficult to perform these tasks [72]. This suggestion has been supported by a study involving several functional balance tests including sit-to-stand and tandem walking tasks [69]. Moving from a sitting to standing position is a task that is repeated with high frequency during daily life. Obese children transferred weight slower and used less leg force when moving from sitting to standing positions. Obese children also had more difficulty in decelerating forward trunk motion when rising, resulting in greater sway velocity once in the standing position [69]. The difficulty of the obese child to perform the sit-to-stand task increases the amount of time spent in sedentary behavior. During a tandem walking task, obese children walked more slowly and with a lower level of performance [69]. The inability to complete simple movement tasks may reduce an obese child's motivation to participate in more complex PA.

Dynamic balance influences many gait parameters. Previous research has found that obese children have a naturally slower walking cadence than normal-weight children [72, 75]. A mathematical model of the effect of adiposity on balance has demonstrated the need for a large ankle torque in order to control and maintain stability [76]. If this ankle torque is not large enough in obese children (after normalization to body weight), then dynamic stability is decreased during gait. The poor balance control is indicated by the greater step width and base of support used by obese children when walking and sitting, respectively [69]. The most common strategy for maintaining stability in obese children is to increase the double support stance phase with an associated decreased swing phase, thereby extending the amount of time the obese child is supported [72, 75]. The slower, more tentative walking pattern indicates the obese child's desire to prevent falls or other disturbances to his or her functional balance. The obese child has a diminished knee and hip flexion displacement, specifically at heel strike, a mechanism that would allow for easier postural control [75]. Previous research has shown that obese children attempt to actively control the vertical fall of their center of gravity at heel strike, but they may not have sufficient muscular force to do so [77]. Because of this strength deficit, many obese children display a lack of knee flexion and a flatter foot at heel strike within the walking pattern. Foot contact patterns also vary more in overweight children, diminishing the toe clearance during the swing phase and giving the obese child a sense of greater stability [75].

Excess mass in overweight children and adolescents results in both an increase in the absolute amount of force applied to the joint as well as the muscular force needed to move the additional mass during ambulation. Hip, knee, and ankle moments are larger in the sagittal, frontal, and transverse planes of obese children [78, 79] and can increase the risk of skeletal malalignment, orthopedic conditions, and injury. In addition to risk of injury, the greater peak joint moments have consequences on the walking pattern of children, and peak ankle joint moments are increased to control for excessive pronation [80]. Specifically, an increased ankle dorsiflexor moment suggests that obese children require a greater braking mechanism in order to remain upright during gait [78]. Combined with the changes in joint kinematics and kinetics, mechanical power is also altered within the gait of obese children [81]. Concentric contraction of hip flexors occurs more frequently in the gait cycle of overweight children than does eccentric contraction, which creates a higher energy transfer ratio [81]. These findings suggest a change in gait style that is mechanically easier to produce but comes at a higher metabolic cost.

Motor Competence in Obese Children

Several studies have investigated the relationship between overweight and fundamental movement skills in children. Cawley and Spiess [82] found that obesity was associated with an 11.1% lower probability of a perfect score in the motor skills of boys at a very young age (2 to 3 years). Similarly, a study of 4- to 8-year-old children showed that obese males were more likely to have impairment in gross motor skills (i.e., standing on one leg; jumping on one leg; clapping hands) than their normal-weight counterparts [83]. Graf et al. [84] also observed poorer performances on different motor tests concerning gross motor development (i.e., balancing backward, one-legged obstacle jumping, jumping from side to side as well as sideway movements) in overweight 6-year-old boys and girls compared to normal-weight peers. Related studies found that, among grade 1 to 10 students, overweight or obese boys and girls performed selected locomotor skills more poorly than their leaner peers [85, 86]. A study in 9- to 12-year-old children found no differences in fundamental movement skills according to weight status; however, the lack of associations in that study might be due to the small sample size [87]. The observed impairment in gross motor skills in overweight or obese children is generally believed to be the mechanical consequence of a greater inertial load on the system caused by the excess mass of body segments participating in the action.

Linked studies in children from grades 1 to 10 showed that body composition was virtually unrelated to skill proficiency for object control (i.e., catch, overarm throw, kick, and forehand strike) [85, 86]. However, a study by D'Hondt et al. [68] found that normal-weight and overweight 5- to 6-year-old children had better ball skills than obese counterparts. The discrepancy in the findings could be the result of differences in evaluation methods (qualitative and quantitative assessments were used, respectively) or the distinction of overweight and obese children as separate categories. Because D'Hondt et al. [68] showed that being obese, but not overweight, appeared to affect ball skills, this suggests that the extent of overweight may be important in understanding motor skill impairment in children. Previous studies have shown that a well-controlled postural balance is beneficial for ball-handling skills in children [88, 89]. The generally lower balance skills of overweight and obese children might explain the poorer ball skills.

Limited data are available concerning the fine motor skills of obese children. Mond et al. [83] found no differences in the prevalence of impairment in fine body coordination (i.e., finger opposition test) or graphomotor coordination (i.e., drawing different figures, drawing of a person) according to overweight status. However, D'Hondt et al. [68] found a trend toward better performances on manual dexterity in normal-weight and overweight children (5 to 12 years) compared to obese peers. In another study [90], obese children performed poorly on a peg-placing task from a seated position compared to overweight and normal-weight peers, suggesting that obesity affects fine motor skills. D'hondt et al. [68, 90] suggested that poorer fine motor skills could partially be explained by a perceptual-motor deficit in obese children, in addition to the mechanical demands related to the movement of the heavier body part. The proposed deficit could affect sensory information that is used for planning and controlling movement so that a lower movement quality in obese children could be expected in both fine and gross movements of body mass and body segments. The occurrence of poorer motor behavior when sensory information is needed to plan and control the ongoing action has been previously suggested in obese children [91, 92]. However, specific evidence is currently lacking to confirm this hypothesis.

It appears that convincing evidence of an inverse association between overweight status and motor competence is restricted to gross motor skills and that the relationship seems to diminish as less body mass is involved in the task. The negative association between overweight and fundamental movement skills is an important finding because lower skill level may impair participation in regular physical activities. Several studies have shown that young and older children with higher levels of motor skill performance tend to be more physically active than peers with less well-developed motor skills [84, 93–98]. However, it is equally plausible that overweight children are less physically active, which reduces their opportunities to improve motor skills. Additionally, children with poorer motor skills may abstain from participating in physical activities and, as a consequence, have greater risk of weight gain. Improved motor skill has the potential to enhance one's motivation to be physically active through improved self-esteem and enjoyment of physical activity (PA) [86] and should be considered in the design of physical activity programs.

PHYSICAL ACTIVITY GUIDELINES FOR OBESE CHILDREN

PA is an integral part of every child's development, regardless of body composition. PA promotes physical and psychological health and well-being during childhood and adolescence, while simultaneously increasing the probability that a child will remain active as an adult [99]. Informal play, the most common type of PA in children under the age of 5 years, can enhance gross motor skills, muscular strength and endurance, and movement economy. As the child grows and develops, an exposure to more formal PA opportunities can also provide settings to influence social development [100]. Regular PA and appropriate nutrition can positively influence the growth and development of body fat, skeletal muscle, and bone, creating a healthy pattern of physical maturation. Regular weight-bearing activity contributes to the health of the musculoskeletal system, controls weight, minimizes body fat, and reduces blood pressure. If patterns of habitual PA are established at early ages and sustained throughout life, the potential health benefits will continue to positively impact longevity [101]. Because of the relationships between PA in youth and likelihood of PA as an adult, it is important to maintain an adequate level of PA during the transition from childhood to adolescence [102].

Several reviews, including a Cochrane Collaboration [103], have evaluated the efficacy of intervention programs that focused on diet, PA, and related aspects of lifestyle modification. The latest Cochrane review identified 22 studies investigating the effects of diet, physical activity, or combination interventions on the ability to prevent weight gain in children. Although none of the interventions significantly improved BMI, several studies investigating a combination of diet and physical activity modifications showed an improvement in BMI status. Additionally, most studies showed an improvement in diet or physical activity behaviors [103]. An increase in knowledge and a positive attitude toward nutrition and physical activity can help to establish sound behavioral practices in children. Multiple-component interventions commonly incorporate an educational aspect to increase knowledge of nutrition, physical activity, and healthy body image [104–110]. The addition of education, as well as increased physical activity, has resulted in more definitive benefits than interventions that only emphasized increased PA. However, because of the range of settings (primary care, community-based, school, after school), durations of the intervention (12 weeks to 3 years), and types of outcome measures (BMI, body composition, PA levels), a direct comparison of intervention studies is difficult.

Clinical Assessment of the Obese Child

Healthcare providers can play a major role in the identification, evaluation, and management of child obesity. On average, U.S. children see their physician three to five times per year, with overweight children having the potential for more visits. The combination of accessibility through patient visits and a willingness by the child to receive body weight advice from the physician creates an opportunity for the healthcare provider to play a pivotal role in the prevention of weight gain in children. During a patient's visit, it is recommended that the healthcare provider assess and identify the patient's current level of PA using clinical assessment tools. However, research by O'Brien et al. [111] found that only a quarter of young obese patients were asked to give a description of PA and inactivity. One of the models for PA counseling is based on successful smoking abatement programs. Within this model, physicians would need to advise the patient on national guidelines, assist the patient in setting PA goals by providing written exercise prescriptions and self-reporting tools, and arrange for a follow-up exam [112]. Unfortunately, pediatric primary care providers have typically focused on nutritional recommendations with less attention given to increasing PA and reducing sedentary behavior [111]. Additionally, although PA discussions should occur during every visit, only 65% of healthcare providers frequently explained the importance of PA with their patients [113]. Other primary care models have a self-management support component such that physicians can train their patients to problem solve and set goals to better manage their health. This type of intervention has shown increased active days in boys and decreased sedentary behavior in boys and girls and supports the positive impact that can be made by the clinician on the health status of overweight children [112].

Physical Activity Characteristics: Mode

The type of activity used in exercise prescription can vary depending on the individual's age, capabilities, and interests. PA as play is emphasized in younger children (1 to 5 years) and recommendations include a focus on gross motor play and locomotor activities as well as interaction with parents, play spaces, and the outdoor environment whenever possible [100]. The very young child is dependent on the adult caregiver to provide opportunity to facilitate movement and activity. Without this opportunity, the development of PA habits can be negatively altered. As the child grows, pleasure in PA must still be maintained, as well as a level of success in the activity. An increase in exposure to activity will increase the level of motor skills in the individual and provide a greater range of PA options [101]. This presents a challenge for overweight children with poorer motor skills who could become discouraged with complex physical activity tasks. A meta-analysis of exercise treatment programs in obese children and adolescents has shown that the most effective exercise treatment for this population is low-intensity, long-duration aerobic exercise combined with high-repetition resistance training [114]. Resistance training has been shown to be well tolerated by this population and results in positive changes to body composition [115, 116]. Additionally, A Pilot Programme for Lifestyle and Exercise (APPLE) project reduced the rate of weight gain and increased activity levels in children (5 to 12 years old) by encouraging those not interested in traditional sporting activities to participate in lifestyle-based activities (e.g., walking) and nontraditional sports (e.g., golf and taekwondo) during extracurricular time at school, after school, and during vacations [117].

Physical Activity Characteristics: Intensity

Moderate-intensity physical activities such as brisk walking, cycling, and outside play are easier for obese children to sustain and are often recommended as initial components of a weight management program. These activities have a metabolic equivalence (MET) within the range of 3 to 6. As fitness improves, intensity can be progressed to more vigorous levels. Vigorous-intensity PA has a MET value greater than 6 and includes jogging, cycling at a faster pace, and participation in sports such as soccer, tennis, and volleyball [118]. To increase compliance by overweight children, vigorous PA should be considered in terms of enjoyment and competency in the activity [101].

Physical Activity Characteristics: Frequency

PA guidelines for children and adolescents recommend at least three sessions per week; most recommend daily PA. Activity sessions do not need to be long in duration (at least in initial stages) but should be sustained at a moderate–intensity. One study has shown that the number of moderate-to-vigorous PA sessions can impact the risk of becoming overweight, independent of the time spent in each session or the total amount of participation time [119].

Physical Activity Characteristics: Duration

The length of time spent in PA is dependent on the ability of the child to maintain the desired intensity. The general recommendation for children and adolescents is at least 1 hour of moderate- to vigorous-intensity PA each day to achieve health benefits [101, 120]. The American College of Sports Medicine recommend that all children and adolescents complete 20 to 30 minutes per day^{-1} at vigorous–intensity [121]. However, some guidelines suggest that PA can still achieve health benefits in increments as small as 15 minutes [120]. Additionally, the incorporation of 10-minute PA sessions within each classroom day has resulted in significant increases in moderate to vigorous PA in preschool and prepubertal children [106]. Completion of at least 105 minutes per week^{-1} of PA can decrease the likelihood of increased BMI by 68% in preschool girls [122] and 60 minutes per week^{-1} of PA can continue to influence BMI 1 and 2 years after the intervention is completed [123]. Guidelines for PA in adolescents have been detailed to a greater extent than those for children. The U.S. Healthy People 2010 Report promotes cardiac fitness at 60 minutes per week^{-1} of vigorous PA [124], whereas the International Consensus on PA Guidelines for Adolescents recommends a minimum of 60 minutes per week^{-1} of moderate to vigorous PA [99], and the Health Education Authority identifies recommendations of moderate PA for active (60 minutes per day^{-1}) and sedentary (30 minutes per day^{-1}) adolescents [125].

Specific recommendations have been created for the purpose of maintaining or preventing weight gain in children. These recommendations are typically modified from available adult data and used in combination with changes in diet and lifestyle. The completion of 45 minutes of moderate-intensity PA and 15 minutes per day^{-1} of vigorous-intensity physical activity has been associated with reduced BMI and body fat [20]. Additionally, previous research has shown that 120 to 180 minutes per week^{-1} of moderate PA can decrease visceral adiposity in children [126–128]. Other recommendations include moderate PA for 40 continuous minutes per day^{-1} [127] or 60 minutes per day^{-1} of activity divided into sessions lasting a minimum of 15 minutes [120]. Expert committees have recommended 210 to 360 minutes per week^{-1} of moderate PA to prevent weight gain in children [129], although research has shown significant effects on body fat percentage at PA levels lower than the recommended dose [130].

CONCLUSION

Overweight and obesity constitute a significant cause of poor health worldwide, particularly in conjunction with low levels of PA [1]. In the late 1990s, a physically active lifestyle was identified as "public health's best buy" [131 p. 264] following landmark publications on PA and health [2, 132]. More recent publications have referenced the "overwhelming evidence that regular PA has important and wide-ranging health benefits" [133 p. 1]. These benefits include reduced risk of obesity, coronary heart disease, type 2 diabetes, and other related health risks such as many forms of cancer, arthritis, sexual dysfunction, depression, anxiety, mood disorders, and cognitive impairment [132, 134]. Additionally, PA results in a wide range of psychological and social health benefits including improved body image [120, 135], perceived health status [120, 136], and enhanced quality of life [137]. In contrast, time spent in sedentary behaviors including watching television and DVDs and playing computer and other screen-based games reduces daily energy expenditure, and interventions suggest a causal relationship between obesity and sedentary behaviors [138]. Although obese children and adolescents have a unique set of physiological, biomechanical, and neuromuscular barriers to PA, it is important to emphasize participation in the widest possible range of physical activity and movement experiences.

References

1. World Health Organization. *"Obesity: Preventing and managing the global epidemic: report of a WHO consultation"*. Geneva: Switzerland; 2000.
2. U.S. Department of Health and Human Services. *Physical Activity and Health: A Report of the Surgeon General*. Atlanta, GA: U.S. Department of Health and Human Services, Centers for Disease Control and Prevention, National Center for Chronic Disease Prevention and Health Promotion; 1996.
3. Swinburn B, Egger G. The runaway weight gain train: too many accelerators, not enough brakes. *BMJ* 2004;**329**:736—9.
4. Brownson RC, Boehmer TK, Luke DA. Declining rates of physical activity in the United States: what are the contributors? *Annu Rev Public Health* 2005;**26**:421—43.
5. Katzmarzyk PT, Janssen I, Ardern CI. Physical inactivity, excess adiposity and premature mortality. *Obes Rev* 2003;**4**:257—90.
6. Janssen I, Katzmarzyk PT, Boyce WF, Vereecken C, Mulvihill C, Roberts C, Currie C, Pickett W. Comparison of overweight and obesity prevalence in school-aged youth from 34 countries and their relationships with physical activity and dietary patterns. *Obes Rev* 2005;**6**:123—32.
7. Yu CW, Sung RY, So R, Lam K, Nelson EA, Li AM, Yuan Y, Lam PK. Energy expenditure and physical activity of obese children: cross-sectional study. *Hong Kong Med J* 2002;**8**:313—17.
8. Mikami S, Mimura K, Fujimoto S, Bar-Or O. Physical activity, energy expenditure and intake in 11 to 12 years old Japanese prepubertal obese boys. *J Physiol Anthropol Appl Human Sci* 2003;**22**:53—60.
9. Mamabolo RL, Kruger HS, Lennox A, Monyeki MA, Pienaar AE, Underhay C, Czlapka-Matyasik M. Habitual physical activity and body composition of black township adolescents residing in the North West Province, South Africa. *Public Health Nutr* 2007;**10**:1047—56.
10. Smith BJ, Phongsavan P, Havea D, Halavatau V, Chey T. Body mass index, physical activity and dietary behaviours among adolescents in the Kingdom of Tonga. *Public Health Nutr* 2007;**10**:137—44.
11. Deforche B, De Bourdeaudhuij I, D'Hondt E, Cardon G. Objectively measured physical activity, physical activity related personality and body mass index in 6- to 10-yr-old children: a cross-sectional study. *Int J Behav Nutr Phys Act* 2009;**6**:25.
12. Haerens L, Deforche B, Maes L, Cardon G, De Bourdeaudhuij I. Physical activity and endurance in normal weight versus overweight boys and girls. *J Sports Med Phys Fitness* 2007;**47**:344—50.
13. Hughes AR, Henderson A, Ortiz-Rodriguez V, Artinou ML, Reilly JJ. Habitual physical activity and sedentary behaviour in a clinical sample of obese children. *Int J Obes (Lond)* 2006;**30**:1494—500.
14. Janz KF, Levy SM, Burns TL, Torner JC, Willing MC, Warren JJ. Fatness, physical activity, and television viewing in children during the adiposity rebound period: the Iowa Bone Development Study. *Prev Med* 2002;**35**:563—71.
15. Jimenez-Pavon D, Kelly J, Reilly JJ. Associations between objectively measured habitual physical activity and adiposity in children and adolescents: Systematic review. *Int J Pediatr Obes* 2010;**5**(1):3—18.
16. Rowlands AV, Eston RG, Ingledew DK. Relationship between activity levels, aerobic fitness, and body fat in 8- to 10-yr-old children. *J Appl Physiol* 1999;**86**:1428—35.
17. Ruiz JR, Rizzo NS, Hurtig-Wennlof A, Ortega FB, Warnberg J, Sjostrom M. Relations of total physical activity and intensity to fitness and fatness in children: the European Youth Heart Study. *Am J Clin Nutr* 2006;**84**:299—303.
18. Treuth MS, Catellier DJ, Schmitz KH, Pate RR, Elder JP, McMurray RG, Blew RM, Yang S, Webber L. Weekend and weekday patterns of physical activity in overweight and normal-weight adolescent girls. *Obesity (Silver Spring)* 2007;**15**:1782—8.
19. Trost SG, Kerr LM, Ward DS, Pate RR. Physical activity and determinants of physical activity in obese and non-obese children. *Int J Obes Relat Metab Disord* 2001;**25**:822—9.
20. Wittmeier KD, Mollard RC, Kriellaars DJ. Physical activity intensity and risk of overweight and adiposity in children. *Obesity (Silver Spring)* 2008;**16**:415—20.
21. Must A, Tybor DJ. Physical activity and sedentary behavior: a review of longitudinal studies of weight and adiposity in youth. *Int J Obes (Lond)* 2005;**29**(Suppl. 2):S84—96.
22. Reichert FF, Baptista Menezes AM, Wells JC, Carvalho Dumith S, Hallal PC. Physical activity as a predictor of adolescent body fatness: a systematic review. *Sports Med* 2009;**39**:279—94.
23. McMurray RG, Harrell JS, Creighton D, Wang Z, Bangdiwala SI. Influence of physical activity on change in weight status as children become adolescents. *Int J Pediatr Obes* 2008;**3**:69—77.
24. Aull JL, Rowe DA, Hickner RC, Malinauskas BM, Mahar MT. Energy expenditure of obese, overweight, and normal weight females during lifestyle physical activities. *Int J Pediatr Obes* 2008;**3**:177—85.
25. Maffeis C, Schutz Y, Schena F, Zaffanello M, Pinelli L. Energy expenditure during walking and running in obese and non-obese prepubertal children. *J Pediatr* 1993;**123**:193—9.
26. Spadano JL, Must A, Bandini LG, Dallal GE, Dietz WH. Energy cost of physical activities in 12-y-old girls: MET values and the influence of body weight. *Int J Obes Relat Metab Disord* 2003;**27**:1528—33.
27. Bandini LG, Schoeller DA, Dietz WH. Energy expenditure in obese and nonobese adolescents. *Pediatr Res* 1990;**27**:198—203.
28. DeLany JP, Harsha DW, Kime JC, Kumler J, Melancon L, Bray GA. Energy expenditure in lean and obese prepubertal children. *Obes Res* 1995;**3**(Suppl. 1):67—72.
29. Grund A, Dilba B, Forberger K, Krause H, Siewers M, Rieckert H, Muller MJ. Relationships between physical activity, physical fitness, muscle strength and nutritional state in 5- to 11-year-old children. *Eur J Appl Physiol* 2000;**82**:425—38.
30. Treuth MS, Figueroa-Colon R, Hunter GR, Weinsier RL, Butte NF, Goran MI. Energy expenditure and physical fitness in overweight vs non-overweight prepubertal girls. *Int J Obes Relat Metab Disord* 1998;**22**:440—7.
31. Bandini LG, Must A, Phillips SM, Naumova EN, Dietz WH. Relation of body mass index and body fatness to energy expenditure: longitudinal changes from preadolescence through adolescence. *Am J Clin Nutr* 2004;**80**:1262—9.
32. Davies PS, Day JM, Lucas A. Energy expenditure in early infancy and later body fatness. *Int J Obes* 1991;**15**:727—31.
33. Goran MI, Shewchuk R, Gower BA, Nagy TR, Carpenter WH, Johnson RK. Longitudinal changes in fatness in white children: no effect of childhood energy expenditure. *Am J Clin Nutr* 1998;**67**:309—16.
34. Johnson MS, Figueroa-Colon R, Herd SL, Fields DA, Sun M, Hunter GR, Goran MI. Aerobic fitness, not energy expenditure, influences subsequent increase in adiposity in black and white children. *Pediatrics* 2000;**106**:E50.
35. Stunkard AJ, Berkowitz RI, Stallings VA, Schoeller DA. Energy intake, not energy output, is a determinant of body size in infants. *Am J Clin Nutr* 1999;**69**:524—30.
36. Goran MI, Hunter G, Nagy TR, Johnson R. Physical activity related energy expenditure and fat mass in young children. *Int J Obes Relat Metab Disord* 1997;**21**:171—8.
37. Ekelund U, Aman J, Yngve A, Renman C, Westerterp K, Sjostrom M. Physical activity but not energy expenditure is

reduced in obese adolescents: a case-control study. *Am J Clin Nutr* 2002;**76**:935–41.
38. Marshall SJ, Biddle SJ, Gorely T, Cameron N, Murdey I. Relationships between media use, body fatness and physical activity in children and youth: a meta-analysis. *Int J Obes Relat Metab Disord* 2004;**28**:1238–46.
39. Burke V, Beilin LJ, Durkin K, Stritzke WG, Houghton S, Cameron CA. Television, computer use, physical activity, diet and fatness in Australian adolescents. *Int J Pediatr Obes* 2006;**1**:248–55.
40. Rey-Lopez JP, Vicente-Rodriguez G, Biosca M, Moreno LA. Sedentary behaviour and obesity development in children and adolescents. *Nutr Metab Cardiovasc Dis* 2008;**18**:242–51.
41. Matheson DM, Killen JD, Wang Y, Varady A, Robinson TN. Children's food consumption during television viewing. *Am J Clin Nutr* 2004;**79**:1088–94.
42. Dixon HG, Scully ML, Wakefield MA, White VM, Crawford DA. The effects of television advertisements for junk food versus nutritious food on children's food attitudes and preferences. *Soc Sci Med* 2007;**65**:1311–23.
43. Wang X, Perry AC. Metabolic and physiologic responses to video game play in 7- to 10-year-old boys. *Arch Pediatr Adolesc Med* 2006;**160**:411–15.
44. Anderson SE, Economos CD, Must A. Active play and screen time in US children aged 4 to 11 years in relation to sociodemographic and weight status characteristics: a nationally representative cross-sectional analysis. *BMC Public Health* 2008;**8**:366.
45. Eisenmann JC, Bartee RT, Smith DT, Welk GJ, Fu Q. Combined influence of physical activity and television viewing on the risk of overweight in US youth. *Int J Obes (Lond)* 2008;**32**:613–18.
46. Laurson KR, Eisenmann JC, Welk GJ, Wickel EE, Gentile DA, Walsh DA. Combined influence of physical activity and screen time recommendations on childhood overweight. *J Pediatr* 2008;**153**:209–14.
47. Monda KL, Popkin BM. Cluster analysis methods help to clarify the activity-BMI relationship of Chinese youth. *Obes Res* 2005;**13**:1042–51.
48. Berndtsson G, Mattsson E, Marcus C, Larsson UE. Age and gender differences in VO2max in Swedish obese children and adolescents. *Acta Paediatr* 2007;**96**:567–71.
49. Zanconato S, Baraldi E, Santuz P, Rigon F, Vido L, De Dalt L, Zacchello F. Gas exchange during exercise in obese children. *Eur J Pediatr* 1989;**148**:614–17.
50. Marinov B, Kostianev S. Exercise performance and oxygen uptake efficiency slope in obese children performing standardized exercise. *Acta Physiol Pharmacol Bulg* 2003;**27**:59–64.
51. Rowland TW. Effects of obesity on aerobic fitness in adolescent females. *Am J Dis Child* 1991;**145**:764–8.
52. Maffeis C, Schena F, Zaffanello M, Zoccante L, Schutz Y, Pinelli L. Maximal aerobic power during running and cycling in obese and non-obese children. *Acta Paediatr* 1994;**83**:113–16.
53. Ara I, Moreno LA, Leiva MT, Gutin B, Casajus JA. Adiposity, physical activity, and physical fitness among children from Aragon, Spain. *Obesity (Silver Spring)* 2007;**15**:1918–24.
54. Goran M, Fields DA, Hunter GR, Herd SL, Weinsier RL. Total body fat does not influence maximal aerobic capacity. *Int J Obes Relat Metab Disord* 2000;**24**:841–8.
55. Deforche B, Lefevre J, De Bourdeaudhuij I, Hills AP, Duquet W, Bouckaert J. Physical fitness and physical activity in obese and nonobese Flemish youth. *Obes Res* 2003;**11**:434–41.
56. Chen LJ, Fox KR, Haase A, Wang JM. Obesity, fitness and health in Taiwanese children and adolescents. *Eur J Clin Nutr* 2006;**60**:1367–75.
57. Blimkie CJ, Ebbeson B, MacDougall D, Bar-Or O, Sale D. Voluntary and electrically evoked strength characteristics of obese and nonobese preadolescent boys. *Hum Biol* 1989;**61**:515–32.
58. Bovet P, Auguste R, Burdette H. Strong inverse association between physical fitness and overweight in adolescents: a large school-based survey. *Int J Behav Nutr Phys Act* 2007;**4**:24.
59. Brunet M, Chaput JP, Tremblay A. The association between low physical fitness and high body mass index or waist circumference is increasing with age in children: the "Quebec en Forme" Project. *Int J Obes (Lond)* 2007;**31**:637–43.
60. Dencker M, Thorsson O, Karlsson MK, Linden C, Eiberg S, Wollmer P, Andersen LB. Daily physical activity related to body fat in children aged 8–11 years. *J Pediatr* 2006;**149**:38–42.
61. Pate RR, Wang CY, Dowda M, Farrell SW, O'Neill JR. Cardiorespiratory fitness levels among US youth 12 to 19 years of age: findings from the 1999–2002 National Health and Nutrition Examination Survey. *Arch Pediatr Adolesc Med* 2006;**160**:1005–12.
62. Byrd-Williams CE, Shaibi GQ, Sun P, Lane CJ, Ventura EE, Davis JN, Kelly LA, Goran MI. Cardiorespiratory fitness predicts changes in adiposity in overweight Hispanic boys. *Obesity (Silver Spring)* 2008;**16**:1072–7.
63. Andersen LB, Sardinha LB, Froberg K, Riddoch CJ, Page AS, Anderssen SA. Fitness, fatness and clustering of cardiovascular risk factors in children from Denmark, Estonia and Portugal: the European Youth Heart Study. *Int J Pediatr Obes* 2008;**3** (Suppl. 1):58–66.
64. Bouziotas C, Koutedakis Y, Nevill A, Ageli E, Tsigilis N, Nikolaou A, Nakou A. Greek adolescents, fitness, fatness, fat intake, activity, and coronary heart disease risk. *Arch Dis Child* 2004;**89**:41–4.
65. Brufani C, Grossi A, Fintini D, Fiori R, Ubertini G, Colabianchi D, Ciampalini P, Tozzi A, Barbetti F, Cappa M. Cardiovascular fitness, insulin resistance and metabolic syndrome in severely obese prepubertal Italian children. *Horm Res* 2008;**70**:349–56.
66. Hue O, Simoneau M, Marcotte J, Berrigan F, Dore J, Marceau P, Marceau S, Tremblay A, Teasdale N. Body weight is a strong predictor of postural stability. *Gait Posture* 2007;**26**:32–8.
67. Arellano CJ, O'Connor DP, Layne C, Kurz MJ. The independent effect of added mass on the stability of the sagittal plane leg kinematics during steady-state human walking. *J Exp Biol* 2009;**212**:1965–70.
68. D'Hondt E, Deforche B, De Bourdeaudhuij I, Lenoir M. Relationship between motor skill and body mass index in 5- to 10-year-old children. *Adapt Phys Activ Q* 2009;**26**:21–37.
69. Deforche BI, Hills AP, Worringham CJ, Davies PS, Murphy AJ, Bouckaert JJ, De Bourdeaudhuij IM. Balance and postural skills in normal-weight and overweight prepubertal boys. *Int J Pediatr Obes* 2009;**4**(3):175–82.
70. Dowling AM, Steele JR, Baur LA. Does obesity influence foot structure and plantar pressure patterns in prepubescent children? *Int J Obes Relat Metab Disord* 2001;**25**:845–52.
71. Dowling AM, Steele JR, Bauer LA. What are the effects of obesity in children on plantar pressure distributions? *Int J Obes Relat Metab Disord* 2004;**28**:1514–19.
72. McGraw B, McClenaghan BA, Williams HG, Dickerson J, Ward DS. Gait and postural stability in obese and nonobese prepubertal boys. *Arch Phys Med Rehabil* 2000;**81**:484–9.
73. Peyrot N, Thivel D, Isacco L, Morin JB, Duche P, Belli A. Do mechanical gait parameters explain the higher metabolic cost of walking in obese adolescents? *J Appl Physiol* 2009;**106**: 1763–70.

74. Mizrahi J, Susak Z. Bi-lateral reactive force patterns in postural sway activity of normal subjects. *Biol Cybern* 1989;**60**:297–305.
75. Hills AP, Parker AW. Gait characteristics of obese children. *Arch Phys Med Rehabil* 1991;**72**:403–7.
76. Corbeil P, Simoneau M, Rancourt D, Tremblay A, Teasdale N. Increased risk for falling associated with obesity: mathematical modeling of postural control. *IEEE Trans Neural Syst Rehabil Eng* 2001;**9**:126–36.
77. Colne P, Frelut ML, Peres G, Thoumie P. Postural control in obese adolescents assessed by limits of stability and gait initiation. *Gait Posture* 2008;**28**:164–9.
78. Shultz SP, Sitler MR, Tierney RT, Hillstrom HJ, Song J. Effects of pediatric obesity on joint kinematic and kinetics during two walking cadences. *Arch Phys Med Rehabil* 2009;**90**(12):2146–54.
79. Gushue DL, Houck J, Lerner AL. Effects of childhood obesity on three-dimensional knee joint biomechanics during walking. *J Pediatr Orthop* 2005;**25**:763–8.
80. Riegger-Krugh C, Keysor JJ. Skeletal malalignments of the lower quarter: Correlated and compensatory motions and postures. *J Orthop Sports Phys Ther* 1996;**23**:164–70.
81. Nantel J, Brochu M, Prince F. Locomotor strategies in obese and non-obese children. *Obesity* 2006;**14**:1789–94.
82. Cawley J, Spiess CK. Obesity and skill attainment in early childhood. *Econ Hum Biol* 2008;**6**:388–97.
83. Mond JM, Stich H, Hay PJ, Kraemer A, Baune BT. Associations between obesity and developmental functioning in pre-school children: a population-based study. *Int J Obes (Lond)* 2007;**31**:1068–73.
84. Graf C, Koch B, Kretschmann-Kandel E, Falkowski G, Christ H, Coburger S, Lehmacher W, Bjarnason-Wehrens B, Platen P, Tokarski W, Predel HG, Dordel S. Correlation between BMI, leisure habits and motor abilities in childhood (CHILT-project). *Int J Obes Relat Metab Disord* 2004;**28**:22–6.
85. Okely AD, Booth ML, Chey T. Relationships between body composition and fundamental movement skills among children and adolescents. *Res Q Exerc Sport* 2004;**75**:238–47.
86. Southall JE, Okely A, Steele JR. Actual and perceived competence in overweight and non-overweight children. *Pediatric Exercise Science* 2004;**16**:15–24.
87. Hume C, Okely A, Bagley S, Telford A, Booth M, Crawford D, Salmon J. Does weight status influence associations between children's fundamental movement skills and physical activity? *Res Q Exerc Sport* 2008;**79**:158–65.
88. Davids K, Bennett S, Kingsbury D, Jolley L, Brain T. Effects of postural constraints on children's catching behavior. *Res Q Exerc Sport* 2000;**71**:69–73.
89. Savelsbergh GJ, Bennett SJ, Angelakopoulos GT, Davids K. Perceptual-motor organization of children's catching behaviour under different postural constraints. *Neurosci Lett* 2005;**373**:153–8.
90. D'Hondt E, Deforche B, De Bourdeaudhuij I, Lenoir M. Childhood obesity affects fine motor skill performance under different postural constraints. *Neurosci Lett* 2008;**440**:72–5.
91. Petrolini N, Iughetti L, Bernasconi S. Difficulty in visual motor coordination as a possible cause of sedentary behaviour in obese children. *Int J Obes Relat Metab Disord* 1995;**19**:928.
92. Bernard PL, Geraci M, Hue O, Amato M, Seynnes O, Lantieri D. [Influence of obesity on postural capacities of teenagers. Preliminary study]. *Ann Readapt Med Phys* 2003;**46**:184–90.
93. Butcher J, Eaton O. Gross and fine motor proficiency in preschoolers: Relationships with free play behavior and activity level. *J Hum Mov Stud* 1989;**16**:27–36.
94. Fisher A, Reilly JJ, Kelly LA, Montgomery C, Williamson A, Paton JY, Grant S. Fundamental movement skills and habitual physical activity in young children. *Med Sci Sports Exerc* 2005;**37**:684–8.
95. Okely AD, Booth ML, Patterson JW. Relationship of physical activity to fundamental movement skills among adolescents. *Med Sci Sports Exerc* 2001;**33**:1899–904.
96. Saakslahti A, Numminen P, Niinikoski H, Rask-Nissila L, Viikari J, Tuominen J, Valimaki I. Is physical activity related to body size, fundamental motor skills, and CHD risk factors in early childhood? *Pediatr Exerc Sci* 1999;**11**:327–40.
97. Williams HG, Pfeiffer KA, O'Neill JR, Dowda M, McIver KL, Brown WH, Pate RR. Motor skill performance and physical activity in preschool children. *Obesity (Silver Spring)* 2008;**16**:1421–6.
98. Wrotniak BH, Epstein LH, Dorn JM, Jones KE, Kondilis VA. The relationship between motor proficiency and physical activity in children. *Pediatrics* 2006;**118**:e1758–1765.
99. Sallis JF, Patrick K. Physical activity guidelines for adolescents: Consensus statement. *Pediatr Exerc Sci* 1994;**6**:302–314.
100. Timmons BW, Naylor PJ, Pfeiffer KA. Physical activity for preschool children—how much and how? *Can J Public Health* 2007;**98**(Suppl. 2):S122–34.
101. Hills AP, King NA, Armstrong TP. The contribution of physical activity and sedentary behaviours to the growth and development of children and adolescents: Implications for overweight and obesity. *Sports Med* 2007;**37**:533–45.
102. Twisk JW. Physical activity guidelines for children and adolescents: a critical review. *Sports Med* 2001;**31**:617–27.
103. Summerbell C, Waters E, Edmunds LD, Kelly S, Brown T, Campbell KJ. Interventions for preventing obesity in children. *Cochrane Database System Reviews*; 2005. CD001871.
104. Chehab LG, Pfeffer B, Vargas I, Chen S, Irigoyen M. "Energy Up": a novel approach to the weight management of inner-city teens. *J Adolesc Health* 2007;**40**:474–6.
105. Coleman KJ, Geller KS, Rosenkranz RR, Dzewaltowski DA. Physical activity and healthy eating in the after-school environment. *J Sch Health* 2008;**78**:633–40.
106. Honas JJ, Washburn RA, Smith BK, Greene JL, Cook-Wiens G, Donnelly JE. The System for Observing Fitness Instruction Time (SOFIT) as a measure of energy expenditure during classroom-based physical activity. *Pediatr Exerc Sci* 2008;**20**:439–45.
107. McCormick DP, Ramirez M, Caldwell S, Ripley AW, Wilkey D. YMCA program for childhood obesity: a case series. *Clin Pediatr (Phila)* 2008;**47**:693–7.
108. Stock S, Miranda C, Evans S, Plessis S, Ridley J, Yeh S, Chanoine JP. Healthy Buddies: a novel, peer-led health promotion program for the prevention of obesity and eating disorders in children in elementary school. *Pediatrics* 2007;**120**:e1059–1068.
109. Tsai PY, Boonpleng W, McElmurry BJ, Park CG, McCreary L. Lessons learned in using TAKE 10! with Hispanic children. *J Sch Nurs* 2009;**25**:163–172.
110. Gutin B, Yin Z, Johnson M, Barbeau P. Preliminary findings of the effect of a 3-year after-school physical activity intervention on fitness and body fat: the Medical College of Georgia Fitkid Project. *Int J Pediatr Obes* 2008;**3**(Suppl. 1):3–9.
111. O'Brien SH, Holubkov R, Reis EC. Identification, evaluation, and management of obesity in an academic primary care center. *Pediatrics* 2004;**114**:e154–159.
112. Huang JS, Sallis J, Patrick K. The role of primary care in promoting children's physical activity. *Br J Sports Med* 2009;**43**:19–21.
113. Boyle M, Lawrence S, Schwarte L, Samuels S, McCarthy WJ. Health care providers' perceived role in changing environments to promote healthy eating and physical activity: baseline findings from health care providers participating in the healthy

eating, active communities program. *Pediatrics* 2009;**123** (Suppl. 5):S293−300.
114. LeMura LM, Maziekas MT. Factors that alter body fat, body mass, and fat-free mass in pediatric obesity. *Med Sci Sports Exerc* 2002;**34**:487−96.
115. McGuigan MR, Tatasciore M, Newton RU, Pettigrew S. Eight weeks of resistance training can significantly alter body composition in children who are overweight or obese. *J Strength Cond Res* 2009;**23**:80−5.
116. Benson AC, Torode ME, Fiatarone Singh MA. The effect of high-intensity progressive resistance training on adiposity in children: a randomized controlled trial. *Int J Obes (Lond)* 2008;**32**:1016−27.
117. Taylor RW, McAuley KA, Williams SM, Barbezat W, Nielsen G, Mann JI. Reducing weight gain in children through enhancing physical activity and nutrition: the APPLE project. *Int J Pediatr Obes* 2006;**1**:146−52.
118. Haskell WL, Lee I-M, Pate RR, Powell KE, Blair SN, Franklin BA, Macera CA, Heath GW, Thompson PD, Bauman A. Physical Activity and Public Health: Updated Recommendation for Adults from the American College of Sports Medicine and the American Heart Association. *Med Sci Sports Exerc* 2007;**39**:1423−34.
119. Mark AE, Janssen I. Influence of bouts of physical activity on overweight in youth. *Am J Prev Med* 2009;**36**:416−21.
120. Strong WB, Malina RM, Blimkie CJ, Daniels SR, Dishman RK, Gutin B, Hergenroeder AC, Must A, Nixon PA, Pivarnik JM, Rowland T, Trost S, Trudeau F. Evidence based physical activity for school-age youth. *J Pediatr* 2005;**146**:732−7.
121. Dishman RK. Increasing and maintaining exercise and physical activity. *Behav Ther* 1991;**22**:345−78.
122. Mo-suwan L, Pongprapai S, Junjana C, Puetpaiboon A. Effects of a controlled trial of a school-based exercise program on the obesity indexes of preschool children. *Am J Clin Nutr* 1998;**68**:1006−11.
123. Fitzgibbon ML, Stolley MR, Schiffer L, Van HL, KauferChristoffel K, Dyer A. Two-year follow-up results for Hip-Hop to Health Jr.: a randomized controlled trial for overweight prevention in preschool minority children. *J Pediatr* 2005;**146**:618−25.
124. US Department of Health and Human Services. *Healthy People 2010. 2nd ed. With understanding and improving health, and objectives for improving health*. Washington, D.C: U.S. Government Printing Office; 2000.
125. Biddle S, Sallis JF, Cavill N. *Young and Active? Young People and Health-Enhancing Physical Activity-Evidence and Implications*. London: Health Education Authority; 1998.
126. Gutin B, Barbeau P, Owens S, Lemmon CR, Bauman M, Allison J, Kang HS, Litaker MS. Effects of exercise intensity on cardiovascular fitness, total body composition, and visceral adiposity of obese adolescents. *Am J Clin Nutr* 2002;**75**:818−26.
127. Maffeis C, Castellani M. Physical activity: an effective way to control weight in children? *Nutr Metab Cardiovasc Dis* 2007;**17**:394−408.
128. Owens S, Litaker M, Allison J, Riggs S, Ferguson M, Gutin B. Prediction of visceral adipose tissue from simple anthropometric measurements in youths with obesity. *Obes Res* 1999;**7**:16−22.
129. Saris WH, Blair SN, van Baak MA, Eaton SB, Davies PS, Di Pietro L, Fogelholm M, Rissanen A, Schoeller D, Swinburn B, Tremblay A, Westerterp KR, Wyatt H. How much physical activity is enough to prevent unhealthy weight gain? Outcome of the IASO 1st Stock Conference and consensus statement. *Obes Rev* 2003;**4**:101−14.
130. Atlantis E, Barnes EH, Singh MA. Efficacy of exercise for treating overweight in children and adolescents: a systematic review. *Int J Obes (Lond)* 2006;**30**:1027−40.
131. Van Mechelen W. A physically active lifestyle—public health's best buy? *Br J Sports Med* 1997;**31**:264−5.
132. Pate RR, Pratt M, Blair SN, Haskell WL, Macera CA, Bouchard C, Buchner D, Ettinger W, Heath GW, King AC, et al. Physical activity and public health. A recommendation from the Centers for Disease Control and Prevention and the American College of Sports Medicine. *JAMA* 1995;**273**:402−7.
133. Blair S. Physical inactivity: the biggest public health problem of the 21st century. *Br J Sports Med* 2009;**43**:1−2.
134. Penedo FJ, Dahn JR. Exercise and well-being: a review of mental and physical health benefits associated with physical activity. *Curr Opin Psychiatry* 2005;**18**:189−93.
135. Strauss RS, Rodzilsky D, Burack G, Colin M. Psychosocial correlates of physical activity in healthy children. *Arch Pediatr Adolesc Med* 2001;**155**:897−902.
136. Aarnio M, Winter T, Kujala U, Kaprio J. Associations of health related behaviour, social relationships, and health status with persistent physical activity and inactivity: a study of Finnish adolescent twins. *Br J Sports Med* 2002;**36**:360−4.
137. Shoup JA, Gattshall M, Dandamudi P, Estabrooks P. Physical activity, quality of life, and weight status in overweight children. *Qual Life Res* 2008;**17**:407−12.
138. DeMattia L, Lemont L, Meurer L. Do interventions to limit sedentary behaviours change behaviour and reduce childhood obesity? A critical review of the literature. *Obes Rev* 2007;**8**:69−81.

CHAPTER 35

Pharmacotherapy in Childhood Obesity

Amélio F. Godoy-Matos, Erika Paniago Guedes, Luciana Lopes de Souza, Mariana Farage

Serviço de Metabologia do Instituto Estadual de Diabetes e Endocrinologia (IEDE/RJ), Rio de Janeiro, RJ, Brazil

INTRODUCTION

Childhood obesity had been viewed as simply a cosmetic problem, and major risks were only considered when the weight excess persisted into adulthood. Recently, however, overweight and obesity in childhood are known to have a significant impact on both physical and psychosocial health [1].

Discussion on strategies of treating childhood and adolescent obesity has been promoted worldwide, and a variety of scientific articles have been published on this topic. Prevention and effective treatment of obese children and adolescents must be a priority. The cornerstone of health promotion in childhood and adolescence is healthy lifestyle behaviors and therapeutic lifestyle change. As emphasized in pediatric guidelines for cardiovascular health and risk reduction, patterns of dietary intake and physical activity for a majority of children and adolescents are not meeting current recommendations. In most studies, adolescents typically remain overweight after conventional therapy [2]. In contrary, short-term pharmacological therapy was found to be beneficial in obese adolescents, according to some studies [3]. These findings have important clinical relevance and may provide additional treatment options for overweight children and adolescents, especially those with a history of unsuccessful weight loss with traditional therapies [4].

It is important to consider that because children and adolescents' bodies are growing and acquiring muscle, bone, and skin, accurately quantifying the effects of weight management therapy in this population requires the use of age- and sex-corrected growth curves and body mass index (BMI) values [5]. (Growth charts offered by the Center for Disease Control are available at www.cdc.gov/growthcharts, in English, Spanish, or French.)

Management of adult obesity relies on a range of options, including diet, physical activity, behavior modification, pharmacotherapy, and surgery [6, 7]. Ultimately, the treatment of obesity in children shares the same fundamental principles as the treatment in adults (i.e., to decrease caloric intake and increase energy expenditure). The primary goal of treatment (i.e., weight reduction or deceleration of weight gain) and the recommended mode of intervention may depend on the child's age and initial level of overweight, among other considerations.

Therapies with pharmacological agents have been suggested for obese adolescents, as long-term evidence from randomized, controlled trials showing maintenance of substantial weight loss with lifestyle changes still remains sparse. Consistent data are available with orlistat and sibutramine [5, 8–10]. Studies with metformin for the treatment of obesity in adolescents have also been done. Nevertheless, there is scanty data to support its indication. Although several antiobesity drugs are on the market, only orlistat is approved for children aged less than 16 years.

A recently published Endocrine Society Clinical Practice Guideline based on expert opinion suggests that pharmacotherapy (in combination with lifestyle modification) is to be considered in (1) obese children only after failure of a formal program of intensive lifestyle modification and (2) overweight children only if severe comorbidities persist despite intensive lifestyle modification, particularly in children with a strong family history of type 2 diabetes or premature cardiovascular disease. Moreover, only those clinicians who are experienced in the use of antiobesity agents and aware of the potential for adverse reactions should provide pharmacotherapy [11].

Evidence from randomized controlled trials showing that lifestyle changes alone can maintain substantial weight loss in the long-term still remains sparse. On the other hand, there is now abundant evidence from clinical trials in adults showing that orlistat and sibutramine can help patients to maintain long-term clinically meaningful weight loss [12]. However, there are no long-term studies with antiobesity drugs in childhood supporting its chronic use. In truth, the longest studies are of no more than 1-year duration. In addition, it should be noted that the majority of evidence comes from studies on children older than 11 years old.

Despite most endocrinologists and pediatricians being conservative in offering drug therapy for this age group, we believe that there is a place for antiobesity drugs in selected cases.

ORLISTAT

Orlistat is a gastrointestinal tract lipase inhibitor that decreases intestinal fat absorption by up to 30%, thereby potentially establishing a negative energy balance [13]. This inhibition of gastrointestinal lipases prevents the breakdown of triglycerides into absorbable fatty acids and monoglycerides, thereby promoting intact excretion of these triglycerides with feces [14]. In adults, it has a good safety profile, is generally well tolerated, has minimal systemic absorption, and produces clinically meaningful and sustained decreases in weight and BMI when combined with a mildly hypocaloric diet and exercise [15–17]. It is approved by Food and Drug Administration (FDA) for use in adolescents aged 12 to 18 years old with BMI more than two units above the 95th percentile for age and gender [5]. Orlistat dosage for adolescents is the same as for adults, 120-mg tid, before meals [14]. Additionally, because orlistat must be consumed at each meal, pediatric patients will require therapy during school hours, which adds logistical complications to the regimen [14].

Pooled meta-analysis in 579 adolescents from two studies, found an additional effect of orlistat over placebo on absolute BMI after 6 months follow-up when given in combination with a lifestyle intervention [5, 18]. In a 1-year study evaluation, orlistat was associated with a decrease in weight of 2.61 kg and in BMI of 0.86. Although the latter is lower than the power goal of the study, it is within the 95% confidence interval of the difference (0.37 to 1.34) [5]. Although it may be considered a small decrease in weight, it was similar to that observed after studies in adults [16, 17].

Studies with orlistat in adults demonstrated additional efficacy in metabolic control, such as in glycemic and lipids profiles [16, 17]. These effects were evaluated as secondary efficacy parameters in adolescents, but orlistat generally demonstrated minimal effects on these metabolic risk factors, compared with placebo [19]. A possible reason for this finding was the fact that lipid and glucose levels and diastolic and systolic blood pressure were mostly normal at baseline [5].

Orlistat is in general well tolerated by adolescents as demonstrated in few studies. Because of its lack of absorption, no systemic side effects have been shown. The most common types of adverse events are those associated with the gastrointestinal tract (GIT). Indeed, they were more prevalent in the orlistat as compared with the placebo intervention [1]. The most common GIT adverse events were fatty/oily stool, oily spotting, increased defecation, cramps, and abdominal pain. These adverse events were generally mild to moderate in intensity and may relate to the mechanism of action of orlistat [5, 20]. Withdrawals resulting from adverse events were higher in the orlistat intervention compared with the placebo/control intervention [1]. In one study, Dual-energy x-ray absorptiometry, obtained from a subset of the study population, demonstrated similar bone mineral content in both groups [5]. In addition, this body composition analysis showed that orlistat did not affect the normal increase in lean body mass physiologically observed in adolescents [5].

There are some concerns regarding possible malabsorption of fat-soluble vitamins (A, D, E, and K) during treatment with orlistat in pediatric population [21]. Plasmatic levels of vitamins A, D, and E have been reported to increase or stay the same, except for one study where vitamin D levels decreased in both the orlistat and placebo interventions [18]. Therefore, a daily multivitamin supplement may be recommended either 2 hours before or after orlistat [13].

SIBUTRAMINE

Sibutramine is an antiobesity agent acting as a nonselective inhibitor of serotonin and noradrenaline reuptake at the presynaptic cleft, thus promoting satiety and reduction in caloric intake [22]. In addition, it has been shown that sibutramine stimulates sympathetic nervous system activity and so could activate thermogenesis [22]. This thermogenic effect could attenuate the expected decline in metabolic rate, maximizing its effect on energy balance, thereby resulting in more weight loss than could be achieved by energy restriction alone. Moreover, the thermogenic activity would allow body weight to become stabilized at a somewhat higher, more acceptable energy intake, and this should aid compliance during long-term weight maintenance [23]. Sibutramine is licensed worldwide for use at 10- to 15-mg qid.

Sibutramine is maybe the most studied drug in young population and has been consistently associated with good results. Indeed, addition of sibutramine to a behavior therapy program in a 12-month placebo-controlled study conducted in obese American adolescents, 12 to 16 years of age, resulted in statistically significant improvements in BMI [9]. At month 12, the estimated mean change in BMI for sibutramine plus behavior therapy was 3.1 kg/m^2 versus 0.3 kg/m^2 for placebo plus behavior therapy (P < 0.001). Additionally, this same group has shown, in a 1 year randomized controlled trial with 498 participants, 12 to 16 years of age, a consistent reduction in BMI and body weight as well as an improved metabolic profile in the sibutramine-treated group [4].

Our group studied 60 Brazilian adolescents, utilizing sibutramine 10 mg a day, in a 6-month randomized, double-blind, placebo-controlled fashion [8]. Patients assigned to the sibutramine group lost an average of 10.3 ± 6.6 kg, and patients in the placebo group lost 2.4 ± 2.5 kg (P < 0.001 for difference between groups). Moreover, more than five times as many adolescents assigned to the sibutramine group (N = 14; 46.6%) reduced their initial body weight by at least 10% in comparison to the placebo group (P < 0.001). Approximately 25% of adolescents assigned to the sibutramine group (N = 7) reduced their initial body weight by at least 15% in comparison to 0% in the placebo group (P < 0 .001) [8].

A subset of obesity in childhood may be more resistant to any kind of treatment, especially to behavioral modification. Within this group, one can include patients with hypothalamic obesity or those accompanied by specific aggravating syndromes like Prader-Willi, Lawrence-Moon-Bardet-Biedl, and others. In general, these patients are not objects for drug studies; however, an interesting study has been done by a Swedish group [24]. They treated 50 such patients with placebo or sibutramine, 10- to 15-mg qid. It was a crossover study, with two periods of 20 weeks each, in a double-blind, randomized fashion, followed by a 28-week open-label period. They clearly demonstrated a clinically and statistical significant weight reduction with sibutramine as compared to placebo. Interestingly, comparing children with hypothalamic (N = 19) versus nonhypothalamic obesity (N = 26), although both exhibited a significant reduction as compared to placebo, the former had a less pronounced effect, thus suggesting a partial resistance to sibutramine treatment [24]. Sibutramine was well tolerated, and adverse events were concordant with the well-known side effects of this drug.

Morbidly obese children and adolescents are also a peculiar subset of patients that nowadays are growing up in incidence [25]. Reisler et al. have shown that sibutramine can be useful in this group of patients, not only to promote weight reduction but also, and maybe most important, to minimize concomitant health problems related to overweight [25]. In this study, 20 adolescents (mean age 15 years 4 months, range 13 to 18 years) with morbid obesity (body mass index above 95th percentile for age or >30 kg/m^2) were treated for 1 year with this behavioral modification plus sibutramine 10 mg. Besides the dropout rate being high (17 patients discontinued the treatment during follow-up period), they could find a significant short-term weight reduction during the first 6 months of treatment. An improvement was observed in patients suffering from concomitant disorders such as severe asthma, hypertension, and obstructive sleep apnea. The main reason for dropout was the slow rate of weight reduction [25]. They had no significant adverse effects, according to what was observed in previous studies with adolescents [4, 8].

Safety of sibutramine has been an issue because of its mechanism of action, and it has been carefully evaluated in adults as well as in adolescents. During adult treatment, consistent side effects of sibutramine therapy included a 0.3 to 2.7 mm Hg increase in systolic blood pressure, a 1.6–3.4 mm Hg increase in diastolic blood pressure, and a two to five beats per minute increase in resting heart rate; other side effects included headache, insomnia, dry mouth, and constipation [26]. Besides constipation and dry mouth the most commonly observed adverse effects in the aforementioned studies with adolescents taking sibutramine was palpitation and tachycardia, which was not reasons for withdrawing from treatment (4, 8, 9). In fact, Berkowitz and collaborators observed mean treatment differences of 1.0 mm Hg, 1.7 mm Hg, and 2.5 beats/min for systolic blood pressure, diastolic blood pressure, and pulse rate respectively. The maximum mean difference in pulse rate (3.7 beats/min) among these patients occurred at month 2 [4]. It should be noted that sibutramine was increased to 15 mg in nearly 50% of patients. This may have contributed to increased side effects. In our hands, sibutramine has been well tolerated. During our study, we performed an echocardiographic evaluation before and after treatment, and no changes were noticed in echocardiographic parameters [8].

One study addressed cardiovascular effects in obese adolescents treated with sibutramine or placebo for 1 year. Curiously, the researchers noticed a similar reduction in blood pressure and heart rate in both groups that was proportional to the amount of weight loss [27].

Sibutramine labeling instructions for adults recommend that all patients taking sibutramine as an ongoing treatment should be monitored for blood pressure and pulse rate. It is important to notice that pulse rate varies throughout childhood and adolescence, but persistent tachycardia (defined by a rate ≥120 beats/minute in older children) should be evaluated as a standard medical care. Sibutramine effects in heart rate and blood pressure in obese adolescents are generally neutralized by the effective reduction in BMI that seems to be even better than that observed in adults [27]. In the United States, sibutramine may be used in adolescents older than 16 years old [10]. Considering the trials where sibutramine was increased to 15-mg qid, it seems that this approach not only did not increase weight loss but also caused more adverse effects. Therefore, it seems reasonable to recommend a dosage of 10-mg qid for the majority of patients.

METFORMIN

Metformin is an insulin sensitizer indicated for treating insulin resistance in type 2 diabetes and polycystic ovary syndrome and is approved for children older than 10 years of age. Metformin reduces hepatic glucose production and plasma insulin levels, inhibits lipogenesis, increases peripheral insulin sensitivity, and may reduce appetite by increasing levels of glucagon-like peptide [28, 29].

Results with metformin, at a daily dose of 1g (0.5g twice daily) or 2g (1g twice daily), as a treatment for obesity in adolescents are contradictories. One study showed a significant improvement in body composition (weight, BMI, waist circumference) and fasting insulin levels in a small number of obese insulin-resistant pediatric patients with metformin therapy versus placebo [30]. A meta-analysis of randomized trials for the treatment of obese children and adolescents gives support for a beneficial metformin effect on obesity outcomes among hyperinsulinemic children and adolescents [31]. Treatment over 6 months has shown to be efficacious in reducing BMI by 1.42 kg/m^2 (equivalent to 0.4 Standard Deviation (SD), based on SD for BMI in U.K. and U.S. adolescents) and Homeostase Model Assessment-Insulin Resistance (HOMA-IR) score by 2.01 (−0.6 SD) [31]. Metformin use was also associated with a small reduction in total cholesterol level (−0.26 SD), but these are unadjusted measures, and it is not possible to determine whether the effects were secondary to reductions in BMI and HOMA-IR or attributable to other factors [32]. However, the effects of metformin on BMI in obese children without diabetes have been synthesized in one published review based on three studies that identified no treatment effect at 6 months (−0.17 kg/m^2 [95% CI −0.62 to −0.28]) [1]. Metformin may not be as effective as behavioral interventions in reducing BMI [1]. When compared with drugs that are licensed for obesity, metformin has moderate effect: meta-analyses of Randomized Clinical Trials (RCTs) reported an orlistat effect of −0.76 kg/m^2 (−1.07 to −0.44) and a sibutramine effect of −1.66 kg/m^2 (−1.89 to −1.43) at 6 months [1]. Nonetheless, the results of this review must be interpreted with caution: studies were of short-term duration and based on small samples; participants were mainly from the United States, and large portions were from ethnic backgrounds known to be at increased risk of metabolic disorders, limiting the generalization of findings; and the studies presented unadjusted measures without intention-to-treat analyses, which may have overestimated treatment effects. Larger, long-term studies across different populations are needed to establish the role of metformin as therapy for obesity and cardiometabolic risk in young people [33].

Metformin has been well tolerated in obese adolescents, with mild and transient adverse events. The most common effects related are abdominal discomfort, diarrhea, and nausea.

CONCLUSION

Children and adolescents may represent a notoriously difficult-to-treat population. In the absence of intervention, overweight and obese adolescents may continue to gain weight rapidly into adulthood. For instance, although only 10% of lean children and adolescents (BMI below the 85th percentile) will become obese adults [34], the majority [83%] of those with a BMI greater than the 95th percentile will [34]. The prevalence of metabolic syndrome among obese children and adolescents has been shown to increase with accelerated weight gain. The onset of cardiovascular complications may also be faster when type 2 diabetes develops in adolescence rather than in adulthood [35]. Nevertheless, even understanding that this is a difficult-to-treat group, adolescents offer the medical community a unique opportunity to hamper the vicious cycle of weight-metabolic disturbance evolution. Adolescents may have more time for physical activity and can be easily motivated and stimulated; therefore, they may obtain better results than adults. Indeed, we treated a group of adults with sibutramine utilizing the same study design and clinical setting used in the adolescent study (Godoy-Matos et al., unpublished results). It was noted that adolescents lost significantly more weight in the placebo as well as in the sibutramine group (Fig. 35.1). This suggests that for the same ethnic population, treated on similar clinical conditions, adolescents may respond much better than adults.

In obese adolescents, slower weight gain has been associated with delayed development of complications such as type 2 diabetes over a 2-year period, suggesting that a therapeutic approach that contributes to

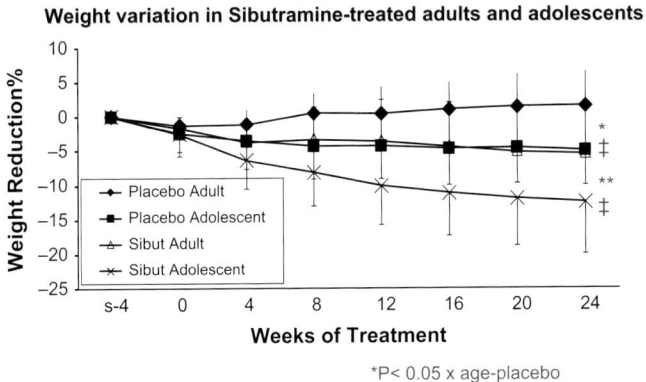

Weight variation in Sibutramine-treated adults and adolescents

*P< 0.05 x age-placebo
**P< 0.001 x age-placebo
‡ p< 0.001 x adol x adults
Godoy-Matos A. et al, unpublished

FIGURE 35.1 Sixty Brazilian adolescents and a similar adult group were assigned to behavioral modification alone or plus sibutramine 10 mg a day, in a 6-month randomized, double-blind, placebo-controlled fashion. The results are shown here.

decreased weight gain is of seminal importance [36]. Numerous factors contribute to obesity, including but not limited to genetic, environmental, metabolic, biochemical, psychological, and physiological factors. These complex causal links make it unlikely that a single intervention will be successful for all obese patients. This would suggest a careful multidisciplinary and multimodality approach [3].

A number of studies, position statements, and guidelines have been published since the late 1990s suggesting that pharmacological intervention is a plausible approach for obesity in this age group [37].

In conclusion, some evidence supports the short-term efficacy and safety of selected pharmacological therapy for children and adolescents; however, the long-term impact of obesity treatments remains unclear.

References

1. Oude Luttikhuis H, Baur L, Jansen H, Shrewsbury VA, O'Malley C, Stolk RP, Summerbell CD. Interventions for treating obesity in children. *Cochrane Database Syst Rev*; 2009. CD001872.
2. Robinson TN. Behavioural treatment of childhood and adolescent obesity. *Int J Obes Relat Metab Disord* 1999;**23**(Suppl. 2):S52−7.
3. McGovern L, Johnson JN, Paulo R, Hettinger A, Singhal V, Kamath C, Erwin PJ, Montori VM. Clinical review: treatment of pediatric obesity: a systematic review and meta-analysis of randomized trials. *J Clin Endocrinol Metab* 2008;**93**:4600−5.
4. Berkowitz RI, Fujioka K, Daniels SR, Hoppin AG, Owen S, Perry AC, Sothern MS, Renz CL, Pirner MA, Walch JK, Jasinsky O, Hewkin AC, Blakesley VA. Effects of sibutramine treatment in obese adolescents: a randomized trial. *Ann Intern Med* 2006;**145**:81−90.
5. Chanoine JP, Hampl S, Jensen C, Boldrin M, Hauptman J. Effect of orlistat on weight and body composition in obese adolescents: a randomized controlled trial. *JAMA* 2005;**293**:2873−83.
6. Fujioka K. Management of obesity as a chronic disease: nonpharmacologic, pharmacologic, and surgical options. *Obes Res* 2002;**10**(Suppl. 2):116S−23S.
7. Clinical Guidelines on the Identification, Evaluation, and Treatment of Overweight and Obesity in Adults: The Evidence Report. National Institutes of Health. *Obes Res* 1998;**6**(Suppl. 2):51S−209S.
8. Godoy-Matos A, Carraro L, Vieira A, Oliveira J, Guedes EP, Mattos L, Rangel C, Moreira RO, Coutinho W, Appolinario JC. Treatment of obese adolescents with sibutramine: a randomized, double-blind, controlled study. *J Clin Endocrinol Metab* 2005;**90**:1460−5.
9. Berkowitz RI, Wadden TA, Tershakovec AM, Cronquist JL. Behavior therapy and sibutramine for the treatment of adolescent obesity: a randomized controlled trial. *JAMA* 2003;**289**:1805−12.
10. Barlow SE. Expert committee recommendations regarding the prevention, assessment, and treatment of child and adolescent overweight and obesity: summary report. *Pediatrics.* 2007;**120**(Suppl. 4):S164−92.
11. August GP, Caprio S, Fennoy I, Freemark M, Kaufman FR, Lustig RH, Silverstein JH, Speiser PW, Styne DM, Montori VM. Prevention and treatment of pediatric obesity: an endocrine society clinical practice guideline based on expert opinion. *J Clin Endocrinol Metab* 2008;**93**:4576−99.
12. Grief SN, Talamayan KS. Preventing obesity in the primary care setting. *Prim Care* 2008;**35**:625−43.
13. Singhal V, Schwenk WF, Kumar S. Evaluation and management of childhood and adolescent obesity. *Mayo Clin Proc.* 2007;**82**:1258−64.
14. Crocker MK, Yanovski JA. Pediatric obesity: etiology and treatment. *Endocrinol Metab Clin North Am* 2009;**38**:525−48.
15. Sjostrom L, Rissanen A, Andersen T, Boldrin M, Golay A, Koppeschaar HP, Krempf M. Randomised placebo-controlled trial of orlistat for weight loss and prevention of weight regain in obese patients. European Multicentre Orlistat Study Group. *Lancet* 1998;**352**:167−72.
16. Davidson MH, Hauptman J, DiGirolamo M, Foreyt JP, Halsted CH, Heber D, Heimburger DC, Lucas CP, Robbins DC, Chung J, Heymsfield SB. Weight control and risk factor reduction in obese subjects treated for 2 years with orlistat: a randomized controlled trial. *JAMA* 1999;**281**:235−42.
17. Torgerson JS, Hauptman J, Boldrin MN, Sjostrom L. XENical in the prevention of diabetes in obese subjects (XENDOS) study: a randomized study of orlistat as an adjunct to lifestyle changes for the prevention of type 2 diabetes in obese patients. *Diabetes Care* 2004;**27**:155−61.
18. Maahs D, de Serna DG, Kolotkin RL, Ralston S, Sandate J, Qualls C, Schade DS. Randomized, double-blind, placebo-controlled trial of orlistat for weight loss in adolescents. *Endocr Pract* 2006;**12**:18−28.
19. Freemark M. Pharmacotherapy of childhood obesity: an evidence-based, conceptual approach. *Diabetes Care* 2007;**30**:395−402.
20. Guerciolini R. Mode of action of orlistat. *Int J Obes Relat Metab Disord* 1997;**21**(Suppl. 3):S12−23.
21. McDuffie JR, Calis KA, Booth SL, Uwaifo GI, Yanovski JA. Effects of orlistat on fat-soluble vitamins in obese adolescents. *Pharmacotherapy* 2002;**22**:814−22.
22. Stock MJ. Sibutramine: a review of the pharmacology of a novel anti-obesity agent. *Int J Obes Relat Metab Disord* 1997;**21**(Suppl. 1):S25−9.
23. Hansen DL, Toubro S, Stock MJ, Macdonald IA, Astrup A. Thermogenic effects of sibutramine in humans. *Am J Clin Nutr* 1998;**68**:1180−6.
24. Danielsson P, Janson A, Norgren S, Marcus C. Impact sibutramine therapy in children with hypothalamic obesity or

obesity with aggravating syndromes. *J Clin Endocrinol Metab* 2007;**92**:4101–6.
25. Reisler G, Tauber T, Afriat R, Bortnik O, Goldman M. Sibutramine as an adjuvant therapy in adolescents suffering from morbid obesity. *Isr Med Assoc J* 2006;**8**:30–2.
26. Weigle DS. Pharmacological therapy of obesity: past, present, and future. *J Clin Endocrinol Metab* 2003;**88**:2462–9.
27. Daniels SR, Long B, Crow S, Styne D, Sothern M, Vargas-Rodriguez I, Harris L, Walch J, Jasinsky O, Cwik K, Hewkin A, Blakesley V. Cardiovascular effects of sibutramine in the treatment of obese adolescents: results of a randomized, double-blind, placebo-controlled study. *Pediatrics* 2007;**120**:e147–57.
28. Zhou G, Myers R, Li Y, Chen Y, Shen X, Fenyk-Melody J, Wu M, Ventre J, Doebber T, Fujii N, Musi N, Hirshman MF, Goodyear LJ, Moller DE. Role of AMP-activated protein kinase in mechanism of metformin action. *J Clin Invest* 2001;**108**:1167–74.
29. Lindsay JR, Duffy NA, McKillop AM, Ardill J, O'Harte FP, Flatt PR, Bell PM. Inhibition of dipeptidyl peptidase IV activity by oral metformin in type 2 diabetes. *Diabet Med* 2005;**22**:654–7.
30. Srinivasan S, Ambler GR, Baur LA, Garnett SP, Tepsa M, Yap F, Ward GM, Cowell CT. Randomized, controlled trial of metformin for obesity and insulin resistance in children and adolescents: improvement in body composition and fasting insulin. *J Clin Endocrinol Metab* 2006;**91**:2074–80.
31. Lee JM, Okumura MJ, Davis MM, Herman WH, Gurney JG. Prevalence and determinants of insulin resistance among U.S. adolescents: a population-based study. *Diabetes Care* 2006;**29**:2427–32.
32. Whincup PH, Cook DG, Adshead F, Taylor S, Papacosta O, Walker M, Wilson V. Cardiovascular risk factors in British children from towns with widely differing adult cardiovascular mortality. *BMJ* 1996;**313**:79–84.
33. Park MH, Kinra S, Ward KJ, White B, Viner RM. Metformin for obesity in children and adolescents: a systematic review. *Diabetes Care* 2009;**32**:1743–5.
34. Whitaker RC, Wright JA, Pepe MS, Seidel KD, Dietz WH. Predicting obesity in young adulthood from childhood and parental obesity. *N Engl J Med* 1997;**337**:869–73.
35. Goran MI, Ball GD, Cruz ML. Obesity and risk of type 2 diabetes and cardiovascular disease in children and adolescents. *J Clin Endocrinol Metab* 2003;**88**:1417–27.
36. Weiss R, Dziura J, Burgert TS, Tamborlane WV, Taksali SE, Yeckel CW, Allen K, Lopes M, Savoye M, Morrison J, Sherwin RS, Caprio S. Obesity and the metabolic syndrome in children and adolescents. *N Engl J Med* 2004;**350**:2362–74.
37. Godoy-Matos AF, Guedes EP, Souza LL, Martins MF. Management of obesity in adolescents: state of art. *Arq Bras Endocrinol Metabol* 2009;**53**:252–61.

CHAPTER 36

Beverage Interventions to Prevent Child Obesity

Rebecca Muckelbauer*, Mathilde Kersting†, Jacqueline Müller-Nordhorn*

**Berlin School of Public Health, Charité University Medical Center, Berlin, Germany and
†Research Institute of Child Nutrition, Dortmund, Germany*

INTRODUCTION

Beverages constitute a significant compound of children's diet, which is, together with physical inactivity, supposed to be a main cause of the obesity epidemic. Beverages are the recommended main source for meeting daily water requirements [1], but they also provide a considerable percentage of about 20% of the dietary energy intake in the habitual diet of children and adolescents [2, 3]. The knowledge about the causing factors of excessive weight gain is indispensable for the development of effective interventions to counteract the rising trend in childhood obesity. The etiology of obesity was shown to be multifactorial, but among the known risk factors, only the environmental and behavioral factors can be influenced. Therefore, previous preventive approaches have focused on the modification of various dietary and physical activity behaviors.

Recently, the dietary factor with the most consistent evidence for an effect on weight gain and obesity was proposed to be the consumption of sugar-containing beverages [4]. These beverages, including soft drinks and fruit juices, are characterized by a high sugar content and their popularity among children and adolescents. Further beverage groups under discussion in the context of body weight regulation and obesity are milk and water. A potentially beneficial role of milk and dairy products in the prevention of obesity in children through several milk components is supposed, but evidence is still equivocal [5–7]. Similarly, total water consumption and the hydration status of the body may affect the regulation of body weight, but this association is controversially discussed [8].

Thus, this chapter describes the current evidence for an effect of the consumption of different beverages and body hydration on the development and prevention of obesity as well as the suggested biological and dietary mechanisms. Finally, an outlook is provided on the future role of beverage interventions against obesity.

BEVERAGES FOR OBESITY INTERVENTIONS

Sugar-Containing Beverages

Definition, Recommendations, and Consumption

In this chapter, the definition of the beverage group "sugar-containing beverages" comprises sugar-sweetened drinks (soft drinks) and fruit juices, but in literature or legislation no consensus exists about terminology and categorization. However, a common characteristic of sugar-containing beverages is the high proportion of sugar that can exceed 10 g per 100 mL resulting in an energy content of 170 kJ or more (Table 36.1). For the subgroup "soft drinks," various terms and definitions have been used in research literature such as "sugar-sweetened beverages" [9] or "energetic drinks" [10]. Definitions also vary between countries; for instance, in the United States only carbonated beverages belong to the group of soft drinks [11], whereas in Germany soft drinks are a heterogeneous group of carbonated and noncarbonated beverages including fruit drinks, lemonades, and soda pop [12]. These different categorizations impede a comparison of the results from studies on the health effects of sugar-containing beverages. The group of fruit juices is often defined by a fruit content of 100%. Beverages with a lower fruit juice content can be called fruit drinks, and their classification to the group of soft drinks is

TABLE 36.1 Content of Energy and Macronutrients in Various Beverages per 100 g[a]

	Drinking water	Soft drink (regular)	Apple juice (100%)	Milk Whole fat (3,5% fat)	Milk Fat reduced (1,5% fat)	Chocolate[b]
Energy (kJ)	0	185	203	272	201	264
Water (g)	100	90	88	87	89	85
Carbohydrates (g)	0	10.9	11.1	4.7	4.8	8.4
Protein (g)	0	0	0.1	3.4	3.4	3.6
Fat (g)	0	0	0	3.6	1.6	1.8

[a]Data are average values obtained from Souci, S. W., Fachmann, W., and Kraut, H. (2008). Die Zusammensetzung der Lebensmittel Nährwert-Tabellen, [The Composition of Food - Tables of Nutrient Contents] 7th ed., Wissenschaftliche Verlagsgesellschaft mbH, Stuttgart.
[b]Milk mixed of 5 g instant cocoa powder per 100 ml fat-reduced milk (1.5% fat) according to German food-based dietary guidelines for children and adolescents [13].

not consistent as well. These difficulties in categorization also favor the use of one beverage group of sugar-containing beverages.

Also in the context of obesity prevention, several national pediatric and dietary institutions as well as international authorities recommend a restricted consumption of soft drinks [13–17]. With regard to 100% fruit juice, recommendations are more differentiated because of its high nutrient density. Currently, the American Academy of Pediatrics recommends that children and adolescents limit juice intake to two servings or half of the recommended fruit servings each day and indicates that an excessive consumption may be associated with overnutrition [18]. Similarly, other national authorities advise against a high consumption of fruit juices because of the probable increased risk for obesity [17].

In several countries, a secular trend has been observed toward increased consumption of sugar-containing beverages among children and adolescents. In the United States, the daily soft drink consumption and percentage of children consuming soft drinks at school rose remarkably within two decades from the late 1970s [3, 19]. This trend was especially pronounced among teenagers, indicated by the percentage of soft drink consumers at school that almost tripled in adolescent boys during this time period [19]. According to a national survey around the year 2000, soft drinks and fruit drinks contributed more than 10% of total energy intake in U.S. children and adolescents and together with juice they provided 13% [3]. However, beverage consumption patterns differ significantly between countries. The current consumption of sugar-containing beverages in German children and adolescents is shown in Figure 36.1. In children aged 6 to 11 years, juices were the second most consumed beverage group with a mean consumption between 200 mL and 270 mL, followed by soft drinks (150 to 230 ml) [20]. Soft drink consumption increased with age from childhood to adolescence and was higher among boys compared with girls [21]. Libuda et al. estimated that in the United States, the average soft drink consumption in adolescent boys was by about 350 g per day higher than in their German counterparts, but, in contrast, juice consumption was lower by about 100 g per day [10].

The Effect on Body Weight

The relation between childhood obesity and the consumption of sugar-containing beverages has been investigated in a number of studies, and several publications reviewed and meta-analyzed their results [9, 22–29]. In 2003, the World Health Organization postulated a high consumption of soft drinks as a "probable" factor that promotes obesity [30]. A later review even considered the strength of evidence with regard to children and adolescents as "strong" [9]. A meta-analysis showed a significant but quite small effect of soft drink consumption on body weight [22]. In contrast, others concluded that more well-designed trials are needed before the evidence can be confirmed [24, 26]. However,

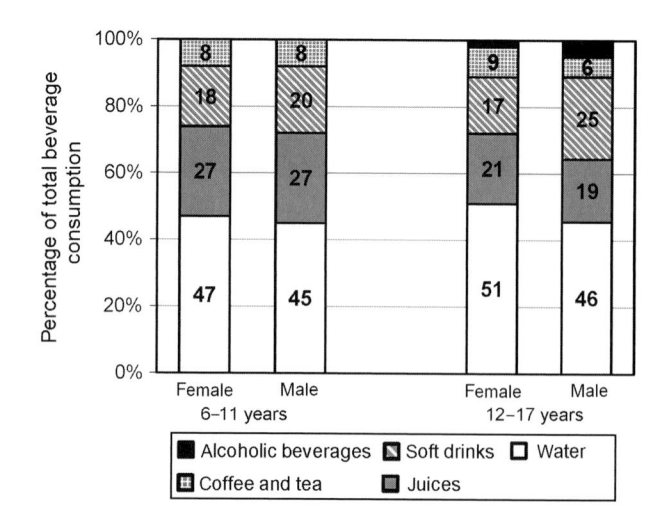

FIGURE 36.1 Consumption of different beverage categories in percentage of total beverage consumption (excluding milk) in two age groups of female and male children in Germany. Figure modified from [20].

some experts even stated that the consumption of sugar-sweetened beverages has become the dietary factor that is most consistently associated with the development of overweight [4], and reducing its consumption should become a major approach in obesity prevention [31].

In contrast to the comprehensive research on the obesogenic effect of soft drinks, only few studies have evaluated the effect of the consumption of fruit juices on obesity. Furthermore, intervention studies on this topic are completely missing. The authors of recent reviews [4, 25, 29] and the American Academy of Pediatrics [18] concluded, because of the contradictory results of the currently available studies, that there is no conclusive evidence for a causal link between 100% fruit juices and childhood obesity. It has to be mentioned that most of the research was conducted in the United States, but there the mean juice consumption is significantly smaller than in Germany [10]. For instance, a German cohort study was able to show an effect of juice consumption on weight gain in girls that was even greater than the effect of soft drink consumption [10].

Mechanisms for an Effect on Body Weight

Several potential biological and dietary mechanisms have been suggested that might underlie the causal link between the consumption of sugar-containing beverages and obesity. Both soft drinks and juices are relatively energy dense because of the high sugar content (Table 36.1). One pathway by which the consumption of sugar-containing beverages could lead to an energy imbalance and to overweight in the long term is an associated increase in total dietary energy intake. There is increasing evidence that energy consumed in the form of beverages is not fully compensated by a reduction in energy intake from solid foods [23, 32]. In a study on children and adolescents, each additional serving (~240 mL) of sugar-sweetened beverage was associated by a daily increase in total energy intake of 106 kcal ($\approx$ 444 kJ) [33]. For example, the average energy content of one serving of soft drink is also about 440 kJ (Table 36.1). One reason for this incomplete compensation might be a weaker satiation effect of beverages compared to solid foods because of a faster gastrointestinal passage [34]. However, the evidence for incomplete energy compensation is not univocal and probably depends on further factors. Libuda and Kersting concluded from a comparison of several experimental studies that the magnitude of incomplete compensation differs by age, the composition of the beverages, and the timing of beverage consumption such as consumed as a snack or during meal [29]. Especially in older children, energy intake from sugar-containing beverages seems to be not adequately compensated [29].

Another potential mechanism for the association between the soft drink consumption and weight gain is the obesogenic effect of high-fructose corn syrup (HFCS). Whereas soft drinks produced in European countries are sweetened with sucrose [9], U.S. soft drinks contain HFCS as added sugar [35]. HFCS might have an obesogenic effect because it is supposed to contain more free fructose [29], which does not induce insulin secretion. Because insulin stimulates satiety signals, fructose is supposed to enhance food intake and weight gain as it does not provide these satiety signals [35]. In addition, fructose promotes lipogenesis in the liver and thereby might cause fat deposition [35]. Libuda and Kersting reviewed the current evidence for the different effects of beverages sweetened with fructose and sucrose on weight gain [29]. They concluded that consumption of HFCS in beverages might be obesogenic but also that it is questionable that HFCS-sweetened beverages are more strongly linked to obesity than beverages sweetened with sucrose [29].

The effect of sugar-containing beverages on obesity could also be mediated by an indirect pathway, as their consumption is known to be associated with other obesity-related dietary and lifestyle factors. One possibility is the replacement of milk with soft drinks in the diet observed among children and adolescents [19, 36, 37]. Soft drink consumption in children and adolescents is also often linked with an unhealthy lifestyle indicated by poor diet quality [36, 38], less favorable dietary habits [39], and increased time spent watching television [40]. Therefore, soft drink consumption may be a proxy for these obesity-related lifestyle factors.

Intervention Studies

Up to now, three randomized controlled intervention trials have investigated the isolated impact of a reduced consumption of sugar-containing drinks on children's body weight. In a cluster trial in elementary schools in the United Kingdom, the prevalence of overweight could be reduced by an educational program to discourage the consumption of carbonated drinks after 12 months [41]. However, no intervention effect on the mean body mass index (BMI) was observed, indicating no overall weight reducing effect of the intervention. This may indicate that children with a body weight status close to the cutoff point for overweight received the greatest benefit from the intervention. However, this isolated educational approach was not able to achieve long-term effects on overweight 2 years after completion of the study [42]. A second intervention trial in the family setting combined behavioral with environmental interventions by weekly home deliveries of noncaloric beverages. After 6 months, this intervention succeeded in reducing energy intake from sugar-sweetened beverages by 82% and had a beneficial effect on BMI in adolescents, but only among the participants with a baseline BMI from the upper BMI tertile (i.e., the already more overweight adolescents) [43]. A similar result was observed in a school-based trial in Brazil among children aged 9 to 12 years who were encouraged by an educational program to exchange sugar-sweetened beverages with water. After 1 school year, consumption of carbonated drinks was reduced, but no overall reduction in BMI was detected. However, among girls who were already overweight at baseline, the intervention succeeded in reducing the BMI compared to the control group [44]. Change in water consumption was not reported.

In contrast to intervention studies that solely focused on the reduction of soft drink consumption, a study conducted in Chile aimed at the replacement of soft drinks by milk. After 4 months the intervention had a beneficial impact on lean body mass among children aged 8 to 10 years, but it did not affect BMI or percentage body fat [45]. Thus, replacement of soft drinks by a caloric beverage such as milk may not be appropriate for obesity prevention.

Water as a Beverage

Definition, Recommendations, and Consumption

The main characteristic of water as a beverage is—in particular against the background of the rising trend of childhood overweight and obesity—that it is free of energy. In Germany, drinking water is the most regularly controlled food available [46] and, together with mineral water and other noncaloric beverages, water is the recommended beverage for children to meet the daily fluid needs [47]. Also according to food-based guidelines of other European countries such as Hungary or Portugal [48, 49] and the United States [50], water is the recommended beverage to fulfill daily fluid needs in a healthy diet.

Since the late 1980s, mineral and drinking water have become the predominant consumed beverages among German children and adolescents, and their proportions have increased in all childhood age groups [51]. A nationwide dietary survey in Germany [20] showed that about half of the total beverage intake, excluding milk, in German children and adolescents came from water, with small variations by sex and age (Fig. 36.1). Unfortunately, representative U.S. data on consumption of water as a beverage are missing as water was not part of the U.S. Department of Agriculture's Food and Nutrient Database categories [52]. One study in Iowa showed that water consumption in young children increased with age, and 5-year-old children drank on average 118 g water per day, which accounted for about one third of the total beverage intake excluding milk [36].

The Effect on Body Weight

In the general population it is widely believed that the plentiful consumption of water can support weight loss in self-management of overweight, but surprisingly few studies have investigated the effect of increased water intake on body weight regulation [8]. Two cross-sectional studies in children did not find a beneficial association between increased water consumption and body weight; they even found a converse relation. According to these data from Germany and the United States, children and adolescents with a high water consumption were more likely to be obese than those with a lower water consumption [53, 54]. However, a causal link cannot be drawn from this association, and the authors suggest that one can interpret water consumption as a proxy for total beverage intake, including energy-containing beverages [54]. Only one prospective study has investigated the effect of water consumption on body weight status in a nonclinical setting. In a secondary analysis of a weight-loss intervention study in adult women, an absolute increase in water consumption was associated with a decrease in body weight, independent of diet and physical activity [55].

Mechanisms for an Effect on Body Weight

There are several speculative mechanisms for a beneficial effect on body weight regulation, but evidence remains contradictory [8]. One postulated pathway for the beneficial effect of water ingestion is a short-term suppression of hunger that might lead to a reduced energy intake. For instance, two experimental studies in women showed that consumption of about two glasses of water (~400 mL) with an *ad libitum* meal increased satiety during the meal [56] and fullness after the meal [57]. Rolls et al. found that reduced hunger after 360 mL of water drunk with the food compared to the hunger perceived by women who ate the food without water [58]. Another study reported that a premeal water consumption (500 mL) decreased meal energy intake significantly in obese, older adults [59]. Further results suggest that this effect depends on the age of the subjects, as water consumption (375 to 500 mL) before a meal was found to reduce energy intake in older adults but not in younger adults [60]. This finding conforms with other studies with younger adults that did not detect an effect on the energy intake at the subsequent meal by the intake of pure water (360 to 470 mL) before or with a meal compared to no water ingestion [57, 58, 61]. A dose-response relationship on the energy intake could also not be found in an experiment with two different volumes of water consumed with a meal [62].

Another potential mechanism by which water consumption might affect body weight is a thermogenic effect of pure, ingested water. In an experimental study with adults, the consumption of 500 mL of water increased the metabolic rate by 30%, resulting in an additional energy expenditure of about 100 kJ [63]. After considering the energy needed for warming the water from its served temperature to body temperature, the energy deficit was still around 60 to 70 kJ. The same research group investigated the effect of the ingestion of 500 mL water among overweight adults and found a mean thermogenic response of about 95 kJ [64]. The authors suggested that the mechanism by which drinking water influenced thermogenesis is through a local decrease in osmolarity in the gastrointestinal tract that may influence energy metabolism by several pathways, such as the sympathetic nervous system [63, 64]. However, this energy-consuming effect of water consumption could not be supported by other studies [65], and no such experiments have been carried out in children.

Water also may have a beneficial effect on the body weight if it replaces the sugar-containing beverages. Increasing water consumption could also lead to an improved hydration status of the body, in particular in population groups with a suboptimal hydration status.

Intervention Studies

To date, only one controlled intervention trial has investigated the effect of increased water consumption on body weight in children. Muckelbauer et al. showed in a large randomized cluster trial that an intervention only promoting water consumption in children of elementary schools in Germany effectively reduced the risk of overweight after 1 school year [66]. The school-based prevention program combined educational and environmental interventions and resulted in an increased water intake of about one glass per day, whereas the concomitant reduction in consumption of sugar-containing beverages, including soft drinks and juices, did not reach significance. The environmental component of the intervention consisted of the installation of water fountains in the schools, providing free access to cool and plain or carbonated water. The educational component was performed by the teachers and comprised classroom lessons dealing with the importance of drinking water. A process evaluation during and beyond the intervention period indicated that the intervention produced sustainable environmental changes in the school setting and also pointed toward a modified long-term behavior in children's beverage consumption [67]. In addition, the intervention was shown to be implementable in the schools and to be widely accepted and supported by teachers and headmasters, which is a prerequisite for the dissemination of the prevention program [67].

Previously, similar interventional approaches on increasing water consumption in schoolchildren have been conducted, but only in studies with designs of lower quality. In a comprehensive program for overweight prevention, which did not use a control group, children were encouraged to drink plain water besides other interventions to improve physical fitness [68]. The program applied nutrition lessons and environmental interventions, also including the installation of water coolers in schools. After 8 years, a decrease in the prevalence of overweight was observed among the schoolchildren. However, because of the study design, it remains unclear to which extent the intervention aiming at the increased water intake accounted for the beneficial effect.

A study with intervention components similar to that of Muckelbauer et al. provided a secondary school with water coolers in combination with lessons on the health benefits of water [69]. The combined approach also resulted in increased water consumption, although the volume of soft drinks purchased by students in schools did not change. However, this study did not report the effect on body weight [69].

Hydration Status and Total Water Intake

Definition, Recommendations, and Hydration Status

Water is quantitatively the most important nutrient in human nutrition [70] and is essential for a number of physiological functions. Consequences of acute water imbalances range from thirst and headache to impaired physical and cognitive performance, and severe losses of about 10% of body water are life threatening [71–73]. In addition, a chronic mild dehydration is potentially associated with various morbidities [74].

Water requirements are often neglected in dietary references [75], with few exceptions such as in the United States and German-speaking countries that defined the adequate intake [72] and guideline values [1] for total water intake. For their correct interpretation, it has to be considered that fluid requirements vary widely among individuals and populations and depend on physical activity and climate, which affect water losses because of perspiration [76]. Therefore, recommendations of total water intake should be understood as values of orientation.

Human water needs are met by water intake from beverages and solid foods and by water generated from the oxidative metabolism of macronutrients. According to German dietary references [1], the recommended total water intake increases during childhood from 1.3 liter in children aged 1 to 3 years to 2.8 liter in adolescents (aged 15 to 18 years). Accordingly, water intake supplied by beverages as the main source of water increases from a recommended amount of 0.8 to 1.5 liter in the respective age groups.

Children are at particular risk for water imbalances because their body surface per unit body weight is larger and their total body water pool related to the water turnover is lower in comparison to adults [73]. A study showed that especially young children in Germany, aged 6 to 11 years, did not reach, on average, this recommended water intake by beverages, whereas adolescents exceeded the recommendations on average [20]. Results from urine osmolality analyses in young children also pointed to an insufficient hydration status on the group level. Therefore, the authors recommended an increase of the usual water intake by about 240 mL to reach a good hydration status in German children [70]. Similarly, in Israel, among a sample of elementary school-aged children about two thirds were found to be moderately to severely dehydrated [77]. However, hydration status depends on multiple factors and therefore it can differ considerably between ethnic groups [77] and countries (e.g., U.S. adults showed a better hydration status compared to the German population) [75].

The Effect on Body Weight

The hydration status of the body is suggested to have an impact on body weight regulation and obesity [78], but there has been little epidemiological research on this topic. Especially for the effect of hydration status on body weight in children, no data are available.

Mechanisms for an Effect on Body Weight

There is some evidence for an association between a poor hydration status and the development of overweight. Results from animal studies indicated that dehydration leads to a preference for a high-fat diet [78]. A preference for dietary fat is perhaps a compensatory mechanism against the water deficit because fat is the best source for metabolic water compared to carbohydrates and protein [78]. This theory is supported by findings of a cross-sectional analysis that found sufficiently hydrated children to have a more desirable diet with a lower energy density in comparison with hypohydrated children [79]. A further pathway by which the hydration status could influence the body weight status is the lipid metabolism. In an experimental study with adults, induced hypoosmolality was found to promote lipolysis that may lead to a reduction of body fat [80].

Milk

Definition, Recommendations, and Consumption

Milk and dairy products are an important part of children's diet because of their significant contribution to daily nutrient requirements of numerous macro- and micronutrients such as protein, calcium, and iodine [47]. Thus, several national food-based guidelines provide amounts or servings of daily consumption. In Germany, a daily intake of 300 to 500 g, depending on age, is recommended [13, 47]. The American Academy of Pediatrics recommends for children aged 1 to 8 years a daily milk and dairy consumption of 2 cups and for older children and adolescents 3 cups [16]. Furthermore, in several Western societies, the recommended milk for school-aged children and adolescents is fat-reduced milk instead of full-fat milk [13, 16, 47]. With regard to the other extreme of fat content, skim milk with a fat content of 0.3% is also not recommended for children because of the low vitamin A and D content [13].

The time trend observed in the past decades toward a decreased milk consumption among children and adolescents—for example, in the United States [3, 19] and in Germany [51]—is worrying. For instance, around 60% of children and adolescents in Germany do not reach the recommended intake of milk and dairy products [81]. In Belgium, young children had a higher consumption of milk and dairy products compared to German children, but according to the Belgian food-based dietary guidelines, also a percentage of 50% to 70%, depending on age and sex, did not reach the recommended daily amount [82]. Another observation was that with increasing age of the children, the consumption of milk products decreased and the gap to the recommended amounts widened [82, 81].

The Effect on Body Weight

Because of the relatively high fat content of milk (Table 36.1) and its fat composition, increased milk consumption used to be associated with a detrimental effect on the development of obesity and coronary heart disease [83]. A more recent opinion is that a moderate consumption of milk and dairy products has no negative effects on health [7]. Even now, a preventive effect of milk, as a proxy for a high calcium intake, on the development of obesity is proposed because of results from animal experiments and epidemiological studies in adults [4]. In children and adolescents, some observational studies showed an inverse association between consumption of dairy products and weight gain or obesity, whereas others did not, and no intervention study has demonstrated an effect on body weight yet [4, 6]. Based on available evidence, experts concluded that the potential role of dairy products in the prevention of obesity in children is still uncertain [4–6, 84].

Mechanisms for an Effect on Body Weight

Several milk components are proposed to have a beneficial effect on the energy or lipid metabolism, and thereby to affect body composition and the development of obesity. One suggested pathway is the calcium content of milk. A high calcium intake could, by the modulation of calcitropic hormones, reduce the influx of calcium into adipocytes, with the consequence of an increase in lipolysis and fat oxidation in adipose tissue [85]. Further, calcium is suggested to inhibit the intestinal fat absorption through the binding of bile and fatty acids. There is also some evidence that calcium affects the appetite regulation as suggested in a review on the effects of milk components on body weight regulation [86]. The fat fraction of milk also contains factors that are supposed to have an impact on body composition. Medium chained triglycerides could impede the fat accumulation in adipocytes, and conjugated linoleic acids may increase the metabolic rate and have a beneficial effect on the serum lipid profile [86]. There is also some evidence that milk substances of the whey fraction have an angiotensin-converting-enzyme (ACE) inhibiting effect, which could lead to an anabolic effect on muscles or to a decreased lipogenesis in adipose tissue, resulting in a more favorable body composition [85]. Other authors have suggested that the two major protein fractions of milk, whey and casein, may have postprandial effects that stimulate protein synthesis and inhibit protein breakdown [87], leading to an increase in lean body mass.

Another mechanism to explain the association between milk consumption and body weight could be a replacement of milk by soft drinks in the diet of children and adolescents that was recently observed [19, 36, 37]. Considering the potential obesogenic effect of sugar-containing beverages, in observational studies it is hard to differentiate between the impacts of the two trends in beverage consumption on the development of obesity.

Some of these suggested pathways for the positive effect of milk consumption on body weight are well documented, but the few intervention studies on this effect in children and adolescents provide inconclusive findings.

Intervention Studies

One randomized controlled trial in Chile investigated the effect of increased milk consumption and concomitantly reduced soft drink consumption in overweight and obese children aged 8 to 10 years [45]. The family-based intervention included instructions provided to the family and the home delivery of milk beverages to replace soft drinks. After 4 months the intervention had a beneficial impact on lean body mass and growth, but it did not affect BMI or percentage body fat [45]. Because of the design and the behavioral aim of the study, it was not possible to distinguish between the effect of the increased milk consumption and the decreased soft drink consumption. Other controlled intervention studies that focused on increased daily consumption of milk or dairy products in children did not find any effect on body weight nor on fat or lean mass [88–90]. Because of the lack of further results from intervention studies, the role of milk and dairy products in the prevention of overweight in children remains controversial.

Other Beverages

Beverages other than water, milk, and sugar-containing beverages are minor contributors to the total beverage intake in children [20, 52]. In German children and adolescents up from the age of 6 years, coffee, tea, and alcoholic beverages together account for 8% to 11% of total beverage intake, excluding milk (Fig. 36.1). Tea contributes with a proportion between 5% and 8% to the beverage intake, and children younger than 12 years rarely drink coffee [91]. Still, among adolescents coffee accounts for less than 2% of the total beverage intake (Fig. 36.1). Especially from the age of 15 years, alcohol consumption is rising in adolescence and reaches an average proportion of about 5% of beverage consumption in German adolescents [91].

Because these beverages play a minor role in children's dietary habits or because there are no clear hints to a direct association with body weight regulation [4], they are not further discussed in this chapter.

PERSPECTIVES ON BEVERAGE INTERVENTIONS FOR OBESITY PREVENTION

Sugar-Containing Beverages

Although the magnitude and the biological mechanisms of the obesogenic effects of sugar-containing beverages in children and adolescents are still controversially discussed, the current evidence is sufficient to recommend a restriction of soft drink consumption. These energy-dense beverages could be regarded as sweets as suggested in food-based dietary guidelines for children in Germany [13]. Thus, future educational programs should communicate to parents as well as to children that sugar-sweetened beverages should be recognized as sweets and, thus, consumption has to be restricted.

Fruit juices are rich in several micronutrients but also contain energy in amounts similar to soft drinks. If consumed in moderate amounts, fruit juices can help to meet the recommended daily fruit consumption in children and adolescents. However, because of the potential detrimental effect on body weight similar to the effect of soft drinks, the consumption of fruit juice should be limited in children and adolescents, especially in population groups at risk for overweight.

Previous intervention studies that focused on decreasing the soft drink consumption were found to have a beneficial impact on body weight, although results of long-term effects are missing. Nevertheless, considering the present findings, beverage interventions may become an important and evidence-based approach in the prevention of child obesity. Interestingly, findings also indicate that the interventions were not equally effective in all groups of children, but specifically in already or nearly overweight children and adolescents. Thus, beverage interventions focusing on a decreased consumption of soft drinks could be particularly suitable for population-based strategies to counteract obesity as they may prevent further weight gain in children at risk for obesity or even can reduce obesity in populations with a high prevalence of obesity. Results of one intervention study that focused on a replacement of soft drinks by milk suggest that the replacement by noncaloric beverages seems to be more promising and is also more plausible for obesity prevention, at least in Western societies with a high proportion of overweight children and a low prevalence of malnutrition.

Settings of effective beverage interventions were found to be the family as well as the school setting, and the combination of behavioral and environmental components seemed to be promising for long-term modifications in beverage consumption. In the school setting, one important environmental intervention is the banning of vending machines for soft drinks [17, 15, 92]. Preventive intervention on a level above the family or school level could be a restricted advertisement of sugar-containing beverages [92], but to date evidence for the effectiveness of those measures is missing.

Although consumption of sugar-containing drinks is only one out of multiple contributors of childhood obesity, the preventive approach on decreasing its consumption is promising. Data have indicated that a total displacement of sugar-sweetened beverages with water would hypothetically result in an average reduction of energy intake of more than 230 kcal ($\approx$ 963 kJ) per day in American children [33]. This cutdown of energy would be quite large, but a total replacement also seems unrealistic. However, even a partial exchange of energy-containing beverages with water could be beneficial as there is evidence that overweight in children is caused by a small but continuous positive energy imbalance between about 125 and 700 kJ per day [93–96]. Thus, small reductions in daily energy intake may be sufficient to prevent the development of overweight.

Water and Hydration Status

To date, observational and intervention studies investigating the effect of increased water intake and hydration status on body weight are scarce and also the underlying biological mechanisms are poorly understood or controversially discussed. However, it seems plausible that promoting water consumption and thereby displacing obesity-associated beverages could have a beneficial effect on body weight. In fact, water, besides other noncaloric beverages, is the recommended beverage for children and adolescents, also in the context of overweight prevention [15, 17, 33, 97].

For school-based programs, a policy of water as the preferred beverage should be implemented as recommended in the Action Plan of the World Health Organization [14, 98]. As shown in one study, the intervention approach only focusing on increasing water consumption only by messages to promote water consumption reduced the risk of overweight in children and therefore could become an effective and feasible component of comprehensive programs for obesity prevention in schools [66, 67]. The promotion of water consumption should be supported by the provision of free access to water because environmental modifications can support educative measures to achieve sustainable modifications in beverage consumption behaviors of children [67].

Increasing water consumption could also contribute to an improved hydration status of the body, in particular in populations with a suboptimal hydration status. A constant good hydration of the body should anyway be aimed at in children. However, the potential role of an improved hydration status in body weight regulation is, to date, very inclusive because of the small number of studies in humans.

Milk

The association between milk consumption and an increased or lower risk for weight gain and body composition remains inconclusive, and research is ongoing. Therefore, no recommendation of milk consumption can be made for interventions to prevent obesity in Western societies, especially as randomized controlled trials on the isolated effect of reduced milk consumption are missing up to now. However, rather than a beverage to cover fluid requirements, milk should be considered as a food item in children's diet that can contribute to the adequate intake of many nutrients thanks to its high nutrient density. Because a trend toward decreased milk consumption has been observed in several countries, a consumption level of milk and dairy products as recommended by age-specific dietary guidelines for children should be an aim of future dietary interventions. However, a population-based intervention on milk consumption seems to be inappropriate; rather, future interventions should focus on groups of children that are identified by the nutrition status and a risk for a too high or too low milk consumption level. In addition, the replacement of whole milk with fat-reduced milk should be forced. On a population level, schools are a practical setting for intervention programs that are tailored to specific age and population groups. The European school milk program is an example for the targeted promotion of milk consumption in schoolchildren.

CONCLUSION

Beverage consumption behaviors were found to impact body weight status in children and adolescents, and therefore they should become a target for the prevention of childhood obesity. According to the available evidence, various interventions that aim for the modification of beverage consumption patterns seem to be promising in the treatment and prevention of childhood overweight and obesity. The replacement of sugar-containing soft drink by water or other noncaloric beverages can be recommended as one behavioral target. Intervention measures should consider educational components together with environmental changes for a sustainable modification of children's individual beverage consumption. School-based programs were shown to be effective in improving beverage consumption patterns in children by increasing water consumption and reducing sugar-containing beverages. Thus, schools as well as other institutions for full-time care may become an important setting for beverage interventions to prevent obesity starting in early childhood. Also interventions in the family setting showed promising results in improving beverage consumption patterns to reduce or prevent obesity.

The potential impact of changed milk consumption on body weight in children remains inconclusive. Thus, dietary interventions should target a consumption of milk and dairy products as recommended in food-based dietary guidelines for children to avoid both over- and underconsumption of milk. A clear recommendation in the context of the obesity prevention is that children should consume fat-reduced milk.

Additionally, it has to be considered that the effect of beverage interventions can differ between subgroups of children, as, for example, a school-based intervention that focused on the promotion of water consumption prevented overweight in German children but failed in the subgroup of children with a migration background [97, 99]. The identification of risk groups can help to save resources by targeting interventions on those children who are at increased risk for overweight and who are especially sensitive for the beverage intervention (e.g., because of their high consumption of sugar-containing beverages). For example, children of a low socioeconomic status showed an increased consumption of soft drinks compared to their counterparts of a higher status in several European countries [98, 100]. Soft drink consumption was especially high among children with a migration background in Germany [21].

Research on the association between weight gain and beverage consumption is still needed on all levels. In experimental studies the biological mechanisms should be enlightened, especially with regard to the impact of water and hydration status on body weight. Prospective observation studies are needed to identify health consequences of beverage consumption habits on population level. Finally, further high-quality intervention trials have to examine the effect of beverage interventions on the body weight in children. Multidisciplinary teams should design effective and implementable interventions on all levels from the home setting to policies and legislation to produce sustained modifications in beverage consumption for obesity prevention in children.

References

1. Deutsche Gesellschaft für Ernährung, Österreichische Gesellschaft für Ernährung, Schweizerische Gesellschaft für Ernährungsforschung, and Schweizerische Vereinigung für Ernährung. [German Nutrition Society, Austrian Nutrition Society, Swiss Society for Nutrition Research, and Swiss Nutrition Association]. *Referenzwerte für die Nährstoffzufuhr [Reference Values for Nutrition Intake]*. Umschau/Braus, Frankfurt am Main; 2000.
2. Storey ML, Forshee RA, Anderson PA. Beverage consumption in the US population. *J Am Diet Assoc* 2006;**106**:1992−2000.
3. Nielsen SJ, Popkin BM. Changes in beverage intake between 1977 and 2001. *Am J Prev Med* 2004;**27**:205−10.
4. Must A, Barish EE, Bandini LG. Modifiable risk factors in relation to changes in BMI and fatness: what have we learned from prospective studies of school-aged children? *Int J Obes (Lond)* 2009;**33**:705−15.
5. Barba G, Russo P. Dairy foods, dietary calcium and obesity: a short review of the evidence. *Nutr Metab Cardiovasc Dis* 2006;**16**:445−51.
6. Huang TT, McCrory MA. Dairy intake, obesity, and metabolic health in children and adolescents: knowledge and gaps. *Nutr Rev* 2005;**63**:71−80.
7. Haug A, Hostmark AT, Harstad OM. Bovine milk in human nutrition—a review. *Lipids Health Dis* 2007;**6**:25.
8. Negoianu D, Goldfarb S. Just Add Water. *J Am Soc Nephrol* 2008;**19**:1041−3.
9. Malik VS, Schulze MB, Hu FB. Intake of sugar-sweetened beverages and weight gain: a systematic review. *Am J Clin Nutr* 2006;**84**:274−88.
10. Libuda L, Alexy U, Sichert-Hellert W, Stehle P, Karaolis-Danckert N, Buyken AE, Kersting M. Pattern of beverage consumption and long-term association with body-weight status in German adolescents: results from the DONALD study. *Br J Nutr* 2008;**99**:1370−9.
11. U.S. Department of Agriculture, Agricultural Research Service. *Food and Nutrient Intakes by Children 1994−96*, 1998. 1999. ARS Food Surveys Research Group, http://www.ars.usda.gov/SP2UserFiles/Place/12355000/pdf/scs_all.pdf, accessed July 23, 2009.
12. Deutsches Lebensmittelbuch. [German Food Book] (2003). Leitsätze für Erfrischungsgetränke. [Guidelines for Softdrinks]. 2002. *BANZ* 2003; **62**.

13. Forschungsinstitut für Kinderernährung. [Research Institute of Child Nutrition]. Empfehlungen für die Ernährung von Kindern und Jugendlichen - optimiX. [Dietary Guidelines for Children and Adolescents]. Forschungsinstitut für Kinderernährung GmbH Dortmund; 2008.
14. World Health Organization. Diet, nutrition and the prevention of chronic diseases. Tech Rep Ser, 916, Geneva; 2003.
15. American Academy of Pediatrics Committee on School Health. Soft drinks in schools. Pediatrics 2004;113:152—4.
16. Gidding SS, Dennison BA, Birch LL, Daniels SR, Gillman MW, Lichtenstein AH, Rattay KT, Steinberger J, Stettler N, Van Horn L. Dietary recommendations for children and adolescents: a guide for practitioners. Pediatrics 2006;117:544—59.
17. Ernährungskommission der Deutschen Gesellschaft für Kinder- und Jugendmedizin [Nutrition Comission of the German Pediatric Association] (DGKJ), Ernährungskommission der Österreichischen Gesellschaft für Kinder- und Jugendheilkunde [Nutrition Comission of the Austrian Pediatric Association] (ÖGKJ), and Ernährungskommission der Schweizerischen Gesellschaft für Pädiatrie [Nutrition Comission of the Swiss Pediatric Association] (SGP). Empfehlungen zum Verzehr zuckerhaltiger Getränke durch Kinder und Jugendliche. [Recommendations on the Intake of Sugar-containing Beverages] Monatsschr Kinderheilkd 2008;156:484—7.
18. American Academy of Pediatrics. The use and misuse of fruit juice in pediatrics. Pediatrics 2001;107:1210—13.
19. Lin B, Ralston K. Competetive Foods: Soft Drinks vs. Milk. Economic Research Service/United States Department of Agriculture, Food Assistance and Nutrition Research Report 2003;34-7:1—3.
20. Mensink GBM, Heseker H, Richter A, Stahl A, Vohmann C. Forschungsbericht Ernährungsstudie als KiGGS-Modul (EsKiMo) [Research Report Nutrition Study as KiGGs-Modul]. Universität Paderborn, Robert Koch-Institut Berlin. 2007. http://www.bmelv.de/SharedDocs/downloads/03-Ernaehrung/EsKiMo Studie.html, accessed December 12, 2007.
21. Mensink GBM, Kleiser C, Richter A. Food consumption of children and adolescents in Germany. Results of the German Health Interview and Examination Survey for Children and Adolescents (KiGGS). Bundesgesundheitsbl - Gesundheitsforsch- Gesundheitsschutz 2007;50:609—23.
22. Vartanian LR, Schwartz MB, Brownell KD. Effects of soft drink consumption on nutrition and health: a systematic review and meta-analysis. Am J Public Health 2007;97:667—75.
23. Bachman CM, Baranowski T, Nicklas TA. Is there an association between sweetened beverages and adiposity? Nutr Rev 2006;64:153—74.
24. Forshee RA, Anderson PA, Storey ML. Sugar-sweetened beverages and body mass index in children and adolescents: a meta-analysis. Am J Clin Nutr 2008;87:1662—71.
25. O'Neil CE, Nicklas TA. A Review of the Relationship Between 100% Fruit Juice Consumption and Weight in Children and Adolescents. American Journal of Lifestyle Medicine 2008;2:315—54.
26. Pereira MA. The possible role of sugar-sweetened beverages in obesity etiology: a review of the evidence. Int J Obes (Lond) 2006;30:S28—36.
27. Gibson S. Sugar-sweetened soft drinks and obesity: a systematic review of the evidence from observational studies and interventions. Nutr Res Rev 2008;21:134—47.
28. Libuda L, Alexy U, Stehle P, Kersting M. Konsum von Erfrischungsgetränken und Entwicklung des Körpergewichts im Kindes- und Jugendalter - Gibt es eine Verbindung? [Softdrink Consumption and Bodyweight Development in Childhood and Adolescence—is there a Relationship?]. Akt Ernähr Med 2008;33:123—31.
29. Libuda L, Kersting M. Soft drinks and body weight development in childhood: is there a relationship? Curr Opin Clin Nutr Metab Care 2009;12(6):596—600.
30. World Health Organization. Diet, Nutrition and the Prevention of Chronic Diseases. World Health Organization and the Food and Agriculture Organization of the United Nations; Geneva; 2003.
31. James J, Kerr D. Prevention of childhood obesity by reducing soft drinks. Int J Obes (Lond) 2005;29(Suppl. 2):S54—7.
32. DiMeglio DP, Mattes RD. Liquid versus solid carbohydrate: effects on food intake and body weight. Int J Obes Relat Metab Disord 2000;24:794—800.
33. Wang YC, Ludwig DS, Sonneville K, Gortmaker SL. Impact of change in sweetened caloric beverage consumption on energy intake among children and adolescents. Arch Pediatr Adolesc Med 2009;163:336—43.
34. Mattes R. Fluid calories and energy balance: the good, the bad, and the uncertain. Physiol Behav 2006;89:66—70.
35. Bray GA, Nielsen SJ, Popkin BM. Consumption of high-fructose corn syrup in beverages may play a role in the epidemic of obesity. Am J Clin Nutr 2004;79:537—43.
36. Marshall TA, Eichenberger Gilmore JM, Broffitt B, Stumbo PJ, Levy SM. Diet quality in young children is influenced by beverage consumption. J Am Coll Nutr 2005;24:65—75.
37. Libuda L, Alexy U, Remer T, Stehle P, Schoenau E, Kersting M. Association between long-term consumption of soft drinks and variables of bone modeling and remodeling in a sample of healthy German children and adolescents. Am J Clin Nutr 2008;88:1670—7.
38. Libuda L, Alexy U, Buyken AE, Sichert-Hellert W, Stehle P, Kersting M. Consumption of sugar-sweetened beverages and its association with nutrient intakes and diet quality in German children and adolescents. Br J Nutr; 2008:1—9.
39. Vagstrand K, Linne Y, Karlsson J, Elfhag K, Karin Lindroos A. Correlates of soft drink and fruit juice consumption among Swedish adolescents. Br J Nutr 2009;101:1541—8.
40. Giammattei J, Blix G, Marshak HH, Wollitzer AO, Pettitt DJ. Television watching and soft drink consumption: associations with obesity in 11- to 13-year-old schoolchildren. Arch Pediatr Adolesc Med 2003;157:882—6.
41. James J, Thomas P, Cavan D, Kerr D. Preventing childhood obesity by reducing consumption of carbonated drinks: cluster randomised controlled trial. BMJ 2004;328:1237.
42. James J, Thomas P, Kerr D. Preventing childhood obesity: two year follow-up results from the Christchurch obesity prevention programme in schools (CHOPPS). BMJ 2007;335:762.
43. Ebbeling CB, Feldman HA, Osganian SK, Chomitz VR, Ellenbogen SJ, Ludwig DS. Effects of decreasing sugar-sweetened beverage consumption on body weight in adolescents: a randomized, controlled pilot study. Pediatrics 2006;117:673—80.
44. Sichieri R, Paula Trotte A, de Souza RA, Veiga GV. School randomised trial on prevention of excessive weight gain by discouraging students from drinking sodas. Public Health Nutr 2009;12:197—202.
45. Albala C, Ebbeling CB, Cifuentes M, Lera L, Bustos N, Ludwig DS. Effects of replacing the habitual consumption of sugar-sweetened beverages with milk in Chilean children. Am J Clin Nutr 2008;88:605—11.
46. Grimm P. Wie gut ist unser Wasser [How good is our water]. Ernährungs-Umschau 2002;49:58—9.
47. Kersting M, Alexy U, Clausen K. Using the concept of Food Based Dietary Guidelines to Develop an Optimized Mixed Diet (OMD) for German children and adolescents. J Pediatr Gastroenterol Nutr 2005;40:301—8.
48. Rodler I. Dietary Guidelines to the Adult Population in Hungary. 2001. ftp://ftp.fao.org/es/esn/nutrition/dietary_guidelines/hun.pdf, accessed August 24, 2009.
49. Instituto do Consumidor Portugal, and Programa Operacional Saude XXI [Portuguese Consumer Institute]. A nova roda dos

50. Popkin BM, Armstrong LE, Bray GM, Caballero B, Frei B, Willett WC. A new proposed guidance system for beverage consumption in the United States. Am J Clin Nutr 2006;83:529−42.
51. Sichert-Hellert W, Kersting M, Manz F. Fifteen year trends in water intake in German children and adolescents: results of the DONALD Study. Dortmund Nutritional and Anthropometric Longitudinally Designed Study. Acta Paediatr 2001;90:732−7.
52. O'Connor TM, Yang SJ, Nicklas TA. Beverage intake among preschool children and its effect on weight status. Pediatrics 2006;118:e1010−18.
53. Fiore H, Travis S, Whalen A, Auinger P, Ryan S. Potentially protective factors associated with healthful body mass index in adolescents with obese and nonobese parents: a secondary data analysis of the third national health and nutrition examination survey, 1988−1994. J Am Diet Assoc 2006;106:55−64. quiz 76−59.
54. Kleiser C, Schaffrath Rosario A, Mensink GB, Prinz-Langenohl R, Kurth BM. Potential determinants of obesity among children and adolescents in Germany: results from the cross-sectional KiGGS Study. BMC Public Health 2009;9:46.
55. Stookey JD, Constant F, Popkin BM, Gardner CD. Drinking Water Is Associated With Weight Loss in Overweight Dieting Women Independent of Diet and Activity. Obesity (Silver Spring) 2008;16:2481−8.
56. Lappalainen R, Mennen L, van Weert L, Mykkanen H. Drinking water with a meal: a simple method of coping with feelings of hunger, satiety and desire to eat. Eur J Clin Nutr 1993;47:815−19.
57. DellaValle DM, Roe LS, Rolls BJ. Does the consumption of caloric and non-caloric beverages with a meal affect energy intake? Appetite 2005;44:187−93.
58. Rolls BJ, Bell EA, Thorwart ML. Water incorporated into a food but not served with a food decreases energy intake in lean women. Am J Clin Nutr 1999;70:448−55.
59. Davy BM, Dennis EA, Dengo AL, Wilson KL, Davy KP. Water consumption reduces energy intake at a breakfast meal in obese older adults. J Am Diet Assoc 2008;108:1236−9.
60. Van Walleghen EL, Orr JS, Gentile CL, Davy BM. Pre-meal water consumption reduces meal energy intake in older but not younger subjects. Obesity (Silver Spring) 2007;15:93−9.
61. Rolls BJ, Kim S, Fedoroff IC. Effects of drinks sweetened with sucrose or aspartame on hunger, thirst and food intake in men. Physiol Behav 1990;48:19−26.
62. Flood JE, Roe LS, Rolls BJ. The effect of increased beverage portion size on energy intake at a meal. J Am Diet Assoc 2006;106:1984−90. discussion 1990−1991.
63. Boschmann M, Steiniger J, Hille U, Tank J, Adams F, Sharma AM, Klaus S, Luft FC, Jordan J. Water-induced thermogenesis. J Clin Endocrinol Metab 2003;88:6015−19.
64. Boschmann M, Steiniger J, Franke G, Birkenfeld AL, Luft FC, Jordan J. Water drinking induces thermogenesis through osmo-sensitive mechanisms. J Clin Endocrinol Metab 2007;92:3334−7.
65. Brown CM, Dulloo AG, Montani JP. Water-induced thermogenesis reconsidered: the effects of osmolality and water temperature on energy expenditure after drinking. J Clin Endocrinol Metab 2006;91:3598−602.
66. Muckelbauer R, Libuda L, Clausen K, Toschke AM, Reinehr T, Kersting M. Promotion and provision of drinking water in schools for overweight prevention: randomized, controlled cluster trial. Pediatrics 2009;123:e661−7.
67. Muckelbauer R, Libuda L, Clausen K, Kersting M. Long-term process evaluation of a school-based programme for overweight prevention. Child Care Health Dev 2009;35(6):851−7.
68. Toh CM, Cutter J, Chew SK. School based intervention has reduced obesity in Singapore. BMJ 2002;324:427.
69. Loughridge JL, Barratt J. Does the provision of cooled filtered water in secondary school cafeterias increase water drinking and decrease the purchase of soft drinks? J Hum Nutr Diet 2005;18:281−6.
70. Manz F, Wentz A, Sichert-Hellert W. The most essential nutrient: defining the adequate intake of water. J Pediatr 2002;141:587−92.
71. Kleiner SM. Water: an essential but overlooked nutrient. J Am Diet Assoc 1999;99:200−6.
72. Food and Nutrition Board. Dietary reference intakes for Water, Potassium, Sodium, Chloride, and Sulfate, Vol. 2009. Washington, D.C: National Academic Press; 2004.
73. Manz F. Hydration in children. J Am Coll Nutr 2007;26:562S−9S.
74. Manz F, Wentz A. The importance of good hydration for the prevention of chronic diseases. Nutr Rev 2005;63:S2−5.
75. Manz F, Wentz A. Hydration status in the United States and Germany. Nutr Rev 2005;63:S55−62.
76. Sawka MN, Cheuvront SN, Carter 3rd R. Human water needs. Nutr Rev 2005;63:S30−9.
77. Bar-David Y, Urkin J, Landau D, Bar-David Z, Pilpel D. Voluntary dehydration among elementary school children residing in a hot arid environment. J Hum Nutr Diet 2009;22(5):455−60.
78. Stookey JD. Another look at: fuel + O2 −> CO2 + H2O. Developing a water-oriented perspective. Med Hypotheses 1999;52:285−90.
79. Stahl A, Kroke A, Bolzenius K, Manz F. Relation between hydration status in children and their dietary profile: results from the DONALD study. Eur J Clin Nutr 2007;61:1386−92.
80. Keller U, Szinnai G, Bilz S, Berneis K. Effects of changes in hydration on protein, glucose and lipid metabolism in man: impact on health. Eur J Clin Nutr 2003;57(Suppl. 2):S69−74.
81. Kersting M, Bergmann K. Calcium and Vitamin D supply to children: Selected results from the DONALD study, focussing on the consumption of milk products. Ernährungs-Umschau 2008;55:523−7.
82. Huybrechts I, Matthys C, Vereecken C, Maes L, Temme EH, Van Oyen H, De Backer G, De Henauw S. Food intakes by preschool children in Flanders compared with dietary guidelines. Int J Environ Res Public Health 2008;5:243−57.
83. Aggett PJ, Haschke F, Heine W, Hernell O, Koletzko B, Lafeber H, Ormisson A, Rey J, Tormo R. Committee report: childhood diet and prevention of coronary heart disease. ESPGAN Committee on Nutrition. European Society of Pediatric Gastroenterology and Nutrition. J Pediatr Gastroenterol Nutr 1994;19:261−9.
84. Nicklas TA. Calcium intake trends and health consequences from childhood through adulthood. J Am Coll Nutr 2003;22:340−56.
85. Zemel MB, Miller SL. Dietary calcium and dairy modulation of adiposity and obesity risk [Milk: the Multi-Talent]. Nutr Rev 2004;62:125−31.
86. de Vrese M. Milch: das Multi-Talent [Milk: the Multi-Talent]. Phoenix 2007;4:6−8.
87. Boirie Y, Dangin M, Gachon P, Vasson MP, Maubois JL, Beaufrere B. Slow and fast dietary proteins differently modulate postprandial protein accretion. Proc Natl Acad Sci U S A 1997;94:14930−5.
88. Chan GM, Hoffman K, McMurry M. Effects of dairy products on bone and body composition in pubertal girls. J Pediatr 1995;126:551−6.
89. Merrilees MJ, Smart EJ, Gilchrist NL, Frampton C, Turner JG, Hooke E, March RL, Maguire P. Effects of diary food supplements on bone mineral density in teenage girls. Eur J Nutr 2000;39:256−62.

90. Cadogan J, Eastell R, Jones N, Barker ME. Milk intake and bone mineral acquisition in adolescent girls: randomised, controlled intervention trial. *BMJ* 1997;**315**:1255–60.
91. Mensink GBM, Heseker H, Richter A, Stahl A, Vohmann C. *Forschungsbericht Ernährungsstudie als KiGGS-Modul (EsKiMo)* [Research Report on the Nutrition Study as KiGGs-Modul], www.bmelv.de/SharedDocs/downloads/03-Ernaehrung/EsKiMo Studie.html, accessed December 12, 2007.
92. Ebbeling CB, Pawlak DB, Ludwig DS. Childhood obesity: public-health crisis, common sense cure. *Lancet* 2002;**360**:473–82.
93. Goran MI. Metabolic precursors and effects of obesity in children: a decade of progress, 1990–1999. *Am J Clin Nutr* 2001;**73**:158–71.
94. Wang YC, Gortmaker SL, Sobol AM, Kuntz KM. Estimating the energy gap among US children: a counterfactual approach. *Pediatrics* 2006;**118**:e1721–33.
95. Butte NF, Ellis KJ. Comment on "Obesity and the environment: where do we go from here?". *Science* 2003;**301**:598. author reply 598.
96. Plachta-Danielzik S, Landsberg B, Bosy-Westphal A, Johannsen M, Lange D. Energy gain and energy gap in normal-weight children: longitudinal data of the KOPS. *Obesity (Silver Spring)* 2008;**16**:777–83.
97. Muckelbauer R, Libuda L, Clausen K, Toschke AM, Reinehr T, Kersting M. Immigrational Background Affects the Effectiveness of a School-based Overweight Prevention Program Promoting Water Consumption. *Obesity (Silver Spring)* 2009;**18**(3):528–34.
98. Vereecken CA, Inchley J, Subramanian SV, Hublet A, Maes L. The relative influence of individual and contextual socio-economic status on consumption of fruit and soft drinks among adolescents in Europe. *Eur J Public Health* 2005;**15**:224–32.

CHAPTER
37

Psychotherapy as an Intervention for Child Obesity

Carl-Erik Flodmark

Childhood and Youth Centre in Malmö Childhood Obesity Unit, Skåne University Hospital
Malmö, Sweden

OBESITY: A DISEASE PUT INTO PERSPECTIVE

How do we discover the cause of a disease? This is a major scientific problem in medicine. Usually we are trying to find *the* cause of a disease. However, a problem arises when a disease is caused by different factors. Suppose five different genes cause obesity and also suppose these genes to be of equal importance. In trying to identify the strongest factor, chance will give us different answers in each study. A debate will arise as to which factor is the strongest. The more equal the factors are, the more difficult it will be to solve the controversy. However, we can accomplish a new understanding if we accept that there are several factors (genetic and social) causing obesity.

A simple way of classifying obesity would be to separate it into two categories: early- and late-onset obesity. Early-onset obesity, predominantly inherited, gives a large body size with a moderate increase in cardiovascular health risks; late-onset obesity, however, is predominantly lifestyle dependent, giving visceral adiposity with a greater increase in cardiovascular health risks. Of course, lifestyle is also important in early-onset obesity, as is inheritance in late-onset obesity.

However, because of the multifactorial causes of obesity, it is necessary to address it in a combined approach with many different components in the treatment program—that is, combining advice about exercise, diets, and training in social skills or even drug treatment or surgery in the most severe cases.

WHY DO WE NEED NEW TREATMENTS?

Many treatments of obesity have been investigated, including diet, exercise, surgery, and medication. None have been found to be effective enough as the sole treatment, e.g., in surgery psychosocial support is needed. It is now also clear that treatment needs to be affirmative and long lasting. Single physical treatments are insufficient because of the accompanying psychological factors, and brief treatments fail to take account of the lifelong genetic influence.

The necessity of a chronic treatment is now more widely recognized. This is due to the increasing knowledge in genetics that many obese people have an inherited susceptibility to developing obesity. Thus, they need lifelong treatment, not merely a short period of training in a good exercise or diet program. After such a period, the problem of obesity used to be thought of as gone and the individual could go back to his or her earlier but somewhat improved lifestyle without risking the development of obesity. If the individual gained weight, it was thought that his or her lifestyle was more unhealthy than the lifestyle of normal-weight persons. Now, the genetic discoveries give room for another interpretation. Furthermore, the concept of programming our genes early in life might explain how genes and environment interact in a more complicated way.

If you have inherited the disease of obesity, it is not enough to live as normal-weight people do regarding exercise and diet—you have to live more than perfectly. This chapter describes the strategies that are available. Of course, if you have no genetic susceptibility for obesity, it is much easier to reduce weight. Just live like other people of normal weight do! However, if you have genes that have been programmed to increase your weight, your lifestyle needs special care.

PSYCHODYNAMIC THERAPY

Psychodynamic therapy is less often used for obesity than for eating disorders. However, Bruch's clinical observations of obesity also included the family [1–3]. The obese child is described as living in a dysfunctional family (i.e., one with a disturbed communication between the parents and the child). The child has difficulties discriminating between emotions and other sensations from the body, such as hunger. Eating is then used as a replacement for other emotional needs. This response is founded early in the mother-child relationship, if the child's need of love, warmth, food and so on is not adequately fulfilled. There are no recent published studies regarding psychodynamic therapy in obesity [4].

BEHAVIORAL AND COGNITIVE THERAPIES

Behavioral therapy has been used in obesity management since first described [5]. The program was based on the belief that obesity is a "learned disease" that was possible to cure by "relearning." However, successful long-term results have not been achieved in adults [6]. Nonetheless, a 10-year follow-up without a control group did show lasting results when booster sessions were given for a period of 4 years. This indicates the difficulties of preserving good results and the need for long-term treatment [7].

Behavioral therapy of obesity is based on the concept of bad eating habits in which an insufficient control of stimulus or rewarding behavior results in increased food intake. These habits can be broken down into small sequences (e.g., the frequency of chewing, of meals, etc.). The parents are regarded as a reinforcement of the children's eating habits. For example, a deposit of money may be paid back to the patient during weight reduction [8].

In 1983, Brownell and co-workers evaluated a program consisting of behavior modification, social support, nutrition, and exercise [9]. They noted that groups in which obese children and their mothers met the group therapist separately gave better results than those in which only the children were seen, or the children were seen together with their mothers.

Others also studied the effects of parent interaction using three groups [10]. The first group consisted of child and parent where parent and child behavior change and weight loss were reinforced by behavioral techniques, the second group consisted of children only and child behavior change and weight loss were reinforced, and in the nonspecific control group families were reinforced for attendance. The best result was achieved in the parent and child group.

Furthermore, cognitive therapy has been used in the treatment of obesity, usually combined with behavioral therapy. This combination is based on the assumption that, through practice and reward, changes in key areas of children's cognitive processing will result in behavioral changes. However, the causal connections between the attempt to influence the child's cognition and the observed behavior changes have not been studied with stringent research designs [11].

Few studies have evaluated cognitive with behavioral therapy. In one such study, 27 children aged 7 to 13 years were randomized to either cognitive therapy or behavioral therapy. No differences were found after 3- and 6-months follow-up, and the therapies were equally effective [12]. The follow-up period was short, however.

In another study, behavioral treatment was combined with either cognitive therapy or nutrition education [13]. The different treatments induced different ways of controlling the weight; for instance, in the cognitive group the weight-related cognitions were more adaptive than in the other groups. However, the analysis showed that there were significant differences regarding the obesity status across time, but not between the different treatments. Finally, another study with a 3-month follow-up also showed that the addition of cognitive therapy to a behavioral program gave no further improvement than behavioral therapy by itself [14].

Finally, Caroline Braet and colleagues showed that cognitive therapy is effective in treating childhood obesity [15]. The treatment was combined with family talks, although regular family therapy was not given. Though it emerged from a different therapeutic background, this program has many similarities with the program based on family therapy [16]. These two studies show that a combined program is effective when using a careful selection of different approaches.

GROUP THERAPY

Many types of therapy can be utilized within the context of a group, and there have been some studies of this approach. For example, a peer group behavior modification program of adolescents gave better results than previous individual contacts [17]. However, the development of group cohesion was tenuous and temporary. Girls who were functioning more independently appeared to do better in weight loss. The study was not randomized, and the patient group was small. In another study, individual dietetic counseling, group dietetic counseling, and group dietetic counseling with behavior modification were compared [18]. The first and last treatments were equally effective at 1-year follow-up and better than group dietetic counseling alone. The general impression has been that group therapy has no decisive advantages over individual therapy [19]. Exceptions may include those groups that we carefully select so that they are strongly homogeneous regarding, for example, gender, age, and social background.

In preschool children, it is probably easier to get the children to accept a group formed by adults. Later on the children need to create their own groups. Probably, activities in groups might be more successful in preschool children than in older children.

However, if you combine the meeting in a group with a more specific method treatment might be effective for some groups. A Family Weight School treatment model was developed within the framework of SOFT (discussed later), setting up a 1-year program consisting of four group meetings [20]. Up to 12 families participated at each 4-hour meeting. A total of 65 out of 72 adolescents completed the program. The participation in the Family Weight School resulted in a significant decrease in degree of obesity in adolescents with body mass index (BMI) z-scores below 3.5 (adult equivalent approximately BMI 40 [21]), but not in adolescents with BMI z-scores above 3.5 compared with a waiting list control group. Thus, the Family Weight School has been shown to be effective in treating adolescents with severe obesity, but not for those with morbid obesity.

This shows that it is not sufficient to set up a group treatment program without adding a specific method. The encounter of a group could be as varied, based on different methods, as an individual meeting would be. Thus, the classification in Medline using group therapy as a specific Mesh term is not clear enough. This is also true for the Mesh term "family therapy," where the meeting of the family is not the only criterion that is important in defining the type of therapy.

The Mesh term "behavioral therapy" does not focus on whether you see an individual, a family, or a group. Thus, "group therapy" and "family therapy" should be given new definitions. Group therapy should be classified according to the psychological technique used. The most common form of family therapy should be called "systemic therapy" (discussed later).

SCHOOL-BASED TREATMENTS AND PREVENTION

It is difficult to give prevention at school without needing to treat the most severe cases. Thus, a good prevention program needs to be backed up by a good treatment program.

Behavioral therapy has also been used in a school setting [22]. The program consisted of behavior modification, nutrition education, and physical activity. Parents and school personnel were involved. Sixty (95%) of the 63 children (5 to 12 years) in the 10-week program lost weight, compared to only 3 (21%) of the 14 control children. The children in the program showed a mean decrease of 15.4% in their percentage overweight and lost an average of 4.4 kg.

Providing treatment in a wider context at school and, furthermore, perhaps not only promoting a good lifestyle to obese children but to *all* children may be a fruitful approach. However, long-term follow-up is difficult in such studies, with so many individuals being treated and so many variables to be controlled for. School-based treatments have been reviewed, but no single program was significantly better than the others, thus no recommendations could be made [23]. Most of the programs are not directed to obese children but instead to groups of all children.

School-based programs often act as a prevention strategy. The Swedish Council on Health Technology Assessment (SBU) did an analysis of prevention studies in childhood obesity [24]. The conclusion was that prevention probably is efficient, although there is no overall identifiable method that could be recommended. This shows the importance of focusing more on the methodological issues.

EARLY TREATMENT

Early treatment (i.e., treatment that started before the major peak incidence of childhood obesity at the age of 10) has shown better results for preschool children than for older children [25]. This type of treatment is in one way similar to school-based treatment as it is common to use groups of children, but it differs in being directed to *obese* children (as discussed earlier). Furthermore, treatment of children seems to be more effective than treatment of adults [26]. Moreover, 50% to 75% of adults in excess of 160% of ideal body weight were obese as children [27]. Thus, early treatment would prevent the most severe cases of obesity in adults.

However, no study has been performed comparing early to late start of treatment. The results could be explained just by including more cases early on that have a better prognosis.

FAMILY THERAPY

The family is regarded as basic to the child's psychological development and a major factor influencing the child's quality of life. Family therapy has been used for children with behavioral or emotional disturbances and for children with chronic diseases. Many studies have been performed, and they have been evaluated in several reviews [28–31]. These show family therapy to be effective in addressing asthma, diabetes, anorexia nervosa, bereavement, and adult schizophrenia. It has also been possible to develop family-based diagnostic tests for those families where a child is showing different symptoms [32].

Psychoeducational family therapy has been used to address schizophrenia. Orhagen and co-workers have studied whether the educational or the therapeutic part of the program was most effective and showed that both are needed [33]. Another Swedish study has shown family therapy to be a cost-effective treatment for childhood asthma [34].

It has also been suggested that family therapy might be helpful for treating obesity [35]. Epstein has shown in several studies the importance of the child's interaction with its parents [8, 10].

The author and co-workers have shown that the use of family therapy in treating obese children in a population screened at school prevents the progression of obesity in older teenagers if treatment is started at the age of 10 [16]. The families were selected from a population-based sample, and three groups were compared. The first group received conventional treatment (i.e., regular visits to a physician and a dietician); the second group underwent six sessions of family therapy. In both groups the duration of treatment was 14 to 18 months. The third group received no treatment.

At follow-up 1 year after the end of treatment, the body mass index was significantly lower in the family therapy group than in the untreated control group. Furthermore, physical fitness was significantly higher in the family therapy group than in the conventionally treated group, and the fat mass (measured by skinfold thickness) was significantly lower. There was no difference between the family therapy group and the conventionally treated group regarding body mass index. This might be due to the better physical fitness in combination with the reduced fat mass leading to a higher muscular mass, thus increasing the body mass index.

SYSTEMIC FAMILY MEDICINE

Family therapy has been tried as treatment for several chronic diseases. However, the techniques are not adapted to the disease. It is important not only to know how to give a message but also to give a message that relates to the problems presented by the disease. Furthermore, the medical condition, in this case obesity, also needs to be addressed. It is better to give the medical treatment as an integrated part of the overall treatment.

Systemic family medicine is a field of medicine that can be defined by an integration of system theory, family therapy, general practice, and modern clinical medicine [36]. In system theory, there is a core that says that one cannot understand the wholeness of any phenomenon by examination, only its component parts. First, psychiatrists applied system theory in clinical practice to treat severe psychiatric cases; later it also became a possibility for clinical medicine. In the field of family therapy today, systemic family medicine is a useful biopsychosocial model that gives the doctors and the team a creative complement to the regular medical/biological model. The traditional paradigms of linear causality are here replaced with a circular model where different factors interact and are connected to each other. Illnesses are, in this perspective, a part of a pattern. Families and networks are often active in a helping process. The therapist is also a part in this ongoing dialogue of communications.

During the decades there have been an increased number of studies concerning the family and its influence on chronic illness [37–39]. In most of these studies, there is a family dysfunction that is associated with poor coping, low adherence, and adverse health outcomes [40–42]. The bodies of research demonstrate that families and their network influence most health-related behavior and bring forward the notion about the limitations to meet the patient alone.

There are several ways of giving family therapy. However, the basic ideas are the same. First, the ambition to change and develop the family structure, based on the needs of the child and the other family members, is important. Second, the family hierarchy, including grandparents, is taken into account. Third, the major way of achieving these goals is to engage the family by gathering them together to discuss the problems or solutions. Finally, the family life cycle is also important, as needs differ as the family evolves. For instance, an additional child requires a changed family structure in which every member has to adapt and yet retain his or her own individuality.

SOLUTION-BASED BRIEF THERAPY

The solution-based brief therapy originally emanated from the field of family therapy. Family therapy has its origin in the schools of interactional, relational, and systemic theory. Since the 1950s, family therapy began to find its roots in the current research about human communication [43–46], and from that point several kinds of schools have developed. During the 1980s, Steve de Shazer [47–50] introduced a kind of therapeutic interaction named solution-based brief therapy. This was an unusual therapy that became famous for its originality and for its simplicity, at least on the surface.

Steve de Shazer was inspired and influenced by poststructuralist philosophers such as Wittgenstein and Derrida who were among the creators of the perspectives of constructivism [51–54], which describes how you in your inner world, and in dialog with significant others, construct an image of the world you are living in. Our relation to language is also like a barrier that can be passed by communication to other people. As human beings, we are using language but the language is also using us. Together this became a map or a construct that is guiding you in life. The construct is continuously changing, or maybe it is not.

In the therapeutic interaction, the therapist begins a kind of language game: "the term language-game is meant to bring into prominence the fact that the speaking of language is a part of an activity, or of a life-form" (p10, item 23) [53]. The language game is in this context a complete system of human communication. The language game is a way to describe that the communication between the therapist and the client has attributes similar to any other language systems.

SOFT

Standardized Obesity Family Therapy (SOFT) is a use of family therapy in a somatic context, treating obesity as is systemic family medicine mentioned earlier. The first study developing this model has been described in detail elsewhere [16]. This is one of the few randomized controlled trials in the treatment of childhood obesity and it was performed in our center after screening a general population of schoolchildren aged 10 to 12. The study was described under the "Family Therapy" section presented earlier in the chapter. This method has now been applied at the Childhood Obesity Unit at Skåne University Hospital, serving children and adolescents in southern Sweden. The method has been further evaluated in the practical setting of this tertiary referral center [55].

SOFT Compared to Other Treatment Models

Although approaches effective in the treatment of childhood and adolescent obesity share many similarities, the models are quite different in their underlying treatment philosophies and implementation strategies [56]. The most distinguishing feature of SOFT is the focus on family interactions as an important source for implementing and maintaining lifestyle changes [36, 57]. SOFT (and also family therapy) focuses on interactions that are not part of psychodynamic, behavioral, or cognitive behavior-based obesity treatment models. Families are often included in the treatment of childhood obesity [58–60]. However, SOFT is the only treatment model for obesity that relies on coherent integration of family systems theory and therapy, developed and evaluated in a medical setting. SOFT integrates systemic [61] and solution-focused theory and principles [49] and is an empirically validated family therapy model for children and adolescents with obesity. The goal of SOFT is to provide an appropriate level of medical and psychosocial support to families of children with obesity.

Research on SOFT

Several studies have tested the efficacy of SOFT in child and adolescent groups. In the first study, family therapy was found to be effective in the treatment of 10- to 12-year-old obese children [62]. Neither systemic family medicine nor SOFT was established at that time. A study description has been given under "Family Therapy."

In a second study, 54 highly obese children and adolescents were offered family therapy by a multidisciplinary treatment team consisting of a pediatrician, a dietician/sports trainer, a pediatric nurse, and a family therapist. This intervention resulted in a significant decrease in the child's degree of obesity, as well as improvement in self-esteem and family functioning [63]. These results were obtained with 3.8 sessions. Eighty-one percent of the families participated in the follow-up. The treatment offered in this study is part of routine clinical practice in the Childhood Obesity Unit and will be described under "Practical Approach" below.

THE PROCESSES IN THERAPY

Approaching the Family

The major problem in obesity is to establish adequate motivation for long-term treatment success. The thoughts and beliefs of the subjects' families will therefore be briefly discussed based mainly on our experiences with the study [16] and the work within the Childhood Obesity Unit using SOFT [64].

In a family in which obesity is frequent, there is a tendency to accept overweight as a positive identification across generation borders. Also, a parent may fear hurting the child physically or mentally by discussing weight control or changes of diet. The therapist had to approach this question with respect.

Different family members showed variations in how they took advantage of the therapy. However, the child was usually the most interested, and therefore most motivated, in regulating his or her weight. This could be related to increasing problems of the preadolescent in relation to finding suitable, well-fitting clothes and his or her desire to look more like other children. Yet few of the obese 10- to 11-year-olds reported any problems regarding bullying by other children. They also reported ordinary relationships with friends.

Even if the child is strongly motivated, he or she is closely dependent on the parent regarding choice of food purchased and served in the home. Usually the families wanted to maintain their habits, and an incongruence arose between this desire and the need for the family to change in order to help the obese child. In this situation, therapy is a means of helping the family to try out other solutions to the problem.

The Strategy in Therapy

The most useful strategy was to recommend small and simple changes rather than more complex ones. The effect of a small change regarding diet or exercise, if allowed to exert its influence for a long time, is much greater than major changes that the family cannot maintain. Indeed, by walking or running 4 km a day (equivalent to 200 kcal in a 40-kg child), the child can lose 1 kg within 35 days, or 5 kg in half a year, even without a reducing diet [65]. Instead, in order to lose 1 kg of adipose tissue in a short period of time and in an unreasonable way, a 40-kg child may have to run 140 km or play tennis for 26 hours. This example is also a metaphor for an efficient change according to Steve de Shazer's model.

The therapist used the structural model (Minuchin) as a frame perspective within which the solution-based model (de Shazer) exerted its influence. Usually the situations that the families wanted to discuss were those in which the child or parents experienced difficulty following the prescribed diet or recommended exercise, not the recommendations per se.

During therapy, adequate information was essential for success in finding solutions. Usually the family was asked to discuss different solutions at home before the next session. The beliefs and thoughts of the obese child were essential to the process.

Family Interaction

How do families communicate their essential needs with regard to feelings, cognitive information, and appreciation? There are indications that the families are not homogenous when their ways of communicating are taken into account. Ways of relating to the obese child cannot easily be generalized, as families are different.

Some general observations will be made, however. The consequences of weight reduction may result in worries about the health and well-being of the child. Often the parents talked about this openly, especially the fear that the child would develop anorexia nervosa. However, the children had much more courage and a more realistic feeling for an appropriate weight goal.

Practical Approach

The treatment lasted for four to six sessions, and sometimes it was even shorter. The clients appreciated this kind of therapy, which clearly differs from traditional psychotherapy. There was a strict focus on solutions, not on problems like the vast majority of psychotherapy suggests (e.g., psychodynamic therapy). Furthermore, the attitude contained a total respect for the patient and his or hers values. However, it was necessary to bring up a goal in therapy; otherwise it was not possible to conduct any therapy.

In solution-focused therapy, small and achievable goals are recommended, as the accomplishment of the first goal may lead to the next. There is also a technique of using scale questions to better visualize how the client approaches a goal. The desired state of change is also a question that brings up a lot of creativity and positive feelings. In order to take small steps, the solution talk becomes realistic and invites a focus on change. "Change is inevitable" is a statement by Bateson that takes advantage of a process that is going on whether we notice it or not. It's a fact of life on this planet [45].

Starting therapy, a process that lasts about 2 years, is initiated with two to four sessions per year. Each session starts with an evaluation of the present situation and, with the help of medical data, ends up with a conclusion. The family takes an active part in this process. This conclusion is always supportive and delivered in a positive manner. The underlying message is always, you're doing your best—and we know it. It also includes an appreciation of valuable achievements by the family and further suggestions for homework.

The Outlining of the Interview

To start with questions like "What has been working well since we met last?" is often very useful throughout therapy. Thus, the family members are given the opportunity to reflect about the favorable circumstances they have contributed to. Furthermore, the therapist appreciates the answers as a sign of positive care by family members. Not only parents but also the child is given credit for these achievements. Thus, positive sequences are initiated. Later on the family's specific problems may be encountered and detailed solutions may be discussed. Usually the family is eager to discuss how to reinforce those aspects of the child that are positive and function well.

The good intentions of the family to maintain results are clarified by discussing what every family member has done in detail and how. This creative process is used as a prophylaxis against future difficulties in maintaining normal weight. How different family members recognize the beginning of a relapse is valuable, as the child can be made aware of the dangerous chain of events that can follow. Usually one or several members of the family are given a task or a question to think over until next time. The therapist finishes the session by complimenting all the members.

At the beginning of the next session, the outcome of the task is checked. Thus, a good cycle of events is created, and the child is considered to function better. This may be expanded to other areas of life with the help of parents and siblings. Finally, the initial problem of good eating behavior is regarded as solved, although the family is aware of the risk of a relapse. By now the family also has a strategy for how to cope with this possibility by reminding the child of the good cycles.

A supervisor and co-therapist were used in the study conducted in 1993 [16]. Before the compliments were given, a short break was taken. Later using SOFT, the treatment team included several professionals (pediatrician, nurse, dietician, sports trainer, psychologist) and a break was not always taken [63].

The therapy included those questions and solutions that the family was ready to discuss. One major topic was the identified patient's (IP) ideal weight and the family's reactions to the beliefs of the child. Often, both the child and the family had unrealistic expectations when it came to achievable goals. After they received information on biological limitations, especially in childhood, most families accepted more realistic goals and time schedules for achieving goals. Another topic was how great a chance the IP had to achieve his or her goal as measured on a visual-analogous scale (VAS; from 0 to 10). All family members were asked to give a value, which might differ from time to time. The kind of support needed for the IP to achieve this goal was discussed. Different suggestions and solutions were listed and discussed. The VAS was also used to measure available resources, and this resulted in many good suggestions for both the IP and other members of the family. It was clear from our observations that the family was eager to solve the problem but they lacked effective solutions.

To summarize, the following items were found to be useful:

- Give the family low-intensity, nonconfrontational contact.
- Identify the resources of the family and acknowledge them.
- Show respect for the family, and use noncondemning interventions.
- Involve important individuals.
- Try to identify the whole system and relate it to its context.

- Accept the individual's definition of the problem.
- Rephrase that definition in a positive context.
- Emphasize the positive solutions.
- Start with the small, simple solutions. Show appreciation.
- Discuss an appropriate and realistic ideal weight.
- Inform the family about the time needed to achieve the goal in the longer term.
- Remind everyone that controlling overweight is hard work.

A CASE

All the family members were seen as being involved and enthusiastic. They all gave many suggestions on how to help the IP. The members asked many questions and were eager to collect information given by the therapist. The father was severely obese and had tried many sorts of treatments. He had an impressive knowledge of nutrition and healthcare issues, although he was not able to use it. The therapist gave him the view that he would know that to do when the time came. He was also given credit for his earlier attempts to lose weight. The mother was also severely obese but more successful in her achievements. She was complimented on this.

The IP showed strong positive feelings toward her parents, which were confirmed by the therapist. This involved all the members of the family in her problem. The difficulty was defined as finding a suitable strategy and a way of knowing when the right time had come to apply it. The family should be convinced that a solution was close at hand before trying once more. The other children in the family and their experiences with weight control were thoroughly discussed and their strengths emphasized. One of the older children had normal weight and stated clearly that she'd had the same difficulties as her little sister up to the age of 15. She did not know how she had succeeded, but this was a turning point for her. The therapist emphasized her own effort in this by complimenting the sister on her achievement.

All the family members, including the IP, stated that this was also what was going to happen in her case. The therapist stated that this was a good example of what strong conviction may achieve and that the IP should be prepared when the time came.

Suggestions were given to the family members as to how to discuss these matters and they were each encouraged to give their personal view to the IP, to increase her readiness to change.

The therapist also asked the IP to mention her ideal weight, so she would be more aware of when her goal was reached. The IP was eager to discuss this, and the family's reactions to her ideal weight were observed.

Complements were given to both the IP and the other family members to reward their good judgment and patience. They were prepared to wait 2 or 3 years for a change to take place.

During therapy, the family started with an intensive program resulting in a substantial weight reduction. The therapist then asked the family how they would notice a relapse as early as possible. Also, a slower rate of increase was recommended (it is not recommended that children lose weight at this age; instead they should gradually approach the normal weight for their height, as an increase in height naturally increases the weight). This view was well received by the family and was also compatible with their beliefs as mentioned earlier.

In another case, interventive interviewing was described [56]. This technique involves using circular and reflexive questions developed by Karl Tomm [66–68]. A practical example is given in the following section.

THE QUESTIONS ARE THE ANSWERS

Here are some examples of how to use the different types of questions in the treatment of obesity in children and adolescents. You are seeing a 15-year boy, along with his mother and father. The setting might be a doctor's office or a room especially set up for conversational therapy.

Linear Questions

>Doctor: How are things going with John's obesity?
>Mother: He is trying to eat less, but I don't know what he is doing when he comes home from school.
>Doctor: Do you follow the lists I have given to you, John?
>John: I have tried to, but I don't know where they are.
>Doctor: When did you see them last?
>John: I don't remember.
>Father: My wife says he is always trying to escape his responsibilities.
>Doctor: Do you remember anything from my lists, John?
>John: No, I don't. Didn't I tell you that a minute ago? I want to go home now.

The linear questions, although not intended, could lead to scapegoating. Here, John is blamed for not being able to follow the diet. This began with the initial complaint of the mother. The doctor used linear questions without the intent of blaming, but this effort was counteracted as the mother got support from the father, who really did not know what was going on at home.

Circular Questions

>Doctor: How are things going with John's obesity?
>Mother: He is trying to eat less, but I don't know what he is doing when he comes home from school.

Now you know that the mother is worried. Instead you use circular questions to investigate the problem.

>Doctor: Who would know that?
>Father: My wife says he is always trying to escape his responsibilities.

Now you know the father also is worried, but he does not know what is happening at home when he is not there.

>Doctor: Who is most worried about your obesity John, your father or your mother?
>John: It is my mother.
>Doctor: How do you know that?
>John: She is always nagging about what I am eating when I get home from school.
>Doctor: Is there any difference in how your mother or how your father reminds you about what you are eating?
>John: Yes, my father reminds me, but my mother is nagging all the time.
>Doctor to mother and father: What can you do to help each other to remind John about his late afternoon snack?

These questions are more neutral, but still you need to be careful. Although you used circular questions, you might need to give the mother more support.

Strategic Questions

Now let us continue the conversation with something more powerful! These questions are used by lawyers and journalists and are *not* recommended for obesity treatment. They could be useful in certain psychiatric conditions, but an example is given here. The doctor wants to increase the father's involvement.

>Father answers: I don't know.
>Doctor to father: Can't you see that you make your wife disappointed by not helping her?
>Father: I have too much to do at work.
>Doctor to father: How is it possible for you to totally abandon your family?
>Father: I am really trying, you know.
>Doctor to father: When do you think your wife will let you choose between your job and your family?

After this exchange, you might never see the family again. Of course, these questions might be efficient, but they are too powerful. Instead, reflexive questions are recommended.

Reflexive Questions

Father answers: I don't know.
Doctor to father: If you would guess, what might you be able to do?
Father: I might call John at home when I have my coffee break and remind him about what he is going to eat.
Doctor to mother: If this was done regularly, do you think this would help John to lose weight?
Mother: Of course, it would. I would be so happy if I didn't have to take all the responsibility for John's eating all the time.

CONCLUSION

Our studies show family therapy to be effective in preventing the development of gross obesity during childhood [16, 55]. Furthermore, behavioral therapy and cognitive behavioral therapy show long-term effects [10, 15, 69].

Many studies in childhood obesity treatment do not focus on the methodological questions. This leaves the outcome up to the skills of the treatment team, which are not described and cannot be conveyed to another study. Moreover, we have the same problem in most prevention trials. Thus, it is of major importance that the methodological issues receive more attention.

The reasons for treating childhood obesity are the negative long-term effects on health. It is not known what is the lowest degree of childhood obesity, expressed in BMI, at which future complications such as cardiovascular disease and diabetes start to be over-represented when compared with the normal-weight population. However, both Mossberg [70] and Must et al. [71] have demonstrated that obesity in childhood is associated with major adverse health effects. Adoption studies involving obese adults [72] have shown how genetic and environmental influences on premature death can be distinguished.

Our studies are good examples of a systemic medical approach integrating psychological methods with medical treatment where the different needs of the individual were taken care of with standard family therapy techniques still gaining a good result. However, the need for urgent action regarding childhood obesity makes further research in this field of knowledge necessary.

References

1. Bruch H. Psychological aspects of overeating and obesity. *Psychosomatics* 1964;**5**:269–74.
2. Bruch H. Eating disorders in adolescence. *Proc Annu Meet Am Psychopathol Assoc* 1970;**59**:181–202.
3. Kaslow FW. The family as background to obesity, *The international book of family therapy*. New York: Bruner; 1974.
4. Porter K. Combined individual and group psychotherapy: a review of the literature 1965-1978. *Int J Group Psychother* 1980;**30**:107–14.
5. Stuart RB. Behavioral control of overeating. *Behav Res Ther* 1967;**5**:357–65.
6. Brownell KD, Wadden TA. The heterogeneity of obesity. *Behavior Therapy* 1991;**22**:153–77.
7. Björvell H, Rössner S. A ten-year follow-up of weight change in severely obese subjects treated in a combined behavioural modification programme. *Int J Obes Relat Metab Disord* 1992;**16**:623–5.
8. Epstein LH, Wing RR, Steranchak L, Dickson B, Michelson J. Comparison of family based behavior modification and nutrition education for childhood obesity. *J Pediatr Psychol* 1980;**5**:25–36.
9. Brownell KD, Kelman JH, Stunkard AJ. Treatment of obese children with and without their mothers: changes in weight and blood pressure. *Pediatrics* 1983;**71**:515–23.
10. Epstein LH, Valoski A, Wing RR, McCurley J. Ten-year follow-up of behavioral, family-based treatment for obese children. *JAMA* 1990;**264**:2519–23.
11. Kendall P, Lochman J. Cognitive-Behavioural Therapies. In: Rutter M, Taylor E, Hersov L, editors. *Child and adolescent psychiatry*. London: Blackwell Science; 1994. pp. 844–57.
12. Duffy G, Spence SH. The effectiveness of cognitive self-management as an adjunct to a behavioural intervention for childhood obesity: a research note. *J Child Psychol Psychiatry* 1993;**34**:1043–50.
13. Kalodner CR, DeLucia JL. The individual and combined effects of cognitive therapy and nutrition education as additions to a behavior modification program for weight loss. *Addict Behav* 1991;**16**:255–63.
14. DeLucia JL, Kalodner CR. An individualized cognitive intervention: does it increase the efficacy of behavioral interventions for obesity? *Addict Behav* 1990;**15**:473–9.
15. Braet C, Mervielde I, Vandereycken W. Psychological aspects of childhood obesity: a controlled study in a clinical and nonclinical sample. *J Pediatr Psychol* 1997;**22**:59–71.
16. Flodmark CE, Ohlsson T, Ryden O, Sveger T. Prevention of progression to severe obesity in a group of obese schoolchildren treated with family therapy. *Pediatrics* 1993;**91**:880–4.
17. Zakus G, Chin ML, Keown M, Hebert F, Held M. A group behavior modification approach to adolescent obesity. *Adolescence* 1979;**14**:481–90.
18. Long CG, Simpson CM, Allott EA. Psychological and dietetic counselling combined in the treatment of obesity: a comparative study in a hospital outpatient clinic. *Hum Nutr Appl Nutr* 1983;**37**:94–102.
19. Aimez P. [Modification of pathogenic dietary behavior. Group techniques]. *Ann Nutr Aliment* 1976;**30**:289–99.
20. Nowicka P, Hoglund P, Pietrobelli A, Lissau I, Flodmark CE. Family Weight School treatment: 1-year results in obese adolescents. *Int J Pediatr Obes* 2008;**3**:141–7.
21. Daley AJ, Copeland RJ, Wright NP, Roalfe A, Wales JK. Exercise therapy as a treatment for psychopathologic conditions in obese and morbidly obese adolescents: a randomized, controlled trial. *Pediatrics* 2006;**118**:2126–34.
22. Brownell KD, Kaye FS. A school-based behavior modification, nutrition education, and physical activity program for obese children. *Am J Clin Nutr* 1982;**35**:277–83.
23. Ward D, Bar-Or E. Role of the Physician and Physical Education Teacher in the Treatment of Obesity at School. *Pediatrician* 1986;**13**:44–51.

24. Flodmark CE, Marcus C, Britton M. Interventions to prevent obesity in children and adolescents: a systematic literature review. *Int J Obes (Lond)* 2006;**30**:579–89.
25. Davis K, Christoffel KK. Obesity in pre-school and school-age children. Treatment early and often may be best. *Arch Pediatr Adolesc Med* 1994;**148**:1257–61.
26. Epstein LH, Valoski AM, Kalarchian MA, McCurley J. Do children lose and maintain weight easier than adults: a comparison of child and parent weight changes from six months to ten years. *Obesity Research* 1995;**3**:411–17.
27. Dietz WH. Childhood obesity: Susceptibility, cause and management. *J Pediatr* 1983;**103**:676–86.
28. Gurman A, Kniskern D. Family therapy outcome research: Knowns and unknowns. In: *Handbook of family therapy*. New York: Branner/Mazel; 1981. pp. 742–51.
29. Hazelrigg M, Cooper H, Bourdin C. Evaluating the effectiveness of family therapy: an integrative review and analysis. *Psychol Bull.* 1987;**101**:428–42.
30. Lask B. Family therapy. *Br Med J* 1987;**294**:203–4.
31. Dare C. Change the family, change the child? *Arch Dis Child* 1992;**67**:643–8.
32. Hansson, K. Familjediagnostik (Family diagnostics.) Lund University, Lund, Sweden; 1989.
33. Orhagen, T. Working with families in schizophrenic disorders: the practice of psycho-educational intervention. Linköping University; 1992.
34. Gustafsson, P. A. Family interaction and family therapy in childhood psychosomatic disease. Linköping University; 1987.
35. Ganley RM. Epistemology, family patterns, and psychosomatics: The case of obesity. *Family Process* 1986;**25**:437–51.
36. Flodmark CE, Ohlsson T. Childhood obesity: from nutrition to behaviour. *Proc Nutr Soc* 2008;**67**:356–62.
37. Gustafsson PA, Cederblad M, Ludvigsson J, Lundin B. Family interaction and metabolic balance in juvenile diabetes mellitus. A prospective study. *Diabetes Res Clin Pract* 1987;**4**:7–14.
38. Gustafsson PA, Kjellman NI, Cederblad M. Family therapy in the treatment of severe childhood asthma. *J Psychosom Res.* 1986;**30**:369–74.
39. Lask B, Matthew D. Childhood asthma. A controlled trial of family psychotherapy. *Arch Dis Child* 1979;**55**:116–19.
40. Larivaara P. Systemic family medicine: a new framework for general practitioners and their interprofessional teams. *Metaforum (Norwegian Association for Family Therapy)* 2008;**25**:33–8.
41. Larivaara P, Taanila A, Aaltonen J, Lindroos S, Väisänen E, Väisänen L. Family-oriented health care in Finland: Background and some innovative projects. *Families, Systems & Health* 2004;**22**:395–409.
42. Larivaara P, Väisänen E, Kiuttu J. Family systems medicine: A new field of medicine. *Nordic Journal of Psychiatry* 1994;**48**:329–32.
43. Bateson G. A theory of play and fantasy; a report on theoretical aspects of the project of study of the role of the paradoxes of abstraction in communication. *Psychiatr Res Rep Am Psychiatr Assoc*; 1955:39–51.
44. Bateson G. Communication in occupational therapy. *Am J Occup Ther* 1956;**10**:188.
45. Bateson G. *Minimal requirements of a theory of schizophrenia. Steps to an ecology of mind*. New York: Jason Aronson; 1972.
46. Bateson G, Jackson DD. Social Factors and Disorders of Communication: Some Varieties of Pathogenic Organization. *Res Publ Assoc Res Nerv Ment Dis* 1964;**42**:270–90.
47. de Shazer S. *Patterns of brief family therapy*. New York: Guilford; 1982.
48. de Shazer S. *Keys to solution in brief therapy*. New York: Norton; 1985.
49. de Shazer S. *Clues: Investigating solutions in brief therapy*. New York: Norton; 1988.
50. de Shazer S. *Putting difference to work*. New York: W.W. Norton & Company, Inc.; 1991.
51. Derrida J. *Writing and difference*. Chicago: University of Chicago Press; 1978.
52. Derrida J. *Positions*. London: Athlone; 1981.
53. Wittgenstein L. *"Philosophical investigations"*. Oxford: Blackwell publishing Ltd; 1953, 1958, 2001.
54. Wittgenstein L. *Philosophical remarks*. Chicago: The University of Chicago Press; 1975.
55. Nowicka P, Pietrobelli A, Flodmark CE. Low-intensity family therapy intervention is useful in a clinical setting to treat obese and extremely obese children. *Int J Pediatr Obes* 2007:1–7.
56. Flodmark CE. Management of the obese child using psychological-based treatments. *Acta Paediatr* 2005;**94**(Suppl):14–22.
57. Flodmark CE. Childhood Obesity. *Clinical Child Psychology and Psychiatry* 1997;**2**:283–95.
58. Kitzmann KM, Beech BM. Family-based interventions for pediatric obesity: methodological and conceptual challenges from family psychology. *J Fam Psychol* 2006;**20**:175–89.
59. Nowicka P, Flodmark CE. Family in pediatric obesity management: a literature review. *Int J Pediatr Obes* 2008;**3**(Suppl. 1):44–50.
60. Young KM, Northern JJ, Lister KM, Drummond JA, O'Brien WH. A meta-analysis of family-behavioral weight-loss treatments for children. *Clinical Psychology Review* 2007;**27**:240–9.
61. Palazolli M, Boscolo L, Cecchin G, Prata G. Hypothesizing-circularity-neutrality: Three guidelines for the conductor of the session. *Family Process* 1980;**21**:3–12.
62. Flodmark CE. *Obesity and hyperlipoproteinaemia in children*. Lund, Sweden: Lund University; 1993.
63. Nowicka P, Pietrobelli A, Flodmark CE. Low-intensity family therapy intervention is useful in a clinical setting to treat obese and extremely obese children. *Int J Pediatr Obes* 2007;**2**:211–17.
64. Nowicka P. *Childhood and adolescent obesity*. Lund: Lund University; 2009.
65. Bar-Or O. *Pediatric Sports Medicine for the Practitioner*. New York: Springer-Verlag; 1983.
66. Tomm K. Interventive interviewing: Part II. Reflexive questioning as a means to enable self-healing. *Fam Process* 1987;**26**:167–83.
67. Tomm K. Interventive interviewing: Part I. Strategizing as a fourth guideline for the therapist. *Fam Process* 1987;**26**:3–13.
68. Tomm K. Interventive interviewing: Part III. Intending to ask lineal, circular, strategic, or reflexive questions? *Fam Process* 1988;**27**:1–15.
69. Epstein LH, Valoski A, McCurley J. Effect of weight loss by obese children on long-term growth. *Am J Dis Child* 1993;**147**:1076–80.
70. Mossberg HO. 40-year follow-up of overweight children. *Lancet* 1989;**2**:491–3.
71. Must A, Jacques PF, Dallal GE, Bajema CJ, Dietz WH. Long-term morbidity and mortality of overweight adolescents. A follow-up of the Harvard Growth Study of 1922 to 1935. *N Engl J Med* 1992;**327**:1350–5.
72. Sørensen TI. Genetic epidemiology utilizing the adoption method: studies of obesity and of premature death in adults. *Scand J Soc Med* 1991;**19**:14–19.

CHAPTER 38

Childhood Obesity
Psychological Correlates and Recommended Therapeutic Strategies

Jennifer E. Phillips*, Ethan E. Hull†, Dana L. Rofey†

*University of Pittsburgh, PA, USA and †Children's Hospital of Pittsburgh, Pittsburgh, PA, USA

INTRODUCTION

The myriad health risks associated with childhood and adolescent obesity include cardiovascular complications such as hypertension, dyslipidemia, insulin resistance, and chronic inflammation [1, 2]. Obesity, along with the accompanying cardiovascular risk factors, has been shown to track from childhood into adulthood [3–5]. In contrast to the many well-established physical health consequences, the psychological correlates of obesity in childhood are less clear [6, 7]. However, overweight and obese youth are often the targets of bias and stereotyping by peers [8–10], teachers [11, 12], and parents [13] and growing evidence documents several psychological comorbidities related to childhood obesity [9, 14–16]. Thus, similar to long-term physical consequences, the negative impact of obesity-related stigma may have lasting effects on emotional well-being.

PSYCHOLOGICAL CORRELATES OF PEDIATRIC OBESITY

In addition to the adverse physical health effects of obesity in youth, a growing body of evidence indicates damaging psychosocial consequences of pediatric obesity. As reviewed here, these include weight-based teasing [14], social isolation and discrimination [9], depression [15], and low self-esteem [14, 16].

Teasing and Social Rejection

Weight-based teasing encountered by overweight and obese youth may take several forms. These include being the subject of verbal remarks such as name calling, being the target of rumors, being ignored, avoided, or otherwise socially excluded, or physical bullying (see the review in [17]). Obese children are rejected more often by peers and are more likely to be socially isolated than their nonoverweight counterparts [18, 19].

Body Dissatisfaction

Reviews conclude that overweight and obese children, particularly girls, exhibit greater body dissatisfaction than their normal-weight peers [7, 20]. Further, body dissatisfaction may have a negative impact on self-esteem in obese children, as indicated by data documenting a mediation effect of body dissatisfaction in the association of obesity and self-esteem in a sample of elementary school children [21].

Self-Esteem

The internalization of weight-based discrimination may have negative implications for self-esteem in obese youth. Weight-based teasing has been associated with poorer self-esteem and an increased likelihood of depression among adolescents [14]. Prospective data support the self-esteem finding and have demonstrated that weight-based peer teasing, along with parental weight criticism, mediates the relationship between overweight and lower self-concept in adolescents [13]. Further, weight-related teasing has been shown to account for associations between weight and body dissatisfaction in youth [22, 23]. This result appears to extend into adulthood as a retrospective study of adults reported an association between childhood weight-based teasing and adulthood body dissatisfaction, which, in turn, covaried with lower self-esteem [24].

Prospective studies examining the development of low self-esteem and obesity generally show that excess weight in children predicts future low self-esteem [13, 25–27]. Epidemiological [28] and clinical data [29] also demonstrate that body mass is inversely related to self-esteem in children, though comprehensive reviews of self-esteem and obesity reveal this relationship to be a modest one [7, 30]. However, the relationship between self-esteem and obesity appears to be stronger when obese children are compared with their nonobese peers specifically on measures of physical self-perception [31] rather than global self-esteem.

Anxiety and Depression

To date, the evidence supporting an association between anxiety-related disorders and pediatric obesity is inconclusive. Some studies demonstrate no significant differences for anxiety symptoms between overweight and normal-weight children [32] and adolescents [33]. In contrast, obese adolescents participating in an inpatient weight-loss program reported higher lifetime prevalence of anxiety disorders as compared to nonobese controls [34], and Buddeburg-Fisher and colleagues [35] found higher rates of anxiety disorders in overweight Swiss high school girls. A longitudinal investigation of childhood psychopathology and body mass in youth aged 8 to 18 showed a significant increase in body mass index (BMI) percentiles for non obese children as compared to controls [36].

Evidence of a relationship between obesity and depression in children and adolescents is also mixed. Research generally shows that community-based samples of obese children do not differ in levels of depression compared to average-weight peers [14, 37, 38], though clinical samples of obese children appear to display higher levels of depression than normal-weight controls [34, 39]. Regarding casual relationships, more research is needed. Two prospective studies did not show that obesity predicted depression in adolescent girls [40, 41], whereas research among boys demonstrates a modest relationship between chronic obesity and higher levels of depression over time [42]. In contrast, other evidence indicates that it is childhood depression that predicts the development of obesity in both children [15] and adults [36, 43, 44]. Thus, no clear association between child psychopathology and obesity has been established, yet the possible long-term negative sequelae of these disorders reinforces the need for future research, particularly regarding the elucidation of any directional relationships.

Suicidal Behaviors

One of the most alarming consequences of obesity in youth may be the increased risk of suicidal behaviors. Several studies have demonstrated that obese adolescents are more likely than their average-weight peers to endorse suicidal ideation and suicide attempts [45–47]. In light of the strong correlation between depression and suicidal behavior [48], these findings lend further credence to the hypothesized link between obesity and depression.

Quality of Life

Taken together, evidence suggests that overweight and obese children may be at increased risk for the development of negative emotional or psychological outcomes. In addition, impairments have been documented in overall quality of life (QOL) scores of obese children and adolescents [49–51], perhaps (in part) because of the negative psychosocial consequences discussed earlier. The high prevalence of childhood and adolescent obesity, along with the potential long-term mental and physical health implications, underscores the need for efficacious obesity-related interventions for children and adolescents.

EMPIRICALLY SUPPORTED TREATMENTS FOR PEDIATRIC OBESITY

Fortunately, a number of strategies have been shown to help to prevent or reduce childhood obesity, and research demonstrates the positive health impacts of weight-loss interventions for pediatric populations [52–54] (see Table 38.1 for key therapeutic components). Similarly, long-term improvements in psychological factors (e.g., anxiety, depression) have been noted in children who have completed a behavioral weight-loss program [55].

The increased prevalence of childhood obesity, though likely the result of a combination of factors, has been largely attributed to the influence of environmental factors (i.e., nutrition and lifestyle) [56], and evidence indicates that some combination of exercise and nutrition instruction, along with dietary restriction, has a greater impact on weight loss than one isolated component [57, 58]. Thus, empirically supported treatments for pediatric obesity typically include nutritional education [57–59] and the promotion of increased physical activity [60, 61]. In addition, findings suggest that the involvement of both children and parents in treatment [62–64] contributes significantly to pediatric weight-loss efforts.

Behavioral Therapy

Ample evidence exists for the efficacy of behavioral treatment strategies in the treatment of pediatric obesity, particularly when parents are involved [65].

TABLE 38.1 Psychotherapeutic Strategies for Pediatric Obesity Treatment

Therapeutic orientation	Key components
Behavioral therapy[a]	Education (dietary, physical activity) Behavioral monitoring (food/activity logging) Contingency contracting and reinforcement programs (praise, tokens) Stimulus control techniques (alternate activities, environmental changes)
Cognitive therapy[b]	Identification of faulty cognitions Recognize connections between thoughts, feelings, behavior Positive self-statements Relaxation training (controlled breathing, progressive muscle relaxation, distraction, imagery) Modeling, role-playing, reinforcement for using CBT skills Problem solving
Motivational interviewing[c]	Collaborative—focus on individual's goals and values Directive—focus on function of ambivalence to elicit motivation Incorporates change talk Non-technical—focus on overall communication, not a specific technique

[a]Wadden, T.A., & Foster, G.D. (2000). Behavioral treatment of obesity. The Medical Clinics of North America, 84, 441–461.
[b]Beck, A. (1997). The past and future of cognitive therapy. Journal of Psychotherapy Practice and Research, 6, 276–284.
[c]Miller, W., & Rollnick, S. (2002). Motivational Interviewing (2nd Ed.), Preparing People for Change. New York: Guilford Press.

Behaviorally-based therapies stress the development of new eating and exercise habits and provide specific strategies for changing the environment. The components used in behavioral weight-management treatment generally include stimulus control strategies, self monitoring of diet and physical activity, and reinforcement of behavior change, [66]. Additionally, parent training is a key element in behavioral pediatric weight management. Parents are asked to engage in several strategies to assist their children in meeting weight-loss goals, including *contingency contracting*, in which parents agree to make behavioral changes alongside those of their children; *functional analysis*, where parents observe and quantify the frequency of a target behavior (i.e., overeating, sedentary behavior) and subsequently note the consequences of the target behavior, and *reinforcement programs*, which use "alternate" behavioral consequences to affect the rate of a specific behavior (i.e., money, praise, tokens, clothing, etc.). Behavioral therapy programs also utilize stimulus control techniques such as teaching individuals to eat more slowly, to delay gratification, to eat in one designated area, and to eat low-calorie snacks.

One such technique developed by Leonard Epstein in the 1970s, teaches a "color-coded" food strategy: high-calorie foods (greater than 5 grams of fat per serving) are coded red and should only be eaten rarely; moderate-calorie foods (between 2 and 5 grams of fat) are coded yellow and can be eaten in moderation; and low-calorie foods (less than 2 grams of fat), including vegetables and some fruits, are coded green and can be consumed freely. Self-monitoring of behavior is also a central strategy of behavioral weight-loss programs, through which the individual maintains records of when and where he or she engages in behaviors that are either supportive of or detrimental to weight-loss efforts. For example, through self-monitoring, individuals note which mood symptoms, with whom, or what times of day may influence eating behavior.

Early research from the 1970s and 1980s [67–71], as well as more recent work from the 1990s [53, 70, 71], support the use of behavioral family-based interventions for pediatric weight loss. In particular, the work of Epstein and colleagues provides compelling evidence for using behavioral interventions in the treatment of pediatric obesity [53, 70]. The results of several of Epstein's randomized clinical trials, in which children ages 6 to 12 years (along with one obese parent) received a 6-month behavioral weight-loss intervention, show that 30% of the children were no longer obese 10 years post-intervention. Overall, behaviorally based family therapy and lifestyle modification appear to be effective in the treatment of obesity in children.

Cognitive Behavioral Therapy

Though some evidence suggests that a behavioral approach to pediatric obesity may be superior to cognitive strategies [72], the inclusion of cognitive treatment components in laboratory-based investigations of childhood and adult weight loss has shown favorable results [70, 71, 73, 74]. Cognitive behavioral therapy (CBT) strategies attempt to address issues that may have been overlooked in early behavioral programs, including cognitive distortions regarding body image and eating, instruction in self-monitoring, problem-solving techniques, motivational issues, and focusing on specific weight-loss goals and barriers to healthy behavior. Similar to behavioral programs, cognitive components are typically used in conjunction with dietary and physical activity education. One early cognitive-behavioral treatment program for children aged 9 to 13 years utilized a 9-week program that included dietary and activity self-monitoring, cognitive strategies for managing negative self-statements, and assertiveness training [75]. Children in the cognitive treatment group lost significantly more weight than controls and retained their weight-loss at 3-month follow-up. Duffy and Spence [76] randomly assigned 27 overweight children (aged 7 to 13 years) to eight sessions of either behavioral management or combined behavioral-cognitive treatment. No differences between treatment groups were noted, and both groups of children demonstrated significant improvements in weight at 6- and 9-month follow-up. Thus, although additional research is needed to establish whether differences in outcome may exist between behavioral treatment and cognitively based strategies, it appears that the two approaches to pediatric weight loss may be equally valuable.

Motivational Interviewing

Research on motivational interviewing for treatment of obesity in pediatric populations is limited, yet promising. Motivational interviewing (MI) is a therapeutic strategy aimed at helping individuals to explore ambivalence about making behavioral changes, and it has been suggested as a possible tool for helping achieve dietary and physical activity modifications [77]. Utilizing reflective listening and methods to elicit "change talk," MI seeks to resolve ambivalence and strengthen the client's reason(s) for engaging in positive behavior change consistent with one's goals and values [78]. Although behavioral modification is considered to be the safest modality for weight loss in youth, compliance issues often lead the families of obese children and adolescents to seek alternate, though riskier, strategies (e.g., pharmacotherapy, bariatric surgery) [56]. Motivational interviewing techniques aimed toward enhancing adherence to dietary and exercise recommendations in children and families could play a key role in promoting safe and effective long-term weight management.

To date, however, little research has been done in the area of MI and pediatric weight loss. Some data suggest that MI assists in promoting more healthful eating habits, increasing physical activity, and improving weight status in adults, but these findings are not consistent [79–81]. Thus far, only two pediatric weight-loss interventions have employed MI techniques, and these are the Healthy Lifestyles Pilot Study [82] and Go Girls [83].

The Healthy Lifestyles Pilot Study, conducted from 2004 to 2005, was aimed at the prevention of overweight among children 3 to 7 years old [82]. Pediatric Research in Office Settings (PROS) clinicians were trained to provide motivational interviewing to patients during office visits. Patients in the control group received usual care, whereas those in the "Minimal" group received one MI session and those in the "Intensive" group received two MI sessions during office visits. At the 6-month follow-up, patients in the Minimal and Intensive groups showed a trend of decreasing BMI-for-age percentiles, though results were not statistically significant. Decreases in families' "eating out" behavior and high-calorie snacking were also noted. Thus, although children's weight changes failed to reach significance, this study demonstrated the feasibility of implementing a physician office-based obesity prevention program using MI.

Go Girls was a church-based nutrition and physical activity program designed for overweight African American adolescent females. In one of the treatment conditions, girls received 4 to 6 MI telephone counseling calls focused on participants' progress. Unfortunately, both 6-month and 1-year post assessments indicated no significant BMI differences between the MI group and controls. Thus, at present, insufficient data exist to determine the efficacy of motivational interviewing for the prevention or treatment of pediatric obesity in children [84].

SUMMARY

The implementation of behavioral, cognitive, and motivational strategies, alongside dietary and physical activity modifications, has proven to be effective in managing the weight status of overweight youth. Underscoring the importance of early intervention for obesity is the finding that long-term weight loss has been shown to be more successful with preadolescents than for adults [85], perhaps because of the higher malleability of behaviors or biological processes earlier in life. However, in their 2006 meta-analytic review of pediatric weight-loss programs, Stice, Shaw, and Marti [86] reported that only 21% of the 64 treatment programs resulted in significant decreases in participants' weight. Thus, though preliminary findings indicate that incorporating the behavioral strategies outlined in this chapter may enhance the outcomes of weight-management programs, substantially more research is needed to provide evidence of their efficacy. It has been suggested that obesity could be considered "a rubric of many diseases, each with a unique etiology, course, and treatment" [84, p. 2030]. Conceivably, if the factors contributing to pediatric obesity are unique to each individual, factors such as age, sex, cultural, and socioeconomic considerations must be taken into account when designing and delivering behavioral obesity treatment. Identification of the core elements of these interventions, as well as specific target ages to maximize the efficacy for certain modalities, may be of particular value when considering how to best treat overweight youth.

RECOMMENDATIONS

Considering the myriad of medical and psychological sequelae related to pediatric obesity, improvements in treatment are essential. Additionally, recent reports estimate the cost of obesity-related healthcare in the United States at $147 billion per year [94]. Thus, the high demand for pediatric obesity treatment necessitates a focus on new and more cost-effective ways of delivering pediatric obesity interventions. Proposed places to start include community programs, schools, or primary care offices [95]. Substantial research is needed to evaluate programs, such as the Healthy Lifestyles Pilot Study, which utilize physician or other community—provider services as additional sources of support and education. Research indicates better weight-loss outcomes with longer treatment duration [96], highlighting the need for more effective ways of helping individuals maintain treatment adherence. Also, in general, sufficient examination of the temporal relationship between affective symptoms and weight gain has not yet occurred.

AREAS OF FOCUS

Although the prevalence of overweight and obesity has risen in all age and ethnic groups [97], evidence from the National Health and Nutrition Examination Survey (NHANES) shows that non-Hispanic black female children and adolescents were more likely to be obese than any other group [98]. Also using NHANES data, Winkleby, Robinson, Sundquist, and Kraemer [99] reported inverse relationships between socioeconomic status and body weight in adolescents, a result supported by similar findings from the National Longitudinal Study of Adolescent Health [100]. Thus, it is imperative that policy programmers, researchers, and interventionists target socioeconomic and racial disparities when planning strategies for delivery of pediatric obesity interventions. Another group of overweight children warranting special consideration, as highlighted in the current chapter, are those with psychological comorbidities. With some exceptions [36], obese youth with psychiatric diagnoses are often excluded from weight-management intervention studies [29], limiting the ability to generalize research findings to pediatric patients with psychological symptomatology. Ultimately, the site of intervention (school, community, primary care, specialty clinic, web-based home programs) and the comorbid conditions (depression, low self-esteem) must be addressed. Evidence suggests that the provision of multidisciplinary, empirically grounded, multilevel obesity treatment may result in the most efficacious interventions for pediatric obesity.

CONCLUSION

Obesity in pediatric and adolescent populations has reached epidemic proportions in the United States. In addition to the increased risk of cardiovascular [87, 88], orthopedic [89], and pulmonary [90] complications faced by overweight youth, the accompanying psychosocial correlates of obesity may adversely affect overall quality of life [49, 50]. Fortunately, several evidence-based pediatric obesity treatments have been successful in promoting weight loss in children and adolescents. As reviewed here, the inclusion of complementary therapeutic strategies has been shown to be effective in enhancing standard pediatric weight-management programs. Behavioral [67–70] and cognitive [73, 74] techniques, used in conjunction with dietary and physical activity change strategies, have demonstrated favorable results for weight loss in obese children and adolescents. By targeting dietary, activity, and other behavioral skills in both children and parents, family-based behavioral programs have been shown to be more effective than targeting children alone [91] and benefit all family members by encouraging reciprocal weight loss between parent and child [92]. Though data supporting the efficacy of motivational interviewing techniques in weight-loss interventions are sparse, these strategies may provide additional safe, cost-effective methods for enhancing motivation for behavior change. Even in more severe cases of obesity, when practitioners may consider additional approaches such as pharmacotherapy or bariatric surgery, these therapies can make a significant contribution to enhancing patients' quality of life and compliance with the weight-loss intervention [93].

References

1. Ford E, Galuska D, Gillespie C, Will J, Giles W, Dietz W. C-reactive protein and body mass index in children: Findings from the Third National Health and Nutrition Examination Survey, 1988–1994. *Journal of Pediatrics* 2001;**138**:486–92.
2. Freedman D, Dietz W, Srinivasan S, Berenson G. The relation of overweight to cardiovascular risk factors among children and adolescents: The Bogalusa heart study. *Pediatrics* 1999;**103**:1175–82.

3. Fuentes R, Notkola I, Shemeikka S, Tuomilehto J, Nissinen A. Tracking of body mass index during childhood: A 15-year prospective population-based family study in eastern Finland. *International Journal of Obesity Related Metabolic Disorders* 2003;**27**:716—21.
4. Hemmingsson T, Lundberg I. How far are socioeconomic differences in coronary heart disease hospitalization, all-cause mortality and cardiovascular mortality among adult Swedish males attributable to negative childhood circumstances and behaviour in adolescence? *International Journal of Epidemiology* 2005;**34**:260—7.
5. Magarey A, Daniels L, Boulton T, Cockington R. Predicting obesity in early adulthood from childhood and parental obesity. *International Journal of Obesity Related Metabolic Disorders* 2003;**27**:505—13.
6. Friedman MA, Brownell KD. Psychological correlates of obesity: Moving to the next research generation. *Psychological Bulletin* 1995;**117**:3—20.
7. Wardle J, Cooke L. The impact of obesity on psychological well-being. *Best Practice & Research Clinical Endocrinology & Metabolism* 2005;**19**:421—40.
8. Kraig K, Keel P. Weight-based stigmatization in children. *International Journal of Obesity* 2001;**25**:1661—6.
9. Latner J, Stunkard A. Getting worse: The stigmatization of obese children. *Obesity Research* 2003;**11**:452—6.
10. Neumark-Sztainer D, Falkner N, Story M, Perry C, Hannan P, Mulert S. Weight-teasing among adolescents: correlations with weight status and disordered eating behaviors. *International Journal of Obesity* 2002;**26**:123—31.
11. Bauer K, Yang Y, Austin S. "How can we stay healthy when you're throwing all of this in front of us?" Findings from focus groups and interviews in middle schools on environmental influences on nutrition and physical activity. *Health Education & Behavior* 2004;**31**:34—46.
12. Neumark-Sztainer D, Story M, Harris T. Perceptions of secondary school staff toward the implementation of school-based activities to prevent weight-related disorders. *American Journal of Health Promotion* 1999;**13**:153—6.
13. Davison K, Birch L. Predictors of fat stereotypes among 9-year-old girls and their parents. *Obesity Research* 2004;**12**:86—94.
14. Eisenberg M, Neumark-Sztainer D, Story M. Associations of weight-based teasing and emotional well-being among adolescents. *Archives of Pediatric and Adolescent Medicine* 2003;**157**:733—8.
15. Goodman E, Whitaker RC. A prospective study of the role of depression in the development and persistence of adolescent obesity. *Pediat rics* 2002;**110**(3):497—504.
16. Pierce JW, Wardle J. Cause and effect beliefs and self-esteem of overweight children. *Journal of Child Psychology & Psychiatry & Allied Disciplines* 1997;**38**:645—50.
17. Puhl R, Latner J. Stigma, obesity, and the health of the nation's children. *Psychological Bulletin* 2007;**133**:557—80.
18. Pearce M, Boergers J, Prinstein M. Adolescent obesity, overt and relational peer victimization, and romantic relationships. *Obesity Research* 2002;**10**:386—93.
19. Strauss R, Pollack H. Social marginalization of overweight children. *Archives of Pediatrics & Adolescent Medicine* 2003;**157**:746—52.
20. Ricciardelli LA, McCabe MP. Children's body image concerns and eating disturbance: A review of the literature. *Clinical Psychology Review* 2001;**21**:325—44.
21. Shin N, Shin M. Body dissatisfaction, self-esteem, and depression in obese Korean children. *Journal of Pediatrics* 2008;**152**:502—6.
22. Lunner K, Werthem EH, Thompson JK, Paxton SJ, McDonald F, Halvaarson KS. A cross-cultural examination of weight-related teasing, body image, and eating disturbance in Swedish and Australian samples. *International Journal of Eating Disorders* 2000;**28**(4):430—5.
23. van den Berg P, Wertheim EH, Thompson JK, Paxton SJ. Development of body image, eating disturbance, and general psychological functioning in adolescent females: A replication using covariance structure modeling in an Australian sample. *International Journal of Eating Disorders* 2002;**32**:46—51.
24. Grilo CM, Wilfley DE, Brownell KD, Rodin J. Teasing, body image and self-esteem in a clinical sample of obese women. *Addictive Behaviors* 1994;**19**(4):443—50.
25. Brown KM, McMahon RP, Biro FM. Changes in self-esteem in black and white girls between the ages of 9 and 14. *Journal of Adolescent Health* 1998;**23**(1):7—19.
26. Hesketh K, Wake M, Waters E. Body mass index and parent-reported self esteem in elementary school children: evidence for a causal relationship. *International journal of obesity and related metabolic disorders* 2004;**28**(10):1233—7.
27. Tiggemann M. Television and adolescent body image: The role of program content and viewing motivation. *Journal of Social and Clinical Psychology* 2005;**24**:193—213.
28. French SA, Perry CL, Leon GR, Fulkerson JA. Self-esteem and change in body mass index over 3 years in a cohort of adolescents. *Obesity Research* 1996;**4**:27—33.
29. Zeller MH, Saelens BE, Roehrig H, Kirk S, Daniels SR. Psychological adjustment of obese youth presenting for weight management treatment. *Obesity Research* 2004;**12**:1576—86.
30. French SA, Story M, Perry CL. Self-esteem and obesity in children and adolescents: A literature review. *Obesity Research* 1995;**3**:479—90.
31. Braet C, Mervielde I, Vandereycken W. Psychological aspects of childhood obesity: A controlled study in a clinical and nonclinical sample. *Journal of Pediatric Psychology* 1997;**22**:59—71.
32. Tanofsky-Kraff M, Yanovski S, Wilfley D, Marmarosh C, Morgan C, Yanovski J. Eating-disordered behaviors, body fat, and psychopathology in overweight and normal-weight children. *Journal of Consulting and Clinical Psychology* 2004;**72**:53—61.
33. Lamertz CM, Jacobi C, Yassouridis A, Arnold K, Henkel AW. Are obese adolescents and young adults at risk for mental disorders? A community survey. *Obesity Research* 2002;**10**:1152—60.
34. Britz B, Siegfried W, Ziegler A, Lamertz C, Herpertz-Dahlmann BM, Remschmidt H, Wittchen H-U, Hebebrand J. Rates of psychiatric disorders in a clinical study group of adolescents with extreme obesity and in obese adolescents ascertained via a population based study. *International Journal of Obesity and Related Metabolic Disorders* 2000;**24**:1707—14.
35. Buddeburg-Fisher B, Klaghofer R, Reed V. Associations between body weight, psychiatric disorders and body image in female adolescents. *Psychotherapy and Psychosomatics* 1999;**68**:325—32.
36. Rofey D, Kolko R, Losif A, Silk J, Bost J, Feng W, Szigethy E, Noll R, Ryan N, Dahl R. A longitudinal study of childhood depression and anxiety in relation to weight gain. *Child Psychiatry and Human Development* 2009;**40**:517—26.
37. Brewis A. Biocultural aspects of obesity in young Mexican schoolchildren. *American Journal of Human Biology* 2003;**15**(3):446—60.
38. Wardle J, Williamson S, Johnson F, Edwards C. Depression in adolescent obesity: cultural moderators of the association between obesity and depressive symptoms. *International Journal of Obesity* 2006;**30**(4):634—43.
39. Erermis S, Cetis N, Tamar M, Bukusoglu N, Akdeniz F, Goksen D. Is obesity a risk factor for psychopathology among adolescents? *Pediatrics International* 2004;**46**:296—301.
40. Stice E, Bearman SK. Body image and eating disturbances prospectively predict growth in depressive symptoms in

adolescent girls: A growth curve analysis. *Developmental Psychology* 2001;**37**:597—607.
41. Stice E, Hayward C, Cameron R, Killen JD, Taylor CB. Body image and eating related factors predict onset of depression in female adolescents: A longitudinal study. *Journal of Abnormal Psychology* 2000;**109**:438—44.
42. Mustillo S, Worthman C, Erkanli A, Keeler G, Angold A, Costello EJ. Obesity and Psychiatric Disorder: Developmental Trajectories. *Pediatrics* 2003;**111**(4):851—9.
43. Anderson SE, Cohen P, Naumova EN, Jacques PF, Must A. Adolescent Obesity and Risk for Subsequent Major Depressive Disorder and Anxiety Disorder: Prospective Evidence. *Psychosomatic Medicine* 2007;**69**(8):740—7.
44. Richardson LP, Davis R, Poulton R, McCauley E, Moffitt TE, Caspi A, Connell F. A longitudinal evaluation of adolescent depression and adult obesity. *Archives of Pediatrics and Adolescent Medicine* 2003;**157**:739—45.
45. Ackard DM, Neumark-Sztainer D, Story M, Perry C. Overeating among adolescents: Prevalence and associations with weight-related characteristics and psychological health. *Pediatrics* 2003;**111**:67—74.
46. Eaton DK, Lowry R, Brener ND, Galuska DA, Crosby AE. Associations of mass index and perceived weight with suicidal ideation and suicide attempts among US high school students. *Archive of Pediatric Adolescent Medicine* 2005;**159**:513—19.
47. Falkner NH, Neumark-Sztainer D, Story M, Jeffery RW, Beuhring T, Resnick MD. Social, educational, and psychological correlates of weight status in adolescents. *Obesity Research* 2001;**9**:32—42.
48. Beck A, Brown G, Berchick R, Stewart B, Steer R. Relationship between hopelessness and ultimate suicide: A replication with psychiatric outpatients. *Focus* 2006;**4**:291—6.
49. Friedlander SL, Larkin EK, Rosen CL, Palermo TM, Redline S. Decreased quality of life associated with obesity in school-aged children. *Archives of Pediatrics and Adolescent Medicine* 2003;**157**:1206—11.
50. Kolotkin RL, Crosby RD, Corey-Lisle P, Li H, Swanson J. Performance of a weight-related measure of quality of life in a psychiatric sample. *Quality of Life Research* 2006;**15**:587—96.
51. Schwimmer JB, Burwinkle TM, Varni JW. Health-related quality of life of severely obese children and adolescents. *Journal of the American Medical Association* 2003;**289**:1813—19.
52. Becque MD, Katch VL, Rocchini AP, Marks CR, Moorehead C. Coronary risk incidence of obese adolescents: Reduction by exercise plus diet intervention. *Pediatrics* 1988;**81**(5):605—12.
53. Epstein L, Valoski A, Kalarchian M, McCurley J. Do children lose and maintain weight easier than adults: A comparison of child and parent weight changes from six months to ten years. *Obesity Research* 1995;**3**:411—17.
54. Katch V, Becque MD, Marks C, Moorehead C, Rocchini A. Basal metabolism of obese adolescents: Inconsistent diet and exercise effects. *American Journal of Clinical Nutrition* 1988;**48**(3):565—9.
55. Levine MD, Ringham RM, Kalarchian MA, Wisniewski L, Marcus MD. Is family-based behavioral weight control appropriate for severe pediatric obesity? *Int J Eat Disord* 2001;**30**:318—28.
56. Miller J, Silverstein J. Management approaches for pediatric obesity. *Nature Clinical Practice Endocrinology & Metabolism* 2007;**3**:810—18.
57. Epstein L, Wing R, Koeske R, Valoski A. Effects of diet plus exercise on weight change in parents and children. *Journal of Consulting and Clinical Psychology* 1984;**52**:429—37.
58. Epstein LH, Wing RR, Penner BC, Kress MJ. The effect of diet and controlled exercise on weight loss in obese children. *Journal of Pediatrics* 1985;**107**:358—61.
59. Emes C, Velde B, Moreau M, Murdoch D, Trussell R. An activity based weight control program. *Adapted Physical Activity Quarterly* 1990;**7**:314—24.
60. Epstein LH. Exercise in the treatment of childhood obesity. *International Journal of Obesity and Related Metabolic Disorders* 19. 1995;**4**(Suppl):S117—21.
61. Epstein LH, Goldfield GS. Physical activity in the treatment of childhood overweight and obesity: current evidence and research issues. *Medicine and Science in Sports and Exercise* 1999;**31**(11 Suppl):S553—9.
62. Brownell KD, Kelman JH, Stunkard AJ. Treatment of obese children with and without their mothers: Changes in weight and blood pressure. *Pediatrics* 1983;**71**:515—23.
63. Kingsley RG, Shapiro J. A comparison of three behavioral programs for the control of obesity in children. *Behavior Therapy* 1977;**8**:30—6.
64. Renjilian DA, Perri MG, Nezu AM, McKelvey WF, Shermer RL, Anton SD. Individual versus group therapy for obesity: effects of matching participants to their treatment preferences. *Journal of Consulting and Clinical Psychology* 2001;**69**:717—21.
65. Epstein LH. Family-based behavioral intervention for obese children. *International Journal of Obesity and Related Metabolic Disorders* 1996;**20**:S14—21.
66. Jelalian E, Saelers BE. Empirically supported treatments in pediatric psychology: pediatric obesity. *Journal of Pediatric Psychiatry* 1994;**24**:223—48.
67. Aragona J, Cassady J, Drabman RS. Treating overweight children through parental training and contingency contracting. *Journal of Applied Behavioral Analysis* 1975;**8**:269—78.
68. Coates TJ, Killen JD, Slinkard LA. Parent participation in a treatment program for overweight adolescents. *International Journal of Eating Disorders* 1982;**1**:37—48.
69. Gross I, Wheeler M, Hess K. The treatment of obesity in adolescents using behavioral self-control. *Clin Pediatr* 1976;**15**(10):920—4.
70. Epstein L, Valoski A, Wing R, McCurley J. Ten year outcomes of behavioral family-based treatment for childhood obesity. *Health Psychology* 1994;**13**:373—83.
71. Flodmark CE, Ohlsson T, Ryden O, Sveger T. Prevention of progression to severe obesity in a group of obese schoolchildren treated with family therapy. *Pediatrics* 1993;**91**:880—4.
72. Herrera E, Johnston CA, Steele RG. Comparison of cognitive and behavioral treatments for pediatric obesity. *Children's Health Care* 2004;**33**:151—67.
73. Senediak C, Spence SH. Rapid versus gradual scheduling of therapeutic contact in a family-based behavioral weight control program for children. *Behavioral Psychotherapy* 1985;**13**:265—87.
74. Williams CL, Bollella M, Carter BJ. Treatment of childhood obesity in pediatric practice. *Ann N Y Acad Sci* 1993;**699**:207—19.
75. Kirschenbaum D, Harris E, Tomarken A. Effects of parental involvement in behavioral weight loss therapy for preadolescents. *Behavior Therapy* 1984;**15**:485—500.
76. Duffy G, Spence S. The effectiveness of cognitive self-management as an adjunct to a behavioural intervention for childhood obesity: A research note. *Journal of Child Psychology and Psychiatry* 1993;**34**:1043—50.
77. DiLillo V, Siegfried N, Smith W. Incorporating motivational interviewing into behavioral obesity treatment. *Cognitive and Behavioral Practice* 2004;**10**:120—30.
78. Miller W, Rollnick S. Preparing People for Change., *Motivational Interviewing*. 2nd ed. New York: Guilford Press; 2002.
79. Dunn C, Deroo L, Rivara F. The use of brief interventions adapted from motivational interviewing across behavioral domains: A systematic review. *Addiction* 2001;**12**:1725—42.

80. Berg-Smith S, Stevens V, Brown K, Van Horn L, Gernhofer N, Peters E, Greenberg R, Snetselaar L, Ahrens L, Smith K. A brief motivational intervention to improve dietary adherence in adolescents. The Dietary Intervention Study in Children (DISC) Research Group. *Health Education Research* 1999;**14**:399–410.
81. Smith D, Heckemeyer C, Kratt P, Mason D. Motivational interviewing to improve adherence to a behavioral weight-control program for older obese women with NIDDM: A pilot study. *Diabetes Care* 1997;**20**:52–4.
82. Schwartz R, Hamre R, Dietz W, Wasseman R, Slora E, Myers E, Sullivan S, Rockett H, Thoma K, Dumitru G, Resnicow K. Office-based motivational interviewing to prevent childhood obesity: A feasibility study. *Archives of Pediatrics & Adolescent Medicine* 1997;**161**:495–501.
83. Resnicow K, Taylor R, Baskin M. Results of go girls: A nutrition and physical activity intervention for overweight African American adolescent females conducted through Black churches. *Obesity Research* 2005;**13**:1739–48.
84. Resnicow K, Davis R, Rollnick S. Motivational Interviewing for Pediatric Obesity: Conceptual Issues and Evidence Review. *J Am Diet Assoc* 2006;**106**:2024–33.
85. Jeffery RW, Drewnowski A, Epstein LH. Long term maintenance of weight loss: current status. *Health Psychology* 2000;**19**(Suppl. 1):5–16.
86. Stice E, Shaw H, Marti C. A meta-analytic review of obesity prevention programs for children and adolescents: The skinny on interventions that work. *Psychology Bulletin* 2006;**132**:667–91.
87. Must A, Strauss R. Risks and consequences of childhood and adolescent obesity. *International Journal of Obesity and Related Metabolic Disorders* 1999;**23**(Suppl 2):S2–11.
88. Reilly JJ, Methven E, McDowell ZC, Hacking B, Alexander D, Stewart L, Kelnar CJH. Health consequences of obesity. *Archives of Disease in Childhood* 2003;**88**:748–52.
89. Dietz W. Health consequences of obesity in youth: Childhood predictors of adult disease. *Pediatrics* 1998;**101**(Suppl):518–24.
90. Lazarus R, Colditz GA, Berkey CS, Speizer FE. Effects of body fat on ventilatory function in children and adolescents: Cross-sectional findings from a random population sample of school children. *Pediatr Pulmonol* 1997;**24**:187–94.
91. Epstein LH, Paluch RA, Roemmich JN, Beecher MD. Family-based obesity treatment, then and now: twenty-five years of pediatric obesity treatment. *Health psychology* 2007;**26**(4):381–91.
92. Wrotniak B, Epstein L, Paluch R, Roemmich J. Parent weight change as a predictor of child weight change in family-based behavioral obesity treatment. *Archives of Pediatric and Adolescent Medicine* 2004;**158**:342–7.
93. Kalarchian M, Marcus M. Management of the bariatric surgery patient: Is there a role for the cognitive behavior therapist? *Cognitive and Behavioral Practice* 2003;**10**:112–19.
94. Centers for Disease Control and Prevention. (July 27, 2009). www.cdc.gov
95. Delamater AM, Jent J, Moine CT, Rios J. Empirically supported treatment of overweight adolescents. In: Jelalian E, Steele R, editors. *Handbook of child and adolescent obesity*. New York: Springer; 2008.
96. Wilfley D, Tibbs T, Van Buren D, Reach K, Walker M, Epstein L. Lifestyle interventions in the treatment of childhood overweight: A meta-analytic review of randomized controlled trials. *Health Psychology* 2007;**26**:521–32.
97. Centers for Disease Control and Prevention. [Youth risk behavior surveillance – United States. 2005]. *Surveillance Summaries, MMWR*; 2006::55 (No. SS-5).
98. Ogden C, Carroll M, Curtin L, McDowell M, Tabak C, Flegal K. Prevalence of overweight and obesity in the United States, 1999–2004. *Journal of the American Medical Association* 2006;**295**:1549–55.
99. Winkleby MA, Robinson TN, Sundquist J, Kraemer HC. Ethnic variation in cardiovascular disease risk factors among children and young adults: findings from the Third National Health and Nutrition Examination Survey, 1988–1994. *JAMA* 1999;**281**(11):1006–13.
100. Goodman E. In: Jelalian E, Steele RG, editors. *Socioeconomic factors related to obesity. Handbook of Childhood and Adolescent Obesity.* New York: Springer; 2008. p. 507.

CHAPTER 39

Dietary Supplements in the Prevention and Treatment of Childhood Obesity

Robert I-San Lin

Chairman, the Certification Board for Nutrition Specialists, Irvine, CA, USA

INTRODUCTION

Dietary supplement treatment of childhood overweight/obesity, in addition to helping the child to regain a normal body weight and composition, aims at enabling the child to build a strong body with normal physical and mental development by improving diets and lifestyles. With a relaxation of food energy restriction, this treatment program can be used for prevention of childhood obesity. This methodology distinguishes dietary supplement treatment from many other methods of treatment of childhood overweight/obesity. Overweight (hereafter denotes increased adiposity, excluding the condition of excessive lean body mass) and obesity are underlying factors of many degenerative diseases. Severely obese adults often have mental deficits and reduced brain tissues. Overweight/obesity is a serious healthcare problem in most affluent countries and in many less affluent ones. In recent decades the incidences of childhood overweight/obesity have been increasing alarmingly worldwide the age of onset younger. Presently, approximately half of American children are overweight, and the trend is moving toward even higher prevalence. Thus, the worst of human suffering and economic loss from overweight/obesity is yet to come. In the long run, proper prevention and treatment of childhood overweight/obesity are more important, meaningful, and cost effective than prevention and treatment of adulthood overweight/obesity because (1) as childhood overweight/obesity continues, a large fraction (>50%) of these children will continue to suffer into adulthood, with a greater portion of their lives being affected; (2) continuing childhood obesity is more likely to result in substantial adipocyte hyperplasia, which is more difficult to correct, then adipocyte hypertrophy, and may be irreversible [1], leading to more serious adulthood obesity later; (3) obese children will have greater risk of developing obesity-associated diseases later in life, with the diseases being more severe; (4) some obesity-related degeneration (e.g., reduced brain tissues) may progressively worsen and not be reversible; (5) there will be a greater cumulative cost of healthcare over their lifetime; and (6) childhood is an important period for building sound dietary habits and lifestyles. Early prevention/treatment of childhood obesity offers a great opportunity to raise a healthy next generation.

Although numerous products and methods of treating adult obesity are available, most of them may be unsafe for obese children. As a result, many parents and healthcare professionals have taken a watch-and-wait approach in dealing with childhood obesity. Presently, >95% of overweight/obesity can be attributed to food energy malnutrition: long-term accumulation of surplus food energy in the body in the form of adipose tissue. Therefore, the most logical, simplistic, and fundamental approach is to subject the affected individuals to a gradual and long-term energy deficit until an ideal or desired body mass index (BMI) is reached. Many supplement methods are based on this principle and are among the safest methods for treating overweight/obesity. These supplement-based methods are in a unique position to help overweight/obese individuals to regain a healthy body with improved physical and, possibly, mental capacities. Because of space limitation, this chapter briefly discusses the basic concerns of treating obese children with dietary supplements and reports on a successful supplement that can also be used, with minor modifications, for prevention.

STRATEGIC CONSIDERATIONS

The basic principle of dietary supplement treatment of childhood obesity is to provide the child with a complete set of essential nutrients (except fat) in proper balance and quantities [2], in conjunction with a mild restriction on food energy intake and increased physical activity, so that the child can experience a gradual weight loss with minimal lean body mass (LBM) loss and without a stunt in physical and mental development. To assure both short- and long-term successes and to further strengthen the children's bodies, they and their parents are guided to acquire healthy dietary habits and physically active lifestyles.

Prevention of Nutritional Deficiencies and Growth Stunt

Deficiencies in essential nutrients can have short- and long-term effects on rapidly growing children, with some damage irreversible. All weight-reduction methods (except surgical removal of adipose tissue, exercise, and induced-metabolic wasting) depend on reduced food energy intake, which often calls for reduced food intake and may lead to nutritional deficiencies. Although overweight/obese children in general have been consuming more foods and are conspicuously taller than their peers and less likely to have nutritional deficiencies, imposing severe food restriction for weight-loss can cause nutritional deficiency and growth stunt. Some obese children are at higher risk of becoming deficient of certain nutrients because their diets comprise primarily high-energy, low-nutrient-dense foods (e.g., starch, sugar, and fat). This is particularly true among East Asian children. Iron deficiency is common among children worldwide and is associated with mental deficit, especially when it occurs at young age. Once a growth stunt has occurred, a remedial nutritional treatment may cause a catch-up growth spurt; however, such catch-up may fall short of making up the full height potential [3] or repairing mental deficit. As taller obese children grow older, frequently there is a natural catch-down process (i.e., slowing down in linear growth rate more than their nonobese peers) and in the end the extra height becomes less conspicuous. Treatment methods that deprive a child of adequate nutritional intake can aggravate the catch-down process [4].

Looking from a historical perspective, since the 1830s, the average height for age of European children has been increasing at about 1 cm per decade. Similar increases have been happening in Japan, Taiwan, and many other East Asian nations. Between 1982 and 1992, the average height of 6-year-old Chinese children increased by 4.4 cm. Children of East Asian families that have immigrated to the United States grow, on average, far taller than their parents. Yet there is no evidence that substantial mutation has occurred in the European population during the past two centuries, in East Asian population during recent decades, or within two generations among the immigrants. Such short periods of time were insufficient to alter the human gene pool significantly. Lifestyle changes cannot explain the increases in height, because the height changes occurred before significant lifestyle changes. Improved nutritional intake must have played a key role in these cases. Thus, many short children of previous generations had to be the result of growth stunt caused by nutritional deficiencies. The seriousness of growth stunt must be taken into consideration when formulating a sound prevention or treatment strategy for childhood obesity.

Protecting Brain and Endocrine Development

Most weight-loss products/programs are based on deprivation of food intake. Whereas a healthy adult can last for almost 2 months on water alone [5–9], growing children are far more susceptible to harm from nutritional deficiencies. Many organs and organ systems can suffer short- or long-term damage from food deprivation. In young children, the brain consumes approximately half of the energy generated from metabolism at the basal rate [10]. Severe undernutrition can affect the developing brain [11], even though it is one of the organs least affected by poor nutritional status. Severe perinatal nutritional deficiency can cause the infant animal's brain to have fewer cells, manifested by low DNA content of the brain. In 1997, Vargas et al. [12] reported on young rats born to nutritionally deprived mothers and fed a deprived diet (50% less than the amount of feed that a normal rat consumed). These rats had brains with 20% lower myelin content. Because myelin is necessary to enable high-speed neuronal signal transmission, this discovery strongly indicates a mental deficit in the deprived young rats and is consistent with mental retardation observed among nutrient-deficient children. Others reported that severe restriction in food intake had caused enlarged intracranial cerebrospinal fluid spaces (i.e., enlargement of ventricles and sulci and shrinkage of both the gray matter and the white matter) [13–24] and cognitive deficits [25]. Some of the alterations do not appear to be completely reversible.

Severe food deprivation alters bone mineral crystalline structures, reduces bone mineral density [26] and strength, and down-regulates the hypothalamic-pituitary-gonadal axis, leading to delayed sexual maturation and amenorrhea. It also up-regulates the hypothalamic-pituitary-adrenal axis, leading to excess cortisol production [27–33]. More alarmingly, a 50% deprivation of food, a degree of restriction that is not as severe as some low-calorie diets (LCD) and all very low calorie diets (VLCD) [34–41] used for slimming, can cause disturbances in brain and endocrine development. Further, severe obese children on VLCDs (406 kcal or 1700 kjoules [kj] daily) can experience plasma amino acid disturbances [42] and immune suppression (e.g., decreased circulating lymphocyte numbers) [43]. These are some readily demonstrable side effects of severe slimming programs. If severe food restrictions were used to treat moderate childhood obesity, the impact on them could be more severe. A sound treatment for overweight/obese children must minimize these side effects.

Building Sound Dietary Habits and Preventing Eating Disorders

A sound treatment for childhood obesity must minimize the risk of eating disorders and help build sound dietary habits. Building sound dietary habits is extremely important for long-term success and for the future wellbeing of the children. Severe food intake restriction for weight loss can lead to eating disorders [44–46], including anorexia nervosa, in susceptible individuals, even though many other factors also contribute to the development of anorexia nervosa [47]. To reduce the risk of eating disorders, obese children must be taught to eat adequate amounts of high-nutrient, low-energy-dense foods (including high-fiber, low-fat foods) to maintain their digestive function and neurological control of appetite. The dietary supplement treatment of obesity is in a pivotal position to help build sound dietary habits.

Building Physically Active Lifestyles and Enhancing Lean Body Mass Accretion

Physical exercise increases metabolic rate and energy expenditure, builds a more perfect and lasting body, and improves physical capacity, including muscular strength, speed, control, and coordination; joint flexibility; and work capacity. Sound dietary supplementation helps maintain the body's ability to perform physical exercise [48]. Increased energy expenditure (a mathematical product of the amount of energy expended per unit time multiplied by the duration of the exercise) is particularly effective for slimming, lowering serum glucose level, and increasing the number of cell surface insulin receptors, leading to normalization of serum insulin level and a reduced risk of diabetes and cardiovascular disease. Aerobic or endurance exercise is important for retaining LBM during slimming. Strength exercise is particularly effective in building LBM, especially skeletal muscles, leading to a shapely body and a high basal metabolic rate [49]; it is also important in preventing LBM loss later as the child grows older. Weight-bearing exercises and physical stresses improve bone density and mineral crystalline structures, enhance bone strength in children and young adults, lead to a greater retention of bone mass [50], and reduce risk of osteoporosis years later. Therefore, a sound treatment for childhood obesity must include physical exercise.

Slimming by severe restriction of food intake can cause rapid weight loss and a substantial LBM loss. An adequate intake of protein and essential micronutrients tends to spare a loss of LBM associated with slimming. A sound dietary supplement treatment of overweight/obese children should enable the children to increase their bodies' LBM percentage or at least should minimize an LBM loss.

Mitigating Risks of Metabolic Syndrome and Cardiovascular Disease

Obese children are at a greater risk of left ventricular hypertrophy, heart enlargement [51–54], and metabolic syndrome (e.g., hypertriglyceridemia, hypercholesterolemia, hypertension, and insulin resistance) [55–62]. Some of these conditions may continue into adulthood, even after the weight problem attenuates [63]. As has been shown with adults, a combination of increased physical activity and a sound diet can lower serum triglycerides level and elevate high density lipoprotein cholesterol (HDL-C) level, leading to a better ratio of HDL-C to total cholesterol [64–77]. These changes can reduce the risk of cardiovascular disease. Moderate- to high-intensity physical exercise activates the adrenaline-noradrenaline-lipoprotein lipase axis and contributes to fat catabolism. Weight loss in conjunction with increased physical activity is particularly helpful in lowering elevated blood pressure in overweight/obese children [78]. Thus, a sound treatment for childhood obesity should also aim at reducing risks or severity of metabolic syndrome, atherosclerosis, and cardiovascular disease.

Promoting Satiety and Reducing Hunger

One of the critical reasons that numerous slimming products/programs have failed is a failure to quench hunger associated with dieting. Consuming a sufficient quantity of protein enhances satiety and reduces hunger [79], particularly when protein and adequate quantities of soluble and insoluble dietary fiber are consumed in proximity. It appears that the following factors may contribute to satiety: (1) the slow intestinal microbial degradation of the fiber (especially the soluble fiber) into short chain fatty acids that enter the circulation, which may have a mild hunger mitigating effect, (2) the bulk-filling mechanical property of fibers, and (3) the elevation of blood (and brain) levels of certain amino acids after a protein-rich meal. However, most amino acids do not enter the brain cells directly because of the blood-brain barrier.

Some substances should be avoided in supplements or diets for overweight/obese children: simple sugars, oligosaccharides, purified flours and starches, and fat. Sugars, oligosaccharides, and starch tend to enhance hunger, perhaps because of their high glycemic effect that induces rapid insulin response. Among macronutrients, fat is the least effective in providing satiation effect [80]. Low-fat foods facilitate lowering of food energy intake and may result in greater weight loss [81]. In laboratory animals, a deficiency in omega-6 essential fatty acids causes inefficient retention of food energy. However, obese children must not be deprived of essential fatty acids to such a severe degree, because metabolites of these fatty acids (e.g., prostaglandins) play important regulatory roles in the body.

THE TREATMENT PROGRAM FOR CHILDHOOD OBESITY

The Dietary Supplement

Since the mid-1970s, we have treated childhood overweight/obesity with a dietary supplement that provides a complete set of essential nutrients (except fat) in proper proportion and quantities (Table 39.1). The supplement is intended for assuring adequate intake of essential nutrients (both macro- and micronutrients, except food energy and essential fatty acids) for all people except infants. It can be conveniently used for treating obesity by partially replacing foods to reduce food energy intake while providing the body with a complete set of essential nutrients in proper amounts and proportion. It can help dieters achieve many key goals, including weight loss, enhanced LBM retention and satiety, reduced hunger, and mitigated development of metabolic syndrome. A serving of this supplement provides all known essential nutrients (except fat) at quantities equaling one third of an adult's U.S. Recommended Daily Allowances (U.S. RDA, later the Daily Values, DV), if the values exist, or one third of the daily requirements based on the best scientific estimates. It has a very low energy density (94 kcal/serving) and a high nutrient density, fortified with vitamins, essential minerals, milk and soy proteins (1: 1 ratio), dietary fiber (soluble and insoluble, 50% each), and soy lecithin. It has three flavors and is made flavorsome by using extracts from fruits, cocoa, or vanilla, together with aspartame. Multiple flavors mitigate the monotony of having one flavor day after day. Each serving (30 g) of the supplement powder is packed in a hermetically sealed 4-inch-by-4-inch pouch made of metallized food-grade packing films so that it has a very long shelf life. To use, simply pull open the pouch, pour the powder into a mixing cup, and mix it with 250 mL room-temperature water to make a serving. The dietary supplement formula was highly acceptable to children and, in most cases, to the family. Often the whole family took this formula, not just the obese/overweight child. If the parents and siblings were within normal weight range, they took the supplement without a restriction on food energy intake. However, if any one of them was overweight, that individual could follow the same program as the child did.

The Childhood Population

Since the mid-1970s, more than 30,000 East Asian overweight/obese children have taken this supplement for weight control for various lengths of time. Among them 600 9-year-old, seemingly healthy obese children (male/female ratio 1:1) and their families were selected randomly at different times for the study. Children with potential confounding conditions were excluded—those with serious psychiatric disorders or serious chronic diseases (e.g., thyroid and other endocrine dysfunctions). Thus, the primary cause of obesity in the children was energy malnutrition. The participating families shared the cost of the supplement, which is moderate, equivalent to approximately one third of a meal cost. For comparison, 600 obese children of similar backgrounds (e.g., classmates or neighbors of comparable weight, height, age, and from families having similar socioeconomical status) were randomly selected as the positive control, and an additional 600 normal-weight children of similar backgrounds were selected as the background control. The positive control and background control children were not given the supplement or asked to follow the dietary and exercise instructions, and they were free to join other weight-control programs if they wished to do so. Their weight and health conditions were monitored similarly.

In preliminary studies, we had collected extensive data on several children populations (including an East Asian children population) and established sets of reference heights and reference (optimal) BMI-for-age for several of these populations; the reference BMI-for-age has an approximate average standard deviation of 16.3% (e.g., Table 39.2). Children having BMI $\geq$ 125% of the reference BMI-for-age (1.53 standard deviations)

TABLE 39.1 Nutrient Contents of the Supplement for Treating Childhood Obesity

Nutrition Facts

SERVING SIZE: 1 pouch (30 g)			SERVINGS PER CONTAINER: 30		
		Amount per Serving			
		Total Calories: 94 kcal			
Total Fat 0 g		Saturate Fat 0 g		Cholesterol: 0 g	
Total Carbohydrate 12 g (4% DV)		Dietary Fiber 4 g (16% DV)			
Protein 13 g					

VITAMINS		% DV			% DV
Vitamin A	1667 I.U.	33%	Vitamin B$_{12}$	2 mcg	33%
Vitamin B$_1$	500 mcg	33%	Folic acid	133 mcg	33%
Vitamin B$_2$	567 mcg	33%	Biotin	100 mcg	33%
Niacin (B$_3$)	6.67 mg	33%	Vitamin C	20 mg	33%
Vitamin B$_5$	3.33 mg	33%	Vitamin D	133 I.U.	33%
Vitamin B$_6$	667 mcg	33%	Vitamin E	10 I.U.	33%

MINERALS		% DV			% DV
Calcium	333 mg	33%	Selenium	23.3 mcg	33%
Chromium	40 mcg	33%	Zinc	5 mg	33%
Copper	667 mcg	33%	Chloride	290 mg	9%
Iodine	56 mcg	33%	Boron	25 mcg	
Iron	6 mg	33%	Nickel	5 mcg	
Magnesium	133 mg	33%	Potassium	620 mg	
Manganese	667 mcg	33%	Silicon	5 mcg	
Molybdenum	25 mcg	33%	Sodium	140 mg	7%
Phosphorus	340 mg	34%	Tin	5 mcg	
			Vanadium	5 mcg	

APPROX. AMINO ACID CONTENT		*Lysine	788 mg
Alanine 433 mg		*Methionine	267 mg
Arginine 736 mg		*Phenylalanine	529 mg
Aspartic acid 1057 mg		Proline	820 mg
Cysteine/cystine 218 mg		Serine	591 mg
Glutamic acid/glutamine 2198 mg		*Threonine	532 mg
Glycine 389 mg		*Tryptophan	199 mg
*Histidine 291 mg		*Tyrosine	458 mg
*Isoleucine 580 mg		*Valine	688 mg
*Leucine 993 mg		*Essential amino acids.	

OTHER NUTRIENTS: Soy Lecithin 1000 mg

TABLE 39.2 East Asian Reference heights (cm) and Reference Body Mass Indexes (kg·m^{-2}), ± Standard Deviations

Age	Male height	Male BMI	Female height	Female BMI
9	130.1 ± 5.8	15.9 ± 2.1	131.2 ± 5.7	16.0 ± 2.7
10	133.8 ± 6.1	16.4 ± 2.3	136.1 ± 5.6	16.5 ± 2.2
11	139.3 ± 5.8	16.8 ± 3.1	143.7 ± 6.1	16.9 ± 2.5
12	146.8 ± 6.5	17.3 ± 3.2	150.3 ± 5.9	17.6 ± 3.1
13	154.9 ± 6.7	17.6 ± 3.3	154.5 ± 5.4	18.2 ± 3.3
14	161.9 ± 6.8	17.9 ± 3.4	156.1 ± 5.8	19.3 ± 3.0
15	166.7 ± 6.3	18.2 ± 3.3	158.2 ± 5.5	19.4 ± 2.9
16	168.2 ± 6.5	18.7 ± 3.2	158.1 ± 5.3	19.6 ± 3.2
17	168.9 ± 5.6	19.3 ± 3.7	158.3 ± 4.9	19.9 ± 2.8
18	169.3 ± 5.7	19.8 ± 3.1	158.4 ± 5.1	20.3 ± 3.1
19	169.7 ± 4.8	20.5 ± 2.9	158.6 ± 4.8	20.9 ± 2.7
20	169.9 ± 4.9	21.2 ± 3.3	158.5 ± 4.5	21.1 ± 3.4

were considered obese. These reference BMI-for-age values were obtained based on the following criteria: lowest frequency of contracting diseases, maximum physical capacity, and minimum risk of accidental injuries or getting involved in accidents [2]. They were used as the target BMI for the overweight/obese children to achieve. The reference heights and reference BMI-for-age as well as a child's height and BMI were plotted as a height or BMI (vertical axis) versus age (horizontal axis) charts. The children's weights were measured daily and averaged weekly to obtain their average weekly weights, and their heights were measured every 2 months; the height and average 2-month weight of a child were converted into BMI and entered on the BMI versus age chart. These charts of height and BMI were used to track the child's progress.

The Weight-Control Program and Results

Enrollment into the Program

As the obese children enrolled into the program with their families, a healthcare professional did the following: (1) performed a physical examination; (2) recorded the child's medical history and current status, vital signs, skinfold thickness, midarm circumference, and other aspects of nutritional assessment; and (3) assessed the child's dietary habit. The family was then loaned (or asked to purchase) a scale that was commonly used in the food and pharmaceutical industries, with capacity from 60 to 100 kg and precision of approximately ± 0.05 kg. The child was instructed to measure his or her weight, with as little clothes on as possible, every morning after passing urine and stools but before doing other things. Their weights, heights, and BMI were recorded as described in the previous section. After 1 year, 288 boys and 283 girls remained, and 4.8% (29) of the children dropped out of the program because their families had moved, because their families did not want to be in the program for the cost, or for other reasons that were unrelated to the efficacy or perceived side effects of the program. At this stage all the remaining children had reduced their BMI (weights) to the acceptable range (discussed later); thereafter their data were related to their weight maintenance when they were free to decide whether or not to take the supplement for nutritional reason, not for slimming, and when they were no longer bound by the instructions of the program. At the end of the second year and the fifth year, 92.7% (282 boys and 274 girls) and 65.2% (206 boys and 185 girls) of the children, respectively, remained trackable. As time passed, the remaining trackable number diminished further: 10th year, 30.6% of the starting children (102 boys/men and 82 girls/women); 15th year, 12.7% of the starting children (41 men and 35 women); and 20th year, 9.5% of the starting children (32 men and 25 women).

Taking the Supplement and Building Healthy Dietary Habits

With their parents' help, these children were instructed to do the following:

1. To take two daily servings of the supplement, one each 15 to 30 minutes before breakfast or dinner.
2. To become more physically active.
3. To estimate the approximate energy contents of foods that they consumed habitually in order to differentiate high-energy-density foods from low ones (based on the approximate macronutrient contents of foods and on energy content of 9, 4, 4, 1.5 kcal per gram for fat, carbohydrate, protein, and dietary fiber, respectively). (The general guideline for macronutrients intake was carbohydrate 53%, protein 30%, and lipid 17% [both omega-3 and -6 fats, from marine species and common vegetable cooking oils, except palm oil] of total food energy, and dietary fiber 25 to 35 g daily.)
4. To control food energy intake to approximately 4604 to 5860 kj (1100 to 1400 kcal) daily, depending on the degree of overweight; the more overweight the more food energy was permitted. (Within this range of food energy intake, the energy deficit would cause a gradual but consistent weight loss of approximately 0.5% to 0.8% of body weight weekly. The greater the degree of overweight, the faster weight loss, which was faster at the beginning but slower after about 2 weeks into the program. The children would achieve this energy-reduction goal

by reducing food consumption moderately and by eating high-nutrient, low-energy-dense foods [e.g., whole grains, lean meat, fish, legumes, and leafy vegetables] and avoiding high-energy, low-nutrient-dense foods [e.g., foods high in fat or sugar, deep-fat-fried foods, and purified starch-based foods].)
5. To use the amount of daily/weekly weight loss to adjust food/food energy intake, because it is impossible to accurately estimate and control energy intake. (If the weight loss was greater than this range, the children were encouraged to consume slightly more food/food energy; contrarily, if the weight loss was below this range, they were encouraged to consume slightly less.)
6. To change snacks from those that were primarily starch, sugar, or fat based to those that were primarily sugar-free, protein or nuts based, lightly salted, or unsalted.
7. To drink primarily sugar-free, aspartame-based beverages or unsalted vegetable juices. (Consumption of fruit juices was not encouraged because of the high sugar and organic acids contents that can induce hunger.)
8. To tolerate slight hunger.
9. To understand that after foods are consumed, the surplus energy is stored as fat in the adipose tissue.
10. To understand that excessive adiposity constitutes obesity.
11. To understand that by consuming less food energy, the body will burn the adipose tissue to make up the energy deficit, leading to weight loss.

The children/parents and their servants were taught (1) how to lower energy content of their meals by using less cooking oil/fat and by using soluble gums or mucilaginous substances as replacements; (2) to use high-nutrient-density foods to prepare tasty meals; (3) to avoid purchasing high-energy, low-nutrient-dense foods and to remove these foods from their household in order to minimize consumption; (4) to use 50% less salt in their cooking (from 7 to 10 g per person per day down to 3.5–5 g) and to choose less salty foods when eating out of the home. Reducing salt intake to 3.5 to 5 g/day reduces the risk of hypertension, which is more likely to occur when overweight/obesity occurs in conjunction with high sodium intake. Excessive salt intake can promptly increase body weight because of subsequent water retention; and high potassium intake has a mildly opposite effect because of its mildly diuretic effect. Unsalted vegetable juices and soups are very rich in potassium and can partially mitigate the effect of high sodium intake.

A healthcare professional visited the child's family once every 2 months to enforce the dietary and physical activity guidelines and to gather health, dietary, and lifestyle data. One year after entering the program, there were significant changes in the children and their families' dietary habits: consumption of high-energy-density foods and of high-salt foods was drastically reduced by 64% and 38%, respectively. Sugar-based beverages were almost totally replaced by aspartame or licorice extract-sweetened drinks, unsalted vegetable juices, fruit juices, or water. Consumption of primarily purified starch-based foods and high starch-high fat-high sugar-based foods was reduced by 48% and 31%, respectively. Whole grain, lean meat, fish, legumes, leafy vegetables, and to a degree fruits became the main constituents of their diets. These trends continued. At the end of the second year larger dietary changes were observed. Many of these changes remained until 20 years later. Thus, the dietary changes took hold for a long time in at least a significant portion of the children.

Building Physically Active Lifestyles

The children and their parents were taught that (1) >90% of the daily energy expenditure is expended in and by LBM; (2) having a large LBM is necessary for burning adipose tissue fast (important for weight control), for building a strong and shapely body, and for longevity; (3) physical exercise is a healthy way to expend extra energy above basal metabolism and to maintain a high metabolic rate [82–83] and is the best way to retain or to grow muscles, which form the bulk of LBM; (4) there are two types of exercise: strength (resistance) exercise, which is highly effective in enhancing muscle accretion, and aerobic exercise, which is easier and, if doing it for a sufficient length of time, is highly effective in burning adipose tissue; and (5) both types of exercise are required for building shapely and strong bodies. These principles were repeatedly indoctrinated every time the healthcare professionals visited the families. They were also taught to avoid a sedentary or physically less active lifestyle (e.g., watching TV/video or playing computer games). They were required to have more physical exercise, in addition to schools' physical education programs. As a result, the children started to participate in various sports and exercises, and adopted physically active lifestyles (e.g., playing basketball, volleyball, baseball, soccer, ping-pong, tennis, jogging, bicycling, hiking, swimming, running, or simply fast walking around a city block). For measuring the children's physical exercise, we used the children's average physical activity rate, defined as the weekly number of engaging in any of the previously mentioned activities for $\geq$ 30 minutes per child. After 2 months, 6 months, and a year in the program, the physical activity rate had increased from baseline 0.6 $\pm$ 0.3 times per child per week to 2.1 $\pm$ 0.9, 3.8 $\pm$ 1.1, and 5.2 $\pm$ 1.8, respectively. These were statistically highly significant

(P < 0.001). Thereafter, the physical activity rate remained high, 5.9 ± 2.1, 5.1 ± 1.7, 4.6 ± 1.4, and 3.6 ± 1.3 times per child per week, for the 5th, 10th, 15th, and 20th year, respectively. Since by the end of the first year all the children had achieved acceptable BMI (weights) (most of them continued to take the supplement for nutritional reasons, not for weight loss) and were not compelled to follow the instructions of the program, these data strongly indicated that the physically active lifestyles that the children had acquired during the 1-year period had lasted for a long time, if not lifelong.

Tracking Height Velocity, BMI, Adiposity, and Lean Body Mass Changes

At the beginning of the program, the boys had an average height of 137.9 cm (Table 39.3); the girls had an average height of 135.9 cm (Table 39.4). The average boys' heights 2 months, 1 year, and 2 years after entering the program were 138.8, 142.5, and 147.2 cm, respectively; and the girls' values were 137.5, 145.7, and 150.3, respectively. There was no loss in height velocity. Rather, their height velocities were slightly but significantly (P < 0.05) faster than the positive and the background control groups. For example, the height velocities for the boys and girls in the program were 4.8% and 3.6%, respectively, greater than those of boys and girls in the background control group. After 1 year, the boys and girls in the program remained 6.5% and 6.1% taller than the boys and girls in the background group, respectively. The height velocities continued even after the first year, when the children achieved their BMI goals and were no longer compelled to follow the instructions.

The goal was to reduce an obese child's BMI down to no more than 7% above the reference BMI-for-age,

TABLE 39.3 Changes in Height (cm), BMI (kg·m^{-2}), and Skinfold Thickness (mm) of the Boys during and post Weight-Control Program

	Number of children	Height	BMI	Triceps skinfold thickness	Subscapular skinfold thickness
Baseline	300	137.9	21.1	21.2	17.3
2 months in the program	300	138.8	19.7	19.2	16.5
End of 1st year	288	142.5	17.8	11.9	10.2
End of 2nd year	282	147.2	18.6	12.1	9.1
End of 5th year	206	167.7	19.3	8.7	9.4
End of 10th year	102	171.1	21.5	10.1	12.2
End of 15th year	41	171.8	23.2	11.7	13.8
End of 20th year	32	170.6	24.7	12.1	14.8

TABLE 39.4 Changes in Height (cm), BMI(kg·m^{-2}), and Skinfold Thickness (mm) of the Girls during and post Weight-Control Program

	Number of children	Height	BMI	Triceps skinfold thickness	Subscapular skinfold thickness
Baseline	300	135.9	21.3	23.3	20.2
2 months in the program	300	137.5	19.9	20.8	18.0
End of 1st year	283	145.7	18.0	12.3	10.1
End of 2nd year	274	150.3	18.8	13.1	11.3
End of 5th year	185	158.9	19.9	14.5	13.1
End of 10th year	82	161.4	22.1	18.2	14.9
End of 15th year	35	160.8	23.1	19.4	17.9
End of 20th year	25	159.6	23.4	15.9	

which was considered acceptable, though at the high end of the normal range. At initiation to the program, the boys had an average BMI 21.1 kg·m^{-2} (Table 39.3). After 2 months, 1 year, and 2 years, the average BMIs were brought down to 19.7, 17.8, and 18.6 kg·m^{-2} (P < 0.05), respectively. Similarly, the values for the girls were brought from 21.3 to 19.9, 18.0, and 18.8 (P < 0.05) (Table 39.4), respectively. Clearly, the program had brought their weights down to the acceptable range during the first year, and they remained in the acceptable range during the second year. These reductions might not appear to be substantial; however, by the end of the first year in the program, the children were 1 year older and would have greater BMI, because children's BMI increase normally with age. Thereafter the tracked children had their BMI increases within the acceptable range into adulthood. For comparison, the tracked children in the positive control and the background control groups had increases in BMI as they aged; the former continued to be obese, and only 76% of the latter remained within normal range. In a very long term treatment of obese children, weight loss is not the most meaningful goal; rather, bringing BMI to the acceptable range is. In mild cases of overweight, just maintaining the weight is sufficient to achieve the goal because of increases in height as the child ages.

The children's triceps and subscapular skinfold thickness is listed in Tables 39.3 and 39.4.

For the first 2 years (i.e., when the children were 9 and 10 years old), the body fat contents were estimated from the following equations [84]:

For boys: Fat % = $100 \times (4.57 \div (1.0879 - 0.00151 \times (T + S)) - 4.142)$
For girls: Fat % = $100 \times (4.57 \div (1.0794 - 0.00142 \times (T + S)) - 4.142)$

where T and S stand for the triceps and subscapular skinfold thickness in mm, respectively.

At the end of the 10th year, when the children were 19 years old, the following equations were used to estimate body fat content:

$$\text{Fat \%} = 100 \times (4.95 \div (C - M \cdot \log S) - 4.50)$$

where C and M are constants from Table 4-11 of Hill and Beddoe [85], the log is 10 based, and S is the skinfold thickness (in mm) for a specific site and gender that C and M refer to.

At the entrance to the program, the baseline fat contents for the boys and girls were 29.6% and 34.9%, respectively. After 1 year in the program, the body fat contents were normalized, 19.2% and 22% for the boys and the girls, respectively. At the end of the 10th year, the average fat contents were 16.9% and 28.4% for the tracked boys and girls (now young men and young women), both within the normal ranges. These values indicated that during the first year in the program, there were substantial losses of body fat; thereafter the fat content remained within the acceptable ranges until the tracked children matured. Because LBM is the body mass minus fat content, there were corresponding substantial increases in LBM.

Other improvements included significantly lowered pulse rate, blood pressure, and levels of serum triglycerides, cholesterol, and glucose. The vital capacity of the lung was measured among a limited number of the children, and there were dramatic improvements.

Some obese children in the positive control group tried to lose weight by taking certain commonly advertised quick-weight-loss products/programs, from one program to the other, and resulted in going through 3.6 ± 1.3 cycles of weight cycling (yo-yo dieting) within 2 years.

DISCUSSIONS

Definition of Childhood Obesity

Experts have used a BMI $\geq 30 \text{ kg} \cdot \text{m}^{-2}$ to define childhood obesity, and the most recent (2006) edition of *Modern Nutrition in Health and Disease* [86] states that "to screen children and adolescent patients for overweight... using a BMI greater than or equal to 30.0....If it is greater than or equal to 30, an in-depth medical assessment is warranted." (p. 979) I strongly disagree with this definition and approach. During past decades, this erroneous definition of childhood obesity in combination with the "watchful waiting" attitude of many pediatricians and parents has permitted a rapid increase in the prevalence of obesity in both children and adults and will continue to do harm. For decades, we have relied on the Lin definition of childhood obesity [2] for screening overweight children. This defines childhood obesity as having a BMI equal to or greater than 125% of the mean (reference) BMI-for-age for a childhood population, applicable to children from 8 to 17 years old. This 25% over-BMI concept derives from my studies on statistical distributions of BMI of childhood populations, which have an average standard deviation approximately 16.3% of the mean. A 25% excess in BMI equals approximately 1.53 standard deviations above the reference BMI. Assuming children's BMI follows the normal (Gaussian) distribution, children having BMI $\geq$ 125% of reference BMI constitute the top 6.25% of the children population.

This definition may appear too stringent; however, it is far less stringent than using BMI 30 to define childhood obesity. Further, considering the substantial risk involved in improper slimming of overweight children, this stringent childhood obesity definition is justified, at least to prevent unwarranted treatment of overweight but not obese children. This "25% over-BMI" definition can be conveniently used in clinical settings, as the average BMI-for-age is available [87, 88]. The matter of defining childhood obesity is further complicated by different children populations having different average heights and BMIs. Presently, the North American child population has a substantially greater average height and BMI than that of the East Asian child population. Child populations from wealthy regions tend to have larger BMI. By using the Lin definition, some obese East Asian children might be classified as overweight only, if the North American reference BMI is relied on. A similar argument can be made that some overweight North American children might be classified as obese if the smaller East Asian reference BMI-for-age is used as the standard. Obviously, there are genetic differences in body size, weight, and shape; however, at the present time and on a population scale, genetic factors appear to be less important in comparison to differences in nutritional intake. This issue of defining childhood obesity will ultimately be decided by what is the best BMI-for-age, which is in turn related to which is more important: growing bigger, having more physical capacity, and potentially having a slightly shorter life span, or growing slower but having less physical capacity and a potentially slightly longer life span. Within the same mammalian species, a larger body size (not just an obese body) is frequently associated with a shorter life span. These issues are interesting subjects for future research.

BMI does not reflect the basic body shape, which is determined primarily by genetic factors. Individual body shape should be taken into account when a more precise evaluation of one's weight-to-height relationship is desired. Sheldon discussed this matter and created "endomorphic" (fat/round), "mesomorphic" (muscular), and "ectomorphic" (thin/slender) to describe differences in body shape [89].

Safety of Slimming Programs for Childhood Obesity

Eating Disorders

Dieting can provoke eating disorders in susceptible individuals. Adolescent girls are particularly vulnerable [90–94]. Many weight-control experts advise eating less food to reduce weight. This advice might have unwanted detrimental consequences in a small fraction of overweight/obese children. A substantial restriction of food intake may increase the risk of developing anorexia nervosa. When children eat too little food, disturbances may develop in their digestive system, the lining, the muscles, the secretory function, appetite, and the neurological control mechanisms. This dietary supplement treatment for obese children emphasizes a reduction of food energy intake, but not so much on the total weight of food consumed, by teaching the children and the family to eat low-energy, high-nutrient-dense foods. For this reason, anorexia nervosa or other eating disorders were not observed among these obese children. Another factor contributing to the prevention of eating disorders was that the amount of food intake was guided by daily/weekly body weight changes.

Quick Slimming, Gout, and Cholelithiasis

Rapid weight loss, especially at a rate >2% body weight per week, can cause the body to burn significant amounts of fat and, to a lesser degree, of protein (LBM). This elevates the serum uric acid level and increases the risks of gout and gallstones in obese adults [95, 96]. Shrinkage of cellular volume and destruction of cells unavoidably leads to a degradation of nucleic acids. The large amounts of purines derived there from are ultimately oxidized by xanthine oxidase into uric acid, which the body can no longer use and must be excreted through the kidneys. Biological burning of fat, and certain amino acids, leads to formation and accumulation of ketone bodies, which competitively inhibit renal secretion of uric acid, and can further elevate serum urate level and increase risk of gout. The mild speed of weight reduction of this program, 0.5% to 0.8% of body weight weekly, did not lead to gout. Furthermore, this supplement program provided large quantities of soluble and insoluble dietary fibers that could help absorb cholesterol and bile for excretion and could attenuate the enterohepatic circulation of bile. The sum of these interacting mechanisms should result in little impact on risk of cholelithiasis; indeed, no such side effect was observed among the children.

Rate of Weight Loss: Preventing Weight Regain and Weight Cycling

At the beginning of dieting, a dieter burns primarily glycogen, leading to a quick weight loss, because glycogen has low energy content (4 kcal/g) and a large amount of water of hydration. As glycogen is burned into carbon dioxide and water, both the water that is produced and the water of hydration are excreted. Thus, to make up the same amount of energy deficit, more than twice the weight of glycogen is burned than fat, and many more times of body water is removed. When glycogen is gradually depleted in about several days to a week after entering a quick-slimming program, the muscles increasingly use fat as the primary fuel and avoid using extra amounts of the remaining protein as an energy source to conserve LBM. Burning fat leads to only about one third to one fourth as much weight loss for the same energy deficit, as compared to burning glycogen. Concurrent to the slowing down in the rate of weight loss caused by switching to fat as the primary fuel, the resting metabolic rate also decreases by 10% to 15%, partly because of an LBM loss and hormonal regulation (e.g., a parallel decrease in blood level of the thyroid hormone triiodothyronine, which regulates metabolic rate and other bodily functions). These two factors lead to a drastic reduction of the slimming rate, commonly known as "hitting the stone wall." There are also disturbances in insulin and glucose metabolism and in other hormonal and electrolyte functions. Opposing to this substantial decrease in metabolic rate, the body often develops an equally dramatic increase in appetite because of the body weight "set point" effect, leading to overeating and rapid weight regain, and causing many dieters to drop out of slimming programs.

Most "crash" or rapid-weight-reduction programs that required the participants, adults or children, to enroll in institutions or to follow rigid weight-loss regimens ended in failures or in almost "instant success" but with very high relapse rates. Even worse, weight cycling often occurs; weight cycling refers to repeated dieting cycles to lose weight then to rapidly regain weight, with ≥10% body weight loss and gain each direction. Fluctuations of body weight less than this amount are not generally considered as weight cycling. The National Institutes of Health's (NIH) asserts that there is no "convincing evidence" supporting the harm in weight cycling [97]. Many experts support this NIH assertion [98]. However, this conclusion is based primarily on results from faulty research methodology—for example, based on (1) too small samples, (2) too short follow-up studies, (3) too small weight fluctuations that were not much different from natural weight loss and regain after acute diseases, trauma, or other causes, or (4) studies that did not control for increased physical activity that some yo-yo cyclers had acquired during cycling. I do not agree with this position that yo-yo weight cycling in an attempt to lower body weight is not unhealthy; rather, it can be harmful, especially when excessive cycling is not accompanied by mitigating measures (e.g., increasing physical activity or having adequate nutritional intake). Our other observations show that weight cycling among adults caused significant LBM losses unless the cycler had adequate nutritional intake and engaged in extra physical exercise to gain or retain LBM. Unfortunately, many dieters, after a failure to maintain reduced weight from taking a quick-slimming product, are unable to resist the attractive advertisements of other magic quick-slimming products or programs and enter into new quick-slimming endeavors, repeating another cycle of yo-yo weight loss/weight regain. Usually, every cycle leads to additional LBM loss and an even faster "fat regain" because the less LBM, the less effectively the body can expend energy, and because the yo-yo cyclers look for the easy way to lose weight without increasing physical activity, leading to more food energy being accumulated in the body as fat. This dietary supplement weight treatment program was successful in helping the children to build sound dietary habits and lifestyles while they were "free living" (not institutionalized), without being subject to severe food restriction and other rigid requirements; this approach helped prevent weight regain after achieving weight-loss goals.

Is Exercise Alone Effective in Weight Loss?

Promoters of quick-slimming products often down play the importance of physical exercise in improving LBM. For example, "Exercise alone has little or no effect on body composition in people with excess body fat" [99]. On the other hand, some experts have promoted slimming by exercise alone or exercise-and-low-fat diets, with little restriction on food energy intake. For example, Foreyt and Goodrick championed a nondieting slimming program that emphasized 1. Development of "therapist and peer support; 2. Cessation of dieting... 3. Gradual increase in exercise; 4. Gradual reduction of fat in eating; and 5. Acceptance of whatever weight is achieved with prudent eating and exercise habits;" (p. 5–6, ref. 100) [100, 101]. My experience indicates that methods like this did not work in most overweight/obese adults and children. Long-term, intense physical activity, without food energy restriction, helps improve body composition substantially by reducing adiposity and increasing LBM, but it has little effect on the body weight or BMI, because neither measures body composition. Often, this method leads to a heavy and muscular body in the short term, but in the long run, when physical activity level decreases as the individuals age, the body also becomes too fat. Exercise-alone methods often fail (e.g., in women). It does not recognize the importance of food energy restriction and assumes a passive view of accepting whatever weight is achieved. Although some experts claim that exercise suppresses appetite, I found that physical exercise at the intensity range commonly practiced did not suppress appetite; rather, it enhanced appetite in the majority. This supplement treatment program for obese children emphasized both food energy restriction and exercise; therefore it was a success.

CONCLUSION

Sound dietary supplements offer the safest ways for prevention and treatment of childhood overweight/obesity; in particular, a supplement that provides a full set of essential nutrients (other than fat) in proper proportions and quantities is highly effective when used in conjunction with increased physical activity and modifications in dietary habit. Parental participation, repeated indoctrination of sound nutritional knowledge and practice, and easiness of compliance to the program are essential to the success. This program also prevented weight regain years later.

References

1. Willard MD. Obesity: types and treatments. *Am. Family Physician* 1991;**43**:2099–108.
2. Lin RIS. *A Comparison between Beautifying-Slimming and Quick-Slimming.* Nutrition International, publisher. Irvine, California, U.S.A. available by, drlin@nutrition-intl.com; 2010.
3. Eisenstein E. Chronic Undernutrition during Adolescence. In "*Adolescent Nutritional Disorders*" (Ann. N.Y. Acad. Sci. vol. 817; M.S. Jacobson, J.M. Rees, N.H. Golden, and C.E. Irwin, Eds., 1997. pp. 138–61.
4. Nuutinen O, Knip M. Long-term weight control in obese children: persistence of treatment and metabolic changes. *International J Obesity* 1992;**16**:279–87.
5. Sapir DG, Owen OE. Renal conservation of ketone bodies during starvation. *Metabolism* 1975;**24**:23–33.
6. Cahill GF. Starvation in man. *N Engl J Med* 1970;**282**:668–75.
7. Felig P, Cummingham J, Levitt M. Energy expenditure in obesity in fasting and postprandial state. *Am J Physiol* 1983;**244**: E45–51.
8. Grande F, Keys A. Body weight, body composition and calorie status. In: Goodhart RS, Shils ME, editors. "*Modern Nutrition in Health and Disease*". Philadelphia: Lea & Febiger; 1980. pp. 3–34.
9. Ravussin E, Burnand B, Schutz. Twenty-four hour energy expenditure and resting metabolic rate in obese, moderately obese, and control subjects. *Am J Clin Nutr* 1982;**35**:566–73.
10. Cahill G. Starvation: some biological aspects. In: Kinney JM, Jeejeebhoy KN, Hill GL, Owen OE, editors. "*Nutrition and Metabolism in Patient Care*". Philadelphia: Saunders Co; 1988. pp. 193–204.

11. Connan F, Campbell IC, Katzman M, Lightman SL, Treasure A. A neurodevelopmental model for anorexia nervosa. *Physiol Behav* 2003;**79**:13–24.
12. Vargas V, Vargas R, Mateu L, and Luzzati V. The effects of Undernutrition on the Physical Organization of Rat Sciatic Myelin Sheaths: An X-ray Scattering Study. In "Adolescent Nutritional Disorders" (Ann. N.Y. Acad Sci vol. 817; Jacobson MS, Rees JM, Golden NH, and Irwin CE, Eds., 1997. pp. 368–71).
13. Kingston K, Szmukler G, Andrewes D, et al. Neuropsychological and structural brain changes in anorexia nervosa before and after re-feeding. *Psychol Med* 1996;**26**:15–28.
14. Golden NH, Ashtari M, Kohn MR, et al. Reversibility of cerebral ventricular enlargement in anorexia nervosa, demonstrated by quantitative magnetic resonance imaging. *J Pediatr* 1996;**128**: 296–301.
15. Enzmann D, Lane B. Cranial computed tomography findings in anorexia nervosa. *J comput Assisted Tomogr* 1977;**1**:410–14.
16. Katzman DK, Lambe EK, Mikulis DJ, et al. Cerebral gray matter and white matter volume deficits in adolescent females with anorexia nervosa. *J Pediatr* 1996;**129**:794–803.
17. Artmann H, Grau H, Adelmann M, et al. Reversible and non-reversible enlargement of cerebrospinal fluid spaces in anorexia nervosa. *Neuroradiol* 1985;**27**:304–12.
18. Palazidou E, Robinson P, Lishman WA. Neuroradiological and neuropsychological assessment in anorexia nervosa. *Psychol Med* 1990;**20**:521–7.
19. Lankenau H, Swigar M, Bhimani S, et al. Cranial CT scans in eating disorder patients and controls. *Compr Psychiatry* 1985;**26**: 136–47.
20. Heinz E, Martinez J, Haenggeli A. Reversibility of cerebral atrophy in anorexia nervosa and Cushing's syndrome. *J comput Assisted Tomogr* 1977;**1**:415–18.
21. Datlof S, Coleman P, Forbes G, et al. Ventricular dilation on CAT scan of patients with anorexia nervosa. *Am J Psychiatry* 1986;**143**: 96–8.
22. Nussbaum M, Shenker I, Marc J, et al. Cerebral atrophy in anorexia nervosa. *J Pediatr* 1980;**96**:867–9.
23. Dolan RJ, Mitchell J, Wakeling A. Structural Brain changes in patients with anorexia nervosa. *Psychol Med* 1988;**18**: 349–53.
24. Fisher M, Golden NH, Katzman DK, et al. Eating Disorder in Adolescents: A background paper. *J Adolesc Health* 1995;**16**: 420–37.
25. Pendleton-Jones B, Duncan CC, Brouwers P, et al. Cognition in eating disorders. *J Clin Exp Neuropsychol* 1991;**13**:711–28.
26. Bachrach LK, Guido D, Katzman DK, et al. Decreased Bone Density in Adolescent Girls with Anorexia Nervosa. *Pediatrics* 1990;**86**:440–7.
27. Kling M, Demitrack M, Whitfield H, et al. Effects of the glucocorticoid antagonist RU 486 on pituitary-adrenal function in patients with anorexia nervosa and healthy volunteers: Enhancement of plasma ACTH and cortisol secretion in underweight patients. *Neuroendocrinol* 1993;**57**:1082–91.
28. Ferrari E, Franschini F, Brambilla F. Hormonal circadian rhythms in eating disorders. *Biol Psychiatry* 1990;**27**: 1007–20.
29. Bockman RS, Weinerman SA. Steroid-induced osteoporosis. *Orthop Clin North Am* 1990;**21**:97–107.
30. Krieg J, Pirke K, Lauer C, et al. Endocrine, metabolic, and cranial computed tomographic findings in anorexia nervosa. *Biol Psychiatry* 1988;**23**:377–87.
31. Kaye W, Gwirtsmam H, George D, et al. Elevated cerebrospinal fluid levels of immunoactive corticotropin-releasing hormone in anorexia nervosa: Relation to state of nutrition, adrenal function, and intensity of depression. *J Clin Endocrinol Metab* 1987;**64**:203–8.
32. Gold PW, Gwirtsman H, Avgerinos PC, et al. Abnormal hypothalamic-pituitary-adrenal function in anorexia nervosa. Pathophysiologic mechanisms in underweight and weight-corrected patients. *N Eng J Med* 1986;**314**:1335–42.
33. Biller BMK, Saxe V, Herzog DB, et al. Mechanism of Osteoporosis in Adult and Adolescent Women with Anorexia Nervosa. *J Clin Endocrinol & Metab* 1989;**68**:548–54.
34. Quaade F, Astrup A. Initial very low calorie diet (VLCD) improves ultimate weight loss. *Internal J Obesity* 1989;**13** (Suppl. 2):107–11.
35. Yanovski SZ, Gormally JF, Leser MS, Gwirtsman HE, Yanovski JA. Binge Eating Disorder affects Outcome of Comprehensive Very-Low-Calorie Diet Treatment. *Obesity Res* 1994;**2**:205–12.
36. Anderson JW, Brinkman VL, Hamilton CC. *Am J Clin Nutr* 1992;**56**:244S–6S.
37. Cox JS, Kreitzman SN, Coxon AY, Walls J. Long-term outcome of a self-help very-low-calorie-diet weight-loss program. *Am J Clin Nutr* 1992;**56**:279S–80S.
38. Richman RM, Steinbeck KS, Caterson ID. Severe obesity: the use of very low energy diets or standard kilojoule restriction diets. *Med J Austral* 1992;**156**:768–70.
39. Yass-Reed EM, Barry NJ, Dacey CM. Examination of pretreatment predictors of attrition in a VLCD and behavior therapy weight-loss program. *Addictive Behaviors* 1993;**18**:431–5.
40. Bleiberg-Daniel F, Fricker J, Dardenne M, Chappuis P, Apfelbaum M. Thymulin activity during very-low-calorie diet. *Europ J Clin Nutr* 1992;**46**:297–9.
41. Pronk NP, Donnelly JE, Pronk SJ. Strength changes induced by extreme dieting and exercise in severely obese female. *J Am College Nutr* 1992;**11**:152–8.
42. Widhalm K, Zwiauer K, Hayde M, Roth E. Plasma concentrations of free amino acids during 3 weeks treatment of massively obese children with a very low calorie diet. *Euro J Pediatrics* 1989;**149**:43–7.
43. Field CJ, Gougeon R, Marliss EB. Change in circulating leukocytes and mitogen responses during very-low-energy all-protein reducing diets. *Am J Clin Nutr* 1991;**54**:123–9.
44. Andronis PT, Kushner R. Orderly dieting and disordered eating: a case report. *Nutr Reviews* 1991;**49**:16–20.
45. Patton GC, Johnson-Sabine E, Wood K, Mann AH, Wakeling A. Abnormal eating attitudes in London schoolgirls—a prospective epidemiological study: outcome at twelve month follow-up. *Psychol Med* 1990;**210**:383–94.
46. Lappalainen R, Sjoden PO, Hurst T, Vesa V. Hunger/craving responses and reactivity to food stimuli during fasting and dieting. *Intern J of Obesity* 1990;**14**:679–88.
47. Wilson GT. Relation of dieting and voluntary weight loss to psychological functioning and binge eating. *Ann Intern Med* 1993;**119**:727–30.
48. Phinney SD. Exercise during and after very-low-calorie dieting. *Am J Clin Nutr* 1992;**56**:190S–4S.
49. Lemons AD, Kreitzman SN, Coxon A, Howard A. Selection of appropriate exercise regimens for weight reduction during VLCD and maintenance. *Internal J Obesity* 1989;**13**(Suppl. 2): 119–23.
50. Snow-Harter CM. Bone health and Prevention of Osteoporosis in active and athletic Women. *Clin Sport Med* 1994;**13**: 389–404.
51. Amad KA, Brennan JC, Alexander JK. The cardiac pathology of chronic exogenous obesity. *Circulation* 1965;**320**:740.
52. Naeye RL, Roode P. The size and number of cells in visceral organs in human obesity. *Am J Clin Pathol* 1970;**54**:251.

53. Ramhamadanig E, Dasgupta P, Brigden G, Lahiri A, Raftery EB, McLean Baird I. Cardiovascular changes in obese subjects on a very low calorie diet. *Int J Obesity* 1989;**13**:95—9.
54. Blake J, Devereux RB, Borer JS, Szulc M, Pappas TW, Laragh JH. Relation of obesity, high sodium intake, and eccentric left ventricular hypertrophy to left ventricular exercise dysfunction in essential hypertension. *Am J Med* 1990;**88**:477—85.
55. MacMahon SW, Blacket RB, MacDonald GJ, Hall W. Obesity, alcohol consumption and blood pressure in Australian men and women: the National Heart Foundation of Australia Risk Factor Prevalence Study. *J Hypertens* 1984;**2**:85—91.
56. Hypertension Detection and Follow-up Program Cooperative Group. Race, education and prevalence of Hypertension. *Am J Epidemiol* 1977;**106**:351—61.
57. Webber LS, Voors AW, Srinivasan SR, Frerichs RR, Berenson GS. Occurrences in childhood of multiple risdk factors for coronary artery disease: the Bogalusa heart Study. *Prev Med* 1979;**8**:407—11.
58. Voors AW, Webber LS, Frerichs RR, Berenson GS. Body weight and body mass: a determinant of basal blood pressure in children: the Bogalusa heart Study. *Am J Epidemiol* 1977;**106**:101—15.
59. Levy RL, Troud WD, White PD. Transient hypertension: its significance in terms of later development of sustained hypertension and cardiovascular-renal diseases. *J Am Med Assoc* 1944;**126**:82—96.
60. Lauer RM, Connor WE, Leaverton PE, Reiter MA, Clarke WR. Coronary heart disease risk factors in school children: the Muscatine Study. *J Pediatr* 1975;**86**:697—708.
61. Stamler R, Stamler J, Reidlinger WF, Algera G, Roberts RH. Weight and blood pressure: findings in hypertension screening of one million Americans. *J Am Med Assoc* 1978;**240**:1607—10.
62. Aristimuno GG, Foster TA, Voors AW, Srinivasan SR, Berenson GS. Influence of persistent obesity in children on cardiovascular risk factors: the Bogalusa Heart Study. *Circulation* 1984;**69**:895—904.
63. Must A, Jacques PF, Dallad GE, Bajema C, Dietz W. Long term morbidity and mortality of overweight adolescents. *N Engl J Med* 1992;**327**(19):1350—5.
64. Atomi Y, Kuroda Y, Asami T, and Kawahara T. HDL$_2$ cholesterol of children (10 to 12 years of age), related to VO$_{2max}$, body fat and sex. In *Children and Exercise XII*. (J. Rutenfranz, R. Mocellin, and F. Klimt, Eds., Champaign, IL.), 1986. pp. 167—72.
65. Craig SB, Bandini LG, Litchtenstein AH, Schaefer EJ, Dietz WH. The impact of physical activity on lipids, lipoproteins, and blood pressure in preadolescent girls. *Pediatrics* 1996;**98**:389—95.
66. DuRant RH, Baranowski T, Rhodes T, et al. Association among serum lipid and lipoprotein concentrations and physical activity, physical fitness, and body composition in young children. *J Pediatr* 1993;**133**:185—92.
67. DuRant RH, Linder CW, Harkness JW, Gray RG. The relationship between physical activity and serum lipids and lipoproteins in black children and adolescents. *J Adolesc Health Care* 1983;**4**:55—60.
68. DuRant RH, Linder CW, Mahoney OM. Relationship between habitual activity and serum lipoprotein levels in white male adolescents. *J Adolesc Health Care* 1983;**4**:235—40.
69. Macek M, Bell D, Rutenfranz. A comparison of coronary risk factors in groups of trained and untrained adolescents. *Eur J Appl Physiol* 1989;**58**:577—82.
70. Nizankowska-blaz T, Abramowicz T. Effects of intensive physical training on serum lipids and lipoproteins. *Acta Pediatr Scand* 1983;**72**:357—9.
71. Perusse L, Despres JP, Tremblay, Leblanc C, Talbot J, Allard C, Bouchard C. Genetic and environmental determinants of serum lipid and lipoproteins in French Canadian families. *Arteriosclerosis* 1989;**9**:308—18.
72. Porkka KVK, Viikari JSA, Taimela S, Dahl M, Akerblom HK. Tracking and predictiveness of serum lipid and lipoprotein measurements in childhood: a 1-year follow-up. *Am J Epid* 1994;**140**:1096—110.
73. Smith BW, Methrey WP, and Sparrow AW. Serum lipid and lipoprotein profiles in elite age group runners. In "Sport for Children and Youth" (1984 Olympic Scientific Congress Proceedings, vol. 10. Weiss MR, and Gould D. Eds., Champaign, IL.) 1986. pp. 269—73.
74. Tell GS, Vellar OD. Physical fitness, physical activity, and cardiovascular disease risk factors in adolescents: the Oslo Youth Study. *Prev Med* 1988;**17**:12—24.
75. Valimaki I, Hursti ML, Pihlakoski L, Viikari J. Exercise performance and serum lipids in relation to physical activity. *Int J Sports Med* 1980;**1**:132—6.
76. Viikari J, Valimaki I, Telama R, et al. Atherosclerosis precursors in Finnish children: physical activity and plasma lipids in 13 and 12-year-old children. In: Ilmarinen J, Vlimaki I, editors. *"Children and Sport"*. New York: Springer-Verlag; 1984. pp. 231—40.
77. Wanne O, Viikari J, Viikari I. Physical performance and serum lipids in 14—16 year old trained normally active and inactive children. In: Ilmarinen J, Vlimaki I, editors. *" Children and Sport"*. New York: Springer-Verlag; 1984. pp. 241—6.
78. Rocchini AP, Katch V, Anderson J, Hinderliter J, Becque D, Martin M, Marks C. Blood pressure and obese adolescents: effect of weight loss. *Pediatrics* 1988;**82**:116—23.
79. Hill AJ, Blundell JE. Macronutrients and satiety: the effects of a high protein or a high carbohydrate meal on subjective motivation to eat and food preferences. *Nutr Behav* 1986;**3**:133—44.
80. Blundell JE, Lawton CL, Cotton JR, Macdiarmid JI. Control of Human appetite: Implications for the intake of dietary fat. *Ann Rev Nutr* 1996;**16**:285—319.
81. Pascale RW, Wing RR, Butler BA, Mullen M, Bononi P. Effects of a behavioral weight loss program stressing calorie restriction versus calorie plus fat restriction in obese individuals with NIDDM or a family history of diabetes. *Diabetes Care* 1995;**18**:1241—8.
82. Mole PA, Stern JS, Schultz CL, Bernauer EM, Holcomb BJ. Exercise reverses depressed metabolic rate produce by severe caloric restriction. *Med Sci Sport Exercise* 1989;**21**:29—33.
83. Frey-Hewitt B, Vranizan KM, Dreon DM, Wood PD. The effect of weight loss by dieting or exercise on resting metabolic rate in overweight men. *Int J Obesity* 1990;**14**:327—34.
84. Cheng Z, Yao HG, Wong GH, Zhan GY. A study on body composition and health conditions of primary school children (in Chinese). *Chinese J of School Health* 1994;**15**:5—6.
85. Hill GL, Beddoe AH. Dimensions of the Human Body and Its Compartments. In: Kinney JM, Jeejeebhoy KN, Hill GL, Owen OE, editors. *Nutrition and Metabolism in Patient Care*. Philadelphia: W.B. Saunders Co; 1988. pp. 89—118.
86. Dietz WH. Childhood Obesity. In: Shils ME, Shike M, Ross AC, Caballero B, Cousins R, editors. *Modern Nutrition in Health and Disease*. Lippincott: Williams & Wilkins, Publ; 2006. Philadelphia pp. 979—90.
87. National Center for Health Statistics (U.S.) 2000 Department of Health and Human Services, Washington, D.C.
88. Frisancho AR. *Anthropometric standards for the assessment of growth and nutritional status*. Ann Arbor, Michigan: University of Michigan Press; 1990.
89. Sheldon WH, Stevens SS, Tucker WB. *The varieties of human physique*. New York: Harper; 1940.

90. Hsu LKG. *Eating Disorders*. New York: Guilford Press; 1990.
91. Polivy J, Herman CP. Undieting: A program to help people stop dieting. *Int J Eating Disorders* 1992;**11**:261–8.
92. Garner DM, Rockert W, Olmsted MP, Johnson C, Coscina DV. Psychoeducational Principles in the Treatment of Bulimia and Anorexia Nervosa. In: Garner DM, Garfinkel PE, editors. *Hand Book of Psychotherapy for Anorexia Nervosa and Bulimia*. New York: Guilford Press; 1985. pp. 513–72.
93. Garner DM, Wooley SC. Confronting the Failure of Behavioral and Dietary Treatments for Obesity. *Clin Psychol Rev* 1991;**11**:729–80.
94. Brownell KD. Personal Responsibility and control over our Body: when expectation exceeds reality. *Health Psychol* 1991;**10**:303–10.
95. Everhart JE. Contributions of obesity and weight loss to gallstone disease. *Ann Intern Med* 1993;**15**:1029–35.
96. Liddle RA, Goldstein RB, Saxton J. Gallstone formation during weight-reduction dieting. *Arch Internal Med* 1989;**149**:1750–3.
97. National Institutes of Health. Weight Cycling. (1995). NIH Publication No. 95-3901, Washington, D.C.
98. The National Task Force on Prevention and Treatment of Obesity. Towards Prevention of Obesity: Research Directions. *Obesity Res* 1994;**2**:571–84. (see p. 577)
99. Ask the Doctor: An interview with Dr. Gill. Hi-Tech Health & Fitness. Feb. 2009, p. 54.
100. Foreyt JP, Goodrick GK. Weight Management without Dieting. *Nutrition Today, March/April*; 1993:4–9.
101. Goodrick GK, Foreyt JP. Why treatments for obesity don't last. *J Am Dietetic Assoc* 1991;**91**:1243–7.

CHAPTER 40

The Role of Arginine for Treating Obese Youth

Catherine J. McNeal*, Guoyao Wu[†], Susie Vasquez[‡], Don P. Wilson[§],
M. Carey Satterfield[†], Jason R. McKnight[†], Hussain S. Malbari*,
Mujtaba Rahman*

*Department of Pediatrics, Scott & White Healthcare, Temple, TX, USA, [†]Faculty of Nutrition, Texas A&M University, College Station, TX, USA, [‡]Department of Pharmacology, Scott & White Healthcare, Temple, TX, USA and [§]Division of Pediatric Endocrinology and Diabetes, Phoenix Children's Hospital, Phoenix, AZ, USA

INTRODUCTION

Failure to diagnose and effectively treat obesity in young individuals misses a major opportunity to prevent or forestall the long-term consequences of this disease. The long-range impact of obesity is very concerning, leading some to speculate that the current epidemic may result in this generation of children being the first who will fail to outlive their parents [1]. Obesity is a significant risk factor for insulin resistance, type 2 diabetes, atherosclerosis, stroke, hypertension, fatty liver disease, and a multitude of additional medical problems that affect nearly every system in the body. Between 1990 and 2000, poor diet and physical inactivity, the cornerstones of obesity, accounted for the second actual cause of death in the United States [2] and contributed to the escalating cost of healthcare worldwide. Unfortunately, many interventions for obesity in children, including lifestyle modification and medical treatment, have been largely ineffective or associated with side effects that limit their use. Thus, identifying new therapeutic interventions to reduce body fat will be extremely beneficial for human health. In animal models, dietary supplementation with L-arginine enhances lipolysis and the expression of key genes responsible for fatty acid oxidation, thereby decreasing body fat. This chapter describes the use of oral L-arginine as a potential therapy to reduce fat mass in obese children.

THE GROWING OBESITY CRISIS WORLDWIDE

Obesity is a major public health problem worldwide [3, 4]. Data from the 2003–2004 National Health and Nutrition Examination Survey (NHANES) show that 66.3% of U.S. adults were overweight (body mass index (BMI) > 25 kg/m^2) or obese (BMI > 30 kg/m^2), and 32.2% were obese [5]. The prevalence of overweight and obesity in adults increased by 16% and 35%, respectively, compared with the survey conducted between 1988 and 1994.

Children and adolescents have not been immune to this epidemic common to their adult counterparts. Overall, 15% of children in the United States (U.S.) are obese as defined by a BMI ≥ 95 percentile for age and gender. This represents a 36% increase over the past decade [6]. The prevalence of obesity is also higher in certain racial-ethnic minorities, particularly Mexican American children in whom the prevalence of obesity reached 23.7% versus 11.8% in non-Hispanic white children [7].

Many other countries are also experiencing the obesity crisis. For example, the prevalence of overweight in China doubled in women and almost tripled in men between 1989 and 1997 [8]. Worldwide, more than 300 million adults are obese and more than 1 billion are overweight. Obesity is a multisystem disease associated with an increased risk for developing insulin resistance, type 2 diabetes, fatty liver disease, atherosclerosis, stroke, hypertension, and cancer among many other conditions [9]. Consequently, obesity claims an increasing number of lives and contributes to tremendous costs of healthcare worldwide [10]. In the United States alone, about 300,000 people die of obesity-related diseases every year, and obesity accounts for 6% to 8% of all healthcare expenditures [9]. The incidence of type 2 diabetes among children has increased over the past decade.

TREATMENT OF OBESITY IN YOUTH

After a careful review, the U.S. Preventative Services Task Force found a paucity of high-quality evidence for effective treatment of obesity in youth [11]. Most research in this field has evaluated the effectiveness of intensive individual, group, and family-based behavioral counseling utilizing specialists in multidisciplinary obesity clinics—therapies that are generally outside the realm of most busy office practices. There is little doubt that lifestyle intervention may be the optimal treatment for obesity, but in practice this is often difficult to implement, especially as a sustainable lifestyle change. For example, Monzavi et al. described the results from a lifestyle intervention program, Kids N Fitness, that was offered free of charge to youth aged 8 to 16 years with a BMI ≥ 25 kg/m^2 or a height-to-weight ratio $>$ the 85th percentile [12]. This was a family-centered 12-week program consisting of 90-minute, weekly modules that included an exercise program for youth participants, education for the parents or caregivers, and parent-child nutritional education. One of the notable observations that the authors reported was a 46% dropout rate of the program participants; half of this group never attended a single session after enrollment. Of those that attended the program, 39% completed the 12-week program and 44% of that group did not return for the final outcome assessment. This program had multiple beneficial effects including weight loss and improved metabolic factors in those that completed the program, but these end points did not meet statistical significance because of the high attrition. Perhaps the strongest evidence for the favorable impact weight loss and exercise have on obesity and the ensuing risk of insulin resistance and diabetes mellitus can be extrapolated from the Diabetes Prevention Program (DPP). In this study 3234 adults were randomized to metformin (850 mg/day) versus intensive therapeutic lifestyle changes (TLC), the latter consisting of $>$150 minutes per week of exercise and a low-fat diet, for up to 4 years. A 4-kg weight loss (~4% change) coupled with an increase in physical activity reduced the onset of 2 diabetes by 58% in the TLC group compared to usual care and compared to a 31% reduction with metformin alone [13]. No comparable data are available in the pediatric population.

The two drugs for weight loss that have been tested in the pediatric population include orlistat, a lipase inhibitor, and sibutramine, a serotonin and norepinephrine uptake inhibitor. Only orlistat has been approved by the Food and Drug Administration (FDA) for youth $\geq$12 years. The largest pediatric study reported by Chanoine et al. was a multicenter randomized, double-blind trial of 539 obese (BMI $\geq$ 2 units above the 95th percentile) 12- to 16-year-old individuals taking orlistat, 120 mg or placebo, three times daily for 1 year plus a hypocaloric diet, exercise, and behavioral therapy [14]. At the end of 1 year, there was a statistically significant 0.5 decrease in BMI with orlistat compared to an increase in BMI by 0.31 with placebo. Dual energy x-ray absorption (DXA) showed that this difference was explained by changes in fat mass, not loss of lean body mass. The maximal weight loss was observed at week 12 and increased thereafter. There were no safety concerns; levels of the fat-soluble vitamins were slightly higher at the end of the study given that the subjects received a daily multivitamin supplement; however, one open-label study did observe a vitamin D deficiency despite multivitamin supplement [15]. Side effects were primarily related to greasy stools, fecal spotting, abdominal pain, nausea, and the like. There was only a 2% discontinuation in the orlistat group, but one in two to three individuals experienced side effects, which usually limits the tolerability of the medication in the standard clinical setting. Several other smaller studies observed small or no effects on weight loss [16]. This medication is now available without a prescription.

Several pediatric studies have evaluated the effects of sibutramine for weight loss in obese adolescents. This medication is FDA-approved for individuals $\geq$ 16 years of age. The largest study, reported by Berkowitz et al., involved 489 individuals aged 12 to 16 years with a BMI $\geq$ 2 units above the 95th percentile for age and gender randomized to 12 months of sibutramine or placebo plus behavioral therapy [17]. Participants were started on a 10 mg dose or placebo for 6 months. If participants failed to lose $>$ 10% of their initial BMI, the dose was increased to 15 mg or placebo. Maximal weight loss occurred at 8 months and was maintained for 1 year, at which time there was a statistically significant 9.4% decrease in BMI in the treatment group compared to a 1.2% decrease in the placebo group. Fasting insulin levels decreased by ~35% in the treatment group compared to a 2% decrease in the placebo group. Insulin sensitivity also significantly improved in the treatment group and other components (fasting glucose, triglycerides, waist circumference, systolic blood pressure [SBP] and waist circumference) decreased more in the group treated with sibutramine compared to placebo. Only SBP failed to reach statistical significance. Change in fat mass was not measured. Hypertension led to the withdrawal of 1.4% of the participants in the sibutramine group and none in the placebo group; withdrawal because of tachycardia was similar in both groups. Other common side effects included headache, constipation, dry mouth, and insomnia. Several smaller studies have also been reported in youth that observed comparable changes [18]. Sibutramine is only available by prescription.

ARGININE SUPPLEMENTATION IN HUMANS: SAFETY, EFFICACY, AND PHARMACOKINETICS

Arginine exists in the L-form in protein and physiological fluid, whereas D-arginine must be synthesized in the laboratory. L-arginine is classified as a semi-essential or conditionally essential amino acid in humans. Although L-arginine can be synthesized in the body, rates are low under certain conditions (e.g., premature births, intestinal dysfunction, overexpression of arginase in tissues, and renal dysfunction), and therefore dietary intake is inadequate to meet requirements [19]. Dietary sources include protein-rich foods such as nuts (peanuts, walnuts, etc.), animal products (milk and milk products, pork, beef, chicken, turkey), seafood, cereals (oats and wheat), chocolate, watermelon, and various legumes particularly soybeans and chickpeas. Castillo et al. [20] studied the in vivo conversion of arginine to nitrate using N^{15}-labeled arginine via continuous intravenous infusion and by intragastric infusion. They observed that 16% ± 2% of the daily nitrate produced in subjects originated from dietary arginine. Approximately 40% of dietary arginine is catabolized in first pass by the human small intestine, and thus 60% of the arginine derived from the enteral diet or drinking water will enter the portal circulation [21]. The peak plasma concentration occurs 90 minutes after oral administration of 6 g of L-arginine; the half-life for this dose is 1.5 to 2 hours. L-arginine is well absorbed orally and is metabolized extensively in the small intestine and extraintestinal tissues. L-arginine is filtered in the renal glomerulus and almost completely reabsorbed in the proximal tubules. On the basis of results from human clinical studies [22], dietary arginine supplementation (maximum of 9 g/day) should increase plasma arginine concentrations in the postabsorptive state by 40% to 80%. L-arginine, the substrate for endothelial nitric oxide synthase (eNOS), is converted to nitric oxide (NO) in animals and humans [19]. As described by Wu and Meininger [21], the beneficial vascular effects of arginine supplementation are mediated through both NO-dependent and NO-independent effects, including membrane depolarization; syntheses of creatine, proline, and polyamines; secretion of insulin, growth hormone, glucagon, and prolactin; plasmin generation and fibrinogenolysis; superoxide scavenging; and inhibition of leukocyte adhesion to a nonendothelial matrix. In support of this role, a meta-analysis of randomized, placebo-controlled trials (12 studies, 492 participants) evaluating short-term (3 to 180 days) L-arginine supplementation (3 to 24 g/d) on endothelial function using flow-mediated dilation (FMD) was recently reported by Yongyi et al. [23]. They concluded that short-term oral L-arginine is effective at improving the fasting vascular endothelial function when the baseline FMD is low. L-arginine supplementation was able to restore dysfunctional endothelium but could not further enhance endothelial function. These results indicate that individuals with impaired endothelial function are likely to benefit from short-term L-arginine supplementation. Borucki et al. also reported that L-arginine supplementation (2.5 grams) is capable of preventing the lipemic-induced endothelial dysfunction after a fatty meal [24].

Arginine also plays important roles in the transport, storage, and excretion of nitrogen; in polyamine synthesis; and in the disposition of ammonia via the urea cycle. Multiple studies in adults suggest that enteral or parenteral administration of arginine can reverse endothelial dysfunction associated with virtually all of the major cardiovascular risk factors (hypercholesterolemia, smoking, hypertension, diabetes, obesity/insulin resistance, and aging) and ameliorate many common cardiovascular disorders (coronary and peripheral arterial disease, ischemia/reperfusion injury, and heart failure) [19, 21]. Thus, arginine supplementation may represent a potentially novel nutritional strategy for preventing and treating many aspects of cardiovascular disease. For example, oral supplementation of L-arginine (7 g three times daily (t.i.d.) for 30 days) improved flow-mediated vasodilatation (FMD) in 27 hypercholesterolemic adults. A study of 13 hypertensive adult subjects who received 3 g t.i.d for 6 months also showed improved FMD, but there was no reduction in blood pressure. Adults with type 2 diabetes mellitus (T2DM) who received oral L-arginine supplementation had improved FMD but no improvement in glucose control [25].

Only one study was found that evaluated the effect of L-arginine on weight loss in obese adults, but to our knowledge none have been carried out in the pediatric population. The adult study was a randomized, placebo-controlled trial in 33 middle-aged, obese (mean BMI 39.1 ± 0.5 kg/m^2) subjects with T2DM receiving no medication. Patients were hospitalized for 21 days [26]. During that time, each received a 1000 kcal/day diet and an exercise training program for

45 minutes twice a day for 5 days/week. They were randomized to 8.3 g/day of L-arginine (average dose was ~80 mg/kg/d) or placebo. As might be expected, both groups lost weight, waist circumference decreased, glucose and fructosamine levels improved, antioxidant capacity improved, adiponectin levels increased, and the leptin-to-adiponectin ratio decreased, yet all improvements were significantly higher in the group treated with arginine (p-values < 0.0001 for most variables). It is particularly noteworthy that fat mass accounted for 100% of the weight loss in the L-arginine group (without any loss of fat-free mass), whereas loss of fat-free mass accounted for 43% of the total weight loss in the placebo group. This led the investigators to conclude that L-arginine supplementation spared lean body mass during weight loss—a conclusion also supported by data in obese rats [27].

Significant adverse effects have been reported when oral L-arginine was used for 6 months (3 g t.i.d) following an acute myocardial infarction [28]. In this case, there was no improvement in the arginine-treated group, and 8.6% of subjects in the treatment group died versus none in the placebo group. However, this study is considered to have significant flaws that call into question the adverse outcomes that were reported [29]. First, there was no significant difference in arginine levels between the two treatment groups, nor was there any significant difference in pre/posttherapy. This could suggest poor compliance but could also be related to the fact that plasma levels of arginine are significantly affected by dietary adherence. Second, the fatal adverse events (two deaths from sepsis and one death of recurrent infarction after discontinuation of arginine) are unlikely to be associated with arginine treatment. Finally, the type of arginine preparation (purity, whether it was a freebase or hydrochloride salt) was not specified—factors that can significantly affect outcomes because of a potentially adverse effect on acid-base balance [21].

One issue that has puzzled investigators is the observation that normal intracellular concentrations of arginine in endothelial cells are about 300- to 500-fold higher than the Michaelis-Menten constant of the isolated, purified eNOS protein [21]. The beneficial response to supplemental L-arginine therapy to promote production of physiological levels of NO despite already high intracellular L-arginine concentrations has been called the "arginine paradox." This paradox may be explained, not by the direct effects of arginine on eNOS but by (1) synthesis of tetrahydrobiopterin, as essential cofactor for NOS [19], and (2) antagonistic effects of arginine on asymmetric dimethylarginine (ADMA), an endogenous NO synthase (NOS) inhibitor [30]. Discrepant results in adults may therefore be related to the fact that L-arginine may only be beneficial in individuals who show (1) a deficiency of tetrahydrobiopterin in endothelial cells and (2) elevated levels of ADMA. Therefore, concentrations of biopterin and the L-arginine/ADMA ratio in the circulation might better identify individuals who benefit from arginine supplementation.

There are very few studies of arginine supplementation in children, and all are relatively short-term studies. However the studies summarized in Table 40.1 support the safety of L-arginine in the pediatric population. Intravenous arginine infusion (up to 0.5 g arginine-HCl/kg body weight for infants or 30 g arginine-HCl for adults over 30 to 60 minutes) or oral arginine administration (9 to 15 g arginine/day for adults) for 7 to 12 weeks has no serious adverse effects on humans. Most adult subjects tolerated higher doses of oral arginine administration (21 g/day for 4 to 12 weeks) or 40 g/day for 1 week [19, 30]. Use of oral L-arginine in published studies of the adult population indicates most common adverse effects are associated with the gastrointestinal tract. These include nausea and diarrhea, abdominal cramps, and bloating (because of a rapid and excess production of NO). Other rare side effects such as flushing and allergic reactions have been reported.

It is worth noting that the pediatric subjects had serious preexisting diseases before participating in these studies. Although the number of children studied was very small, the side effects reported are similar to those in adults. As noted previously, the peak plasma arginine concentration occurs 90 minutes after oral administration of 6 g of L-arginine; the half-life for this dose is 1.5 to 2 hours [22]. L-arginine is well absorbed orally and is metabolized extensively in the body. L-arginine is filtered in the renal glomerulus and almost completely reabsorbed in the proximal tubules.

There has been some skepticism about the utility of arginine supplementation for weight loss in adults despite favorable findings in animal models. Several points in this regard merit discussion. First, humans are not arginine deficient based on nitrogen balance—there is plenty of arginine in most foods; some animal experiments were flawed in this regard because they used arginine-deficient species. However, both Zucker diabetic fatty (ZDF) rats and diet-induced obese rats in our experiments (described later) were not deficient in arginine on the basis of nitrogen balance [27, 34]. Second, it should be recognized that arginine plays an important role in regulating oxidative metabolism of key nutrients, particularly lipids and glucose in animals [27] and possibly in humans [26]. These changes can result in loss of fat mass and a favorable metabolic profile. Finally, all prior experiments to demonstrate the effects of arginine on insulin sensitivity were carried out in adults. Children may be more sensitive to arginine

TABLE 40.1 Clinical Studies of Oral L-arginine (Arg) in Children or Adolescents

Reference	Study design	Study population	Age range (average)	Treatment	Relevant safety issues
1. Lim et al. [31]	Randomized, double-blind; placebo controlled, crossover	12 transplant patients; 15 healthy controls	9-29 yo; 7-26 yo; average age n/a	6 g/d b.i.d. × 2 weeks	8 out of 12 patients completed the study. 1 patient could not swallow Arginine tablets; 2 were dropped because of noncompliance; 1 had sudden death on placebo before Arginine was initiated; all the healthy controls completed the study. Per authors, no major side effects noted by any control or transplant subject; 1 female transplant patient noted a minor increase in menstrual flow while on arginine therapy.
2. Bennett-Richards et al. [32]	Randomized, double-blind; placebo controlled, crossover	25 normotensive children with chronic renal failure	7-17 yo (11.5 ± 3 years)	2.5 g/m^2 or 5g/m^2 t.i.d. × 4 weeks; 4-week washout b/t crossover; (average dosing of 2.275 g t.i.d.)	21 out of 25 children completed the study; 1 child received renal transplant; 3 were unable to tolerate Arginine because of unpleasant taste in 2 and nausea in 1. After 3 children with low GFR c/o nausea, dose adjusted to 2.5 g/m2 TID in those with GFR < 35 mL/min/1.73 m^2
3. Amin et al. [33]	Randomized, double-blind; placebo controlled	152 premature infants with birth weight ≤ 1250 g and gestational age ≤ 32 weeks		261 mg/kg/d or placebo during the first 28 days of life	No side effects reported.

treatment because they are in a formative stage. There is a particularly high requirement of arginine for tissue protein synthesis in young mammals [19]. Thus, we believe that the burden of new evidence regarding arginine supplementation in an animal model is compelling and that the potential risk-benefit ratio in obese children is favorable given the safety profile and minimal side effects. Given the epidemic of obese children and the dire impact obesity has on future health, it behooves us to evaluate such an inexpensive and widely available treatment for pediatric obesity in a randomized, placebo-controlled trial, even if only small improvements are found.

ROLE OF NITRIC OXIDE (NO) IN FAT METABOLISM

NO is produced from L-arginine by NO synthases (NOS) in virtually all mammalian cells, including adipocytes, hepatocytes, and muscle fibers [35]. Increasing extracellular levels of arginine from 0.1 to 5 mM dose-dependently increases NO synthesis in cells [35–37]. Studies demonstrate that through an increase in the expression of peroxisome proliferator-activated receptor γ co-activator 1α (PGC-1α), a master regulator of mitochondrial biogenesis [38, 39], endogenous NO triggers mitochondrial biogenesis in diverse cell types [40]. Thus, NO may stimulate the oxidation of energy substrates (including fatty acids and glucose) in adipocytes, liver, skeletal muscle, heart, and the whole body. Consistent with this view is the finding that mice with the knockout of endothelial NOS had higher body fat weight than wild-type mice with normal expression of the NOS protein although food intake was similar between the two groups of animals [40]. Similarly, an inhibition of systemic NO synthesis increased plasma levels of triglycerides and elevated body fat in rats [41]. Although exogenous NO donors may either inhibit or increase lipolysis (measured as the release of glycerol) in incubated adipocytes depending on their doses and experimental conditions [42, 43], there is strong evidence that endogenous NO increases lipolysis in white adipose tissue, fatty acid oxidation in hepatocytes, and glucose utilization in skeletal muscle [44–47]. Additionally, results from our studies indicate that an increase in NO availability within physiological ranges through arginine provision markedly increased lipolysis as well as the oxidation of fatty acids and glucose in rat adipose tissue [34]. Similar results were obtained from studies with growing pigs, which naturally gain a large amount of fat [48, 49].

DIETARY ARGININE SUPPLEMENTATION REDUCES FAT MASS IN ADULT ZUCKER DIABETIC FATTY RATS

We (G.W.) have a long-standing interest in arginine nutrition and diabetes, particularly in the regulation of NO synthesis in mammalian cells [35, 37, 48, 49]. Most recently, we turned our attention to the Zucker diabetic fatty (ZDF) rat [50] [a genetically obese animal model] [51], which lacks functional leptin receptors [52]. In the course of our study to determine the effect of 10-week dietary arginine supplementation (1.25% in drinking water) on vascular function, we found that the arginine treatment reduced the body weight of adult ZDF rats by 16% compared with alanine-treated ZDF rats (isonitrogenous control), even though food intake was the same [34]. The subsequent dissection of tissues revealed that the arginine treatment reduced epididymal and abdominal (retroperitoneal) fat weights by 25% and 45%, respectively [34]. The weights of other tissues, including brain, skeletal muscle (gastrocnemius muscle, extensor digitorum longus muscle, and soleus muscle), heart, kidney, liver, lung, spleen, small intestine, and testes, did not differ between arginine-treated and control ZDF rats [48]. Our serendipitous findings suggest that arginine is a potentially novel, effective fat-reducing amino acid in obese animals.

To provide a molecular basis for the antiobesity action of arginine, we conducted a preliminary study to determine gene expression in the abdominal adipose tissue of ZDF rats using microarray analysis. Our results indicated that expression of adenosine monophosphate (AMP)-activated protein kinase, NOS-1, and PGC-1α increased by 123%, 145%, and 500%, respectively, in the adipose tissue of arginine-treated ZDF rats [34]. As noted earlier, PGC-1α is a master regulator of mitochondrial biogenesis [38, 39]. In addition, AMP-activated protein kinase is known to trigger the oxidation of energy substrates in skeletal muscle, heart, liver, and adipose tissue [53, 54]. Furthermore, cGMP stimulates the mitochondrial oxidation of acetyl-CoA in cells [55]. Thus, the increases in expression of the genes for PGC-1α, NOS-1, and AMP-activated protein kinase in adipose tissue are expected to promote the mitochondrial oxidation of energy substrates, thereby decreasing the availability of long-chain fatty acyl-CoA for triglyceride synthesis and of acetyl-CoA for fatty acid synthesis. This outcome reduces fat mass in the body.

DIETARY ARGININE SUPPLEMENTATION REDUCES FAT MASS IN DIET-INDUCED OBESE RATS

Because the gene pool of the human population has not changed sine the early 2000s and yet the prevalence of obesity has increased 35%, high-dietary intake of fat is likely a major factor contributing to the current epidemic worldwide [3, 4, 8, 9]. Thus, we conducted a preliminary study to determine whether dietary arginine supplementation will reduce fat mass in a diet-induced obese rat model [27]. Obesity in rats was induced with a high-fat (24% fat) diet. Feeding the high-fat diet to rats for 16 weeks increased the mass of fat tissues (Table 40.2). Remarkably, dietary arginine supplementation reduced the mass of all fat depots in both lean and obese rats (Table 40.2). Strikingly, the arginine treatment

TABLE 40.2 Dietary Arginine Supplementation Reduces Fat Mass in Diet-Induced Obese Rats

Rats	Treatment	Fat depots (g)			
		Retroperitoneal	*Epididymal*	*Mesenteric*	*Inguinal*
LF-Fed	Control	7.41 ± 0.69 [b]	7.45 ± 0.63 [c]	3.16 ± 0.35 [b]	6.78 ± 0.46 [c]
LF-Fed	Arginine	4.51 ± 0.33 [c]	5.89 ± 0.33 [d]	1.75 ± 0.16 [c]	4.54 ± 0.27 [d]
HF-Fed	Control	11.2 ± 1.34 [a]	11.0 ± 0.86 [a]	4.57 ± 0.63 [a]	13.3 ± 1.18 [a]
HF-Fed	Arginine	7.44 ± 0.46 [b]	8.79 ± 0.60 [b]	2.84 ± 0.18 [b]	8.83 ± 0.76 [b]

Data are mean ± SEM, n = 8. Beginning at 4 weeks of age, male Sprague-Dawley rats had free access to diets containing 4% or 24% fat for 15 weeks. After this 15-week period of feeding, rats continued to be fed the low- or high-fat diet, but rats in each dietary group started to receive drinking water supplemented daily with either 1.25% L-arginine-HCl or 2.04% L-alanine (isonitrogenous control) for 12 weeks. At the end of the 12-week arginine treatment, fat tissues were obtained for each rat. LF, low-fat fed; HF, high-fat fed. a–d: Means with different superscript letters within a column differ (P < 0.05). Adapted from Jobgen et al. [27].

reduced the mass of retroperitoneal, epididymal and mesenteric fat tissues in obese rats to the levels observed for the control lean rats. Results of microarray studies have indicated that dietary Arg supplementation enhances expression of key genes that promote lipolysis, oxidation of energy substrates, and removal of oxidants in adipose tissue [56].

ARGININE INCREASED IN VITRO LIPOLYSIS IN HUMAN ADIPOCYTES

To ascertain the relevance of the findings from rats to human fat cells, we conducted a preliminary study using commercially available human adipocytes. We found that increasing extracellular concentrations of arginine from 0.4 to 2 mM increased (P < 0.01) the oxidation of 1 mM palmitate and 5 mM glucose by 32% and 51%, respectively, in cultured human adipocytes (N = 4). Further, we found that the arginine treatment decreased (P < 0.01) the incorporation of palmitate and glucose into triglycerides in adipocytes by 35% and 39% (N = 4), respectively. The addition of N^G-monomethylarginine (0.5 mM, an inhibitor of NOS) blocked NO production by the cells and partially prevented the effects of arginine on palmitate and glucose metabolism. These preliminary findings suggest that NO mediates, in part, the stimulatory action of arginine on the mitochondrial oxidation of energy substrates in adipocytes. Modulation of the arginine-NO pathway can beneficially ameliorate insulin resistance in obesity and diabetes [57].

In an initial attempt to determine a role for arginine in regulating lipid metabolism in adipose tissues of obese humans, we incubated subcutaneous and omental fat tissues from obese subjects in the presence of 0, 0.5, or 2 mM L-arginine [58], using established procedures [59]. Our results indicated that increasing extracellular arginine concentrations from 0 to 2 mM dose-dependently increased lipolysis in both subcutaneous and omental fat tissues (Table 40.3). Likewise, the addition of 5 μM 8-bromo cGMP (a cell-permeable cGMP analog) or sodium nitroprusside (an NO donor) stimulated lipolysis in the human fat tissues (Table 40.3). These results show that NO stimulates lipolysis in human adipose tissue as in rat adipose tissue [60].

CONCLUSION

In summary, we are now facing a global crisis of obesity of epidemic proportions. Innovative research is needed to identify therapies to effectively combat obesity. To our knowledge, there is no published information regarding the effect of arginine supplementation on weight loss in obese youth. Results of our

TABLE 40.3 Arginine, cGMP, or NO Donor-Stimulated in vitro Lipolysis In Human Adipose Tissues

Addition to incubation medium	Subcutaneous fat	Omental fat
	Glycerol release (pmol/3 h/mg lipids)	
None	303 ± 16 [c]	212 ± 11 [c]
0.5 mM L-Arginine	367 ± 21 [b]	272 ± 15 [b]
2 mM L-Arginine	449 ± 20 [a]	319 ± 16 [a]
5 μM 8-Bromo cGMP	402 ± 15 [a]	338 ± 13 [a]
5 μM Sodium nitroprusside (NO donor)	458 ± 26 [a]	326 ± 12 [a]

Data are mean ± SEM, n = 8. Subcutaneous and omental fat tissues were obtained from adult women with BMI between 30 and 40 kg/m². Means sharing different letters (a−b) within a column differ (P < 0.01). Adapted from Wu et al. [57].

preliminary study indicate that dietary arginine supplementation, *even if started in adult life,* markedly reduced body fat mass in both genetically obese and diet-induced obese rats. Arginine also increased the

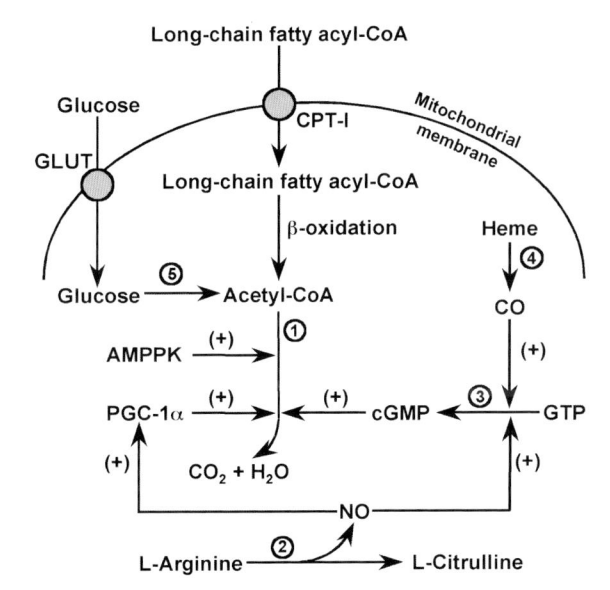

FIGURE 40.1 A proposed mechanism for the role of dietary arginine supplementation in enhancing substrate oxidation in ZDF rats. Enzymes that catalyze the indicated reactions are (1) Krebs cycle enzymes, (2) nitric oxide synthase, (3) guanylyl cyclase, (4) heme oxygenase, and (5) enzymes of glycolysis and pyruvate dehydrogenase. NO, produced from L-arginine by NO synthase, enhances expression of PGC-1α (a master regulator of oxidative phosphorylation and mitochondrial biogenesis). Both NO and CO (a product of heme oxygenase) activate guanylyl cyclase to generate cGMP, which stimulates the mitochondrial oxidation of acetyl-CoA via inhibition of acetyl-CoA carboxylase. AMPPK, AMP-activated protein kinase; CO, carbon monoxide; CPT-1, carnitine palmitoyltransferase-1; GLUT, glucose transporters; NO, nitric oxide; PGC-1α, peroxisome proliferator-activated receptor γ co-activator-1α. The symbol "+" denotes stimulation. Reproduced from Fu et al. [34].

oxidation of fatty acid and glucose in cultured human adipocytes, and it stimulated lipolysis in incubated adipose tissues from obese humans. Emerging evidence shows that oral administration of arginine can selectively promote fat loss and improve whole-body insulin sensitivity in obese adults with non-insulin-dependent diabetes mellitus. Future studies are warranted to evaluate the effects of dietary arginine supplementation on obese youth. New knowledge about the nutrition, physiology, and pharmacology of arginine will promote its worldwide use as a potential nutraceutical for improving human health.

References

1. Olshansky SJ, Passaro DJ, Hershow RC, Layden J, Carnes BA, Brody J, Hayflick L, Butler RN, Allison DB, Ludwig DS. A potential decline in life expectancy in the United States in the 21st century. *N Engl J Med* 2005;**352**:1138–45.
2. Mokdad AH, Marks JS, Stroup DF, Gerberding JL. Actual causes of death in the United States, 2000. *JAMA* 2004;**291**:1238–45.
3. Hill JO, Wyatt HR, Reed GW, Peters JC. Obesity and the environment: where do we go from here? *Science* 2003;**299**:853–5.
4. Abelson P, Kennedy D. The obesity epidemic. *Science* 2004;**304**:1413.
5. Ogden CL, Carroll MD, Curtin LR, McDowell MA, Tabak CJ, Flegal KM. Prevalence of overweight and obesity in the United States, 1999–2004. *JAMA* 2006;**295**:1549–55.
6. Williams CL, Gulli MT, Deckelbaum RJ. Prevention and treatment of childhood obesity. *Atheroscler Rep* 2001;**3**:486–97.
7. Ogden CL, Carroll MD, Flegal KM. Epidemiologic trends in overweight and obesity. *Endocrinol Metab Clin North Am* 2003;**32**:741–60.
8. Bell AC, Ge K, Popkin BM. Weight gain and its predictors in Chinese adults. *Int J Obes* 2001;**25**:1079–86.
9. Pi-Sunyer X. A clinical view of the obesity problem. *Science* 2003;**299**:859–60.
10. Finkelstein EA, Fiebelkorn IC, Wang G. (2003). National medical spending attributable to overweight and obesity: how much, and who's paying? Health Aff (Millwood) Suppl Web Exclusives: W3-219-26.
11. US Preventive Services Task Force. Screening and interventions for overweight in children and adolescents: recommendation statement. *Pediatrics* 2005;**116**:205–9.
12. Monzavi R, Dreimane D, Geffner ME, Braun S, Conrad B, Klier M, Kaufman FR. Improvement in risk factors for metabolic syndrome and insulin resistance in overweight youth who are treated with lifestyle intervention. *Pediatrics* 2006;**117**:e1111–8.
13. Knowler WC, Barrett-Connor E, Fowler SE, Hamman RF, Lachin JM, Walker EA, and Nathan DM. Diabetes Prevention Program Research Group. Reduction in the incidence of type 2 diabetes with lifestyle intervention or metformin. *N Engl J Med* 2002;**346**:393–403.
14. Chanoine JP, Hampl S, Jensen C, Boldrin M, Hauptman J. Effect of orlistat on weight and body composition in obese adolescents: a randomized controlled trial. *JAMA* 2005;**293**:2873–83.
15. McDuffie JR, Calis KA, Booth SL, Uwaifo GI, Yanovski JA. Effects of orlistat on fat-soluble vitamins in obese adolescents. *Pharmacotherapy* 2002;**22**:814–22.
16. Maahs D, de Serna DG, Kolotkin RL, Ralston S, Sandate J, Qualls C, Schade DS, Ozkan B, Bereket A, Turan S, Keskin S. Addition of orlistat to conventional treatment in adolescents with severe obesity. *Eur J Pediatr* 2004;**163**:738–41.
17. Berkowitz RI, Fujioka K, Daniels SR, Hoppin AG, Owen S, Perry AC, Sothern MS, Renz CL, Pirner MA, Walch JK, Jasinsky O, Hewkin AC, and Blakesley VA. Sibutramine Adolescent Study Group. Effects of sibutramine treatment in obese adolescents: a randomized trial. *Ann Intern Med* 2006;**145**:81–90.
18. Godoy-Matos A, Carraro L, Vieira A, Oliveira J, Guedes EP, Mattos L, Rangel C, Moreira RO, Coutinho W, Appolinario JC. Treatment of obese adolescents with sibutramine: a randomized, double-blind, controlled study. *J Clin Endocrinol Metab* 2005;**90**:1460–5.
19. Wu G, Bazer FW, Davis TA, Kim SW, Li P, Rhoads JM, Satterfield MC, Smith SB, Spencer TE, Yin YL. Arginine metabolism and nutrition in growth, health and disease. *Amino Acids* 2009;**37**:153–68.
20. Castillo L, deRojas TC, Chapman TE, Vogt J, Burke JF, Tannenbaum SR, Young VR. Splanchnic metabolism of dietary arginine in relation to nitric oxide synthesis in normal adult man. *Proc Natl Acad Sci USA* 1993;**90**:193–7.
21. Wu G, Meininger CJ. Arginine nutrition and cardiovascular function. *J Nutr* 2000;**130**:2626–9.
22. Boger RH, Bode-Boger SM. The Clinical Pharmacology of L-Arginine. *Annu Rev Pharmacol Toxicol* 2001;**41**:79–99.
23. Yongyi B, Sun L, Yang T, Sun K, Chen J, Hui R. Increase in fasting vascular endothelial function after short-term oral L-arginine is effective when baseline flow-mediated dilation is low: a meta-analysis of randomized controlled trials. *Am J Clin Nutr* 2009;**89**:77–84.
24. Borucki K, Aronica S, Starke I, Luley C, Westphal S. Addition of 2.5g L-arginine in a fatty meal prevents the lipemia-induced endothelial dysfunction in healthy volunteers. *Atherosclerosis* 2009;**205**:251–4.
25. Maxwell AJ, Cooke JP. L-Arginine: its role in cardiovascular function. In: Loscalzo J, Vita JA, editors. "Nitric Oxide and the Cardiovascular System". Totowa, NJ: Humana; 2001. pp. 547–85.
26. Lucotti P, Setola E, Monti LD, Galluccio E, Costa S, Sandoli EP, Fremo I, Rabaiotti G, Gatti R, Piatti P. Beneficial effects of a long-term oral L-arginine added to a hypocaloric diet and exercise training program in obese, insulin-resistant type 2 diabetic patients. *Am J Physiol* 2006;**291**:E906–12.
27. Jobgen WJ, Meininger CJ, Jobgen SC, Li P, Lee MJ, Smith SB, Spencer TE, Fried SK, Wu G. Dietary L-arginine supplementation reduces white-fat gain and enhances skeletal muscle and brown fat masses in diet-induced obese rats. *J Nutr* 2009;**139**:230–7.
28. Schulman SP, Becker LC, Kass DA, Champion HC, Terrin ML, Forman S, Ernst KV, Kelemen MD, Townsend SN, Capriotti A, Hare JM, Gerstenblith G. L-arginine therapy in acute myocardial infarction: the Vascular Interaction With Age in Myocardial Infarction (VINTAGE MI) randomized clinical trial. *JAMA* 2006;**295**:58–64.
29. Abumrad NN, Barbul A. Arginine therapy for acute myocardial infarction. *JAMA* 2006;**295**:2138–9.
30. Maxwell AJ, Cooke JP. L-Arginine: its role in cardiovascular function. In: Loscalzo J, Vita JA, editors. "Nitric Oxide and the Cardiovascular System". Totowa, NJ: Humana; 2001. pp. 547–85.
31. Lim DS, Mooradian SJ, Goldberg CS, Gomez C, Crowley DC, Rocchini AP, Charpie JR. Effect of oral L-arginine on oxidant stress, endothelial dysfunction, and systemic arterial pressure in young cardiac transplant recipients. *Am J Cardiol* 2004;**94**:828–31.
32. Bennett-Richards KJ, Kattenhorn M, Donald AE, Oakley GR, Varghese Z, Bruckdorfer KR, Deanfield JE, Rees L. Oral L-arginine does not improve endothelial dysfunction in children with chronic renal failure. *Kidney Int* 2002;**62**:1372–8.

REFERENCES

33. Amin HJ, Zamora SA, McMillan DD, Fick GH, Butzner JD, Parsons HG, Scott RB. Arginine supplementation prevents necrotizing enterocolitis in the premature infant. *J Pediatr* 2002;**140**:425–31.
34. Fu WJ, Haynes TE, Kohli R, Hu J, Shi W, Spencer TE, Carroll RJ, Meininger CJ, Wu G. Dietary L-arginine supplementation reduces fat mass in Zucker diabetic fatty rats. *J Nutr* 2005;**135**:714–21.
35. Wu G, Morris Jr SM. Arginine metabolism: nitric oxide and beyond. *Biochem J* 1998;**336**:1–17.
36. Morris Jr SM. Recent advances in arginine metabolism. *Curr Opin Clin Nutr Metab Care* 2004;**7**:45–51.
37. Kohli R, Meininger CJ, Haynes TE, Yan W, Self JT, Wu G. Dietary L-arginine supplementation enhances endothelial nitric oxide synthesis in streptozotocin-induced diabetic rats. *J Nutr* 2004;**134**:600–8.
38. Wu ZD, Puigserver P, Andersson U, Zhang CY, Adelmant G, Mootha V, Troy A, Cinti S, Lowell B, Scarpulla RC, Spiegelman BM. Mechanisms controlling mitochondrial biogenesis and respiration through the thermogenic coactivator PGC-1. *Cell* 1999;**98**:115–24.
39. Lehman JJ, Barger PM, Kovacs A, Saffitz JE, Medeiros DM, Kelly DP. Peroxisome proliferator-activated receptor γ coactivator-1 promotes cardiac mitochondrial biogenesis. *J Clin Invest* 2000;**106**:847–56.
40. Nisoli E, Clementi E, Paolucci C, Cozzi V, Tonello C, Sciorati C, Bracale R, Valerio A, Francolini M, Moncada S, Carruba MO. Mitochondrial biogenesis in mammals: the role of endogenous nitric oxide. *Science* 2003;**299**:896–9.
41. Khedara A, Goto T, Morishima M, Kayashita J, Kato N. Elevated body fat in rats by the dietary nitric oxide synthase inhibitor, L-N$^{\omega}$-nitroarginine. *Biosci Biotech Biochem* 1999;**63**:698–702.
42. Gaudiot N, Jaubert AM, Charbonnier E, Sabourault D, Lacasa D, Giudicelli Y, Ribiere C. Modulation of white adipose tissue lipolysis by nitric oxide. *J Biol Chem* 1998;**273**:13475–81.
43. Lincova D, Misekova D, Kmonickova E, Canova N, Farghali H. Effect of nitric oxide donors on isoprenaline-induced lipolysis in rat epididymal adipose tissue: studies in isolated adipose tissues and immobilized perfused adipocytes. *Physiol Res* 2002;**51**:387–94.
44. Khedara A, Kawai Y, Kayashita J, Kato N. Feeding rats the nitric oxide synthase inhibitor, L-N$^{\omega}$-nitroarginine, elevates serum triglyceride and cholesterol and lowers hepatic fatty acid oxidation. *J Nutr* 1996;**126**:2563–7.
45. Kurowska EM, Carroll KK. Hypochelesterolemic properties of nitric oxide: in vivo and in vitro studies using nitric oxide donors. *Biochim Biophys Acta* 1998;**1392**:41–50.
46. Gaudiot N, Ribiere C, Jaubert AM, Giudicelli Y. Endogenous nitric oxide is implicated in the regulation of lipolysis through antioxidant-related effect. *Am J Physiol* 2000;**279**:C1603–10.
47. Fruhbeck G, Gomez-Ambrosi G. Modulation of the leptin-induced white adipose tissue liposis by nitric oxide. *Cell Signal* 2001;**13**:827–33.
48. Tan BE, Yin YL, Liu ZQ, Li XG, Xu HJ, Kong XF, Huang RL, Tang WJ, Shinzato I, Smith SB, Wu G. Dietary L-arginine supplementation increases muscle gain and reduces body fat mass in growing-finishing pigs. *Amino Acids* 2009;**37**:169–75.
49. He QH, Kong XF, Wu G, Ren PP, Tang HR, Hao FH, Huang RL, Li TJ, Tan BE, Li P, Tang ZR, Yin YL, Wu YN. Metabolomic analysis of the response of growing pigs to dietary L-arginine supplementation. *Amino Acids* 2009;**37**:199–208.
50. Meininger CJ, Cai S, Parker JL, Channon KM, Kelly KA, Becker EJ, Wood MK, Wu G. GTP cyclohydrolase I gene transfer increases nitric oxide synthesis in endothelial cells and isolated vessels from type I and type II diabetic rats. *FASEB J* 2004;**18**:1900–2.
51. Clark J, Palmer CJ, Shaw WN. The diabetic Zucker fatty rat. *Proc Soc Exp Biol Med* 1983;**173**:68–75.
52. Lee WNP, Bassilian S, Lim S, and Boros LG. Loss of regulation of lipogenesis in the Zucker diabetic fatty (ZDF) rat. *Am J Physiol* 2000;**279**:E425–E432.
53. Hardie DG, Pan DA. Regulation of fatty acid synthesis and oxidation by the AMP-activated protein kinase. *Biochem Soc Trans* 2002;**30**:1064–70.
54. Tomas E, Kelly M, Xiang XQ, Tsao TS, Keller C, Keller P, Luo ZJ, Lodish H, Saha AK, Unger R, Ruderman NB. Metabolic and hormonal interactions between muscle and adipose tissue. *Proc Nutr Soc* 2004;**63**:381–5.
55. Garcia-Villafranca J, Guillen A, Castro J. Involvement of nitric oxide/cyclic GMP signaling pathway in the regulation of fatty acid metabolism in rat hepatocytes. *Biochem Pharmacol* 2003;**65**:807–12.
56. Jobgen W, Fu WJ, Gao H, Li P, Meininger CJ, Smith SB, Spencer TE, Wu G. High fat feeding and dietary L-arginine supplementation differentially regulate gene expression in rat white adipose tissue. *Amino Acids* 2009;**37**:187–98.
57. Wu G, Meininger CJ. Nitric oxide and vascular insulin resistance. *BioFactors* 2009;**35**:21–7.
58. Wu G, Lee MJ, Fried SK. The arginine-NO pathway modulates lipolysis in adipose tissues of obese human subjects. *FASAB J* 2007;**21**:A1052.
59. Trujillo ME, Sullivan S, Harten I, Schneider SH, Greenberg AS, Fried SK. Interleukin-6 Regulates Human Adipose Tissue Lipid Metabolism and Leptin Production in vitro. *JCEM* 2004;**89**:5577–82.
60. Jobgen WS, Fried SK, Fu WJ, Meininger CJ, Wu G. Regulatory role for the arginine-nitric oxide pathway in energy-substrate metabolism. *J Nutr Biochem* 2006;**17**:571–88.

CHAPTER
41

Prevention of Childhood Obesity with Use of Natural Products

Jin-Taek Hwang*, Dae Young Kwon*, Joohun Ha†

*Department of Biogeron Food Technology, Korea Food Research Institute, Kyongki-do, Republic of Korea and
†Department of Biochemistry and Molecular Biology, Medical Research Center for Bioreaction to Reactive Oxygen Species and Biomedical Science Institute, School of Medicine, Seoul, Republic of Korea

Abbreviations: AMPK, amp-activated protein kinase; BMI, body mass index; LKB1(also called STK11), serine/threonine kinase 11; AICAR, aminoimidazole carboxamide ribonucleotide; mTOR, mammalian target of rapamycin; eEF2, eukaryotic elongation factor2; ACC, acetyl-CoA carboxylase; HMGR, 3-hydroxy-3-methylglutaryl coenzyme A reductase; TSC, tuberous sclerosis; SIRT1, sirtuin-1; PGC-1α, Peroxisome proliferator-activated receptor gamma co-activator 1-alpha; ROS, reactive oxygen species; PKA, protein kinase A; ERK, extracellular signal-regulated kinase; AS160, Akt substrate of 160 kDa; NRF-1, nuclear respiratory factor 1; MEF2, myocyte enhancer factor 2; HCF, host cell factor; mTORC1, mammalian target of rapamycin complex-1; ADD1, Alpha aducing-1; ATGL, adipose triglyceride lipase; L-PK, liver-type pyruvate kinase; IKKβ, inhibitor of nuclear factor kappa-B; CD163, cluster of Differentiation 163; TNF, tumor necrosis factor; HFD, high-fat diet; NOS, nitric oxide synthases; IL-1beta, interleukin1 beta; IL-6, interleukin 6; MCP-1, monocyte chemoattractant protein-1; iNOS, inducible nitric oxide synthase; COX-2, cyclooxygenase-2; SREBP, sterol regulatory element binding protein; FAS, fatty acid synthase; C/EBP, CCAAT/enhancer-binding protein; PPAR, peroxisome proliferator-activated receptor; UCP, uncoupling protein; NAFLD, nonalcoholic fatty liver disease; VAT, visceral adipose tissue; JNK, c-jun N-terminal kinase; 4EBP1, 4E-binding protein 1.

INTRODUCTION

Obesity is a serious problem for normal growth in children, with primary and secondary health risks such as insulin resistance, high blood pressure, cardiovascular diseases, hypertension, and even cancer [1–3]. Childhood obesity is determined on the basis of body mass index (BMI), but BMI is not a diagnostic parameter. There are two types of mammalian adipose tissues: white adipose tissue (WAT) and brown adipose tissue [4]. WAT stores excess energy and has receptors for insulin, growth hormones, norepinephrine, and glucocorticoids [5]. Brown adipose tissue contains mitochondria-rich adipose cells and generates body heat via a gradient of protons in mitochondrial inner membranes [6].

Fat accumulation is caused by excessive food intake and low levels of daily exercise, which affect fatty acid synthesis and beta-oxidation [7–9]. Compounds to treat obesity should target these cellular mechanisms. Adipocytes are derived from mesenchymal stem cells and pass through different stages, including alteration in cell shape, growth arrest, clonal expansion, lipid storage, lipid oxidation, and eventually cell death [10, 11], with changes in gene expression at each stage. For example, Pref-1, a preadipocyte-expressed protein marker, is a growth factor for preadipocytes but disappears during adipocyte differentiation [12]. Growth arrest is necessary for differentiation of preadipocytes into adipocytes, which involves transcription factors such as peroxisome proliferator-activated receptor γ (PPARγ) and CCAAT/enhancer-binding protein α (C/EBPα) [13–15], and these factors represent promising targets for antiobesity agents. The final stage of differentiation produces increases in triacylglycerol (TAG) metabolism enzymes such as fatty acid synthase (FAS) and glyceraldehyde-3-phosphate dehydrogenase [16, 17]. In addition, lipolysis, or the breakdown of triglycerides (TGs), is necessary to regulate energy homeostasis [18, 19]. Several protein kinase families, such as protein kinase A (PKA) and extracellular signal-regulated kinases (ERKs), are involved in lipolysis [20, 21]. Furthermore, adipocyte apoptosis can reduce fat content under the control of proapoptotic and antiapoptotic proteins [22, 23].

The oxidation of fatty acids produced by mature adipocytes is important for thermogenesis and maintaining energy homeostasis, and this is regulated by enzymes such as carnitine palmitoyltransferase 1 (CPT-1), a regulatory enzyme involved in fatty acid oxidation in the mitochondrial outer membrane, and uncoupling protein (UCP), a mitochondrial transporter family protein involved in thermogenesis [24–26]. The stages of adipocyte development are regulated by the master metabolic protein kinase, AMP-activated protein kinase (AMPK). AMPK inhibits proteins involved in preadipocyte-to-adipocyte differentiation, such as PPARγ, C/EBPα, and sterol regulatory element-binding protein 1 (SREBP-1), and regulates the expression of lipolysis or fatty acid oxidation genes [27–30]. AMPK is activated by energy deprivation, hypoxia, ischemia/reperfusion, the presence of reactive oxygen species (ROS), and exercise [31, 32]. AMPK is activated by changes in the cellular AMP/ATP ratio to stimulate process such as glucose uptake and fatty acid oxidation [32, 33]. Thus, AMPK is a potential target for preventing obesity and obesity-induced metabolic disorders.

IMPORTANCE OF AMPK IN CONTROLLING OBESITY AND METABOLIC DISORDERS

AMPK helps maintain energy homeostasis by controlling metabolic pathways and is sensitive to changes in the cellular AMP/ATP ratio under energy stress [34, 35]. Active AMPK down-regulates anabolic pathways such as protein synthesis, DNA synthesis, gluconeogenesis, fatty acid synthesis, and cholesterol biosynthesis to reduce energy consumption. Active AMPK also up-regulates catabolic pathways such as glycolysis and beta-oxidation to generate ATP [32, 33, 36].

AMPK inhibits 3-hydroxy-3-methylglutaryl (HMG)-coenzyme A (CoA) reductase (HMGR), a rate-limiting enzyme of cholesterol biosynthesis that converts HMG-CoA into mevalonic acid in the mevalonate pathway [37]. AMPK also regulates fatty acid metabolism by directly phosphorylating and inactivating acetyl-CoA carboxylase (ACC), an enzyme that converts acetyl-CoA to malonyl-CoA—the first committed step in fatty acid synthesis [38, 39]. Malonyl-CoA inhibits CPT-1, which transports fatty acids from the cytosol to the mitochondria [40]. AMPK inhibits ACC to inhibit malonyl-CoA formation, as well as stimulating CPT-1 expression, to trigger fatty acid oxidation [41]. Fatty acid oxidation begins with fatty acid activation by fatty acyl-CoA ligase to produce fatty acyl-CoA in the cytosol. CPT-1 on the inner surface of the outer mitochondrial membrane then transports fatty acyl-CoA by binding it to an acylcarnitine molecule [42], which is transported into the mitochondria by carnitine-acylcarnitine translocase to be oxidized [42]. AMPK stimulates the CPT-1 expression [41].

AMPK activation also contributes to glucose metabolism by promoting glucose uptake and glycolysis. Activators of AMPK can up-regulate the glucose transporter 4 (*Glut-4*) gene in muscle, which improves type 2 diabetes [43, 44]. Similarly, AMPK stimulates the glucose transport mediated by Akt substrate of 160 kDa (AS160), a Rab GTPase-activating protein [45, 46]. A specific activator of AMPK, 5-aminoimidazole-4-carboxamide ribonucleoside (AICAR), increased AS160 phosphorylation by insulin-independent mechanisms in skeletal muscle, suggesting that AS160 is a downstream target of AMPK [45, 46]. Moreover, AICAR-stimulated AS160 phosphorylation was restored to normal levels in AMPK subunit-deficient mice, indicating that AMPK subunits are necessary for AICAR-stimulated AS160 phosphorylation [46]. AMPK also induces PPARγ co-activator 1α (PGC-1α), a member of the PGC-1 family, which is important in mitochondrial biogenesis, glucose metabolism, and thermogenesis [47]. PGC-1α functions as a co-regulator of nuclear receptors and stimulates the activation of transcription factors such as nuclear respiratory factor 1 (NRF1), myocyte enhancer factor 2 (MEF2), host cell factor (HCF), and others to regulate energy metabolism pathways [48–50]. MEF2 or cyclic AMP response element (CRE) is essential for muscle contraction-induced PGC-1α promoter activity [51, 52]. Interestingly, PGC-1α mRNA and protein levels are increased by exercise in rats and humans, and these levels are regulated by AMPK activation [53]. Exercise activates calcineurin, AMPK, and protein kinase C (PKC) pathways to exert beneficial effects against diseases [54]. For example, AMPK regulates PGC-1α expression in response to exercise [53, 54]. AMPK is required for increased PGC-1α expression in the skeletal muscle in response to creatine depletion, and deficiency of LKB1, an upstream regulator of AMPK, blocks the expression of PGC-1α and mitochondrial proteins [47, 55]. Thus, AMPK may regulate the therapeutic effects of exercise via PGC-1α and is an interesting target for exercise-mimicking compounds (Fig. 41.1).

Metabolic abnormalities, including obesity and diabetes, are significant risk factors for cancers such as colorectal cancer [56, 57]. Several studies suggested that AMPK signaling contributes cancer development. LKB,

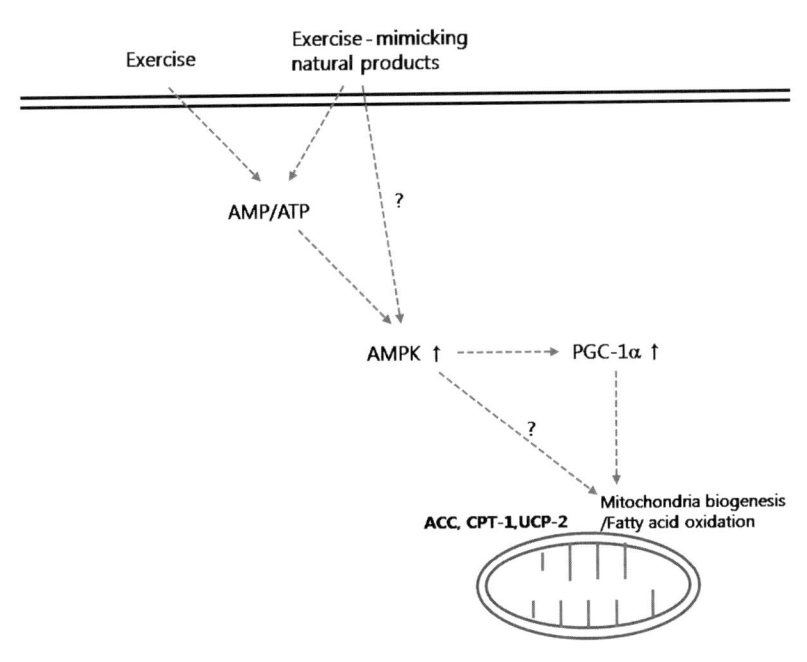

FIGURE 41.1 Putative mechanism of natural product-induced fatty acid oxidation. Exercise or exercise-mimicking natural products can activate AMP-activated protein kinase (AMPK) both via AMP/ATP ratio-dependent or independent mechanisms, increasing the expression of peroxisome proliferator-activated receptor γ co-activator 1α (PGC-1α) to trigger mitochondrial biogenesis and fatty acid oxidation.

a tumor-suppressor protein, is an upstream kinase of AMPK, suggesting that AMPK is involved in cancer development [58]. Other proteins such as phosphatase and tensin homolog (PTEN), tuberous sclerosis (TSC), and mammalian target of rapamycin (mTOR) complex 1 (mTORC1) play important roles in cell growth, and mutations in these proteins can promote cancer development [59]. AMPK regulates mTORC1 activity and activates TSC2 to inhibit mTORC1 as well as cell growth under energy stress condition [60, 61]. Similarly, p53 inhibits mTOR activity via AMPK activation in response to cancer chemotherapeutic drug: Sestrin1 and Sestrin2, two p53 target genes activate AMPK and phosphorylate TSC2, thereby resulting in inhibition of mTOR [62, 63].

STRUCTURE AND EXPRESSION OF AMPK

AMPK is a heterotrimer consisting of α, β, and γ subunits [64]. The α subunit is a catalytic subunit that contains a serine/threonine kinase domain at the N terminus, and AMPK is activated by phosphorylation at threonine-172 by an upstream AMPK kinase (AMPKK) [65, 66]. The α subunit has two isoforms, α1 and α2, with the α1 isoform expressed throughout the body and the α2 isoform highest in muscles and liver [65, 66]. These two isoforms are phosphorylated by the upstream kinase, AMPKK, and are dephosphorylated and inactivated by protein phosphatase 2C (PP2C) and PP2A [67, 68]. Dephosphorylation of α2, in particular, is mediated by PP2A. The β subunit acts as a scaffold between the α and γ subunits and has two isoforms (β1 and β2). This subunit contains an association with SNF1 complex (ASC) domain and a carbohydrate-binding module (CBM) for detecting glycogen particles. The γ subunit has three isoforms (γ1, γ2, and γ3) and contains cystathionine beta synthase (CBS) domains for detecting changes in the ATP/AMP ratio [69]. A set of 2 CBS domains is termed a Bateman domain. AMP binds to the two Bateman domains present in the γ subunit to induce a conformational change in the γ subunit and expose the catalytic domain of the α subunit [69, 70]. The γ1, α1, and β1 isoforms are widely expressed, whereas the γ2 and γ3 isoforms are expressed in muscles.

ANTIOBESITY ACTION OF A PHARMACOLOGICAL AMPK ACTIVATOR

AICAR, an AMPK activator, inhibits adipocyte differentiation and reduces neutral lipid content by suppressing adipogenic genes such as PPARγ, C/EBPα, and adducin 1 (ADD1)/SREBP-1 in 3T3-L1 adipocytes [71]. AICAR treatment also dramatically reduced body weight and insulin resistance in high-fat diet-fed (HFD) mice by activating PGC-1α. PGC-1α regulates adaptive thermogenesis and induces the expression of UCP1, a key molecule involved in body heat production [72, 73]. AMPK activation thus induces PGC-1α expression, mitochondrial biogenesis, as well as NRF1 expression [74]. AICAR treatment also inhibited lipogenesis and increased fatty acid oxidation by changing the mRNA expression of PPARα, PPARδ, and PGC-1α, and it also increased adipose triglyceride lipase (ATGL) content and fatty acid release, indicating that AMPK works via induction of mitochondrial biogenesis by PGC-1α [75].

AMPK can also suppress the expression of glycolytic and lipogenic genes in the liver. AICAR or a constitutively active form of AMPK, AMPKα1, inhibits insulin- or glucose-induced expression of liver-type pyruvate kinase (L-PK), FAS, Spot14, and ACC genes [76]. In addition, AMPK regulates the nuclear hormone receptor, hepatocyte nuclear factor 4α (HNF4α), which is involved in *L-PK* gene transcription [77].

The hypothalamus integrates peripheral signals such as insulin and leptin to regulate food intake [78]. Hypothalamic neurons regulate energy and metabolic homeostasis by regulating fatty acid metabolism. Thus, C75, a synthetic FAS inhibitor and CPT-1 stimulator, reduces food intake by regulating neuropeptides [79]. AMPK not only acts the expression of both FAS and SREBP-1c in hepatocytes and pancreatic islets but also regulates food intake in the hypothalamus [80, 81].

Adipocytes secrete several cytokines, termed adipokines, such as adiponectin, tumor necrosis factor α (TNF-α), and resistin to modulate immune responses. Adiponectin enhances insulin action and relates to AMPK activity in the liver, skeletal muscles, and adipocytes [82, 83]. The globular domain of adiponectin (gAd) significantly increases AMPK activity in endothelial cells [84]. Moreover, AMPK activation can inhibit TNF-α activity or high glucose-induced activity of inhibitor of κB kinase β (IKKβ) in endothelial cells; AMPK inhibition by a pharmacological inhibitor or via gene knockdown abolishes the effect of gAd on AMPK, leading to inhibition of TNF-α or high glucose-stimulated IKKβ activity [85, 86]. Thus, AMPK appears to regulate the inflammatory signaling pathways induced by adipocytes.

Adiponectin also suppresses the cellular and surface expression of CD163, a cysteine-rich scavenger receptor that takes up native hemoglobin (Hb) and haptoglobin (Hp)-Hb complexes in monocytes [87, 88]. Under the same conditions, metformin and AICAR also suppress CD163 expression [87]. Because CD163 is elevated in type 2 diabetes and obesity, AMPK activators such as adiponectin, metformin, and AICAR can treat diabetes or obesity by reducing CD163 levels in vitro.

Metformin, a derivative of guanidine, is clinically used for the treatment of obesity-induced type 2 diabetes [89]. Metformin and AICAR activate AMPK and suppress the expression of ACC, lipogenic enzymes, and SREBP-1, a key transcription factor in lipogenesis that increases fatty acid oxidation [90]. In a model of alcoholic fatty liver disease, ethanol increased the protein expression and transcription of SREBP-1, but AICAR and metformin blocked this increase, suggesting a role in the development of alcoholic fatty liver disease [91]. Ethanol consumption significantly decreases the circulation of adiponectin, an adipokine associated with AMPK activity [92], and AICAR attenuates ethanol consumption-induced fatty liver disease by suppressing hepatic SREBP-1c and FAS expression as well as inhibiting TG synthesis [91]. Thus, an AMPK activator may help prevent the development of alcoholic fatty liver disease. Erectile dysfunction is a sexual dysfunction associated with obesity. Penile nitric oxide synthase (NOS) expression is reduced by obesity-induced erectile dysfunction [93]. AMPK can regulate neuronal (n) NOS and endothelial (e) NOS, and metformin treatment reversed the fat accumulation and restored NOS expression in 5-month-old HFD obese rats, a model of obesity-induced erectile dysfunction [94].

PREVENTION OF OBESITY BY AMPK ACTIVATORS FOUND IN NATURAL PRODUCTS

Berberine, a quaternary ammonium salt found in the Chinese herb *Coptis chinensis*, has been widely used to prevent various diseases [95]. Berberine can activate AMPK signaling by increasing both the AMP/ATP and ADP/ATP ratios in cell culture systems, producing an antiobesity effect [96]. Berberine activates AMPK to reduce cholesterol and TG synthesis in both cell and animal experiments, and it also induces fatty acid oxidation by inhibition of ACC via a mitogen-activated protein kinase (MAPK)-/ERK-dependent mechanism [97, 98]. Berberine also improves lipid dysregulation and fatty liver disease through central and peripheral actions in mice [97, 98]. Berberine treatment reduces liver weight, hepatic and plasma TG levels, and cholesterol levels by promoting AMPK activation, fatty acid oxidation, and expression of lipid metabolism-related genes [96, 97]. Moreover, berberine reduces obesity-induced inflammation via blocking the expression of proinflammatory genes such as TNF-α, interleukin 1β (IL-1β), IL-6, monocyte chemoattractant protein 1 (MCP-1), inducible (i) NOS, and cyclooxygenase-2 (COX-2) in the adipose tissues of obese db/db mice [99].

α-Lipoic acid (α-LA), an essential cofactor of many enzymes, is a naturally occurring short-chain fatty acid that has an antiobesity effect [100]. α-LA reduces weight and food intake and increases energy expenditure by decreasing hypothalamic AMPK activity [101]. α-LA also increases AMPK and ACC phosphorylation levels [102] and reduces threonine phosphorylation of p70 ribosomal protein S6 kinase (p70S6K) and 4E-binding protein 1 (4EBP1) in the MIN6 beta cells [102]. α-LA treatment of aged mice improved body composition and glucose tolerance and reduced energy expenditure via enhanced AMPK phosphorylation and expression of PGC-1α in the skeletal muscle. Palmitate beta-oxidation, by decreasing protein synthesis, is associated with enhanced AMPK phosphorylation and expression of PGC-1α and GLUT4, but it attenuated the phosphorylation of protein synthesis-related proteins such as mTOR and p70S6K [103]. Thus, α-LA improves muscle energy metabolism by enhancing AMPK-PGC-1α-mediated mitochondrial biogenesis and increases lean body mass loss by inhibiting protein synthesis via mTOR inhibition.

AMPK activation plays an important role in obesity-induced endothelial dysfunction (e.g., atherosclerosis), which can also be overcome by α-LA [104]. α-LA treatment restored normal heart size, echocardiogram recordings, and TG content in mice overexpressing the acyl-CoA synthase (ACS), by enhancing AMPK activation and PGC-1α expression but blocking SREBP-1c and FAS expression [105].

Resveratrol is a polyphenolic compound found in the skin of red grapes that is beneficial in treating various diseases [106]. Resveratrol activates sirtuin 1 (SIRT1), a protein that regulates energy homeostasis, as well as PGC-1α to induce oxidative mitochondrial enzymes [107]. Resveratrol treatment reduces HFD-induced obesity, nonalcoholic fatty liver disease, and insulin resistance in mice and also inhibits TAG accumulation in HepG2 cells through a mechanism that involves increased AMPK phosphorylation [108], suggesting that the beneficial effect of resveratrol against fatty liver disease is related to AMPK activation. Moreover, resveratrol lowers obesity-induced proinflammatory responses; it increases the concentration of adiponectin and lower TNF-α production in the visceral adipose tissue (VAT) of obese rats [109]. This effect was also associated with AMPK activation.

Epigallocatechin-3-gallate (EGCG), a gallic acid ester of the catechins found in green tea, has antiobesity effect [110]; reduces food intake and blood levels of TG, cholesterol, and leptin; and promotes energy expenditure and fat oxidation in vivo [111, 112]. ECGC can activate AMPK signaling [110], and we previously showed that EGCG significantly inhibited adipocyte differentiation and rapidly activated AMPK in 3T3-L1 adipocytes [113].

Curcumin is a major polyphenol found in turmeric used to treat obesity and other diseases [114]. In cell culture systems, curcumin reduces fat accumulation and glycerol-3-phosphate acyltransferase 1 expression, whereas it enhances AMPK phosphorylation and CPT-1 expression, resulting in the acceleration of fatty acid oxidation [115]. Curcumin significantly reduces serum cholesterol levels and the expression of PPARγ and C/EBPα to reduce body fat and body weight gain [115]. We also showed that curcumin inhibited adipocyte differentiation and growth, activated AMPK, and suppressed PPARγ expression in 3T3-L1 adipocytes [116]. In those studies, a synthetic AMPK activator inhibited adipocyte differentiation as well as PPARγ expression. Plasma FFA levels are associated with an increased low frequency (LF)/high frequency (HF) ratio, an index of disturbance in sympathovagal balance; this was also improved by curcuminoid supplementation in HFD obese rats [117]. Curcumin also inhibits obesity-induced diabetes and inflammation in murine models of insulin-resistant obesity. Dietary curcumin significantly reduces macrophage infiltration of WAT, hepatic nuclear factor κB activity, hepatomegaly, and hepatic inflammation marker levels, whereas it increases adipose tissue adiponectin production [118]. Obesity-induced hypercholesterolemia is associated with nonalcoholic steatohepatitis, resulting in hepatic fibrosis. Curcumin reduced cellular cholesterol levels and low-density lipoprotein receptor (LDLR) gene expression by activating PPARγ and differentially regulating SREBPs expression in hepatic stellate cells, which suggests that curcumin may help prevent hypercholesterolemia-associated hepatic fibrogenesis [119].

Ginseng is widely used for the prevention of metabolic disorders and obesity in Asian countries [120]. Ginsenosides, the active components of ginseng, can activate or inhibit signaling molecules [121]. Ginsenoside Rg3 (Rg3), which is derived from ginseng radix, significantly reduces body weight and insulin resistance by altering the expression of glucose metabolism or fatty acid metabolism genes [122]. We previously observed that ginsenoside Rh2 (Rh2) from Korean red ginseng root inhibits adipocyte differentiation via the activation of AMPK signaling and inhibition of PPARγ [123]. Similarly, Rg3 inhibited adipocyte differentiation of 3T3-L1 cells via PPARγ inhibition and AMPK activation [124].

Ginsenoside Rb2 (Rb2) reduces the increase in total cholesterol and TAG levels caused by high cholesterol and fetal bovine serum, together with up-regulation of SREBP and leptin mRNA, suggesting that Rb2 can prevent fat accumulation [125]. Compound K (20-O-(β-D-glucopyranosyl)-20(S)-protopanaxadiol), an intestinal bacterial metabolite of protopanaxadiol ginsenosides, inhibits nonesterified fatty acid (NEFA)-induced pancreatic beta-cell death in MIN6N8 mouse insulinoma beta cells by modulating stress-activated protein kinase (SAPK)/c-Jun N-terminal kinase (JNK) activation, suggesting that Compound K has therapeutic potential for obesity-induced diabetes [126]. We also showed that genistein, an isoflavone abundant in soy products, inhibits adipocyte differentiation, causes apoptosis via the release of intracellular ROS, as well as activates AMPK [113].

Quercetin, a flavonoid found in plants, is an antioxidant that reduces total cholesterol, TG, FFA, and insulin levels in obese Zucker rats [127]. Moreover, quercetin improved obesity-induced inflammation via increases in adiponectin levels and reductions in both NO_x levels and VAT TNF-α production in obese Zucker rats [127]. Quercetin further inhibited adipogenesis by suppressing the expression of PPARγ and C/EBPα [128]. Quercetin is proapoptotic for adipocytes by decreasing mitochondrial membrane potential and increasing caspase-3 activity [129]. Quercetin activates AMPK in HepG2 cells via SIRT1, an NAD(+)-dependent histone/protein deacetylase associated with the longevity caused by caloric restriction [130]. Quercetin treatment also inhibits adipogenesis and adipogenesis-related enzymes via phosphorylation of AMPK and its substrate, ACC, and induces apoptosis in mature adipocytes via modulating the ERK and JNK pathways [131].

Other natural products modulate obesity via AMPK. For example, a fish oil supplement reduced total cholesterol and lowered lipids in lean $LDLR^{-/-}$ mice by activating hepatic AMPK [132]. Similarly, AMPK activation by n-3 polyunsaturated fatty acids (PUFAs) increases AMPKα1 and CPT-1 activity in the liver and skeletal muscle of obese diabetic rats, leading to reduced body weight [133]. Biotransformation of blueberry juice by the bacterium *Serratia vaccinii* activates AMPK in muscle cells and adipocytes, which inhibits adipogenesis [134].

BPG obtained from *Balanophora polyandra* Griff, decreased blood glucose and TG levels as well as TG content in skeletal muscle of HFD C57BL/6 mice via AMPK activation [135]. Sulfated glucosamine (SGlc) dose-dependently reduced TG content and activated both AMPKα and AMPKβ in 3T3-L1 adipocytes [136]. Eicosapentaenoic acid (EPA), an n-3 PUFA, modulates adipokine production by adipocytes via AMPK activation [137]. *Juniperus chinensis* hot water extract (JCE) reduces body weight gain, visceral fat-pad weight, and blood levels of lipid, insulin, and leptin in HFD rats via AMPK activation. Further, theaflavins extracted from black tea significantly reduce fatty acid synthesis and stimulate fatty acid oxidation by activating AMPK through the LKB1 and ROS pathways [138]. Taken together, AMPK signaling mediates the antiobesity effect of natural products, at least in part, by inhibiting the expression of fatty acid synthesis proteins and enhancing fatty acid oxidation.

CONCLUSION

Natural products to treat obesity must be safe and effective, preferably with clear mechanisms of action to aid further testing. Natural products such as berberine, α-LA, resveratrol, EGCG, curcumin, ginsenosides, quercetin, fish oil, PUFAs, blueberry juice, and JCE can activate AMPK in cultured cells or rodents (Fig. 41.2).

AMPK plays a central role in inhibiting protein synthesis via protein synthesis proteins such as mTOR, p70S6K, eukaryotic elongation factor 2 (eEF-2), and 4EBP1. The natural products highlighted in this chapter also influence protein synthesis in other disease models, including cancer, via AMPK activation, similar to fatty acid synthesis. AMPK also regulates energy homeostasis in response to energy stress conditions such as exercise. Exercise training stimulates genes such as PGC-1α, a transcriptional co-activator, to regulate oxidative metabolism. Natural products also stimulate PGC-1α gene expression via AMPK activation, providing a molecular mechanism of the beneficial effects of exercise. Thus, AMPK activation by natural products seems to mimic the effects of exercise.

Fatty acid synthesis and oxidation are complex processes that involve signaling molecules such as ACC, FAS, SREBP, PPARγ, SIRT1, CPT-1, C/EBP, PGC-1α, and UCP2. Several natural products modulate these processes putatively via AMPK activation, but a direct link between AMPK and fatty acid metabolism remains to be established. Further work on the molecular events involved in preventing obesity, including childhood obesity, will provide new mechanisms for regulating AMPK signaling and subsequently new therapeutic agents from natural compounds or ingredients.

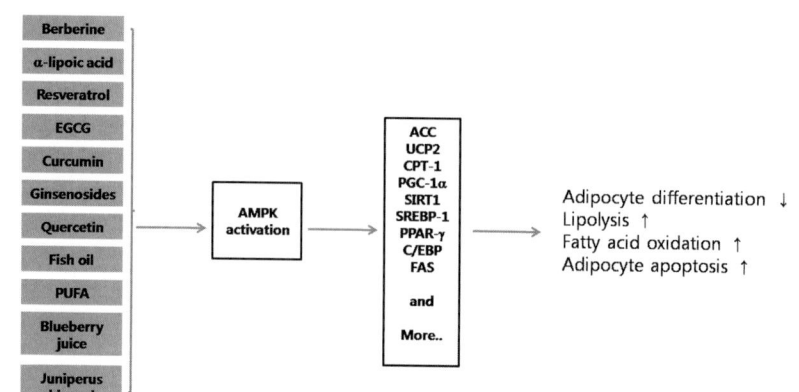

FIGURE 41.2 AMPK activators in natural products exert beneficial effects against obesity via modulating fatty acid metabolism. Berberine, α-lipoic acid (α-LA), resveratrol, epigallocatechin-3-gallate (EGCG), curcumin, ginsenosides, quercetin, fish oil, n-3 polyunsaturated fatty acids (PUFAs), blueberry juice, and *Juniperus chinensis* hot water extract (JCE) can modulate the expression or activation of fatty acid metabolism-related proteins, putatively via AMPK activation, thereby exerting beneficial effects against obesity.

References

1. Chia DJ, Boston BA. Childhood obesity and the metabolic syndrome. *Advances in Pediatrics* 2006;**53**:23−53.
2. Gardner M, Gardner DW, Sowers JR. The cardiometabolic syndrome in the adolescent. *Pediatric Endocrinology Reviews* 2008;(Suppl. 4):964−8.
3. Schlienger JL, Luca F, Vinzio S, Pradignac A. Obesity and Cancer. *La Revue de Medecine Interne* 2009;**30**:776−82.
4. Fonseca-Alaniz MH, Takada J, Alonso-Vale MI, Lima FB. Adipose tissue as an endocrine organ: from theory to practice. *Jornal de Pediatria (Rio de Janeiro)* 2007;**83**:S192−203.
5. Avram A, Avram M, James W. Subcutaneous fat in normal and diseased states: Anatomy and physiology of white and brown adipose tissue. *Journal of the American Academy of Dermatology* 2005;**53**:671−83.
6. Ricquier D, Bouillaud F. Mitochondrial uncoupling proteins: from mitochondria to the regulation of energy balance. *Journal of Physiology* 2000;**529**:3−10.
7. Wlodek D, Gonzales MJ. Decreased energy levels can cause and sustain obesity. *Journal of Theoretical Biology* 2003;**225**:33−44.
8. Doucet E, Tremblay A. Food intake, energy balance and body weight control. *European Journal of Clinical Nutrition* 1997;**51**:846−55.
9. Robinson JR, Niswender KD. What are the risks and the benefits of current and emerging weight-loss medications? *Current Diabetes Reports* 2009;**9**:368−75.
10. Xie H, Sun Y, Lodish HF. Targeting microRNAs in obesity. *Expert Opinion on Therapeutic Targets* 2009;**13**:1227−38.
11. Rosen ED, Spiegelman BM. Molecular regulation of adipogenesis. *Annual Review of Cell and Developmental Biology* 2000;**16**:145−71.
12. Sul HS, Smas C, Mei B, Zhou L. Function of pref-1 as an inhibitor of adipocyte differentiation. *International Journal of obesity* 2000;**24**(Suppl. 4):S15−19.
13. Morrison RF, Farmer SR. Hormonal signaling and transcriptional control of adipocyte differentiation. *Journal of Nutrition* 2000;**130**:3116S−21S.
14. Kirkland JL, Tchkonia T, Pirtskhalava T, Han J, Karagiannides I. Adipogenesis and aging: does aging make fat go MAD? *Experimental Gerontology* 2002;**37**:757−67.
15. Rosen ED. The transcriptional basis of adipocyte development. *Prostaglandins Leukotrienes and Essential Fatty Acids* 2005;**73**:31−4.
16. Rolland V, Dugail I, Le Liepvre X, Lavau M. Evidence of increased glyceraldehyde-3-phosphate dehydrogenase and fatty acid synthetase promoter activities in transiently transfected adipocytes from genetically obese rats. *Journal of Biological Chemistry* 1995;**270**:1102−6.
17. Halleux CM, Servais I, Reul BA, Detry R, Brichard SM. Multihormonal control of ob gene expression and leptin secretion from cultured human visceral adipose tissue: increased responsiveness to glucocorticoids in obesity. *The Journal of Clinical Endocrinology and Metabolism* 1998;**83**:902−10.
18. Large V, Arner P, Regulation of lipolysis in humans. Pathophysiological modulation in obesity, diabetes, and hyperlipidaemia. *Diabetes and Metabolism* 1998;**24**:409−18.
19. Owen OE, Reichard GA, Patel MS, Boden G. Energy metabolism in feasting and fasting. *Advances in Experimental Medicine and Biology* 1979;**111**:169−88.
20. Cho KJ, Shim JH, Cho MC, Choe YK, Hong JT, Moon DC, Kim JW, Yoon DY. Signaling pathways implicated in alpha-melanocyte stimulating hormone-induced lipolysis in 3T3-L1 adipocytes. *Journal of Cellular Biochemistry* 2005;**96**:869−78.
21. Robidoux J, Kumar N, Daniel KW, Moukdar F, Cyr M, Medvedev AV, Collins S. Maximal beta3-adrenergic regulation of lipolysis involves Src and epidermal growth factor receptor-dependent ERK1/2 activation. *Journal of Biological Chemistry* 2006;**281**:37794−802.
22. Park HJ, Rayalam S, Della-Fera MA, Ambati S, Yang JY, Baile CA. Withaferin A induces apoptosis and inhibits adipogenesis in 3T3-L1 adipocytes. *Biofactors* 2008;**33**:137−48.
23. Xiao Y, Yuan T, Yao W, Liao K. 3T3-L1 adipocyte apoptosis induced by thiazolidinediones is peroxisome proliferator-activated receptor-gamma-dependent and mediated by the caspase-3-dependent apoptotic pathway. *FEBS Journal* 2010;**277**:687−96.
24. Cameron-Smith D, Burke LM, Angus DJ, Tunstall RJ, Cox GR, Bonen A, Hawley JA, Hargreaves M. A short-term, high-fat diet up-regulates lipid metabolism and gene expression in human skeletal muscle. *American Journal of Clinical Nutrition* 2003;**77**:313−18.
25. Kondo T, Kishi M, Fushimi T, Kaga T. Acetic acid upregulates the expression of genes for fatty acid oxidation enzymes in liver to suppress body fat accumulation. *Journal of Agricultural and Food Chemistry* 2009;**57**:5982−6.
26. Argyropoulos G, Harper ME. Uncoupling proteins and thermoregulation. *Journal of Applied Physiology* 2002;**92**:2187−98.
27. Giri S, Rattan R, Haq E, Khan M, Yasmin R, Won JS, Key L, Singh AK, Singh I. AICAR inhibits adipocyte differentiation in 3T3L1 and restores metabolic alterations in diet-induced obesity mice model. *Nutrition and Metabolism* 2006;**3**:31.
28. Yang J, Craddock L, Hong S, Liu ZM. AMP-activated protein kinase suppresses LXR-dependent sterol regulatory element-binding protein-1c transcription in rat hepatoma McA-RH7777 cells. *Journal of Cellular Biochemistry* 2009;**106**:414−26.
29. Winder WW, Taylor EB, Thomson DM. Role of AMP-activated protein kinase in the molecular adaptation to endurance exercise. *Medicine and Science in Sports and Exercise* 2006;**38**:1945−9.
30. Saha AK, Ruderman NB. Malonyl-CoA and AMP-activated protein kinase: an expanding partnership. *Molecular and Cellular Biochemistry* 2003;**253**:65−70.
31. Fujii N, Jessen N, Goodyear LJ. AMP-activated protein kinase and the regulation of glucose transport. *American Journal of Physiology Endocrinology and Metabolism* 2006;**291**:E867−77.
32. Daval M, Foufelle F, Ferre P. Functions of AMP-activated protein kinase in adipose tissue. *Journal of Physiology* 2006;**574**(Pt 1):55−62.
33. Hardie DG. AMPK: a key regulator of energy balance in the single cell and the whole organism. *International Journal of Obesity* 2008;**32**:S7−12.
34. Steinberg GR, Macaulay SL, Febbraio MA, Kemp BE. AMP-activated protein kinase-the fat controller of the energy railroad. *Canadian Journal of Physiology and Pharmacology* 2006;**84**:655−65.
35. Hardie DG, Hawley SA, Scott JW. AMP-activated protein kinase-development of the energy sensor concept. *Journal of Physiology* 2006;**574**(Pt 1):7−15.
36. Hue L, Rider MH. The AMP-activated protein kinase: more than an energy sensor. *Essays in Biochemistry* 2007;**43**:121−37.
37. Pallottini V, Montanari L, Cavallini G, Bergamini E, Gori Z, Trentalance A. Mechanisms underlying the impaired regulation of 3-hydroxy-3-methylglutaryl coenzyme A reductase in aged rat liver. *Mechanisms of Ageing and Development* 2004;**125**:633.
38. Ruderman NB, Park H, Kaushik VK, Dean D, Constant S, Prentki M, Saha AK. AMPK as a metabolic switch in rat muscle, liver and adipose tissue after exercise. *Acta Physiologica Scandinavica* 2003;**178**:435−42.
39. Hardie DG, Pan DA. Regulation of fatty acid synthesis and oxidation by the AMP-activated protein kinase. *Biochemical Society Transaction* 2002;**30**(Pt 6):1064−70.

40. Foster DW. The role of the carnitine system in human metabolism. *Annals of the New York Academy of Sciences* 2004;**1033**:1–16.
41. Saha AK, Ruderman NB. Malonyl-CoA and AMP-activated protein kinase: an expanding partnership. *Molecular Cellular Biochemistry* 2003;**253**:65–70.
42. Kerner J, Hoppel C. Fatty acid import into mitochondria. *Biochimica et Biophysica Acta* 2000;**1486**:1–17.
43. Winder WW. AMP-activated protein kinase: possible target for treatment of type 2 diabetes. *Diabetes Technology and Therapy* 2000;**2**:441–8.
44. McGee SL, van Denderen BJ, Howlett KF, Mollica J, Schertzer JD, Kemp BE, Hargreaves M. AMP-activated protein kinase regulates GLUT4 transcription by phosphorylating histone deacetylase 5. *Diabetes* 2008;**57**:860–7.
45. Jing M, Cheruvu VK, Ismail-Beigi F. Stimulation of glucose transport in response to activation of distinct AMPK signaling pathways. *American Journal of Physiology Cell Physiology* 2008;**295**:C1071–82.
46. Treebak JT, Glund S, Deshmukh A, Klein DK, Long YC, Jensen TE, Jørgensen SB, Viollet B, Andersson L, Neumann D, Wallimann T, Richter EA, Chibalin AV, Zierath JR, Wojtaszewski JF. AMPK-mediated AS160 phosphorylation in skeletal muscle is dependent on AMPK catalytic and regulatory subunits. *Diabetes* 2006;**55**:2051–8.
47. Winder WW, Taylor EB, Thomson DM. Role of AMP-activated protein kinase in the molecular adaptation to endurance exercise. *Medicine and Science in Sports and Exercise* 2006;**38**:1945–9.
48. Baar K. Involvement of PPAR gamma co-activator-1, nuclear respiratory factors 1 and 2, and PPAR alpha in the adaptive response to endurance exercise. *Proceedings of the Nutrition Society* 2004;**63**:269–73.
49. Czubryt MP, McAnally J, Fishman GI, Olson EN. Regulation of peroxisome proliferator-activated receptor gamma coactivator 1 alpha (PGC-1 alpha) and mitochondrial function by MEF2 and HDAC5. *Proceeding of the National Academy of Science* 2003;**100**:1711–16.
50. Vercauteren K, Gleyzer N, Scarpulla RC. PGC-1-related coactivator complexes with HCF-1 and NRF-2beta in mediating NRF-2(GABP)-dependent respiratory gene expression. *Journal of Biological Chemistry* 2008;**283**:12102–11.
51. Akimoto T, Li P, Yan Z. Functional interaction of regulatory factors with the Pgc-1_ promoter in response to exercise by in vivo imaging. *American Journal of Physiology Cell Physiology* 2008;**295**:288–92.
52. Schuler M, Ali F, Chambon C, Duteil D, Bornert JM, Tardivel A, Desvergne B, Wahli W, Chambon P, Metzger D. PGC1alpha expression is controlled in skeletal muscles by PPARbeta, whose ablation results in fiber-type switching, obesity, and type 2 diabetes. *Cell Metabolism* 2006;**4**:407–14.
53. Kuhl JE, Ruderman NB, Musi N, Goodyear LJ, Patti ME, Crunkhorn S, Dronamraju D, Thorell A, Nygren J, Ljungkvist O, Degerblad M, Stahle A, Brismar TB, Andersen KL, Saha AK, Efendic S, Bavenholm PN. Exercise training decreases the concentration of malonyl-CoA and increases the expression and activity of malonyl-CoA decarboxylase in human muscle. *American Journal of Physiology Endocrinology and Metabolism* 2006;**290**:E1296–303.
54. Rockl KS, Witczak CA, Goodyear LJ. Signaling mechanisms in skeletal muscle: acute responses and chronic adaptations to exercise. *IUBMB Life* 2008;**60**:145–53.
55. Zong H, Ren JM, Young LH, Pypaert M, Mu J, Birnbaum MJ, Shulman GI. AMP kinase is required for mitochondrial biogenesis in skeletal muscle in response to chronic energy deprivation. *Proceedings of the National Academy of Sciences* 2002;**99**:15983–7.
56. Stürmer T, Buring JE, Lee IM, Gaziano JM, Glynn RJ. Metabolic abnormalities and risk for colorectal cancer in the physicians' health study. *Cancer Epidemiology Biomarkers and Prevention* 2006;**15**:2391–7.
57. Pais R, Silaghi H, Silaghi AC, Rusu ML, Dumitrascu DL. Metabolic syndrome and risk of subsequent colorectal cancer. *World Journal of Gastroenterology* 2009;**15**:5141–8.
58. Motoshima H, Goldstein BJ, Igata M, Araki E. AMPK and cell proliferation-AMPK as a therapeutic target for atherosclerosis and cancer. *Journal of Physiology* 2006;**574**(Pt 1):63–71.
59. Krymskaya VP, Goncharova EA. PI3K/mTORC1 activation in hamartoma syndromes: therapeutic prospects. *Cell Cycle* 2009;**8**:403–13.
60. Wang J, Whiteman MW, Lian H, Wang G, Singh A, Huang D, Denmark T. A non-canonical MEK/ERK signaling pathway regulates autophagy via regulating Beclin 1. *Journal of Biological Chemistry* 2009;**284**:21412–24.
61. Beevers CS, Chen L, Liu L, Luo Y, Webster NJ, Huang S. Curcumin disrupts the Mammalian target of rapamycin-raptor complex. *Cancer Research* 2009;**69**:1000–8.
62. Hay N. p53 strikes mTORC1 by employing sestrins. *Cell Metabolism* 2008;**8**:184–5.
63. Budanov AV, Karin M. P53 target genes sestrin 1 and sestrin2 connect genotoxic stress and mTOR signaling. *Cell* 2008;**134**:451–60.
64. Winder WW, Hardie DG. AMP-activated protein kinase, a metabolic master switch: possible roles in type 2 diabetes. *American Journal of Physiology* 1999;**277**:E1–10.
65. Hardie DG. The AMP-activated protein kinase pathway—new players upstream and downstream. *Journal of Cell Science* 2004;**117**(Pt 23):5479–87.
66. Carling D. The AMP-activated protein kinase cascade–a unifying system for energy control. *Trends in Biochemical Sciences* 2004;**29**:18–24.
67. Marley AE, Sullivan JE, Carling D, Abbott WM, Smith GJ, Taylor IW, Carey F, Beri RK. Biochemical characterization and deletion analysis of recombinant human protein phosphatase 2C alpha. *Biochemical Journal* 1996;**320**(Pt 3):801–6.
68. Li Q, Li J, Ren J. UCF-101 Mitigates Streptozotocin-Induced Cardiomyocyte Dysfunction: Role of AMP-Activated Protein Kinase. *American Journal of Physiology Endocrinology and Metabolism* 2009;**297**:E965–73.
69. Day P, Sharff A, Parra L, Cleasby A, Williams M, Hörer S, Nar H, Redemann N, Tickle I, Yon J. Structure of a CBS-domain pair from the regulatory gamma1 subunit of human AMPK in complex with AMP and ZMP. *Acta Crystallographica Section D: Biological Crystallography* 2007;**63**(Pt 5):587–96.
70. Rudolph MJ, Amodeo GA, Iram SH, Hong SP, Pirino G, Carlson M, Tong L. Structure of the Bateman2 domain of yeast Snf4: dimeric association and relevance for AMP binding. *Structure* 2007;**15**:65–74.
71. Giri S, Rattan R, Haq E, Khan M, Yasmin R, Won JS, Key L, Singh AK, Singh I. AICAR inhibits adipocyte differentiation in 3T3L1 and restores metabolic alterations in diet-induced obesity mice model. *Nutrion Metabolism* 2006;**3**:31.
72. Lee WJ, Kim M, Park HS, Kim HS, Jeon MJ, Oh KS, Koh EH, Won JC, Kim MS, Oh GT, Yoon M, Lee KU, Park JY. AMPK activation increases fatty acid oxidation in skeletal muscle by activating PPARalpha and PGC-1. *Biochemical and Biophysical Research Communications* 2006;**340**:291–5.
73. Suwa M, Nakano H, Kumagai S. Effects of chronic AICAR treatment on fiber composition, enzyme activity, UCP3, and PGC-1 in rat muscles. *Journal of Applied Physiology* 2003;**95**:960–8.
74. Bergeron R, Ren JM, Cadman KS, Moore IK, Perret P, Pypaert M, Young LH, Semenkovich CF, Shulman GI. Chronic activation of

75. Gaidhu MP, Fediuc S, Anthony NM, So M, Mirpourian M, Perry RL, Ceddia RB. Prolonged AICAR-induced AMP-kinase activation promotes energy dissipation in white adipocytes: novel mechanisms integrating HSL and ATGL. *Journal of Lipid Research* 2009;**50**:704−15.
76. Leclerc I, Kahn A, Doiron B. The 5'-AMP-activated protein kinase inhibits the transcriptional stimulation by glucose in liver cells, acting through the glucose response complex. *FEBS Letters* 1998;**431**:180−4.
77. Li T, Chanda D, Zhang Y, Choi HS, Chiang JY. Glucose stimulates cholesterol 7{alpha}-hydroxylase gene (CYP7A1) transcription in human hepatocytes. *Journal of Lipid Research*; 2009. In press.
78. Gerozissis K. Brain insulin, energy and glucose homeostasis; genes, environment and metabolic pathologies. *European Journal of Pharmacology* 2008;**585**:38−49.
79. Ronnett GV, Kim EK, Landree LE, Tu Y. Fatty acid metabolism as a target for obesity treatment. *Physiology & Behavior* 2005;**85**:25−35.
80. Viollet B, Athea Y, Mounier R, Guigas B, Zarrinpashneh E, Horman S, Lantier L, Hebrard S, Devin-Leclerc J, Beauloye C, Foretz M, Andreelli F, Ventura-Clapier R, Bertrand L. AMPK: Lessons from transgenic and knockout animals. *Frontier in Bioscience* 2009;**14**:19−44.
81. Rutter GA, Da Silva Xavier G, Leclerc I. Roles of 5'-AMP-activated protein kinase (AMPK) in mammalian glucose homoeostasis. *Biochemical Journal* 2003;**375**(Pt 1):1−16.
82. Misra P. AMP activated protein kinase: a next generation target for total metabolic control. *Expert Opinion on Therapeutic Targets* 2008;**12**:91−100.
83. Steinberg GR, Jorgensen SB. The AMP-activated protein kinase: role in regulation of skeletal muscle metabolism and insulin sensitivity. *Mini-Reviews in Medicinal Chemistry* 2007;**7**:519−26.
84. Deng G, Long Y, Yu YR, Li MR. Adiponectin directly improves endothelial dysfunction in obese rats through the AMPK-eNOS Pathway. *International Journal of Obesity* 2010;**34**:165−71.
85. Huang NL, Chiang SH, Hsueh CH, Liang YJ, Chen YJ, Lai LP. Metformin inhibits TNF-alpha-induced IkappaB kinase phosphorylation, IkappaB-alpha degradation and IL-6 production in endothelial cells through PI3K-dependent AMPK phosphorylation. *International Journal of Cardiology* 2009;**134**:169−75.
86. Wu X, Mahadev K, Fuchsel L, Ouedraogo R, Xu SQ, Goldstein BJ. Adiponectin suppresses IB kinase activation induced by tumor necrosis factor-α or high glucose in endothelial cells: role of cAMP and AMP kinase signaling. *American Journal of Physiology Endocrinology and Metabolism* 2007;**293**:E1836−44.
87. Sporrer D, Weber M, Wanninger J, Weigert J, Neumeier M, Stogbauer F, Lieberer E, Bala M, Kopp A, Schaffler A, Buechler C. Adiponectin downregulates CD163 whose cellular and soluble forms are elevated in obesity. *European Journal of Clinical Investigation* 2009;**39**:671−9.
88. Moestrup SK, Moller HJ. CD163: a regulated hemoglobin scavenger receptor with a role in the anti-inflammatory response. *Annals of Medicine* 2004;**36**:347−54.
89. Saenz A, Fernandez-Esteban I, Mataix A, Ausejo M, Roque M, Moher D. Metformin monotherapy for type 2 diabetes mellitus. *Cochrane Database of Systematic Reviews* 2005;**20**:CD002966.
90. Zhou G, Myers R, Li Y, Chen Y, Shen X, Fenyk-Melody J, Wu M, Ventre J, Doebber T, Fujii N, Musi N, Hirshman MF, Goodyear LJ, Moller DE. Role of AMP-activated protein kinase in mechanism of metformin action. *The Journal of Clinical Investigation* 2001;**108**:1167−74.
91. You M, Matsumoto M, Pacold CM, Cho WK, Crabb DW. The role of AMP-activated protein kinase in the action of ethanol in the liver. *Gastroenterology* 2004;**127**:1798−808.
92. You M, Rogers CQ. Adiponectin: a key adipokine in alcoholic fatty liver. *Experimental Biology and Medicine* 2009;**234**:850−9.
93. Traish AM, Feeley RJ, Guay A. Mechanisms of obesity and related pathologies: androgen deficiency and endothelial dysfunction may be the link between obesity and erectile dysfunction. *FEBS Journal* 2009;**276**:5755−67.
94. Kim YW, Park SY, Kim JY, Huh JY, Jeon WS, Yoon CJ, Yun SS, Moon KH. Metformin restores the penile expression of nitric oxide synthase in high-fat-fed obese rats. *Journal of Andrology* 2007;**28**:555−60.
95. Yin J, Zhang H, Ye J. Traditional chinese medicine in treatment of metabolic syndrome. *Endocrine, Metabolic & Immune Disorders—Drug Targets* 2008;**8**:99−111.
96. Lee YS, Kim WS, Kim KH, Yoon MJ, Cho HJ, Shen Y, Ye JM, Lee CH, Oh WK, Kim CT, Hohnen-Behrens C, Gosby A, Kraegen EW, James DE, Kim JB. Berberine, a natural plant product, activates AMP-activated protein kinase with beneficial metabolic effects in diabetic and insulin-resistant states. *Diabetes* 2006;**55**:2256−64.
97. Kim WS, Lee YS, Cha SH, Jeong HW, Choe SS, Lee MR, Oh GT, Park HS, Lee KU, Lane MD, Kim JB. Berberine improves lipid dysregulation in obesity by controlling central and peripheral AMPK activity. *American Journal of Physiology Endocrinology and Metabolism* 2009;**296**:E812−19.
98. Brusq JM, Ancellin N, Grondin P, Guillard R, Martin S, Saintillan Y, Issandou M. Inhibition of lipid synthesis through activation of AMP kinase: an additional mechanism for the hypolipidemic effects of berberine. *Journal of Lipid Research* 2006;**47**:1281−8.
99. Jeong HW, Hsu KC, Lee JW, Ham M, Huh JY, Shin HJ, Kim WS, Kim JB. Berberine suppresses proinflammatory responses through AMPK activation in macrophages. *American Journal of Physiology Endocrinology and Metabolism* 2009;**296**:E955−64.
100. Shay KP, Moreau RF, Smith EJ, Smith AR, Hagen TM. Alpha-lipoic acid as a dietary supplement: molecular mechanisms and therapeutic potential. *Biochimica et Biophysica Acta* 2009;**1790**:1149−60.
101. Kim MS, Lee KU. Role of hypothalamic 5'-AMP-activated protein kinase in the regulation of food intake and energy homeostasis. *Journal of Molecular Medicine* 2005;**83**:514−20.
102. Targonsky ED, Dai F, Koshkin V, Karaman GT, Gyulkhandanyan AV, Zhang Y, Chan CB, Wheeler MB. Alpha-lipoic acid regulates AMP-activated protein kinase and inhibits insulin secretion from beta cells. *Diabetologia* 2006;**49**:1587−98.
103. Wang Y, Li X, Guo Y, Chan L, Guan X. Alpha-Lipoic acid increases energy expenditure by enhancing adenosine monophosphate-activated protein kinase-peroxisome proliferator-activated receptor-gamma coactivator-1alpha signaling in the skeletal muscle of aged mice. *Metabolism* 2009;**59**(7):967−76.
104. Lee WJ, Lee IK, Kim HS, Kim YM, Koh EH, Won JC, Han SM, Kim MS, Jo I, Oh GT, Park IS, Youn JH, Park SW, Lee KU, Park JY. Alpha-lipoic acid prevents endothelial dysfunction in obese rats via activation of AMP-activated protein kinase. *Arteriosclerosis Thrombosis and Vascular Biology* 2005;**25**:2488−94.
105. Lee Y, Naseem RH, Park BH, Garry DJ, Richardson JA, Schaffer JE, Unger RH. Alpha-lipoic acid prevents lipotoxic cardiomyopathy in acyl CoA-synthase transgenic mice. *Biochemical and Biophysical Research Communications* 2006;**344**:446−52.
106. Marques FZ, Markus MA, Morris BJ. Resveratrol: cellular actions of a potent natural chemical that confers a diversity of

107. Lagouge M, Argmann C, Gerhart-Hines Z, Meziane H, Lerin C, Daussin F, Messadeq N, Milne J, Lambert P, Elliott P, Geny B, Laakso M, Puigserver P, Auwerx J. Resveratrol improves mitochondrial function and protects against metabolic disease by activating SIRT1 and PGC-1alpha. *Cell* 2006;**127**:1109−22.
108. Shang J, Chen LL, Xiao FX, Sun H, Ding HC, Xiao H. Resveratrol improves non-alcoholic fatty liver disease by activating AMP-activated protein kinase. *Acta Pharmacologica Sinica* 2008;**29**:698−706.
109. Rivera L, Moron R, Zarzuelo A, Galisteo M. Long-term resveratrol administration reduces metabolic disturbances and lowers blood pressure in obese Zucker rats. *Biochemical Pharmacology* 2009;**77**:1053−63.
110. Moon HS, Lee HG, Choi YJ, Kim TG, Cho CS. Proposed mechanisms of (-)-epigallocatechin-3-gallate for anti-obesity. *Chemico-Biological Interactions* 2007;**167**:85−98.
111. Lin JK, Lin-Shiau SY. Mechanisms of hypolipidemic and antiobesity effects of tea and tea polyphenols. *Molecular Nutrition and Food Research* 2006;**50**:211−17.
112. Wolfram S, Wang Y, Thielecke F. Anti-obesity effects of green tea: from bedside to bench. *Molecular Nutrition and Food Research* 2006;**50**:176−87.
113. Hwang JT, Park IJ, Shin JI, Lee YK, Lee SK, Baik HW, Ha J, Park OJ. Genistein, EGCG, and capsaicin inhibit adipocyte differentiation process via activating AMP-activated protein kinase. *Biochemical and Biophysical Research Communications* 2005;**338**:694−9.
114. Edwards T. Inflammation, pain, and chronic disease: an integrative approach to treatment and prevention. *Alternative Therapies in Health and Medicine* 2005;**11**:20−7.
115. Ejaz A, Wu D, Kwan P, Meydani M. Curcumin inhibits adipogenesis in 3T3-L1 adipocytes and angiogenesis and obesity in C57/BL mice. *Journal of Nutrition* 2009;**139**:919−25.
116. Lee YK, Lee WS, Hwang JT, Kwon DY, Surh YJ, Park OJ. Curcumin exerts antidifferentiation effect through AMPKalpha-PPAR-gamma in 3T3-L1 adipocytes and antiproliferatory effect through AMPKalpha-COX-2 in cancer cells. *Journal of Agricultural and Food Chemistry* 2009;**57**:305−10.
117. Pongchaidecha A, Lailerd N, Boonprasert W, Chattipakorn N. Effects of curcuminoid supplement on cardiac autonomic status in high-fat-induced obese rats. *Nutrition* 2009;**25**:870−8.
118. Weisberg SP, Leibel R, Tortoriello DV. Dietary curcumin significantly improves obesity-associated inflammation and diabetes in mouse models of diabesity. *Endocrinology* 2008;**149**:3549−58.
119. Kang Q, Chen A. Curcumin suppresses expression of low-density lipoprotein (LDL) receptor, leading to the inhibition of LDL-induced activation of hepatic stellate cells. *British Journal of Pharmacology* 2009;**157**:1354−67.
120. Hasani-Ranjbar S, Nayebi N, Larijani B, Abdollahi M. A systematic review of the efficacy and safety of herbal medicines used in the treatment of obesity. *World Journal of Gastroenterology* 2009;**15**:3073−85.
121. Lu JM, Yao Q, Chen C. Ginseng compounds: an update on their molecular mechanisms and medical applications. *Current Vascular Pharmacology* 2009;**7**:293−302.
122. Lim S, Yoon JW, Choi SH, Cho BJ, Kim JT, Chang HS, Park HS, Park KS, Lee HK, Kim YB, Jang HC. Effect of ginsam, a vinegar extract from Panax ginseng, on body weight and glucose homeostasis in an obese insulin-resistant rat model. *Metabolism* 2009;**58**:8−15.
123. Hwang JT, Kim SH, Lee MS, Kim SH, Yang HJ, Kim MJ, Kim HS, Ha J, Kim MS, Kwon DY. Anti-obesity effects of ginsenoside Rh2 are associated with the activation of AMPK signaling pathway in 3T3-L1 adipocyte. *Biochemical and Biophysical Research Communications* 2007;**364**:1002−8.
124. Hwang JT, Lee MS, Kim HJ, Sung MJ, Kim HY, Kim MS, Kwon DY. Antiobesity effect of ginsenoside Rg3 involves the AMPK and PPAR-gamma signal pathways. *Phytotherapy Research* 2009;**23**:262−6.
125. Kim EJ, Lee HI, Chung KJ, Noh YH, Ro Y, Koo JH. The ginsenoside-Rb2 lowers cholesterol and triacylglycerol levels in 3T3-L1 adipocytes cultured under high cholesterol or fatty acids conditions. *Biochemistry and Molecular Biology Reports* 2009;**42**:194−9.
126. Kim K, Kim DH, Kim HY. Compound K protects MIN6N8 pancreatic beta-cells against palmitate-induced apoptosis through modulating SAPK/JNK activation. *Cell Biology International* 2009;**34**:75−80.
127. Rivera L, Morón R, Sánchez M, Zarzuelo A, Galisteo M. Quercetin ameliorates metabolic syndrome and improves the inflammatory status in obese Zucker rats. *Obesity (Silver Spring)* 2008;**16**:2081−7.
128. Yang JY, Della-Fera MA, Rayalam S, Ambati S, Hartzell DL, Park HJ, Baile CA. Enhanced inhibition of adipogenesis and induction of apoptosis in 3T3-L1 adipocytes with combinations of resveratrol and quercetin. *Life Science* 2008;**82**:1032−9.
129. Hsu CL, Yen GC. Induction of cell apoptosis in 3T3-L1 pre-adipocytes by flavonoids is associated with their antioxidant activity. *Molecular Nutrition and Food Research* 2006;**50**:1072−9.
130. Suchankova G, Nelson LE, Gerhart-Hines Z, Kelly M, Gauthier MS, Saha AK, Ido Y, Puigserver P, Ruderman NB. Concurrent regulation of AMP-activated protein kinase and SIRT1 in mammalian cells. *Biochemical and Biophysical Research Communications* 2009;**378**:836−41.
131. Ahn J, Lee H, Kim S, Park J, Ha T. The anti-obesity effect of quercetin is mediated by the AMPK and MAPK signaling pathways. *Biochemical and Biophysical Research Communications* 2008;**373**:545−9.
132. Saraswathi V, Morrow JD, Hasty AH. Dietary fish oil exerts hypolipidemic effects in lean and insulin sensitizing effects in obese LDLR-/- mice. *Journal of Nutrition* 2009;**139**:2380−6.
133. Motawi TM, Hashem RM, Rashed LA, El-Razek SM. Comparative study between the effect of the peroxisome proliferator activated receptor-alpha ligands fenofibrate and n-3 polyunsaturated fatty acids on activation of 5′-AMP-activated protein kinase-alpha1 in high-fat fed rats. *Journal of Pharmacy and Pharmacology* 2009;**61**:1339−46.
134. Vuong T, Benhaddou-Andaloussi A, Brault A, Harbilas D, Martineau LC, Vallerand D, Ramassamy C, Matar C, Haddad PS. Antiobesity and antidiabetic effects of biotransformed blueberry juice in KKA(y) mice. *International Journal of Obesity* 2009;**33**:1166−73.
135. Tao R, Ye F, He Y, Tian J, Liu G, Ji T, Su Y. Improvement of high-fat-diet-induced metabolic syndrome by a compound from Balanophora polyandra Griff in mice. *European Journal of Pharmacology* 2009;**616**:328−33.
136. Kong CS, Kim JA, Kim SK. Anti-obesity effect of sulfated glucosamine by AMPK signal pathway in 3T3-L1 adipocytes. *Food and Chemical Toxicology* 2009;**47**:2401−6.
137. Lorente-Cebrian S, Bustos M, Marti A, Martinez JA, Moreno-Aliaga MJ. Eicosapentaenoic acid stimulates AMP-activated protein kinase and increases visfatin secretion in cultured murine adipocytes. *Clinical Science* 2009;**117**:243−9.
138. Kim SJ, Jung JY, Kim HW, Park T. Anti-obesity effects of Juniperus chinensis extract are associated with increased AMP-activated protein kinase expression and phosphorylation in the visceral adipose tissue of rats. *Biological and Pharmaceutical Bulletin* 2008;**31**:1415−21.

SECTION VI

COMMENTARY AND RECOMMENDATIONS

CHAPTER
42

The Role of United States Law to Prevent and Control Childhood Obesity

Jennifer L. Pomeranz

Rudd Center for Food Policy and Obesity, Yale University, New Haven, CT, USA

INTRODUCTION

In the United States, 32% of children are overweight, 16% of children are obese, and 11% are extremely obese [1]. Since 1980, the prevalence of childhood obesity has tripled, making this generation the first expected to have a shorter life expectancy than that of their parents [2]. Serious action is needed on multiple levels and across various sectors to address this public health crisis. Public health experts, including those at the Centers for Disease Control (CDC) and the Institute of Medicine (IOM), recommend policy changes at the environmental level to address obesity in the United States. Change is required in several settings, including communities, schools, childcare, worksites, and healthcare facilities [3]. The government can facilitate and support such changes by enacting legislation and regulation at the federal, state, tribal, and local levels.

At the federal level, Congress has the power to enact laws to address obesity and also require federal agencies to do the same within their administrative authority. The U.S. Department of Agriculture (USDA) is responsible for much of the nations food supply through its agricultural programs, including administering the Food, Conservation, and Energy Act (commonly referred to as the Farm Bill), emergency feeding programs, and commodity distribution and other nutrition-assistance programs to low-income families, American Indian reservations, and the elderly [4]. The USDA is also responsible for the National School Lunch and Breakfast Programs and the Child Nutrition and WIC Reauthorization Act of 2004, which addresses summer food services, child and adult care food programs, and the special nutrition program for women, infants, and children. Additional agencies that directly influence the health of the nation's youth include the Food and Drug Administration (which has the primary authority over the safety and labeling of food) [5], the Department of Education, the Department of Transportation, and the CDC.

There is an emerging understanding that health needs to be considered in all policies in order to address health disparities in general and the significant public health issue of obesity [6]. Government agencies whose primary mission does not necessarily include health can positively influence public health by considering the impact their policy making has on health. The federal government has concrete opportunities to do this in the upcoming years. The most significant opportunity will be in 2013 when the Farm Bill is up for reauthorization. The Child Nutrition and WIC Reauthorization Act of 2004 and the federal transportation act, SAFETEA-LU, are also up for reauthorization in 2010. If government seriously considers health issues during these reauthorization processes, there would be great potential to improve the public's health, especially that of the nation's children.

In terms of media, the Federal Communications Commission (FCC) is in charge of regulating all communication on radio, television, wire, satellite, and cable. Until recently, the FCC has not been very active in regulating marketing directed at children aside from establishing time limitations on commercials during children's programming and a prohibition against host selling [7]. However, the commission recently published a notice of inquiry, "In the Matter of Empowering Parents and Protecting Children in an Evolving Media Landscape" [8], indicating that it intends to become more involved in this arena. The primary agency responsible for regulating marketing directed at children is the Federal Trade Commission (FTC), which has authority over false, deceptive, and unfair advertisements [9]. In 2007, Congress directed the FTC to report on food marketing directed at children and adolescents [10]. The FTC found that in 2006, approximately $870 million was spent on child-directed marketing and $1 billion on marketing to adolescents, with roughly $300 million overlapping between the two age groups [11]. At the time of this writing, the FTC is in the process of following up on this study by collecting and reviewing recent industry information on expenditures, activities, and voluntary regulations of food marketing practices to children and adolescents [12].

Federal law generally preempts, or trumps, state and local law that conflicts with it [13]. However, public health has traditionally been a state and local concern, as states and locales historically have exercised primary jurisdiction over matters related to the public's health, safety, and welfare [14]. Thus, there is much room at the state and local levels to address childhood obesity.

States and locales have a unique ability and role to play in devising solutions to public health issues that require culturally sensitive considerations. Obesity is a complex problem that will require legal interventions in multiple settings. Along these lines, state legislatures have proposed bills on various topics such as farm-to-school programs [15], increased physical education [16] and nutrition standards in schools [17], anticommercialization of schools [18], soda taxes [19], trans fat bans [20], and menu labeling laws [21]. These are all promising strategies to address childhood obesity.

In addition, all states and many locale jurisdictions have boards of health that have the primary responsibility to protect the public health of their citizens [22]. States also have their own departments of agriculture, education, housing, and transportation that can work independently or in unison to devise solutions to decrease the incidence and prevalence of childhood obesity in their communities.

In 2008, the Centers for Disease Control convened a National Summit on Legal Preparedness for Obesity Prevention and Control to review the current state of the law for obesity prevention and control and to identify gaps and develop legal action options to address obesity in the United States. The *Journal of Law, Medicine and Ethics* created a supplemental issue in 2009, reporting the proceedings. Many recommendations in the article "Improving Laws and Legal Authorities for Obesity Prevention and Control" are directly applicable to addressing childhood obesity [23]. Excerpts are reprinted here with permission.

Access to Healthy Food

The overarching contributors to choosing healthy foods are the cost, quantity, and quality of the food supply. One factor to the general make-up and relative pricing of food in the U.S. is due in large part to the farm subsidies established and maintained under the Farm Bill. Under this crucial piece of legislation, the USDA provides substantial agricultural subsidies,[4] primarily for major commodity crops such as corn, soy, wheat, and cotton.[5] As a result, these crops are available in a relative abundance, and this drives down their price as well as that of the foods and beverages manufactured with them and livestock reared on them. The overabundance and economic incentives to eat calorie-dense, nutrient-poor foods have proven to be obesogenic and a contributor to the public health problems in the country. From 1985 to 2000, the price of fruits and vegetables in the U.S. rose 117%, compared to 46% for sweets and desserts and 20% for soft drinks.[6]

Reconsideration of farm subsidies has been raised fervently in recent years and Summit participants advocated subsidizing a variety of vegetables and fruits, and foods such as nuts, legumes, and animals raised on food they naturally eat (instead of corn), in order to shift the U.S. diet in a healthier direction. Studies in Iowa show that farmers who produce commodity crops operate at a net loss[7] and that both farmers and the state's economy would benefit from increasing the production of fruit and vegetables,[8] which could also result in decreased produce prices and increased consumption.

However, states and local governments need not wait on the reauthorization of the federal Farm Bill to encourage healthy lifestyles in their communities. The food environment—i.e., the ratio of fast food restaurants to grocery stores to convenience stores, access to and availability of fresh food, prevalence of liquor stores and food desserts—contributes to, or is a barrier to healthy eating and a healthy weight.[9] Low-income communities have one-third to one-half the number of supermarkets found in more affluent neighborhoods, but twice as many small markets or corner stores that are less likely to carry produce and other healthy items and are often relatively more expensive.[10] Studies show that the proximity one lives to stores that carry fresh vegetables is positively related to the person's intake of vegetables.[11] Conversely,

(Continued)

Access to Healthy Food (cont'd)

fast-food outlets across neighborhoods are negatively associated with residents' health outcomes, in that a greater distribution of fast-food restaurants is associated with a greater prevalence of overweight/obesity among neighborhood residents.[12]

The built environment is composed of several relevant variables including the land-use mix, street connectivity, the accessibility of fast-food outlets, grocery stores, farmers' markets, public transit stations, and green and open spaces—all malleable by local governments.[13] Applicable legal action items are discussed further in the Healthy Places section.

Healthy Places

Laws and policies targeting Healthy Places address the main locus of intervention, including community, workplace, business, and transportation.[27] This paper provides selected examples in different settings to recommend action items intended to ensure individuals can make healthy lifestyle choices where they are.

Zoning and the Built Environment

The United States Supreme Court upheld zoning to protect public health as a proper exercise of the government's traditional police power.[28] Government officials can alter the built environment through zoning to advance their community's public health. Possible zoning ordinances to improve the availability of fresh foods at lower prices include zoning land-use for grocery stores and farmers' markets.[29] Zoning strategies to reduce the availability of unhealthy options include banning fast food outlets, drive-through service and/or formula restaurants, or zoning the density of fast food outlets through per unit space or through spacing requirements, and zoning fast-food outlets into or out of certain districts.[30] For example, despite the nearly universal availability of school-provided lunch in schools, a significant percentage of high school students go off-campus to eat lunch.[31] Zoning fast-food establishments away from high schools could have an impact on the quality of foods and beverages accessible and thus, consumed by these students during the school day.

The built environment also contributes to the ability of residents to engage in physical activity, for necessity, recreation, and play.[32] For children, this means more safe routes to school, safe playgrounds and open green spaces to play. For adults, the Surgeon General recommends they engage in at least 30 minutes of moderate physical activity daily. Notwithstanding these recommendations, research reveals that at least half of American adults do not meet the guidelines[33] and that many in fact lead sedentary lifestyles.[34]

Researchers and Summit participants identified societal factors that affect levels of physical activity, which include individual characteristics (demographics, household, and lifestyle characteristics, culture, time allocation, etc.); the built environment (land use patterns, transportation systems, and design features); and the social environment (societal values and preferences, public policies, and economic forces).[35] Adult physical activity levels have declined in large part due to reduced demand for daily physical activity in leisure and in travel. The modern reliance on automobiles is being challenged by rising gas prices, environmental concerns, road congestion, increasing obesity, and decreasing physical fitness. Thus, a shift to more ubiquitous and affordable public transportation is necessary. Increased access to public transportation often provides opportunities for physical activity because most transit trips begin and/or end with walking.[36]

The "walkability" of a community is a key index of its healthiness. Results from a CDC study suggest that Americans who walk to and from public transit obtain an appreciable amount of daily transit-related physical activity (median of 19 minutes), with 29% of transit walkers achieving 30 or more minutes of daily physical activity solely during the commute.[37] Importantly, it has been shown that walking and other less vigorous forms of physical activity are easier to sustain over time.[38] Pedestrian improvements—e.g., sidewalks, marked crosswalks, and street amenities—encourage both walking and transit use. Local governments can also require that all new construction accommodate pedestrians, and also wheelchairs, bicycles, and strollers.

Schools

School should be a place where students can buy and eat nutritious foods and engage in meaningful physical activity. Public schools must respond to directives from federal, state, and local authorities. The federal government can set standards for school nutrition and exercise and condition the receipt of funding on a school system's attainment of those standards.[55] States can also mandate nutrition and physical activity standards.[56]

Nutrition

The National School Lunch Program and the National School Breakfast Program (collectively, the NSLP)[57] provide per-meal cash reimbursements to schools that

(Continued)

Access to Healthy Food (cont'd)

offer meals to students ostensibly meeting certain nutritional standards.[58] However, despite the availability of lunch in most schools, the percentage of students who actually eat lunch offered by the school is only about 70 percent for middle school students and 60 percent for high school students.[59] Whether or not students purchase or eat the school provided meal, many students also purchase products from vending machines, school stores, and snack bars.

Foods sold in competition with the NSLP in food-service areas during the lunch periods, or "competitive foods," are allowed at the discretion of state and local authorities,[60] unless they are on the list of "foods of minimal nutritional value" (FMNV).[61] However, the only foods recognized as FMNV are the following: soda water, water ices, chewing gum, hard candy, jellies and gums, marshmallow candy, fondant, licorice, spun candy, and candy coated popcorn.[62] This is because many products are considered exempt,[63] the definition does not cover an abundance of non-nutritious foods, and the sales of FMNV are only prohibited in the food service areas during the lunch periods.[64] Thus, schools can avoid this restriction by placing vending machines beyond the food service area and allow the sale of FMNV before and after the meal period.[65] The federal government must expand the scope of its FMNV provision to include the whole school campus not just the cafeteria and to cover all hours during which school activities are being held whether before or after the normal school day. State and local laws can also prohibit permissive practices and include meaningful monitoring and enforcement provisions in schools' wellness policies.

State and local authorities are authorized to impose additional restrictions on the sale of competitive food.[66] Many locations strengthened the nutrition standards for their school districts in response to the federal mandate to local educational agencies to establish wellness policies.[67] The mandate directed local agencies to develop "goals for nutrition education, physical activity, and other school-based activities that are designed to promote student wellness."[68] The federal directives were broad recommendations and districts around the country responded in a variety of ways.[69] As a result, most secondary schools still allow competitive foods and have student-accessible vending machines.[70] A recent study of the food in schools revealed that foods of lower nutritional value are more available than healthier foods in the nation's schools and students in low socio-economic areas have less access to healthier snacks.[71]

Districts should strengthen the nutritional guidelines for meals and snacks sold in their schools. Researchers found that "the most effective policies are those that prohibit sales of all beverages with caloric sweeteners (except for certain milk products), impose portion limits, apply throughout the school day, and apply to all grade levels, with age adjustments only for container sizes."[72] Similarly, restrictions on food should be based on content (i.e., sugar, fat, and/or sodium) and fruits and vegetables should be made available.[73] Experience shows that by restricting what is allowed in schools, industry will work with the districts to provide products that meet the healthier criteria.[74]

Competitive foods and beverages are supplied by companies through individual contracts with schools or districts. States and school districts have the ability to limit what the companies can supply through limitations in the contracts. For example, when Philadelphia School District changed its beverage policy to only permit 100 percent juice, water, and milk for younger students and these same beverages, plus electrolyte replacement drinks, in high schools, their supplier was contractually obligated to comply with these guidelines.[75] Another option, of course, is to ban competitive food and beverages entirely.

Moreover, schools have the power to restrict some or ban all marketing on their campuses. First Amendment analysis leads to the conclusion that school districts have broad constitutional authority to control marketing in their facilities, including restricting the marketing of all foods and beverages, or just those foods and beverages not allowed to be sold in the school according to school or district policies.[76] [This will be discussed further later in the chapter in the section titled "Marketing in Schools."]

Physical Activity and Physical Education

Some local physical education and physical activity efforts were derailed by schools simultaneously trying to comply with the No Child Left Behind Act of 2001 (NCLB). NCLB was designed to improve achievement in education through standardized testing in schools across the country. As such, physical education, health education, and physical activity requirements are not being mandated by most states.[77] The National Association for Sport and Physical Education (NASPE) Shape of the Nation report found that nearly a third of the states do not mandate physical education for elementary and middle school students, and 12 states allow students to earn required physical education credits through online physical education courses.[78] Moreover, while most states require some sort of physical education (P.E.), how often students actually engaged in physical activity varies widely. Between 17 and 22 percent of students attended P.E. each school day. Another 11 to 14 percent scheduled

(Continued)

Access to Healthy Food (cont'd)

P.E. three or four days a week and 22 percent scheduled P.E. one day a week.[79] A way to counteract this trend is for the federal government to include support for, and require, physical education, physical activity, and health education on a regular and routine basis so all school-aged children achieve the recommended 60 minutes or more of physical activity each day. This can be achieved through revisions to the authorizing language in No Child Left Behind.

<Endnotes from "Improving Laws and Legal Authorities for Obesity Prevention and Control">

[4] Editorial, "Harvesting Cash," *Washington Post*, available at <http://www.washingtonpost.com/wp-srv/nation/interactives/farmaid/> (last visited March 18, 2009).

[5] Editorial, "Making the Most of a Subsidy," *Washington Post*, available at <http://www.washingtonpost.com/wp-dyn/content/graphic/2006/07/03/GR2006070300057.html> (last visited March 18, 2009).

[6] J. J. Putnam, J. E. Allhouse, and L. S. Kantor, "U.S. Per Capita Food Supply Trends: More Calories, Refined Carbohydrates, and Fats," *Food Review* 25, no. 3 (2002): 2-15.

[7] Leopold Center for Sustainable Agriculture, Iowa State University, *Food Facts: Results from Marketing and Food Systems Research*, March 2008, at 8, available at <http://www.leopold.iastate.edu/research/marketing_files/food/Food_Facts_0308.pdf> (last visited March 18, 2009).

[8] D. Swenson, Leopold Center for Sustainable Agriculture, Iowa State University, *The Economic Impacts of Increased Fruit and Vegetable Production and Consumption in Iowa: Phase II*, 2006, available at <http://www.leopold.iastate.edu/pubs/staff/files/health_0606.pdf> (last visited March 18, 2009).

[9] A. F. Brown, R. B. Vargas, A. Ang, and A. R. Pebley, "The Neighborhood Food Resource Environment and the Health of Residents with Chronic Conditions: The Food Resource Environment and the Health of Residents," *Journal of General Internal Medicine* 23, no. 8 (2008): 1137-1144.

[10] *Id.*

[11] J. N. Bodor, D. Rose, T. A. Farley, C. Swalm, and S. K. Scott, "Neighbourhood Fruit and Vegetable Availability and Consumption: The Role of Small Food Stores in an Urban environment," *Public Health Nutrition* 11, no. 4 (2008): 413-420.

[12] F. Li, P. A. Harmer, B. J. Cardinal, M. Bosworth, A. Acock, D. Johnson-Shelton, and J. M. Moore, "Built Environment, Adiposity, and Physical Activity in Adults Aged 50-75," *American Journal of Preventative Medicine* 35, no. 1 (2008): 38-46.

[13] *Id.*

[27] See Gostin and Pomeranz, *supra* note 1. [L. O. Gostin and J. L. Pomeranz, "The Vital Domains of Obesity Prevention and Control: Healthy Lifestyles, Healthy Places, and Healthy Societies," *Assessing Laws and Legal Authorities for Obesity Prevention and Control*. Journal of Law Medicine and Ethics Supp. 2009)]

[28] *Village of Euclid v. Ambler Realty*, 272 U.S. 365 (1926).

[29] .K. Hodgson, Regulation of Food Access through Comprehensive Planning and Zoning," Virginia Tech, Urban Affairs and Planning, Alexandria Center, April 17, 2008 (unpublished manuscript).

[30] J. S. Mair, M. W. Pierce, and S. P. Teret, *The Use of Zoning to Restrict Fast Food Outlets: A Potential Strategy to Combat Obesity*, October 2005, available at <http://www.publichealthlaw.net/Zoning%20Fast%20Food%20Outlets.pdf> (last visited March 18, 2009).

[31] J. Delva, P. M. O'Malley, and L. D. Johnston, "Availability of More-Healthy and Less-Healthy Food Choices in American Schools: A National Study of Grade, Racial/Ethnic, and Socioeconomic Differences," *American Journal of Preventive Medicine* 33, no. 4, Supplement (2007): S226-S239.

[32] W. C. Perdue, L. A. Stone, and L. O. Gostin, The Built Environment and Its Relationship to the Public's Health: The Legal Framework," *American Journal of Public Health* 93, no. 9 (2003): 1390-1394.

[33] L. M. Besser and A L. Dannenberg, "Walking to Public Transit Steps to Help Meet Physical Activity Recommendations," *American Journal of Preventive Medicine* 29, no. 4 (2005): 273-280.

[34] F. Li, P. A. Harmer, B. J. Cardinal, M. Bosworth, A. Acock, D. Johnson-Shelton, J. M. Moore, "Built Environment, Adiposity, and Physical Activity in Adults Aged 50-75," *American Journal of Preventive Medicine* 35, no. 1 (2008): 38-46.

[35] R. J. Stokes, J. MacDonald, and G. Ridgeway, Estimating the Effects of Light Rail Transit on Health Care Costs," *Health Place* 14, no. 1 (2008): 45-58.

[36] See Besser and Dannenberg, *supra* note 33.

[37] *Id.*

[38] See Stokes, MacDonald, and Ridgeway, *supra* note 35.

[56] P. Moran, J. Pomeranz, and M. M. Mello, *Policies Affecting Access to Sugar-Sweetened Beverages in Schools: A Legal and Regulatory Review*, Report to the Robert Wood Johnson Foundation, 2006.

[57] The National School Lunch Program and the National School Breakfast Program have identical "competitive food" standards and thus are, for purposes of this paper, treated as one program. See 7 C.F.R. § 210.12 (National School Lunch Program Competitive Food rules) and 7 C.F.R. § 220.12 (National School Breakfast Program Competitive Food rules).

[58] USDA Memorandum, *National School Lunch Program/ School Breakfast Program*, January 16, 2001.

[59] See Delva, O'Malley, and Johnston, *supra* note 31.

[60] 7 CFR 210.11(a)(1).

[61] 7 CFR 210.11 (b).

[62] 7 CFR 210 Appendix B (a).

[63] 7 CFR 210 Appendix B (b).

[64] 7 CFR 210.11(a).

[65] S. Fox, A. Meinen, M. Pesik, M. Landis, P. L. Remington, Competitive Food Initiatives in Schools and Overweight in Children: A Review of the Evidence," *WMJ* 104 (2005): 38-43.

[66] 7 CFR 210.11(b).

[67] Public Law 108-265 [S. 2507], June 30, 2004.

[68] Public Law 108-265 [S. 2507], June 30, 2004 § 204 (a)(1).

[69] See Moran, Pomeranz, and Mello, *supra* note 56.

[70] H. Patrick and T. A. Nicklas, A Review of Family and Social Determinants of Children's Eating Patterns and Diet Quality," *Journal of the American College of Nutrition* 24, no. 2 (2005): 83-92.

[71] See Delva, O'Malley, and Johnston, *supra* note 31.

[72] M. M. Mello, J. Pomeranz, and P. Moran, "The Interplay of Public Health Law and Industry Self-regulation: The Case of Sugar-Sweetened Beverage Sales in Schools," *American Journal of Public Health* 98, no. 4 (2008): 595-604.

[73] M. Story, K. M. Kaphingst, and S. French, "The Role of Schools in Obesity Prevention," *Future of Children* 16, no. 1 (2006): 109-142.

[74] See Moran, Pomeranz, and Mello, *supra* note 56. J. E. Whatley Blum, A. M. Davee, R. L. Devore, C. M. Beaudoin, P. L. Jenkins, L. A. Kaley, D. A. Wigand, "Implementation of Low-Fat, Low-Sugar, and Portion-Controlled Nutrition Guidelines in Competitive Food Venues of Maine Public High Schools," Journal of School Health 77, no. 10 (2007): 687-693.

[75] See Moran, Pomeranz, and Mello, *supra* note 56.

[76] S. K. Graff, "First Amendment Implications of Restricting Food and Beverage Marketing in Schools," *ANNALS of the American Academy of Political and Social Science* 615 (2008): 157-177.

[77] H. Trickey, "No Child Left Out of the Dodgeball Game?" CNN.com (Health), August 24, 2006, available at <http://www.cnn.com/2006/HEALTH/08/20/PE.NCLB/index.html> (last visited March 18, 2009).

[78] National Association for Sport and Physical Education (NASPE), "2006 Shape of the Nation Report," available at <http://www.aahperd.org/naspe/ShapeOfTheNation/> (last visited March 18, 2009).

[79] *Id.*

MARKETING IN SCHOOLS

In its 2008 report to Congress, the FTC found that $186 million was spent on in-school food and beverage marketing expenditures [24]. Ninety percent of in-school marketing was for carbonated beverages, and juice and non-carbonated beverages, with quick-service restaurants accounting for most of that remaining 10% [25]. The IOM found that the "competitive multifaceted marketing of high-calorie and low nutrient food and beverage products in school settings is widely prevalent and appears to have increased steadily" over the decade leading up to 2006 [26]. In fact, the General Accounting Office (GAO) reported that although some states have enacted laws both supporting and limiting commercial activities in schools, most laws address only one discreet practice (e.g., ads on buses) [27]. Significantly, the GAO reported that the amount and type of commercial activity in schools has either remained steady or increased from 2000 to 2004, depending on the district [28]. The issue remains unaddressed for most of the public schools around the country.

State and local boards of education can insert marketing restriction clauses in their contracts with vendors that ban or otherwise limit the amount, type, or placement of advertising on school campuses. Legislatures and school boards can also institute legal bans or restrictions on food and beverage marketing in their districts. Unless the board of education or school itself indicates otherwise, a public school is considered a nonpublic forum [29]. This means that "the government 'may reserve the forum for its intended purposes, communicative or otherwise, as long as the regulation on speech is reasonable and not an effort to suppress expression merely because public officials oppose the speaker's view'" [30].

The Supreme Court consistently confirms that the school board has the authority to determine what speech is appropriate for public schools [31]. Thus, marketing restrictions in schools will survive judicial scrutiny under the First Amendment if they are reasonable and viewpoint neutral [32]. Unambiguous examples of viewpoint-neutral restrictions include banning all advertising on campus, banning all food and beverage advertising on campus, and banning the marketing of foods and beverages not allowed to be sold in the schools [33]. These are reasonable restrictions that would further the schools' interest in protecting children from commercialization and advancing their students' health.

CONCLUSION

The ability of lawmakers to address childhood obesity is impressive and far-reaching. All levels of government have been increasing their efforts on this front, and this proclivity must continue in order to tackle the enormity of the public health problem. Legislative and regulatory bodies can implement the legal interventions discussed earlier to improve the food and built environment for children whether they are at home, in school, or in the community. The goal is to change the environment to make access to healthy food, clean water, green space, and safe communities available to all children in the United States. Only by addressing this public health problem in all environments and through various measures across disciplines can we tackle childhood obesity in the United States.

References

1. Center for Disease Control and Prevention. *Obesity at a Glance*. Available at, www.cdc.gov/NCCdphp/publications/AAG/obesity.htm; 2009 (accessed November 19, 2009).
2. Olshansky SJ, Passaro DJ, Hershow RC, Layden J, Carnes BA, Brody J, Hayflick L, Butler RN, Allison DB, Ludwig DS. "A Potential Decline in Life Expectancy in the United States in the 21st Century". *NEJM* 2005;**352**:1138–45.
3. Dietz WH, Hunter AS. Legal Preparedness for Obesity Prevention and Control: The Public Health Framework for Action. *Journal of Law, Medicine & Ethics* Summer 2009;(Supp):9–14.
4. U.S. Department of Agriculture Laws and Regulations (10/22/09) Available at www.usda.gov/wps/portal/!ut/p/_s.7_0_A/7_0_1OB?navid=FOOD_DISTRIB&;parentnav=LAWS_REGS&navtype=RT (accessed November 19, 2009).
5. The Federal Food, Drug, and Cosmetic Act of 1938; 21 U.S.C. §301 et seq.
6. Ståhl T, Wismar M, Ollila E, Lahtinen E, Leppo K. Health in All Policies: Prospects and Potentials. 2006. at 4–5. Finnish Ministry of Social Affairs and Health. Available at www.euro.who.int/document/e89260.pdf (accessed November 21, 2009).
7. Federal Communications Commission Commercial Limits in Children's Programming. Available at www.fcc.gov/parents/commercials.html (accessed November 19, 2009).
8. See Notice of Inquiry: "In the Matter of Empowering Parents and Protecting Children in an Evolving Media Landscape" (adopted October 23, 2009). Available http://hraunfoss.fcc.gov/edocs_public/attachmatch/FCC-09-94A1.pdf (accessed November 19, 2009).
9. Federal Trade Commission Act of 1938, 15 U.S.C. §45(a)(1); 15 U.S.C. §52.
10. Food Industry Marketing to Children Report; Orders to File Special Report; FTC Matter No.: P064504. Available www.ftc.gov/os/6b_orders/foodmktg6b/index.shtm (accessed December 7, 2008).
11. Federal Trade Commission Report: Marketing Food to Children and Adolescents. July 2008. Available at: www.ftc.gov/os/2008/07/P064504foodmktingreport.pdf (accessed December 7, 2008).
12. Federal Trade Commission's Notice of Agency Information Collection Activities, 74 Fed. Reg. 48072 (Sept. 21, 2009).
13. The Supremacy Clause of the United States Constitution, article VI, paragraph 2.
14. L.O. Gostin. Public Health Theory and Practice in the Constitutional Design. 11 Health Matrix 265, 282–3 (2001).
15. Illinois: HB 78 (2009); Massachusetts: SD 1637(2009); Nebraska: SB 130 (2009); Oregon: HB 2800 (2009); South Carolina: HB 3179 (2009).
16. Minnesota: HB 439 and SB 61(2009).

REFERENCES

17. Massachusetts: SB 1639 (2009); Mississippi: HB 1262 (2009); Minnesota: HB 252 (2009).
18. Massachusetts: HB 450 (2009).
19. Hawaii: HB 438 and SB 185 (2009).
20. Washington: SB 5857 (2009).
21. Rhode Island: HB 5520 and SB 534 (2009); Florida: SB 2590 (2009).
22. Association of State and Territorial Health Officials (ASTHO). Profile of State Public Health Volume One. 2009. Available at www.astho.org/Research/Major-Publications/Profile-of-State-Public-Health-Vol-1/ (accessed December 7, 2009).
23. Pomeranz JL, Gostin LO. Improving Laws and Legal Authority to Prevent Obesity. *Journal of Law Medicine and Ethics* 2009;**37**(Supp):62–75.
24. *See* Federal Trade Commission Report: Marketing Food to Children and Adolescents. July 2008, at 23. Available at www.ftc.gov/os/2008/07/P064504foodmktingreport.pdf (accessed December 7, 2009).
25. Federal Trade Commission Report: Marketing Food to Children and Adolescents. July 2008, at 23. Available at www.ftc.gov/os/2008/07/P064504foodmktingreport.pdf (accessed December 7, 2009).
26. Institute of Medicine. *Food marketing to children and youth: threat or opportunity?*. Washington, D.C: National Academies Press; 2006. at 190.
27. General Accounting Office. Report to Congress: Commercial Activities in Schools. 2004, at 14; Available at www.gao.gov/new.items/d04810.pdf (accessed December 7, 2009).
28. General Accounting Office. Report to Congress: Commercial Activities in Schools. 2004, at 9; Available at www.gao.gov/new.items/d04810.pdf (accessed December 7, 2009).
29. *Hazelwood School District v. Kuhlmeier*, 484 U.S. 260, 270 (1988); Planned Parenthood of Southern Nevada v. Clark County School District, 941 F.2d 817, 822–9 (9th Cir. 1991).
30. *Planned Parenthood of Southern Nevada v. Clark County School District*, 941 F.2d 817, 822 n.5 (9th Cir. 1991) (quoting *Perry Education Association v. Perry Local Educators Association*, 460 U.S. 37, 46 (1983)).
31. *Hazelwood School District v. Kuhlmeier*, 484 U.S. 260, 267 (1988).
32. Graff SK. First Amendment Implications of Restricting Food and Beverage Marketing in Schools. *ANNALS of the American Academy* 2008;**615**:158–77.
33. Graff SK. First Amendment Implications of Restricting Food and Beverage Marketing in Schools. *ANNALS of the American Academy* 2008;**615**:158–77.

CHAPTER 43

Childhood Obesity as an Amplifier of Societal Inequality in the United States

Stanley J. Ulijaszek

Institute of Social and Cultural Anthropology, University of Oxford, United Kingdom

INTRODUCTION

Social and economic factors are important in the production of population obesity [1], contributing to widely differing rates among similarly economically developed nations [2]. In addition, cultural factors contribute to differences in obesity rates by way of perceptions of appropriate, healthy, and beautiful body size [3]. In industrialized society, obesity is a characteristic of lower social and economic classes [1], having been once associated with higher classes prior to widespread economic prosperity [4]. The potential influences of social and economic forces on the production of obesity are well known [1, 5]. Inequality has been associated with population obesity [6], and Sobal [7] has suggested pathways whereby obesity can influence socioeconomic status (SES). In his formulation, the perception of obesity by oneself and others is central to the attainment of education, occupation, and income by way of values and behaviors that result in prejudice, bias, discrimination, and stigma (Fig. 43.1). Sobal's [7] formulation places education, income, and occupation equal in the production of SES among obese people. However, education and occupation condition income, and income must therefore play a dominant role in the production of SES.

Obesity and low SES are tied in a transgenerational vicious circle, such that obesity leads to low SES, and low SES produces obesity. According to Sobal [7], obesity in childhood and adolescence

> may exert a strong influence on socioeconomic status. Most adults have largely attained their final educational, occupational, and marital status. For them, the values, types of behavior, and resources associated with their socioeconomic position influence their weight more strongly. Thus, obesity causes status and status causes obesity, each under different conditions of the life cycle. (p.241)

Children and adolescents in households enmeshed in a physical and social environment configured by the low SES of their parents and caregivers are more likely to develop obesity that persists into adulthood [8], increasing and accelerating the risks of ill health [9, 10] as well as psychiatric disorders [11, 12]. Given the rapid and continuing rise in obesity rates in the United States [13], the most striking prediction concerning the long-term effect of obesity is demographic, through reduced life expectancy because of increased mortality from chronic disease [14]. This may in part be attributed to the long-term health risks of developing obesity in childhood [15]. Childhood obesity is also socially stigmatized [16, 17], and in the United States such stigma transcends ethnic and racial categories [18] but is more pronounced in some groups than others. Obese children then go on to face social disadvantages in employment, education, healthcare, and interpersonal relationships [19, 20].

In industrialized nations, obesity, high dietary energy intake, and low physical activity levels cluster among low-income groups [7, 21]. Social class is also negatively associated with diet quality, primarily through the mechanism of cost [22], although economic factors alone cannot explain variation in nutritional health within communities [23] or across nations [6]. Although the relationships among SES and obesity are powerful and synergistic, the SES construct is insufficient to describe some of the cultural influences on status production in society, and therefore on obesity production. Socioeconomic status has two closely related dimensions. The economic one is represented by financial wealth,

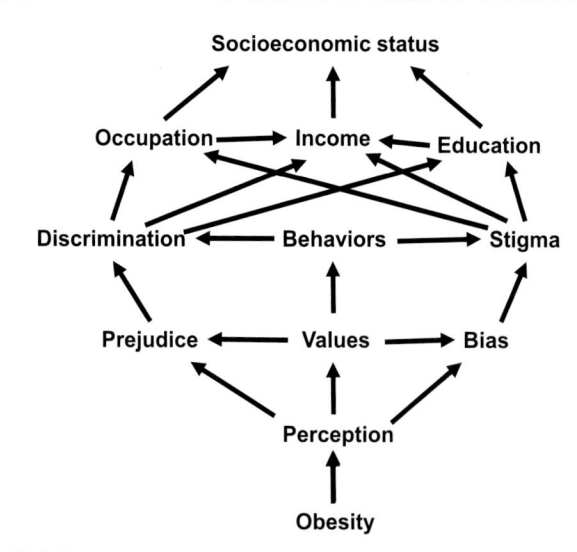

FIGURE 43.1 Social and behavioral factors that mediate the influence of obesity on socioeconomic status (adapted from Sokal 1991).

whereas the social one can incorporate education, occupational prestige, authority, and community standing. Whereas economic status is easy to measure (assuming that someone will accurately reveal his or her income in survey), occupational prestige, authority, and community standing are more difficult to estimate. Cultural factors overlap with social ones, values that help confer status in society include forms of knowledge, skills, and education [24]. Although the SES construct can be made numerically tractable, there is no consensus definition of SES, nor is there a widely accepted SES measurement tool [25, 26]. And although prestige is a component of social distance [27], ethnicity is not a consistent predictor of household prestige [28]. Measures of economic status may differ in their meaning across ethnic groups because of different cultural valuation of material goods and services. Similarly, measures of social status may vary culturally. Thus, it is important to separate the effects of SES from ethnicity or race [27]. Oakes and Rossi [26] have proposed a material, social, and human capital model of SES that omits race, as there is no easy way to quantify it. However, race and ethnicity remain important but imperfect markers of cultural variation that may carry health consequences that are independent of SES [29, 30].

A way of addressing the issue of race in considering inequality and obesity is put forward here, using Bourdieu and Boltanski's [31] "theory of practice." This links economic, social, and cultural forms of capital (or value) in an overarching category of symbolic capital. These represent categories through which power relationships within society are negotiated. This construct permits a more complete examination of societal stratification and its human biological consequences and amplifiers, including ethnicity, because it incorporates the notion of cultural value of, for example, preferences in body size and shape, which shows variation within and between groups.

In this chapter, I examine ways in which obesity in childhood and adolescence is structured by symbolic capital both inherited from parents and caregivers and formed by individuals across life. The focus is primarily on the United States, although it draws on literature from elsewhere in the industrialized world where appropriate. Differences in obesity rates across major ethnic groups are discussed, because this is an area in which social and cultural forms of capital differ and may offer insights into obesity and its associated traits as a form of symbolic capital. Although classifications of ethnicity can obscure as much as they can reveal, they are dominant categories that structure the thinking of those involved in obesity policy, research, and practice and are therefore used here to describe major differences in obesity rates within the U.S. population. It is argued that if obesity carries embodied capital in a low SES or particular group, it may be one of the few forms of capital they have. If branded fast-food outlets surround them, the selection, purchase, and consumption of fast food may be another achievable form of cultural capital, that of objectified capital where other forms of bought status are out of reach. Given that children, adolescents, and adults have become increasingly segregated by media use in current society and that food choices are plastic, it is argued that children's food choices have become increasingly influenced by corporate interests and not solely their family, caregivers, or social group.

Rates of childhood and adolescent obesity have risen dramatically in the United States since the 1970s [32] across a period of steady expansion of economic inequality only reversed briefly and marginally during the years of the Clinton administration [33]. With the current political administration avowed to a reduction in societal inequalities, it is perhaps timely to examine how childhood obesity may be an inadvertent amplifier of societal inequality. First, it is important to elaborate the concept of symbolic capital and why it is appropriate for framing the problem in hand.

SYMBOLIC CAPITAL AND OBESITY

Although there are many ways of thinking about population obesity [34], when genetic determinism is removed from the frame, the problem is reduced to the role of individual agency in negotiating societal structures that are obesogenic in the production of appropriate (or inappropriate) body size. In "Structure and agency," Bourdieu and Boltanski [31] examine the relationship between these two forces in shaping the personal character, ways of thinking and bodily comportment of individuals. Collectively, the development of correct dispositions (or habitus) within society are framed in different social fields: the kin group, social networks, and organizations such as school, university, the workplace, and activity groupings. Habitus formation is influenced by the social field one is born to or (in the case of social mobility) aspires to. The building and maintenance of habitus involves the accrual and retention of symbolic capital, which is built out of economic, social, and cultural capital. Figure 43.2 places Sobal's [7] scheme for the influence of obesity on SES within Bourdieu and Boltanski's [31] framework of symbolic capital. Economic and social capital are the disaggregated components of SES, whereas the three types of cultural capital (embodied, objectified, and institutional) are shown as linked to occupation, education, and income, but also to obesity itself.

The SES inversion of obesity in Western societies has been explained by generally increased purchasing power, a decline in food price, and the low material quality of food available to people of low SES [22]. A more nuanced explanation comes from Sobal [7], who places income, education, and occupation as separate but interactive predictors of obesity. Neither explanation is complete, as they do not accommodate cultural capital in, for example, differences in food choices and perceptions in ideal body size. A further explanation is put forward here, one that locates SES within Bourdieu and Boltanski's [31] framework.

Economic capital allows the purchase of adequate food supply and the technological means of transport and recreation, and some types of cultural capital. Social capital is a characterization of group cohesion through social intercourse that facilitates cooperation for mutual benefit [35]. Groups considered of either high or low social status when compared with each other may possess equal levels of social capital, if they have equal levels of within-group social cohesion. Although social capital can explain why obesity can persist within class formations—for example, through obesity networks [36]—economic capital can help explain why overall obesity levels should rise with increasing economic prosperity, but only to levels where average individual food security is good. Three subtypes of cultural capital have been elaborated [31]. Embodied cultural capital consists of properties of the self that are either consciously acquired or inherited through socialization within the family and its social networks. Given differences in the cultural valuation of body size among different ethnic groups in the United States, obesity may carry greater embodied cultural capital in groups that value greater body weight than among groups that do not. Objectified cultural capital is represented by physical objects that can convey status symbolically and can include such things as works of art, prestigious brands of car, and designer-labeled clothes. If such objects carry monetary value, they may be bought and sold, and therefore economic and cultural capital may be traded. Institutionalized cultural capital consists of recognition of individuals by the state, usually in terms of academic credentials, qualifications, and honors. Such capital can to some extent be bought, if the state places a financial cost on education, for example.

Cultural capital is acquired over time as it becomes part of one's habitus. Different societies and social fields vary in the value they place on different types of capital. For example, the field of business places higher value on economic capital than social or cultural capital. In the field of education, greater value is placed on the cultural capital that is embodied in knowledge and its generation. If obesity and fatness carry cultural capital in a society or ethnic group, as, for example, among African Americans, this may represent embodied capital that is valued in a context where other forms of capital are hard to acquire.

Different forms of capital flow into each other, and there are upper levels to the amount of different types of capital that can be accrued. In major universities and arts organizations, for example, large endowments usually come from those whose symbolic capital cannot be furthered by an increase in economic capital and for whom economic contribution to knowledge or arts organizations with high cultural capital raises their own cultural capital and overall symbolic worth. The limits of embodied capital probably lie in socially exposed extreme pathologies. Low body mass associated with anorexia nervosa to an extent that is externally visible becomes socially stigmatizing, as does high body mass when associated with extreme obesity. When set in a broader frame of symbolic capital, the relationships

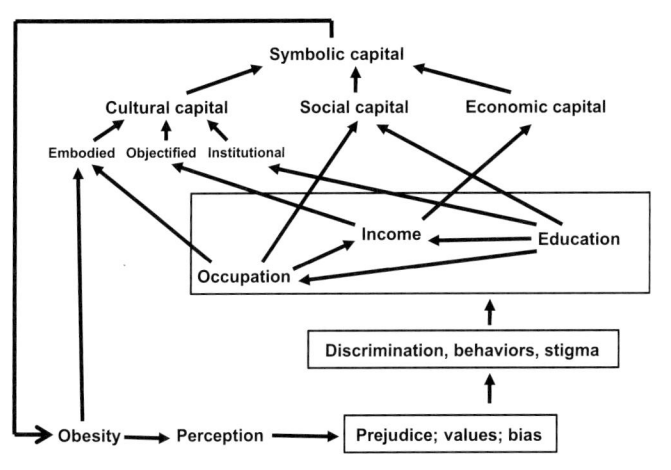

FIGURE 43.2 Links between obesity, socioeconomic capital, and cultural capital in the formation of symbolic capital.

between obesity and SES are opened up to cultural factors such as embodied capital, a component of habitus, which is constituted differently by different groups as defined, for example, by national, ethnic, racial or migratory characteristics and which is formed across the life span with the acquisition of symbolic capital.

INEQUALITY, ETHNICITY, AND OBESITY

In most industrialized nations, the economic growth of recent decades has benefited the rich more than the poor. In some countries, including Canada, Finland, Germany, Italy, Norway, and the United States, the gap has also increased between the rich and the middle classes [33]. In the United States, income inequality has grown at a much faster rate than the Organization for Economic Cooperation and Development average from the mid-1970s until the mid-2000s [33]. Social inequality has been shown to contribute to illness independently of income level [37, 38], suggesting that hierarchy has effects that can act across large populations and not just within discrete groups, across all income levels [39].

In the United States, Zhang and Wang [40] found that SES inequality in the distribution of obesity among over 10,000 adults in the nationally representative National Health and Nutrition Examination Survey III (1988–1994) varied enormously according to gender and ethnicity. This is confirmed by data from the United States 2006–2008 Behavioral Risk Surveillance System on over a million adults, which shows obesity rates to vary much more by ethnicity than gender [41] (Fig. 43.3). In nationally representative surveys carried out in the United States, ethnicity is self-identified within broad census categories, such as Hispanic, Mexican American, African American, and skin color, of which a choice of white and black is offered [42]. These do not map onto any precise genetic typologies [29] and often lead to misunderstanding, as, for example, when 42% of people of Latin American ancestry did not recognize the category of "Hispanic" as representing them, whereupon they ignored the specified racial categories and identified themselves as "some other race" [43].

Data on more than 46,000 children and adolescents from the U.S. 2003 National Survey of Children's Health indicate that race/ethnicity, SES, and behavioral factors are independently related to childhood and adolescent obesity [44]. This is supported by Zhang and Wang's [40] analysis, which found a consistent inverse association between SES and obesity among European Americans of both genders, but not among non-European Americans. For example, a positive relationship between SES and obesity was found for African American and Mexican American men, but not for women. Among adolescents, the highest inverse gradient among socioeconomic status and obesity has been found among the highest income nations, the United States and Germany in particular [45]. In the United States, analyses of nationally representative data on children and adolescents, including the National Health and Nutrition Examination Surveys I, II, and III, the BRFSS, the Youth Risk Behavior Surveillance System, and the National Longitudinal Survey of Adolescent Health [32] show relationships between SES and obesity in childhood and adolescence also to vary by age, gender and ethnicity (Fig. 43.4).

Among African American children and adolescents, SES is positively associated with obesity in both boys and girls [40], this effect persisting into adult life for males. Among European Americans, a negative association between SES and obesity in childhood disappears in adolescence and reappears in adult life for males, whereas for females a positive association between SES

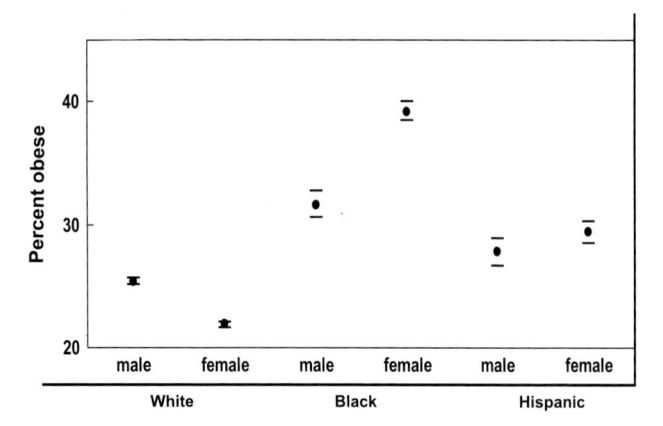

FIGURE 43.3 Prevalence of obesity among black, white, and Hispanic adults, United States, 2007–2008, 95% confidence intervals given as bars below and above the average (data from Centers for Disease Control [41]).

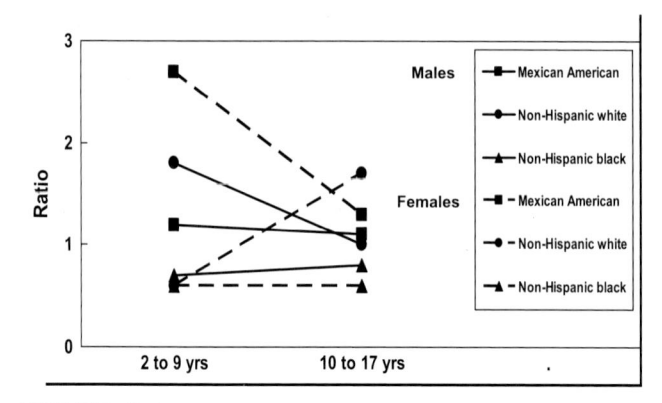

FIGURE 43.4 Ratio of obesity rates among children and adolescents by socioeconomic status (low status divided by high), United States, 1999–2002 (data from Wang and Beydoun [32]).

and obesity in childhood becomes inverted in adolescence, remaining so into adult life. Among Mexican Americans, more children of lower SES are obese than those of higher SES, these differences largely disappearing in adolescence (Fig. 43.5). A positive association between SES and obesity emerges among adult male Mexican Americans, but not among females [32, 40]. What these disparities reveal is that either the socioeconomic environment affects different ethnic and age groups differently or that low SES means different things in different groups. Some of the ethnic variation in obesity rates by SES among children and adolescents has been attributed to disparities in the availability of food stores across neighborhoods inhabited by different groups [32], with African Americans and Mexican Americans generally having access to fewer chain supermarkets than Europeans [46], and lower SES and minority groups having restricted access to physical activity facilities [47].

Childhood obesity has been linked to neighborhood of residence, with characteristics such as walkability [48, 49], differentials in socioeconomic mix [39], and disadvantage and relative safety [50] being cited as the dominant environmental causes. Structural factors make susceptibility to obesity greater in some communities than others. Swinburn et al. [51], who coined the term "obesogenic environments," argued that the physical, economic, social, and cultural environments of the majority of industrialized nations encourage positive energy balance in their populations. Obesogenicity was defined by them as "the sum of influences that the surroundings, opportunities, or conditions of life have on promoting obesity in individuals or populations." (p. 564). In the context of inner city United States, this would include poor access to food of good nutritional quality and low access to exercise facilities. But this is an incomplete picture, because individual exposure to obesogenic environments is mediated socially, politically, and economically [34] and does not explain why there should be an inverse SES association with obesity among African American children but a positive one among Mexican American children.

Social class differences in obesity-relevant health behaviors have been invoked to explain relationships between SES and obesity [52, 53]. However, they do not explain the variation in SES differences in obesity rates by ethnicity shown in the analysis of Wang and Beydoun [32]. In part, the problem may lie with the measurement of SES itself. Although the National Health and Nutrition Examination Surveys, the Behavioral Risk Factor Surveillance System Survey, and the National Longitudinal Study of Adolescent Health all construct SES from measures of poverty, income, and education, they each do so slightly differently [54]. Across ethnicity, a particular attainment in education level may not reflect differences in the quality of that education, whereas the recording of occupation does not give any measure of the extent of control over one's work [54], an aspect of inequality with demonstrable health consequences [37]. Furthermore, immediate income is not a proxy for wealth, which may have time depth. And none of these measures reflect changing life circumstances [54].

Life-course differences in obesity rates and variation by SES among Mexican Americans and European Americans may reflect the inadequacies of the SES construct in capturing ethnicity factors [55]. They may also suggest that either social life in childhood, adolescence, and adulthood takes place in discrete social fields or cultures, or that the social groupings embedded in particular ethnic groups are in transition. Media representations in the United States encourage a separation of social fields between childhood, adolescence, and adult life, although the boundaries across such fields is porous and varying according to how much of everyday life is negotiated among people of different ages within the intersecting fields of the household, school, and social and religious groupings. Mexican American

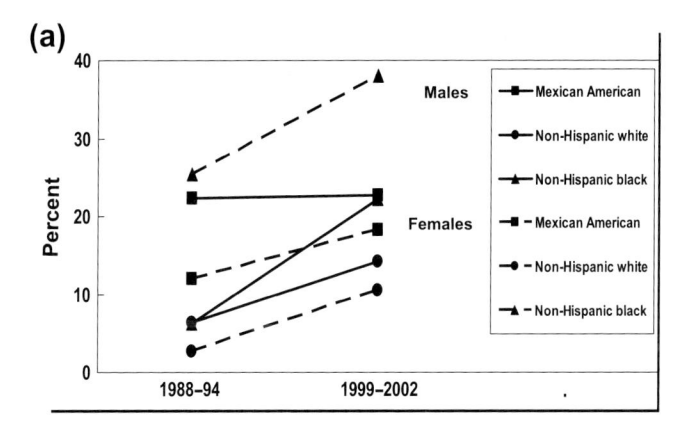

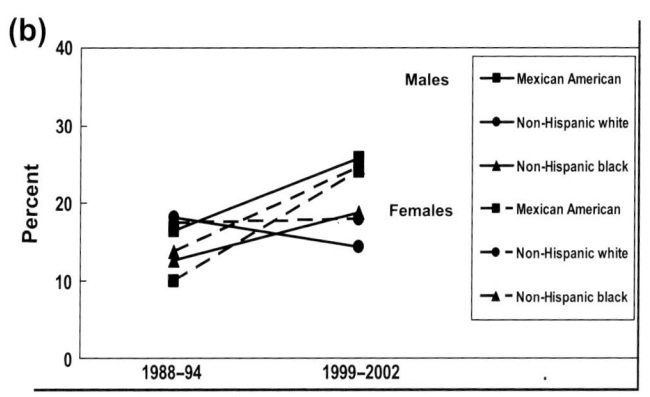

FIGURE 43.5 (a) Obesity rates of high-socioeconomic-status adolescents, by ethnic group, United States, 1988–2002 (adapted from Wang and Beydoun [32]). (b) Obesity rates of low-socioeconomic-status adolescents, by ethnic group, United States, 1988–2002 (data from Wang and Beydoun [32]).

society is much more in demographic and geographical transition than that of the majority of European American or African American society, with the number of people of Latin American origins in the United States more than doubling between 1980 and 2000 [56].

The symbolic capital framework can offer reasons for these differences. In childhood, the social and economic capital of an individual is largely that of the social grouping and of parents and caregivers, and children of low SES carry much less of either type of capital than do children of high SES. In adolescence, some children of low SES may acquire more economic capital than their high SES equivalents simply because they may leave school early and take on jobs. And in the absence of paid employment, higher engagement in criminal activity by low SES adolescents serves the same ends. Among African American men, obesity adversely affects wages and labor force participation and increases incentives for participating in criminal activity [57]. Whereas children and adolescents of higher SES are also likely to attain more institutional cultural capital than their lower SES counterparts, if embodiment ideals are toward larger body size among the low SES group, then they can acquire more embodied cultural capital in this way. And although objectified cultural capital may depend on the economic circumstances of parents and caregivers, some forms of such capital can also be acquired relatively cheaply in industrialized society, for example, through the purchase of branded fast food. Embodied capital reflects the values of the dominant forces in society. Thus, bodily ideals of greater body weight might come to carry less embodied capital among migrants, for example, in the United States than in their country of origin, as cultural ideals of thinness are promoted more heavily in the United States.

In an obesogenic environment, one way to avoid obesity is to exercise resistance behaviorally, through cognitive restraint of food intake, and culturally, by way of practices that restrict food intake and encourage physical activity. Alternatively, groups that seek to resist a dominant ideology, as perhaps among some African American groups, may favor obesity. Among African American children and adolescents, embodied capital associated with larger body size (stopping at the level of pathological obesity) has persisted even among those of higher SES [32], and this may reflect resistance and the maintenance of ethnically dominant cultural capital ascriptions to large body size. Adult African American women prefer body size that is larger, on average, than similar groups of European American women [58]. This preference has been identified in older [59] and low SES African American women also [60]. Furthermore, overweight and obese African American women perceive themselves to be healthier, more attractive, and more attractive to the opposite sex than white women of similar weight and age (58, 59, 60). European Americans, on the other hand, experience dissatisfaction with their own body size at lower BMI than either Mexican or African Americans [61]. Obesity rates among African American children and adolescents are similar to those of African Americans and higher than those of European Americans [32]. Among Hispanic groups, for example, women are more satisfied (or less dissatisfied) with their bodies than are white women despite having higher weights [62], are less concerned with weight than whites [63], and are more likely to rate themselves as attractive [64]. Furthermore, whereas white women report body dissatisfaction below the criterion for overweight, Hispanic women do not do so until they are overweight [61], nor do they endorse thin beauty ideals [65]. Furthermore, Mexican Americans, while being heavier than whites, engage in less dieting behavior [66] and report higher desired body weights than whites [67].

Various groups in which obesity has risen across recent decades and that previously were shown to desire or accept larger bodies and obesity have moved to prefer thinner bodies [68]. In the United States, this has taken place among African American girls [69, 70] and African American women with diabetes [71]. Among European Americans, the desire for thinner body size is increasingly observed in children and adolescents and is not confined to females of upper socioeconomic status [70]. Thus, the high cultural capital that high body fatness has carried may have contributed to the rise of obesity among such groups, but it may cease to be an important contributor in subsequent generations [2]. Against this, in-migration and migrant valuation of large body size may lead to ambivalence about appropriate body size in communities such as Mexican American ones. In Mexico, relationships between SES and obesity are positively directed, with obesity rates among children from private schools being higher than among those in state schools [72] and greater income being associated with higher levels of obesity among older Mexican adults [73]. However, overweight or obese Mexican children are more likely to be stigmatized than those who are not [74], indicating that attitudes might be changing, at least in the playground.

FOOD AND THE BODY AS TWO TYPES OF CULTURAL CAPITAL

Obesity is a multifactorial, systemic problem [9] whose complex political ecology resists any single action, whether at the individual or societal level. Most approaches to childhood obesity fail to acknowledge that the body is not just a machine for living in, as medicine would place it, but also an object for negotiating the world and an individual's social identity. If obesity carries cultural capital in a low SES group, it may be one of the few forms of capital these individuals have. If branded fast-food outlets surround them, the selection, purchase, and consumption of fast food may be another achievable form of cultural capital.

If embodied capital is what particular ethnic groups or social classes have most of, and if large body size is valued, then the health implications of obesity may be peripheral to their struggle for what social position they can get. Within ethnic or class group, larger body size may endow status, when in a broader societal context, little else is available by which to mark status or symbolic capital. And within-group, childhood obesity may be a direct outcome of a socially sanctioned formation of appropriate habitus. Where, among migrants, slimmer body size ideals emerge, as among Pacific Islanders in New Zealand [75] and young Mexican American girls [76], this may reflect a realignment of habitus to minimize rejection, ostracism, and negative social relations in the intersecting social fields of school and the workplace. In the United States, overweight and obesity has been stigmatized across the past hundred years or so [77-79], the prevalence of such stigma having almost doubled since the mid-1990s [80]. Obesity stigma among adolescents shows similar patterns to that among adults. In a social networking study of 2728 American adolescents, Crosnoe et al. [81] found that larger body size constrained the size of adolescents' friendship circles in high school, primarily because of the stigma attached to larger bodies and because larger adolescents sought the company of the numerically fewer people that were like them.

The symbolic coding of food has been elaborated to a high degree across history in industrialized and industrializing nations, a process that continued at breakneck pace with the development of global food cultures and of diverse supermarkets and restaurants to deliver them. Using Europe as his example, Bourdieu [82] elaborated the view that social capital can be gained through food by using it as a vehicle for reproducing social class distinctions. As social class groupings are determined by a combination of varying degrees of social, economic, and cultural capital, they incorporate symbolic goods, especially those regarded as having the attributes of excellence, as tools for creating distinction [82]. Excellence is shaped by the dominating class and is driven by cultural capital, which marks differences between the classes and which is gained by learning the aesthetic dispositions of the class one is born to. Thus, tastes in food are indicators of class, and trends in their consumption vary by class, with lower classes opting for cheaper, fat-rich foods that can be eaten plentifully and higher classes opting for foods marked by originality and exoticism.

How can people of low SES acquire cultural capital through food? Not through buying expensive luxury items, because price and local availability prohibits it; rather, fast-food provides such an outlet. The United States and other industrialized nations have seen growth of fast-food consumption to a significant proportion of daily intake. For example, the proportion of daily dietary energy intake from restaurants and fast-food providers by U.S. adolescents increased three-fold between the late 1970s and late 1990s, from 6.5% to 19.3% [83], with one third or more of them consuming some fast food on any given day [84]. In a nationally representative dietary survey (the 1994-1996 and 1998 Continuing Survey of Food Intakes by Individuals), fast-food consumption was reported for the day before the survey among 42% of children and adolescents and 37% of adults [85]. In Australia, 22% of adolescents consume fast food every day [86], such consumption being associated with a cultural shift in eating practices in Australian society [87]. Fast-food manufacturers have developed product lines that carry images of originality, exoticism, and often global power. These products have valency as cultural capital through branding and advertising, and objectified status can be accrued by an individual for at least the time it takes them to think about fast food, choose the brand, choose the items, and eat them. Such capital is price sensitive for adolescents but not for younger children (largely because parents do the buying), with the probability of obesity being lower where fast food is more expensive for the former age group [88].

Although the use of food in the quest for status is universal among all societies, high-status foods vary enormously across societies [89]. Bourdieu [82] suggested that class distinction and preferences are most marked in ordinary choices of everyday life, with cooking and tastes in food. These, he suggested, are primarily learned in childhood. In the industrialized world, children identify the symbolic value of foods from an early age. For example, preschool children in the United States are aware of and can identify advertised food brands, and by the age of 7 years, can shop independently, find information about what they want to buy, and show what they have bought to other children [90]. Again, where options for building cultural capital are limited, branded fast foods are an affordable option for the children of poorer groups in the United States and elsewhere.

In industrialized nations, food choices are shaped by income and the food industry. An example of how cultural capital may be attributed to foods and their consumption is that of meat. Fiddes [91] has written extensively about the symbolic value of meat, particularly among elites, for whom it has been a means for demonstrating authority [92]. By acknowledging meat to be a symbol of earthly power, Fiddes [92] has demonstrated the logic of denying access to it to lower social classes and has shown how abstinence from it by some religious orders represents the shunning of earthly power for spiritual control. Starting from very low levels, per capita consumption of meat in the developing world more than doubled from 1967 to 1997 as demand rose with increasing prosperity [93]. In the United States, where consumption levels were among the highest on earth in the mid-1960s, they rose by 16% between 1967 and 1997 [94]. And while globally the demand for meat remains impossible to meet, it remains a prestige good and a form of objectified cultural capital through consumption. When, in industrialized societies, everyone can eat meat, the higher classes can distinguish themselves by consuming only the most aesthetically desirable types and cuts of meat or by shunning it altogether and consuming other types of prestige foods.

The effort by fast-food companies to brand and advertise otherwise low-grade meat and animal tissue into meat products such as burgers and sausages separates them from their source within an animal, elevates their status, and influences their consumption among lower SES groups [95] by keeping the price low. Analysis of data from the United States 2000–2002 Multi-Ethnic Study of Atherosclerosis shows that fast-food consumption and neighborhood fast-food exposure are associated with poorer diet [96]. Childhood food choices are malleable [97] and are shaped primarily by parents and caregivers [98]. However, media use influences consumption of media-promoted foods [99] and through branding and advertising on television and the Internet. With respect to the latter, advertising is both viral and by association with fast-food games (advergaming) [100]. Thus, children's food choices are increasingly influenced by corporate interests and not solely their familial or local social fields.

THE IMPACTS OF CHILDHOOD OBESITY ON SOCIETY

The likelihood that significant proportions of the population of obese children and adolescents will become obese adults suggests that negative correlates of large body size, including stigma, poor educational opportunities, and occupational prospects, are likely to persist into the next generation. Obesity also limits upward social mobility. Evidence for this consequence in the United States comes from the National Longitudinal Survey of Labor Market Experience, Youth Cohort in the 1980s, which shows that both women and men who had been overweight in late adolescence or early adulthood in 1981 were less likely to have married, and had completed fewer years of education, lower household incomes, lower self-esteem, and higher rates of poverty 7 years later than those who had not been overweight [101]. In the United Kingdom, downwardly mobile women are more satisfied with their appearance than their peers in their social class of origin [102], indicating that incongruity between an individual's large body size and his or her SES can be resolved by downward social migration as well as by losing weight. Obesity in the United States is linked through social networks [36] as well as following an inverse gradient of SES. Social networks are driven by the maintenance and acquisition of symbolic capital, among which body size has valency. Data from the National Longitudinal Study of Adolescent Health show that the factors most associated with having strong social networks were low body mass index and abilities in athletic and academic performance [81]. These social networks were not influenced by parental education (which can be taken as a proxy for social class), within-school friendships, or ethnicity. Children in the United States are stratified by social status according to various criteria, including the school they attend [103, 104], and the lack of effects of social class and ethnicity on friendship network size is probably caused by the social homogeneity that may exist within schools in the United States.

CONCLUSION

The economic growth that the United States has enjoyed since the 1970s has come with increased economic inequality, which is now greater than it is in most other industrialized nations [33]. On average, African Americans and Mexican Americans continue to earn far less than European Americans [103]. I argue that exacerbated economic differences contribute to the growth of obesity in the United States as poorer groups seek to create symbolic capital in the ways open to them, through embodied and objectified capital (Fig. 43.2). Whereas bias, prejudice, discrimination, and stigma limit the opportunities available to obese people in terms of education, occupation, and income, the low symbolic capital they hold may lead them to use obesity as a form of cultural capital within-group and to consume fast food as their only affordable objectified status marker. Across the broader population, however, obesity makes it difficult for individuals to break out of particular constellations of inequality as bounded by ethnicity and SES. For example, whereas obese African Americans (especially females) experience more obesity-related stigma than European Americans [105], those who have achieved professional work status experience more perceived interpersonal mistreatment compared to those of lower SES [106]. Furthermore, relative to other forms of bias, weight bias is stronger than two other forms of xenophobia, gay and Islam bias in the present-day United States [107]. Among children, fat stigmatization is stronger against girls than boys [108]. The recognition that obesity is one of the major social stigmas in the United States at present has led advocates to appeal for change in existing models of employment discrimination [109].

At the individual level, there need to be cultural motivators to resist obesity beyond those related to aspirations for material and social status. For anthropologists, relationships between inequality and illness, of whatever kind, are forms of structural violence enacted through cultures and rationalities [110]. Structural violence represents ways in which given social structures or institutions injure people by preventing them from meeting their basic needs. Life spans are reduced when people are socially dominated, politically oppressed, or economically exploited. Differences in economic inequality across nations, though largely associated with globalization, are also influenced by governmental policies, either in relation to redistribution of wealth or investment in infrastructure that promotes self-reliance [33]. Although this might not yet be enough, the message for obesity control at the population level is that reducing inequality between people and peoples matters. If inequality cannot be reduced, then among its effects will be the persistence and increase in obesity rates. And, to paraphrase Tanner [111] when he talked of child growth in communities, childhood obesity will continue to be a mirror of inequality in society.

Acknowledgments

I thank Dr Caroline Potter for her comments on an earlier draft of this manuscript.

References

1. McLaren L. Socioeconomic status and obesity. *Epidemiol Rev* 2007;**29**:29–48.
2. Ulijaszek SJ, Lofink H. Obesity in biocultural perspective. *Annu Rev Anthropol* 2006;**35**:337–60.
3. de Garine I, Pollock N. *"Social Aspects of Obesity and Fatness"*. New York: Gordon and Breach; 1995.
4. Ulijaszek SJ. Social aspects of obesity and fatness: a critique. In: de Garine I, Pollock N, editors. *"Social Aspects of Obesity and Fatness"*. New York: Gordon & Breach; 1995. pp. 291–9.
5. Sobal J, Stunkard AJ. Socioeconomic status and obesity: a review of the literature. *Psychol Bull* 1989;**105**:260–75.
6. Pickett KE, Kelly S, Brunner E, Lobstein T, Wilkinson RG. Wider income gaps, wider waistbands? An ecological study of obesity and income inequality. *J Epidemiol Comm Health* 2005;**59**:670–4.
7. Sobal J. Obesity and socioeconomic status: a framework for examining relationships between physical and social variables. *Med Anthropol* 1991;**13**:231–47.
8. Wardle J, Brodersen NH, Cole TJ, Jarvis MJ, Boniface DR. Development of adiposity in adolescence: five year longitudinal study of an ethnically and socioeconomically diverse sample of young people in Britain. *Br Med J* 2006;**332**:1130–5.
9. World Health Organization. *"Obesity: Preventing and Managing the Global Epidemic."* World Health Organization Technical Report Series 894. Geneva: World Health Organization; 2000.
10. Daniels SR. The consequences of childhood overweight and obesity. *Future of Children* 2006;**16**:47–67.
11. Van Vlierberghe L, Braet C, Goossens L, Mels S. Psychiatric disorders and symptom severity in referred versus non-referred overweight children and adolescents. *Eur Child Adolescent Psych* 2009;**18**:164–73.
12. Carpiniello B, Pinna F, Pillai G, Nonnoi V, Pisano E, Corrias S, Orru MG, Orru W, Velluzzi F, Loviselli A. Psychiatric comorbidity and quality of life in obese patients. Results from a case-control study. *Int J Psych Med* 2009;**39**:63–78.
13. Centers for Disease Control. *Data and Statistics. Overweight and Obesity Trends Among Adults*, www.cdc.gov/obesity/data/index.html; 2009a. Accessed August 21, 2009.
14. Olshansky SJ, Passaro DJ, Hershow RC, Layden J, Carnes BA, Brody J, Hayflick L, Butler RN, Allison DB, Ludwig DS. A potential decline in life expectancy in the United States in the 21st century. *N Eng J Med* 2005;**352**:1138–45.
15. Schuster DP. Changes in physiology with increasing fat mass. *Seminars Pediatr Surg* 2009;**18**:126–35.
16. Hansson LM, Karnehed N, Tynelius P, Rasmussen F. *Prejudice against obesity among 10-year-olds: a nationwide population-based study Acta Paediatrica* 2009;**98**:1176–82.
17. Puhl RM, Latner JD. Stigma, obesity, and the health of the nation's children Psychol. *Bull* 2007;**133**:557–80.
18. Greenleaf C, Chambliss H, Rhea DJ, Martin SB, Morrow JR. Weight stereotypes and behavioral intentions toward thin and fat peers among White and Hispanic adolescents. *J Adolescent Health* 2006;**39**:546–52.
19. Brownell KD, Puhl R, Schwartz MB, Rudd L. *Weight bias: Nature, consequences, and remedies*. New York: Guilford Press; 2005.
20. Puhl R, Brownell KD. Bias, discrimination, and obesity. *Ob Res* 2001;**9**:788–805.
21. Sundquist J, Johansson SE. The influence of socioeconomic status, ethnicity and lifestyle on body mass index in a longitudinal study. *Int J Epidemiol* 1998;**27**:57–63.
22. Darmon N, Drewnowski A. Does social class predict diet quality? *Am J Clin Nutr* 2008;**87**:1107–17.
23. Karp RJ. Malnutrition among children in the United States. The impact of poverty. In: Shils ME, Shike M, Ross AC, Caballero B, Cousins RJ, editors. *"Modern Nutrition in Health and Disease"*. 10th edition. Baltimore, Maryland: Williams Wilkins Lippincott; 2005. pp. 860–74.
24. Bourdieu P. The forms of capital. In: Richardson J, editor. *"Handbook of Theory and Research for the Sociology of Education"*. New York: Greenwood Press; 1986. pp. 241–58.
25. Campbell RT. Substantive and statistical considerations in the interpretation of multiple measures of SES. *Social Forces* 1983;**62**:450–66.
26. Oakes JM, Rossib PH. The measurement of SES in health research: current practice and steps toward a new approach. *Soc Sci Med* 2003;**56**:769–84.
27. Farley R, Jackson WR. *"The Color Line and the Quality of Life in America"*. New York: Russell Sage; 1987.
28. Sampson W, Rossi PH. Race and family social standing. *Am Sociol Rev* 1975;**40**:201–14.
29. The Race, Ethnicity and Genetics Working Group. The use of racial, ethnic, and ancestral categories in human genetics research. *Am J Hum Genet* 2005;**77**:519–32.

30. Lillie-Blanton M, Parsons PE, Gayle H, Dievler A. Racial differences in health: not just black and white, but shades of gray. *Annu Rev Public Health* 1996;**17**:411–48.
31. Bourdieu P, Boltanski L. La production de l'idéologie dominante. *Actes de la Recherche en Sciences Sociales* ; 1976:2–3. 3-73.
32. Wang Y, Beydoun MA. The obesity epidemic in the United States—gender, age, socioeconomic, racial/ethnic, and geographical characteristics: a systematic review and meta-regression analysis. *Epidemiol Rev* 2007;**29**:6–28.
33. Organization for Economic Cooperation and Development. *"Growing Unequal? Income Distribution and Poverty in OECD Countries"*. Paris: Organization for Economic Cooperation and Development; 2008.
34. Ulijaszek SJ. Seven models of population obesity. *Angiology* 2008;**59**:34S–8S.
35. Baron S, Field J, Schuller T. *"Social Capital: Critical Perspectives"*. Oxford: Oxford University Press; 2000.
36. Christakis NA, Fowler JH. The spread of obesity in a large social network over 32 years. *N Engl J Med* 2007a;**357**:370–9.
37. Marmot M. *"Status Syndrome: How Your Social Standing Directly Affects Your Health and Life Expectancy.rldquo;*. London: Bloomsbury Press; 2004.
38. Isaacs JD, Stephen L, Schroeder SA. Class: the ignored determinant of the nation's health. *N Eng J Med* 2004;**351**:1137–42.
39. Donohoe M. Causes and health consequences of environmental degradation and social injustice. *Soc Sci Med* 2003;**56**:573–87.
40. Zhang Q, Wang Y. Socioeconomic inequality of obesity in the United States: do gender, age, and ethnicity matter? *Soc Sci Med* 2004;**58**:1171–80.
41. Centers for Disease Control. *Differences in prevalence of obesity among black, white, and Hispanic adults: United States, 2007–2008*, www.cdc.gov/mmwr/preview/mmwrhtml/mm5827.htm; 2009b. Accessed August 12, 2009.
42. Grieco EM, Cassidy RC. *Overview of race and Hispanic origin. Census 2000 Brief*, www.census.gov/prod/2001pubs/centbr01-1.pdf; 2001. Accessed August 12, 2009.
43. Mays VM, Ponce NA, Washington DL, Cochran SD. Classification of race and ethnicity: implications for public health. *Annu Rev Public Health* 2003;**24**:83–110.
44. Singh GK, Kogan MD, van Dyck PC, Siahpush M. Racial/ethnic, socioeconomic, and behavioral determinants of childhood and adolescent obesity in the United States: analyzing independent and joint associations. *Ann Epidemiol* 2008;**18**: 682–95.
45. Due P, Damsgaard MT, Rasmussen M, Holstein BE, Wardle J, Merlo J, Currie C, Ahluwalia N, Sørensen TIA, Lynch J, plus the HBSC obesity writing group. Socioeconomic position, macroeconomic environment and overweight among adolescents in 35 countries. *Int J Obes*; 2009. doi: 10.1038/ijo.2009.128.
46. Powell LM, Slater S, Mirtcheva D, Bao Y, Chaloupka FJ. Food store availability and neighbourhood characteristics in the United States Prev. *Med* 2007;**44**:189–95.
47. Gordon-Larsen P, Nelson MC, Page P, Popkin BM. Inequality in the built environment underlies key health disparities in physical activity and obesity. *Pediatr* 2006;**117**. 417-124.
48. Spence JC, Cutumisu N, Edwards J, Evans J. Influence of neighbourhood design and access to facilities on overweight among preschool children. *Int J Pediatr. Obes* 2008;**3**:109–16.
49. Oliver LN, Hayes MV. Neighbourhood socio-economic status and the prevalence of overweight Canadian children and youth. *Canadian J Publ Health* 2005;**96**:415–20.
50. Pagani LS, Huot C. Why are children living in poverty getting fatter? *Paediatr Child Health* 2007;**12**:698–700.
51. Swinburn BA, Egger G, Raza F. Dissecting obesogenic environments: the development and application of a framework for identifying and prioritizing environmental interventions for obesity. *Prev Med* 1999;**29**:563–70.
52. Jeffrey RW, French SA, Firster JL, Spry VM. Socioeconomic status differences in health behaviors related to obesity: the healthy worker project. *Int J Obes* 1991;**15**:689–96.
53. Stamatakis E, Primatesta P, Chinn S, Rona R, Falascheti E. Overweight and obesity trends from 1974 to 2003 in English children: what is the role of socioeconomic factors? *Arch Dis Childh* 2005;**90**:999–1004.
54. Braveman PA, Cubbin C, Egerter S, Chideya S, Marchi KS, Metzler M, Posner S. Socioeconomic status in health research. One size does not fit all. *J Am Med Assoc* 2005;**294**:2879–88.
55. Williams DR. Race/ethnicity and socioeconomic status: measurement and methodological issues. *Int J Health Serv* 1996;**26**:483–505.
56. Saenz R. Latinos and the Changing Face of America. Population Reference Bureau, Washington DC, (2009).
57. Price GN. Obesity and crime: Is there a relationship? *Economics Letters* 2009;**103**:149–52.
58. Flynn KJ, Fitzgibbon M. Body images and obesity risk among black females: a review of the literature. *Ann Behav Med* 1998;**20**: 13–24.
59. Stevens J, Kumanyika SK, Keil JE. Attitudes toward body size and dieting: differences between elderly black and white women. *Am J Publ Health* 1994;**84**:1322–5.
60. Becker DM, Yanek LR, Koffman DM, Bronner YC. Body image preferences among urban African Americans and whites from low income communities. *Ethn Dis* 1999;**9**:377–86.
61. Fitzgibbon ML, Blackman LR, Avellone ME. The relationship between body image discrepancy and body mass index across ethnic groups. *Obes Res* 2000;**8**:582–9.
62. Crago M, Shisslak CM, Estes LS. Eating disturbances among American minority groups: a review. *Int J Eating Disorders* 1996;**19**:239–48.
63. Harris MB, Koehler KM. Eating and exercise behaviors and attitudes of Southwestern Anglos and Hispanics. *Psychol Health* 1992;**7**:165–74.
64. Altabe M. Ethnicity and body image: Quantitative and qualitative analysis. *Int J Eating Disorders* 1998;**23**:153–9.
65. Rubin LR, Fitts ML, Becker AE. Whatever feels good in my soul: Body ethics and aesthetics among African American and Latina women. *Cult Med Psychiatr* 2003;**27**:49–75.
66. Stern MP, Pugh JA, Gaskill SP, Hazuda HP. Knowledge, attitudes, and behavior related to obesity and dieting in Mexican Americans and Anglos: The San Antonio Heart Study. *Am J Epidemiol* 1982;**115**:917–28.
67. Winkleby MA, Gardner CD, Taylor CB. The influence of gender and socioeconomic factors on Hispanic/white differences in body mass index. *Prev Med* 1996;**25**:203–11.
68. Anderson LA, Eyler AA, Galuska DA, Brown DR, Brownson RC. Relationship of satisfaction with body size and trying to lose weight in a national survey of overweight and obese women aged 40 and older, United States. *Prev Med* 2002;**35**:390–6.
69. Sherwood NE, Story M, Beech B, Klesges L, Mellin A, Neumark-Sztainer D, Davis M. Body image perceptions and dieting among African-American preadolescent girls and parents/caregivers. *Ethn Dis* 2003;**13**:200–7.
70. Katz ML, Gorden-Larsen P, Bentley ME, Kelsey K, Shields K, Ammerman A. Does skinny mean healthy? Perceived ideal, current, and healthy body sizes among African-American girls and their female caregiver. *Ethn Dis* 2004;**14**:533–41.
71. Anderson LA, Janes GR, Ziemer DC, Phillips LS. Diabetes in urban African Americans. Body image, satisfaction with size, and weight change attempts. *Diab Educ* 1997;**23**:301–8.

72. Bacardi-Gascon M, Jimenez-Cruz A, Jones E, Perez IV, Martinez JAL. Trends of Overweight and Obesity Among Children in Tijuana, Mexico. *Ecol Food Nutr* 2009;**48**:226—36.
73. Smith KV, Goldman N. Socioeconomic differences in health among older adults in Mexico. *Soc Sci Med* 2007;**65**:1372—85.
74. Bacardi-Gascon M, Leon-Reyes MJ, Jimenez-Cruz A. Stigmatization of overweight Mexican children. *Child Psych Human Dev* 2007;**38**:99—105.
75. Brewis AA, McGarvey ST, Jones J, Swinburn BA. Perceptions of body size in Pacific Islanders. *Int J Obes* 1998;**22**:185—9.
76. Hall SK, Cousins JH, Power TG. Self-concept and perceptions of attractiveness and body size among Mexican-American mothers and daughters. *Int J Obes* 1991;**15**:567—75.
77. Forth CE, Carden-Coyne A. *Cultures of the Abdomen. Diet, Digestion, and Fat in the Modern World*. Basingstoke, Hampshire: Palgrave Macmillan; 2005.
78. Dejong W. The stigma of obesity: the consequences of naïve assumptions concerning the causes of physical deviance. *J. Health Soc Behav* 1980;**21**:75—87.
79. Puhl R, Brownell KD. Bias, discrimination, and obesity. *Obes Res* 2001;**9**:788—805.
80. Andreyeva T, Puhl RM, Brownell KD. Changes in perceived weight discrimination among Americans, 1995—1996 through 2004—2006. *Obesity* 2008;**16**:1129—34.
81. Crosnoe R, Frank K, Strassmann A. Gender, body size and social relations in American high schools. *Social Forces* 2008;**86**:1189—216.
82. Bourdieu P. *Distinction: a Social Critique of the Judgment of Taste (R. Nice, translator)*. Cambridge, Massachusetts: Harvard University Press; 1984.
83. Nielsen J, Siega-Riz AM, Popkin BM. Trends in food locations and sources among adolescents and young adults. *Prev Med* 2002;**35**:107—13.
84. United States Department of Agriculture. *RDA's, Food Away, and Use of Supplements, 1994—96*. Agricultural Research Service, Food Surveys Research Group, www.ars.usda.gov/Services/docs.htm?docid=14531; 1999. Accessed August 17, 2009.
85. Paeratakul S, Ferdinand MN, Champagne CM, Ryan DH, Bray GA. Fast-food consumption among US adults and children: Dietary and nutrient intake profile. *J Am Dietet Assoc* 2003;**103**:1332—8.
86. Savige GS, Ball K, Worsley A. Food intake patterns among Australian adolescents. *Asia Pacific J Clin Nutr* 2007;**16**:738—47.
87. Mohr P, Wilson C, Dunn K, Brindal E, Wittert G. Personal and lifestyle characteristics predictive of the consumption of fast foods in Australia. *Publ Health Nutr* 2007;**12**:1456—63.
88. Powell LM, Bao YJ. Food prices, access to food outlets and child weight. *Econ Hum Biol* 2009;**7**:64—72.
89. Wiessner P, Schiefenhovel W. *"Food and the Status Quest"*. Oxford: Berghahn Books; 1996.
90. Nestle M. *"Food Politics: How the Food Industry Influences Nutrition and Health"*. University of California Press; Berkeley 2002.
91. Fiddes N. *"Meat. A Natural Symbol."* London: Routledge; 1991.
92. Fiddes N. Social aspects of meat eating. *Proc Nutr Soc* 1994;**53**:271—80.
93. Rosegrant MW, Paisner MS, Meijer S, Witcover J. *2020 Global Food Outlook, Trends, Alternatives, and Choices. A 2020 Vision for Food, Agriculture, and the Environment Initiative*. Washington, D.C: International Food Policy Research Institute; 2001.
94. Food and Agriculture Organization. *Food consumption*, www.faostat.org; 2009 (accessed July 15, 2009).
95. Gronhaug KG, Trapp PS. Perceived social class appeals of branded goods. *J Consumer Marketing* 1988;**5**:25—30.
96. Moore LV, Roux AV, Nettleton JA, Jacobs DR, Franco M. Fast-Food Consumption, Diet Quality, and Neighborhood Exposure to Fast Food. *Am J Epidemiol* 2009;**170**:29—36.
97. Mela D. Eating behaviour, food preferences and dietary intake in relation to obesity and body-weight status. *Proc Nutr Soc* 1996;**55**:803—16.
98. Falciglia G, Pabst S, Couch S, Goody C. Impact of parental food choices on child food neophobia. *Children's Health Care* 2004;**33**:217—25.
99. Borzekowski DL, Robinson TN. The 30-second effect: an experiment revealing the impact of television commercials on food preferences of preschoolers. *J Am Dietetic Assoc* 2001;**101**:42—6.
100. Moore ES. *Its child's play: advergaming and the online marketing of food to children. Kaiser Family Foundation Report*. Menlo Park, California: Henry J. Kaiser Family Foundation; 2006.
101. Gortmaker SL, Must A, Perrin JM, Sobol AM, Dietz WH. Social and Economic Consequences of Overweight in Adolescence and Young Adulthood. *N Engl J Med* 1993;**329**:1008—12.
102. McLaren L, Kuh D. Women's body dissatisfaction, social class, and social mobility. *Soc Sci Med* 2004;**58**:1575—84.
103. Rose SJ. *Social Stratification in the United States: The American Profile Poster Revised and Expanded*. New York: The New Press; 2007.
104. Kendall D. Class in the United States: Not only alive but reproducing. Research in Soc. *Stratification Mobility* 2006;**24**:89—104.
105. Puhl RM. Perceptions of weight discrimination. *Int J Obes* 2008;**32**:992—1000.
106. Carr D, Jaffe KJ, Friedman MA. Perceived interpersonal mistreatment among obese Americans: do race, class, and gender matter? *Obesity* 2008;**16**:S60—8.
107. Latner JD, O'Brien KS, Durso LE, Brinkman LA, MacDonald T. Weighing obesity stigma: the relative strength of different forms of bias. *Int J Obes* 2008;**32**:1145—52.
108. Tang-Peronard JL, Heitman BL. Stigmatization of obese children and adolescents, the importance of gender. *Obes Rev* 2008;**9**:522—34.
109. Wang L. Weight discrimination: one size fits all remedy? *Yale Law Rev* 2008;**117**:1900—45.
110. Galtung J. Violence, peace and peace research. *J Peace Res* 1969;**6**:167—91.
111. Tanner JM. Growth as a mirror of the condition of society: secular trends and class distinctions. In: Demirjian A, editor. *Human Growth. A Multidisciplinary Review*. London: Taylor & Francis; 1986. pp. 3—34.

CHAPTER 44

Childhood Obesity, Food Choice and Market Influence

Jane Kolodinsky, Amanda Goldstein, Erin Roche

University of Vermont, Department of Community Development and Applied Economics and the Food Systems Research Collaborative at the Center for Rural Studies and Burlington, VT, USA

INTRODUCTION: THE DGA AND THEN SOME, OR SMALL FRIES AND A COKE, PLEASE

French fries are the most common vegetable fed to toddlers [1]. A french fry is classified as a vegetable according to the Dietary Guidelines for Americans (DGA), but one small fast-food serving of fries contains 290 calories, half (142 calories) of which come from added fats. This small serving of french fries contains about a tablespoon of fat, the equivalent of the daily requirement of added fats and oils for toddlers [2].

Even counting french-fried potatoes as a vegetable, between 78% and 90% of children ages 2 and older still do not meet the recommended intake for vegetables on any given day. The average across all children is about 1 cup per day, whereas 1.5 cups is recommended [2, 3]. Further, there is evidence that Americans' preference for fruits and vegetables is on the decline [4]. More troubling is that the most common fruits and vegetables consumed by adolescents, such as french fries, are not the nutrient-dense ones that correlate with decreased risk for multiple chronic diseases [3].

At the same time, children's consumption of milk has been declining since 1965, while consumption of soda and fruit-flavored beverages has been increasing [5]. On average, adolescents meet only 74% of their daily calcium requirements [6]. The substitution of sweetened beverages for milk both decreases protein and calcium intakes and increases the intake of added sugars. This is particularly troubling because calcium has been shown to play a role in energy metabolism [6].

More evidence pointing to increased consumption of dietary fats and sugars is the trend toward eating meals away from home. Away-from-home food expenditures accounted for approximately 44% of all food expenditures in 2007, and it has been estimated that in 2010, 53% of money allocated toward food will be spent away from home [7, 8]. Restaurant sales have increased 312% since the late 1980s and in 2006 represented $511 billion in sales [8]. Away-from-home food accounts for nearly half of all food dollars spent, up 25% since 1995 [9]. Both industry and government estimates indicate continued growth [8, 10]. In addition, food purchased at restaurants is reported to be at least 1.4 times higher in energy density as compared to food prepared at home, higher in sodium and saturated fat, and lower in fiber and calcium [11–13].

Restaurants and food manufacturers capitalize on Americans' love of a good value and offer increasingly larger portions at low prices [14]. Especially in fast-food outlets, larger sizes are used as selling points and as enticement to customers [15]. For example, spending only $1.57 more on a cheeseburger buys 600 extra calories, 64 more cents spent on french fries buys 330 more calories, and 37 cents can buy 450 more soft drink calories [16]. Although much of the research focuses on adults, there are data that show children are also moving toward higher intakes from food away from home [17]. Furthermore, many adults are caregivers, and children often eat what their caregivers eat.

The number of children and adolescents specifically eating at fast-food restaurants has increased over time [17]. Fast-food outlets are popular among adolescents such that, on average, they eat at a fast-food restaurant twice a week [18]. On a typical day, 30% of youth aged 4 to 19 consume fast food [19]. With fast food being higher in fat and energy, children get a disproportionate number of their recommended daily calories at these establishments. Plus, consumption of fast foods has been linked with decreased consumption of fruits, vegetables, and milk; higher total energy, and an increase in relative body mass index (BMI) in adolescents [20–22]. Even among toddlers, 57.4% consume at least a single meal or snack away from home in a typical day [23].

Because dietary patterns are formed early in childhood and persist into adolescence and adulthood, facts about childhood food behaviors should sound alarm bells for professionals, government officials, and family members alike [24–26]. We are seeing patterns: increases in consumption of energy-dense but nutrient-poor foods, decreases in fruit and vegetable consumption, increases in food away-from-home consumption higher in fat and calories, decreases in fluid milk consumption, and preferences moving away from vegetables. All these point to "more calories in than out" at younger ages. The obesity epidemic can have negative consequences not only for individuals, but also for the many social, medical, and economic systems in which they interact.

OBESITY AS A PROBLEM

Obesity is clearly a public health concern in the United States. Comparing data since the 1980s, the prevalence of obesity has increased for children aged 6 to 11 years from 6.5% to 17% and for those aged 12 to 19 years from 5% to 17.6% [27–29]. From 2000 to 2005 alone, the nationwide prevalence of obesity for all age groups increased by 24%, with the largest weight increases occurring within heaviest BMI groups [30]. Between 2003 and 2006, 11.3% of children and adolescents aged 2 through 19 years were at or above the 97th weight percentile of the 2000 BMI-for-age growth charts, 16.3% were at or above the 95th percentile, and 31.9% were at or above the 85th percentile [28]. Further, 2007 National Youth Risk Behavior Survey data indicate that among high school students, 13% were obese.

The relationship between food choice and obesity in both youth and adults is well documented, and food choice patterns associated with adult obesity develop in youth [31–34]. What one learns and does as a child and young adult influences how one acts in adulthood. In addition, overweight and obese children are likely to remain so throughout adulthood. Overweight adolescents have a 70% chance of becoming overweight or obese adults [35]. If one or more of their parents are overweight or obese, that likelihood increases to 80%. So a logical entry point to addressing obesity is to direct interventions toward children and adolescents.

Not merely an aesthetics problem, obesity is costly in terms of health and economics. As evidence of its magnitude, in 2008 the Centers for Disease Control and Prevention (CDC) reported approximately 300,000 obesity-related deaths compared to 38,000 new AIDS diagnoses in each of the previous 5 years (and 16,000 deaths from AIDS-related causes in the same time frame) [36]. Traditionally seen as "adult" problems, obesity-related chronic diseases are increasingly diagnosed at younger and younger ages [37]. Specifically, type 2 diabetes has emerged as a critical health issue in overweight children, with one study reporting a 10-fold increase between 1982 and 1994 [38–40]. Overweight and obesity in youth are also associated with various risk factors for cardiovascular disease (i.e., hypertension, development of arthrosclerotic lesions, and accelerated coronary arthrosclerosis) [41–45].

The cost in dollars resulting from obesity-related health conditions is large and growing. Almost 10% of all healthcare expenditures in the United States are attributable to being overweight [46, 47]. The rate of hospitalizations among adolescents alone for obesity-related diagnoses rose dramatically during the 1980s, while the cost of inpatient care tripled [48]. These trends are potentially devastating to an already overburdened healthcare system because they add an entire new generation to the health bill while another generation is still living. There must be a tipping point; with that comes the possibility of "breaking the bank." The average annual family health insurance premium in 2009 was 34% higher than the average family premium was in 2004 and 131% higher than in 1999 [49].

WHAT YOUNG PEOPLE EAT: SOFAAS, NOT FRUIT 'N' VEG

How did we reach the current level of obesity, and what role does nutrition and food choice play? We must look at what people are eating and then assess what makes them eat such foods. Only then can we begin to address the behaviors that make individuals obese.

Much attention has been paid to fruit and vegetable consumption by adolescents based on ethnicity, health status, gender, and income level [50–54]. The 2005 Youth Risk Behavior Survey results indicated that only 18% of twelfth grade students consumed the recommended amount of fruits and vegetables, a decline in the percentage since ninth grade. For children aged 2 to 11, mean numbers of daily servings were below minimum recommendations for all food groups except the dairy group [55]. In fact, 16% of youth did not meet any recommendations, and only 1% met all recommendations. Numerous studies have found that overweight children demonstrate less desirable food habits [3, 56, 57]. Nutrient-dense foods have been replaced with diets deriving many calories from solid fats, alcohol, and added sugars. The U.S. Department of Agriculture (USDA) now specifically guides people to stay away from these foods called SoFAAS [58].

Research confirms that young adults also do not eat a healthy diet. One study found that just 30% of first-year college students reported getting the recommended five daily servings of fruits and vegetables, and half of these college students ate high-fat foods more frequently than recommended [59, 60]. Further, their eating habits did not generally improve by their second year [60]. Especially troubling, many college students reported eating no servings of fruits or vegetables [60–62]. Other studies have found that college women eat less than one serving of fruit and 2.4 servings of vegetables per day, and only one quarter of all college students report getting the recommended servings of fruits and vegetables [63, 64]. Another study found that half or more of college students on a meal plan report eating at least the recommended amount of fruits and vegetables; however, the purchase data show that students are not buying amounts of fruits and vegetables equal to the DGA recommendations in the dining hall [65]. On average, the students in this study were about $^3/_4$ cup short of making purchases that meet the recommendations for fruit and more than $1^1/_2$ cups short for vegetables, similar to the findings of others who researched college student eating patterns and used serving size measures [62, 65].

Dairy consumption, especially among young women, was also below the recommended levels [64]. Only 14% drank more than three glasses of milk [66]. College women consumed just 1.3 servings of dairy [63]. On the other hand, 33.8% of high school students drink soda at least one time a day [67].

Consumption of energy-dense snack foods that are high in solid fats and added sugar is likely contributing to a diet that does not meet DGA recommendations. Research shows that snacking among young adults aged 19 to 29 increased dramatically between 1977–1978 and 1994–1996 [68]. Not only did the amount of energy consumed per snacking occasion increase, but the number of snacks per day as well as the caloric density of each snack also increased. Sebastian et al. found that foods consumed as snacks provided 35% of the day's total discretionary calorie intake and 43% of total added sugar intake [69].

With increased snacking, there is greater overall daily caloric intake and a propensity toward obesity, because despite the energy density, people consume the same volume of food. Therefore, high consumption of energy-dense foods is associated with high-energy intakes [70, 71]. However, caloric value is not synonymous with nutrition, and consuming energy does not ensure good nutrition. While rich in calories, energy-dense foods are typically low in nutrients and can dilute the overall quality, or nutrient density, of the diet [72, 73].

The news isn't all bad, however. Weight gain among college freshmen has been documented, but on average it is much more modest than the mythical "freshman fifteen" [74, 75]. College-age students who live on campus or are on a meal plan may have better eating habits than their peers, but most still do not meet the Food Pyramid guidelines [34, 62]. Another study found that more students met the recommended amounts who participated in a university meal plan than those who did not, especially for fruits and meat, suggesting the importance of access and availability in achieving healthy choices [62]. Furthermore, college students and graduates ate more foods high in dietary fiber, more grains and dark green vegetables, and more lower-fat milk and meat than nonstudents [64].

INFLUENCES ON DIETARY CONSUMPTION

Why are children not eating a healthy diet? There are numerous factors related directly to food that contribute to food choice behaviors, such as price, availability, taste, value, knowledge, nutrition, and time [71, 77–84]. There are also other factors, including demographic characteristics, region of residence, cultural heritage, and parental influence [85–88]. Furthermore, it is impossible to ignore the intervening effects of the marketplace.

Food group consumption has been shown to vary by age, income, education, and ethnicity [85–88]. Many studies have concluded that lower-income households spend less per person for food than higher-income households [89-93]. Of the total spent on food by individuals receiving food assistance, only 9% was spent on vegetables and 7% on fruits [90, 91]. Those small expenditure shares translate into low-cost spending on fresh foods and do not allow individuals to meet the 1999 Dietary Guidelines [83].

Compounding the effects of less income for food purchase is decreased access to and availability of cheaper foods for poor people. Types and sizes of grocery stores differ by geographical location and region. In low-income areas, smaller groceries and convenience stores selling fewer large-size or bulk items are more prevalent than large supermarkets [78, 79, 81]. Poorer people are more likely to shop at those local smaller stores because they may lack convenient transportation [77]. However, those local stores do not provide a great variety of options and offer few large-item choices, leading people of lower socioeconomic status to not only pay more for their food, but to receive lower-quality items [77, 88].

When shopping at any location, purchasing energy-dense foods is employed as a money-saving strategy; it allows people to consume a high amount of energy at a low cost [76]. Energy-dense foods, including those higher in SoFAAS, are those with little water content and tend to be high in fat, sugar, and starch. Energy density is inversely linked to energy cost such that dietary energy intake can be maintained at a lower cost to the consumer [93]. However, it is not just those in poverty who are affected. Affluent consumers also face increasing prevalence and affordability of such foods in the marketplace [15].

Furthermore, foods that are nutritious are relatively costly, as calories provided by whole grains, fresh produce, and lean meats are more expensive than calories from refined grains, added sugars, and added fats [96]. In addition, raw food items can require significant time input (in the forms of meal preparation time and kitchen labor) to create a meal, and people increasingly do not have excess time in a day [95]. Time-saving tactics can be observed in people's food choices, eating behaviors, and food provisioning. Mothers, in particular, have reported employing the following strategies to combat time constraints: replacing home-cooked meals with fast food, restaurant takeout, "meals in a box," or microwave dinners; sacrificing nutrition for a quick meal; eating faster; and shortening food consumption periods [96–99]. As dependents, children eat what their parents provide regardless of the meal's nutritive value.

Relying on packaged and away-from-home foods might also stem from decreased knowledge of how to cook. Home economic courses teaching food preparation skills are no longer required classes throughout primary and secondary education. Perhaps such programs are still necessary because several studies have shown increased fruit and vegetable consumption and vitamin intake resulting from learning cooking skills [100–103]. Stookey and Barker also reported a negative association between cooking skills and convenience food consumption [100]. Evidence exists that suggest food skills interventions may be a useful starting point for initiating dietary change [103].

Whether due to lack of knowledge, lack of time, or affordability and availability of convenience foods, it is apparent that people do not prepare meals as much as they used to. The amount of time spent preparing food and cleaning up since the 1960s has dropped by nearly 50% for women [95, 104]. Supermarkets have reacted by increasing their selection of prepared convenience foods, catalyzing a consumer response. Individuals currently spend 35% of their total food-eaten-at-home dollars on packaged, prepared goods [7, 107]. One result of this trend is that food preparation is not modeled for children and they do not learn how to prepare food for themselves. As evidence of that, per capita consumption of at-home fresh vegetables has experienced slower growth rates among younger consumers [106].

The cycle of buying increasing amounts of packaged foods and food away from home is self-perpetuating. Technological innovations and agricultural policy have allowed food manufacturers to increase the available amount and variety of processed high-fat snack foods [7, 106, 108]. That has led to the increase in snacking mentioned earlier. Not only has the frequency of snacking increased, but there has also been a marked increase in the portion sizes of foods being consumed [15, 109].

As portions have grown, they have become more dissociated from government-recommended serving sizes for healthful eating [14]. Specifically, foods with the highest excess above USDA standard portion sizes are those in the cookies (700%), pasta (480%), muffins (333%), steaks (224%), and bagels (195%) categories [15]. Children are becoming confused and fail to recognize correct portion sizes [110]. They report preferences for portions of french fries, meats, and potato chips that are larger and vegetable portions that are smaller than what is recommended. As with increasing consumption of energy-dense food, larger portions do not result in eating fewer meals. Instead, growing portions result in people eating more [111–113].

Furthermore, chronic exposure to large portions and the ensuing overeating does not deter one from continuing to eat more. Jeffery et al. found that even over time, people sustained increases in energy intake due to snacking [114]. To such an extent that the "effects of portion size may be powerful enough to affect rate of weight gain over time" [114]. Further leading to the potential for weight gain is lack of compensation for larger portion sizes by decreased consumption at other times in the day [115].

MEDIATING EFFECTS ON FOOD CHOICE

Although they have just been discussed in detail in isolation, the variables that impact food choice (Fig. 44.1) are moderated by the influence of the market and home environment on individuals. The marketplace, through both sponsored and nonsponsored information, seeks to influence choices made by consumers. However, knowledge of nutrition passed down through culture and parental transfer can allow consumers to interpret and counteract marketing messages.

The hierarchical model used in fields of marketing and consumer behavior identifies three phases of behavior. The first stage is cognitive including actions

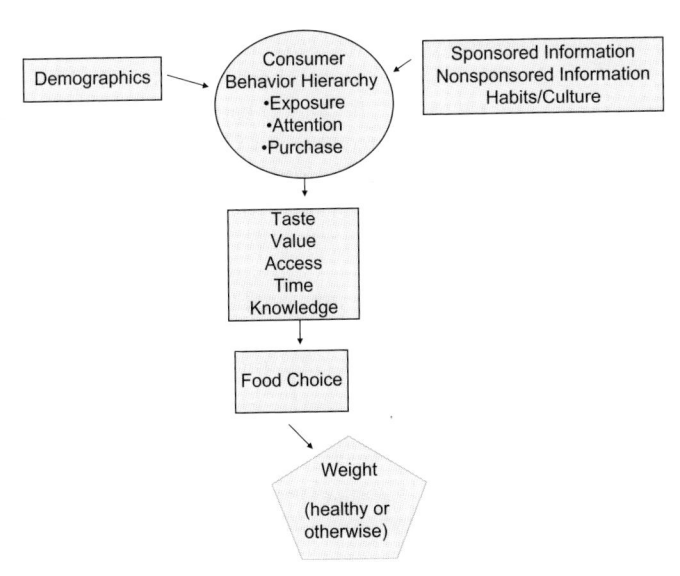

FIGURE 44.1 Consumer behavior model of food choice and obesity-mediating effects of sponsored and nonsponsored information.

such as attention, exposure, and awareness [116]. The second stage is affective and incorporates interest, knowledge, and evaluation. The third stage is behavior including intent and action. This model provides a useful lens to better understand food choice behavior, especially among children and young adults who have not yet formed habits regarding food choice. Understanding how preferences are established is an important element to predicting food choice behavior.

Private and public industry information affects the cognition and attitudinal stages. The goal of private advertisement campaigns, or sponsored information, is to convince consumers to buy specific products. In 2008, the food and beverage sector spent approximately $7.8 billion on advertising, which is 5.5% of all U.S. measured media advertising [117]. However, the money spent on soft drink advertising has increased at a faster rate than overall food-related advertising [118]. Spending for advertising soft drinks rose from $541 million in 1995 to $799 million in 1999 (50%), whereas overall food-related advertising over the same period increased less than 20%. Currently, advertising budgets are much higher, as Coca Cola Company alone spent $752.1 million in 2008 and PepsiCo spent $1.29 billion [117].

Not only do food and beverage manufacturers directly target children and adolescents, advertising has been found to affect food preferences for children even as young as 2 years [119, 120]. Powell et al. found that in 2003, 27.2% of children's exposure to total nonprogram content time was for food-related product advertising [121]. Cereal accounted for 27.6%, sweets and snacks for 19.9%, fast-food restaurants for 12%, beverages for 8.8%, non-fast-food restaurants for 5.4% and other foods such as beef, bread, cheese, and hot dogs accounted for 16.3%. On the other hand, only 0.8% of total nonprogram content time exposure was for all public service announcements combined.

Industry-sponsored advertisements are not the only types of information available to consumers. The U.S. government provides dietary guidelines and various government agencies and nonprofit organizations sponsor educational public service announcements. However, the amount of money spent by industry dwarfs that spent by federal and state governments to promote nutrition and other healthy behaviors. For example, "5 a day for better health" is a social marketing campaign that encourages more positive nutrition behaviors among American consumers. The "5 a day" campaign is a partnership between government, industry, and nonprofit organizations and has helped increase the percentage of Americans consuming five or more servings of fruits and vegetables per day from 23% in 1991 to 35% in 2003 [122]. In 2004, $9.55 million was spent on communications for the federal and California "5 a day" programs to encourage eating five or more servings of fruit and vegetables each day [123]. During that same year, $11.26 billion was spent on advertising by the food, beverage, and restaurant industries. In other words, industry expenditures for food, beverage, and fast-food advertising were 1178 times greater than the budgets for the California and federal "5 a day" campaigns.

Other behavior change programs include the U.S. *Got milk?* campaign, the U.S. Department of Health and Human Services' Centers for Disease Control and Prevention's (CDC) VERB™ Campaign, and a recent attempt by New York City's public health officials to encourage individuals to replace sugary drinks with lower-calorie beverages. The *Got milk?* ad campaign cost $110 million and ran over 5 years, yet it did not increase milk sales [124]. However, there is 90% awareness among teenagers and a report of college students meeting dietary guidelines for dairy but no other food group [125, 126].

The CDC launched a national, multicultural, social marketing campaign in 2002 that ran through 2006 to increase and maintain physical activity among youth aged 9 to 13. The VERB campaign encouraged children and adolescents to be physically active every day through paid advertising, marketing strategies, and partnership efforts to reach the distinct audiences of 9- to 13-year-olds. It achieved high levels of awareness in its first year with higher levels of physical activity reported for subgroups of U.S. children [127]. New York City public health officials spent $277,000 over 3 fiscal years (including money for creative work and focus groups) to develop advertisements discouraging viewers from consuming sugary sodas and juice drinks. The ads, which graphically portray negative the effects of sugar-sweetened beverage consumption and provide text promoting lower-calorie substitutes, will run in 1500 subway cars for 3 months.

Recognizing that getting attention through witty tag lines and intriguing imagery is only part of the solution, the U.S. government provides detailed recommendations and advice concerning food behaviors and consumption amounts in its Dietary Guidelines for Americans (DGA). These guidelines are jointly issued and updated every 5 years by the Departments of Agriculture and Health and Human Services to provide authoritative advice for people 2 years and older about how good dietary habits can promote health and reduce risk for major chronic diseases. The DGA recommendations also advocate the importance of physical activity in combination with quality dietary consumption as a means of achieving optimal health. The DGA recommendations are not tailored to specific individuals but generally encourage consumption of a healthy diet as defined by ample amounts of fruits and vegetables, whole grains, and fat-free or low-fat dairy products; inclusion of lean meats, poultry, fish, beans, eggs, and nuts; and limited intake of saturated fats, trans fats, cholesterol, salt (sodium), and added sugars [128]. The 2005 edition of the Dietary Guidelines remain current until the next edition is released in 2010.

MyPyramid (Fig. 41.2) accompanies the DGA and provides a memorable graphical representation that reminds individuals to make smart choices from every food group; find balance between food and physical activity; get the most nutrition out of calories; and stay within daily calorie needs. The various colors represent the food groups (orange is for grains; green, vegetables; red, fruits; yellow, oils; blue, milk; and purple, meat and beans) and correspond in width to the proportion of entire diet they should comprise. MyPyramid and the DGA make recommendations for people to get necessary nutrients and avoid foods with low nutritional value, but they do not implicitly address how to ensure the right number of calories. Mypyramid.gov provides an interactive platform for preschoolers and older children through interactive games, posters, and exercises designed to acquaint them with the DGA.

Nutrition labels are required on most packaged foods and, in conjunction with MyPyramid, provide nutrition information about specific food products. Numerous studies have shown a link between use of nutrition labels on packaged food and consumer attitudes and preferences [129]. Some studies have shown links between nutrition label use and general changes in dietary patterns as well as decreases in intake of fat [130–134]. Studies have also shown links between education interventions and nutrition knowledge and improved choices [135–138]. Further, there is some indication that the labeling of food products along with educational campaigns have a positive effect on consumer choice, though these studies have not specifically included labels on restaurant menus, but examined labels in the context of the National Labeling and Education Act (NLEA) for packaged foods [139–142].

There is some evidence that simple labels highlighting lower-fat choices can make a positive difference and that reading food labels is associated with self-reported lower intakes of fat [133, 139, 143, 144]. A study of fast-food restaurants in New York City, before the 2008 labeling regulations took effect, suggests a connection between seeing calorie information and purchase behavior [145]. However, unless consumers understand the information that is provided in restaurants, it will not be useful [146]. A limited number of studies show that menu labels combined with an education intervention improve food choices [147–149].

Nutrition labeling requirements only apply to packaged foods. Foods purchased in raw form, such as fresh produce, and food purchased in restaurants or other away-from-home food outlets are typically not labeled. The FDA does currently require some restaurant labeling under the Nutrition Labeling and Education Act of 1990, but these regulations only apply to menu items specifically claimed to be healthy. The regulation also allows nutrition information to be provided by any "reasonable means," not requiring information to be on menus, nor to use the U.S. packaged-food standard "Nutrition Facts" format [144].

However, communities are increasingly concerned about obesity and see new labeling on restaurant menus as a weapon to combat obesity. Despite the gap in the academic literature and lack of guidance from the FDA, legislation has been introduced at the local, state, and national levels that would give consumers additional information on restaurant menu items [150]. In September 2008, the LEAN Act was introduced in the U.S. Senate, and California became the first state to

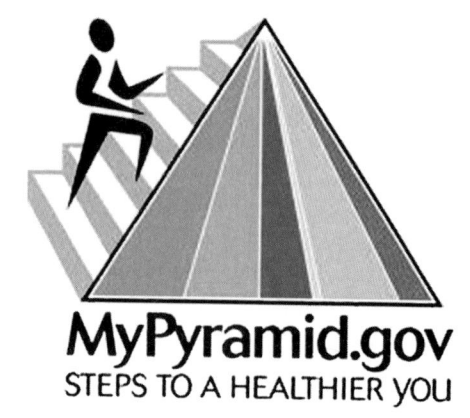

FIGURE 41.2 Pyramid tracker.

pass menu labeling legislation though many other states have legislation pending [150–152]. Menu labeling regulations adopted in 2006 in New York City have withstood legal tests and were finally enacted in 2008, meaning that New York City joins other local communities like King County, Washington, and the city of San Francisco in regulating menu information [145, 153, 154]. In 2010, many other states introduced menu labeling legislation.

RECENT STEPS IN THE RIGHT DIRECTION

The U.S. Department of Agriculture Food and Nutrition Service released the interim rules on a new Women, Infants, and Children (WIC) food package in 2007. The ruling states the following: The new food packages align with the 2005 Dietary Guidelines for Americans and infant feeding practice guidelines of the American Academy of Pediatrics. The food packages better promote and support the establishment of successful, long-term breast-feeding, provide WIC participants with a wider variety of foods including fruits and vegetables and whole grains, and provide WIC state agencies greater flexibility in prescribing food packages to accommodate the cultural food preferences of WIC participants [155]. Providing a wider variety of fruits, vegetables, and whole grains in packages available to low-income mothers with children is a step in the right direction with regard to increasing exposure to healthier food choices.

The 2010 Dietary Guidelines for Americans is currently in the early comment stage. Many of the early comments are from industry representatives who continue to urge a science-based approach to the final guidelines. The 2005 DGA process can be characterized as a battle between industry and academics. The final language of the 2005 DGA was moderate in scope, including phrases such as "don't sugarcoat it" and "make smart choices from every group" [156]. Banter at professional meetings throughout the development period for the 2005 DGA included discussions about nutritionists wanting stronger language about limiting added sugars and fats. Perhaps these discussions, along with the continued increase in childhood obesity, have paved the way for more transparent language in the 2010 DGA.

Government regulations and mandates aside, communities and other stakeholders are testing creative solutions to address obesity in children. Recognizing the need to catch the problem at its onset, the following programs are directed at youth. The overarching goal is to intervene when children are forming dietary habits so they gain nutrition knowledge and grow into healthy adolescents and adults. It is children who are the most capable warriors in the war against obesity.

In 2009, Whole Foods launched a national initiative to improve nutritional content of school meals. Called the "School Lunch Revolution," it provides resources to food service directors to help them replace frozen, processed foods with fresh, made-from-scratch foods. The initiative asks Congress to support stronger nutritional requirements in the National School Lunch Program, a part of the Child Nutrition Act being considered for reauthorization in 2010.

The state of Texas has passed legislation requiring that schools not provide students with access to foods of minimal nutritional value, including carbonated beverages, sweetened waters, chewing gum, and candy. School cafeterias are also prohibited from frying meals [157]. At the federal level, the USDA Fresh Fruit and Vegetable Program introduces children to fresh fruit and vegetables and provides funds to states to support programs aimed at this goal and to purchase fresh fruit and vegetables.

Farm-to-School (F2S) initiatives have been shown to improve children's eating habits on multiple levels. Using more locally produced foods in school meal and snack programs directly increases students' consumption of fresh fruits and vegetables; this impact is particularly important for students from low-income families who are often dependent on the National School Lunch and Breakfast Programs for daily nutritional intake. As a boon to school lunch programs, F2S programs consistently show increases (between 4% and 16%) in school meal participation rates [158–160]. Furthermore, one California school meal cost analysis showed that participation rate increases of merely 8% or more can offset additional costs of labor related to an F2S salad bar program [159].

Experiential education that connects children to the sources of their food—such as school gardens, field trips to farms, classroom visits from farmers, and cooking projects that teach about nutrition using local ingredients—improve students' food preferences and eating behaviors in meaningful ways that will nourish them throughout their lives [161].

Recent private/public partnerships including Smart Choices, guiding stars, and NuVal rate the nutritional quality of foods on supermarket shelves using nutritional guidelines. Although some individuals and groups are quite critical of these programs, products participating in any of the programs must meet at least minimal nutritional standards. Guiding stars and NuVal are proprietary and do not reveal their nutritional grading methods [162, 163]. Smart Choices reveals the minimum standards any product must meet in order to qualify for a front-of-package label [164]. However, the Center for Science in the Public Interest (CSPI) has questioned industry-led initiatives and has urged the Food and Drug Administration (FDA) to initiate federal standards about front-of-package "summary" labels [165].

First Lady Michelle Obama's recent "Let's Move" campaign may be just what the public needs with regard to balancing the responsibility of childhood obesity among government, industry, and the individual [166]. Its three-pronged approach to giving parents information, improving school food choices, and encouraging physical activity is a commonsense approach with wide appeal.

Overall, a variety of efforts are under way to help children and families make healthier food choices that keep their calorie and nutrient intakes in line with the DGA. Evaluation research is needed to determine which, if any, program is successful in stemming the rising tide of childhood obesity.

CONCLUSION

Obesity is a growing problem in children of all ages. It is clear that children are not meeting the DGA recommendations for several food categories and, in general, consume too many added sugars and solid fats. The solution to the obesity epidemic is not as easy as giving advice to "change what you eat," however. A large number of variables are at work that contribute to keeping the energy balance equation out of balance. At the organizational level, the food industry has used techniques including sponsored communication, value menus with distorted portion sizes, and large promotional budgets to move children's food choice preferences toward higher-calorie, less nutrient rich options. Families are increasingly faced with pressures of both time and money and are also swayed into purchasing convenience foods and restaurant meals as a way to be more efficient in their meal preparation. The federal government and public service spending to promote DGA guidelines and healthier choices is dwarfed by the resources of the private sector used to persuade children and the "food gatekeepers" in their households to spend on other types of foods. Although less quantified when compared to adult obesity, there is little doubt that excess weight is leading to increases in the rate of chronic disease at younger ages, with an undeniable impact on the cost of healthcare. A number of community-based, and public/private partnerships are emerging to develop programs that help households make healthier choices. Clearly, a multifaceted approach is necessary to curb the growth in obesity in U.S. children.

References

1. Morin KH. Update on what and how much infants and toddlers eat. *The Am J Mat Child Nurs* 2006;**31**(4):269.
2. US Department of Agriculture. MyPyramid.gov: Steps to a Healthier You. www.mypyramid.gov. Published April 19, 2005. Updated June 18, 2008. Accessed June 15, 2006.
3. Lorson BA, Melgar-Quinonez HR, Taylor CA. Correlates of fruit and vegetable intakes in US children. *J Am Diet Assoc* 2009; **109**(3):474–8.
4. Stewart H, Blisard N. Are younger cohorts demanding less fresh vegetables? *Rev Ag Econ* 2008;**30**(1):43–60.
5. Cavadini C, Siega-Riz AM, Popkin BM. US adolescent food intake trends from 1965 to 1996. *BMJ* 2000;**83**(1):18–24.
6. Zemel MB, Miller SL. Dietary calcium and dairy modulation of adiposity and obesity risk. *Nutr Rev* 2004;**62**(4):125–31.
7. Bureau of Labor Statistics. *Consumer Expenditures in 2007*. Washington, DC: US Department of Labor; 2009.
8. National Restaurant Association. *Restaurant Industry Facts At a Glance*. Available at, www.restaurant.org/research/ind_glance.cfm; 2008. Accessed June 23, 2008.
9. Stewart H, Blisard N, Bhuyan S, Nayga Jr RM. *The Demand for Food Away From Home: Full Service or Fast-Food?* Washington, DC: Economic Research Service/USDA, Agriculture Economics Report No. 33953; 2004. Available at: http://purl.umn.edu/33953.
10. Blissard N, Lin B-H, Cromartie J, Ballenger N. America's Changing Appetite: Food Consumption and Spending to 2020. *Food Review* 2002;**25**(1):2–9.
11. Variyam JN. *Nutrition Labeling in the Food-Away-From-Home Sector: An Economic Assessment*. Washington, DC: Economic Research Service/USDA, Economic Research Report No. 7235; 2005. Available at: http://purl.umn.edu/7235.
12. Lin B-H, Frazao E. *Away-From-Home Foods Increasingly Important to Quality of American Diet*. Washington, D.C: Economic Research Service/USDA, Agriculture Information Bulletin No. 749; 1999.
13. Guthrie JF, Smallwood DM. Evaluating the effects of the Dietary Guidelines for Americans on consumer behavior and health: Methodological challenges. *J Am Diet Assoc* 2003;**2**:S42–9.
14. Rolls BJ. The supersizing of America: Portion size and the obesity epidemic. *Nutrition Today* 2003;**38**(2):42.
15. Young LR, Nestle M. The contribution of expanding portion sizes to the US obesity epidemic. *Am J Pub Health* 2002;**92**(2):246–9.
16. The National Alliance for Nutrition and Activity (NANA). *From Wallet to Waistline: The Hidden Costs of Super Sizing*. Washington, DC: NANA; 2002.
17. Lin BH, Frazao E, Guthrie J. *Away-From-Home Foods Increasingly Important to Quality of American Diet*. Washington, D.C: Economic Research Service/USDA, Agriculture Information Bulletin No. 749; 1999.
18. Jekanowski MD. Causes and consequences of fast food sales growth. *Food Review* 1999;**22**:11–16.
19. Bowman SA, Vinyard BT. Fast Food Consumption of U.S. Adults: Impact on Energy and Nutrient and Overweight Status. *J Am CollNutr* 2004;**23**(2):163–8.
20. Sebastian RS, Goldman JD, U.S. Department of Agriculture, A. US adolescents and MyPyramid: Associations between fast-food consumption and lower likelihood of meeting recommendations. *J Am Diet Assoc* 2009;**109**(2):226–35.
21. French SA, Story M, Jeffery RW. Environmental influences on eating and physical activity. *Ann Rev Pub Health* 2001;**22**(1):309–35.
22. Thompson OM, Ballew C, Resnicow K. Food purchased away from home as a predictor of change in BMI Z-score among girls. *Int J Obes* 2004;**28**:282–9.
23. Ziegler P, Briefel R, Ponza M, Novak T, Hendricks K. Nutrient intakes and food patterns of toddlers' lunches and snacks: Influence of location. *J Am Diet Assoc* 2006;**106**:124–34.
24. Birch LL. Development of food acceptance patterns in the first years of life. *Proc Nutr Soc* 1998;**57**(4):617–24.
25. Lytle P, Seifert MPH, Greenstein MS, McGovern P. How do children's eating patterns and food choices change over time? Results from a cohort study. *Am J Health Prom* 2000;**14**(4):222–8.

REFERENCES

26. Nader PR, Stone EJ, Lytle LA, Perry CL, Osganian SK, Kelder S. Three-year maintenance of improved diet and physical activity: The CATCH cohort. *Arch PedAdol Med* 1999;**153**(7):695–704.
27. Centers for Disease Control and Prevention. NHANES data on the Prevalence of Overweight among Children and Adolescents: United States, 2003–2004. *National Center for Health Statistics*. Available at, www.cdc.gov/nchs/products/pubs/pubd/hestats/overweight/overwght_child_03.htm; 2009.
28. Ogden CL, Carroll MD, Flegal KM. High body mass index for age among US children and adolescents, 2003–2006. *J Am Med Assoc* 2008;**299**(20):2401–5.
29. Eaton DK, Kann L, Kinchen S. Youth Risk Behavior Surveillance—United States, 2007. *Centers for Disease Control and Prevention*. Available at, www.cdc.gov/HealthyYouth/yrbs/pdf/yrbss07_mmwr.pdf; 2008.
30. Sturm R. Increases in morbid obesity in the USA: 2000–2005. *Pub Health* 2007;**121**(7):492–6.
31. Hancox RJ, Milne BJ, Poulton R. Association between child and adolescent television viewing and adult health: A longitudinal birth cohort study. *The Lancet* 2004;**364**:257–62.
32. Jackson DM, Djafarian K, Stewart J, Speakman JR. Increased television viewing is associated with elevated body fatness but not with lower total energy expenditure in children. *Am J ClinNutr* 2009;**89**(4):1031–6.
33. Yang X, Telama R, Viikari J, Raitakari OT. Risk of obesity in relation to physical activity tracking from youth to adulthood. *Med Science Sports Ex* 2006;**38**(5):919–25.
34. Brunt AR, Rhee YS. Obesity and lifestyle in US college students related to living arrangements. *Appetite* 2008;**51**(3):615–21.
35. US Surgeon General. *Overweight and Obesity: Health Consequences*. Available at, www.surgeongeneral.gov/topics/obesity/calltoaction/fact_consequences.htm; 2001. Accessed June 25, 2008.
36. CDC. *Obesity and Overweight Trends*. Available at, www.cdc.gov/nccdphp/dnpa/obesity/trend/index.htm; 2008. Accessed June 15, 2008.
37. Katz L, Abraham M, Dominant Western health care: Type 2 diabetes mellitus. *J Trans Nurs* 2006;**17**(3):230–3.
38. American Diabetes Association. Type 2 diabetes in children and adolescents. *Pediatrics* 2000;**105**(3):671–80.
39. Pinhas-Hamiel O, Zeitler P. The global spread of type 2 diabetes mellitus in children and adolescents. *J Peds* 2005;**146**(5):693–700.
40. Pinhas-Hamiel O, Dolan LM, Daniels SR, Standiford D, Khoury PR, Zeitler P. Increased incidence of non-insulin-dependent diabetes mellitus among adolescents. *J Peds* 1996;**128**:608–15.
41. Berenson GS, Srinivasan SR, Wattigney W, Harsha D. Obesity and cardiovascular risk in children. *Ann NY Ac Sci* 1993;**699**:93–103.
42. Freedman DS, Dietz WH, Srinivasan SR, Berenson GS. The relation of overweight to cardiovascular risk factors among children and adolescents: The Bogalusa Heart Study. *Pediatrics* 1999;**103**(6):1175–82.
43. Urrutia-Rojas X, Egbuchunam CU, Bae S. High blood pressure in school children: prevalence and risk factors. *BMC Pediatrics* 2006;**6**(1):3238.
44. Berenson GS, Wattigney WA, Tracy RE. Atherosclerosis of the aorta and coronary arteries and cardiovascular risk factors in persons aged 6 to 30 years and studied at necropsy (The Bogalusa Heart Study). *Am J Cardio* 1992;**70**(9):851–8.
45. McGill HC, McMahan CA, Herderick EE. Obesity accelerates the progression of coronary atherosclerosis in youth. *Circulation* 2002;**105**:2712–18.
46. Finkelstein E, French F, Variyam JN, Haines PS. Pros and Cons of Proposed Interventions to Promote Healthy Eating. *Am J Prev Med* 2004;**27**(3S):163–71.
47. Sweeney NM, Glaser D, Tedeschi C. The eating and physical activity habits of inner-city adolescents. *J PedHlth Care* 2007;**21**(1):13–21.
48. Wang G, Dietz WH. Economic burden of obesity in youths aged 6 to 17 years: 1979–1999. *Pediatrics* 2002;**109**(5):e81.
49. The HenryKaiser Family Foundation J. *KaiserEDU: An online health policy resource for faculty and students*. Available at, www.kaiserEDU.org; 2009. Accessed September 28, 2009.
50. Larson N, Neumark-Sztainer D, Hannan P, Story M. Trends in Adolescent Fruit and Vegetable Consumption, 1999–2004 Project EAT. *Am J Prev Med* 2007;**32**(2):147–50.
51. Rasmussen M, Krolner R, Klepp K-I, Lytle L, Brug J, Bere E, Due P. Determinants of Fruit and Vegetable Consumption Among Children and Adolescents: A Review of the Literature. Part I: Qualitative Studies. *Int JBehavNutr Phys Act* 2006;**3**:22.
52. deIrala-Estevez J, Groth M, Johansson L, Oltersdorf U, Prattala R, Martinez-Gonzalez MA. A Systematic Review of Socio-Economic Differences in Food Habits in Europe: Consumption of Fruit and Vegetables. *Eu J ClinNutr* 2000;**54**(9):706–14.
53. Pereira MA, Kartashov AI, Ebbeling CB, Van Horn L, Slattery ML, Jacobs DR, Ludwig DS. Fast-Food Habits, Weight Gain, and Insulin Resistance (the CARDIA Study): 15-Year Prospective Analysis. *The Lancet* 2005;**365**:36–42.
54. Rose D, Richards R. Food Store Access and Household Fruit and Vegetable Use Among Participants in the US Food Stamp Program. *Pub Health Nutr* 2004;**7**:1081–8.
55. Munoz KA, Krebs-Smith SM, Ballard-Barbash R, Cleveland LE. Food intakes of US children and adolescents compared with recommendations. *Pediatrics* 1997;**100**(3):323–9.
56. Dehghan M, Akhtar-Danesh N, Merchant AT. Childhood obesity, prevalence and prevention. *Nutr J* 2005;**4**(1):24–31.
57. Ludwig DS, Peterson KE, Gortmaker SL. Relation between consumption of sugar-sweetened drinks and childhood obesity: A prospective, observational analysis. *The Lancet* 2001;**357**:505–8.
58. US Department of Agriculture. Americans consume too many calories from SoFAAS (saofas?!). *US Food Policy: A public interest perspective*. Available at, http://usfoodpolicy.blogspot.com/2006/06/usda-americans-consume-too-many.html; 2009. Accessed September 25, 2009.
59. Racette SB, Deusinger SS, Strube MJ, Highstein GR, Deusinger RH. Weight Changes, Exercise, and Dietary Patterns During Freshman and Sophomore Years of College. *J Am College Health* 2005;**53**(6):245–51.
60. Schuette LK, Song WO, Hoerr SL. Quantitative use of the Food Guide Pyramid to evaluate dietary intake of college students. *J Am Diet Assoc* 1996;**96**(5):453–7.
61. Patterson BH, Block G, Rosenberger WF, Pee D, Kahle LL. Fruit and vegetables in the American diet: data from the NHANES II survey. *Am J Public Health* 1990;**80**(12):1443–9.
62. Brown LB, Dresen RK, Eggett DL. College Students can Benefit by Participating in a Prepaid Meal Plan. *J Am Diet Assoc* 2005;**105**(3):445–8.
63. Anding JD, Suminski RR, Boss L. Dietary Intake, Body Mass Index, Exercise, and Alcohol: Are College Women Following the Dietary Guidelines for Americans? *J Am College Health* 2001;**49**(4):167–75.
64. Georgiou CC, Betts NM, Hoerr SL, Keim K, Peters PK, Stewart B. Among young adults, college students and graduates practiced more healthful habits and made more healthful food choices than did nonstudents. *J Am Diet Assoc* 1997;**97**:754–9.
65. Richards A, Kattelmann K, Ren C. Motivating 18- to 24-Year-Olds to Increase Their Fruit and Vegetable Consumption. *J Am Diet Assoc* 2006;**106**(9):1405–11.

66. Eaton DK, Kann L, Kinchen S, Ross J, Hawkins J, Harris WA. Youth Risk Behavior Surveillance—United States 2005. *J School Health* 2006;**76**(7):353–72.
67. Eaton DK, Kann L, Kinchen S. Youth Risk Behavior Surveillance—United States, 2007. *Centers for Disease Control and Prevention*. Available at, www.cdc.gov/HealthyYouth/yrbs/pdf/yrbss07_mmwr.pdf; 2008.
68. Zizza C, Siega-Riz AM, Popkin BM. Significant increase in young adults' snacking between 1977–1978 and 1994–1996 represents a cause for concern! *Prev Med* 2001;**32**(4):303–10.
69. Sebastian RS, Cleveland LE, Goldman JD. Effect of snacking frequency on adolescents' dietary intakes and meeting national recommendations. *J Adoles Health* 2008;**42**(5):503–11.
70. Rolls BJ, Barnett RA. In: *"The volumetrics weight-control plan: Feel full on fewer calories"*. New York: Harper Paperbacks; 2000.
71. Drewnowski A, Specter SE. Poverty and obesity: The role of energy density and energy costs. *Am J ClinNutr* 2004;**79**(1):6–16.
72. Nestle M. Soft drink "pouring rights": Marketing empty calories to children. *Public Health Reports* 2000;**115**(4):308–19.
73. Livingstone MBE, Rennie KL. Added sugars and micronutrient dilution. *Obes Rev* 2009;**10**(S1):34–40.
74. Wengreen HJ, Moncur C. Change in diet, physical activity, and body weight among young-adults during the transition from high school to college. *Nutr J* 2009;**8**:32–8.
75. Hoffman DJ, Policastro P, Quick V, Lee SK. Changes in body weight and fat mass of men and women in the first year of college: A study of the "Freshman 15". *J Am Coll Health* 2006;**55**(1):41–6.
76. Drewnowski A, Specter SE. Poverty and obesity: The role of energy density and energy costs. *Am J ClinNutr* 2004;**79**(1):6–16.
77. Caraher M, Dixon P, Lang T, Carr-Hill R. Access to healthy foods: part I. *Barriers to accessing healthy foods: Differentials by gender, social class, income and mode of transport. Health Ed J* 1998;**57**(3):191–201.
78. Chung C, Myers Jr SL. Do the poor pay more for food? An analysis of grocery store availability and food price disparities. *J Cons Affairs* 1999;**33**(2):276–96.
79. Kunreuther H. Why the poor may pay more for food: Theoretical and empirical evidence. *J Bus* 1973;**46**(3):368–83.
80. Powell LM, Slater S, Mirtcheva D, Bao Y, Chaloupka FJ. Food store availability and neighborhood characteristics in the United States. *Prev Med* 2007;**44**(3):189–95.
81. Stevens C. Food Prices are Higher in the City, Study Shows. *Detroit News* May 16 1995;**A2**.
82. Glanz K, Basil M, Maibach E, Goldberg J, Snyder D. Why Americans eat what they do: Taste, nutrition, cost, convenience, and weight control concerns as influences on food consumption. *J Am Diet Assoc* 1998;**98**(10):1118–26.
83. Cassady D, Jetter KM, Culp J. Is price a barrier to eating more fruits and vegetables for low-income families? *J Am Diet Assoc* 2007;**107**(11):1909–15.
84. French SA, Story M, Hannan P, Breitlow KK, Jeffery RW, Baxter JS. Cognitive and demographic correlates of low-fat vending snack choices among adolescents and adults. *J Am Diet Assoc* 1999;**99**(4):471–4.
85. Kant AK. Dietary patterns and health outcomes. *J Am Diet Assoc* 2004;**104**:615–35.
86. Deshmukh-Taskar P, Nicklas TA, Yang SJ, Berenson GS. Does food group consumption vary by differences in socioeconomic, demographic, and lifestyle factors in young adults? The Bogalusa Heart Study. *J Am Diet Assoc* 2007;**107**(2):223–34.
87. Solheim R, Lawless HT. Consumer purchase probability affected by attitude towards low-fat foods, liking, private body consciousness and information on fat and price. *Food QualPref* 1996;**7**(2):137–43.
88. Cullen K, Baranowski T, Watson K, Nicklas T, Fisher J, O'Donnell S. Food category purchases vary by household education and race/ethnicity: Results from grocery receipts. *J Am Diet Assoc* 2007;**107**(10):1747–52.
89. Kaufman P, MacDonald J, Lutz S, Smallwood D. *Do the poor pay more for food? Item selection and price differences affect low-income household food costs*. Washington, DC: U.S. Department of Agriculture Economic Research Service; 1997.
90. Smallwood DM, Blaylock JR, Lutz S, Blisand N. Americans spending a smaller share of income on food. *Food Review* 1996;**18**(2):16–19.
91. Lutz SM, Smallwood DM, Blaylock JR. Limited financial resources constrain food choices. *Food Review* 1995;**18**(1):13–17.
92. Smallwood DM, Kuhn B, Hanson K, Vogel S, Blaylock JR. Economic effects of refocusing national food-assistance efforts. *Food Review* 1995;**18**(1):2–12.
93. Basiotis P. Validity of the Self-Reported Food Sufficiency Status Item in the U.S. Department of Agriculture's Food Consumption Surveys. In: *The Proceedings*. Columbia, MO: Presented at the American Council on Consumer Interests 38th Annual Conference; 1992.
94. Rolls BJ, Drewnowski A, Ledikwe JH. Changing the energy density of the diet as a strategy for weight management. *J Am Diet Assoc* 2005;**105**(5S):98–103.
95. Rose D. Food stamps, the Thrifty Food Plan, and meal preparation: The importance of the time dimension for US nutrition policy. *J Nutr Ed Behav* 2007;**39**(4):226–32.
96. Guthrie JF, Lin BH, Frazao E. Role of food prepared away from home in the American diet, 1977–78 versus 1994–96: Changes and consequences. *J Nutr Ed Behav* 2002;**34**(3):140–50.
97. Jabs J, Devine CM. Time scarcity and food choices: An overview. *Appetite* 2006;**47**(2):196–204.
98. Jabs J, Devine CM, Bisogni CA, Farrell TJ, Jastran M, Wethington E. Trying to find the quickest way: Employed mothers' constructions of time for food. *J Nutr Ed Behav* 2007;**39**(1):18–25.
99. Hessing M. More than clockwork: Women's time management in their combined workloads. *Socio Perspect* 1994;**37**(4):611–33.
100. Stookey J, Barker M. The diets of low-income women: The role of culinary knowledge. *Appetite* 1995;**24**:286.
101. Cresswell J. *Get Cooking Project Report*. Glasgow: Greater Glasgow Health Board Health Promotion Department; 1995.
102. Dobson B, Kellard K, Talbot D. *A Recipe for Success? An Evaluation of a Community Food Project*. Loughborough: Centre for Research in Social Policy; 2000.
103. Wrieden WL, Anderson AS, Longbottom PJ. The impact of a community-based food skills intervention on cooking confidence, food preparation methods and dietary choices—an exploratory trial. *Pub Health Nutr* 2007;**10**(2):203–11.
104. Cutler DM, Glaeser EL, Shapiro JM. Why have Americans become more obese? *J Econ Perspect* 2003;**17**(3):93–118.
105. Perman S. The joy of not cooking: Americans spend less time cooking every year; yet the $100 billion "home-meal replacement" market has produced few winners. *Time*; June 1998;66–9.
106. Stewart H, Lucier G. *Younger Consumers Exhibit Less Demand for Fresh Vegetables*. Washington, DC: Economic Research Service/USDA, Outlook report No.VGS-333-01; 2009. Available at: http://www.ers.usda.gov/publications/vgs/2009/08Aug/vgs33301.
107. Nestle M. *Food Politics*. Berkeley, CA: University of California Press; 2002.
108. Pollan M. The (Agri) Cultural Contradictions of Obesity. *NY Times*: October 12, 2003. Available at: http://www.nytimes.com/2003/10/12/magazine/12WWLN.html?scp=1&sq=agricultural%20contradictions%20of%20obesity&st=cse.

109. Smiciklas-Wright H, Mitchell DC, Mickle SJ, Goldman JD, Cook A. Foods commonly eaten in the United States, 1989–1991 and 1994–1996: Are portion sizes changing? *J Am Diet Assoc* 2003;**103**(1):41–7.
110. Colapinto CK, Fitzgerald A, Taper LJ, Veugelers PJ. Children's Preference for Large Portions: Prevalence, Determinants, and Consequences. *J Am Diet Assoc* 2007;**107**:1183–90.
111. French SA. Pricing effects on food choices. *J Nutr* 2003;**133**(3):841S–843.
112. Wansink B. *"Mindless eating: Why we eat more than we think."* New York: Bantam-Dell; 2006.
113. Wansink B, Park S. Accounting for taste: Prototypes that predict preference. *J Database Mktg* 2000;**7**:308–20.
114. Jeffery RW, Rydell S, Dunn CL, Harnack LJ, Levine AS, Pentel PR. Effects of portion size on chronic energy intake. *Int J BehavNutr Phys Act* 2007;**4**(1):27–31.
115. American Dietetic Association. Position of the American Dietetic Association: Weight management. *J Am Diet Assoc* 2009;**109**:330–46.
116. Lavidge RJ, Steiner GA. A model for predictive measurements of advertising effectiveness. *J Mktg* 1961;**25**:59–62.
117. Advertising Age. 100 Leading National Advertisers: 2009 edition index. 2008. Available at: http://adage.com/datacenter/article?article_id=136308. Accessed June 7, 2009.
118. Harris JM, Kaufman PR, Martinez SW, Price C. *The US Food Marketing System, 2002*. Washington, DC: Economic Rsearch Service/USDA, Agricultural Economic Report No. 811; 2002. Available at http://www.ers.usda.gov/publications/aer811/.
119. Story M, French S. Food advertising and marketing directed at children and adolescents in the US. *Int J BehavNutr Phys Act* 2004;**1**(1):3–19.
120. Borzekowski DL, Robinson TN. The 30-second effect: An experiment revealing the impact of television commercials on food preferences of preschoolers. *J Am Diet Assoc* 2001;**101**(1):42–6.
121. Powell LM, Szczypka G, Chaloupka FJ. Exposure to food advertising on television among US children. *Arch PedAdoles Med* 2007;**161**(6):553–60.
122. National Institutes of Health National Cancer Institute. *5 a day for better health program evaluation report*. Washington, DC: US Government Printing Office; 2000.
123. California Pan-Ethnic Health Network and Consumers Union. *Out of Balance: Marketing of soda, candy, snacks and fast foods drowns out healthful messages*. California: Consumers Union. Available at, www.consumersunion.org/pdf/OutofBalance.pdf. www.consumersunion.org/pdf/OutofBalance.pdf; 2005.
124. Smith WA. Social marketing: an overview of approach and effects. *Injury Prev* 2006;**12**:38–43.
125. Kyllo R. *2002 Milkpep Annual Report*. Available at, www.milkdelivers.org/about/2002annualrpt_advertising.cfm?printPage=1&; 2003. Accessed July 30 2006.
126. Holben DH, Hassell JT, Holcomb JP. College Freshmen Do Not Eat Within Food Pyramid Guidelines. *J Am Diet Assoc* 1998;**98**(9):A51.
127. Huhman M, Potter LD, Wong FL, Banspach SW, Duke JC, Heitzler CD. Effects of a mass media campaign to increase physical activity among children: Year-1 results of the VERB campaign. *Pediatrics* 2005;**116**(2):277–84.
128. US Department of Agriculture. *Dietary Guidelines for Americans*. Washington, DC: Department of Health and Human Services and the Department of Agriculture. Available at, www.health.gov/dietaryguidelines/dga2005/document/html; 2005.
129. Drichoutis AC, Lazaridis P, Nayga RM. Consumers' use of nutritional labels: a review of research studies and issues. *AcadMktgSci Rev* 2006;**9**:1–22.
130. Derby BM, Levy AS. (1991). Consumer Use of Food Labels: Where Are We? Where Are We Going? Annual meeting of the American Dietetic Association, Orlando, FL.
131. Variyam JN, Blaylock J, Smallwood DM. *Diet-Health Information and Nutrition. The Intake of Dietary Fats and Cholesterol*. Washington, DC: Economic Research Service/USDA, Technical Bulletin No. 1842; 1997.
132. Huang TTK, Kaur H, McCarter KS, Nazir N, Choi WS, Ahluwalkia JS. Reading nutrition labels and fat consumption in adolescents. *J Adolesc Health* 2004;**35**(5):399–401.
133. Neuhouser ML, Kristal AR, Patterson RE. Use of Food Nutrition Labels is Associated with Lower Fat Intake. *J Am Diet Assoc* 1999;**99**(1):45–53.
134. Shepherd R, Towler G. Nutrition knowledge, attitudes and fat intake: application of the theory of reasoned action. *J Human NutrDietet* 2007;**20**(3):159–70.
135. Manios Y, Moschonis G, Katsaroli I, Grammatikaki E, Tanagra S. Changes in diet quality score, macro-micronutrients intake following a nutrition education intervention in postmenopausal women. *J Hum NutrDietet* 2007;**20**:126–31.
136. Kelley E, Ashley B, Getlinger M, Nitzke S. A Lesson on How Much Should I Eat Helps Learners Understand and Apply MyPyramid Recommendations. *J Nutr Ed Behav* 2008;**40**(2):116–17.
137. Anderson AS. Achieving dietary guidelines the naturally nutrient rich approach. *J Hum NutrDietet* 2005;**18**:335–6.
138. Robroek SJ, Bredt FJ, Burdorf A. The cost-effectiveness of an individually tailored long-term worksite health promotion programme on physical activity and nutrition: design of a pragmatic cluster randomised controlled trial. *BMC Pub Health* 2007;**7**:259.
139. Teisl MF, Bockstael NE, Levy A. Measuring the welfare effects of nutrition information. *Am J Agric Econ* 2001;**83**(1):133–49.
140. Teisl MF, Levy AS. Does nutrition labeling lead to healthier eating? *J Food Distrib Res* 1997;**28**:18–27.
141. Kreuter MW, Brennan LK, Scharff DP, Lukwago SN. Do nutrition label readers eat healthier diets? Behavioral correlates of adults' use of food labels. *Am J Prev Med* 1997;**13**(4):277–83.
142. United States Food and Drug Administration. *Nutritional Labeling and Education Act Requirements*. Washington, D.C: U.S. Department of Health and Human Services. Available at, www.fda.gov/ICECI/Inspections/InspectionGuides/ucm074948.htm; 1994.
143. Davis-Chervin D. Influencing Food Selection with Point-of-Choice Nutrition Information. *J Nutr Ed Behav* 1985;**17**(1):18–22.
144. Schmitz MF, Fielding JE. Point-of-choice nutritional labeling: evaluation in a worksite cafeteria. *J Nutr Ed Behav* 1986;**18**(Suppl 2):S65–8.
145. Bassett MT, Dumanovsky T, Huang C, Silver LD, Young C, Nonas C, Matte TD, Chideya S, Frieden TR. Purchasing Behavior and Calorie Information at Fast-Food Chains in New York City, 2007. *Am J Public Health* 2008;**98**(8):1457–9.
146. Krukowski R, Harvey-Berino J, Kolodinsky J, Narsana R, DeSisto TP. Consumers May Not Use or Understand Calorie Labeling in Restaurants. *J Am Diet Assoc* 2006;**106**(6):917–20.
147. Yamamoto JA, Yamamoto JB, Yamamoto BE, Yamamoto LG. Adolescent fast food and restaurant ordering behavior with and without calorie and fat content menu information. *J Adolesc Health* 2005;**37**:397–402.
148. Fiske A, Cullen KW. Effects of Promotional Materials on Vending Sales of Low-Fat Items in Teachers' Lounges. *J Am Diet Assoc* 2004;**104**:90–3.

149. Liddell JA, Lockie GM, Wise A. Effects of a nutrition education programme on the dietary habits of a population of students and staff at a centre for higher education. *J Hum Nutr Diet* 1992; **5**(1):23—33.
150. Center for Science in the Public Interest (CSPI). (2007—2008). Nutrition Labeling in Chain Restaurants, State and Local Bills/Regulations. Available at www.cspinet.org/menulabeling Accessed November 11, 2008.
151. Carper TA. *Sen. Carper & Murkowski introduce bill to help Americans make smart and healthy choices when dining out*. Available at, http://carper.senate.gov/press/record.cfm?id=303597; 2008. Accessed November 7, 2008.
152. National Conference of State Legislatures. *Trans Fat and Menu Labeling*. Available at, www.ncsl.org/programs/health/transfatmenulabelingbills.htm; 2008. Accessed May 27, 2008.
153. Metropolitan King County Council. *Restaurant industry agrees to post nutritional information for diners*. Available at, www.kingcounty.gov/council/news/2008/March/JP_menu.aspx; 2008. Accessed May 27, 2008.
154. Allday E. S.F. super require posting of nutrition info. *San Francisco Chronicle*; March 12, 2008. Available at: http://articles.sfgate.com/2008-03-12/bay-area/17165891_1_nutrition-labels-fight-obesity-menus.
155. U.S. Department of Agriculture Food and Nutrition Service. *Special Supplemental Nutrition Program for Women, Infants and Children (WIC): Revisions in the WIC Food Packages; Interim Rule*. Available at, www.fns.usda.gov/wic/regspublished/wicfoodpkginterimrulepdf.pdf; 2007.
156. US Department of Agriculture. *Dietary Guidelines*. Available at, www.mypyramid.gov/guidelines/index.html; 2009. Accessed September 25, 2009.
157. Texas Department of Agriculture. *Texas Public School Nutrition Policy*. Available at, www.squaremeals.com/vgn/tda/files/2348/13440_TPSNP%20SY_09-10.pdf; 2009.
158. Feenstra G, Ohmart J. *Yolo County Farm to School Evaluation Report Year 4 Annual Report*. Davis, CA: UC Sustainable Agriculture Research and Education Program; 2005.
159. Center for Food and Justice, Occidental College. *Riverside Farm to School Demonstration Project, Final Grant Report, December 1, 2004—November 30, 2006*. Riverside, CA: The California Endowment; 2006.
160. Flock P, Petra C, Ruddy V, Peterangelo J. *A salad bar featuring organic choices: revitalizing the school lunch program*. Washington, D.C.: Olympia School District. Available at, http://agr.wa.gov/marketing/smallfarm/saladbarorganicchoices.pdf; 2003.
161. Robinson-O'Brien R, Story M, Heim S. Impact of garden-based youth nutrition intervention programs: A review. *J Am Diet Assoc* 2009;**109**(2):273—80.
162. Price Chopper Corporation. *NuVal: Ingredients for a Healthy Lifestyle*. Available at, www2.pricechopper.com/nuval/index2.shtml; 2009. Accessed September 30, 2009.
163. Corporation Hannaford. *Nutritious shopping made simple*. Available at, www.hannaford.com/Contents/Healthy_Living/Guiding_Stars/index.shtml; 2009. Accessed September 30, 2009.
164. Choices Smart. *Helping Guide Smart Food and Beverage Choices*. Available at, www.smartchoicesprogram.com/index.html; 2009. Accessed September 28, 2009.
165. Silverglade B, Heller IR. *Food Labeling Chaos: The Case for Reform, Center for Science in the Public Interest (March)*. Available at, http://cspinet.org/new/pdf/food_labeling_chaos_report.pdf; 2010.
166. The White House. *First Lady Michelle Obama Launches Let's Move: America's Move to Raise a Healthier Generation of Kids*, www.LetsMove.gov; 2010. Accessed March 22, 2010.

CHAPTER 45

The Role of Media in Childhood Obesity

Amy B. Jordan*, Ariel Chernin†

*The Annenberg Public Policy Center, University of Pennsylvania, Philadelphia, PA, USA

CHILDREN'S MEDIA USE PATTERNS

The American Academy of Pediatrics (AAP) recommends that children's screen media use be limited to no more than 2 hours per day in children over the age of 2 and that media use be avoided altogether for children under the age of 2 [1]. Surveys of U.S. parents find that most families do not adhere to these recommendations, however. These studies find that school-age children spend, on average, 3 hours per day watching television; and when other "screen media" such as video games and computers are factored in, that number climbs closer to 5 hours per day [2–3].

One reason children spend so much of their leisure time watching television may lie in the ubiquity of television throughout American homes. The average family owns four working television sets, the majority subscribe to cable or satellite services that provide hundreds of channels, more than two thirds of children have a television set in the bedroom, and four in ten families have a TV in the dining room or kitchen [2]. Children's increased access to television—particularly in the bedroom—has been linked to heavier viewing [4–5].

A second reason children spend so much time with electronic media may lie in the fact that for some there may be fewer free-time alternatives. Family income is negatively related to children's television time [6]. This may be due to the lack of income needed to afford activities that might limit children's viewing time—for example, dues necessary to play in community-organized sports or membership costs of local youth-serving organizations such as the YMCA. The link between low socioeconomic status and heavy viewing may also be related to the quality of the neighborhood environment and parents' comfort level in sending their children "out to play." In one study, parents were asked about the challenges they might face in bringing their child's viewing in line with the AAP recommendations. Those from lower-income communities worried that without the TV and video games to keep them indoors and occupied, their children might be less safe or more likely to get into trouble [2]. Another longitudinal survey, which tracked children from kindergarten through fourth grade, found that children who watched more television lived in neighborhoods that were perceived by parents as less safe [7].

A third reason for children's heavy media use may lie in the notion that patterns of media use are passed on from parents to children. Children are socialized regarding their attitudes toward television viewing (e.g., it is a waste of time versus a pleasurable activity) and their preferences for media content (e.g., educational versus entertainment oriented), and they may adopt media use habits that provide a tempo to their day [8]. Several studies have found that a strong predictor of children's heavy media use is parents' heavy media use [9–11].

THE RELATIONSHIP BETWEEN CHILDREN'S HEAVY MEDIA USE AND CHILDHOOD OVERWEIGHT

Though researchers have long studied the effect of television viewing, video game playing, and even computer use on academic and social outcomes, they have only relatively recently turned their attention to the impact of media use on children's physical well-being. The evidence for a relationship between children's heavy media use and childhood obesity has been mounting, however. Cross-sectional surveys indicate that as the number of hours children spend watching television rises, so too does their body fat percentage and risk of overweight [12–14]. Prospective studies also find childhood television viewing to be a risk factor for subsequent adiposity [7, 15]. Perhaps most persuasive are randomized controlled trials (RCTs), which have linked the reduction of television and other screen media use to decreased body mass index (BMI), waist circumferences, and triceps skinfold thickness in elementary school age children [16]; decreased overweight in middle school girls [17]; and weight loss among overweight 8- to 12-year-old children [18].

Although television remains the medium with which children spend the most time [19], the use of other sedentary media has risen since the late 1990s (Kaiser Family Foundation). Several studies suggest that the role of nontelevision media in childhood overweight should not be overlooked. Findings of a significant relationship between adolescent weight status and electronic game play [20–21] and heavy computer use [19–22] indicate that the focus should not remain exclusively with television. Indeed, an Australian study found that though there was no association between heavy television viewing and children's physical well-being, adolescents who reported a high level of video game use reported poorer health/well-being [22].

MECHANISMS FOR EXPLAINING THE ASSOCIATION

If we accept the evidence that heavy media use is a contributing factor to childhood overweight, it is critical to understand the mechanisms that underlie the relationship. Building on Robinson's [23] framework, we propose three potential pathways, which are likely independent contributors though not necessarily mutually exclusive.

Media Influence on Physical and Sedentary Activity

One might intuitively believe that children's heavy use of media displaces time spent in physical activity. One might also assume that children who are more physically active are less likely to be overweight. These relationships, however, are not always that straightforward. Although television viewing prevents physical activity in that moment, there is little evidence to suggest that, over the course of a day or week, the amount of time children spend watching TV is associated with the amount of time they spend engaged in physical activity. A systematic review by Marshall et al. [27] on the relationship between media use and physical activity showed little support for the displacement hypothesis. The association between physical activity and weight status is also complex. Research with adolescents has found that, as expected, physical activity is inversely associated with overweight status [24], but other studies have found an inconsistent relationship [25] or no relationship [26].

It is possible that the lack of relationship between physical activity, media use, and overweight is due to unreliable measures of physical activity in children. More likely, however, there are distinct behavioral pathways to obesity for physical activity and inactivity [28–30]. Several studies have found that decreasing sedentary behaviors (i.e., television viewing and video game playing) is a more successful strategy for helping overweight children reduce BMI than increasing physical activity [18]. Epstein found that reductions in the targeted sedentary behavior (in this study, television viewing and computer use in overweight children aged 4 to 7) resulted in less energy intake and weight loss but did not lead to increased physical activity. That said, the best possible scenario for preventing overweight may be a combination of screen time reduction and frequent moderate-to-vigorous physical activity [29, 31, 32].

Media Influence on Dietary Habits

The media may shape children's food choices and caloric intake by exposing children to persuasive messages about food, cuing them to eat, and depressing satiety cues of eating while viewing.

According to estimates by the Federal Trade Commission, children between the ages of 2 and 11 are exposed to 25,600 advertisements per year, of which 5500 (or 15 per day) are for food or beverages [33]. These advertisements are predominantly for foods that are high in salt, sugar, and fat and low in nutritional value [34]. Clearly children's food consumption affects their weight status. But does children's exposure to junk food advertisements affect their diets? A large body of research indicates that advertising influences children's food preferences, their eating behaviors, and the purchase requests they direct to parents [35–38]. In one study, children watched a television show with or without food commercials and then participated in a simulated shopping trip with their mothers. Children exposed to the commercials requested significantly more products than children who did not see the commercials and requested a greater number of products that had been featured in the ads [38].

A study of children's intake of meals where food brands were present or absent found that overweight children show greater responsiveness to food branding than nonoverweight children [39]. In another study, elementary school age children watched a cartoon that contained either food advertising or advertising for other products and received a snack while watching. Results indicated that children consumed 45% more when exposed to food advertising, regardless of prior report of hunger or whether the food offered was the food advertised. The authors hypothesized that food advertisements prime children to eat while viewing and concluded that snacking while watching commercial TV with food advertisements for only 30 minutes per day would lead to a weight gain of almost 10 pounds per year if not compensated [40].

Researchers have found an association between heavy television viewing and more frequent snacking [41, 42], the consumption of sugary beverages [42, 43], and more frequent visits to fast-food chains [42]. Heavy television viewing is also negatively associated with the consumption of fruits and vegetables [44]. Although much of this research is cross-sectional, it is possible that the heavy advertising of fast-food restaurants and highly sugared cereals and drinks contributes to youths' belief that these are appropriate foods to eat as meals and snacks [45]. In addition, the practice of "product placement"—in which food companies pay to feature their product in children's movies and general audience television shows—is becoming more frequent but its effects are not well understood. How are the young viewers of the program *American Idol* affected by the ubiquitous Coca-Cola cups in front of the judges?

Some scholars suggest that television affects weight status because children consume higher-calorie, nutritionally poor foods while viewing TV. Saelens et al. [46] found cross-sectional and longitudinal associations between the number of meals children ate while viewing TV and the number of hours spent watching TV. When television viewing is combined with eating, whether during mealtime [47] or snack time [48], children eat fewer fruits and vegetables and consume more calories, even when potential covariates such as socioeconomic factors are controlled. As mentioned earlier, food advertising during the television programs children watch could be priming young viewers to consume more and lower-quality food. However, other researchers suggest that television viewing decreases internal signals of satiety or the feeling of fullness. Blass and colleagues [49], for example, found that TV viewing, in contrast to music listening, significantly increased the amount of pizza and macaroni and cheese college students consumed in the experimental setting in which there were no advertisements at all.

Media Influence on Sleep Behaviors

A third potential mechanism underlying the connection between media use and childhood overweight may lie in the influence of media on sleep patterns. Though the empirical base is too limited to confirm the relationship between heavy television viewing and childhood overweight through the causal pathway of inadequate sleep, recent data are intriguing. An estimated 20% to 30% of young children have some type of sleep difficulty, including bedtime resistance, sleep onset delay, anxiety around sleep, and shortened sleep duration [50]. Snell, Adam, and Duncan [51] found that 13% of the 3- to 7-year-old children in their nationally representative sample slept less than 9 hours per night (11 hours is recommended). Researchers have found short sleep duration to be an independent risk factor for overweight and obesity in children [52]. Data from the Avon Longitudinal Study of parents and children in the United Kingdom found that short sleep duration at the age of 30 months predicted obesity at age 7 [53]. In a Japanese sample of 10,000 3-year-olds, the frequency of sleeping less than 10 hours a night was greater in obese children than nonobese children (29.3% versus 13.7%) [54]. In addition, short sleepers in this sample were significantly more likely to be overweight 3 years later than children who slept the recommended time.

There is evidence that children's media use may be causing or exacerbating children's sleep problems. Owen and colleagues [55] found that bedtime television viewing by 4- to 10-year-olds was significantly associated with bedtime resistance, sleep onset delay, and decreased sleep duration. Paavonen et al. [56] similarly found that watching TV at bedtime was associated with sleeping difficulties for 5- to 6-year-olds. Children themselves report using television as a sleep aid. More than one third of a sample of 5th to 10th grade Dutch youth reported that they turn on the TV to help them fall asleep; however, nighttime TV viewing was negatively related to their number of hours of sleep per week [57].

What is not clear from the existing body of research is whether television viewing creates sleep problems or whether those suffering from sleep problems turn to media as a sleep aid [55]. A national telephone survey of parents of 6-month-olds to 6-year-olds found that 53% said that television viewing can help calm their child [58]. In this study, 30% of parents said that a motivation for putting a TV in the child's bedroom was because it helps the child fall asleep. More research is needed to understand parents' beliefs about their children's use of media, what shapes whether they direct children toward or away from media, and whether bedtime is a period when parents can feasibly shift their child to other sleep-inducing activities, such as book reading.

CAN MEDIA BE A PART OF THE SOLUTION?

Though it may be ironic to create mass media-based interventions to encourage physical activity and more healthful eating, evaluations of such campaigns have found some success. In 2001, Congress allocated $125 million to the Centers for Disease Control and

Prevention (CDC) to design a national campaign to help children foster good habits over a lifetime. One of the most notable elements of the funding allocation was the directive to use methods that are employed by the best youth marketers. The CDC ultimately focused on encouraging "tweens" (9- to 12-year-olds) to become more physically active, and they branded their effort the VERB campaign [59]. By encouraging adolescents to find their "verb"—activities that might define them or that they most enjoy—campaign designers aimed to help children develop more positive attitudes about exercise and participate more frequently in physical activities. An evaluation of the campaign over time found that youth who were more aware of the VERB campaign and reported being exposed to more of the campaign's messages were more likely to feel self-efficacy in their ability to exercise, were more likely to find social support in their efforts to exercise, and were more likely to participate in regular physical activity. This held true even after their initial physical activity beliefs and behaviors before the start of the campaign were factored in, although it was more evident after 2 years of campaign exposure than it was after only 1 year [60].

Another campaign, aimed at encouraging consumers to switch from whole or 2% to 1% or skim milk as an easy way to reduce intake of saturated fat, used paid advertisements, press conferences, and school-based educational programs in an intervention city and tracked milk consumption against a matched control city [61]. Sales of high-fat milk in the intervention cities decreased from 82% of overall milk sales at baseline to 59% in the month following the campaign. In the comparison city, sales of high-fat milk were 72% of overall milk sales at baseline and 67% in the month following. The authors argued that the paid campaign was cost effective—approximately 9 cents for each person reached by the campaign.

RECOMMENDATIONS

The good news about research on the impact of children's media use on childhood obesity is that we are closer to identifying behaviors that are potentially modifiable. An expert panel on children, television viewing, and weight status published what it believes are the most promising strategies for reducing the negative effects of media use on children's weight status based on evidence addressing potential mechanisms and the existing experimental research [62]:

1. *Eliminate TV from children's bedrooms.* The panel recommends that TVs be eliminated completely from children's bedrooms. In addition, it must be recognized that with the growing convergence of media platforms, parents must beware that children might simply substitute one screen medium for another (for example, watching TV programs on the computer). Eliminating bedroom media use may reduce overall screen time and may help to limit nighttime media use that may interfere with children's healthy sleep.
2. *Encourage mindful viewing by monitoring screen media watched, budgeting TV time, and fostering media literacy.* The panel recommends that parents begin by monitoring the screen media their children use before they make a decision on budgeting, as many parents are not aware of just how much time their children spend with media [2]. Moreover, the committee encourages parents to collaborate with children on establishing appropriate amounts of screen media use and sharing and discussing the content to which children are exposed.
3. *Turn off the TV while eating.* Disconnecting food from TV viewing may increase awareness of food consumption while also increasing family communication, and decreasing total TV watching time. One important first step may be to remove television sets from those areas of the house where meals and snacks are normally consumed (such as the dining room and kitchen).
4. *Use school-based curricula to reduce children's screen time.* The panel noted that schools are an excellent forum for efficiently and effectively reaching a large number of youth with a focused curriculum. School-based interventions in preschool [63], elementary schools [16], and middle schools [17] have been found to be successful in reducing television viewing and, in some cases, reducing weight gain.
5. *Provide training for healthcare professionals to counsel them on reducing children's media use.* About three quarters of U.S. newborn to eighteen-year-olds are seen regularly (once a year or more) by a medical care provider [64]. The panel recommends training and support for healthcare professionals on issues related to reducing children's use of media.

IS THERE A ROLE FOR PUBLIC POLICY?

In 2005, the Institute of Medicine declared that food and beverage marketing to children and youth in the United States is out of balance with healthful diets [45]. The response to this report has been a call to increase industry self-regulation and, if progress is not made, to move toward increased government regulation. Other national governments have moved to prohibit advertising to children (for example, Norway and Sweden ban ads aimed at children aged 12 and younger) and have specifically banned junk-food advertising on television programs designed for children or that have children as a large part of its audiences (for example, the United Kingdom has strict nutritional criteria that must be met for food advertised to children under the age of 16). However, in the United States, policy makers are loath to interfere with the marketplace economy or impose restrictions on the First Amendment rights of broadcasters. Broadcasters have instead pledged to increase their "healthy lifestyle" messages and, according to one study, seem to be doing so [65]; however, it is not clear how such messages are received. If a child watches an advertisement in which Ronald McDonald and children ride their bikes to McDonald's, are child viewers more likely to want to exercise and less likely to consume fast food? In addition, the Council of Better Business Bureaus' Children's Advertising Review Unit (CARU) has asked its members to encourage "responsible use" of food and beverages. There are no sanctions for noncompliance if CARU determines a member violates its voluntary code [66].

Another public policy that has been considered involves limiting the use of television and other "passive" or "sedentary" media use in federally funded schools and childcare centers. Christakis and Garrison [67] conducted a telephone survey of licensed childcare programs in four states across the United States and found that nearly 70% of home-based daycare and almost 36% of center-based childcare programs reported using television with preschool-aged children. The mean time of daily television use for preschoolers in a daycare setting in which television was used was 3.4 hours in home-based programs and 1.2 hours in center-based programs. Jordan's [65] observations of the use of television in a low-income, federally subsidized daycare center indicates that there is much opportunity to educate teachers and caregivers about ways to extend the educational potential of viewing, including tying favorite TV characters and programs to hands-on experiences and using TV lessons as teachable moments. In addition to educating teachers and providers about appropriate screen media use, daycare centers and schools have been effective settings for delivering interventions to reduce screen time. In a preschool setting, Dennison and colleagues [63] were effective in reducing children's television/video viewing with a health promotion curriculum that consisted of seven interactive 20-minute sessions. In an elementary school setting, children were encouraged to participate in a 10-day TV turnoff period and their families were provided with a device called a TV Allowance, which automatically turns off the electronic device once the maximum preset time has been reached. Children participating in this intervention decreased television viewing by about one third of their baseline viewing and significantly reduced the number of meals and snacks consumed while watching TV [16].

Another school-based approach involves media literacy training designed to increase children's understanding of the functions and purposes of various media forms (e.g., the primary purpose of advertising is to persuade) and to encourage the critical evaluation of media messages. Not surprisingly, research suggests that children easily learn the content of media literacy curricula [68–70]. There is less evidence, however, that children apply these lessons while using media [71]. Thus, a child may understand that food commercials intend to persuade, but this knowledge may not mitigate the influence of the ads. More research is needed to identify the types of media literacy training that are most likely to stimulate critical thinking skills. Curricula that combine media literacy and media reduction may prove to be the most effective.

CONCLUSION

Children who watch a lot of television have an increased risk of overweight during childhood and are more likely to be overweight as adults. Indeed, in a longitudinal study of 1037 New Zealand men followed between the ages of 5 and 32, childhood television viewing was a better predictor of adult BMI and fitness than adult viewing and remained a significant predictor of these outcomes even after adjusting for adult viewing [72]. The research reviewed in this chapter highlights the need to educate parents and children about healthy media diets when children are still quite young. Although much remains to be understood about exactly how children's heavy media use contributes to childhood obesity, there is now a solid evidence base that can be used to design screen time reduction interventions. Healthcare providers, moreover, can suggest simple steps that families can implement to limit screen time to 3 hours per day or less as a strategy for combating overweight, including removing televisions from children's bedrooms, becoming more aware of children's screen media time, and disconnecting eating from viewing.

References

1. American Academy of Pediatrics (AAP). Children, adolescents, and television. *Pediatrics* 2001;**107**:423–6.
2. Jordan A, Hersey J, McDivitt J, Heitzler C. Reducing children's television-viewing time: A qualitative study of parents and their children. *Pediatrics* 2006;**18**(5):e1303–10.
3. Rideout V, Hamel E. *The media family: Electronic media in the lives of infants, toddlers, preschoolers and their parents*. Rep. no 7500. Menlo Park, CA: Henry J. Kaiser Family Foundation; 2006.

4. Jordan A, Bleakley A, Manganello J, Hennessy M, Stevens R, Fishbein M. The role of television access in the viewing time of U.S. adolescents. *Journal of Children and Media* forthcoming 2010;**4**(4).
5. Dennison BA, Erb TA, Jenkins PL. Television viewing and television in bedroom associated with overweight risk among low-income preschool children. *Pediatrics* 2002;**109**: 1028–35.
6. Grund A, Krause H, Siewers M, Rieckert H, Muller MJ. Is TV viewing an index of physical activity and fitness in overweight and normal weight children? *Public Health Nutrition* 2001;**4**: 1245–51.
7. Gable S, Chang Y, Krull JL. Television watching and frequency of family meals are predictive of overweight onset and persistence in a national sample of school-aged children. *American Dietetic Association* 2007;**107**(1):53–61.
8. Jordan A. The role of media in children's development: An ecological perspective. *Journal of Developmental and Behavioral Pediatric* June 2004;**25**(3):196–207.
9. Woodard E, Gridina N. *Media in the home 2000*. Philadelphia, PA: The Annenberg Public Policy Center of the University of Pennsylvania; 2000.
10. Francis LA, Lee Y, Birch LL. Parental weight status and girls' television viewing, snacking, and body mass index. *Obesity Research* 2003;**11**(1):143–51.
11. Delva J, Johnston LD, O'Malley PM. The epidemiology of overweight and related lifestyle behaviors: Racial/ethnic and socioeconomic status differences among American Youth. *American Journal of Preventive Medicine* 2007;**33**:178–86.
12. Gortmaker SL, Must A, Sobol A, Peterson K, Colditz G, Dietz WH. Television viewing as a cause of increasing obesity among children in the United States, 1986–1990. *Archives of Pediatrics and Adolescent Medicine* 1996;**150**(4):356–63.
13. Hancox RJ, Poulton R. Television is associated with childhood obesity: But is it clinically important? *International Journal of Obesity* 2006;**30**:171–5.
14. Montgomery-Reagan K, Bianco JA, Heh V, Rettos J, Huston RS. Prevalence and correlates of high body mass index in rural Appalachian children aged 6–11 years. *Rural and Remote Health* 2009;**9**(1234):1–11.
15. Dietz WH, Gortmaker SL. Do we fatten our children at the television set? *Pediatrics* 1985;**75**(5):807–11.
16. Robinson TN. Reducing children's television viewing to prevent obesity: A randomized controlled trial. *Journal of the American Medical Association* 1999;**282**:151–67.
17. Gortmaker SL, Peterson K, Weicha J, Sobol AM, Dixit S, Fox MK, Laird N. Reducing obesity via a school-based interdisciplinary intervention among youth: Planet Health. *Archives of Pediatrics and Adolescent Medicine* 1999;**153**:409–18.
18. Epstein LH, Paluch RA, Gordy CC, Dorn J. Decreasing sedentary behaviors in treating pediatric obesity. *Archives of Adolescent and Pediatric Medicine* 2000;**154**:220–6.
19. Russ SA, Larson K, Franke TM, Halfon N. Associations between media use and health in US children. *Academic Pediatric Association* 2009;**9**(5):300–6.
20. Vandewater EA, Shim M, Caplovitz AG. Linking obesity and activity level with children's television and video game use. *Journal of Adolescence* 2004;**27**(1):71–85.
21. McMurray RG, Harrell JS, Deng S, Bradley CB, Cox LM, Bangdiwala SI. The influence of physical activity, socioeconomic status, and ethnicity on the weight status of adolescents. *Obesity Research* 2000;**8**(2):130–9.
22. Epstein LH, Roemmich JN, Robinson JL, Paluch RA, Winiewicz DD, Fuerch JH, Robinson TN. A randomized trial of the effects of reducing television viewing and computer use on body mass index in young children. *Archives of Pediatrics and Adolescent Medicine* 2008;**162**(3):239–45.
23. Robinson T. Television viewing and childhood obesity. *Pediatric Clinics of North America* 2001;**48**:1017–25.
24. Dowda M, Ainsworth BE, Addy CL, Saunders R, Riner W. Environmental influences, physical activity, and weight status in 8- to 16-year olds. *Archives of Pediatrics and Adolescent Medicine* 2001;**155**(6):711–17.
25. Stovitz SD, Steffen LM, Boostrom A. Participation in physical activity among normal- and overweight Hispanic and Non-Hispanic White adolescents. *Journal of School Health* 2008;**78**(1):19–25.
26. Lioret S, Maire B, Volatier JL, Charles MA. Child overweight in France and its relationship with physical activity, sedentary behavior and socioeconomic status. *European Journal of Clinical Nutrition* 2007;**61**(4):509–16.
27. Marshall SJ, Biddle SJ, Gorely T, Cameron N, Murdey I. Relationships between mass media use, body fatness and physical activity in children and youth: A meta-analysis. *International Journal of Obesity Related Metabolic Disorders* 2004;**28**(10):1238–46.
28. Gordon-Larsen P, McMurray RG, Popkin BM. Adolescent physical activity and inactivity vary by ethnicity: The national longitudinal study of adolescent health. *The Journal of Pediatrics* 1999;**135**(3):301–6.
29. Eisenmann JC, Bartee RT, Smith DT, Welk GJ, Fu Q. Combined influence of physical activity and television viewing on the risk of overweight in US youth. *International Journal of Obesity* 2008;**32**:613–18.
30. Mark AE, Janssen I. Relationship between screen time and metabolic syndrome in adolescents. *Journal of Public Health* 2008;**30**(2):153–60.
31. Robinson TN, Killen JD, Kraemer HC, Wilson DM, Matheson D, Haskell WL, Pruitt LA, Powell TM, Owens AS, Thompson NS, Flint-Moore NM, Davis GJ, Emig KA, Brown RT, Rochon J, Green S, Varady A. Dance and reducing television viewing to prevent weight gain in African American girls: The Stanford GEMS pilot study. *Ethnicity and Disease* 2003;**13**:S65–77.
32. Laurson KR, Eisenmann JC, Welk GJ, Wickel EE, Gentile DA, Walsh DA. Combined influence of physical activity and screen time recommendations on childhood overweight. *The Journal of Pediatrics* 2008;**153**:209–14.
33. Holt D, Ippolito P, Desrochers D, Kelley C. *Children's Exposure to TV Advertising in 1977 and 2004: Information for the obesity debate.* Washington, DC: Federal Trade Commission; 2007.
34. Gantz W, Schwartz N, Angelini J, Rideout V. *Food for thought: Television food advertising to children in the United States.* Menlo Park, CA: Kaiser Family Foundation; 2007.
35. Borzekowski DLG, Robinson TN. The 30-second effect: An experiment revealing the impact of television commercials on food preferences of preschoolers. *Journal of the American Dietetic Association* 2001;**101**:42–6.
36. Goldberg ME, Gorn GJ, Gibson W. TV messages for snack and breakfast foods: Do they influence children's preferences? *Journal of Consumer Research* 1978;**5**:73–81.
37. Gorn GJ, Goldberg ME. Behavioral evidence of the effects of televised food messages on children. *Journal of Consumer Research* 1982;**9**:200–5.
38. Stoneman Z, Brody GH. The indirect impact of child-oriented advertisements on mother-child interactions. *Journal of Applied Developmental Psychology* 1982;**2**:369–76.
39. Forman J, Halford JCG, Summe H, MacDougall M, Keller KL. Food branding influences ad libitum intake differently in children depending on weight status: Results of a pilot study. *Appetite* 2009;**53**:76–83.

REFERENCES

40. Harris JL, Bargh JA, Brownell KD. Priming effects of television food advertising on eating behavior. *Health Psychology* 2009;**28**(4):404–13.
41. Snoek HM, Van Strien T, Janssens JM, Engels RC. The effect of television viewing on adolescents' snacking: individual differences explained by external, restrained and emotional eating. *Journal of Adolescent Health* 2006;**3**:448–51.
42. Utter J, Neumark-Sztainer D, Jeffery R, Story M. Couch potatoes or French fries: Are sedentary behaviors associated with body mass index, physical activity, and dietary behaviors among adolescents? *Journal of the American Dietetic Association* 2003;**103**(10):1298–305.
43. Miller SA, Taveras EM, Rifas-Shiman SL, Gillman MW. Association between television viewing and poor diet quality in young children. *International Journal of Pediatric Obesity* 2008;**3**(3):168–76.
44. Dubois L, Farmer A, Girard M, Peterson K. Social factors and television use during meals and snacks is associated with higher BMI among pre-school children. *Public Health Nutrition* 2008;**11**(12):1267–79.
45. Institute of Medicine. *Preventing childhood obesity: Health in the balance*. Washington, DC: The National Academies Press; 2005.
46. Saelens BE, Sallis JF, Nader PR, Broyles SL, Berry CC, Taras HL. Home environmental influences on children's television watching from early to middle childhood. *Developmental and Behavioral Pediatrics* 2002;**23**(3):127–32.
47. Coon KA, Goldberg J, Rogers BL, Tucker KL. Relationships between use of television during meals and children's food consumption patterns. *Pediatrics* 2001;**107**:E7.
48. Matheson DM, Wang Y, Klesges M, Beech BM, Kraemer HC, Robinson TN. African-American girls' dietary intake while watching television. *Obesity Research* 2004;**12**(Suppl. 1):32S–7S.
49. Blass EM, Anderson DR, Kirkorian HL, Pempek TA, Price I, Koleini MF. On the road to obesity: Television viewing increases intake of high-density foods. *Physiology and Behavior* 2006;**88**:597–604.
50. Zimmerman F. *Children's media use and sleep problems: Issues and unanswered questions*. Menlo Park, CA: The Henry J. Kaiser Family Foundation; June 2008.
51. Snell E, Adam E, Duncan G. Sleep and the body mass index and overweight status of children and adolescents. *Child Development* 2007;**78**(1):309–23.
52. Nixon GM, Thompson J, Han DY, Becroft DM, Clark PM, Robinson E, Waldie KE, Wild CJ, Black PN, Mitchell EA. Short sleep duration in middle childhood: risk factors and consequences. *Sleep* 2008;**31**(1):71–8.
53. Taheri, S. The link between short sleep duration and obesity: We should recommend more sleep to prevent obesity. *Archives of Disease in Childhood*, 91, 881–4.
54. Kagamimori S, Yamagami T, Sokejima S. The relationship between lifestyle, social characteristics and obesity in 3-year-old Japanese children. *Child: Care, Health and Development* 1999;**25**(3):302–10.
55. Owens J, Maxim R, McGuinn M, Nobile C, Msall M, Alario A. Television viewing habits and sleep disturbance in school children. *Pediatrics* 1999;**104**:e27.
56. Paavonen E, Pennonen M, Roine M, Valkonen S, Lahikainen A. TV exposure associated with sleep disturbances in 5- to 6-year old children. *Journal of Sleep Research* 2006;**15**(2):154–61.
57. Eggermont S, van den Bulck J. Nodding off or switching off? The use of popular media as a sleep aid in secondary school children. *Journal of Paediatric Child Health* 2006;**42**(7–8):428–33.
58. Rideout V, Vandewater E, Wartella E. *Electronic media in the lives of infants, toddlers, and preschoolers*. Menlo Park, CA: The Henry J. Kaiser Family Foundation; Fall 2003.
59. Asbury LD, Wong FL, Price SM, Nolin MJ. The Verb campaign: applying a branding strategy in public health. *American Journal of Preventive Medicine* 2008;**34**(6S):S183–7.
60. Huhman ME, Potter LD, Duke JC, Judkins DR, Heitzler CD, Wong FL. Evaluation of a national physical activity intervention for children: VERB campaign, 2002–2004. *American Journal of Preventive Medicine* 2007;**32**(1):38–43.
61. Reger B, Wootan MG, Booth-Butterfield S, Smith H. 1% or less: a community-based nutrition campaign. *Public Health Reports* 1998;**113**:410–19.
62. Jordan A, Robinson T. Children, television viewing, and weight status. *Annals of the American Academy of Political and Social Sciences* January 2008;**615**(January):119–32.
63. Dennison BA, Russo TJ, Burdick PA, Jenkins PL. An intervention to reduce television viewing by preschool children. *Archives of Pediatrics and Adolescent Medicine* 2004;**158**:170–6.
64. Dey AN, Schiller JS, Tai DA. Summary health statistics for U.S. children: National Health Interview Survey, 2002. *Vital Health Statistics* 2004;**10**:1–78.
65. Jordan A. *Food marketing on children's television: A multi-year comparison*. Boston, MA: Paper presented at the biennial meeting of the Society for Research on Child Development; April 2007.
66. Wilde P. Self-regulation and the response to concerns about food and beverage marketing to children in the United States. *Nutrition Reviews* 2009;**67**(3):155–66.
67. Christakis DA, Garrison MM. Preschool-aged children's television viewing in child care settings. *Pediatrics* 2009;**124**(6):1627–32.
68. Christenson PG. Children's perceptions of TV commercials and products: The effects of PSAs. *Communication Research* 1982;**9**:491–524.
69. Donohue TR, Henke LL, Meyer TP. Learning about television commercials: The impact of instructional units on children's perceptions of motive and intent. *Journal of Broadcasting* 1983;**27**:251–61.
70. Feshbach S, Feshbach ND, Cohen SE. Enhancing children's discrimination in response to television advertising: The effects of psychoeducational training in two elementary school-age groups. *Developmental Review* 1982;**2**:385–403.
71. Livingstone S, Helsper E. Does advertising literacy mediate the effects of advertising on children?: A critical examination of two linked research literatures in relation to obesity and food choice. *Journal of Communication* 2006;**56**:560–84.
72. Lanhuis CE, Poulton R, Welch D, Hancox RJ. Programming obesity and poor fitness: the long-term impact of childhood television. *Obesity* 2008;**16**:1457–9.

CHAPTER 46

Evaluation and Management of Childhood Obesity in Primary Care Settings

Goutham Rao

Weight Management and Wellness Center, Children's Hospital of Pittsburgh (of UPMC),
University of Pittsburgh School of Medicine, Pittsburgh, PA, USA

INTRODUCTION

The well-publicized epidemic of obesity affects both adults and children. In the United States, 31.9% of children are either overweight or obese, 16.3% are obese [1]. Many other developed countries are similarly affected. The combined prevalence of overweight and obesity is higher than 15% in Canada, the United Kingdom, and several Mediterranean countries [2]. Childhood obesity is now a significant problem in many developing countries as well. Roughly 11% of middle-class Indian children, for example, are obese [3]. Among adults, obesity is strongly associated with type 2 diabetes, hypertension, dyslipidemia, cardiovascular disease, biliary tract disease, and asthma [4]. There is also a strong association between obesity and cancer of the colon, breast in postmenopausal women, endometrium, esophagus, and kidney [5]. Disturbingly, childhood obesity has become so serious that some of these problems are now emerging in children. A generation ago, type 2 diabetes was rare among children. Today, in some settings, it constitutes nearly half of all new cases of diabetes diagnosed among children [6].

The purpose of this chapter is to provide practical recommendations for busy primary care physicians for the evaluation and management of common obesity-related illnesses among overweight and obese children and to offer strategies for helping children achieve or maintain a healthy weight. The chapter makes use of a case study to describe a stepwise approach to the problem.

CURRENT PHYSICIAN PRACTICES AND ATTITUDES

There is ample evidence that physicians are ill equipped to tackle obesity, in both adults and children. A 1999 study, for example, revealed that only 42% of obese adults recall being advised to lose weight during the past year [7]. Among children, the rate of nutrition and physical activity counseling by physicians did improve between 1993 and 2002, but the quality and effectiveness of this counseling is unknown [8]. Pediatricians consistently report a lack of self-efficacy in providing obesity-related counseling [9, 10]. A recent survey by Perrin et al. revealed that only 12% of pediatricians report high self-efficacy in managing obesity, even though 39% feel that treatment of obesity by physicians has the potential to be effective. Physicians felt much more comfortable treating asthma, attention deficit hyperactivity disorder, and sexually transmitted diseases than obesity. When asked what resources would help them better treat obesity, 96% of the pediatricians surveyed thought that better counseling tools to guide patients toward lifestyle modification would be somewhat or definitely helpful [11]. A lack of research specifically in primary care settings has been cited as one reason why physicians lack the skills to tackle obesity. The U.S. Preventive Services Task Force (USPSTF) has pointed out that "that there is very limited evidence for behavioral or other overweight treatment that is feasible for primary care delivery or referral," and that "few studies have taken place in primary care settings." It calls for "pragmatic clinical and public health prevention strategies" [12 p. e139].

CASE STUDY

Samantha is a 14-year-old Caucasian girl who comes to your office approximately 1 week after you saw her for a mild ankle sprain. She has completely recovered. Samantha lives at home with her mother, father, and 17-year-old brother. Both her parents are obese and have hypertension and dyslipidemia. Her father is 51 years old and has also had type 2 diabetes for approximately 10 years. She has no significant medical or surgical history. She has no allergies and takes no medications. She began menstruating at age 13 and has normal periods every 28 days. Samantha is 5'6" (168 cm) tall and weighs 189 lbs (86 kg). Her waist circumference is 36" (91 cm), approximately at the 90th percentile for girls her age [16]. Her blood pressure is 130/85 mmHg. The remainder of her physical examination is normal. She has never had laboratory tests of any kind.

Physicians also demonstrate an inability to identify and treat obesity-related illness in children. Roughly 11% of obese children in general and 31% of obese minority children are hypertensive [13, 14]. Hansen, Gunn, and Kaelber found that among 507 children identified as hypertensive through chart reviews from a network of outpatient clinics, just 26% were diagnosed as hypertensive by their physicians [15].

CORE MEDICAL EVALUATION

Samantha is obese with a BMI of $30.5 kg/m^2$, which is at the 97.5th percentile for girls her age. Initial medical evaluation includes assessment of components of the metabolic syndrome—an aggregation of multiple cardiovascular risk factors such as impaired glucose metabolism and lipid disturbances, whose development is promoted by obesity and insulin resistance. In addition to obesity, risks for metabolic syndrome include genetics, ethnicity, increased visceral adiposity, oxidative stress, and different lifestyle factors [17]. The International Diabetes Federation (IDF) has recently developed a set of criteria for the definition of metabolic syndrome to be used in children of all ages (Table 46.1). Note that metabolic syndrome cannot be diagnosed in children under 10 but that evaluation should be considered in such children when a family history suggests increased cardiovascular risk. For adolescents age 16 and older, the IDF adult criteria can be used. The criteria are used not to make a diagnosis of metabolic syndrome for its own sake but to guide medical and laboratory evaluation. Samantha clearly has a high probability of having metabolic syndrome, even without knowing her glucose or lipid levels, given her obesity, high waist circumference, elevated blood pressure, and strong family history of cardiovascular risks.

Hypertension

The National High Blood Pressure Education Program (NHBPEP) Working Group has developed and disseminated blood pressure standards for children and adolescents that depend on height, sex, and age [18]. Samantha's height is at the 86th percentile. Both her systolic and diastolic blood pressures are at approximately the 95th percentile for girls her age. This is in the hypertensive range. Detailed recommendations for management of hypertension can be found in the NHBPEP guidelines and are summarized in Table 46.2. In Samantha's case, her blood pressure should be rechecked in 1 to 2 weeks. Weight-management counseling should be provided. Pharmacotherapy is indicated in children with coexistent diabetes or end-organ damage, those with secondary hypertension, and those whose blood pressure remains elevated despite non-pharmacological measures.

Dyslipidemia

The American Academy of Pediatrics (AAP) recommends initial screening for lipid disorders in children with a family history of dyslipidemia or premature heart disease, and in children with obesity, hypertension, diabetes, or a history of smoking. Screening should be completed between 2 and 10 years of age [19]. Testing should be repeated every 3 to 5 years if results are normal. Screening is appropriate for Samantha, given her obesity, family history, and elevated blood pressure (at least at her initial visit). She is likely to manifest a pattern typical of adolescents with the metabolic syndrome of elevated triglycerides (>150 mg/dL) and low HDL cholesterol (< 35 mg/dL) [20]. Aggressive diet therapy and weight management is the most appropriate treatment in that case. Omega-3 fatty acid supplements (EPA and DHA) have also been shown to be effective in lowering triglycerides [21]. Children age 10 or older with elevated levels of LDL cholesterol, despite aggressive attempts at dietary and weight management, are candidates for drug therapy. Statin therapy should be considered first-line if LDL remains at or above 190 mg/dL (4.90 mM) or at or above 160 mg/dL (4.10 mM) in children with a family history of premature cardiovascular disease and those with two or

TABLE 46.1 IDF Criteria for Metabolic Syndrome

Age group (years)	Obesity (WC)	Triglycerides	HDL-C	Blood pressure	Glucose (mmol/l) or known T2DM
6 to < 10	≥90th percentile	Metabolic syndrome cannot be diagnosed, but further measurements should be made if there is a family history of metabolic syndrome, T2DM, dyslipidaemia, cardiovascular disease, hypertension and/or obesity.			
10 to < 16	≥90th percentile or adult cut-off if lower	≥1.7 mmol/l (≥150 mg/dl)	<1.03 mmol/l (<40 mg/dl)	Systolic ≥130 mm Hg or diastolic ≥85 mm Hg	≥5.6 mmol/l (100 mg/dl) or known T2DM (if ≥5.6 mmol/l recommend an OGTT)
16+	Use existing IDF criteria for adults[2]				

WC: waist circumference; HDL-C: high-density lipoprotein cholesterol; T2DM: type 2 diabetes; OGTT: oral glucose tolerance test.
From Alberti G, Zimmet P, Kaufman F, Tajima N, Silink M, Arslanian S, Wong G, Bennett P, Shaw J, Caprio S. The IDF consensus definition of the metabolic syndrome in children and adolescents; www.idf.org/home/index.cfm?node=1611. Accessed February 13, 2009.

more other cardiovascular risk factors that are not under control [20, 22].

Identifying Impaired Glucose Metabolism/Type 2 Diabetes

The American Diabetes Association (ADA) recommends screening for type 2 diabetes in overweight and obese children age 10 and older with any two of the following risks: family history of type 2 diabetes in first- or second-degree relative, high-risk ethnicity (non-European origin), or signs of insulin resistance (acanthosis nigricans, polycystic ovaries syndrome, hypertension) [23]. Samantha is therefore a candidate for screening. Screening should be carried out every 2 years in high-risk children. The ADA recommends fasting plasma glucose (FPG) due to its low cost and convenience. A 2-hour, 75-gm oral glucose tolerance test (OGTT), however, has been shown to be more sensitive. Recommendations for management of impaired fasting glucose, impaired glucose tolerance, and type 2 diabetes in adolescents can be found elsewhere [24].

TABLE 46.2 NHBPEP Guidelines for Evaluation, Follow-up and Treatment of Elevated Blood Pressure in Children and Adolescents

	SBP or DBP percentile[a]	Frequency of BP measurement	Therapeutic lifestyle changes	Pharmacological therapy
Normal	<90th	Recheck at next scheduled physical examination	Encourage healthy diet, sleep, and physical activity	
Prehypertension	90th to <95th or if BP exceeds 120/80 even if <90th percentile up to <95th percentile[b]	Recheck in 6 mo	Weight-management counseling if overweight; introduce physical activity and diet management[c]	None unless compelling indications such as chronic kidney disease, diabetes mellitus, heart failure, or LVH exist
Stage 1 hypertension	95th–99th percentile plus 5 mm Hg	Recheck in 1–2 weeks or sooner if the patient is symptomatic; if persistently elevated on two additional occasions, evaluate or refer to source of care within 1 mo	Weight-management counseling if overweight; introduce physical activity and diet management[c]	Initiate pharmacotherapy in cases of symptomatic hypertension, secondary hypertension end-organ damage, or persistent hypertension despite non-pharmacologic therapy or compelling indications as shown above
Stage 2 hypertension	>99th percentile plus 5 mm Hg	Evaluate or refer to source of care within 1 wk or immediately if the patient is symptomatic	Weight-management counseling if overweight; introduce physical activity and diet management[c]	Initiate therapy[d]

[a] For gender, age, and height measured on at least three separate occasions; if systolic and diastolic categories are different, categorize by the higher value.
[b] This occurs typically at 12 years old for SBP and at 16 years old for DBP.
[c] Parents and children trying to modify the eating plan to the Dietary Approaches to Stop Hypertension Study eating plan could benefit from consultation with a registered or licensed nutritionist to get them started.
[d] More than one drug may be required.
From the National High Blood Pressure Education Program Working Group on High Blood Pressure in Children. The fourth report on the diagnosis, evaluation, and treatment of high blood pressure in children and adolescents; www.nhlbi.nih.gov/health/prof/heart/hbp/hbp_ped.htm. Accessed February 23, 2009.

EVALUATION FOR OTHER PROBLEMS

An Expert Committee convened by the American Medical Association (AMA) recommends measurement of alanine transaminase (ALT) and aspartate transaminase (AST) to detect fatty liver disease and measurement of BUN and creatinine to detect renal impairment in obese children (from longstanding hypertension or diabetes) [25]. Clinicians need to be aware of a number of other medical and psychosocial problems in obese children. Polycystic ovary syndrome (PCOS), characterized by hyperandrogenemia and menstrual irregularities in addition to polycystic ovarian morphology, is common in obese, adolescent girls [26]. Obese children are more likely than their normal-weight peers to suffer from a wide range of musculoskeletal problems including pain [27]. Clinicians should recognize sleep problems in obese children. Sleep-disordered breathing, especially obstructive sleep apnea, is common and should be suspected in children with loud snoring, daytime somnolence, and restless sleep.

Obese children are frequently the victims of discrimination. Many suffer from low self-esteem, social isolation, and overall poorer psychological well-being [28]. Clinicians should be alert to the presence of depression and other psychological problems.

WEIGHT-MANAGEMENT COUNSELING

Specialized centers and research programs offer effective intensive counseling programs for obese children that promote behavior modification. Unfortunately, such programs can at best accommodate a tiny fraction of obese children. The widespread availability of safe, effective, and inexpensive medications for the treatment of obesity is likely many years away. Significant environmental and societal change holds the promise of reversing the problem. This will likely require change in public policy that affects, for example, how certain foods are marketed and how our communities are structured (e.g., making it easier to walk from one place to another). Environmental changes take a long time to bring about and even longer to have a substantial impact on people's health. Today, settings in which identification, prevention, and treatment of obesity is practical and rational include schools where children spend much of their time and primary care practices, through which they receive much of their care.

As discussed, primary care physicians lack practical tools with which to provide counseling. They also have limited time. Physician contact in annual preventive medicine visits, during which a number of issues are discussed, is just 17 to 20 minutes long [29]. Physicians are therefore often charged with addressing the issue of weight along with other problems. The challenge is to provide useful counseling in an efficient way. The "5As" (ask, advise, agree, assist, and arrange) is a simple and useful paradigm for delivery of preventive services originally developed as the "4As" by the National Cancer Institute for smoking cessation counseling [30]. The 5As are described in more detail in Table 46.3 [31]:

TABLE 46.3 5As Organizational Construct for Clinical Counseling

Assess: Ask about/assess behavioral health risk(s) and factors affecting choice of behavior change goals/methods.

Advise: Give clear, specific, and personalized behavior change advice, including information about harms and benefits.

Agree: Collaboratively select appropriate goals and methods based on the patient's interest in and willingness to change the behavior.

Assist: Using behavior change techniques (self-help or counseling), aid the patient in achieving agreed-upon goals by acquiring the skills, confidence, and social/environmental supports for behavior change, supplemented with adjunctive medical treatments when appropriate (e.g., pharmacotherapy for tobacco dependence, contraceptive drugs/devices).

Arrange: Schedule follow-up contacts to provide ongoing assistance/support and to adjust the treatment plan as needed, including referral to more intensive or specialized treatment.

From Whitlock EP, Orleans CT, Pender N, Allan J. Evaluating primary care behavioral counseling interventions. An evidence-based approach. Agency for Healthcare Research and Quality. U.S. Preventive Services Task Force; www.ahrq.gov/clinic/3rduspstf/behavior/behavintr.pdf. Accessed February 23, 2009.

With respect to obesity, the first step is to raise the issue of weight in a respectful way (e.g., by explaining BMI and the health risks of obesity) and to *ask* about common obesity-related behaviors, such as those listed in Table 46.4 [32]. Tools are available to make gathering this information easier [25]. Let's assume that an inquiry into her habits reveals that Samantha drinks approximately 1.5 liters of regular soft drinks per day. She rarely has fast food. She has several hours of "screen time" per day in the form of using her computer and is not

TABLE 46.4 Useful Questions for Identifying Common Obesity-Related Behaviors in Children

Do you eat regular fast food (burgers, fries, etc.) more than once per week?

Do you consume more than one serving of sweet beverage (fruit juice, fruit drink/punch, regular soft drink, energy drink, etc.) a day?

Do you participate in a minimum of 30 minutes of physical activity per day?

Do you eat dinner together with at least one parent on most days of the week?

Do you watch television, play video games, or use a computer (other than for schoolwork) for more than 2 hours a day?

involved in any significant physical activity. She usually eats with her family. It's important to ask about her interest in changing some of her habits. An appropriate message could take the following form:

> Samantha, by asking you a few questions, I've picked up that there are some behaviors that you need to change to achieve a healthier weight and to prevent gaining too much weight in the future. Are you interested in working on making changes over a period of time?

Assuming she is interested in making changes, the next step is to provide her with appropriate *advice:*

> There are many different causes of obesity. In your case, there are at least three important things you need to work on: First, the amount of soft drink you are consuming is a big part of the problem. Soft drinks are a major cause of obesity. Second, it sounds like you don't get any regular physical activity. This can be simple things like walking or riding a bike for 30 to 60 minutes on most days of the week. Finally, the amount of time you spend playing video games is a problem. Spending less time playing video games and more time being physically active would help you achieve a healthier weight.

The next step is to *agree* on a plan for change. This involves setting goals that are realistic and take into consideration the patient's own readiness to change behavior. Change in behavior should be promoted incrementally:

> Let's work on changing some of these behaviors, Samantha. Do you think you could cut down to two cans of regular soda per day? I realize this is a big step. I'd like you to try to do this. Try water instead of soft drinks whenever you can. Also, do you think you could take a walk for 10 minutes every day after school?

One can *assist* children with behavior changes by making useful suggestions:

> You've been drinking lots of soft drinks for a long time. Cutting back may not be easy. Have you tried other sorts of refreshments? If water isn't what you like, how about low-fat milk? This might be worth trying.

Finally, it's important to provide reinforcement and encouragement by *arranging* follow-up visits. Let's assume that over the course of a couple of months, Samantha has cut down on soft drink consumption (and lost about 5 pounds) but has made little progress in walking regularly. An appropriate message can be offered during a follow-up visit:

> Samantha, I think it's wonderful that you've cut out so much soda from your diet. It's great that you've lost weight. You told me the walking hasn't gone that well. Are you willing to try again? Let's try and find out why walking has been hard. Maybe another activity might be better for you.

The process continues with repeated inquiry into behaviors whenever possible, reinforced advice, setting new goals, and providing assistance over time.

ADVANTAGES AND LIMITATIONS OF 5AS APPROACH

The approach described earlier has four important advantages. First, it is relatively simple to deliver. Second, because it is delivered through primary care physicians whenever the opportunity allows, it is accessible to most children. More intensive approaches may be more effective, but because they reach a smaller proportion of children in need, their impact on public health is significantly less [31]. Third, it is customizable to individual patients and practices. Skipping breakfast, for example, is a common behavior associated with obesity among some children. Incorporating a question about skipping breakfast into the "ask" component is easy to do. Finally, because it emphasizes healthy behaviors rather than actual weight, it does not stigmatize overweight and obese children. A thin child with unhealthy habits is still at risk for obesity and therefore can be counseled in the same way as an overweight or obese child.

Among its disadvantages, it can be argued that the 5As paradigm, though useful in smoking cessation counseling and for other problems, is not a proven approach for weight management. Bear in mind, however, that though clinical guidelines for management of obesity have been available for some time, the widespread adoption of obesity guidelines has not taken place, nor has implementation yet been shown to be effective in controlling obesity. Furthermore, the Institute of Medicine emphasizes the need to act even in the absence of high-quality evidence: "Knowing that it is impossible to produce an optimal solution a priori, we more appropriately adopt surveillance, trial, measurement, error, success, alteration, and dissemination as our course, *to be embarked upon immediately.* Given that the health of today's children and future generations is at stake, we must proceed with all due urgency and vigor" [33 p. 137].

References

1. Ogden CL, Carroll MD, Flegal KM. High body mass index for age among US children and adolescents, 2003–2006. *JAMA* 2008;**299**(20):2401–5.
2. Janssen I, Katzmarzyk PT, Boyce WF, Vereecken C, Mulvihill C, Roberts C, Currie C, Pickett W. Comparison of overweight and obesity prevalence in school-aged youth from 34 countries and their relationships with physical activity and dietary patterns. *Obes Reviews* 2005;**6**(2):123–32.

3. Chhatwal J, Verma M, Riar SK. Obesity among pre-adolescents and adolescents of a developing country (India). *Asia Pac J Clin Nutr* 200;13(3):231−5.
4. Mokdad AH, Ford ES, Bowman BA, Dietz WH, Vinicor F, Bales VS, Marks JS. Prevalence of obesity, diabetes, and obesity-related health risk factors, 2001. *JAMA* 2003;**289**(1):76−9.
5. Bianchini F, Kaaks R, Vainio H. Overweight, obesity, and cancer risk. *Lancet Oncol* 2002;**3**(9):565−74.
6. Hannon TS, Rao G, Arslanian SA. Childhood obesity and type 2 diabetes. *Pediatrics* 2005;**116**(2):473−80.
7. Galuska DA, Will JC, Serdula MK, Ford ES. Are health care professionals advising obese patients to lose weight? *JAMA* 1999;**282**(16):1576−8.
8. Rao G. Pediatric obesity-related counseling in the outpatient setting. *Amb Pediatr* 2005;**5**:377−9.
9. Story MT, Neumark-Stzainer DR, Sherwood NE, et al. Management of child and adolescent obesity: attitudes, barriers, skills, and training needs among health care professionals. *Pediatrics* 2002;**110**:210−14.
10. Kolagotla L, Adams W. Ambulatory management of childhood obesity. *Obes Res* 2004;**12**:275−83.
11. Perrin EM, Flower KB, Garrett J, Ammerman AS. Preventing and treating obesity: Pediatricians' self-efficacy, barriers, resources, and advocacy. *Amb Pediatr* 2005;**5**:150−6.
12. Whitlock EP, Williams SB, Gold R, Smith PR, Shipman SA. Screening and interventions for childhood overweight: a summary of evidence for the US Preventive Services Task Force. *Pediatrics* 2005;**116**(1):e125−44.
13. Sorof JM, Lai D, Turner J, Poffenbarger T, Portman RJ. Overweight, ethnicity, and the prevalence of hypertension in school-aged children. *Pediatrics* 2004;**113**:475−82.
14. Puri M, Flynn JT, Garcia M, Nussbaum H, Freeman K, DiMartino-Nardi JR. The frequency of elevated blood pressure in obese minority youth. *J Clin Hypertens* 2008;**10**(2):119−24.
15. Hansen ML, Gunn PW, Kaelber DC. Underdiagnosis of hypertension in children and adolescents. *JAMA* 2007;**298**(8):874−9.
16. Alberti G, Zimmet P, Kaufman F, Tajima N, Silink M, Arslanian S, Wong G, Bennett P, Shaw J, Caprio S. The IDF consensus definition of the metabolic syndrome in children and adolescents. www.idf.org/home/index.cfm?node=1611 Accessed 13 February 2009.
17. Steinberger J, Daniels SR, Eckel RH, Hayman L, Lustig RH, McCrindle B, Mietus-Snyder ML. Progress and challenges in metabolic syndrome in children and adolescents. AHA scientific statement. *Circulation* 2009;**119**:628−47.
18. National High Blood Pressure Education Program Working Group on High Blood Pressure in Children. The fourth report on the diagnosis, evaluation, and treatment of high blood pressure in children and adolescents. *Pediatrics* 2004 Aug;**114**(Suppl. 2): 555−76.
19. Daniels SR, Greer FR. the Committee on Nutrition. Lipid screening and cardiovascular health in childhood. *Pediatrics* 2008;**122**:198−208.
20. Kavey RE, Daniels SR, Lauer RM, et al. American Heart Association guidelines for primary prevention of atherosclerotic cardiovascular disease beginning in childhood. *Circulation* 2003;**107**(11):1562−6.
21. Balk E, Chung M, Lichenstein A, et al. Effects of omega-3 fatty acids on cardiovascular risk factors and intermediate markers of cardiovascular disease. *Evid Rep Technol Assess (Summ)* 2004 Mar; (93):1−6.
22. McCrindle BW, Urbina EM, Dennison BA, Jacobson MS, Steinberger J, Rocchini AP, Hayman LL, Daniels SR. American Heart Association Atherosclerosis, Hypertension, and Obesity in, American Heart Association Council of Cardiovascular Disease in the Young, American Heart Association Council on Cardiovascular Nursing. Drug therapy of high-risk lipid abnormalities in children and adolescents: a scientific statement from the American Heart Association Atherosclerosis, Hypertension, and Obesity in Youth Committee, Council of Cardiovascular Disease in the Young. *Circulation* 2007 Apr 10;**115**(14): 1948−67.
23. American Diabetes Association. Screening for type 2 diabetes. *Diabetes Care* 2004;**27**(Suppl. 1):S11−14.
24. Hannon TS, Rao G, Arslanian SA. Childhood obesity and type 2 diabetes mellitus. *Pediatrics* 2005;**116**(2):473−80.
25. Rao G. Childhood obesity: Highlights of AMA Expert Committee recommendations. *Am Fam Physician* 2008;**78**(1):56−66.
26. Blank SK, Helm KD, McCartney CR, Marshall JC. Polycystic ovary syndrome in adolescence. *Ann NY Acad Sci* 2008;**1135**: 76−84.
27. Stovitz SD, Pardee PE, Vazquez G, Duval S, Schwimmer JB. Musculoskeletal pain in obese children and adolescents. *Acta Paediatr* 2008;**97**(4):489−93.
28. Wardle J, Cooke L. *Best Pract Res Clin Endocrinol Metab* 2005; **19**(3):421−40.
29. American Academy of Pediatrics. *Division of Health Policy Research. Periodic Survey of Fellows #56. Executive Summary. Pediatricians' Provision of Preventative Care and Use of Health Supervision Guidelines.* Elk Grove Village, IL: American Academy of Pediatrics; 2004.
30. Glynn TJ, Manley MW. *How to help your patients stop smoking: a manual for physicians.* (NIH publication no. 89-3064.). Bethesda, MD: National Cancer Institute; 1989.
31. Whitlock EP, Orleans CT, Pender N, Allan J. Evaluating primary care behavioral counseling interventions. An evidence-based approach. Agency for Healthcare Research and Quality. U.S. Preventive Services Task Force. www.ahrq.gov/clinic/3rduspstf/behavior/behavintr.pdf Accessed 23 February 2009.
32. Obesity Rao G. *FP Essentials Monograph, Edition No. 349. AAFP Home Study.* Leawood, KS: American Academy of Family Physicians; June 2008.
33. Koplan JP, Liverman CT, Kraak VI. IOM Committee on Prevention of Obesity in Children and Youth. Preventing childhood obesity: Health in the balance: Executive summary. *J Am Diet Assoc* 2005;**105**(1):131−8.

CHAPTER 47

The Future Directions and Clinical Management of Childhood Obesity

Clodagh S. O'Gorman, Jonathan Cauchi, Jill K. Hamilton, Denis Daneman

Division of Endocrinology, Department of Pediatrics, The Hospital for Sick Children and University of Toronto, Toronto, Ontario, Canada

INTRODUCTION

The purpose of this chapter is to evaluate current approaches to the management of childhood obesity, while at the same time attempting to predict future directions in this field. We have divided this chapter into sections called "Knowledge Gaps" to highlight areas of research which we feel deserve particular attention: etiology, screening and non-modifiable risk factors, lessons from medical models of obesity, and interventions. At various intervals in this chapter, we make suggestions regarding future possible directions for clinical care and research in childhood obesity. A review of available data suggests that the current epidemic of childhood obesity has occurred too rapidly and too widely to be caused by genetic drift alone. Rather it is likely related to modifiable risk factors, providing the potential to reverse the present trend.

It is widely accepted that obesity is complex and multifactorial with significant short-term morbidity and long-term morbidity and mortality. It is unlikely that a single approach to the investigation and management will be applicable to all overweight individuals. Therefore, in order to impact on this condition, a multifaceted approach, encompassing research from bench to bedside to backyard is essential. Furthermore, everyone with a vested interest in mitigating the impact of childhood obesity needs to play an active role, including: governmental and nongovernmental agencies; international, national, and local policy makers; school and physical education teachers; providers of extracurricular activities to schoolchildren; the media; producers of food and exercise or leisure equipment; pharmaceutical manufacturers; as well as parents, families, and community groups.

Lustig proposed that Newton's first law of thermodynamics be used to explain the etiology of obesity, to patients, parents and families, and health professionals [1]. This law states: "Within a closed system, energy is neither created nor destroyed, but is transformed from one form to another." Using this law to conceptualize obesity, the implication is that energy taken in must be equal to energy expended plus energy stored [1]. This is a simple explanation of the etiology of obesity; however, in practice, obesity is far more complex. Fore*sight* is an agency funded by the government of the United Kingdom that "creates challenging visions of the future to ensure effective strategies now." One of its challenges has been to address the issue of obesity (www.foresight.gov.uk). Its report, "Fore*sight* Tackling Obesity: Future Choices—Project Report" summarizes the associations in eight thematic clusters between published studies on obesity, and these thematic clusters are centered around the central "engine" of obesity studies (Fig. 47.1). The seven thematic clusters include societal influences, food production, individual psychology, food consumption, biology, individual activity, and activity environment. The Fore*sight* group mapped studies to each other, dependent on what influenced each study and what each domain each study affected. One of the striking features of this map is that food production influences many of the other thematic clusters, without evidence from published literature that the other thematic clusters influence food production.

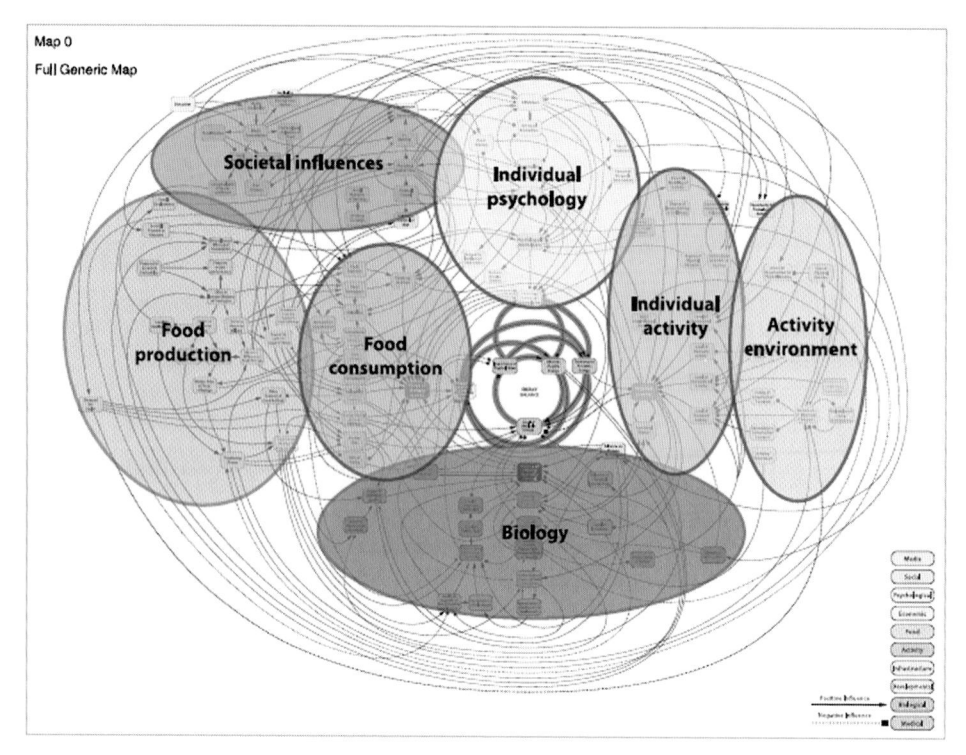

FIGURE 47.1 The full obesity system map, with thematic clusters, reproduced with permission from "Tackling obesity: Future choices," available at www.foresight.gov.uk.

KNOWLEDGE GAP 1: ETIOLOGY OF CHILDHOOD OBESITY

Study the past if you would define the future. —Confucius, *Chinese philosopher and reformer (551 BC–479 BC)*

Activity

When energy intake exceeds energy required for both basal metabolism and physical activity (exercise) combined, the excess is net energy gain, and this is stored as adipose tissue. Childhood obesity is considerably more complex and multifactorial than suggested by this simple formula. But it is clear that net energy gain contributes to childhood obesity. Exercise increases energy expenditure, but it also increases the basal metabolic rate, which contributes to increased energy expenditure after and between bouts of physical activity. The health benefits of exercise are many and varied, including improved self-esteem and mood, probably moderated by release of endorphins [2], enhanced insulin sensitivity [3], and a direct positive effect on the vasculature, even in children and youth, reducing the risk of atherosclerosis later in life [4]. Thus, the benefits of exercise extend beyond weight control or weight loss. It is also important to note that the health benefits of exercise are independent of weight loss. Therefore, it is possible to be heavy but still physically fit and thus to benefit from exercise—the so-called fat-but-fit phenomenon.

Sedentary behavior is increasingly viewed as distinct from activity or inactivity [5]. Examples of sedentary behavior include taking the elevator rather than the stairs or getting a car ride rather than walking to the bus stop. Sedentary behavior is positively associated with increased body mass index (BMI) [6] and more recently with increased blood pressure [7]. Sedentary behavior, like activity, may be measured by accelerometers. Some data suggest that not all sedentary behavior is the same, with some sedentary states (e.g., television watching) being more obesogenic than others [7]. Further studies are required to evaluate this theory. Additionally, reducing sedentary behavior rather than increasing activity may be an easier aim for patients enrolled in weight-loss intervention studies. Some studies in children suggest that reducing television and computer use contributes to decreasing the BMI, but this change is mediated by decreased caloric intake rather than increased activity [8]. Future interventions to address the prevention and treatment of obesity may be more successful if they aim to decrease sedentary behavior rather than or in addition to increasing exercise. Further long-term studies are required.

Current Canadian guidelines recommend that children and adolescents participate in at least 90 minutes of daily physical activity [9]. As recently as 2005, 90% of Canadian youth aged 12 years failed to achieve this level of activity [9, 10]. Furthermore, physical activity in adolescents tends to decline as they approach adulthood [10, 11]. In 2007, physical activity declined 1.8% to 2.7% per year in boys aged 10 to 17 years and 2.6% to 7.4% per year in girls aged 10 to 17 years [11]. This trend of reducing physical activity almost certainly continues throughout adulthood.

BMI correlates positively with conditions such as type 2 diabetes and atherosclerosis. Although weight loss may improve outcomes, prevention of weight gain is likely to be more effective in preventing the development of these conditions and so facilitate improved health. Prevention of further weight gain, or decreasing the trajectory of weight gain, may be a more achievable aim of weight control regimes for many individuals. More studies are required to address the relationships between body weight at different ages and obesity-related morbidity and mortality.

For children with decreased exercise tolerance compared to their peers, engaging in competitive team-based sports may be discouraging. Solo sports, such as martial arts or dance, might lead to less comparison with peers, while also reducing or eliminating the amount of "bench time" a child may be subject to in a team sport. Nonetheless, solo sports can be equally as fun and rewarding, and ultimately as competitive, as organized team sports. Not all team sports are equally physically demanding either: team sports that are spontaneous may offer children less bench time and more activity than organized team sports [12]; but organized competitive team sports may offer increasing levels of competition, with greater opportunity to gradually increase performance and physical fitness. Most weight-loss interventions utilize behavior modification or cognitive behavior therapy but in children, these tools may be more complex, given the stage of cognitive development [13]. Finally, children may be more willing to participate in lifestyle exercise (defined as exercise that is achieved during the activities of daily living) than programmed aerobic exercise because it is more integrated into a person's day and has a more social flavor [14].

Clinicians, policy makers, and educators must be sensitive to the specific needs of overweight children and adapt exercise and activity programs accordingly, without allowing them to appear different or receive special attention in front of their peers. One aspect of the multifaceted approach to reversing the obesity trend in children should be a focus on physical activity, incorporating both organized and casual opportunities for reducing sedentariness and increasing physical activity. Team sports may benefit some children, but they are not always the answer for increasing activity. For children who are obese and who do not participate in any regular activities, it may be easier to decrease sedentary behavior in the short term with perhaps phased introduction of increased activity in the long term. Studies that separate the effects of increasing activity versus decreasing sedentary behavior are difficult to conduct but are required.

Screen Time

Screen time includes time spent watching television, playing computer games, and other computer uses. Screen time is positively associated with increased BMI. But not all screen time is equally obesogenic [7]. It is recommended currently that total screen time should be less than 2 hours daily for children over 2 years of age [15] and that children under 2 years should not have any screen exposure [11]. Although these recommendations were originally designed to promote early neurocognitive development, they should be fortuitous in obesity prevention.

In children, there is a positive association between screen time and increased weight [16]. There are several postulated reasons why screen time increases weight gain. First, children consume high-calorie snacks during screen time [11]. Second, children are exposed to multiple food commercials during this time, which is likely to further increase the child's consumption of energy-dense food. This is likely to be more significant while watching television than while watching prerecorded movies, without breaks for commercials. Third, during television watching, the basal metabolic rate falls to very low levels, lower than that during sleeping.

Introducing computer games that require active physical involvement, a concept recently termed "exergaming," can attenuate the decline in activity as a result of increased screen time [17]. Currently, exergaming has been the subject of very few and very small randomized controlled trials [18–20]. In the future, larger trials will be needed to assess whether these can actually be recommended to parents as part of the approach to decreasing or preventing childhood obesity.

Food Choices

Other ways to reduce net energy gain include decreasing energy consumed or altering the quality or type of energy consumed. Reduced energy intake can be achieved by replacing high-energy but relatively nutritionally deficient foods with lower-energy but nutritionally rich foods. In the past, dieting strategies tried to eliminate high-fat foods from the diet. However, when reduced fat consumption is accompanied by increased carbohydrate consumption, to maintain satiety, then weight loss is often not achieved [16]. Increased carbohydrate intake promotes positive energy gain and excess ingested carbohydrates are converted for storage to fatty acids [21]. Reduced energy gain may be better affected by replacing fat and carbohydrate intake with increased intake of vegetables, fruits, legumes, and whole grains. It is known that many adults with low BMIs have low-energy but highly nutritious diets [21]. In addition to weight benefits, there are significant data suggesting that vegetables, fruits, legumes, and whole grains are associated with decreased risk of cardiovascular and other chronic diseases [22]. These data are generally only available in adults and are extrapolated to children. Further research into altering children's nutritional intake is required.

Children's eating habits are changing rapidly. In the 1970s, children ate 17% of their meals outside the home, including eating fast food totaling 2% of their diet [23]. In the 1990s, 30% of dietary intake was eaten outside the home, with fast food comprising 10% of daily food intake [23]. Children today consume smaller amounts of milk, vegetables, eggs, and whole-grain breads and more poultry, fruit and fruit juices, softdrinks, cheeses, and salty snacks in their diets [16]. The Canadian Community Health Survey in 2004 reported that one in five children aged 4 to 13 years and one in three adolescents aged 14 to 18 years consumed a fast food meal the day before their interview [16].

The eating habits and consequent BMI of children tend to reflect those of the adult caregivers with whom the children live and spend their time [24]. Children learn from and model themselves on these caregivers [25]. Therefore, children tend to have the same attitudes to food and affinity for energy-dense foods as the adults in their families or social circles. It is likely that altering the food choices of caregivers will simultaneously alter the food choices of children. However, studies are required to evaluate whether or not this is true and whether or not the effects of altering the children's food choices are long lasting. If so, it may be more effective to target adults for food choice educational programs. Some pediatric weight-maintenance programs focus on family-based dietary interventions, with varying degrees of success [26, 27]. One study in particular showed benefit from education programs to either increase fruit and vegetables or to decrease high-fat foods, but results showed relatively greater weight loss in the group that was encouraged to increase fruit and vegetables [26]. It must be remembered that adults are generally the purchasers of food for households, and much of the food that the children eat is eaten in the home.

Furthermore, when a caregiver restricts a food that a child enjoys, the child is likely to consume increased quantities of this restricted food [28] and to consume it in the absence of hunger. Several studies have demonstrated the consequences of food restriction in long- and short-term eating behaviors in Caucasian girls [29, 30]. Eating in the absence of hunger also appears to be a learned trait. Francis and Birch in 2005 found that daughters of overweight mothers displayed increased gains in BMI and increased eating in the absence of hunger at 5 years of age [31]. Future studies should explore the impact on children of food restriction and eating without hunger in caregivers and the field should be extended to study other ethnicities. This may help to define cultural, social, and genetic differences in childhood obesity.

Taste

It has been suggested that individuals with higher bitter taste sensitivity might choose to avoid antioxidant-rich vegetables because of their perceived bitterness, and they might instead consume sweeter or fattier foods, which are frequently more obesogenic. Similarly, choosing sweet foods may be influenced by polymorphisms in sweet taste receptors. Finally, it has been suggested that a so-called fat taste perception may have evolved to recognize energy-dense foods and to select foods containing fat-soluble vitamins and essential fatty acids [32]. If genetic factors explain partly food selection, it is possible that targeted interventions for susceptible individuals will be developed in the future. These hypotheses and relationships warrant further investigation [32].

Maternal Employment and Food Choices

Many studies have established that mothers influence food restriction and food monitoring more than fathers [29]. Many of the factors influencing weight and food selection will confound each other, as many of these factors are inter-related complexly, including socioeconomic status, employment, urban versus rural living, influence of extended family, and the like. However, there are many research opportunities for exploring the influence of family, caregivers, and parents on children's weight.

A Japanese study [33] demonstrated that maternal employment status (full time, part time, or unemployed) is associated with the BMI of children aged 12 to 13 years. The children of mothers in full-time employment had the highest BMI, followed by the mothers in part-time employment, and the children of unemployed mothers had the lowest BMI. Furthermore, the children of mothers in full-time employment snacked more frequently, the children of mothers in part-time employment ate larger meal portions, and the children of unemployed mothers ate meals faster [33]. This study illustrates the importance of parental supervision in educating children about healthy eating practices.

The reasons for the variations in a child's food intake with the mother's work practices may include the amount of supervision available to influence or educate children on healthy food choices. Other possible confounders include the reasons why a mother is unemployed or in part-time employment, level of education of both parents, income of the father (if he is the primary breadwinner in the family), and socioeconomic status. These confounders are not necessarily universal in different societies. Although it has been established that mothers more than fathers influence food restriction and food monitoring [29], similar studies should be conducted to explore the effects of paternal employment on children's food choices and eating patterns.

Breast-Feeding

Current guidelines recommend breast-feeding until at least 6 months old, as this significantly reduces the probability of overweight at 4 to 5 years of age [34]. A German study of 9357 children aged between 5 and 6 years found that breast-fed children had significantly lower rates of overweight and obesity compared to non-breast-fed children (9.2% versus 12.6% and 2.8% versus 4.5%, respectively) [35]. This reduction in risk of obesity may occur through metabolic programming, a mechanism in which metabolic factors that are active during prenatal and postnatal development influence health and disease risk in later life [35].

There are other suggested benefits of breast-feeding. First, the constituents of breast milk vary considerably with the metabolic state of the mother, the maternal diet, the duration of lactation, the volume of milk consumed by the infant, and the degree of breast milk expression [35]. This variety in the constituents of breast milk may explain why adults who were breast-fed as infants eat a more varied diet than adults who were formula-fed infants. Second, bottle-fed babies drink more calories than breast-fed babies. It is postulated that breast-fed babies learn satiety signals, whereas the intake volume of bottle-fed babies is determined largely by their parents. This satiety effect may be mediated through the effect of leptin on the hypothalamus, or through epigenetic factors, which are not well understood to date but are being explored [36, 37]. Third, formula is typically higher in protein content than breast milk, and higher levels of protein consumption in early life favor weight gain in both rodent and human studies [35]. Additionally, a high protein intake may result in higher secretion of insulin and Insulin-like growth factor-1 (IGF-1), which may lead to higher levels of insulin resistance in later life [35]. Fourth, breast-feeding mothers show a reduced incidence of neuroendocrine responses to stressors, lower perceived stress levels, and fewer symptoms of depression compared to formula-feeding mothers [35]. Of course, there are indications for choosing formula over breast-feeding or for supplementing breast-feeding with formula feeding. There are also emerging data that breast milk from mothers with diabetes or other metabolic disturbances actually increases the child's risk of obesity, rather than decreasing it [38, 39]. Nonetheless, the evidence supporting breast-feeding is substantial, and many pediatric societies worldwide advocate breast-feeding infants for at least 6 months.

Fast-Food Product Television Marketing

Evidence shows that children are especially susceptible to marketing, possibly attributable to their reduced judgment compared to adults [40]. A study reported in 2006 found that 36% of advertisements during commercial breaks were for fast-food restaurants [41]. Marketing has a primary effect on demand for fast-food products [42]. Television influences the requests children aged 2 to 11 years make to their parents to purchase goods [43]. There is a deficit in evidence for teenagers, and this area should be explored by further research. In society today, where many children have screen time in excess of recommendations and are exposed to television adverts for high-energy, nutritionally deficient foods, the potential impact on excess weight gain is clear.

In 2007, the Institute of Medicine determined that there was too little evidence to firmly establish that television advertisement is a direct influence on childhood obesity [16], but it did provide recommendations for bans or restrictions on the use of cartoon characters, celebrity endorsements, health claims, stealth marketing, and marketing in schools. Health claims are reasonable to include, given that of 367 products not classified as confectionery, soft drinks, or bakery items, 89% were of poor nutritional quality [44]. The aim of reducing fast-food advertising aimed at children is to prevent the negative health effects of these foods. This is reminiscent of the smoking ban in most advertising media several decades ago. However, studies are required to further evaluate the effects of reducing fast-food advertisements aimed at children. There are some suggestions that fast-food companies may include addictive nutrients in their products [45] and price the addictive products lower than other products [45]. Potentially, this makes their product more accessible and promotes lifetime consumers, mirroring another tactic utilized by tobacco companies. We suggest that physicians, policy makers, and those who care for children should consider adopting the Institute of Medicine's stance and support the restriction of fast-food advertisements aimed at children.

School Contributions

The influence of schools on healthy eating behavior is significant. Both the Center for Disease Control (CDC) and the World Health Organization (WHO) have supported proposals that encourage offering healthier food programs in all schools. It is thought that these school-based programs will promote lifelong healthy eating habits [46]. Other approaches to improving healthy food options at school include reducing the availability of foods with saturated fats, sweetened beverages, and snacks and increased availability of fruits and vegetables and improved dietary intake. The presence of sweetened beverages and snacks in vending machines and other school vendors has not yet declined sufficiently [47]. Based on the surplus of evidence that sweetened beverages promote increasing BMI and metabolic syndrome and the endorsement of the WHO and CDC to improve the nutritional situation in schools, policy makers should seriously consider banning sweetened beverages in schools internationally [48, 49].

KNOWLEDGE GAP 2: SCREENING AND NON-MODIFIABLE RISK FACTORS

Body Mass Index and Other Anthropometric Measures of Adiposity

Calculation of BMI, based on measurement of height and weight, is a powerful tool for calculating risk of overweight and obesity, and extrapolating this calculation to predict the risk of other conditions, such as cardiovascular disease, in adult populations. The accepted definitions of overweight and obesity in adult populations are based on BMI cutoffs [50]. However, the use of BMI has limitations. At a population level, it is a simple tool that can generate significant amounts of data. At an individual level, any two people with the same BMI might have significantly different body shapes, with significantly different areas of deposition of body fat, and significantly different risks of cardiovascular or other diseases. So BMI alone does not provide any indication of fat partitioning. Some authors have proposed the supplementation of BMI with a grading system to provide additional information about the complications of obesity in adult populations [51]. This proposed staging system is currently being evaluated in a clinical setting. Dependent on the level of success with this staging system, it is reasonable to consider researching and adapting it for use in childhood obesity in the future.

There are additional difficulties comparing BMI measurements across different populations. Studies have shown that Caucasians have more visceral adiposity and African Americans more subcutaneous adiposity, at the same BMI, and, therefore, Caucasians are likely to be at higher cardiovascular risk than African Americans at the same BMI [50, 52]. In studies of adults, it has been suggested that the combined use of BMI and serum measurement of triglycerides provides a much better tool for predicting risk. Future research studies in children should utilize other factors combined with BMI to establish cumulative risk in children with obesity.

The BMI of children changes as they age. Therefore, BMI centiles or standard deviation scores (SDS) are used, and overweight and obesity are based on these centile or SDS scores, and they vary depending on the age and gender of the child. These are more cumbersome than using simple standard BMI cutoff levels for defining overweight and obesity in adults.

It is evident that supplementary or replacement measures of screening for adiposity and risk in children are required. Examples of attributes of an ideal screening tool for screening for obesity include that the tool is inexpensive, quick to perform, accessible to all healthcare professionals without the need for expensive equipment or training, easily reproducible, reliable, able to provide information that is specific to the individual (related to age, gender, and body fat partitioning, subcutaneous versus visceral fat deposition), amenable to collection and collation to generate useful information about populations, and applicable to an individual serially over time to monitor for changes. Several measures have been proposed. These include waist circumference, waist:height ratio and waist:hip ratio measurements. In 2007, age- and gender-specific cutoffs for pediatric waist circumferences were proposed [53], based on the National Cholesterol Education Program Adult Treatment Panel and International Diabetes Federation adult criteria. Since then, the waist:height ratio has been shown to correlate well with BMI [54], and it has been proposed that a ratio greater than 0.5 should be used as a simple marker of excess adiposity in children [55]. Finally, in a study by Garnett and colleagues, a waist:height ratio >0.5 has been shown to be associated strongly with increased clustering of cardiovascular risk factors, compared with waist:height ratio <0.5 (odds ratio 11.14) [56].

In the future, studies will be required that address the applicability, reproducibility, generalizability, and validity of these suggested measures as screening tools for obesity in various populations of children, both ethnic and medical populations. Studies comparing the data collected from these simple measures to data collected from Dualenergy X-ray absorptiometry (DEXA) scans or Magnetic resonance imaging (MRI) of abdominal and subcutaneous adipose tissue will also be required, to compare the value of these new measures in predicting not just risk of obesity but risk of metabolically active adiposity and consequent metabolic and cardiovascular risk. It is possible that some combination of these or other measures will prove to be strongly predictive of overweight and obesity and, more importantly, body fat partitioning in children.

Lifelong Aging: The Barker Hypothesis and the Thrifty Genotype

The concept of fetal programming, or metabolic programming, has its origins in the theory and consequent epidemiological study, now known as the Barker hypothesis. The study, which Barker originally designed to test his hypothesis, was an epidemiological study in Hertfordshire, an affluent region in the United Kingdom, which traced the causes of death of more than 5000 men born between 1911 and 1930. As predicted by the hypothesis, men with the lowest birth weights had the highest death rates from cardiovascular disease [57].

Although the Barker hypothesis does not predict obesity risk in later life based on birth weight, a related concept is the thrifty genotype. This concept suggests that later health, including weight, of a baby is dependent in part on the uterine environment to which it is exposed. For example, one study found that maternal insulin resistance during pregnancy is associated with increased infant weight gain and adiposity over the first year of life, independent of maternal glucose tolerance [58]. Studies on Dutch families following the Dutch famine from 1944–1945 show that babies' birth weights are affected adversely by maternal undernutrition during pregnancy and that the specific trimester of undernutrition also impacts birth weights [59]. Therefore, an expectant mother who is poorly nourished is likely to deliver a baby who, in later life, will gain weight more rapidly in a nutrient-rich environment, compared to the later life health of offspring whose mother was nourished in a nutrient-rich environment during pregnancy. This nutrient-rich antenatal uterine environment has been termed "obesogenic." There is also the concept of lifelong aging, which would suggest that the aging process is commenced during the neonatal period, if not programmed during the neonatal period. Therefore, the intrauterine environment and birth weight are examples of nonmodifiable risk factors for an individual's future risk of obesity and cardiovascular risk factors.

Many questions remain unanswered. Does weight loss in women that occurs before pregnancy prevent the thrifty genotype and later obesity risk in offspring? Similarly, does prevention of excess weight gain in obese pregnant women prevent the thrifty genotype and later obesity risk in offspring? What are the contributions of nature and nurture to the Barker hypothesis and to the thrifty genotype? What will be the effect of population level interventions by policy makers? Can the increasing rate of obesity in developing countries be stemmed by education about healthy food and lifestyle choices? What will be the implications of the introduction of "obesogenic" food and lifestyle choices to some countries in the developing world, particularly so soon after the extreme food shortages during the 1980s?

KNOWLEDGE GAP3: LESSONS FROM MEDICAL MODELS OF OBESITY

Certain groups of children are particularly susceptible to the development of obesity. In this section we highlight some of these groups and important features in each.

Childhood Cancer Survivors

Long-term survivors of childhood cancer therapy have an increased lifetime risk of obesity, diabetes, and the metabolic syndrome [60, 61]. Additionally, some studies identify increased visceral adiposity, which confers increased metabolic risk, without increased BMI in childhood cancer survivors compared with controls [62]. There are data to suggest that obesity occurs predominantly in those with panhypopituitarism or dysregulated hypothalamic-pituitary axes and is mediated by a relative deficiency of IGF-1 [63]. However, this does not explain all cases of obesity and metabolic syndrome in survivors of childhood cancer, and further investigations are required.

IUGR and Child Abuse Survivors

Other children also at increased risk of obesity related to medical therapy include children who were previously treated for intra-uterine growth restriction (IUGR) [64] and those who were previously victims of child abuse [65]. It is possible that the increased risk of obesity in those children who were treated for IUGR is a natural phenomenon, as explained by the Barker hypothesis. It is also possibly mediated by increased attention to and awareness of caloric intake by both parents and, ultimately, the child. Similarly, in grownup children who were victims of child abuse, obesity could be mediated by depression, other psychological or psychiatric disorders, dysregulated hypothalamic-pituitary-adrenal axis, or overeating as either a coping mechanism or as a mechanism of self-protection from further unwanted attention [25].

Craniopharyngioma and Hypothalamic Obesity

Craniopharyngioma is a central nervous system tumor, with low proliferative potential, which occurs in the hypothalamic-pituitary area and results in morbid postoperative obesity in 25% to 60% of affected children. Hypothalamic obesity is a syndrome of intractable weight gain associated with hyperphagia, and it develops following surgery or cranial irradiation for pituitary or hypothalamic tumors, including craniopharyngioma [65, 66]. Children and adolescents with craniopharyngioma and hypothalamic obesity have been demonstrated to have increased insulin secretion without impaired insulin sensitivity on oral glucose tolerance testing [66]. They also have demonstrated delayed and submaximal suppression of the appetite-stimulating hormone ghrelin following oral glucose tolerance testing, which may partly explain their increased appetite and diminished satiety [67]. Finally, children and adolescents with craniopharyngioma and hypothalamic obesity have very abnormal sleep patterns with increased hypoxia during sleep and increased sleep fragmentation compared with obese controls [68]. Detailed investigation of children with craniopharyngioma in these studies may have provided some insights into the physiology of function and control of various mechanisms in adolescents with exogenous obesity.

Similarly, interventions in children with craniopharyngioma may provide insights into potential therapies of other conditions also. For example, a trial of metformin (for improving insulin sensitivity) and diazoxide (for decreasing insulin secretion) resulted in increased weight loss in children with craniopharyngioma and hypothalamic obesity [69]. Some authors believe that hyperinsulinemia may be an independent risk factor for further weight gain [1].

Prader-Willi Syndrome and Hypothalamic Obesity

Prader-Willi syndrome (PWS), which occurs in 1/15,000 live births, is the most common genetic cause of obesity [70]. Patients with PWS generally have hypotonia and failure to thrive in the neonatal period, followed by hyperphagia and intractable obesity from the age of approximately 2 to 4 years onward [71]. Typically, the hyperphagia of PWS is characterized by stealing food, hiding food, binge eating, nighttime eating, and eating non-nutritive substances as well as food. In addition to hyperphagia and obesity, patients with PWS also have hypogonadism, cognitive delay, growth hormone deficiency, sleep disordered breathing with sudden death [71], and, in more recent studies, central adrenal insufficiency [72]. To date, studies of children with PWS have demonstrated increased levels of the appetite-stimulating hormone ghrelin, but with appropriate decreases in ghrelin following food intake [73–75]. Furthermore, somatostatin appropriately suppresses ghrelin in PWS but without any effect on appetite or weight [74, 75]. PWS patients also have reduced levels of the appetite-suppressing gut hormone pancreatic polypeptide Y [76]. To date, pharmacological interventions for obesity [71] and restrictive bariatric surgery [77] in individuals with PWS have been largely disappointing. However, novel medications for obesity intervention have not yet been trialed in PWS patients [71], and ongoing research is required.

KNOWLEDGE GAP 4: INTERVENTIONS

Pharmacotherapy

Only two drugs are approved by the U.S. Food and Drug Administration (FDA) for use in adolescents to treat obesity: orlistat and sibutramine. The earliest age that has FDA approval for pharmacological treatment of childhood obesity is 10 years (orlistat). Orlistat blocks 30% of ingested dietary fats by inhibiting pancreatic, gastric, and carboxylester lipases [78]. Sibutramine reduces weight gain by inhibiting norepinephrine and serotonin reuptake, which causes increased satiety and thermogenesis. Common side effects of sibutramine include dry mouth, anorexia, insomnia, constipation, and headache. Tachycardia and hypertension have also been noted with sibutramine use. Patients using this medication should be monitored throughout therapy [78].

There are a number of other drugs that have not been approved yet by the FDA for treatment of childhood obesity or in some cases even in adult obesity. Metformin reduces hepatic glucose production and plasma insulin, inhibits lipogenesis, increases peripheral insulin sensitivity, and may increase satiety, but the mechanism of action of satiety increase is currently unknown and this is not currently an indication for its use in obesity treatment [34]. Topiramate is an anticonvulsant that produces its physiological effects by enhancing the γ-aminobutyric acid-A (GABA$_a$) receptor and inhibiting sodium channels and a glutamate receptor other than the N-methyl-D-aspartate receptors [34]. The hormone leptin is secreted by adipocytes in response to energy accumulation. Leptin receptors are located in the hypothalamus and anterior pituitary and communicate the availability of energy [13]. When it was initially discovered, leptin was thought to be a potential miracle cure for obesity. However, data now show that leptin levels are increased in most individuals with obesity, consistent with leptin resistance rather than leptin deficiency. Leptin treatment is only beneficial in obesity treatment in the exceptionally rare cases of leptin deficiency resulting from leptin gene mutation [34]. Untreated growth hormone deficiency and other forms of hypopituitarism, hypothyroidism, Cushing's disease/syndrome, and hypoparathyroidism may result in weight gain, which may respond to adequate hormone replacement therapy [34]. Overall, most patients with obesity do not have hormone deficiencies, and hormone supplementation has not been shown to be beneficial and is not recommended. These drugs are selected on the basis of reducing BMI; however, they may have differential effects on BMI and obesity-associated comorbidities. Metformin, for example, has more significant effects on glucose tolerance and insulin production compared to body weight. Current recommendations are that children with BMIs below the 95th percentile should not be treated with antiobesity drugs.

Pharmacogenetics

Pharmacogenetics is a quickly expanding field concerned with the interaction between drugs and an individual's genes that affect the efficacy of the drugs being administered. Genetic variation is a factor related to increased risk of obesity. For example, patients with an insertion at the Leptin receptor gene (LEPR) locus lose more weight than patients with a deletion at the same locus when treated with acarbose [79]. As with all genetics studies, large sample sizes are required to detect weak or moderate genetic predisposition to obesity [80]. In addition, given the size and complexity of the genome, it is difficult to have confidence that the loci being studied truly represent all the contributing genes relevant to obesity. Moreover, interactions between different gene products influence the up-/down-regulation of these loci, which further complicates our understanding of interactions between drugs and genes. It is clear from the complexity of these questions that genetically driven therapy for obesity, and for all other diseases, is still in its infancy and further research is required.

Bariatric Surgery

Until recently, bariatric surgery in childhood has been avoided because of concerns about the unforeseen consequences of altering the anatomical and physiological conditions in the growing child, the potential iatrogenic lifelong consequences of this procedure, and the risk of perioperative complications [34]. Recently, bariatric surgery has been performed in some teens with severe obesity, most commonly in large centers and in the context of clinical trials. Current recommendations for bariatric surgery in children include (1) only following achievement of pubertal Tanner stage 4 or 5; (2) BMI > 50 kg/m^2 without comorbidities or BMI > 40 kg/m^2 with severe comorbidities; (3) severe comorbidities, which persist despite more than 6 months of medically supervised and medically advised lifestyle modification [34] with or without a pharmacotherapy course; (4) psychological evaluation that demonstrates a stable and competent home life; (5) to be performed only by an experienced surgical team in a surgical center that is involved with or contributes to studies on the outcome of bariatric surgery in pediatric patients; and (6) that the patient should demonstrate commitment to healthy dietary and activity habits prior to consideration for surgery [34].

There exists a need for large, multicenter studies to evaluate current pediatric bariatric surgical procedures. In studies to date, the resolution of type 2 diabetes after bariatric surgery ranged from 64% to 100%, with higher remission rates following earlier surgery [17]. Postoperative complication rates are similar in adolescents compared to adults (4.2% and 6.5%), with the caveat that adolescents had fewer comorbidities [17]. In the future, it is possible that bariatric surgery will become increasingly accepted in young people and at increasingly younger ages and may be performed for obesity alone, not only obesity with associated comorbidities. However, much more research is required. Currently, it is recommended that pediatric bariatric surgical procedures should only be performed in the context of large multicenter research studies.

The Exercise Pill

The advantages of exercise both in the prevention and treatment of many diseases are well documented [81]. Unfortunately, many people are physically unable to exercise adequately because of injury or a debilitating disease, or are not willing to put in the effort, or do not gain sufficient benefit from exercise to reverse negative health effects. For these individuals, the prospect of a pill that could provide the benefits of exercise without the work is very attractive. A study of sedentary mice treated with an activator of peroxisome-proliferator-activated receptor delta (PPAR-delta) and an adenosine monophosphate (AMP)-activated protein kinase called AICAR described an improvement in exercise performance by 44% compared to sedentary untreated controls. The mechanism of improvement appears to be increased levels of glucose transporter-4 (GLUT-4) transporters and mitochondrial enzymes in skeletal muscles.

This compound may prove to be a potential new pharmacotherapy agent used in performance enhancement and in treating obesity and type 2 diabetes [82].

However, AMP-activating protein kinase has also been associated with naturally occurring mutations that have been linked with ventricular pre-excitation and hypertrophic cardiomyopathy. Furthermore, it has also been associated with the regulation of apoptosis, which in the hypothalamus could stimulate eating [83]. Although there is consensus among scientists that this pharmacological agent and its derivatives may be promising leads toward the treatment of obesity and diabetes, it is unlikely that a single pill will replace the surplus of physiological benefits of exercise. There are many research opportunities—bench, bedside, and translational—to evaluate the exercise pill.

Personalized Medicine

The concept of personalized medicine is one that will inevitably become more important in the future of many areas of medicine. Given its complexity, it is likely that obesity is one area that stands to benefit tremendously from personalized medicine. Personalized medicine means that advances in science will be utilized to choose optimum therapies for *specific patients* with a given condition. This contrasts with historical, and many current, therapeutic choices, in which the selection is driven by therapies available for a *specific condition* and the past history of therapies trialled by a specific patient with that condition. This tailoring of therapeutic options to an individual, with that person's individual genetic traits, implies that it might be possible to select therapies that will have the most efficacy and the fewest and mildest side effects for an individual.

Specific to the ongoing difficulties with clinical care of obesity, studies report inconsistent responses between both individuals and interventions. It is likely that the more successful approach to obesity management will be a multifactorial intervention, and this will reflect the multifactorial complex nature of the disease. However, the use of personalized medicine to select the optimum therapy for each individual among the various available therapies in each of the multifactorial choices will possibly improve patient outcomes.

Genetics/Epigenetics

Extensive studies have been performed on the interactions between genes and diet and genes and exercise. "The human gene map for performance and health-related fitness phenotypes" is one example. In 2000, Rankinen et al. initially summarized the available literature reporting the variation in response to exercise, based on genetics [83]. Since then, this report has been updated regularly. The report of published studies concerning genetic variation and exercise or performance to the end of 2007 includes 239 gene entries and quantitative trait loci, including 7 located on the X-chromosome and 18 located on the mitochondria [84].

The challenges in utilizing genetic information to enhance obesity treatment are summarized by Bray [84]. It is likely that these challenges will need to be addressed before genetic studies become an accepted tool in the choices of interventions for obesity management. These challenges include (1) the establishment of biomarkers that will predict outcomes in response to applied interventions, (2) the development of affordable and practical methods to characterize these biomarkers, (3) the public and medical acceptability of measurement of these biomarkers in the general population, and (4) the assurance that information gained from personalized medicine will be used responsibly or monitored to prevent the opportunity to abuse this information.

Nutrigenomics and Nutrigenetics

The Human Genome project contributed to the possibility of personal medicine by identifying single nucleotide polymorphisms that can significantly predict drug response [85]. The acknowledgment that nutrition can influence the genome, and therefore the transcriptome, proteome, and metabolome, is an exciting development and has prompted numerous new avenues of study. It has been determined that consumption of nutrients has an immediate effect on the up-/down-regulation of many genes and protein translation in the fed and fasting states [86]. In addition, early nutrition has also been seen to provoke epigenetic changes that can influence adult chronic diseases.

Nutrigenomics builds on the idea of genome-centered medicine by observing the interaction of nutrition with the genome and resultant proteome and metabolome changes [85]. Nutrigenetics on the other hand looks at the differences between genes resulting from nutrition and how to develop and use nutriceuticals that are tailored to a person's genome [87]. It has been proposed that a personalized medicine approach could contribute to better health gains when following general dieting guidelines. Even though this field of research is expanding rapidly, it is still relatively young.

Contribution of City Planners and Policy Makers: Walkability

In 2006, ecological models suggested that children's weight from age 6 months to 5 years was influenced positively by maternal prepregnancy body size, maternal smoking during pregnancy, and children's television/media use, and influenced negatively by breast-feeding and children's physical activity. There was limited research on community-level factors, policies, and interventions. The authors suggested that future policies and interventions should be subject to evaluation and aimed to support parents and young children to develop health-related behaviors that may prevent early childhood overweight [88]. We agree that more emphasis needs to be placed on research at community level, with the subsequent development of community-level policies and interventions to address future pediatric obesity.

Some data already exists about the concept of "walkability," which is a measure of the built environment. The walkability of the area in which a child lives is defined by the system of road networks, intersections, amenities, facilities for activity, and the population density of that area. Studies performed when children presented for routine vaccinations suggest that there is a direct correlation between the BMI of females and the walkability of the neighborhood in which they live. So in areas that are highly walkable, girls have lower BMI (Influence of neighborhood design and access to facilities on overweight among preschool children) [89]. To date, similar correlations have not been established in boys. This may be a reflection of the increased likelihood of girls to decrease their participation in activities after the start of puberty. It is also possible that the concept of walkability is confounded, in at least some studies, by socioeconomic status. In a study of urban environments examining more than 42,000 adolescents enrolled in the National Longitudinal Study of Adolescent Health, it was found that groups of adolescents with higher socioeconomic status had a significantly greater relative odds ratio of having facilities for activity, and that more facilities for activity was associated with decreased overweight and increased relative odds of achieving more weekly moderate or vigorous physical activity [90].

Regardless of whether walkability and the built environment affect health and weight independently or whether this is confounded by socioeconomic status, urban planners need to consider the implications of walkability to children and families, the implications of the relative ease with which they can walk from place to place in their own neighborhoods, and the implications that urban planning policies have on children's long-term weight and health. The future of pediatric obesity research, intervention, and management must be multidisciplinary and collaborative. This includes the necessary and important input of urban planners and the realization that they can bring about changes in children's health by paying due attention to issues such as walkability and access to activity facilities. This also includes the input of healthcare workers and policy makers, however, who can be responsible for bringing these data to the attention of urban planners.

Contribution of City Planners and Policy Makers: The "Twinkie Tax" Revisited

The infamous "Twinkie Tax," a tax levy of 8.25% applied to "nonessential food" in California in 1991, resulted in net tax revenue increases of $200 million and a decrease of 10% in snack sales. Objections at the local level—including the arbitrary and unequal nature of the tax, the implied penalties to those without access to fresh foods, and the difficulties implementing the tax—contributed to its repeal in 1992 [91]. Similar taxes on "nonessential" or non-nutritive foods have been implemented in other jurisdictions. Despite the mixed reactions, there are still some proponents for similar taxations to be applied in other countries and jurisdictions. Some authors suggest that lower socioeconomic status and lower-income families are those most likely to purchase non-nutritive foods, and therefore those most likely to be penalized by these taxes, and that for this reason these taxes discriminate against the more vulnerable in society. Nonetheless, when the concept of the Twinkie tax was first introduced by researchers at Stanford University, the increased revenue from taxation was supposed to be redirected toward lowering food prices of healthier choice, and frequently more expensive, foods. It is our opinion that unilateral taxation is insufficient, but taxation coupled with other incentives to increase the purchase of nutrient-rich, energy-low foods and to improve education surrounding the approach to food and lifestyle choices in general might be more effective than simple taxation. Conversely, education strategies and incentives to increase consumption of nutrient-rich, energy-low foods alone, without the implementation of Twinkie taxes, may be sufficient to redress the socioeconomic imbalance.

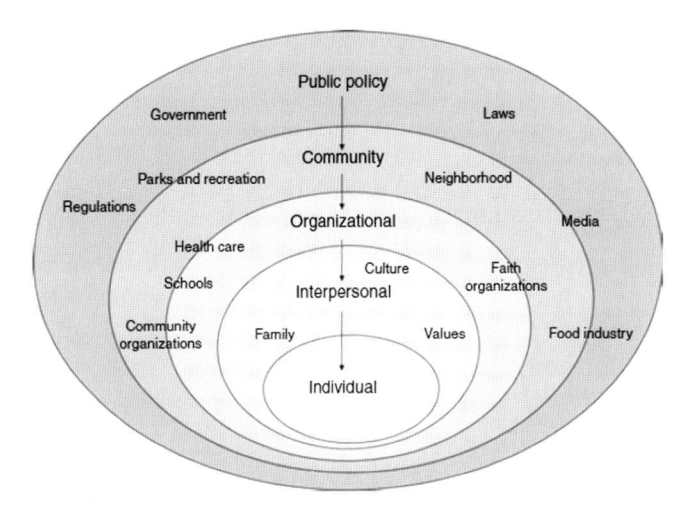

FIGURE 47.2 Reproduced with permission from "Tackling obesity: Future choice," available at www.foresight.gov.uk.

CONCLUSION

Foresight.gov suggests that the future of obesity interventions and management will require large-scale projects for the prevention of obesity, population-based solutions, including studies of the built environment, diet, and activity; a greater focus on prevention with particular attention to those at risk of obesity; an improved understanding of human behavior and values and the influences of these on food and lifestyle choices; and policy initiatives (figure 47.2). Clearly, this will not be the task of a single research group but will require multidisciplinary collaboration, likely at an international level, as well as innovative approaches.

The future of childhood obesity includes improvements in clinical care, accelerated research efforts, and careful monitoring of the prevalence of obesity. In this chapter we have tried to highlight research questions and clinical questions that are important for the future of childhood obesity. Many approaches to clinical care and research of childhood obesity have been unsuccessful. Therefore, looking to the future, the approach to this vexing problem needs to be innovative.

Weight loss for an individual person is a laudable goal, but it is difficult to attain and difficult to maintain. As one obesity expert has stated: "In 20 years of medical practice, I have yet to meet anyone who chose to be fat" [92 p.371]. Society needs to strive to support, and not to stigmatize, every individual with obesity. But the lessons of that individual's past need to be learned and applied to the future so that obesity prevention for future generations becomes a priority. Obesity, like other diseases, has a complex, interrelated etiology that includes genetic, lifestyle, physiological, environmental, and other contributors. Obesity must be accepted as a chronic disease and resources appropriately contributed to it [92].

References

1. Lustig RH. Childhood obesity: behavioral aberration or biochemical drive? Reinterpreting the first law of thermodynamics. *Nature Clinical Practice Endocrinology and Metabolism* 2006;**2**:447–58.
2. Paluska S, Schwnk T. Physical activity and mental health: current concepts. *Sports Medicine* 2000;**29**:167–80.
3. van der Heijden GJ, Toffolo G, Manesso E, Sauer PJ, Sunehag AL. Aerobic Exercise Increases Peripheral and Hepatic Insulin Sensitivity in Sedentary Adolescents. *J Clin Endocrinol Metab* 2009;**94**(11):4292–9.
4. Watts K, Jones T, Davis E, Green D. Exercise training in obese children and adolescents: Current concepts. *Sports Medicine* 2005;**35**:375–92.
5. Taveras E, Field A, Berkey C, Rifas-Shiman S, Frazier A, Colditz G, Gillman M. Longitudinal relationship between television viewing and leisure-time physical activity during adolescence. *Pediatrics* 2007;**119**:E314–19.
6. Heelan KA, Eisenmann JC. Physical activity, media time, and body composition in young children. *Journal of Physical Activity and Health* 2006;**3**:200–209.
7. Martinez-Gomez D, Tucker J, Heelan KA, Welk GJ, Eisenmann JC. Associations between sedentary behavior and blood pressure in young children. *Archives of Pediatrics and Adolescent Medicine* 2009;**163**:724–730.
8. Epstein LH, Roemmich JN, Robinson JL, Paluch RA, Winiewicz DD, Fuerch JH, Robinson TN. A randomized trial of the effects of reducing television viewing and computer use on body mass index in young children. *Arch Pediatr Adolesc Med* 2008;**162**:239–245.
9. Cameron C, Craig CL, Bull FC, Bauman A. Canada's physical activity guides: has their release had an impact? *Applied Physiology, Nutrition, and Metabolism* 2007;**32**:S161–9.
10. Belanger M, Gray-Donald K, O'Loughlin J, Paradis G, Hanley J. When adolescents drop the ball: sustainability of physical activity in youth. *American Journal of Preventative Medicine* 2009;**37**:41–9.
11. Krebs NF, Himes JH, Jacobson D, Nicklas TA, Guilday P, Styne DM. Assessment of child and adolescent overweight and obesity. *Pediatrics* 2007;**120**:S193–228.
12. Anderson CB, Hughes SO, Fuemmeler BF. Parent-child attitude congruence on type and intensity of physical activity: Testing multiple mediators of sedentary behavior in older children. *Health Psychology* 2009;**28**:328–438.
13. Jasik CB, Lustig RH. Adolescent obesity and puberty: The "Perfect Storm". *Menstrual Cycle and Adolescent Health* 2008;**1135**:265–79.
14. Singhal V, Schewnk WF, Kumar S. Evaluation and management of childhood and adolescent obesity. *Mayo Clinic Proceedings* 2007;**82**:1258–64.
15. Krebs NF, Himes JH, Jacobson D, Nicklas TA, Guilday P, Styne D. Assessment of child and adolescent overweight and obesity. *Pediatrics* 2007;**120**(Suppl 4):S193–228.
16. Roblin L. Childhood obesity: food, nutrient, and eating-habit trends and influences. *Applied Physiology Nutrition and Metabolism* 2007;**32**:635–45.
17. Spanakis E, Gragnoli C. Bariatric surgery, safety and type 2 diabetes. *Obes Surg* 2009;**19**:363–8.
18. Chin A, Paw MJ, Jacobs WM, Vaessen EP, Titze S, van Mechelen W. The motivation of children to play an active video game. *J Sci Med Sport* 2008;**11**:163–6.
19. Madsen KA, Yen S, Wlasiuk L, Newman TB, Lustig R. Feasibility of a dance videogame to promote weight loss among overweight children and adolescents. *Arch Pediatr Adolesc Med* 2007;**161**:105–7.
20. Ni Mhurchu C, Maddison R, Jiang Y, Jull A, Prapavessis H, Rodgers A. Couch potatoes to jumping beans: A pilot study of the effect of active video games on physical activity in children. *Int J Behav Nutr Phys Act* 2008;**5**:8.
21. Palou A, Bonet M, Pico C. On the role and fate of sugars in human nutrition and health. Introduction. *Obesity Reviews* 2009;**10**:1–8.
22. Mann J. Dietary carbohydrate: relationship to cardiovascular disease and diorders of carbohydrate metabolism. *European Journal of Clinical Nutrition* 2007;**61**:S100–11.
23. Maziak W, Ward KD, Stockton MB. Childhood obesity: are we missing the big picture? *Obesity Reviews* 2008;**9**:35–42.
24. Hood MY, Moore LL, Sundarajan-Ramamurti A, Singer M, Cupples LA, Ellison RC. Parental eating attitudes and the development of obesity in children. The Framingham Children's Study. *Int J Obes Relat Metab Disord* 2000;**24**:1319–25.

25. Bentley T, Widom CS. A 30-year follow-up of the effects of child abuse and neglect on obesity in adulthood. *Obesity* 2009;**10**: 1038–53.
26. Epstein LH, Paluch RA, Beecher MD, Roemmich JN. Increasing healthy eating vs. reducing high energy-dense foods to treat pediatric obesity. *Obesity (Silver Spring)* 2008;**16**:318–26.
27. Epstein LH, Paluch RA, Roemmich JN, Beecher MD. Family-based obesity treatment, then and now: twenty-five years of pediatric obesity treatment. *Health Psychol* 2007;**26**: 381–91.
28. Ventura A, Birch L. Does parenting affect children's eating and weight status? *International Journal of Behavioral Nutrition and Physical Activity* 2008;**5**:15.
29. Blissett J, Haycraft E. Are parenting style and controlling feeding practices related? *Appetite* 2008;**50**:477–85.
30. Joyce JL, Zimmer-Gembeck MJ. Parent feeding restriction and child weight. The mediating role of child disinhibited eating and the moderating role of the parenting context. *Appetite* 2009;**52**: 726–34.
31. Francis LA, Birch LL. Maternal weight status modulates the effects of restriction on daughters' eating and weight. *Int J Obes (Lond)* 2005;**29**:942–9.
32. Garcia-Bailo B, Toguri C, Eny KM, El-Sohemy A. Genetic variation in taste and its influence on food selection. *OMICS* 2009;**13**: 69–80.
33. Gaina A, Sekine M, Chandola T, Marmot M, Kagamimori S. Mother employment status and nutritional patterns in Japanese junior high schoolchildren. *International Journal of Obesity* 2009;**33**: 753–7.
34. August GP, Caprio S, Fennoy I, Freemark M, Kaufman FR, Lustig RH, Silverstein JH, Speiser PW, Styne DM, Montori VM. Prevention and treatment of pediatric obesity: An endocrine clinical practice guideline based on expert opinion. *Journal of Clinical Endocrinology and Metabolism* 2008;**93**:4576–99.
35. Koletzko B, von Kries R, Monasterolo RC, Subias JE, Scaglioni S, Giovannini M, Beyer J, Demmelmair H, Anton B, Gruszfeld D, Dobrzanska A, Sengier A, Langhendries JP, Cachera MFR. Can infant feeding choices modulate later obesity risk? *American Journal of Clinical Nutrition* 2009;**89**:S1502–8.
36. Plagemann A, Harder T. Hormonal programming in perinatal life: leptin and beyond. *Br J Nutr* 2009;**101**:151–2.
37. Plagemann A, Harder T, Brunn M, Harder A, Roepke K, Wittrock-Staar M, Ziska T, Schellong K, Rodekamp E, Melchior K, Dudenhausen JW. Hypothalamic proopiomelanocortin promoter methylation becomes altered by early overfeeding: an epigenetic model of obesity and the metabolic syndrome. *J Physiol* 2009;**587**: 4963–76.
38. Plagemann A, Harder T. Breast feeding and the risk of obesity and related metabolic diseases in the child. *Metab Syndr Relat Disord* 2005;**3**:222–32.
39. Plagemann A, Harder T, Franke K, Kohlhoff R. Long-term impact of neonatal breast-feeding on body weight and glucose tolerance in children of diabetic mothers. *Diabetes Care* 2002;**25**:16–22.
40. Richards TJ, Patterson PM, Tegene A. Obesity and nutrient consumption: A rational addiction? *Contemporary Economic Policy* 2007;**25**:309–24.
41. Outley CW, Taddese A. A content analysis of health and physical activity messages marketed to African American children during after-school television programming. *Archives of Pediatrics and Adolescent Medicine* 2006;**160**:432–5.
42. Richards TJ, Padilla L. Promotion and fast food demand. *American Journal of Agricultural Economics* 2009;**91**:168–83.
43. McGinnis JM, Gootman J, Kraak VJ, editors. *Food marketing to children and youth: Threat or opportunity?* Washington, DC: Institute of Medicine of the National Academies; 2006.
44. Elliott C. Assessing "fun foods": nutritional content and analysis of supermarket foods targeted at children. *Obesity Reviews* 2008;**9**: 368–77.
45. Richards TJ, Patterson PM, Hamilton SF. Fast food, addiction, and market power. *Journal of Agricultural and Resource Economics* 2007;**32**:425–47.
46. Jaime PC, Lock K. Do school based food and nutrition policies improve diet and reduce obesity? *Preventive Medicine* 2009;**48**: 45–53.
47. Cullen KW, Watson KB. The impact of the Texas public school nutrition policy on student food selection and sales in Texas. *American Journal of Public Health* 2009;**99**:706–12.
48. Nguyen S, Choi HK, Lustig RH, Hsu CY. Sugar-sweetened beverages, serum uric acid, and blood pressure in adolescents. *Journal of Pediatrics* 2009;**156**:807–13.
49. Fung TT, Malik V, Rexrode KM, Manson JE, Willet WC, Hu FB. Sweetened beverage consumption and risk of coronary heart disease in women. *American Journal of Clinical Nutrition* 2009;**89**: 1037–42.
50. Caprio S, Daniels SR, Drewnowski A, Kaufman FR, Palinkas LA, Rosenbloom AL, Schwimmer JB. Influence of race, ethnicity, and culture on childhood obesity: implications for prevention and treatment: a consensus statement of Shaping America's Health and the Obesity Society. *Diabetes Care* 2008;**31**:2211–21.
51. Sharma AM, Kushner RF. A proposed clinical staging system for obesity. *International Journal of Obesity* 2009;**33**:289–95.
52. Liska D, Dufour S, Zern TL, Taksali S, Cali AM, Dziura J, Shulman GI, Pierpont BM, Caprio S. Interethnic differences in muscle, liver and abdominal fat partitioning in obese adolescents. *PLoS One* 2007;**2**:e569.
53. Jolliffe CJ, Janssen I. Development of age-specific adolescent metabolic syndrome criteria that are linked to the Adult Treatment Panel III and International Diabetes Federation criteria. *J Am Coll Cardiol* 2007;**49**:891–8.
54. Kahn HS, Imperatore G, Cheng YJ. A population-based comparison of BMI percentiles and waist-to-height ratio for identifying cardiovascular risk in youth. *J Pediatr* 2005;**146**:482–8.
55. McCarthy HD, Ashwell M. A study of central fatness using waist-to-height ratios in UK children and adolescents over two decades supports the simple message—"keep your waist circumference to less than half your height." *Int J Obes (Lond)* 2006;**30**:988–92.
56. Garnett SP, Baur LA, Cowell CT. Waist-to-height ratio: a simple option for determining excess central adiposity in young people. *Int J Obes (Lond)* 2008;**32**:1028–30.
57. Barker DJP, Winter PD, Osmond C, Margetts B, Simmonds SJ. Weight in infancy and death from ischemic heart-disease. *Lancet* 1989;**2**:577–80.
58. Hamilton JK, Odrobina E, Yin J, Hanley AJ, Zinman B, Retnakaran R. Maternal Insulin Sensitivity During Pregnancy Predicts Infant Weight Gain and Adiposity at 1 Year of Age. *Obesity (Silver Spring)* 2010;**18**(2):340–6.
59. Stein AD, Lumey LH. The relationship between maternal and offspring birth weights after maternal prenatal famine exposure: the Dutch Famine Birth Cohort Study. *Hum Biol* 2000;**72**:641–54.
60. Kourti M, Tragiannidis A, Makedou A, Papegeorgiou T, Rousso I, Athanassiandou F. Metabolic syndrome in children and adolescents with acute lymphoblastic leukemia after the completion of chemotherapy. *Journal of Pediatric Hematology Oncology* 2005;**27**: 499–501.
61. Oeffinger KC, Buchana GR, Eschelman DA, Denke MA, Andrews TC, Germak JA, Tomlinson GE, Snell LE, Foster BM. Cadriovascular risk factors in young adult survivors of childhood acute lymphoblastic leukemia. *Journal of Pediatric Hematology Oncology* 2001;**23**:424–30.

62. Neville KA, Cohn RJ, Steinbeck KS, Johnston K, Walker JL. Hyperinsulinemia, impaired glucose tolerance, and diabetes mellitus in survivors of childhood cancer: Prevalence and risk factors. *Journal of Clinical Endocrinology and Metabolism* 2006;**91**: 4401−7.
63. Talvensaari KK, Lanning M, Tapanainen P, Knip M. Long-term survivors of childhood cancer have an increased risk of manifesting the metabolic syndrome. *Journal of Clinical Endocrinology and Metabolism* 1996;**81**:3051−5.
64. Evensen KAI, Steinshamn S, Tjonna AE, Stolen T, Hoydal MA, Wisloff U, Brubakk AM, Vik T. Effects of preterm birth and fetal growth retardation on cardiovascular risk factors in young adulthood. *Early Human Development* 2009;**85**:239−45.
65. Ahmet A, Blaser S, Stephens D, Guger S, Rutkas JT, Hamilton J. Weight gain in craniopharyngioma−a model for hypothalamic obesity. *J Pediatr Endocrinol Metab* 2006;**19**:121−7.
66. Simoneau-Roy J, O'Gorman C, Pencharz P, Adeli K, Daneman D, Hamilton J. Insulin sensitivity and secretion in children and adolescents with hypothalamic obesity following treatment for craniopharyngioma. *Clin Endocrinol (Oxf)* 2010;**72**(3):364−70.
67. O'Gorman CS, Simoneau-Roy J, Adeli K, Hamilton J. Appetite-Related Hormone Levels in Patients with Craniopharyngioma and Hypothalamic Obesity. In *Pediatric Academic Societies & Asian Society for Pediatric Research Joint Meeting*, Hawaii, USA; 2008.
68. O'Gorman CS, Simoneau-Roy J, MacFarlane J, MacLusky I, Daneman D, Hamilton J. Sleep disordered breathing in patients with craniopharyngioma and hypothalamic obesity. In *Lawson Wilkins Pediatric Endocrine Society and Pediatric Academic Societies Annual Joint Meeting*, Baltimore, Maryland, May 2nd, 2009.
69. Hamilton J, Conwell L, Ahmet A, Jeffery A, Daneman D. Hypothalamic obesity following craniopharyngioma surgery: Results of a pivotal trial of combined diazoxide and metformin therapy. In *International Society of Pediatric and Adolescent Diabetes*, Ljubjana, Slovenia, September 4th, 2009.
70. Cassidy SB. Prader-Willi Syndrome. *Journal of Medical Genetics* 1997;**34**:917−23.
71. Goldstone AP, Holland AJ, Hauffa BP, Hokken-Koelega AC, Taber M. Recommendations for the diagnosis and management of Prader-Willi syndrome. *Journal of Clinical Endocrinology and Metabolis* 2008;**93**(11):4183−97.
72. de Lind van Wijngaarden RF, Siemensma EP, Festen DA, Otten BJ, van Mil EG, Rotteveel J, Odink RJ, Bindels-de Heus GC, van Leeuwen M, Haring DA, Bocca G, Mieke Houdijk EC, Hoorweg-Nijman JJ, Vreuls RC, Jira PE, van Trotsenburg AS, Bakker B, Schroor EJ, Pilon JW, Wit JM, Drop SL, Hokken-Koelega AC. Efficacy and Safety of Long-Term Continuous Growth Hormone Treatment in Children with Prader-Willi Syndrome. *J Clin Endocrinol Metab* 2009;**94**(11):4205−15.
73. Goldstone AP, Patterson M, Kalingag N, Ghatei MA, Brynes AE, Bloom SR, Grossman AB, Korbonits M. Fasting and postprandial hyperghrelinemia in Prader-Willi syndrome is partially explained by hypoinsulinemia, and is not due to peptide YY3-36 deficiency or seen in hypothalamic obesity due to craniopharyngioma. *Journal of Clinical Endocrinology and Metabolism* 2005;**90**:2681−90.
74. De Waele K, Ishkanian SL, Bogarin R, Miranda CA, Ghatei MA, Bloom SR, Pacaud D, Chanoine JP. Long-acting octreotide treatment causes a sustained decrease in ghrelin concentrations but does not affect weight, behaviour and appetite in subjects with Prader-Willi syndrome. *European Journal of Endocrinology* 2008;**159**:381−8.
75. Tan TMM, Wanderpump M, Khoo B, Patterson M, Ghatei MA, Goldstone AP. Somatostatin infusion lowers plasma ghrelin wihout reducing appetite in adults with Pradi-Willi syndrome. *Journal of Clinical Endocrinology and Metabolism* 2004;**89**:4162−5.
76. Goldstone AP. Prader-Willi syndrome: advances in genetics, pathophysiology and treatment. *Trends Endocrinol Metab* 2004;**15**: 12−20.
77. Scheimann AO, Butler MG, Gourash L, Cuffari C, Klish W. Critical analysis of bariatric procedures in Prader-Willi syndrome. *J Pediatr Gastroenterol Nutr* 2008;**46**:80−3.
78. Dunican KC, Desilets AR, Montalbano JK. Pharmacotherapeutic options for overweight adolescents. *Annals of Pharmacotherapy* 2007;**41**:1445−55.
79. Adamo KB, Tesson F. Genotype-specific weight loss treatment advice: how close are we? *Applied Physiology, Nutrition, and Metabolism* 2007;**32**:351−66.
80. Vella A, Camilleri M. Pharmacogenetics: potential role in the treatment of diabetes and obesity. *Expert Opinion on Pharmacotherapy* 2008;**9**:1109−19.
81. Imbeault P. The unswallowed pill: physical activity. *Applied Physiology Nutrition and Metabolism* 2007;**32**:305−6.
82. Goodyear LJ. The exercise pill—too good to be true? *N Engl J Med* 2008;**359**:1842−4.
83. Rankinen T, Perusse L, Rauramaa R, Rivera MA, Wolfarth B, Bouchard C. The human gene map for performance and health-related fitness phenotypes: the 2001 update. *Medicine and Science in Sports and Exercise* 2001;**34**. 1219−123.
84. Bray MS, Hagberg JM, Perusse L, Rankinen T, Roth SM, Wolfarth B, Bouchard C. The human gene map for performance and health-related fitness phenotypes: the 2006-2007 update. *Med Sci Sports Exerc* 2009;**41**:35−73.
85. Subbiah MT. Nutrigenetics and nutraceuticals: the next wave riding on personalized medicine. *Transl Res* 2007;**149**:55−61.
86. Roche HM. Nutrigenomics: new approaches for human nutrition research. *Journal of the Science of Food and Agriculture* 2006;**86**: 1156−63.
87. Lovegrove JA, Gitau R. Personalized nutrition for the prevention of cardiovascular disease: a future perspective. *J Hum Nutr Diet* 2008;**21**:306−16.
88. Hawkins S, Law C. A review of risk factors for overweight in preschool children: A policy perspective. *International Journal of Pediatric Obesity* 2006;**1**:195−209.
89. Spence JC, Cutumisu N, Edwards J, Evans J. Influence of neighbourhood design and access to facilities on overweight among preschool children. *Int J Pediatr Obes* 2008;**3**:109−16.
90. Gordon-Larsen P, Nelson M, Page P, Popkin B. Inequality in the built environment underlies key health disparities in physical activity and obesity. *Pediatrics* 2006;**117**:417−24.
91. Zuck R. What balancing acts follow tax on snacks? *Paper, Film and Foil Converter* 1992;**66**:4.
92. Sharma AM. Obesity is not a choice. *Obesity reviews* 2009;**10**: 371−72.

Index

Acanthosis nigricans (AN)
  diabetes type 2 risks, 100
  insulin resistance association, 59
ADHD, see Attention deficit hyperactivity disorder
Adipocyte
  arginine supplementation and lipolysis induction, 439
  mature cell features, 183
  precursor cell features, 184
Adiponectin, bone regulation, 300
Adipose tissue
  endothelial cells, 184–185
  hormones and bone health, 300
  immune cells
    macrophages, 185–186
    overview, 185
    T cells, 186–187
  insulin effects, 202–203, 209–211
  nitric oxide and fat metabolism, 437–438
  stromal cells, 184
Advertising, see Marketing; Media
Advocacy
  nurse, 66
  pediatrician, 9
AICAR, antiobesity action, 445–446, 509–510
AMP-activated protein kinase (AMPK)
  activators and antiobesity action
    AICAR, 445–446, 509–510
    metformin, 446
    natural products, 446–448
  dysregulation and cancer, 444–445
  obesity and metabolic disorder regulation, 444–445
  regulation, 445
  structure, 445
AMPK, see AMP-activated protein kinase
Amylin, bone regulation, 300
AN, see Acanthosis nigricans
Antipsychotic drug-induced weight gain
  mechanism, 270–271
  overview, 267–270
  prospects for study, 272
  treatment, 271–272
Anxiety, obese children
  confounding factors in study, 247–248
  epidemiology, 266
  evidence against causal relationship, 246–247
  evidence for causal relationship, 247, 412
  management, 248–250, 252
  prospective studies, 247
Apiprazole, weight gain, 269–270
ARC, see Arcuate nucleus

Arcuate nucleus (ARC), sleep loss impact on energy balance, 174–175
Arginine supplementation
  adipocyte lipolysis induction, 439
  animal studies of fat loss
    diet-induced obese rat, 438–439
    Zucker diabetic fatty rat, 438
  efficacy for weight loss, 435–436
  metabolism, 435
  nitric oxide
    endothelial function, 435–436
    fat metabolism role, 437–438
  prospects, 439–440
  safety, 436–437
Attention deficit hyperactivity disorder (ADHD)
  epidemiology, 266
  gestational obesity and offspring risks, 158–159, 161–163
  management, 266–267

BA, see Behavioral activation
Balance, obese children features, 373–374
Balance Project, community-based prevention, 313
Baptist Lui Ming Choi Primary School, Hong Kong
  employee wellness, family, and community involvement, 349
  physical education promotion, 348–349
Bariatric surgery
  nonalcoholic fatty liver disease management, 227
  nurse's viewpoint, 65–66
  recommendations, 509
Barker hypothesis, 507
Be Active, Eat Well, community-based prevention, 312
Behavioral activation (BA), depression management in obesity, 253
Behavioral therapy, obesity management, 402, 412–413
Berberine, antiobesity action, 446
Beverages
  hydration status, see Hydration status
  milk
    body weight effects, 394–395
    consumption, 394
    intervention studies, 395–397
  soft drink taxation, 285
  sugar-containing beverages
    body weight effects, 390–391
    content, 390
    definition, 389

  intervention studies, 391–392, 395–396
  recommendations, 390
  water as beverage
    body weight effects, 392–393
    intervention studies, 393, 396
    overview, 392
BIA, see Bioelectrical impedance analysis
Bias
  healthcare bias, 66–67
  obese children, 233–234
Bioelectrical impedance analysis (BIA), body composition assessment, 34
BMI, see Body mass index
Body compositionBody fat; Lean body mass
Body dissatisfaction, obese children, 236, 260, 411
Body fat, see also Adipose tissue
  assessment, 34–35, 507
  body mass index
    identification of excess body fat, 38–39
    relationship, 32–34
  bone mineral density relationship, 298–299
  classification of excess, 37–38
  dietary supplement response, 426–427
  heritability, 147–148
  school-based obesity prevention outcomes, 324, 336–339
Body mass index (BMI)
  body fat
    identification of excess, 38–39
    relationship, 32–34
  bone mineral density relationship, 298
  calculation, 4
  classification, 35–36, 61, 427–428
  dietary supplement response, 426–427
  heritability, 147–148
  limitations in children, 506
  metabolic syndrome in youth prevalence analysis, 110–111
  prevention of childhood obesity, 153
  recommendations for young women, 153–154
  weight status tracking, see Weight status
Bone
  body composition effects, 298–299
  bone mineral density
    body weight relationship, 298
    fracture risk in diabetes, 299
    obese children, 299
    surrogate marker for strength, 297–298
  hormonal regulation
    adipose tissue, 300
    pancreas, 300
  vitamin D status, 299

515

Breast feeding
    duration in obese mothers, 152–153
    recommendations, 505
Bulimia, obesity as risk factor, 16
Bullying, obese children, 238–239, 259, 411

Calorie labeling, menus, 284–285
Cancer
    AMP-activated protein kinase role, 444–445
    craniopharyngioma and hypothalamic obesity, 508
    obesity in survivors, 507
Capital, see Socioeconomic status
CARU, see Children's Advertising Review Unit
CBT, see Cognitive behavioral therapy
CDC, see Centers for Disease Control
Centers for Disease Control (CDC), body mass index classification, 35–36
CHANGE study, community-based prevention, 313
ChEDE, see Child Eating Disorder Examination
Child abuse, obesity association, 507–508
Child Eating Disorder Examination (ChEDE), 236–237
Children's Advertising Review Unit (CARU), 491
Cholelithiasis, slimming program safety, 428
Choline, maternal obesity and child behavior problem pathophysiology, 161–162
Clozapine, weight gain, 267
Cognitive behavioral therapy (CBT)
    anxiety management, 252
    depression management, 251–252
    obesity management, 250–251, 402, 413–414
Cognitive restraint
    factors affecting
        mother-child relationship, 15–16
        parenting style, 16
        stress, 15
    overview, 15
Cognitive therapy, obesity management, 402
College, see School
Communication, effective communication and prosocial coping, 49–50
Community-based prevention, childhood obesity
    definition, 305
    examples
        Balance Project, 313
        Be Active, Eat Well, 312
        CHANGE study, 313
        FLVS study, 312
        Pathways study, 310–311
        Shape up Somerville, 311–313
        SWITCH study, 313
    prospects, 315–316
    rationale, 306, 314

    recommendations, 313
    research
        analysis, 308, 310
        community-based participatory research, 306
        community-placed research, 305
        design, 307–308
        measures, 308–309
        strategy elements, 310–311
    theory
        ecological models of health behavior, 306
        social change models, 307
Comorbidity, obesity evaluation, 8–9
Coping
    coping-competence model, 47
    effective communication and prosocial coping, 49–50
    parenting, coping, and self-regulation
        good-enough parenting, 48–49
        healthy environment, 48
        secured attachment, 39
Craniopharyngioma, hypothalamic obesity, 508
C-reactive protein (CRP), sleep loss impact on energy balance, 175
CRP, see C-reactive protein
Cultural differences
    culinary cultures and food consumption practices, 130–131
    culture overview, 127–129
    diabetes type 2, 99–100
    familial contexts, 133
    global context of cultured bodies, 129–130
    interventions in childhood obesity, 135–136
    metabolic syndrome in youth prevalence analysis, 112
    national health survey analysis of racial/ethic and socioeconomic differences in childhood obesity
        joint effects of disparities, 80–83
        National Health and Nutrition Examination Survey, 75, 415
        National Survey of Children's Health, 72–74
        prevalence trends, 76
        racial/ethic differences, 76, 78–79, 81, 83
        socioeconomic status differences, 76–77
        statistical analysis, 75–76
    national sociocultural trends influencing body weight, 132–133
    nurse's viewpoint, 58, 67–68
    physical activity, 131–132
    practices related to food consumption and physical activity, 130
    school-based obesity prevention intervention, see Healthier Options for Schoolchildren
    socioeconomic status, see Socioeconomic status
    taste preference development in childhood, 130
Curcumin, antiobesity action, 447

Depression, obese children
    depression predicting obesity, 246
    epidemiology, 251, 266
    evidence against causal relationship, 245–246
    evidence for causal relationship, 246, 412
    management, 248–252, 266–267
    obesity predicting depression, 246
    overview, 235–236, 260
DGA, see Dietary Guidelines for Americans
Diabetes type 1
    complications in obese children and adolescents, 292–293
    fracture risk, 299
    weight, weight gain, and risk
        children and adolescents, 290–292
        overview, 289–290
Diabetes type 2
    assessment, 497
    complications, 101
    epidemiology
        family history of type 2 diabetes, 89
        general youth population, 88
        gestational diabetes, 89–90
        obese children, 89
    follow-up in youth, 101
    fracture risk, 299
    inflammation and cardiovascular risk, 203–205
    longitudinal studies
        adults, 98
        youth, 98–99
    nonalcoholic fatty liver disease association, 224–226
    prediabetes, see Prediabetes
    presentation, 101
    prevalence
        global prevalence, 95–96
        youth, 96–98
    prevention, 101–102
    risk factors, 99–102
    screening, 99, 101–103
Diet, see Nutrition
Dietary Guidelines for Americans (DGA)
    french fry classification, 475
    recommendations, 480
    revision, 481
Dietary supplement, obesity treatment
    arginine, see Arginine supplementation
    composition, 422–423
    physical activity promotion, 425–426
    physiological changes, 426–427
    study design
        enrollment, 424
        instructions, 424–425
        population characteristics, 422, 424
Dieting
    hunger reduction, 421–422
    insulin resistance studies in children
        low-carbohydrate diet, 213–215
        low-glycemic index diet, 213
Discrimination, obese children, 233–234
Dyslipidemia, screening, 102, 496–497

Eating disorders
    interpersonal psychotherapy, 251
    obese children, 236–237
    obesity as risk factor, 16
    prevention, 421
    slimming program safety, 428
Economic impact, childhood obesity, 282, 476
EGCG, see Epigallocatechin-3-gallate
Endothelial cell, adipose tissue, 184–185
Epigallocatechin-3-gallate (EGCG), antiobesity action, 447
Epigenetics
    maternal obesity and child behavior problems, 161
    prospects for study, 510
Ethnicity, see Cultural differences
Exercise
    definition, 371
    physical activity, see Physical activity

F2S, see Farm-to-School
Family history, see also Maternal obesity; Parenting
    contexts in childhood obesity, 133
    diabetes type 2, 99
    functioning, 51–52
    nurse's viewpoint on obesity impact, 57–58
    nutritionist's viewpoint on obesity impact, 13–14, 17
    obesity evaluation, 6
Family therapy
    case study, 407–408
    overview, 403–404
    process
        approach, 405–406
        family interaction, 406
        interview, 406–409
        practical approach, 406
        strategy, 406
    solution-based brief therapy, 404–405
    Standardized Obesity Family Therapy, 405
    systemic family medicine, 404, 409
Farm subsidies, legislation, 456–457
Farm-to-School (F2S), 481
Fast food
    marketing, 505–506
    preferences of children, 475–476
Fat, see Adipose tissue; Body fat
Fatty liver disease, see Nonalcoholic fatty liver disease
FCC, see Federal Communications Commission
Federal Communications Commission (FCC), marketing regulation, 455
Federal Trade Commission (FTC), marketing regulation, 456
Fish oil, antiobesity action, 448
Fitness, see Physical fitness
Five A's approach, obesity prevention, 498–499
FLVS study, community-based prevention, 312

Folate, maternal obesity and child behavior problem pathophysiology, 160–162
Food choice
    dairy, 477
    fast food preferences of children, 475–476
    fruits and vegetables, 476–477
    influences, 477–478
    marketing, 478–479
    maternal employment status effects, 504–505
    mediation, 478–481
    obesity relationship, 476
    personal responsibility, 283
    policy and legislation, 481–482
    snacks, 477
    taste perception, 504
    trends, 504
French fry, Dietary Guidelines for Americans classification, 475
Fruit juice, see Beverages
FTC, see Federal Trade Commission
FTO
    polymorphisms and child mental health problems, 162
    variants and obesity, 148–149, 217

Gait, obese children features, 374
Gestational diabetes, diabetes type 2 risks in offspring, 100
Gestational obesity, see Maternal obesity
GH, see Growth hormone
Ghrelin, Prader-Willi syndrome levels, 194–195
Ginseng, antiobesity action, 447
Global Forum for Physical Education Pedagogy (GoFPEP), 353
GMM, see Group mixture modeling
GoFPEP, see Global Forum for Physical Education Pedagogy
Go Girls, 251
Got Milk? campaign, 479
Gout, slimming program safety, 428
Group mixture modeling (GMM), weight status tracking, 24–25
Group therapy, obesity management, 402–403
Growth curve
    non-normative growth curves, 24–27
    normative growth curves, 23–24
Growth hormone (GH), deficiency in Prader-Willi syndrome, 192
Grundy Center
    overview, 351
    partnership building, 351–352

HDL, see High-density lipoprotein
Healthcare bias, nurse's viewpoint, 66–67
Healthier Options for Schoolchildren (HOPS)
    academic measures, 336
    data analysis
        measures, 336
        two-stage approach, 336
    dietary intervention, 334–335

free and reduced-price meal subsample analysis, 339–340
    intervention components, 334
    limitations, 341
    nutrition and healthy living curricula, 336
    outcomes
        academics, 339
        physiological parameters, 337–339
    overview, 361
    physical activity component, 335–336
    strengths, 341
    study design, 334
Healthy Options for People through Extension (HOPE), 362–364
Healthy Places, law and policy, 457
High-density lipoprotein (HDL), metabolic syndrome in youth prevalence analysis, 110
HOPE, see Healthy Options for People through Extension
HOPS, see Healthier Options for Schoolchildren
Hormone-sensitive lipase (HSL), insulin effects, 209
HSL, see Hormone-sensitive lipase
Hydration status
    body weight effects, 394
    water requirements, 393–394
Hypertension
    arginine supplementation effects, 435–436
    assessment, 496
    guidelines, 497
    sibutramine risks, 434–435

Impaired fasting glucose, see Prediabetes
Impaired glucose tolerance, see Prediabetes
Insulin, bone regulation, 300
Insulin resistance, see also Diabetes type 2; Metabolic syndrome
    adipose tissue effects, 202–203, 209–211
    assessment, 211
    diet studies in children
        low-carbohydrate diet, 213–215
        low-glycemic index diet, 213
    energy intake regulation, 205
    evolutionary perspective, 215–216
    inflammation and cardiovascular risk, 203–205
    metformin and weight gain mechanisms, 212–213
    obese children, 212
    overview, 201
    pathophysiology, 203
    Prader-Willi syndrome, 193–194
    prevention, 205
    signaling pathways, 201–202
    weight gain in children, 211–212
Insulin resistance syndrome, see Metabolic syndrome
International Obesity Task Force (IOTF), body mass index classification, 35–36
Interpersonal psychotherapy (IPT)
    depression management, 252

Interpersonal psychotherapy (IPT) (*Continued*)
    eating disorder management, 251
Intrauterine growth retardation (IUGR), treatment and obesity association, 507
IOTF, *see* International Obesity Task Force
IPT, *see* Interpersonal psychotherapy
IUGR, *see* Intrauterine growth retardation

Juvenile diabetes 1, *see* Diabetes type

Kids N Fitness, 434

Labeling
    calorie labeling on menus, 284–285
    nutritional labeling requirements, 480
Laboratory findings, obesity evaluation, 7
Latent transitions analysis (LTA), weight status tracking, 24–25
Lateral hypothalamus area (LHA), sleep loss impact on energy balance, 173, 175
LBM, *see* Lean body mass
Lean body mass (LBM)
    bone mineral density relationship, 298–299
    dietary supplement response, 426–427
    physical activity and accretion, 421, 429
    school-based obesity prevention outcomes, 324, 336–338
Leptin
    bone regulation, 300
    maternal obesity and child behavior problem pathophysiology, 159–160
    sleep loss impact on energy balance, 174
    therapy, 508–509
LHA, *see* Lateral hypothalamus area
α-Lipoic acid, antiobesity action, 446–447
LTA, *see* Latent transitions analysis

Macrophage, adipose tissue, 185–186
Marketing, *see also* Media
    Children's Advertising Review Unit, 491
    fast foods, 505–506
    regulation, 455–456
    school regulation, 460
Maternal employment status, dietary effects, 504–505
Maternal obesity
    breast feeding duration, 152–153
    complications, 163
    distress and development, 163
    family environment
        dietary habits, 152
        physical activity, 152
    gestational obesity
        behavioral problems in offspring
            confounding factors, 163
            mechanisms, 159–163
            overview, 158–159
            prenatal programming, 159
        generational effects, 153
        gestational weight gain studies, 150–151
        neurodevelopmental impact, 157–158
        offspring risks for obesity, 149–150
        overnutrition effects on fetus, 151–152
    heritability, 147–148

Media
    child use patterns
        overview, 487
        overweight relationship, 487–488
        recommendations, 490
    influences
        dietary habits, 488
        physical activity, 488
        sleep behavior, 489
    obesity interventions, 489
    public policy, 490–491
Medical history
    obesity evaluation, 6
    weight gain, 5
Metabolic syndrome
    cardiovascular manifestations, 142–143
    clinical relevance for later life, 143–144
    definition for children, 143
    pathophysiology in childhood, 139–143
    prevalence in youth
        cultural differences, 112
        National Health and Nutrition Examination Survey analysis, 108–111
        pathophysiology and secular trends, 112–113
        projections, 113
        regional-based sample estimates, 111–112
    prevention, 421
    risk factors, 107, 203
    assessment, 497
Metformin
    AMP-activated protein kinase activation, 446
    antipsychotic drug-induced weight gain management, 271–272
    obesity management, 386, 508
    prediabetes management, 91–92
    weight gain mechanisms, 212–213
Methylenetetrahydrofolate reductase (MTHR), gene polymorphisms and child mental health problems, 162
MI, *see* Motivational interviewing
Milk, *see* Beverages
Mitochondria, regulation of fatty acid entry, 210–211
Motivational interviewing (MI), obesity management, 251, 414
Motor competence, obese children, 374–375
MTHR, *see* Methylenetetrahydrofolate reductase
MyPyramid, 480

NAFLD, *see* Nonalcoholic fatty liver disease
National Health and Nutrition Examination Survey (NHANES)
    analysis of racial/ethic and socioeconomic differences in childhood obesity, 75, 415
    metabolic syndrome in youth prevalence analysis, 108–111
National School Lunch Program (NSLP), 285, 339–340, 457–458, 481

National Survey of Children's Health (NSCH), analysis of racial/ethic and socioeconomic differences in childhood obesity, 72–74
NHANES, *see* National Health and Nutrition Examination Survey
Nitric oxide (NO)
    arginine supplementation and endothelial function, 435–436
    fat metabolism role, 437–438
NO, *see* Nitric oxide
Nonalcoholic fatty liver disease (NAFLD)
    cardiovascular disease and diabetes association, 224–226
    diagnosis, 223–224
    epidemiology, 221
    pathogenesis, 222–223
    screening, 60, 102
    treatment, 226–227
North Vista Primary School, Singapore
    community as partners, 350–351
    overview, 350
    teachers as researchers, 350–351
NSCH, *see* National Survey of Children's Health
NSLP, *see* National School Lunch Program
Nurse viewpoint, obesity
    factors influencing, 57–58
    impact, 59–60
    prevention, 62–63
    screening, 60–62
    treatment, 63–68
Nutrigenomics, prospects for study, 510
Nutrition, *see also* Food choice
    calorie labeling on menus, 284–285
    dietary trends, 346–347
    family environment, 152
    insulin resistance diet studies in children
        low-carbohydrate diet, 213–215
        low-glycemic index diet, 213
    labeling requirements, 480
    maternal obesity and child behavior problem pathophysiology, 160–161
    nurse's viewpoint, 64
    prevention of deficiency and stunting, 420
Nutritionist viewpoint, obesity
    cognitive restraint in children, 15–16
    eating disorders, 16
    genetics and family aspects, 13–14
    physical activity, 17
    prevention and treatment, 17–18

Obesity hypoventilation syndrome (OHS), features and management, 178
Obesogenic environment, obesity induction, 283–284
Obestatin, Prader-Willi syndrome levels, 194–195
Obstructive sleep apnea syndrome (OSAS), features and management, 167, 177–178
OGTT, *see* Oral glucose tolerance test
OHS, *see* Obesity hypoventilation syndrome

Olanzapine, weight gain, 267–270
Oral glucose tolerance test (OGTT)
  diabetes diagnosis, 87
  Prader-Willi syndrome, 194
  prediabetes, 88
OrganWise Guys Comprehensive School Program (OWG CSP), 360–365, 367
Orlistat
  mechanism of action, 384
  nurse's viewpoint, 65
  obesity management, 384, 434, 508
OSAS, see Obstructive sleep apnea syndrome
Osteocalcin, bone regulation, 300
OWG CSP, see OrganWise Guys Comprehensive School Program

Paraventricular nucleus (PVN), sleep loss impact on energy balance, 174–175
Parenting
  coping, and self-regulation
    good-enough parenting, 48–49
    healthy environment, 48
    secured attachment, 39
  family functioning, 51–52
  modeling, 52
  perception of child's weight, 67
  style, 16, 50–52
  time pressure, convenience, and child-centered parenting, 133–135
Pathways study, community-based prevention, 310–311
PCOS, see Polycystic ovarian syndrome
Pediatrician viewpoint, obesity
  advocacy, 9
  assessment, 5–8, 496–498
  attitudes, 495–496
  identification, 4–5
  prevention, 3–4
  screening, 4
  treatment, 8–11
  weight-management counseling, 498–499
Perifornical area (PFA), sleep loss impact on energy balance, 173, 175
Perilipin, insulin effects, 209
Personalized medicine, prospects, 510
Personal responsibility, dietary choices, 283
PFA, see Perifornical area
Pharmacogenetics, obesity drugs, 509
Physical activity
  cultural differences, 131–132
  definition, 371
  family environment, 152
  guidelines for obese children
    clinical assessment, 376
    exercise prescription
      duration, 377
      frequency, 377
      intensity, 377
      mode, 376
      overview, 375–376
    lean body mass accretion, 421, 429

  media influences, 488
  nurse's viewpoint, 64–65
  nutritionist's viewpoint, 17
  obese children features, 371–372
  prediabetes management, 91
  promotion through law and policy, 458–459
  recommendations, 502–503
  school-based obesity prevention outcomes, 322–323, 335–336, 348–349
  screen time and inactivity, 347, 503
  trends in physical inactivity, 347
Physical examination, obesity evaluation, 7–8
Physical fitness
  definition, 371
  obese children features
    balance and gait, 373–374
    motor competence, 374–375
    overview, 372–373
Pioglitazone, nonalcoholic fatty liver disease management, 227
POLAR Scholar program, 352
Polycystic ovarian syndrome (PCOS)
  depression association, 253
  evaluation, 498
  insulin resistance, 203
Portion size, food preferences, 477–478
Prader-Willi syndrome (PWS)
  clinical features, 191–193
  genetics, 191
  ghrelin levels, 194–195
  glucose metabolism–ghrelin linkage, 195–196
  hypothalamic obesity, 508
  incidence, 191
  obestatin levels, 194–195
Prediabetes
  epidemiology
    family history of type 2 diabetes, 89
    general youth population, 88
    gestational diabetes, 89–90
    obese children, 89
  impaired fasting glucose, 87–88
  impaired glucose tolerance, 87–88
  pathophysiology, 87–88
  progression, 90–91
  screening, 88, 90
  treatment, 91–92
Pregnancy, see Gestational diabetes; Maternal obesity
Preptin, bone regulation, 300
Preschoolers, obesity interventions, 403
Prevalence
  diabetes type 2
    global prevalence, 95–96
    youth, 96–98
  epidemic of childhood obesity, 346
  global epidemic of obesity, 345–346, 433–434
  metabolic syndrome in youth
    cultural differences, 112
    National Health and Nutrition Examination Survey analysis, 108–111

    pathophysiology and secular trends, 112–113
    projections, 113
    regional-based sample estimates, 111–112
  national health survey analysis trends in childhood obesity, 76, 281
  trends in overweight and obesity, 31–32, 282
Prevention
  diabetes type 2, 101–102
  eating disorders, 421
  insulin resistance, 205
  metabolic syndrome, 421
  obesity, see also Community-based prevention; School-based obesity prevention
    five A's approach, 498–499
    nurse's viewpoint, 62–63
    pediatrician's viewpoint, 3–4
    weight cycling, 428–429
Primary care, see Pediatrician viewpoint, obesity
Project SPARK, 320
Psychodynamic therapy, obesity, 402
Psychological history, obesity, 258
PVN, see Paraventricular nucleus
PWS, see Prader-Willi syndrome

QoL, see Quality of life
Quality of life (QoL), obese children, 237–238, 412
Quercetin, antiobesity action, 447–448
Quetiapine, weight gain, 267–268

Race, see Cultural differences
Readiness for change, obesity evaluation, 6–7
Resistin, bone regulation, 300
Resveratrol, antiobesity action, 447
Risk assessment, pediatrician's viewpoint, 4–5
Risperidine, weight gain, 267–270

Safe Routes to School (SR2S), 320
Schizophrenia
  pediatric epidemiology, 267
  weight gain on antipsychotics
    mechanism, 270–271
    overview, 267–270
    prospects for study, 272
    treatment, 271–272
School
  college weight gain, 477
  eating behavior influences, 506
  food policy, 285–286
  legislation for obesity prevention, 457
  marketing regulation, 460
  problems of obese children, 260–261
School-based obesity prevention
  Baptist Lui Ming Choi Primary School of Hong Kong
    employee wellness, family, and community involvement, 349
    physical education promotion, 348–349

School-based obesity prevention (Continued)
  barriers to delivery, 327–328
  behavioral therapy, 403
  evidence-based tools for improvement, 367–368
  Global Forum for Physical Education Pedagogy, 353
  Grundy Center
    overview, 351
    partnership building, 351–352
  Healthier Options for Schoolchildren
    academic measures, 336
    data analysis
      measures, 336
      two-stage approach, 336
    dietary intervention, 334–335
    free and reduced-price meal subsample analysis, 339–340
    intervention components, 334
    limitations, 341
    nutrition and healthy living curricula, 336
    outcomes
      academics, 339
      physiological parameters, 337–339
    overview, 361
    physical activity component, 335–336
    strengths, 341
    study design, 334
  Healthy Options for People through Extension, 362–364
  integrated approach, 347–348
  international perspectives, 325
  North Vista Primary School of Singapore
    community as partners, 350–351
    overview, 350
    teachers as researchers, 350–351
  OrganWise Guys Comprehensive School Program, 360–365, 367
  outcomes
    body fat, 324
    dietary intake, 323–324
    factors influencing effectiveness, 324–325
    physical activity, 322–323
  overview of strategies, 320–321
  POLAR Scholar program, 352
  prospects, 341–342, 353–354
  public-private partnerships, 363–366, 368
  rationale, 319–320, 359
  recommendations, 328
  research
    gaps, 325–326
    limitations, 326
  success components, 366
  Supplemental Nutrition Assistance Education Program, 362–363, 366
  theory, 321–322
  WISERCISE!, 360–361
Screen time, physical inactivity indicator, 347, 503
Screening
  diabetes type 2, 99, 101–103
  fatty liver disease, 60, 102
  hyperlipidemia, 102
  obesity
    nurse's viewpoint, 60–62
    pediatrician's viewpoint, 4
Self-esteem, obese children, 234–235, 259–260, 411–412
Self-regulation
  overview, 45–47
  parenting, coping, and self-regulation
    good-enough parenting, 48–49
    healthy environment, 48
    secured attachment, 39
  weight-related problems, 44–45
Serotonin transporter, gene polymorphisms and child mental health problems, 162–163
SES, see Socioeconomic status
Sex differences, diabetes type 2, 100
Shape up Somerville (SUS), community-based prevention, 311–313
Sibutramine
  mechanism of action, 384
  nurse's viewpoint, 65
  obesity management, 384–386, 434, 508
SIRT1, caloric restriction effects, 205
Skin, nurse's viewpoint for care, 60
Skinfold thickness, body composition assessment, 34–35
Sleep disorders
  behavioral impact in obesity, 176–177
  energy balance impact in obesity, 173–176
  epidemiology
    obesity and sleep loss studies
      adolescents, 171–172
      children, 169–171
    prevalence
      obesity in children and adolescents, 167–168
      short sleep in children and adolescents, 168–169
  laboratory studies of obesity and sleep loss correlation, 172–173
  media influences, 489
  obesity hypoventilation syndrome, 178
  obstructive sleep apnea syndrome, 167, 177–178
  treatment, 178
Snacks, taxation, 285
SNAP-Ed, see Supplemental Nutrition Assistance Education Program
Social functioning, obese children, 238–239, 260–261, 411
Socioeconomic status (SES)
  diabetes type 2 prevalence, 95
  food and body as cultural capital, 468–470
  inequality, ethnicity, and obesity, 466–468
  maternal obesity, 163
  national health survey analysis of racial/ethic and socioeconomic differences in childhood obesity
    joint effects of disparities, 80–83
    National Health and Nutrition Examination Survey, 75
    National Survey of Children's Health, 72–74
    prevalence trends, 76
    racial/ethic differences, 76, 78–79, 81, 83
    socioeconomic status differences, 76–77
    statistical analysis, 75–76
  social and behavioral factors influencing obesity, 463–464
  societal impact of childhood obesity, 470
  symbolic capital and obesity, 464–466
Soda, see Beverages
Soft drink, see Beverages
SOFT, see Standardized Obesity Family Therapy
SR2S, see Safe Routes to School
Stages of Change model, 6–7
Standardized Obesity Family Therapy (SOFT), 405
Suicidal behavior, obese children, 261, 412
Supplemental Nutrition Assistance Education Program (SNAP-Ed), 362–363, 366
SUS, see Shape up Somerville
SWITCH study, community-based prevention, 313
Syndrome X, see Metabolic syndrome
Systems review, obesity evaluation, 6

Taste perception, food choice influences, 504
T cell, adipose tissue, 186–187
Teasing, see Bullying
TEE, see Total energy expenditure
Television, physical inactivity correlation, 347, 372, 503
Thrifty genotype, 507
TNF-α, see Tumor necrosis factor-α
Total energy expenditure (TEE), sleep loss impact on energy balance, 176
Treatment stages, obesity, 9–11
Triglyceride, metabolic syndrome in youth prevalence analysis, 110
Tumor necrosis factor-α (TNF-α), nonalcoholic fatty liver disease pathogenesis, 223
Twinkie tax, 511

UDCA, see Ursodeoxycholic acid
Ursodeoxycholic acid (UDCA), nonalcoholic fatty liver disease management, 227

VERB campaign, 479
Very-low calorie diet (VLCD), risks in children, 421
Visceral fat, insulin resistance correlation, 202–203
Vitamin D, bone health, 299
Vitamin E, nonalcoholic fatty liver disease management, 227
VLCD, see Very-low calorie diet

Waist circumference
  diabetes type 2 risks, 100
  metabolic syndrome in youth prevalence analysis, 110
Walkability, environment planning, 510–511

Water, *see* Beverages; Hydration status
Weight cycling, prevention, 428–429
Weight goals, obesity management, 11
Weight status
    developmental trajectories, 21
    non-normative growth curves, 24–27
    normative growth curves, 23–24
    nurse's viewpoint, 61
    tracking in childhood and adolescence, 21–23
    weight regain prevention, 428–429
WHO, *see* World Health Organization
WIC, *see* Women, Infants, and Children
WISERCISE!, 360–361
Women, Infants, and Children (WIC), 481
World Health Organization (WHO), body mass index classification, 36

Ziprasidone, weight gain, 267–268
Zoning, law and policy, 457